Pulmonary Pathology

Other books in this series:

Prayson: Neuropathology

Iacobuzio-Donahue & Montgomery: Gastrointestinal and Liver Pathology

Thompson: Head and Neck Pathology

O'Malley & Pinder: Breast Pathology

Thompson: Endocrine Pathology

Zhou & Magi-Galluzzi: Genitourinary Pathology

Hsi: Hematopathology

Sidawy & Ali: Fine Needle Aspiration Cytology

Other books coming soon in this series:

Busam: Dermatopathology

Folpe & Inwards: Bone and Soft Tissue Pathology

Nucci & Oliva: Gynecologic Pathology

Tubbs & Stoler: Cell and Tissue Based Molecular Pathology

Pulmonary Pathology

A Volume in the Series
Foundations in Diagnostic Pathology

Edited by

Dani S. Zander, M.D.

Professor and Chair of Pathology
University Chair in Pathology
Department of Pathology
Penn State Milton S. Hershey Medical Center and
Penn State University College of Medicine
Hershey, Pennsylvania

Carol F. Farver, M.D.

Director, Pulmonary Pathology
Vice-Chair of Education
Division of Pathology and Laboratory Medicine
Cleveland Clinic
Cleveland, Ohio

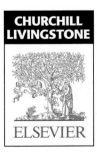

CHURCHILL
LIVINGSTONE

ELSEVIER

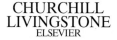

1600 John F. Kennedy Blvd.
Ste 1800
Philadelphia, Pennsylvania 19103-2899

PULMONARY PATHOLOGY
A Volume in the Series Foundations in Diagnostic Pathology   ISBN: 978-0-443-06741-9

Notice

Knowledge and best practice in this field are constantly changing. As new research and experience broaden our knowledge, changes in practice, treatment and drug therapy may become necessary or appropriate. Readers are advised to check the most current information provided (i) on procedures featured or (ii) by the manufacturer of each product to be administered, to verify the recommended dose or formula, the method and duration of administration, and contraindications. It is the responsibility of the practitioner, relying on their own experience and knowledge of the patient, to make diagnoses, to determine dosages and the best treatment for each individual patient, and to take all appropriate safety precautions. To the fullest extent of the law, neither the Publisher nor the Editors assume any liability for any injury and/or damage to persons or property arising out of or related to any use of the material contained in this book.

The Publisher

Library of Congress Cataloging-in-Publication Data

Pulmonary pathology / [edited by] Dani S. Zander, Carol F. Farver. — 1st ed.
   p. ; cm. — (Foundations in diagnostic pathology)
   Includes bibliographical references.
   ISBN 978-0-443-06741-9
  1. Lungs—Pathophysiology. 2. Lungs—Diseases—Diagnosis. I. Zander, Dani S. II. Farver, Carol F. III. Series.
   [DNLM: 1. Lung Diseases—diagnosis. 2. Lung Diseases—pathology. 3. Pleural Diseases—diagnosis. 4. Pleural Diseases—pathology. WF 600 P98374 2008]
   RC711.P832 2008
   616.2'4—dc22

                2007034369

Acquisitions Editor: Bill Schmitt
Developmental Editor: Nicole DiCicco
Publishing Services Manager: Joan Sinclair
Project Manager: Bryan Hayward
Design Coordinator: Karen O'Keefe

Printed in China

Last digit is the print number: 9 8 7 6 5 4 3 2 1

My thanks to my husband, Dr. Erik Zander, who has been an unwavering source of encouragement and goodwill, and to my children, Brianne and Paul Zander, for their kindness and patience during the preparation of this book.
— *Dani S. Zander, MD*
My thanks to my husband, Dr. Robert Needlman, for his love, support and infinite optimism that carried me through this and many other projects and to our daughter, Grace Needlman, whose true joy of learning inspires me each and every day.
— *Carol F. Farver, MD*

Ashley W. Allison, M.D.
Fellow in Dermatopathology, Department of Dermatology,
The University of Texas Medical Branch, Galveston, Texas

Sadir J. Alrawi, M.D.
Chief of Surgical Oncology, University of Florida
at Jacksonville, Jacksonville, Florida

Richard L. Attanoos, M.D.
Consultant Histopathologist, Department of Histopathology,
Llandough Hospital, Cardiff and Vale NHS Trust, Wales,
United Kingdom

Marie Christine Aubry, M.D.
Associate Professor of Pathology, Division of Anatomic
Pathology, Mayo Clinic, Laboratory Medicine and Pathology,
Rochester, Minnesota

Roberto J. Barrios, M.D.
Professor of Pathology and Laboratory Medicine, Weill Medi-
cal College of Cornell University; Department of Pathology,
The Methodist Hospital, Houston, Texas

Mary Beth Beasley, M.D.
Assistant Professor of Pathology, Department of Pathology,
Mount Sinai School of Medicine, New York, New York

Jennifer Brainard, M.D.
Section Head, Cytopathology, Department of Anatomic
Pathology, Cleveland Clinic Foundation, Cleveland, Ohio

Elisabeth Brambilla, MD, Ph.D.
Professor of Pathology, Département d'Anatomie et Cytolo-
gie Pathologiques, CHU Albert Michallon, INSERM U823,
Université J. Fourier, Grenoble, France

Kelly J. Butnor, M.D.
Assistant Professor of Pathology, Department of Pathology,
Fletcher Allen Health Care/University of Vermont Burlington,
Burlington, Vermont

Omar R. Chughtai, M.D.
Director of Operations, Chughtai's Lahore Lab, Lahore, Pakistan

Carlyne D. Cool, M.D.
Associate Clinical Professor, Department of Pathology,
University of Colorado Health Sciences Center; Associate
Professor, Department of Medicine, National Jewish Medical
and Research Center, Denver, Colorado

Michael H. Covinsky, M.D., Ph.D.
Assistant Professor of Pathology, University of Texas Health
Science Center at Houston Medical School, Department of
Pathology and Laboratory Medicine, Houston, Texas

Gail H. Deutsch, M.D.
Assistant Professor of Pathology, Pathology and Laboratory
Medicine, Cincinnati Children's Hospital Medical Center,
Cincinnati, Ohio

Megan K. Dishop, M.D.
Assistant Professor, Department of Pathology, Texas
Children's Hospital, Baylor College of Medicine,
Houston, Texas

Carol F. Farver, M.D.
Director, Pulmonary Pathology; Vice-Chair of Education,
Division of Pathology and Laboratory Medicine, Cleveland
Clinic, Cleveland, Ohio

Douglas B. Flieder, M.D.
Department of Pathology, Fox Chase Cancer Center,
Philadelphia, Pennsylvania

Armando E. Fraire, M.D.
Professor, Department of Pathology, University of
Massachusetts Medical School, Worcester, Massachusetts

Anthony A. Gal, M.D.
Professor of Pathology, Department of Pathology and
Laboratory Medicine, Emory University School of Medicine,
Atlanta, Georgia

Allen R. Gibbs, M.D.
Llandough Hospital, Department of Histopathology, Penarth,
Cardiff and Vale NHS Trust, United Kingdom

Linda K. Green, M.D.
Professor of Pathology, Baylor College of Medicine, and
Director of Cytology, Flow Cytometry and FISH, Michael E.
DeBakey Veterans Affairs Medical Center, Houston, Texas

Ulrike Gruber-Mösenbacher, M.D.
Staff Pathologist, Institute of Pathology, Academic
Teaching Hospital, Feldkirch, Austria

Donald G. Guinee, Jr., M.D.
Virginia Mason Medical Center, Department of Pathology,
Seattle, Washington

Abida K. Haque, M.D.
Professor of Pathology, Weill Medical School of Cornell
University; Department of Pathology, The Methodist
Hospital, Houston, Texas

Aliya N. Husain, M.D.
Professor of Pathology, Department of Pathology, University
of Chicago, Chicago, Illinois

Diana N. Ionescu, M.D., FRCPC
Consultant Pathologist, BC Cancer Agency, Clinical Assistant
Professor, Department of Pathology, University of British
Columbia, Vancouver, British Columbia, Canada

Jaishree Jagirdar, M.D.
Professor of Pathology and Director of Anatomic Pathology,
University of Texas Health Science Center at San Antonio,
Department of Pathology, San Antonio, Texas

Keith M. Kerr, BSc, MB ChB, FRCPath, FRCPEd
Consultant Pathologist, Department of Pathology, Aberdeen
Royal Infirmary, Professor of Pulmonary Pathology, Aberdeen
University School of Medicine, Foresterhill, Aberdeen,
Scotland, United Kingdom

Andras Khoor, M.D.
Chair, Department of Laboratory Medicine and Pathology,
Mayo Clinic, Jacksonville, Florida

Claire Langston, M.D.

Professor, Department of Pathology, Baylor College of
Medicine, Texas Children's Hospital, Houston, Texas

Sylvie Lantuejoul, M.D., Ph.D.

Professor of Pathology, Département d'Anatomie et Cytologie
Pathologiques, CHU Albert Michallon, INSERM U823,
Université J. Fourier, Grenoble, France

Kevin O. Leslie, M.D.
Consultant and Vice Chair for Anatomic Pathology Services,
Department of Laboratory Medicine and Pathology, Mayo
Clinic Arizona, Scottsdale, Arizona; Professor of Pathology,
Mayo Clinic College of Medicine, Rochester, Minnesota

Cynthia M. Magro, M.D.
Professor of Pathology and Laboratory Medicine and Director of
Dermatopathology, Weill Medical College of Cornell University,
New York Presbyterian Hospital–Cornell Campus, Department
of Pathology and Laboratory Medicine, New York, New York

Andre L. Moreira, M.D., Ph.D.
Assistant Attending, Department of Pathology, Memorial
Sloan Kettering Cancer Center, New York. New York

Bruno Murer, M.D.
Ospedale dell' Angelo, AULSS 12 Veneziana, Veneziana,
Anatomic Pathology Department, Mestre-Venice, Italy

Ronald C. Neafie, M.D.
Chief, Parasitic Disease Pathology Branch, Department of
Environmental and Infectious Disease Sciences, Armed
Forces Institute of Pathology, Washington, D.C.

Christopher D. Paddock, M.D., M.P.H.T.M
Staff Pathologist/Research Medical Officer, Infectious Disease
Pathology Branch, Centers for Disease Control and Prevention,
Atlanta, Georgia

Helmut H. Popper, M.D.
Professor of Pathology, Laboratories for Molecular Cytogenetics,
Environmental, and Respiratory Tract Pathology, Institute of
Pathology, Medical University of Graz, Graz, Austria

Gary W. Procop, M.D., M.S.
Chairman, Department of Clinical Pathology; Director,
Molecular Microbiology, Mycology, and Parasitology,
Cleveland Clinic Pathology and Laboratory Medicine
Institute, Cleveland, Ohio

Semyon A. Risin, M.D., Ph.D.
Professor, Department of Pathology and Laboratory Medi-
cine, University of Texas Health Science Center–Houston
Medical School; Director of Clinical Immunology, Memorial
Herrmann Hospital, Houston, Texas

Anna E. Sienko, M.D., FRCP(C)
Department of Pathology, The Methodist Hospital, Houston,
Texas

Thomas A. Sporn, M.D.
Assistant Professor of Pathology, Duke University
Medical Center, Department of Pathology, Durham,
North Carolina

Dongfeng Tan, M.D.
Associate Professor, Department of Pathology, MD Anderson
Cancer Center, Houston, Texas

William D. Travis, M.D.
Attending Thoracic Pathologist, Department of Pathology,
Memorial Sloan Kettering Cancer Center; Professor of
Pathology, Weill Medical College of Cornell University,
New York, New York

David H. Walker, M.D.
The Carmage and Martha Walls Distinguished University
Chair in Tropical Diseases, Professor and Chairman, Department of Pathology, Executive Director, Center for Biodefense
and Emerging Infectious Disease, University of Texas Medical Branch at Galveston, Galveston, Texas

Joanne L. Wright, M.D., FRCP
University of British Columbia, Department of Pathology,
Vancouver, British Columbia, Canada

Sherif R. Zaki, M.D., Ph.D.
Chief, Infectious Diseases Pathology Branch DVRD,
NCZVED Centers for Disease Control and Prevention,
Atlanta, Georgia

Dani S. Zander, M.D.
Professor and Chair of Pathology, University Chair in Pathology, Department of Pathology, Penn State Milton S. Hershey
Medical Center and Penn State University College of Medicine, Hershey, Pennsylvania

Foreword

The study and practice of anatomic pathology is both exciting and overwhelming. Surgical pathology, with all of the subspecialties it encompasses, and cytopathology have become increasingly complex and sophisticated, and it is not possible for any individual to master the skills and knowledge required to perform all of these tasks at the highest level. Simply being able to make a correct diagnosis is challenging enough, but the standard of care has far surpassed merely providing a diagnosis. Pathologists are now asked to provide large amounts of ancillary information, both diagnostic and prognostic, often on small amounts of tissue, a task that can be daunting even to the most experienced pathologist.

Although large general surgical pathology textbooks are useful resources, they by necessity could not possibly cover many of the aspects that pathologists needs to know and include in their reports. As such, the concept behind Foundations in Pathology was born. This series is designed to cover the major areas of surgical and cytopathology, and each edition is focused on one major topic. The goal of every book in this series is to provide the essential information that any pathologist, whether general or subspecialized, in training or in practice, would find useful in the evaluation of virtually any type of specimen encountered.

Dr. Dani Zander, Professor and Chair of Pathology at Penn State Milton S. Hershey Medical Center, and my valued colleague at the Cleveland Clinic, Dr. Carol Farver, both outstanding and renowned pulmonary pathologists, have edited what I believe to be an outstanding state-of-the-art book covering the essential aspects of pulmonary pathology. Although there are other outstanding and comprehensive pulmonary pathology textbooks available, I know of no other book that so effectively gets to the core of what practicing surgical pathologists want and need to know about this challenging topic. The list of contributors is a virtual Who's Who of pulmonary pathology, including authors who have not only contributed to the literature in this field, but, more importantly, have been practicing pulmonary pathology for many years, acquiring invaluable diagnostic experience. As with all of the other editions in the Foundations in Diagnostic Pathology series, the information presented in this book is organized into headings, covering the essential clinical and pathologic features of each entity. There are a large number of practical tables and high-quality photomicrographs, which similarly capture the essence of the topics being discussed, with bullet points to allow a quick summary of the information. Where applicable, the authors thoroughly integrate ancillary diagnostic techniques, including immunohistochemistry, immunofluorescence, electron microscopy, and molecular diagnostics.

This edition is organized into 40 chapters encompassing the full spectrum of pulmonary pathology. The first three chapter focus on normal pulmonary anatomy and tissue artifacts, the uses (and abuse) of the lung biopsy, and a pattern-based approach to the diagnosis of pulmonary diseases. The remaining chapters examine congenital/pediatric, vascular, infectious, idiopathic, and neoplastic conditions. Separate chapters are also provided to include fibroinflammatory and neoplastic diseases of the pleura.

I wish to extend my heartfelt appreciation to Drs. Zander and Farver, who took on this project despite innumerable other clinical and administrative responsibilities. Their organizational and editorial skills have truly made this edition outstanding. I would also like to extend my appreciation to the many authors who have also taken the time from their busy lives to provide their knowledge and expertise. It is my sincerest hope that you find this volume of Foundations in Diagnostic Pathology to be a valuable addition to your library and, more importantly, to your everyday practice of pulmonary pathology.

JOHN R. GOLDBLUM, M.D.

Although other books focused on pulmonary pathology exist, we hope that this volume will occupy a favored spot on the reader's bookshelf. In planning, writing, and editing this book, we have sought to equip the student of pulmonary pathology with the necessary tools to feel confident in the interpretation of most lung and pleural samples and to be able to assist other physicians in applying knowledge of disease pathology to its diagnosis and treatment. The spectrum of lung and pleural pathology is quite broad, and the varied natures and presentations of the disorders that arise in these locations offer many challenges to the pathologist. In this book, we have attempted to create integrated depictions of these fascinating processes. Information about recent molecular genetic advances and applications of immunohistochemistry, immunofluorescence, ultrastructural analysis, and clinical laboratory testing is presented to supplement the clinical, radiologic, and morphologic information that forms the basis for disease diagnosis, classification, prognosis, and treatment. Diagnosis of lung and pleural diseases goes far beyond pattern recognition, in most cases. To be accurate and sure of ourselves, we must usually consider the pathology in the context of the whole patient. This book is intended to assist you in this process by providing the information you need in an appealing format and concentration. We hope that you will find this book to be more than just a diagnostic aid, but also a valued consultative "friend."

DANI S. ZANDER, M.D.
CAROL F. FARVER, M.D.

Contents

1

Normal Anatomy, Tissue Artifacts, and Incidental Structures

Douglas B. Flieder

NORMAL ANATOMY

The lungs occupy most of the volume of the thoracic cavity. The average weights of male and female lungs are approximately 850 grams and 750 grams, respectively. The right lung is composed of ten distinct segments, which comprise three lobes (upper, middle, and lower) while the left lung has ten segments organized into two lobes (upper and lower). Each lobe is covered with pleura (visceral pleura) and is separated from the other lobes by fissures. At the microscopic level, the lungs feature distinct yet integrated components including conducting airways, air spaces, blood vessels and lymphatics, and other cellular constituents (Table 1-1).

AIRWAYS

Not only do conducting airways form the passageways through which air enters and exits the lungs, but they also warm, humidify, and aid in sterilizing incoming air. The trachea bifurcates into the left and right mainstem bronchi, which bifurcate into additional bronchi that undergo further bifurcations into smaller bronchi and then bronchioles. Airways in adult lungs usually undergo twenty-three divisions, to finally merge with the gas exchange units, the alveoli.

Airways are classified as either bronchi or bronchioles. Bronchi have cartilaginous walls and measure more than 0.1 cm in diameter, while bronchioles measure less than 0.1 cm in diameter and lack cartilage. In the mainstem bronchi, hyaline cartilage is C-shaped, but as the airways enter the lung tissue, the cartilage becomes discontinuous. As the bronchial diameter decreases, the cartilage plates become smaller. Unlike bronchioles, bronchi also have submucosal salivary-type glands with both serous and mucous cells (Figure 1-1).

Terminal bronchioles are the smallest pure conducting airways; about 30,000 terminal bronchioles are found within the lungs. The terminal bronchioles bifurcate into respiratory bronchioles, whose walls consist partially of alveoli (Figure 1-2). Bronchioles also give rise to alveolar ducts, which terminate in alveolar sacs.

Airways are composed of mucosa, submucosa, muscularis propria, and adventitia. Bronchial epithelium lines the airway lumen and includes pseudostratified ciliated columnar epithelial cells, interspersed goblet cells and neuroendocrine cells, and underlying basal cells. The ciliated respiratory epithelial cells and goblet cells are specialized cells that function in mucociliary clearance mechanisms. Goblet cells secrete mucus, which is important for trapping inhaled particles, and the cilia propel the mucus and entrapped particles toward the pharynx, where they can be eliminated. Bronchi also feature basal cells, pluripotential reserve cells that can regenerate a damaged bronchial mucosa. Scattered neuroendocrine cells are also interspersed in the respiratory epithelium. Clusters of neuroendocrine cells can occasionally be found at airway bifurcations and are termed neuroepithelial bodies. Neuroendocrine cells may not be recognizable in routine hematoxylin- and eosin-stained tissue sections, but can be highlighted by immunohistochemical staining using antibodies directed against chromogranin or synaptophysin antigens. Neuroendocrine cells may play a role in lung development and/or ventilation/perfusion regulation.

In bronchioles, goblet cells are replaced by nonciliated columnar cells with prominent apical cytoplasm (Clara cells). Clara cells produce surfactant-like material, accumulate and detoxify inhaled toxins, and serve as progenitor cells for regeneration of damaged bronchiolar epithelium.

1

TABLE 1-1

Structural and Cellular Components of the Lungs

Parts of the Lung	Structural Components	Cellular Components
Bronchi	Epithelium	Ciliated columnar cells
		Goblet cells
		Basal cells
		Neuroendocrine cells
	Subepithelial connective tissue	
	Submucosal serous and mucinous acini with myoepithelial cells	
	Smooth muscle	
	Hyaline cartilage	
	Autonomic nervous system components	
	Vasculature and lymphatics	
Bronchioles	Epithelium	Ciliated columnar cells
		Clara cells
	Subepithelial connective tissue	
	Smooth muscle	
	Autonomic nervous system components	
	Vasculature and lymphatics	
Alveoli	Epithelium	Type I pneumocytes
		Type II pneumocytes
	Alveolar macrophages	
	Interstitium	Fibroblasts
		Myofibroblasts
		Monocytes/macrophages
		Mast cells
		Collagen and elastic fibers
	Alveolar capillaries	Endothelial cells
		Pericytes
Interlobular septa	Connective tissue	
	Veins and lymphatics	
Visceral pleura	Mesothelial cells	
	Connective tissue with blood vessels and lymphatics	

All airways feature a basement membrane, composed of type IV collagen and laminin, and underlying elastic fibers and smooth muscle bundles. Airways are richly innervated by parasympathetic and sympathetic nerves. Blood vessels and lymphatics also course through the airway submucosa.

GAS EXCHANGE UNITS

An average lung contains approximately 300 million alveoli and has 140 m² of gas-exchanging alveolar surface. Several terminal bronchioles and associated air spaces form each pulmonary lobule, which is bounded by a fibrous septum (Figure 1-3). The lobules function semiautonomously, with neural controls to regulate air and blood flow. Lobules consist of up to 30 individual gas exchange compartments, termed acini. An acinus is an anatomic unit that consists of multiple respiratory bronchioles, alveolar ducts, and alveoli that are supplied by a single terminal bronchiole.

Individual alveolar sacs are lined by two types of epithelium joined by well formed tight junctions (Figure 1-4). Type I pneumocytes have flattened nuclei and inconspicuous cytoplasm. They constitute 40% of the lining cells, yet cover 90% of the alveolar surface owing to their abundant (up to 50 microns long) and thin (as little as 0.1 micron thick) cytoplasm. Type I pneumocytes facilitate O_2 and CO_2 exchange across

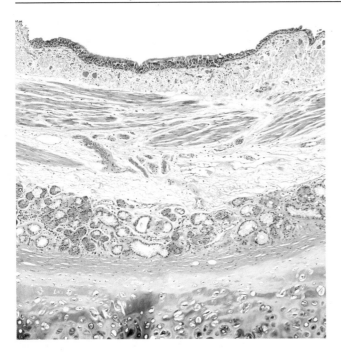

FIGURE 1-1
Bronchus
The bronchial wall features pseudostratified ciliated columnar epithelium with goblet cells, submucosal seromucinous glands, bronchial vessels and lymphatics, smooth muscle, and hyaline cartilage.

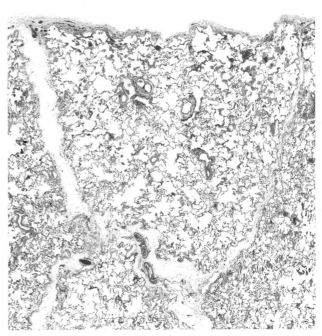

FIGURE 1-3
Pulmonary lobule
The pulmonary lobule is bounded by interlobular septa and visceral pleura, which contain pulmonary veins and lymphatics.

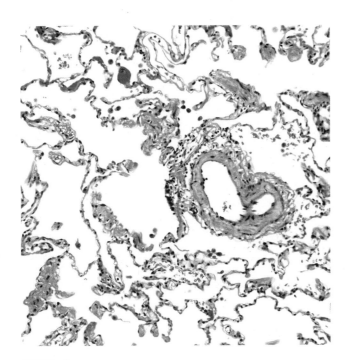

FIGURE 1-2
Respiratory bronchiole and peribronchiolar structures
The respiratory bronchiole travels with a small branch of the pulmonary artery. This airway opens into an alveolar duct as well as individual alveolar sacs. Scattered intra-alveolar macrophages are a common finding, and may be increased in smokers.

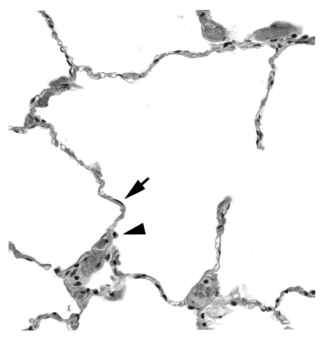

FIGURE 1-4
Alveoli
Alveolar walls seem to consist only of capillaries, and are lined by flattened type I cells (arrow) and occasional type II cells (arrowhead). The air space is free of debris or cells.

their cytoplasm. Type II pneumocytes are cuboidal cells with large basally located nuclei, variably prominent nucleoli, and granular or vacuolated cytoplasm. These epithelial cells constitute 60% of the alveolar lining cells but cover only 5% of the air space surface. In addition to secreting surfactant, a phospholipid that lowers surface tension and prevents alveolar collapse at low intra-alveolar pressures, type II pneumocytes are alveolar stem cells capable of dividing and terminally differentiating into type I cells after alveolar injury.

Communications between alveoli are not present at birth, but appear shortly thereafter and increase in number throughout life. Pores measuring up to 10 microns in diameter, termed pores of Kohn, are rarely seen in histologic sections and may contain surfactant or be open and involved in collateral ventilation. Pores larger than 15 microns, between alveoli, are called fenestrae and are considered abnormal. Communications between terminal bronchioles and alveoli, termed canals of Lambert, also aid in collateral ventilation and probably play a part in lambertosis, the covering of alveolar walls by respiratory epithelium that occurs after some episodes of airway injury.

Pulmonary capillaries in alveolar walls are vitally important for gas exchange. Incredibly, the intricate alveolar capillary meshwork yields an air–blood interface of 125 m^2, a surface area approximately 70 times that of the skin. At many points, the basal lamina underlying type I pneumocytes fuses with the basal lamina underlying pulmonary capillary endothelial cells. Endothelial cells are easily recognized in histologic sections and participate in regulating gas, water, and solute transport, converting angiotensin I to angiotensin II, inactivating bradykinin, and taking part in a variety of other metabolic functions.

Alveolar walls also contain small numbers of mesenchymal cells including fibroblasts, smooth muscle cells, pericytes, and myofibroblasts. The mesenchymal cells maintain the septal elastic and collagen fibers and proteoglycans, while the contractile cells control capillary blood flow. Scattered mast cells, and occasional lymphocytes and monocytes, are also normally present, but large numbers of inflammatory cells in the alveolar interstitium indicate a pathological process.

VASCULATURE

The lungs have dual blood supplies. The bronchial circulation is part of the systemic circulation and has a high pressure and high oxygen content. Bronchial arteries most often arise from the descending aorta and "feed" the bronchial tree as far as the respiratory bronchiole. Branches also nourish most of the mediastinal visceral pleura. Large bronchial arteries can be seen in the bronchial adventitia and usually demonstrate only

one elastic lamina, the internal elastic lamina. Bronchial veins travel in the bronchial adventitia and feed into either the azygos or hemiazygos vein, or they empty into the pulmonary venous system.

The pulmonary circulation originates from the right ventricle. The main pulmonary arteries branch into lobar arteries and enter the lungs with the lobar bronchi. The arteries branch in tandem with the airways and additionally feature right-angle bifurcations in order to reach peribronchiolar alveoli. It is useful to keep in mind that arteries accompanying airways in histologic sections should have approximately the same diameters as the airways. Differences indicate the existence of a pathologic process. Compared to systemic arteries, pulmonary arteries feature more elastic and less smooth muscle, resulting in relatively increased luminal diameters. Two or more elastic laminae are found in arteries greater than 0.1 cm in diameter, yet as arteries become smaller, the smooth muscle layer becomes thinner and the elastic laminae fuse and fragment. Pulmonary venules are inconspicuous but coalesce to form small veins within the interlobular septa. These lobular veins diverge into larger veins at subsegmental septa and eventually join the bronchi and pulmonary arteries at the segmental level. The large veins proceed to the hilum and drain oxygenated blood into the left atrium for systemic distribution.

LYMPHATICS AND IMMUNE EFFECTOR CELLS

Two separate inconspicuous lymphatic systems drain extracellular fluid, debris, and inflammatory cells from the lung. A centriacinar system resides within the bronchovascular bundles, starting at the level of the respiratory bronchioles. Lymphatics associated with pulmonary arteries extend deeper into the acinus than those associated with airways, but the two components of this system intersect often as they course through the lung to the hilum. The peripheral acinar system associated with pulmonary veins begins at the edge of the acinus and tracks through the interlobular septa and pleura. Although the two lymphatic systems communicate at lobar, lobular, and pleural boundaries, they drain separately into hilar lymph nodes. While the right lung and left lower lobe usually drain into the right lymphatic duct, and the remainder of the left lung drains into the left thoracic duct, interconnecting mediastinal lymphatic channels allow for cross-drainage. Flat endothelial cells line lymphatic channels, and larger lymphatics contain adventitial smooth muscle and collagen. Alveolar walls do not have lymphatics, yet the interstitial space is capable of draining extracellular fluid.

Small submucosal lymphoid aggregates are termed bronchus-associated lymphoid tissue (BALT) and are most commonly seen at bronchial bifurcations and near respiratory bronchioles. While these structures have little known significance in children, the presence of BALT in adults suggests a pathologic process. Approximately 60% of the lymphoid cells are B-cells, generally small lymphocytes with a centrocyte-like appearance, and the remainder are T-cells. There are occasional HLA-DR$^+$ interdigitating cells and follicular dendritic cells. Germinal centers can form in the BALT. Overlying attenuated epithelium, so-called lymphoepithelium, facilitates antigen processing. Lymphoid aggregates involving other locations in the lung should be considered abnormal.

Intrapulmonary lymph nodes are found in all age groups but are more common in tobacco smokers and individuals with occupational exposures to asbestos and nonfibrous silicates. Two-thirds are solitary, and most measure less than 2.0 cm in diameter. The lymph nodes usually lie in subpleural areas, along interlobular septa, or within the major fissures of the lung, and resemble normal lymph nodes with the additional frequent findings of anthracosilicotic pigment deposition and silicotic nodules.

Alveolar macrophages are bone marrow-derived phagocytes that enter the air spaces from the systemic circulation. Resident interstitial monocytes also contribute to alveolar macrophages. After engulfing debris, macrophages can persist in the alveolar sacs or be eliminated from the lung, primarily via airway clearance mechanisms and lymphatic drainage. When particle burdens are very high and macrophages are overwhelmed, particles accumulate in the visceral pleura, alveolar septa, and connective tissues around airways. Particles derived from tobacco smoke and air pollution are particularly prominent around respiratory bronchioles.

PLEURA

The visceral pleura has five layers. A single layer of mesothelial cells without a basement membrane rests on a submesothelial layer of loose connective tissue approximately as thick as the mesothelial cell layer. The third layer is a well defined elastic layer, and the fourth is the interstitial or loose connective tissue layer containing lymphatics, blood vessels, and collagen. The final layer is composed of elastic fibers and fibrous tissue that merge with the underlying lung. This architecture is often disturbed in settings of inflammatory or neoplastic disorders. Parietal pleurae are similar to visceral pleurae, but the layers are less distinct. The mesothelial cells lie on a connective tissue plane containing a single elastic layer and scattered blood vessels and lymphatics. The parietal pleura interdigitates with chest wall adipose tissue overlying dense collagen. This endothoracic fascia fuses with either skeletal muscle or rib periosteum. It should be noted that the presence of fat in a pleural biopsy does not necessarily indicate that a biopsy is from the parietal pleura, since fatty metaplasia of visceral pleurae and

subpleural lung tissue is a common finding in many disease states.

ARTIFACTS

Variations in normal histology and tissue distortions resulting from specimen procurement often present challenges for pathologists evaluating the lung specimens (Table 1-2). Tissue from apical segments of lung features larger alveoli and fewer blood vessels than basal segment specimens, and often shows fibrosis and elastosis ("apical cap"). Visceral pleura is thicker at the lung bases and in fissures than over smooth lung surfaces. Lung tips, especially the lingula and right middle lobe tips, often demonstrate non-specific scarring and honeycomb change even in individuals without clinical pulmonary disease. Peribronchial alveolar septa are thicker and slightly fibrotic, so samples from these regions should not be overinterpreted as representing fibrosing interstitial lung disease. Age-associated changes, including bronchial wall submucosal elastosis, bronchial seromucinous gland hyperplasia or oncocytic metaplasia, intimal thickening of vessel walls, senile vascular sclerosis, and alveolar space enlargement (senile emphysema), do not represent pathologic processes.

Biopsy and resection specimens may feature atelectasis secondary to compression associated with the biopsy

---

TABLE 1-2

Common Artifacts in Lung Tissues

Artifacts	Challenges
Atelectasis and mechanical compression	Can mimic interstitial fibrosis
	Can mimic exogenous lipoid pneumonia
	Can mimic or obscure malignancies, especially small cell carcinoma (crush artifact)
Overinflation	Can mimic lymphatic dilatation
	Can mimic emphysema
	Can wash out intra-alveolar cells
Procedure-associated hemorrhage	Can mimic pulmonary hemorrhage syndromes
Mechanical displacement of tissue	Can mimic malignancy
Air-dry artifact	
Sponge artifact (due to use of sponge in processing)	

procedure (Figure 1-5). Atelectatic areas may not be interpretable, and one should be wary of attempting to diagnose interstitial lung diseases in these samples. Compression can produce a rounding of alveoli, suggesting lipoid change and a diagnosis of exogenous lipoid pneumonia. The absence of alveolar macrophages and fibrosis, however, should argue against this diagnosis. Injection of formalin into surgical lung biopsies can be done to inflate them and facilitate evaluation of interstitial abnormalities. Overinflation of lung tissue, however, can expand interlobular septa and pulmonary lymphatics or overexpand alveoli, leading to erroneous considerations of lymphangiectasia and emphysema.

Surgical clamping of lung tissue may also lead to septal edema and distortion of alveolar spaces not unlike that produced by pathology laboratory-induced specimen overinflation. Lung specimens extensively handled by surgeons may feature visceral pleural mesothelial cell sloughing with dense intracapillary neutrophils and surface fibrin strands.

Due to the biopsy procedure, alveoli may fill with blood, but in the absence of hemosiderin-laden macrophages, intra-alveolar fibrin, and/or alveolar septal neutrophils, a pulmonary hemorrhage syndrome is less likely. Smokers' macrophages contain tan-brown pigment that will stain with an iron stain, but the particles are finer than coarse hemosiderin.

Transbronchial biopsies can also show procedure-related artifacts. Crush artifact is common in endoscopic biopsies, particularly those obtained from small cell carcinomas and lymphoid processes. Caution is advisable when making a diagnosis on severely crushed tissue (Figure 1-6) and well preserved diagnostic areas should be sought to ensure the accuracy of the interpretation. Circumferential strips of bronchial wall with partially denuded respiratory epithelium should be recognized as such, and clumps of displaced ciliated epithelium with prominent goblet cells should not be mistaken for malignancy.

INCIDENTAL FINDINGS

A large variety of incidental findings can be seen in the lung, and can involve any anatomic compartment. Some abnormalities discovered unexpectedly can have clinical relevance (e.g., granuloma containing mycobacteria, pulmonary embolus), and although incidental, these findings can represent important diagnostic entries. Most incidental findings, however, do not have potential clinical significance, and the main importance of recognizing many of these entities lies in not confusing them with another more significant process (Table 1-3, Figures 1-7 through 1-9).

FIGURE 1-5

Artifactual atelectasis

Artifactual atelectasis can interfere with morphologic interpretation of lung samples. This biopsy is actually unremarkable, but could be misconstrued as showing a fibrosing process. Surgical lung biopsies and resection specimens are frequently compressed during surgery or in the pathology laboratory, but specimen inflation with formalin can improve one's ability to assess tissue architecture and evaluate for subtle pathologic changes.

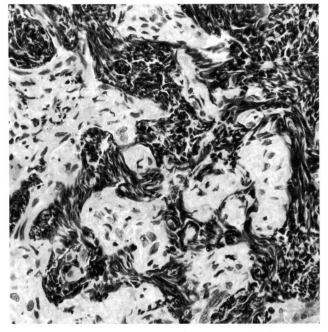

FIGURE 1-6

Crush artifact

Crush artifact interferes with morphologic assessment. Small cell carcinomas are particularly susceptible to this artifact, but other benign and malignant processes can also show this change. In this case, the concomitant cytology specimen and immunohistochemical stains were diagnostic of malignant lymphoma.

TABLE 1-3

Common Incidental Findings in Lung Tissues

Large Airways	Alveolar Parenchyma	Vascular
Ossification of bronchial cartilage	Scar	Megakaryocyte
Oncocytic metaplasia of bronchial submucosal glands	Apical cap	Small embolus
Bronchial submucosal elastosis	Focus of smooth muscle hyperplasia	Calcification of elastic fibers
	Metaplastic bone	Senile venous sclerosis
	Corpora amylacea	
	Blue body	
	Schaumann's body	
	Asteroid body	
	Calcium oxalate crystal	
	Mallory's hyaline-like material in type II pneumocytes	
	Ferruginous body	
	Foreign body, including aspirated material	
	Cholesterol cleft	
	Carcinoid tumorlet	
	Minute meningothelial-like nodule	
	Isolated granuloma	
	Anthracotic pigment deposit	
	Silicotic nodule	

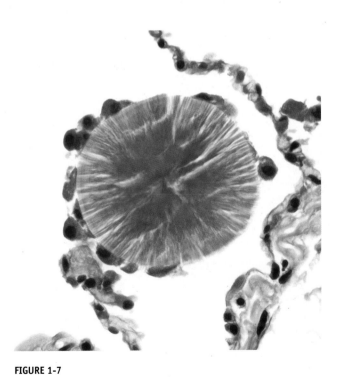

FIGURE 1-7

Corpus amylaceum

Corpora amylacea are common incidental findings in air spaces. These 30- to 200-micron diameter spherical structures are composed of glycoproteins and may have prominent radiations. Although they are PAS-positive, they should not be mistaken for fungal organisms.

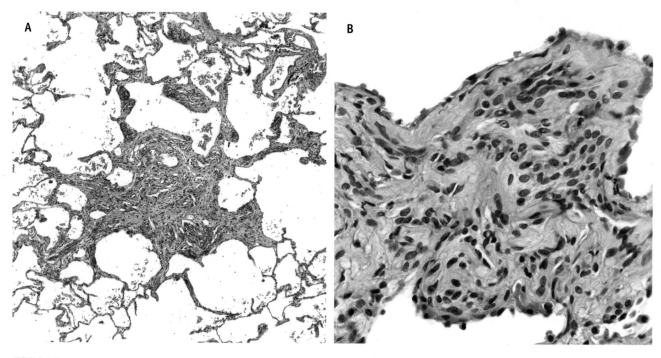

FIGURE 1-8

Minute meningothelial-like nodule

A, B. Minute meningothelial-like nodules usually measure less than 3 mm and are nodular perivenular interstitial proliferations of meningothelial-like cells. They consist of nests and streams of cells with uniform oval nuclei, homogeneous chromatin, and lightly basophilic cytoplasm. Intranuclear inclusions can be seen, and cells show immunoreactivity with anti-EMA antibodies. These common incidental proliferations should not be confused with malignancy.

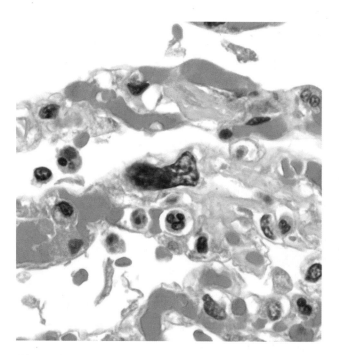

FIGURE 1-9

Megakaryocyte

Megakaryocytes travel through the pulmonary circulation and can be mistaken for metastatic tumor cells or virally infected cells. They can be especially prominent in settings of significant blood loss and acute inflammatory conditions.

SUGGESTED READINGS

1. Nagaishi C. *Functional Anatomy and Histology of the Lung*. 1st ed. Baltimore: University Park Press; 1972.

2. Aguayo S, Schuyler W, Murtagh J, et al. Regulation of branching morphogenesis by bombesin-like peptides and neutral endopeptidase. *Am J Respir Cell Mol Biol*. 1994;10:635-42.

3. Wang NS. Anatomy. In: Dail DH, Hammar SP, eds. *Pulmonary Pathology*. 2nd ed. New York, NY: Springer-Verlag, 1994:21–44.

4. Crapo JD, Barry BE, Gehr P, et al. Cell number and cell characteristics of the normal human lung. *Am Rev Respir Dis*. 1982;125:740-5.

5. Bienenstock J. Bronchus-associated lymphoid tissue. *Int Arch Allergy Immunol*. 1985;76:62-9.

6. Okada Y, Ito M, Nagaishi C. Anatomical study of the pulmonary lymphatics. *Lymphology*. 1979;12:118-24.

7. Kradin RL, Spirn PW, Mark EJ. Intrapulmonary lymph nodes. *Chest*. 1985;87:662-7.

8. Van Haarst J, de Wit H, Drexhage H, et al. Distribution and immunophenotype of mononuclear phagocytes and dendritic cells in the human lung. *Am J Respir Cell Mol Biol*. 1994;10:487-92.

9. Colby TV, Leslie KO, Yousem SA. Lungs. In: Mills SE, ed. *Histology for Pathologists,* 3rd ed. Philadelphia: Lippincott, Williams and Wilkins, 2007:473-504.

2

The Uses and Abuses of the Lung Biopsy

Anthony A. Gal

INTRODUCTION

The lung biopsy is widely recognized as a valuable tool for the diagnosis and management of diverse pulmonary disorders. The various procedures currently in use such as the open lung biopsy (OLBx), video-assisted thoracoscopic (VATS) biopsy, and transbronchial lung biopsy (TBBx) can be diagnostic when performed under appropriate circumstances and if evaluated by the pathologist with several caveats in mind. Although the morphological findings seen in lung biopsy specimens may represent a specific disease entity, in many circumstances these changes may be non-specific findings that will need to be correlated with the clinical and radiographical presentations.

HISTORY

The lung biopsy is a relatively new tool for the diagnosis of lung diseases. Although rigid bronchoscopy was introduced just before the end of the 19th century, it was primarily used for visualization of the large airways without pathological confirmation. Later refinements in procedures led to its use for the evaluation of central lesions, but peripheral lesions were poorly visualized and seldom biopsied.

In the early 1960s, refinements in optical technology led to the first flexible fiber-optic bronchoscope. The introduction of this new equipment and its application in a variety of clinical situations led to increased use of the TBBx. Thereafter, numerous studies examined the role of fiberoptic bronchoscopy and the diagnostic yield of TBBx in a spectrum of clinical settings.

Following World War II, major advances in surgical technique, anesthesia, and antibiotic therapy led to the development of the OLBx. During the 1950s and into the 1970s, there were several clinical and pathological studies that evaluated the diagnostic efficacy of OLBx in various types of non-neoplastic diseases. However, thoracotomy with OLBx can be associated with significant morbidity and mortality.

Video-assisted thoracoscopic surgery (VATS) allows the thoracic surgeon to procure tissue via a less invasive means and potentially minimize post-operative complications. In capable hands, several studies have shown that the ability to procure tissue via VATS is equivalent to that of open thoracotomy.

EFFICACY OF THE TRANSBRONCHIAL LUNG BIOPSY

In common practice, the TBBx is performed by the bronchoscopist in the hopes of arriving at a definitive diagnosis and avoiding the use of a more invasive procedure such as an OLBx or VATS biopsy. Various cytological specimens such as bronchial washings, bronchial brushings, and bronchoalveolar lavages are usually collected during the bronchoscopy procedure to improve overall diagnostic yield. Although TBBx can be a highly effective tool for the diagnosis of certain lung diseases, its role in most other circumstances is quite limited (see Table 2-1). Moreover, the prudent pathologist should not fall into the trap of being forced into rendering a diagnosis from the TBBx outside of certain clinical and pathological settings.

Transbronchial lung biopsy is particularly effective for the diagnosis of primary lung carcinomas; the addition of cytological specimens increases the overall yield. Other less common primary lung tumors, such as carcinoid tumors, sclerosing hemangiomas, or bronchial gland tumors, could be potentially diagnosed by TBBx, in appropriate circumstances. TBBx is less effective in the setting

TABLE 2-1

Reliability of Transbronchial Biopsy*

High Utility	Probably Diagnostic	Possibly Diagnostic	Unreliable
Lung cancer and some metastases	Alveolar hemorrhage	Wegener's granulomatosis	Usual interstitial pneumonia
Sarcoidosis	Capillaritis in anti-neutrophil cytoplasmic antibody-related disorders	Eosinophilic pneumonia	Desquamative interstitial pneumonia
Opportunistic infections in immunocompromised patients	Goodpasture's disease	Lymphoid interstitial pneumonia	Respiratory bronchiolitis interstitial lung disease
Lung transplantation	Lupus pneumonitis	Obliterative bronchiolitis	Nonspecific interstitial pneumonia
	Alveolar proteinosis	Drug toxicity	
	Lymphangioleiomyomatosis	Hypersensitivity pneumonitis	
	Unusual tumors	Langerhans cell histiocytosis	

*Adapted from reading option 4.

of metastasis to the lungs, particularly when solitary and peripheral in location. In addition, morphologic features of metastases can sometimes mimic those of primary lung carcinomas, so the pathologist must be careful to consider the possibility of a metastasis when evaluating a carcinoma. Immunohistochemical staining can be helpful for this purpose (Chapter 38). Sarcoidosis is another disorder that can be readily diagnosed by TBBx and endobronchial biopsies, assuming that other granulomatous disorders have been excluded. However, the presence of non-necrotizing granulomas in TBBx always bears consideration of a broad differential diagnosis (Figure 2-1). In immunocompromised patients, certain opportunistic infections, such as *Pneumocystis jiroveci*, or viral or other fungal infections can be diagnosed by TBBx. Finally, in lung transplant recipients, TBBx is highly effective for the diagnosis of acute allograft rejection, sometimes effective for obliterative bronchiolitis, and less effective for some of the other entities that occur in this clinical setting such as post-transplant lymphoproliferative disorders.

The TBBx can provide useful information in certain non-neoplastic lung diseases. The presence of diffuse alveolar hemorrhage with necrotizing capillaritis may suggest the diagnosis of an anti-neutrophil cytoplasmic antibody-related lung disease or another autoimmune disorder. For other rare disorders such as pulmonary alveolar proteinosis or lymphangioleiomyomatosis the TBBx may be diagnostic, but histochemical and immunohistochemical stains should be employed for confirmation.

For many other disorders, it is unlikely that the TBBx will be effective. In pulmonary Wegener's granulomatosis, it is essential to find both the necrotizing granulomata and vasculitis; however, it is quite exceptional to receive adequate tissue with these pathological findings in small biopsy specimens. Moreover, caution is advised since vasculitis-like changes can be seen in blood vessels which are adjacent to necrotizing granulomas due to various infectious disorders. When the TBBx shows tissue eosinophilia, it may not be possible to further characterize this infiltrate. For lymphoproliferative disorders, the biopsy may not provide sufficient tissue to separate lymphoid interstitial pneumonia from low-grade malignant lymphoma or other disorders in this category.

The TBBx is essentially unreliable for the diagnosis and classification of the diffuse idiopathic interstitial lung diseases. The distinct and somewhat characteristic findings are based on pathological criteria that were derived from open lung biopsies. Although some clinicians attempt to use TBBx as a first-step diagnostic procedure, the limited sample size, the inability to evaluate various regions of the lung, and potential tissue artifacts render it essentially useless for the diagnosis of these disorders.

PROBLEMS WITH LUNG BIOPSY

ISSUES OF TISSUE

The morphologic changes that are present in lung biopsies of inflammatory diseases are seldom specific for a single entity and can be the result of various causes.

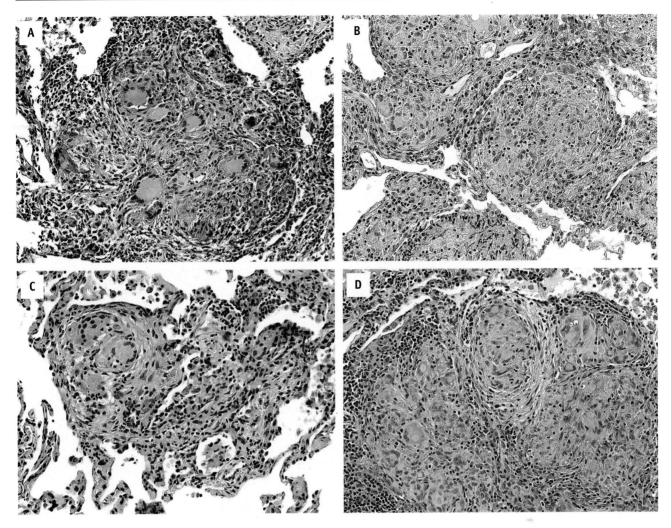

FIGURE 2-1

Non-necrotizing granulomas in biopsy specimens
The presence of a non-necrotizing granuloma should lead to the consideration of several disease processes, which can have similar morphologies:
(A) Sarcoidosis; **(B)** Beryllosis; **(C)** Chronic hypersensitivity pneumonitis; **(D)** Tuberculosis.

This is particularly true of the interstitial lung diseases, in which the pathological findings frequently overlap. For example, each of the key histological features seen in usual interstitial pneumonia (UIP) [i.e., fibroblast foci, patchy chronic interstitial inflammation, variation in degree and extent of fibroconnective tissue ("temporal heterogeneity"), and honeycombing fibrosis] are not specific for UIP and may not be present in limited biopsy samples (Figure 2-2). Alternatively, when a nonspecific feature such as chronic interstitial inflammation is seen in a biopsy, it may or may not be of diagnostic significance. Other features such as blood, edema, fibrosis, or chronic bronchiolitis are commonly present in specimens, and it may be difficult to decide if these changes have true pathologic significance.

As would be expected, a TBBx procured by rigid or fiberoptic bronchoscopy typically yields a limited number of lung tissue fragments. While a small biopsy may be sufficient for the diagnosis of malignancy, it may not be sufficient for other disorders. For example, in

the setting of lung transplantation, it has been suggested that at least five pieces of alveolated lung tissue containing greater than 100 alveoli be present for a proper evaluation. Another major problem with TBBx is the inability to evaluate the low-power architectural features that are essential for differentiating the various interstitial lung diseases.

Larger specimens such as OLBx and VATS biopsies generally provide more generous samples, but there may also be problems in obtaining adequate lung tissue for diagnosis. Specimens taken from the lingula, or from a markedly fibrotic or elastotic lung may not be representative of the underlying disease process. The term "end-stage lung" should be reserved for situations in which there is radiographic evidence of extensive disease.

A number of artifacts may occur in lung biopsies (Chapter 1), potentially interfering with interpretation. Inflation techniques can be used to obviate artifactual atelectasis in OLBx and VATS biopsies. A small gauge needle is inserted into the lung to inflate

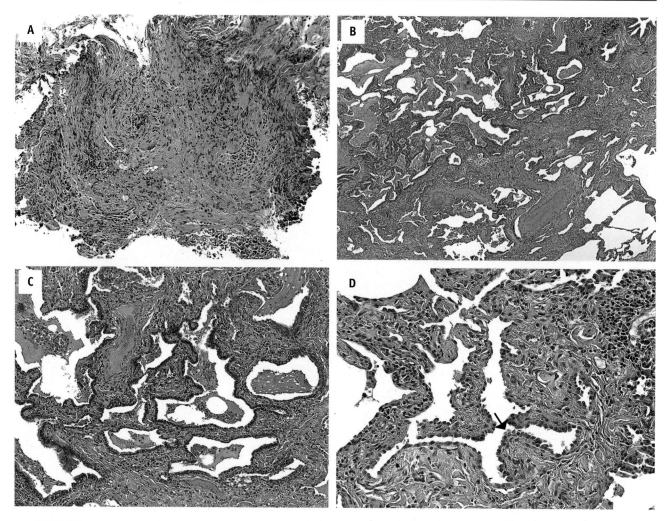

FIGURE 2-2

Limited use of transbronchial biopsy in idiopathic pulmonary fibrosis

(A) The transbronchial biopsy discloses some fibrosis, but is otherwise non diagnostic; **(B)** The subsequent open lung biopsy clearly discloses the low-power architectural features of usual interstitial pneumonia (UIP); **(C)** The honeycombing fibrosis, which is an important feature in diagnosing UIP, is clearly established in the open lung biopsy, but was not seen in the transbronchial biopsy; **(D)** The fibroblastic focus, which consists of young basophilic collagen underneath the alveolar epithelium, is evident at the arrow in the open lung biopsy. This feature was also not appreciated in the transbronchial lung biopsy.

the lung with formalin. This procedure expands the alveolar spaces and eliminates collapse. For the frozen section, this technique can be easily modified by using a slightly larger gauge needle; the OCT embedding medium can inflate the small sample, and this technique will facilitate cryosectioning and avoid atelectasis (Figure 2-3).

INTERPRETIVE ISSUES

The histological evaluation and interpretation of lung biopsies is often a challenging task for the pathologist. There are several explanations for this: the level of experience and confidence level of the pathologist, the quality and number of specimens evaluated, and whether appropriate clinical, radiographic, or other pertinent information is

readily available. Yet, there seems to be substantial variance in the interpretation of lung biopsies.

A presurgical biopsy by TTBx or cytology of a primary lung carcinoma usually results in accurate tumor classification. In most instances, the tumor can be readily classified as either "small cell carcinoma" or "non-small cell carcinoma." However, further classification into pathological subgroups of non-small cell lung cancer (i.e., squamous cell carcinoma, adenocarcinoma, or large cell carcinoma) may not always be feasible. Reproducibility studies of lung tumor pathological classification have demonstrated significant problems in inter-observer and in intra-observer variability.

A well-studied example of this inter-observer variability is duly noted for pulmonary neuroendocrine tumors. Although the recent "World Health Organization Classification of Tumors of the Lung" defines distinct histopathological criteria for each of these

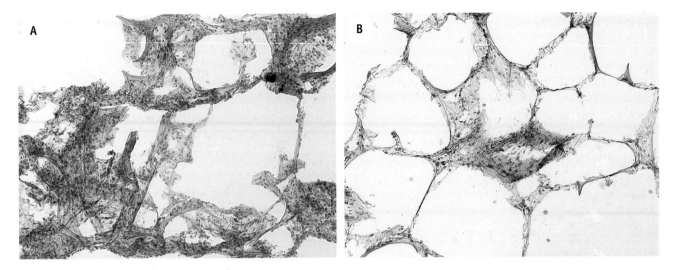

FIGURE 2-3

Inflation of lung during frozen section

(A) This piece of lung is structurally normal, but the artifactual atelectasis could lead to a misinterpretation of pulmonary fibrosis; **(B)** Injecting the lung tissue with OCT-embedding material prevents the artifactual atelectasis and facilitates cryosectioning.

tumors, there are persistent difficulties in accurate tumor classification in high-grade tumors (Figure 2-4). There is considerable disagreement and inability to reach a consensus diagnosis amongst experienced lung pathologists; this variability can be as high as 50% in the case of large cell neuroendocrine carcinoma.

Sophisticated imaging technology using morphometric optical imaging techniques has shown that certain descriptive cytological and histological criteria once proposed in classification schemata may not be reliable criteria for the classification of pulmonary neuroendocrine tumors.

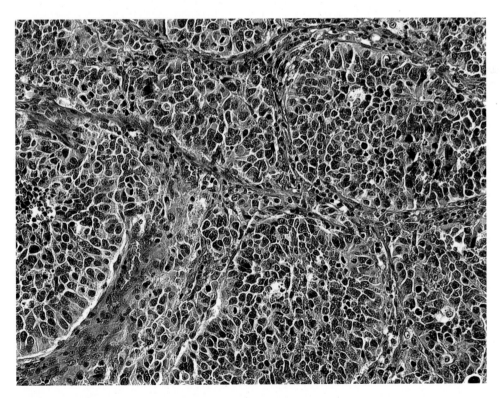

FIGURE 2-4

Problematic high-grade neuroendocrine carcinoma of the lung

Classification of this high-grade neuroendocrine carcinoma would be difficult: large cell neuroendocrine carcinoma versus combined small cell carcinoma with large cell neuroendocrine carcinoma.

There are many pitfalls for making an accurate diagnosis of a pulmonary neuroendocrine tumor in TBBx. A carcinoid tumor could be overdiagnosed as small cell carcinoma and vice versa. Not infrequently, small cell carcinoma in TBBx exhibits significant crush artifact or a subpopulation of larger cells, which makes it difficult to separate from other entities in the differential diagnosis. Judicious use of immunohistochemical stains (keratins, TTF-1, p63, CD-56, or other neuroendocrine markers) may be helpful in some circumstances, but the findings could complicate matters, particularly if the results are not conclusive. Correlation of the TBBx with cytology specimens is strongly recommended for problematic cases.

Another significant example of inter-observer variability in lung pathology is in the classification of the diffuse interstitial lung diseases. It is common knowledge that many general surgical pathologists have difficulties in this endeavor, yet this can also be challenging for the expert. Amongst pulmonary pathologists who have expertise in interstitial lung diseases there is a high degree of diagnostic accuracy for some disorders (e.g., sarcoidosis), but poorer degrees of concordance for others (e.g., usual interstitial pneumonia versus nonspecific interstitial pneumonia).

CONCLUSION

Transbronchial lung biopsies offer a low-risk approach to acquiring tissue that is more likely to be diagnostic in some clinical settings than others. Open lung and VATS biopsies are sensitive and specific tests that should be utilized when a specific diagnosis cannot be gleaned from available clinical and radiographic data and TBBx. It cannot be overemphasized that the morphologic findings must be correlated with the clinical and radiographical presentations. A first-hand knowledge of the indications and limitations of lung biopsies is necessary for proper patient care and diagnosis.

SUGGESTED READINGS

1. Churg A. Transbronchial biopsy: nothing to fear. *Am J Surg Pathol.* 2001;25:820-2.
2. Colby TV, Churg AC. Patterns of pulmonary fibrosis. *Pathol Annu.* 1986. 21(Pt 2):277-309.
3. Ferson PF, Landreneau RJ. Thoracoscopic lung biopsy or open lung biopsy for interstitial lung disease. *Chest Surg Clin N Am.* 1998;8: 749-62.
4. Gal AA. The use and abuse of the lung biopsy. *Adv Anat Pathol.* 2005;12:195-202.
5. Jones AM, Hanson IM, Armstrong GR, et al. Value and accuracy of cytology in addition to histology in the diagnosis of lung cancer at flexible bronchoscopy. *Respir Med.* 2001;95:374-8.
6. Katzenstein AL, Askin FB. Interpretation and significance of pathologic findings in transbronchial lung biopsy. *Am J Surg Pathol.* 1980;4: 223-34.
7. Marchevsky AM, Gal AA, Shah S, et al. Morphometry confirms the presence of considerable nuclear size overlap between "small cells" and "large cells" in high-grade pulmonary neuroendocrine neoplasms. *Am J Clin Pathol.* 2001;116:466-72.
8. Nicholson AG, Addis BJ, Bharucha H, et al. Inter-observer variation between pathologists in diffuse parenchymal lung disease. *Thorax.* 2004;59:500-5.
9. Wilson RK, Fechner RE, Greenberg SD, et al. Clinical implications of a "nonspecific" transbronchial biopsy. *Am J Med.* 1978;65:252-6
10. Wall CP, Gaensler EA, Carrington CB, et al. Comparison of transbronchial and open biopsies in chronic infiltrative lung diseases. *Am Rev Respir Dis.* 1981;123:280-5.

3 A Pattern-Based Approach to Diagnosis

Diana N. Ionescu • Kevin O. Leslie

INTRODUCTION

Each of us follows well established patterns as we go about our daily lives, and in turn we interact with our world through the recognition of patterns: in the people we know, the places we live, and the structures that form our physical environment. Similarly, the specialty of anatomic pathology relies heavily on pattern recognition, especially given the observational nature of this medical discipline. The experienced anatomic pathologist quickly recognizes the pattern of disease and, without dwelling on the initial overview, very often has already moved on instinctively to glean additional qualitative and quantitative information to arrive at a diagnosis. This initial observation forms the basis for this chapter and the basic patterns of pulmonary disease that will be discussed here. In addition, we will explore how additional specific morphologic findings at higher magnification contribute to the construction of a specific diagnosis or limited differential diagnosis.

The lung is an organ open to the environment, and with every breath it is exposed to a large number of potential injuries. Despite superb dynamics and adaptability, the lung responds to injury with a limited repertoire of inflammatory and reparative reactions. These reactions can be grouped based on their acuity (e.g., acute, subacute, and chronic) and by the distribution of abnormalities spatially or in relation to underlying lung anatomy (e.g., alveolar space-filling, nodule formation). Some lung diseases are characterized by quite subtle changes at the microscopic level, and these are grouped together as a pattern we refer to as "minimal changes" (at scanning magnification). Through these foundation patterns, we present a practical approach to pulmonary pathology.

A journey through the true three-dimensional microanatomy of the lung, even today, is still mainly an imaginative one. A histology slide prepared from lung tissue presents the lung anatomy in two dimensions. To the inexperienced eye, the structure appears at first overly simple, yet translating what is seen in two dimensions to its corollary in three-dimensional anatomy takes considerable practice and repeated exposure. As a reasonable starting point, a schematic representation may be helpful (Figure 3-1). This relationship is also very important in correlating the histopathology with the radiologic changes, particularly those seen in high-resolution computed tomography (HRCT) scans. A radiology-pathology correlation of anatomic distribution in lung pathology is summarized in Table 3-1.

The clinical and radiological information and a low-magnification evaluation of a lung wedge biopsy should immediately suggest a short differential diagnosis. When looking at a lung biopsy, the first question to ask is: what is the dominant pattern on this slide? Is the pattern acute lung injury (pattern 1), fibrosis (pattern 2), chronic cellular interstitial infiltrates (pattern 3), alveolar filling (pattern 4), or nodules (pattern 5), or does the biopsy look nearly normal through the 2x objective (pattern 6)? In this chapter we will present these 6 patterns by describing the essential elements that comprise each of them, followed by a diagnostic algorithm by which individual disease entities within each pattern can be discerned. This pattern-based diagnostic approach is most helpful in the assessment of surgical wedge lung biopsies for non-neoplastic disease—the most difficult and challenging samples in pulmonary pathology. By following the pattern-based approach we can be certain that all histological entities from the most common to the most esoteric are acknowledged and, therefore, unlikely to be missed.

Detailed clinical and radiological features of the specific lung diseases, along with treatment and prognosis, are presented throughout the chapters of this book. Here we will emphasize the pathologic features helpful in narrowing the differential diagnosis and provide cross-references to other chapters for more detailed discussion wherever appropriate.

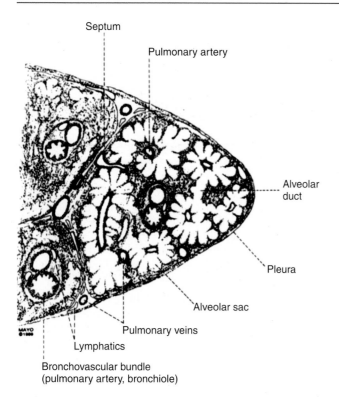

Septum

Pulmonary artery

Alveolar duct

Pleura

Alveolar sac

Pulmonary veins

Lymphatics

Bronchovascular bundle
(pulmonary artery, bronchiole)

FIGURE 3-1

Schematic representation of microscopic lung anatomy
(Reproduced with permission from Colby, T, et al. Atlas of Pulmonary Surgical Pathology. Philadelphia: W.B. Saunders Co., 1991)

TABLE 3-1

Anatomic Distribution in Diffuse Lung Disease

Histologic	Radiologic (HRCT)
Broncho/bronchiolocentric	Centrilobular
	Bronchovascular
Angiocentric	Bronchovascular (arterial)
	Interlobular septal (venous)
Pleural/subpleural	Pleural/subpleural
Lymphatic	Bronchovascular
	Interlobular septal
	Pleural/subpleural
Peripheral acinar	Subpleural peripheral distribution (paraseptal)
Septal	Septal (interlobular septal)
Random nodular	Random nodular
Parenchymal consolidation	Consolidation
Diffuse interstitial	Diffuse interstitial, ground-glass attenuation
Mixed and unclassified	Mixed/unclassifiable

With permission from B.C. Dekker Inc. (reference 4).

ACUTE LUNG INJURY (PATTERN 1)

ELEMENTS OF THE PATTERN

The lung biopsy is involved by varying amounts of alveolar wall edema, intra-alveolar edema and fibrin, and has reactive alveolar lining cells (Figure 3-2). Acute lung injury typically has a short clinical evolution and often a rapid onset of symptoms. When the pattern of diffuse lung injury is noted, the biopsy should be searched for specific histological features that will help to suggest a more specific etiology. Infectious diseases should always lead the differential diagnosis in Pattern 1, and therefore special stains for organisms are a requirement, along with close correlation with clinical history and microbiologic findings.

I. ACUTE LUNG INJURY WITH EDEMA, FIBRIN, AND REACTIVE TYPE 2 CELLS

Many systemic medical conditions can affect the lung, especially cardiovascular diseases, but also shock, trauma, sepsis, etc. Many of these conditions are rarely biopsied, and when they are, it is to assess the presence, extent, and severity of the lung injury and to rule out the possibility of atypical infection. The earliest changes seen in acute lung injury are interstitial (alveolar septal) edema, followed by intra-alveolar edema and fibrin, and then accumulation of cellular alveolar debris. A search for necrosis or granulomas is essential in this setting.

II. ACUTE LUNG INJURY WITH FIBRIN AND ORGANIZATION ONLY

A new entity has recently been described with some similarities to diffuse alveolar damage (DAD) discussed below, termed acute fibrinous and organizing pneumonia (AFOP). AFOP lacks hyaline membranes but is rich in fibrinous alveolar exudates (Figure 3-3). By definition, AFOP lacks evidence of infection or extravascular eosinophils as might be expected of acute eosinophilic pneumonia.

III. ACUTE LUNG INJURY WITH HYALINE MEMBRANES

Hyaline membranes are accumulations of proteinaceous alveolar exudates at the periphery of the alveoli. These become adherent to the alveolar septa and are seen to outline the alveolar spaces (Figure 3-4). The diagnosis of

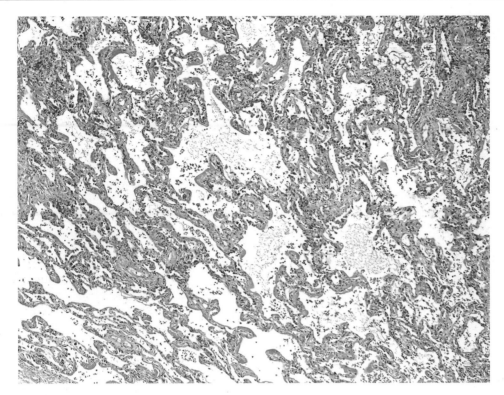

FIGURE 3-2

Acute lung injury (pattern 1)
The lung biopsy demonstrates alveolar wall edema, intra-alveolar edema and fibrin, and reactive alveolar lining cells.

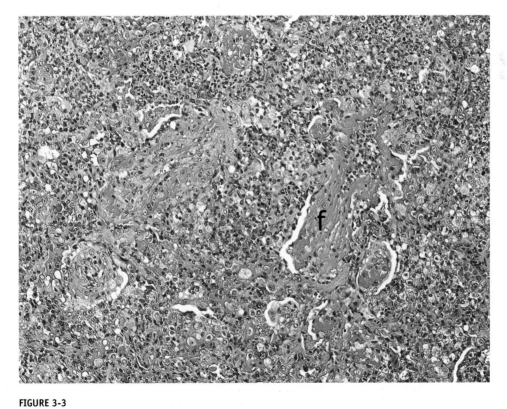

FIGURE 3-3

Acute fibrinous and organizing pneumonia (pattern 1)
AFOP shares many features with diffuse alveolar damage. However, instead of hyaline membranes, AFOP is characterized by aggregated fibrin (**f**) in alveolar spaces and variable degrees of organization.

ACUTE LUNG INJURY (PATTERN 1)—FACT SHEET AND PATHOLOGIC FEATURES

Definition

➤➤ Lung biopsies are diffusely involved by interstitial and alveolar edema, intra-alveolar fibrin, and reactive type 2 cell hyperplasia

Potential Etiologies

➤➤ Infections
➤➤ Sepsis
➤➤ Shock, trauma
➤➤ Radiation
➤➤ Drugs or toxins
➤➤ Aspiration
➤➤ Many others (see other chapters)

Histologic Characteristics

➤➤ Edema: interstitial and alveolar
➤➤ Reactive type 2 pneumocytes
➤➤ Hyaline membranes or fibrin deposition in alveoli
➤➤ Variably present:
   ➤➤ Necrosis
   ➤➤ Neutrophils
   ➤➤ Eosinophils
   ➤➤ Siderophages
   ➤➤ Vacuolated macrophages

DAD is appropriate when hyaline membranes are present. As the time between the insult and the biopsy becomes longer, the hyaline membranes become more organized (cellular) and distinct (thicker), a phenomenon seen three to seven days after injury. During this phase, fibrin thrombi can be seen in the small pulmonary arteries, and the interstitium shows a mononuclear cell inflammatory infiltrate. When reactive type 2 cell hyperplasia is seen, the injury is usually about one week old, and the proliferative phase of DAD has started. This phase is characterized by fibroblastic proliferation, seen mainly in the interstitium, but also in the alveoli (Figure 3-5). By late proliferative phase, most hyaline membranes have been reabsorbed. Mitotic activity can be prominent, and immature squamous metaplasia can be seen. Acute lung injury is often a repetitive event (i.e., drugs or systemic connective tissue disease manifesting in the lung), and therefore changes characteristic of the exudative and proliferative phases of DAD can be seen in the same biopsy.

Among lung infections, viral infections are a recognized trigger of DAD (Chapter 13). Bacterial and fungal infections can also occassionally present as DAD, either in the setting of a pneumonia or a systemic infection (sepsis).

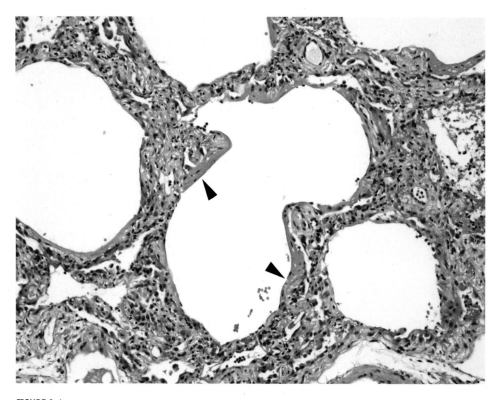

FIGURE 3-4

Diffuse alveolar damage—exudative phase (pattern 1)
Proteinaceous alveolar exudates (hyaline membranes—arrowheads) can be seen lining alveolar spaces in this example of exudative phase DAD.

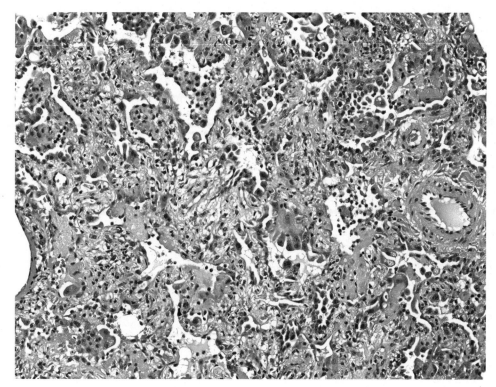

FIGURE 3-5
Diffuse alveolar damage—proliferative phase (pattern 1)
The proliferative phase of DAD is heralded by the presence of increased cellularity in both the interstitium and alveolar spaces, the latter typically in the form of intra-alveolar fibroblasts (organizing pneumonia).

IV. Acute Lung Injury with Necrosis

Necrosis in the setting of acute lung injury can be seen in infections, infarction, acute aspiration, and even malignant tumors. Necrosis can involve lung parenchyma alone or occur with necrosis of airway epithelium (Figure 3-6).

Influenza, herpes simplex, varicella-zoster, and adenovirus pneumonias are all infections characterized by DAD with necrosis, and some can be easily recognized by characteristic viral cytopathic effects such as intranuclear inclusions (herpes simplex, varicella-zoster), or smudge cells (adenovirus). Some bacterial and fungal infections can also produce necrosis.

Although lung infarction and acute aspiration pneumonia are localized rather than diffuse processes, they can be seen in a background of DAD and demonstrate necrosis. Malignancies can also present with associated areas of DAD, and necrosis can be prominent in these cases.

V. Acute Lung Injury with Neutrophils

The presence of neutrophils in the alveolar spaces should always raise the possibility of infection (e.g., acute bronchopneumonia) (Figure 3-7). In addition, a careful search for capillaritis is always warranted as this finding, with hemosiderin-laden macrophages, carries strong implications for immediate therapeutic intervention (immunosuppression for immune-mediated alveolar hemorrhage).

Influenza pneumonia can present with fibrinous and focally neutrophilic DAD. Identification of bacteria by Gram or silver stain in predominantly neutrophilic DAD is indicative of bacterial pneumonia, and fungi should also be sought with a silver stain.

VI. Acute Lung Injury with Eosinophils

Several different conditions have been described in which the air spaces contain eosinophils. This could represent a manifestation of an idiopathic or a secondary form of eosinophilic pneumonia, due to an infection, drug, tumor, or systemic disease. Peripheral blood and bronchoalveolar lavage eosinophils are commonly elevated in these conditions.

Eosinophilic pneumonia shows airspaces filled with variable numbers of eosinophils and plump eosinophilic macrophages (Figure 3-8). Eosinophilic microabscesses and multinucleation of macrophages can also be observed. Atypical type II cell hyperplasia can accompany these changes, raising a concern about viral infection or tumor. If the patient is treated with corticosteroids, eosinophils are reduced considerably.

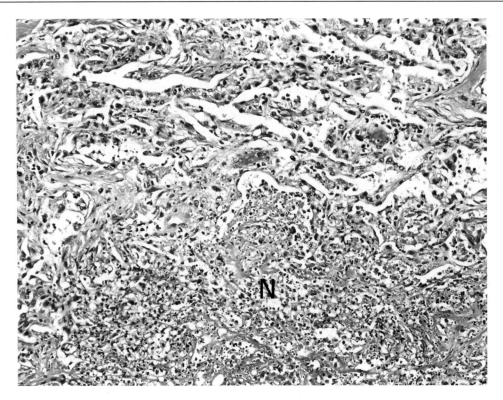

FIGURE 3-6

Necrosis in diffuse alveolar damage is a sign of infection (pattern 1)
Necrosis (N) in the setting of acute lung injury is usually an indication of infection. Necrosis can also be seen in Wegener's granulomatosis, lung infarction, acute aspiration, and malignant tumors. Necrosis can involve lung paren-chyma alone or primarily involve airway epithelium.

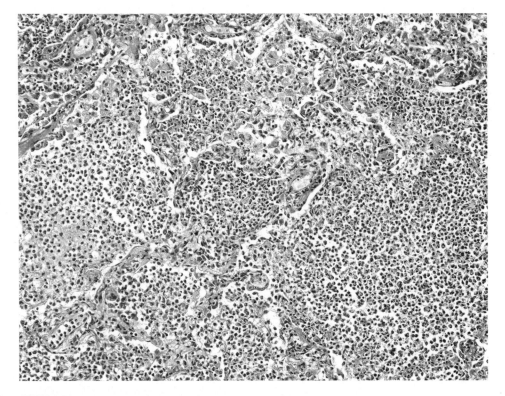

FIGURE 3-7

Acute injury with alveolar neutrophils (pattern 1)
The presence of many neutrophils in the alveolar spaces is characteristic of acute bronchopneumonia, and should always raise the consideration of infection.

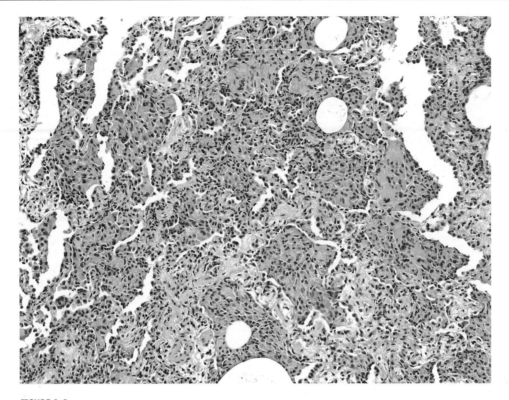

FIGURE 3-8

Acute eosinophilic pneumonia (pattern 1)
Acute injury accompanied by air space filling with variable numbers of eosinophils, plump eosinophilic macrophages, and reactive type 2 cell hyperplasia is characteristic of acute eosinophilic pneumonia. There is often variation in lobular intensity.

VII. Acute Lung Injury with Siderophages

Identification of hemosiderin-laden macrophages (with coarsely granular, brown-golden, refractile pigment) in the setting of Pattern 1 raises a differential diagnosis to include lung infarction, drug toxicity, and a condition referred to as diffuse alveolar hemorrhage (DAH). Diffuse alveolar hemorrhage of immune origin shows fresh hemorrhage and hemosiderin-laden macrophages in the alveolar spaces (Figure 3-9), and often small vessel vasculitis. Attention should be given to distinguish it from the artifactual hemorrhage, which appears as fresh hemorrhage without associated siderophages, fibrin, or capillaritis. It must also be distinguished from a hemorrhagic infectious pneumonia.

VIII. Acute Lung Injury with Vacuolated Macrophages

The presence of intra-alveolar macrophages with prominently vacuolated cytoplasm and associated alveolar fibrin accumulation (Figure 3-10) should raise the differential diagnosis of drug toxicity. Drug toxicity in the lung has many manifestations, from DAD to fibrosis (Chapter 19). Cytotoxic drugs often cause DAD, most commonly bleomycin, busulfan, and carmustine. An anti-arrhythmic drug, amiodarone, is well recognized to cause pulmonary toxicity, characterized microscopically by acute and organizing lung injury with vacuolated macrophages.

FIBROSIS (PATTERN 2)

Elements of the Pattern

The lung architecture is distorted by varying degrees of collagen deposition, giving the biopsy an overall eosinophilic appearance (Figure 3-11). A large number of lung diseases can lead to permanent structural lung remodeling with fibrosis, very often with alveolar loss. As with the other patterns presented, radiological findings are extremely helpful for suggesting specific diagnoses.

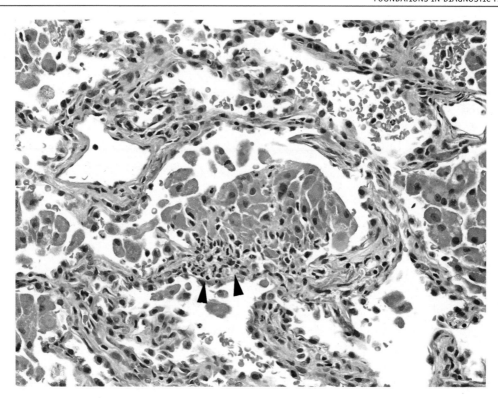

FIGURE 3-9

Diffuse alveolar hemorrhage with capillaritis (pattern 1)
Alveolar hemorrhage of immune origin is characterized by both fresh hemorrhage and hemosiderin-laden macrophages in the alveolar spaces. In this case of Wegener's granulomatosis, capillaritis is present focally (arrowheads).

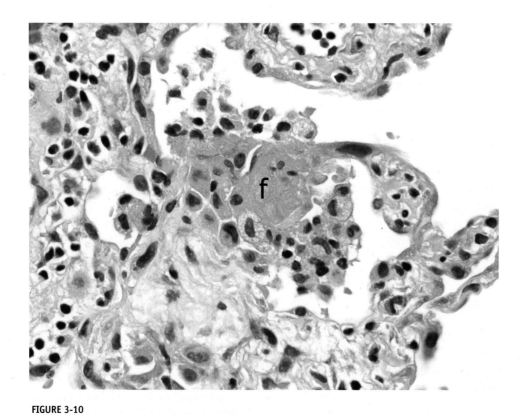

FIGURE 3-10

Acute injury with vacuolated alveolar macrophages (pattern 1)
The presence of intra-alveolar macrophages having a prominently vacuolated cytoplasm and associated alveolar fibrin (f) accumulation (attesting to acute injury) raises a differential diagnosis to include drug toxicity. This is a case of bleomycin toxicity.

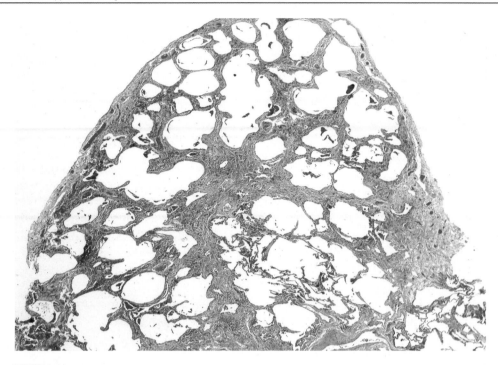

FIGURE 3-11
Fibrosis (pattern 2)
The lung architecture is distorted by varying degrees of collagen deposition, giving the biopsy an overall eosinophilic (pink) appearance.

I. FIBROSIS WITH TEMPORAL HETEROGENEITY (HONEYCOMBING TO NORMAL)

USUAL INTERSTITIAL PNEUMONIA PATTERN

Usual interstitial pneumonia (UIP) is the prototype of pulmonary fibrosis with so-called "temporal heterogeneity." Temporal heterogeneity refers to the variegated appearance of the lung biopsy in UIP, where areas of advanced fibrosis are seen adjacent to entirely normal lung, with interspersed areas of active fibroblastic proliferation known as "fibroblastic foci." The UIP pattern tends to have fibrosis at the periphery of the lung lobules, with centrilobular (i.e., peribronchovascular) sparing (Figure 3-12). Honeycomb changes eventually develop.

When a UIP pattern is identified and no cause can be found (e.g., chronic hypersensitivity, systemic connective tissue disease), the process is considered idiopathic, and the clinical term for this condition is idiopathic pulmonary fibrosis (IPF). HRCT typically shows abnormalities mostly present at the periphery of the lung and in the lung bases in IPF.

Honeycombing is the final common pathway for many types of severe lung injuries (Figure 3-13), and is characterized by focal or diffuse replacement of alveolar architecture by cystic spaces surrounded by thick fibrous septa, with mucous or air-filled air spaces. Thick, irregular bundles of smooth muscle can be present around these cysts within areas of fibrosis, presumably due to progressive parenchymal collapse with incorporation of native airway and vascular smooth muscle into the fibrosis. Honeycombing is not specific for UIP/IPF, and can develop with other interstitial lung diseases, as well.

II. FIBROSIS WITH UNIFORM ALVEOLAR SEPTAL SCARRING

NON-SPECIFIC INTERSTITIAL PNEUMONIA PATTERN

Non-specific interstitial pneumonia (NSIP) was described in 1994 by Katzenstein and Fiorelli as a constellation of disorders with an overall significantly better prognosis than UIP (90% survival at 5 years). Patients with NSIP were often found to have resolving infection, collagen vascular disease (CVD), or hypersensitivity pneumonitis. Many of the CVDs have an NSIP-pattern of lung injury.

FIBROSIS (PATTERN 2)—FACT SHEET AND PATHOLOGIC FEATURES

Definition
➤ Lung biopsies in which there is variable fibrosis

Diseases to Be Considered
➤ Fibrosis and microscopic honeycombing
  ➤ Usual interstitial pneumonia (UIP)
  ➤ Connective tissue diseases
    ➤ Rheumatoid arthritis (RA)
    ➤ Progressive systemic sclerosis (PSS)
    ➤ Mixed connective tissue disease (MCTD)
    ➤ Dermatomyositis/polymyositis (DM/PM)
    ➤ Sjögren's Syndrome (SS)
  ➤ Hypersensitivity pneumonitis
  ➤ Chronic eosinophilic pneumonia
  ➤ Erdheim-Chester disease
  ➤ Sarcoidosis (advanced)
  ➤ Chronic drug reactions
  ➤ Healed infectious pneumonias, DAD, and other inflammatory processes,
➤ Prominent bronchiolization and/or bronchiolocentric scarring
  ➤ Pulmonary Langerhans cell histiocytosis
  ➤ Respiratory bronchiolitis
  ➤ Connective tissue diseases
  ➤ Chronic hypersensitivity pneumonitis
  ➤ Small airways diseases
  ➤ Chronic aspiration
➤ Intra-alveolar vacuolated cells
  ➤ Chronic obstruction
  ➤ Drug toxicity
  ➤ Metabolic diseases
  ➤ Hermansky-Pudlak syndrome
➤ Hyaline membranes
  ➤ Connective tissue diseases (acute, subacute)
  ➤ Acute exacerbation of IPF
➤ Intra-alveolar siderophages
  ➤ Chronic cardiac congestion/chronic interstitial pulmonary edema
  ➤ Chronic alveolar hemorrhage
  ➤ Pneumoconiosis

On scanning magnification, biopsies with an NSIP pattern show preserved lung architecture with interstitial fibrosis having a "temporally homogeneous" appearance. Three forms of NSIP were originally proposed: a cellular inflammatory form, a mixed inflammatory and fibrotic form, and a purely fibrotic form (Figure 3-14).

III. FIBROSIS WITH AIRWAY-CENTERED SCARRING

Peribronchiolar metaplasia (Figure 3-15) also referred to as "bronchiolization" or "Lambertosis", consists of a proliferation of cuboidal epithelial cells over a scaffolding of interstitial fibrosis. It is considered a nonspecific reactive/reparative reaction to chronic injury of the terminal and respiratory bronchiole, often due to cigarette smoking or various inhaled agents or toxins. Connective tissue diseases, chronic hypersensitivity pneumonitis, small airways diseases with constrictive bronchiolitis, and chronic aspiration can also show prominent peribronchiolar metaplasia, and this finding can occur idiopathically as an isolated abnormality. Many of these disorders also show other histologic features of airway disease such as mucostasis, bronchiolar smooth muscle hyperplasia, and the presence of variable numbers of lightly pigmented air space macrophages within bronchiolar lumens and in the immediate surrounding alveoli. Langerhans cell histiocytosis also classically affects the small airways, producing bronchiolocentric stellate scors.

IV. FIBROSIS WITH INTRA-ALVEOLAR VACUOLATED CELLS

Accumulation of intra-alveolar macrophages in the air spaces is a nonspecific phenomenon. Intra-alveolar macrophages characterized by fine vacuolation in their cytoplasm can be observed with drug toxicity (i.e., Amiodarone), chronic obstruction ("golden pneumonia"), genetic storage diseases, and the Hermansky-Pudlak syndrome (HPS). HPS is a group of autosomal recessive genetic disorders associated with Golgi apparatus abnormalities. The largest cohort of HPS (400-500 individuals) resides in northwest Puerto Rico. The phenotype is characterized clinically by oculocutaneous albinism, platelet storage pool deficiency, and variable tissue lipofuscinosis. Histopathologically, broad zones of fibrosis are seen, either pleural based or centered on the airways. Alveolar septal thickening is present and associated with prominent, clear, vacuolated type II pneumocytes (Figure 3-16).

V. FIBROSIS WITH HYALINE MEMBRANES

The presence of hyaline membranes in a lung biopsy dominated by fibrosis suggests an acute event superimposed on a chronic lung disease with scarring. When the background fibrosis is peripherally accentuated and associated with honeycombing (UIP pattern), then the acute process may be exacerbation of the underlying disease (Figure 3-17).

Acute exacerbations of IPF are characterized clinically by sudden development of acute respiratory distress and new alveolar infiltrates in radiological studies in a patient being followed for IPF. On microscopic examination, acute lung injury is seen, superimposed on background fibrosis that can be highlighted by a Masson trichrome stain. An acute infectious process or drug

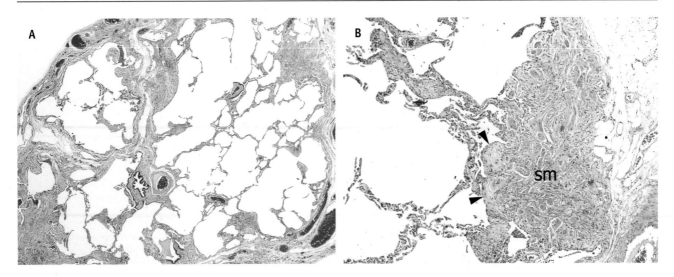

FIGURE 3-12

Usual interstitial pneumonia (pattern 2)

The "UIP pattern" tends to have fibrosis at the periphery of the lung lobules, with centrilobular (i.e., peribronchovascular) sparing **(A)**, fibroblastic foci (arrowheads) at the interface of fibrosis and normal lung, and smooth muscle "hyperplasia" (sm) in fibrosis **(B)**. Microscopic honeycombing is frequently present, even if honeycomb cysts are not visible on HRCT scan.

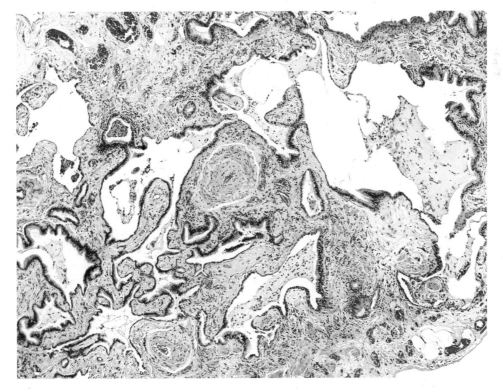

FIGURE 3-13

Microscopic honeycombing (pattern 2)

Microscopic honeycombing is not a specific finding; it represents the end stage of multiple types of severe lung injury.

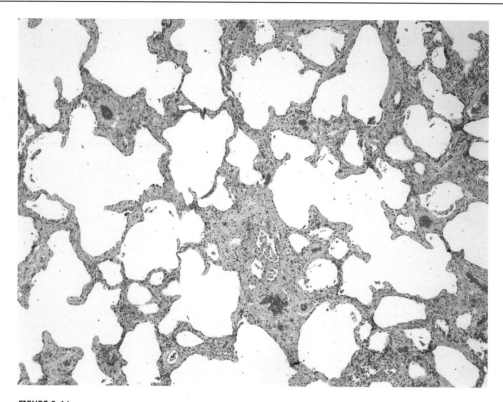

FIGURE 3-14

Nonspecific interstitial pneumonia (pattern 2)
Note the diffuse, inactive appearance of the interstitial fibrosis illustrated here. The expected temporal heterogeneity of UIP is not a feature of fibrotic NSIP.

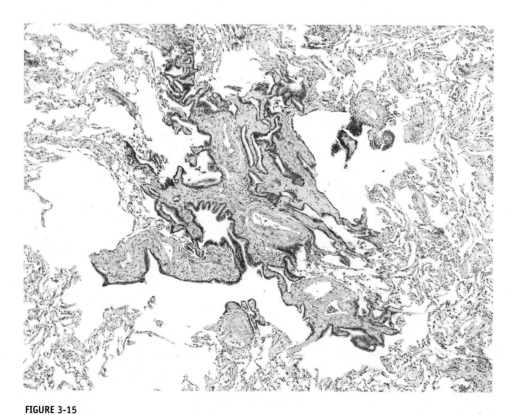

FIGURE 3-15

Peribronchiolar metaplasia and fibrosis (pattern 2)
Scarring around the terminal airways often is related to chronic inhalational injury (e.g., asbestosis, smoking-related lung diseases). When localized to the immediate vicinity of the airway, epithelial metaplasia may accompany the fibrosis, producing complex branching patterns sometimes referred to as "Lambertosis" (for the canal of Lambert).

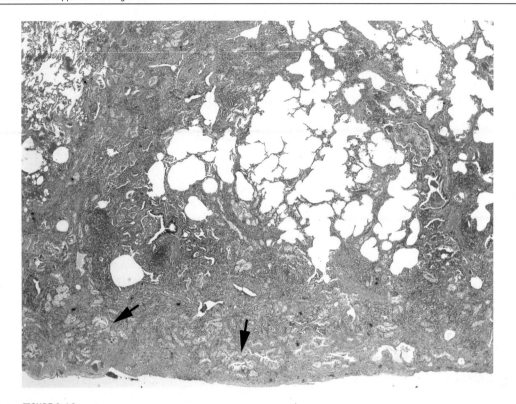

FIGURE 3-16

Hermansky-Pudlak syndrome (pattern 2)
This genetic disorder results in broad irregular zones of fibrosis as seen here. Some of the fibrosis is pleural-based and some is airway-centered. Note the "clear cells" of HPS even at low magnification (arrows).

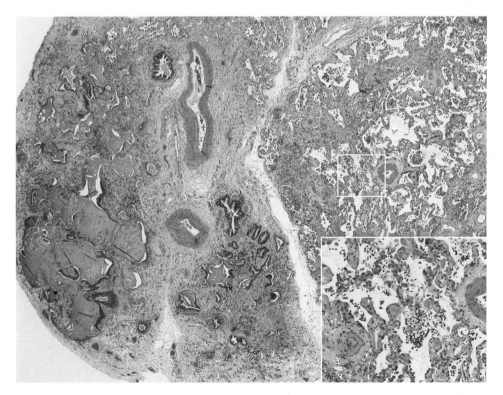

FIGURE 3-17

Acute on chronic disease (pattern 2)
Acute presentation of chronic lung disease is not uncommon. When the background fibrosis is peripherally accentuated and associated with honeycombing (UIP pattern), then the acute process may be an exacerbation of the underlying disease, superimposed infection, or an unrelated acute drug toxicity. Here, note microscopic honeycombing on the left and acute lung injury on the right (inset).

reaction superimposed on an unrelated chronic lung disease is also in the differential diagnosis.

VI. Fibrosis with Intra-Alveolar Siderophages

Chronic passive congestion, chronic immune-mediated alveolar hemorrhage, pneumoconiosis, and idiopathic hemosiderosis can present in lung biopsies with fibrosis and accumulation of intra-alveolar siderophages. Both hemosiderin and exogenous iron in siderosis stain with Prussian blue, but hemosiderin lacks the black cores within particles, characteristic of iron oxide seen in exogenous siderosis.

VII. Other Patterns of Fibrosis

Other patterns of fibrosis can help suggest an underlying disease. For example, fibrosis in sarcoidosis will follow the subpleural areas, interlobular septa, and bronchovascular bundles. In Erdheim-Chester disease, a distinctive pattern of subpleural and septal fibrosis with lymphatic distribution is seen (Figure 3-18).

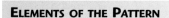

CHRONIC CELLULAR INTERSTITIAL INFILTRATES (PATTERN 3)

Elements of the Pattern

The lung is involved by varying types and distributions of chronic inflammation (Figure 3-19). Inflammatory infiltrates occupy the interstitium and are composed primarily of mononuclear inflammatory cells (lymphocytes, plasma cells, and histiocytes).

I. Chronic Cellular Interstitial Infiltrates with Mononuclear Cells and Granulomas

A. Hypersensitivity Pneumonitis

Hypersensitivity pneumonitis (HP) represents the prototype disease of Pattern 3, most often biopsied in the subacute form. The histologic picture is that of a chronic bronchiolocentric interstitial pneumonia characterized by the accumulation of lymphocytes and variable numbers of plasma cells in the interstitium. At scanning

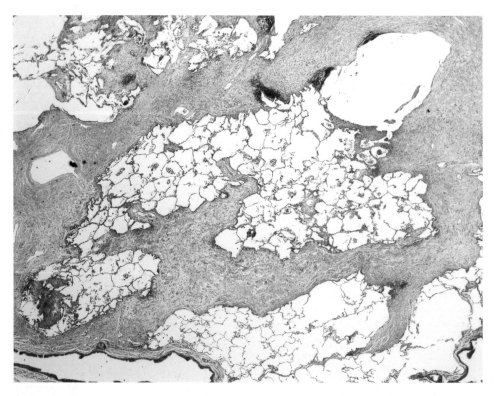

FIGURE 3-18

Erdheim-Chester disease (pattern 2)
A prominent pattern of subpleural and septal fibrosis with a distinctive lymphatic distribution is seen in Erdheim-Chester disease. Characteristic osteosclerosis is usually present on radiographs, typically involving the long tubular bones.

CHRONIC CELLULAR INFILTRATES (PATTERN 3)—FACT SHEET AND PATHOLOGIC FEATURES

Definition

▸▸ The lung biopsy is dominated by variable amounts of chronic inflammation and reactive type 2 pneumocyte hyperplasia

Diseases to Be Considered

▸▸ Hypersensitivity pneumonitis
▸▸ Nonspecific interstitial pneumonia (NSIP)
▸▸ Lymphoid interstitial pneumonia (LIP)
▸▸ Lymphoma
▸▸ Diffuse lymphoid hyperplasia
▸▸ Follicular bronchiolitis
▸▸ Collagen vascular diseases
▸▸ Infections

Histologic Characteristics

▸▸ Mononuclear inflammatory cell infiltrates
   ▸▸ Inflammatory infiltrate in the alveolar wall
   ▸▸ Preserved lung architecture
   ▸▸ Lymphocytes, plasma cells, plasmacytoid lymphocytes, histiocytes
▸▸ Lymphoid aggregates/germinal centers
   ▸▸ Mature lymphocytes
   ▸▸ Invasion into bronchial epithelium
   ▸▸ Spatial distribution: along airways, bronchovascular sheaths, lymphatics, or subpleurally
▸▸ Other findings
   ▸▸ Viral inclusions
   ▸▸ Granulomas and multinucleated giant cells
   ▸▸ Food particles
   ▸▸ Eosinophils and macrophages

---

magnification, the lung structure is preserved. Small, poorly formed granulomas can be seen in the interstitium (Figure 3-20). Scattered giant cells of the foreign body type can be seen around the terminal airways and may contain cleft-like clear spaces or small particles, which appear refractile under polarized light. Eventually, some cases progress to fibrosis (Pattern 2).

B. Atypical Mycobacterial Infection/Hot Tub Lung

The nontuberculous mycobacteria (NTM) include species such as *M. kansasii*, *M. avium* complex, and *M. xenopi*. A distinctive and recently highlighted manifestation of NTM can mimic hypersensitivity pneumonitis. Here, NTM infection occurs in the normal host as a result of bioaerosol exposure (so called "hot tub lung"). The characteristic histopathologic findings are a chronic cellular bronchiolitis accompanied by non-necrotizing or minimally necrotizing granulomas in the terminal airways and adjacent alveolar spaces (Figure 3-21).

C. Lymphoid Interstitial Pneumonia

The histopathologic hallmark of the lymphoid interstitial pneumonia (LIP) pattern is an exclusively interstitial and expansile lymphocytic or lymphoplasmacytic infiltrate that must be proven to be polyclonal. Granulomas commonly accompany the interstitial lymphocytic infiltrates. LIP is distinguished from the cellular form of NSIP mainly by the intensity of the lymphoid infiltrate

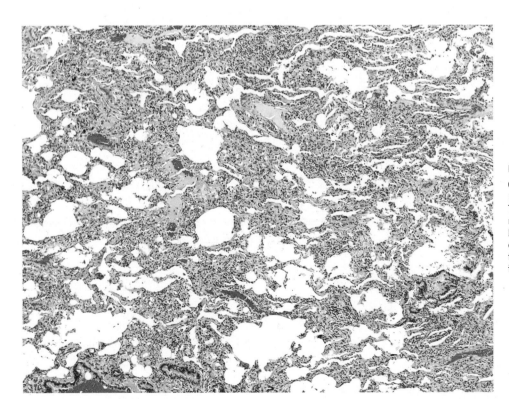

FIGURE 3-19

Chronic cellular infiltrates (pattern 3)

The lung demonstrates chronic inflammation, and the biopsy has an overall blue appearance at scanning magnification. This example is a case of bird fanciers' lung (a form of hypersensitivity pneumonia).

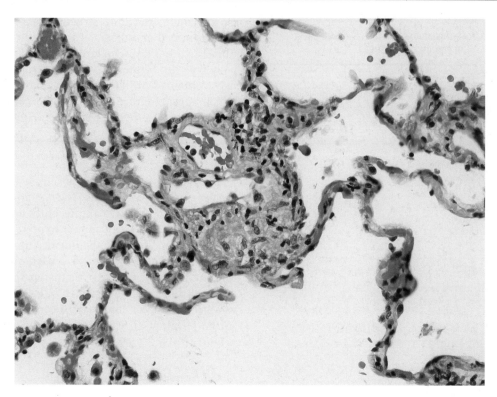

FIGURE 3-20

Hypersensitivity pneumonia (pattern 3)

A cellular interstitial pneumonia with scattered, poorly formed interstitial granulomas is typical of hypersensitivity pneumonia.

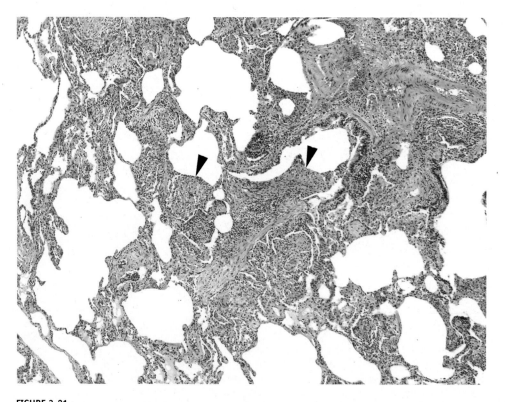

FIGURE 3-21

Hot tub lung (pattern 3)

The characteristic histopathologic findings include a chronic cellular bronchiolitis accompanied by non-necrotizing or minimally necrotizing granulomas in the terminal airways and adjacent alveolar spaces (arrowheads).

(Figure 3-22). In difficult cases, gene rearrangement studies may be necessary to rule out low-grade lymphoma. An LIP pattern can be seen in adults and children with immunodeficiency syndromes or connective tissue diseases.

D. Lymphomas

Lymphomas involving the lung can also present with dense mononuclear cell infiltration and sometimes granulomas. The cellular infiltrate is homogenous and extends along the lymphatic routes of the lungs (bronchovascular bundles, pleura and interlobular septa).

II. Chronic Cellular Interstitial Infiltrates with or without Lymphoid Aggregates

A. Lymphoid Interstitial Pneumonia/Diffuse Lymphoid Hyperplasia

Some cases of LIP also show germinal centers along airways and lymphatic routes, and when these are prominent, diffuse lymphoid hyperplasia is the preferred term.

B. Follicular Bronchiolitis

A specific subtype of chronic bronchiolitis, this process is characterized by the presence of lymphoid follicles with well formed germinal centers, in bronchiolar walls (Figure 3-23). Follicular bronchiolitis can be part of the pulmonary manifestations of CVDs, immunodeficiencies, chronic infections, and airway disease associated with inflammatory bowel disease. The lymphoid infiltrate in the bronchovascular bundle is composed of small mature lymphocytes, which show a tendency to invade airway epithelium raising the differential diagnosis of lymphoepithelial lesions as seen in low-grade lymphomas of BALT/MALT type. Follicular bronchiolitis can also be seen in association with various occupational exposures.

C. Non-Specific Interstitial Pneumonia Pattern

This pattern is discussed above.

D. Other Findings

Cellular changes can be seen in infections with the herpesviruses and respiratory viruses (Chapter 13). Multinucleated giant cells can be a part of a chronic cellular infiltrate. They are rather nonspecific, and intravenous

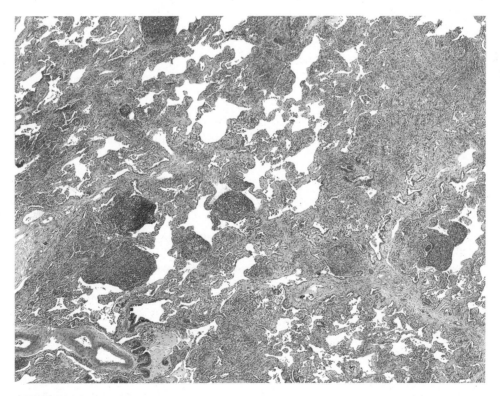

FIGURE 3-22
Lymphoid interstitial pneumonia (pattern 3)
LIP is distinguished from the cellular form of NSIP by the intensity of lymphoid infiltration. Lymphoma must be rigorously excluded.

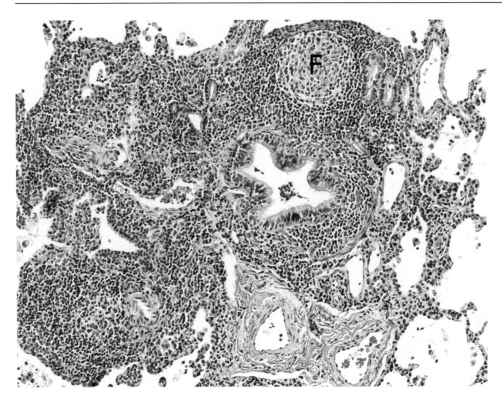

FIGURE 3-23
Follicular bronchiolitis (pattern 3)
Follicular bronchiolitis is characterized by lymphoid follicles with well formed germinal centers (F) in bronchiolar walls.

drug abuse, aspiration pneumonia, eosinophilic pneumonia, hard metal disease, and other pneumoconioses can present with prominent multinucleated giant cells. When eosinophils are part of a chronic cellular infiltrate, the differential diagnosis includes eosinophilic lung diseases and smoking-related diseases, which have been described in more detail as part of the other patterns (Pattern 1, Pattern 4, Pattern 5).

ALVEOLAR FILLING (PATTERN 4)

ELEMENTS OF PATTERN

The alveoli are filled with cells or noncellular elements.

I. ALVEOLAR FILLING WITH CELLS

A. ALVEOLAR FILLING BY FIBROBLASTS—ORGANIZING PNEUMONIA

The prototype for the alveolar filling pattern is organizing pneumonia (OP) in which immature fibroblasts (myofibroblasts) grow within the terminal airways and alveoli, forming polypoid structures (Figure 3-24). OP represents a nonspecific reaction to lung injury and requires a search for an etiology. The lung responds to many insults by air space organization. In cases where an etiology cannot be determined, the correct clinical term is cryptogenic organizing pneumonia (COP).

B. ALVEOLAR FILLING BY NEUTROPHILS

Alveolar filling by neutrophils indicates an acute process, and the leading entity in the differential diagnosis is acute bacterial pneumonia (Figure 3-25). Gram stains for bacteria, as well as acid fast and Grocott methenamine silver stains for mycobacteria and fungi, respectively, are needed to evaluate for an infectious etiology. Correlation with BAL or sputum cultures is also recommended.

C. DIFFUSE ALVEOLAR HEMORRHAGE

Diffuse alveolar hemorrhage has many immunologic and non-immunologic causes (Chapter 8). Histologically, alveoli are filled with red blood cells and often hemosiderin-laden macrophages, depending on the longevity of the process. Immunologically-mediated pulmonary hemorrhage (also discussed in Pattern 1) can manifest by brisk episodes of neutrophilic capillaritis with shedding of neutrophils into the alveolar spaces, mimicking acute bronchopneumonia. The presence of alveolar fibrin, acute hemorrhage, and hemosiderin-laden macrophages is an important clue to look for the small vessel vasculitis.

ALVEOLAR FILLING (PATTERN 4)—FACT SHEET AND PATHOLOGIC FEATURES

Definition
» Lung biopsies in which there is filling of alveolar spaces by cells or noncellular elements

Diseases
» Fibroblasts
  » Organizing pneumonia (OP)
» Neutrophils
  » Acute infectious (usually bacterial) pneumonia
» Blood
  » Diffuse alveolar hemorrhage
» Macrophages
  » Desquamative interstitial pneumonia
  » Desquamative interstitial pneumonia-like pattern
  » Respiratory bronchiolitis-interstitial lung disease (RB-ILD)
  » Post-steroid-treated eosinophilic pneumonia
  » Drug reactions
  » Obstructive pneumonia
  » Histiocytic infectious pneumonias (immunosuppressed hosts)
  » Malakoplakia
  » Exogenous lipoid pneumonia
  » Storage diseases
» Eosinophils
  » Eosinophilic pneumonia, chronic and acute
  » Churg-Strauss syndrome
» Non-cellular elements
  » Pneumoconiosis
  » Pulmonary alveolar proteinosis
  » *Pneumocystis jiroveci* infection
  » Acute pulmonary edema
  » Mucostasis of airway disease
  » Bronchioloalveolar carcinoma
  » Pulmonary alveolar microlithiasis (PAM)

D. Alveolar Filling with Macrophages

Macrophages are encountered in relatively large numbers in many lung biopsies, partly because they are an integral part of the lung's defensive system, and partly because many patients who undergo lung biopsy are smokers.

1. Desquamative Interstitial Pneumonia (DIP)

This interstitial lung disease usually develops in smokers and is characterized by diffuse accumulation of intra-alveolar macrophages (Figure 3-26). At low magnification, the lung architecture is preserved and the alveolar spaces are filled by lightly brown-pigmented macrophages. Multinucleated cells are commonly present. The interstitium shows a variably intense mononuclear inflammatory infiltrate, and sometimes lymphoid follicles are present. Significant fibrosis or honeycombing is usually absent.

2. Desquamative Interstitial Pneumonia-Like Pattern

A pattern similar to DIP is also seen in several unrelated diseases, including respiratory bronchiolitis-interstitial lung disease (RB-ILD) and post-steroid-treated eosinophilic pneumonia. Any area of decreased lung compliance can show accumulation of alveolar macrophages.

3. Respiratory Bronchiolitis—Interstitial Lung Disease (RB-ILD)

A smoking-related airway disease, RB-ILD is also discussed later under small airways disease, as part of Pattern 6 (nearly normal lung biopsy). RB is a lesion of the respiratory bronchiole characterized by mild chronic inflammation, minimal peribronchiolar fibrosis, and the accumulation of smokers' macrophages in the lumen of the airway (Figure 3-27). Smokers macrophages should be distinguished from siderophages (see Pattern 1), which contain coarser granules of stainable iron. RB-ILD is distinguished from DIP microscopically by the more limited and bronchiolocentric extent of macrophage accumulation in the former. Correlation with HRCT is required.

4. Post-Steroid-Treated Eosinophilic Pneumonia (EP)

Eosinophilic pneumonia (EP), especially post-steroid treatment, can appear as an accumulation of intra-alveolar macrophages accompanied by only rare eosinophils.

5. Other Diseases

Other processes that can manifest with prominent alveolar macrophage accumulation include drug reactions, such as amiodarone effects. The macrophages show fine cytoplasmic vacuolization, which is also observed in the adjacent reactive type II pneumocytes. Post-obstructive pneumonia is seen distal to obstruction due to intrinsic or extrinsic factors, mainly tumors or fibrosis. It consists of accumulations of foamy macrophages filled with lipids, which give them a yellowish color on gross examination.

In immunocompromised patients, infectious pneumonias may manifest predominantly as histiocytic alveolar reactions, without the classic neutrophilic infiltrates. Malakoplakia-like reactions to *Rhodococcus equi* infection (Figure 3-28) and cryptococcal pneumonia in the form of mucoid pneumonia are two examples of macrophage-rich pneumonias. Histoplasmosis can also present with loose macrophage infiltrates in alveoli in immunocompromised patients.

Exogenous lipoid pneumonia and storage diseases can also cause a similar pattern and are discussed in other chapters.

E. Alveolar Filling by Eosinophils

In chronic and acute eosinophilic pneumonias, large numbers of eosinophils fill alveoli and are accompanied by variable numbers of macrophages and multinucleated

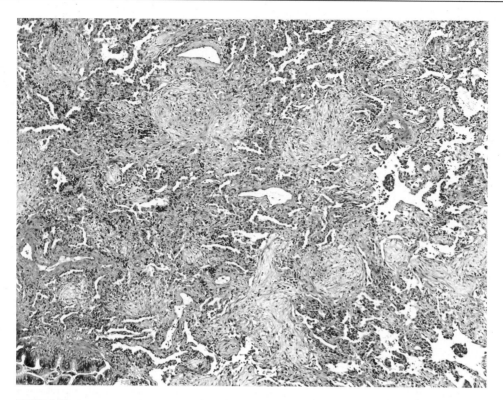

FIGURE 3-24

Organizing pneumonia (pattern 4)
Alveolar space organization, characterized by immature fibroblast proliferation, represents a nonspecific reaction to lung injury and requires a search for an etiology.

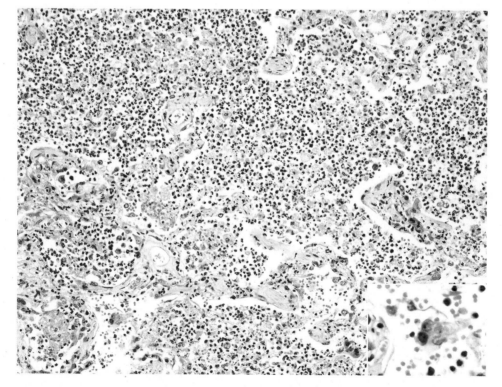

FIGURE 3-25

Acute bronchopneumonia (pattern 4)
Alveolar filling by neutrophils most often represents an acute bacterial pneumonia. Here, acute bronchopneumonia accompanies a rare case of free-living pulmonary amebiasis. Many amoeba are present, highlighted in the inset.

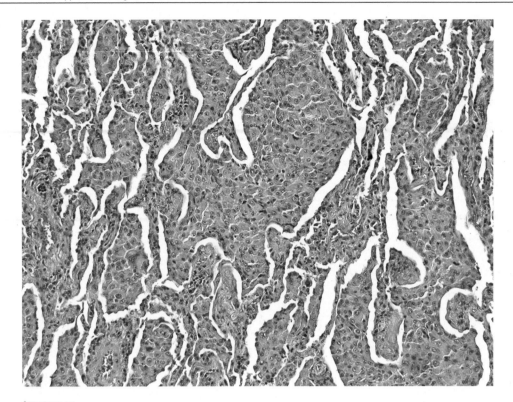

FIGURE 3-26

Desquamative interstitial pneumonia (pattern 4)
This idiopathic interstitial pneumonia is characterized by diffuse accumulation of intra-alveolar macrophages and mild interstitial fibrosis.

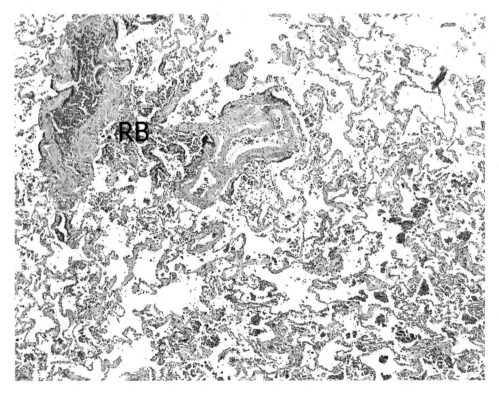

FIGURE 3-27

Respiratory bronchiolitis-interstitial lung disease (pattern 4)
RB is a lesion of the respiratory bronchiole characterized by mild chronic inflammation, minimal peribronchiolar fibrosis, and the accumulation of smokers' macrophages in the vicinity of the respiratory bronchiole. In RB-ILD, the macrophage reaction is more extensive, involving peribronchiolar alveoli, although less diffuse than that of DIP.

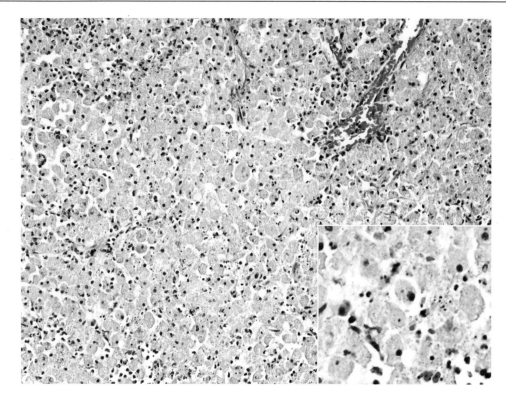

FIGURE 3-28

Malakoplakia-like reaction to *R. equi* (pattern 4)
Immunocompromised patients infected with *Rhodococcus equi* develop dense lung consolidation with a prominent histiocytic reaction. Organisms are plentiful and are present within the histiocytes.

giant cells, and variable degrees of interstitial fibrous or organizing pneumonia. A similar pattern may be seen as a component of Churg-Strauss syndrome.

II. ALVEOLAR FILLING WITH NON-CELLULAR MATERIAL

Non-cellular material that can fill the alveolar spaces may be fibrinous, proteinaceous, mucinous, and even osseous.

A. ALVEOLAR FILLING WITH PROTEINACEOUS MATERIAL

1. PULMONARY ALVEOLAR PROTEINOSIS (PAP)

PAP can present in a primary idiopathic form, but can also be encountered as a secondary phenomenon. The histologic pattern of PAP is distinctive at low magnification. There is pink eosinophilic material filling the alveoli which appears granular and sporadically "chunky" at higher magnification (Figure 3-29). Cholesterol clefts may also be seen in the exudates. The eosinophilic material is PAS-positive and diastase resistant, and is reactive with antibodies against surfactant. There is usually a lack of inflammation in the interstitium or the alveoli. The presence of inflammatory changes suggests a coexisting disease, especially infection. *Nocardia* infection is particularly known to be associated with PAP.

2. PNEUMOCYSTIS INFECTION

In *Pneumocystis jiroveci* pneumonia, the alveolar exudate is foamier, has a honeycomb appearance, and lacks the cholesterol clefts and globular material seen in PAP (Figure 3-30).

3. PULMONARY EDEMA

Intra-alveolar edema is rather non-specific and can be the earliest manifestation of acute lung injury. The eosinophilic material encountered in a case of pulmonary edema lacks the granularity and cellular debris described in PAP. Edema is a diagnosis of exclusion, in cases were the proteinaceous material is less dense, PAS negative, and the methenamine silver stain fails to reveal *Pneumocystis* infection.

B. ALVEOLAR FILLING WITH MUCUS

1. MUCOSTASIS IN SMALL AIRWAY DISEASES

Mucostasis is a common finding associated with small airway diseases. It can be observed in settings of chronic obstructive pulmonary disease, asthma, localized airway

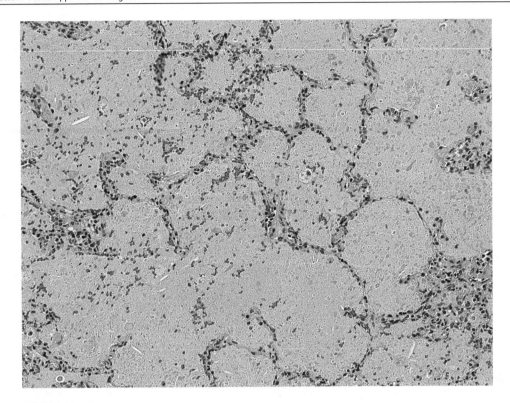

FIGURE 3-29

Alveolar proteinosis (pattern 4)
The histologic pattern of alveolar proteinosis is distinctive at low magnification. There is pink eosinophilic material filling the alveoli which appears granular and sporadically "chunky" at higher magnification.

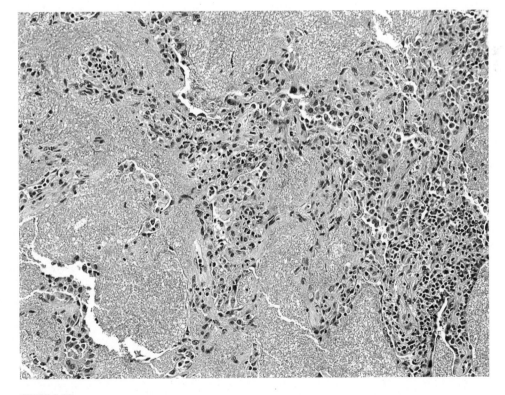

FIGURE 3-30

***Pneumocystis* pneumonia (pattern 4)**
This infection is associated with a higher degree of inflammation in the lung biopsy than that seen in PAP. The protein-aceous material is also foamier, finely vacuolated, and lacks the cholesterol clefts and globular material seen in PAP.

obstruction, bronchiectasis, and bronchiolitis. It consists of accumulation of amphophilic mucus in dilated airways, sometimes with extrusion into the surrounding alveolar spaces.

2. BRONCHIOLOALVEOLAR CARCINOMA

The presence of extensive intra-alveolar mucin, especially in the absence of other pathology on biopsy, should always raise some concern for bronchioloalveolar carcinoma.

C. ALVEOLAR FILLING WITH CALCIFICATION AND BONE

Dystrophic calcification and ossification occur frequently in localized scars and granulomas. More diffuse interstitial "metastatic" calcifications can develop with calcium imbalances, and nodular calcification can be related to forms of pulmonary venous hypertension. The presence of numerous tiny calcified bodies in the alveolar spaces raises the possibility of pulmonary alveolar microlithiasis (PAM), a rare autosomal recessive lung disease. The microliths are concentrically laminated and contain calcium and phosphorus with a composition similar to bone (Figure 3-31). They need to be distinguished from corpora amylacea, which are smaller and lack calcifications.

D. ALVEOLAR FILLING WITH EXOGENOUS MATERIALS

In pneumoconioses (chapter 18), a variety of exogenous materials can be observed in air spaces and can stimulate a variety of histologic reactions.

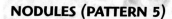

NODULES (PATTERN 5)

ELEMENTS OF THE PATTERN

At low magnification, nodules usually have a sharp, discernible interface with the adjacent lung parenchyma (Figure 3-32). Microscopic classification can be pursued at higher power and lead to a more specific differential diagnosis. Observation of the distribution of the nodules is also important, since particular disorders can present with particular patterns of distribution: lymphatic, bronchocentric, angiocentric, and random.

I. NODULES COMPOSED OF GRANULOMAS

A. NODULES COMPOSED OF GRANULOMAS WITH NECROSIS

1. GRANULOMATOUS INFECTIONS

Well-formed granulomas are often the dominant finding in mycobacterial and fungal infections, and should prompt special stains and cultures for these microorganisms. Negative stains do not exclude infections.

2. WEGENER'S GRANULOMATOSIS (WG)

At low magnification, these granulomas consist of areas of nodular consolidation with necrosis that is often geographic (Figure 3-33). At the edge of the

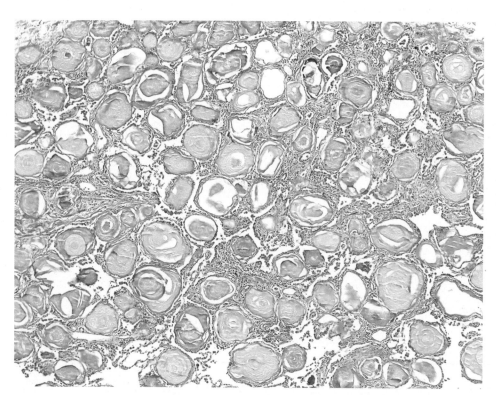

FIGURE 3-31

Alveolar microlithiasis (pattern 4)
The intra-alveolar microliths of pulmonary alveolar microlithiasis are concentrically laminated, show radial striations, and are composed of calcium and phosphorus with a composition similar to normal bone.

NODULES (PATTERN 5)—FACT SHEET AND PATHOLOGIC FEATURES

Definition

▸▸ Lung biopsies in which there are sharp, easily discernible nodules

Diseases to Be Considered

▸▸ Granulomatous infections
▸▸ Wegener's granulomatosis
▸▸ Sarcoidosis
▸▸ Aspiration pneumonia
▸▸ Pneumoconioses
▸▸ Pulmonary Langerhans cell histiocytosis
▸▸ Healed or healing infections
▸▸ Diffuse panbronchiolitis
▸▸ Reactive lymphoid proliferations
▸▸ Lymphomas

Histologic Characteristics

▸▸ Granulomas
  ▸▸ With necrosis
  ▸▸ Without necrosis
▸▸ Fibrotic, hypocellular nodules
▸▸ Lymphocytic nodular lesions
▸▸ Nodules of atypical/neoplastic cells

necrosis, there is a peripheral zone of palisading histiocytes. The necrosis in WG is basophilic as compared to the eosinophilic necrosis typically seen in infections. Neutrophilic microabscesses are a very helpful diagnostic feature and can be found in the centers of granulomas or in a background of chronic inflammation and fibrosis. Neutrophilic microabscesses can also be seen in infections such as blastomycosis and nocardiosis, however. In WG, vasculitis is also seen, as well as other histologic changes which are discussed in more detail in chapter 8.

WG must be distinguished from infection. The nodules in WG are usually multiple and bilateral, and those of infection are usually solitary. WG shows the characteristic blue necrosis and vasculitis described above, but approximately 87% of mycobacterial and 57% of fungal lung infections with necrotizing granulomas can be associated with vasculitis. ANCA testing is often helpful and should be performed and correlated with the clinical, radiologic, and histopathologic findings.

3. Other Diseases to Be Considered

When the necrosis shows admixed atypical cells, the differential diagnosis should include lymphomatoid granulomatosis, lymphoma and carcinoma.

B. Nodules Composed of Granulomas without Necrosis

Non-necrotizing granulomatous nodules are more likely to be of non-infectious etiology than necrotizing ones. Sarcoidosis and berylliosis can produce non-necrotizing granulomas. In sarcoidosis, granulomas are classically distributed along lymphatic channels of the bronchovascular bundles, interlobular septa, and pleura. Adjacent small granulomas can coalesce to form larger nodules, and the area between granulomas is frequently sclerotic (Figure 3-34). Distinctive inclusions may be

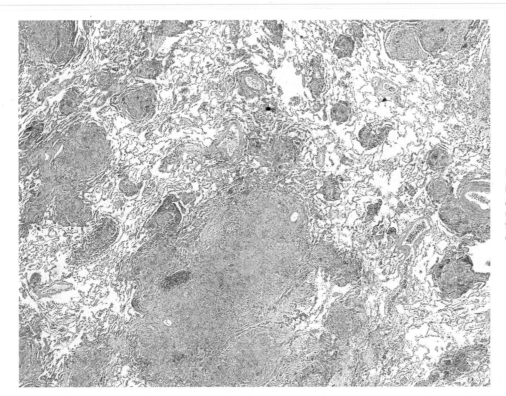

FIGURE 3-32

Nodules (pattern 5)

At scanning magnification, nodules usually have a sharp, discernible interface with the adjacent lung parenchyma.

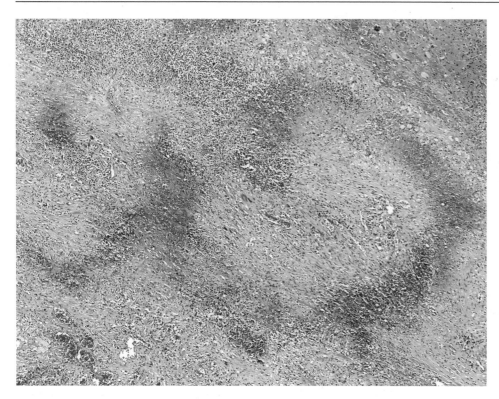

FIGURE 3-33

Wegener's granulomatosis (pattern 5)
The nodules of classical Wegener's granulomatosis consist of areas of nodular consolidation with necrosis (typically geographic and basophilic), and associated mixed inflammatory infiltrates (including eosinophils and plasma cells).

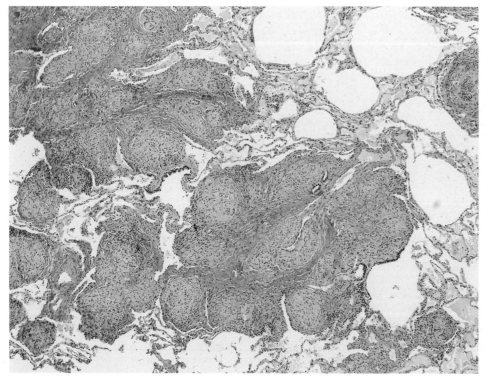

FIGURE 3-34

Sarcoidosis (pattern 5)
Adjacent small granulomas coalesce to form larger nodules.

present within giant cells, such as asteroid and Schaumann bodies, but they are not specific.

The chronic form of berylliosis can have granulomas indistinguishable from those of sarcoidosis. Granulomatous infections should also be included in the differential diagnosis and appropriate staining and cultures performed. In some disorders, nodules may consist of aggregates of multinucleated giant cells rather than granulomas. This can be seen in aspiration pneumonia (often bronchocentric distribution), pneumoconioses, and intravenous talcosis (angiocentric distribution).

II. FIBROTIC NODULES WITH VARIABLE INFLAMMATORY INFILTRATES

A. SILICOSIS/SILICATOSIS

Fibrotic and hyalinized nodules seen along the lymphatics or in a random distribution are characteristically seen in pulmonary disease related to silica exposure (Chapter 18). Nodules also include macrophages containing the particulate matter. Silicate particles appear birefringent in the histiocytes and/or at the periphery of the nodules. Pure silica is poorly birefringent in plane-polarized light.

B. PULMONARY LANGERHANS CELL HISTIOCYTOSIS (PLCH)

PLCH (Chapter 23) is characterized by stellate-shaped nodules (Figure 3-35) in a bronchiolocentric (early) or random (late) distribution and associated with cysts. The nodules are variably cellular and fibrotic, depending upon age, and often contain Langerhans cells with folded nuclei having grooves. Adjacent to the nodules, a DIP pattern is typically seen.

C. HEALED OR HEALING INFECTIONS

Resolving or resolved abscesses, pneumonias, and granulomas can have this appearance. It may be difficult to define an etiology for these lesions.

III. NODULES COMPOSED OF LYMPHOID CELLS

Nodular lymphohistiocytic lesions have a specific differential diagnosis, which includes follicular bronchiolitis, diffuse lymphoid hyperplasia, malignant lymphoma, lymphomatoid granulomotosis (LYG) and even the possibility of a benign intraparenchymal lymph node. These entities are discussed in chapter 22. Immunohistochemical studies, flow cytometry, and molecular diagnostic

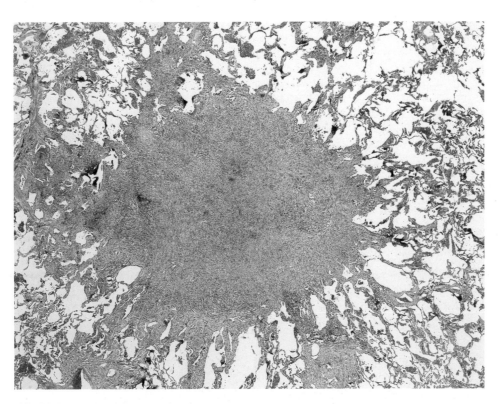

FIGURE 3-35

Pulmonary Langerhans cell histiocytosis (pattern 5)
The nodules of PLCH lesions have a stellate appearance and variable degrees of cellularity and fibrosis, depending upon age.

techniques may be useful for assessing clonality and distinguishing lymphoma from reactive proliferations.

Nodular lymphoid infiltrates showing central necrosis and prominent vascular infiltration are characteristic of lymphomatoid granulomatosis (Figure 3-36). Atypical lymphocytes and mixed inflammatory infiltrates comprise the nodules and necrosis is commonly present. This lymphoma is now accepted as an EBV-related B-cell lymphoma.

Diffuse panbronchiolitis (DPB) is a distinctive form of chronic bronchiolitis seen almost exclusively in people of East Asian descent (Japan, Korea, China). This disease entity can produce a dramatic diffuse nodular pattern in lung biopsies, with severe chronic inflammation centered on respiratory bronchioles early in the disease, followed by involvement of distal membranous bronchioles and peribronchiolar alveolar spaces as the disease progresses. A characteristic low magnification appearance is that of nodular bronchiolocentric lesions (Figure 3-37).

IV. NODULES COMPOSED OF ATYPICAL/NEOPLASTIC CELLS

Nodules composed of atypical neoplastic cells are seen in a wide variety of primary and metastatic carcinomas, sarcomas, lymphomas, and melanomas. These entities are discussed in other chapters.

NEARLY NORMAL BIOPSY (PATTERN 6)

Lung biopsies showing little or no disease at scanning magnification fit into Pattern 6. In this situation, attention should be given to the airways and blood vessels, and to the possibility of a cyst. The possibility of a sampling error should also be considered, but only after a thorough evaluation.

When a lung biopsy appears nearly normal, the first entities to consider are small airway diseases (SAD) and diseases affecting the pulmonary vasculature. When examining the small airways, determine if they are dilated, constricted or collapsed, absent, or markedly reduced in number. Evaluate for inflammation and fibrosis (obliterative bronchiolitis). Bronchiolitis produces thickening of the bronchiolar walls that may be subtle. Collections of foamy alveolar macrophages are a clue to look for airway obstruction. The etiologies and presentations of small airway diseases are covered in chapter 21.

With pulmonary hypertension, the spectrum of changes may also be quite subtle and includes muscular hypertrophy, intimal proliferation, concentric laminar intimal fibrosis, necrotizing vasculitis, and plexiform lesions. Pulmonary veno-occlusive disease (PVOD) causes fibrous obliteration of the pulmonary veins, which can be highlighted by using trichrome and elastic stains. The parenchyma appears congested, with hemosiderin-laden

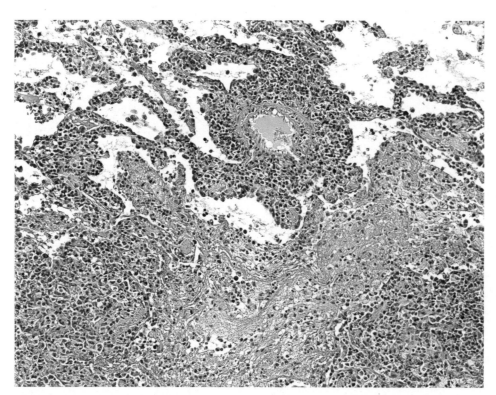

FIGURE 3-36

Angiocentric immunoproliferative disorder (lymphomatoid granulomatosis) (pattern 5)

When a nodular lymphoid infiltrate shows areas of necrosis and prominent vascular infiltration, LYG should be a strong consideration. Epstein-Barr virus detection by in situ hybridization plays a critical diagnostic role in LYG today.

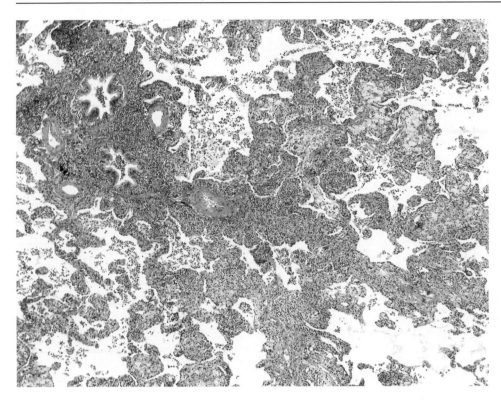

FIGURE 3-37

Diffuse panbronchiolitis (pattern 5)
The characteristic feature of DPB is the accumulation of many pale vacuolated macrophages in the walls of terminal airways and in surrounding alveolar spaces, accompanied by lymphoid infiltrates.

NEAR-NORMAL LUNG (PATTERN 6)—FACT SHEET

Definition

▸ Lung biopsies in which there is little or no disease evident at scanning magnification

Main Considerations

▸ Small airway diseases
▸ Pulmonary vascular diseases
▸ Sampling error

---

macrophages. Repeated hemorrhages causes deposition of iron and calcium on the elastic fibers with formation of structures resembling ferruginous bodies (i.e., endogenous pneumoconiosis). Arterial changes consisting of intimal fibrosis and muscular hypertrophy can also be seen.

A normal biopsy (all previously mentioned possibilities excluded) in a clinically symptomatic patient should tentatively raise the possibility of sampling error. Correlation with clinical and radiographic findings can be helpful for assessing the probability of a sampling error.

SUGGESTED READINGS

1. American Thoracic Society/European Respiratory Society international multidisciplinary consensus classification of the idiopathic interstitial pneumonias. *Am J Resp Crit Care Med*. 2002;165:277-304.
2. Colby TV. Bronchiolitis. Pathologic considerations. *Am J Clin Pathol*. 1998;109:101-9.
3. Leslie KO, Wick M, eds. *Practical Pulmonary Pathology: A Diagnostic Approach*. 1st ed. Philadelphia: Churchill-Livingstone; 2005.
4. Leslie KO, Colby TV, Swenson SJ. Anatomic distribution and histopathologic patterns of interstitial lung disease. In: Schwarz M, King T, eds. *Interstitial Lung Disease*. 4th ed. Hamilton, Ontario: B.C. Dekker Inc., 2003.
5. Leslie KO. Pathology of interstitial lung disease. *Clin Chest Med*. 2004;25:657-703.
6. Ryu JH, Colby TV, Hartman TE, Vassallo R. Smoking-related interstitial lung diseases: a concise review. *Eur Respir J*. 2001;17:122-32.
7. Tansey D, Wells AU, Colby TV, et al. Variations in histological patterns of interstitial pneumonia between connective tissue disorders and their relationship to prognosis. *Histopathology*. 2004;44:585-96.
8. Travis WD, Colby TV, Lombard C, Carpenter HA. A clinicopathologic study of 34 cases of diffuse pulmonary hemorrhage with lung biopsy confirmation. *Am J Surg Pathol*. 1990;14:1112-25.

4

Congenital, Developmental, and Inherited Disorders

Megan K. Dishop • Claire Langston

- Diffuse Developmental Disorders
- Surfactant Dysfunction Disorders
- Developmental "Cystic" Lesions
- Disorders with Abnormal Bronchial Connection: Bronchial Atresia, Intralobar Sequestration, and Extralobar Sequestration
- Primary Pulmonary Lymphatic Disorders
- Primary Ciliary Dyskinesia
- Cystic Fibrosis

Congenital and developmental disorders of the lung manifest almost exclusively in pediatric patients, and include a wide array of disorders resulting from abnormalities of lung architecture, cellular function, and metabolism. Although this list is not exhaustive, these disorders may be subdivided as follows: (1) disorders with inherent abnormalities of lung structure, (2) inherited disorders of surfactant metabolism, (3) focal developmental "cystic" lesions, (4) disorders of abnormal bronchial connection, (5) lymphatic disorders in infancy, (6) ciliary abnormalities, and (7) cystic fibrosis. All of these disorders are uncommon, and most are rarely encountered in clinical practice; however, together they account for significant morbidity and mortality in the pediatric population and can often be a diagnostic challenge for the pathologist.

DIFFUSE DEVELOPMENTAL DISORDERS

CLINICAL FEATURES

Diffuse developmental disorders of lung architecture are rare entities which typically present in the neonate. Babies with acinar dysplasia have an early arrest of lung development resulting in respiratory distress and death in the first few hours of life (Figures 4-1, 4-2). Most reported cases have occurred in otherwise normal female infants at or near term. Although the pathogenesis is not known, an abnormality of epithelial-mesenchymal interaction during development has been proposed. Congenital alveolar dysplasia refers to a poorly characterized disorder with arrest in lung development at a later stage and thus with a somewhat less severe presentation (Figure 4-3). Similar to acinar dysplasia, affected infants have respiratory difficulty at birth but may be sustained for some time with ventilatory support. Alveolar capillary dysplasia with misalignment of pulmonary veins (ACD/MPV) typically causes respiratory symptoms and persistent pulmonary hypertension in term or near-term infants in the first days of life. Initially identified only at autopsy, increasing clinical suspicion has resulted in diagnostic lung biopsies to exclude the diagnosis in recent years (Figure 4-4). Although there are exceptions, most affected infants die in the first month of life despite intensive supportive measures. ACD/MPV is associated with other often minor malformations, particularly involving the cardiac, gastrointestinal, and genitourinary systems. Hypoplastic left heart syndrome is the most frequently associated cardiac malformation. Sibling pairs have been reported, suggesting autosomal recessive disease.

DIFFERENTIAL DIAGNOSIS

Acinar dysplasia should be distinguished from other less severe forms of pulmonary hypoplasia. Congenital alveolar dysplasia may be difficult to separate from the changes seen in the lungs of infants with respiratory failure who have been intensively supported for long periods of time. The typical history of respiratory failure in a term infant and the uniformity of the histologic changes are key observations in this situation. Unlike ACD/MPV, congenital alveolar dysplasia shows normal location and course of veins. Normally, the pulmonary veins arise in interlobular septa from small veins draining pulmonary lobules and travel centrally within these septa, positioned adjacent to bronchi and large pulmonary arteries near the hilum; these small septal veins are reduced or absent in ACD/MPV but are present in congenital alveolar dysplasia.

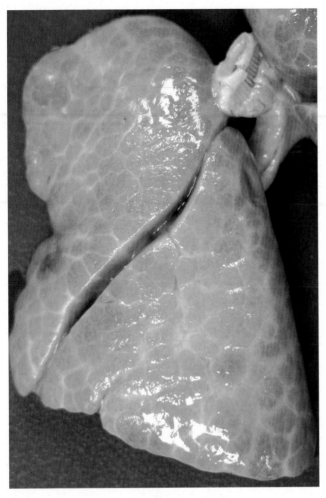

FIGURE 4-1
Acinar dysplasia
The lungs are small and show accentuated lobules with thickened interlobular septa.

PROGNOSIS AND THERAPY

These diffuse developmental disorders are universally fatal. Lung transplantation may be an option for babies with ACD/MPV if recognized early.

SURFACTANT DYSFUNCTION DISORDERS

CLINICAL FEATURES

As a group, genetic mutations in proteins affecting surfactant metabolism are an important cause of respiratory distress in otherwise healthy term or near-term infants, as well as an emerging cause of chronic lung disease in older children and adults. Tremendous progress has been made in this area in just the last few years, as mutations in three genes are now recognized to cause surfactant dysfunction disorders. Surfactant protein B (Sp-B) mutations were the first to be recognized in 1993, followed by mutations in surfactant protein C (Sp-C). Since the association was described by Nogee and colleagues in 2004, mutations in the ATP-binding cassette transporter ABCA3 have emerged as the most common cause of such disorders presenting in infancy.

PATHOLOGIC FEATURES

In infants, mutations of Sp-B and ABCA3 typically manifest as pulmonary alveolar proteinosis (Figure 4-5), while Sp-C mutations typically have more lobular remodeling and less alveolar proteinosis material, yielding a pattern of chronic pneumonitis of infancy (Figure 4-6). Sp-C mutations are also recognized as a cause of idiopathic and familial pulmonary fibrosis in older children and adults, and ABCA3 mutations have also been identified in a few older children with chronic and fibrosing lung disease. It should be noted that there are cases with morphology consistent with surfactant dysfunction in which no mutation has been identified in any of these three genes. Other genes and clinical patterns of disease will almost certainly be identified as more is learned about this complex set of metabolic disorders. Mutations in surfactant proteins and related proteins may also be genetic modifiers affecting the natural history and prognosis of various forms of acquired lung disease.

DEVELOPMENTAL "CYSTIC" LESIONS

CLINICAL AND PATHOLOGIC FEATURES

Congenital cystic adenomatoid malformations (CCAM) have been classified by Stocker according to cyst size and histomorphologic resemblance to segments of the developing bronchial tree and air spaces, from proximal (CCAM, type 0) to distal (CCAM, type 4). More recently, the term congenital pulmonary airway malformation (CPAM) has been proposed for this group of lesions, as not all are cystic, and only one type has "adenomatoid" morphology. The two most common of these are more simply described as the large cyst type (Stocker type 1) and the small cyst type (Stocker type 2) CCAMs. The other three morphologic types are all thought to represent different pathogenetic processes: acinar dysplasia (type 0), pulmonary hyperplasia (type 3), and low-grade cystic pleuropulmonary blastoma (type 4).

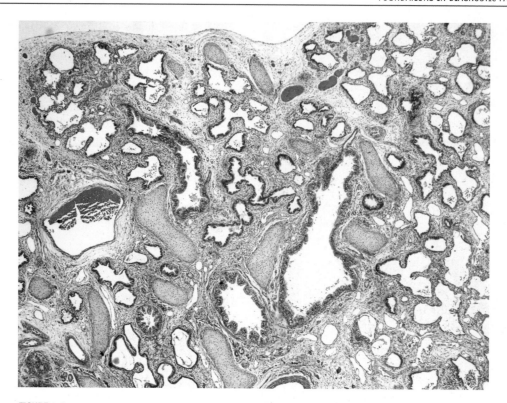

FIGURE 4-2

Acinar dysplasia
Microscopically, the lobules contain dilated branching airways and large air spaces resembling growth arrest at the pseudoglandular stage of development. No saccular structures or alveoli are present.

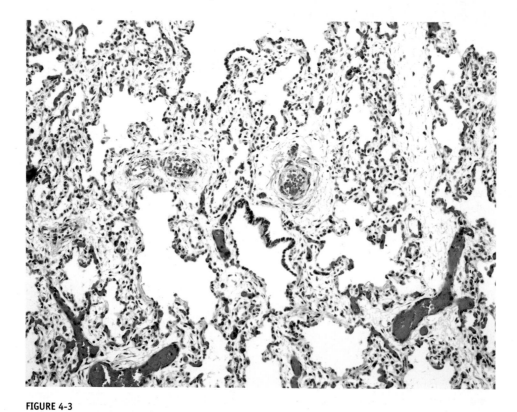

FIGURE 4-3

Congenital alveolar dysplasia
The lung development appears arrested at a later stage in development than acinar dysplasia, in this case resembling early saccular development in a term neonate.

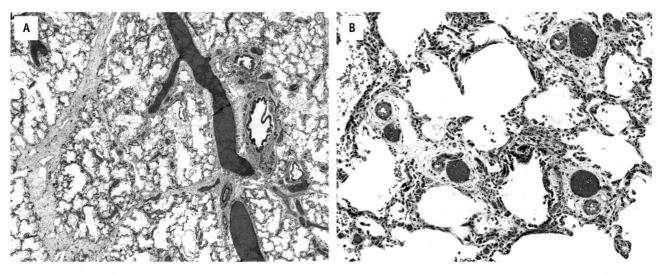

FIGURE 4-4

Alveolar capillary dysplasia with misalignment of pulmonary veins
The congested pulmonary veins are malpositioned, accompanying the pulmonary artery branches and airways **(A).** Within the lobules, the dilated venules accompany the hyperplastic lobular arterioles and the alveolar capillary bed is deficient **(B).** (Movat pentachrome stain)

DIFFUSE DEVELOPMENTAL DISORDERS—FACT SHEET

Definition
‣ A group of developmental disorders with abnormal parenchymal development and sometimes abnormal vasculature

Incidence
‣ Rare
‣ ACD/MPV most common

Morbidity and Mortality
‣ Uniformly lethal

Gender and Age Distribution
‣ Term or near-term neonates
‣ Marked female predominance in acinar dysplasia

Clinical Features
‣ Acinar dysplasia—immediate respiratory distress; cannot be supported
‣ Congenital alveolar dysplasia—early respiratory distress; can be supported
‣ ACD/MPV—respiratory symptoms and persistent pulmonary hypertension in a term infant in the first days to weeks of life; may be associated with other malformations

Radiologic Features
‣ Acinar dysplasia—small hazy lungs; often air leak with resuscitation
‣ Congenital alveolar dysplasia and ACD/MPV—diffusely hazy lungs

Prognosis and Treatment
‣ Fatal despite maximal supportive measures.
‣ Survival is limited to hours in acinar dysplasia and weeks in congenital alveolar dysplasia
‣ Death usually in the first month in ACD/MPV, although longer survivals are reported
‣ Lung transplantation may be an option for some

DIFFUSE DEVELOPMENTAL DISORDERS—PATHOLOGIC FEATURES

Gross Findings
Acinar dysplasia:
‣ Small lungs with small lobules and thickened white interlobular septa

Congenital alveolar dysplasia:
‣ Normal to increased lung weight

ACD/MPV:
‣ Deeply congested
‣ Normal to increased lung weight

Microscopic Findings
Acinar dysplasia:
‣ Developmental arrest in pseudoglandular phase, with normal cytodifferentiation but nearly absent acinar development
‣ Sometimes prominent airway smooth muscle and ectopic cartilage

Congenital alveolar dysplasia:
‣ Developmental arrest in late canalicular/early saccular phase
‣ Reduced alveolar wall capillaries in some cases
‣ May have arterial hypertensive changes

ACD/MPV:
‣ Malpositioned pulmonary veins accompany arterioles in the lobules and small pulmonary arteries adjacent to bronchioles
‣ Striking muscularization of small pulmonary arteries and arterioles
‣ Dilated and congested veins and venules
‣ Dilated central channels in alveolar walls, but deficient alveolar capillaries
‣ Normal position of larger veins adjacent to proximal bronchi
‣ Lobular architectural simplification (variable)
‣ Lymphangiectasia (1/3 of cases)

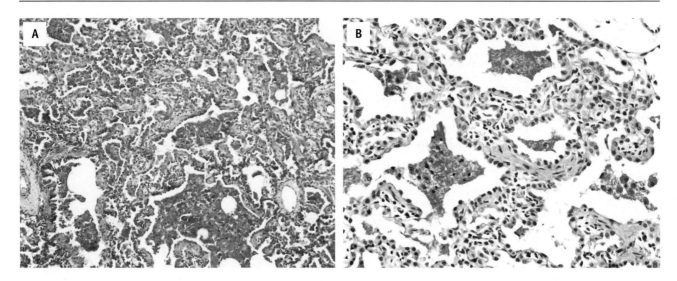

FIGURE 4-5

Pulmonary alveolar proteinosis pattern (surfactant protein B, ABCA3 mutations)
Mutations in the surfactant protein B gene **(A)** and ABCA3 gene **(B)** typically result in a pulmonary alveolar proteinosis pattern in infants, with slightly granular abundant eosinophilic proteinosis material in air spaces, occasional foamy histiocytes, and diffuse alveolar epithelial hyperplasia (periodic acid Schiff).

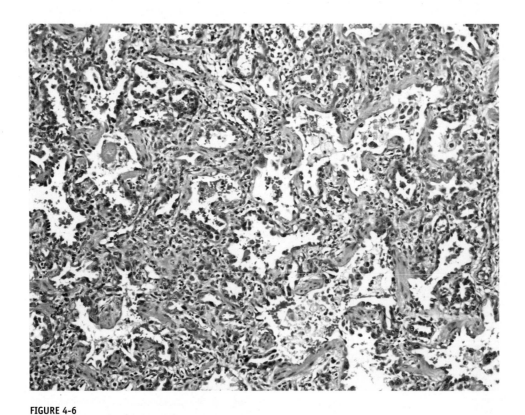

FIGURE 4-6

Chronic pneumonitis of infancy pattern (surfactant protein C mutation)
Mutations in surfactant protein C result in variable morphology depending in part on age at diagnosis. In infants, the lung typically has a pattern of chronic pneumonitis of infancy, characterized by lobular remodeling, diffuse prominent alveolar epithelial hyperplasia, scattered globular eosinophilic proteinosis material, and foamy histiocytes, often with occasional cholesterol cleft formation.

SURFACTANT DYSFUNCTION DISORDERS —FACT SHEET

Definition

▸ Heterogenous group of inherited disorders of surfactant metabolism

Incidence

▸ Rare

Morbidity and Mortality

▸ Death in infancy (Sp-B, Sp-C, ABCA3)
▸ Chronic lung disease in infants and older children (ABCA3, SP-C)
▸ Chronic lung disease and fibrosis in adults (SP-C)

Age Distribution

▸ Infancy—Sp-B
▸ Infants, older children, and adults—Sp-C
▸ Infants, older children, and possibly adults—ABCA3

Clinical Features

▸ Term infants with respiratory difficulty in first weeks and months of life (Sp-B, Sp-C, ABCA3)
▸ Chronic lung disease in older children (Sp-C, ABCA3)
▸ Sp-B and ABCA3 mutations—autosomal recessive
▸ Sp-C mutation—autosomal dominant loss of function
▸ May have family history. Parents and grandparents sometimes affected with Sp-C
▸ Clinical manifestations milder for Sp-C than SP-B

Radiologic Features

▸ "Crazy paving" pattern on chest CT (SP-B)
▸ Diffuse ground-glass opacity similar to hyaline membrane disease
▸ Chronic interstitial disease (SP-C)

Prognosis and Treatment

▸ Variable prognosis
▸ Treatment with supportive measures, steroids, and hydroxychloroquine may delay the need for lung transplantation in Sp-C

SURFACTANT DYSFUNCTION DISORDERS—PATHOLOGIC FEATURES

Gross Findings

▸ In infancy, heavily consolidated-appearing lungs. Some with pulmonary alveolar proteinosis pattern may have yellow material visibly distending airspaces

Microscopic Findings

▸ In infancy, all show diffuse prominent alveolar epithelial hyperplasia with at least focal PAS-positive globular or granular proteinaceous material in alveoli
▸ Histologic patterns:
  ▸ Classic pulmonary alveolar proteinosis pattern—associated most commonly with Sp-B mutations
  ▸ Variant pulmonary alveolar proteinosis pattern with some lobular remodeling, interstitial widening, foamy macrophages, and granular proteinosis—more commonly associated with Sp-B and ABCA3 mutations
  ▸ Chronic pneumonitis of infancy pattern with lobular remodeling, interstitial widening, abundant foamy macrophages, few cholesterol clefts, mild interstitial inflammation, and sparse proteinosis—usually associated with Sp-C mutations
  ▸ Desquamative interstitial pneumonia pattern—usually associated with Sp-C mutations
  ▸ Nonspecific interstitial pneumonia—associated with Sp-C and ABCA3 mutations in infants and older children
  ▸ Idiopathic pulmonary fibrosis—associated with Sp-C mutations in older children and adults

Ancillary Studies

▸ Electron microscopy
  ▸ Sp-B—absence of normal lamellar bodies with hybrid lamellar/multivesicular bodies and absent tubular myelin
  ▸ ABCA3—distinctive tiny lamellar body-like structures with electron dense inclusion "fried egg"; sometimes absence of lamellar bodies
  ▸ Sp-C—No known ultrastructural abnormalities
▸ Surfactant protein and precursor protein quantitation on bronchoalveolar lavage fluid
▸ Immunohistochemistry for surfactant protein B, pro-B, and pro-C; diagnostic pattern only for Sp-B mutations
▸ Surfactant gene mutation studies (SP-B, SP-C, ABCA3) on blood or frozen lung tissue

Pathologic Differential Diagnosis

▸ Pulmonary alveolar proteinosis pattern—acquired proteinosis in immunodeficient patients or those with antibodies to GM-CSF. These patients are typically older and do not have the diffuse marked alveolar epithelial hyperplasia seen in the setting of congenital alveolar proteinosis
▸ Chronic pneumonitis of infancy—Other forms of chronic interstitial lung disease with endogenous lipoid pneumonia

The large cyst type CCAM is the most common of these (Figures 4-7, 4-8). While it is said to usually present in infancy with progressive respiratory difficulty, age at presentation is variable. Identification of these lesions by fetal ultrasound has led to the recognition of cases which regress in utero, as well as other cases which remain asymptomatic until early childhood. There have also been cases not detected until late childhood or adulthood. An association has been described between large cyst type CCAM and bronchioalveolar carcinoma, typically in incompletely resected cases or with late identification in older children.

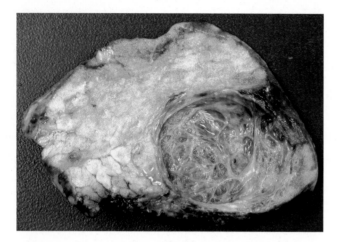

FIGURE 4-7

Congenital cystic adenomatoid malformation, large cyst type (Stocker type 1)
The large cyst type CCAM may be unilocular with thick trabeculations or multilocular with septations. It has been defined as having cysts greater than 2 cm in diameter, but is often larger, as in this 4 cm lesion from the right middle lobe of a 4-month-old infant.

The small cyst type CCAM is typically seen in the setting of in utero airway obstruction as part of a malformation sequence, as in extralobar sequestration and bronchial atresia with or without abnormal vascular connection. While it was initially described in association with other developmental abnormalities, this is now less typical, as isolated asymptomatic cases can now be identified by in utero ultrasound.

DIFFERENTIAL DIAGNOSIS

The differential diagnosis of large cyst CCAM includes bronchogenic cyst, pneumatocele, lymphatic cyst, and lymphangioma. A bronchogenic cyst is a solitary unilocular cyst filled with fluid or mucus, usually attached to the trachea or a major bronchus, but sometimes intrapulmonary (Figure 4-9). Origin is from an aberrant or supernumerary bud of primitive foregut. It is most common in the mediastinum above the carina, but may be seen in the hilum of lung, and paramidline. When intrapulmonary, the distal parenchyma may show air space enlargement due to the mass effect of the cyst. Clinical presentation in infancy is due to respiratory distress from mass effect. Later there may be supervening infection, but many remain asymptomatic. A pneumatocele is an acquired air-filled cyst resulting from leakage of air via an airway into a region of parenchymal injury, for example, resolving pneumonia. A pneumatocele is not lined by respiratory epithelium and usually shows evidence of organization at the periphery. A pulmonary lymphatic cyst may have a similar gross appearance as a large cyst CCAM, but it is histologically distinct, with a lymphatic rather than respiratory-type lining. It may contain protein-rich lymph fluid. Intrapulmonary lymphangioma has a similar radiologic appearance, but is clearly interstitial on gross examination and has typical histology of lymphangioma in other locations. Low-grade (type 1)

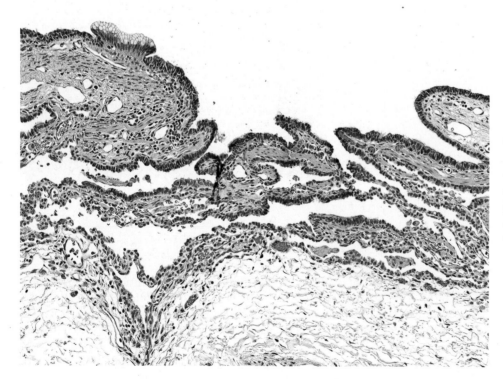

FIGURE 4-8

Congenital cystic adenomatoid malformation, large cyst type (Stocker type 1)
The wall of the cyst shows areas of continuity between the lumen and adjacent smaller alveolar duct-like structures and alveoli. Focal mucigenic epithelium resembling gastric foveolar epithelium is a frequent finding.

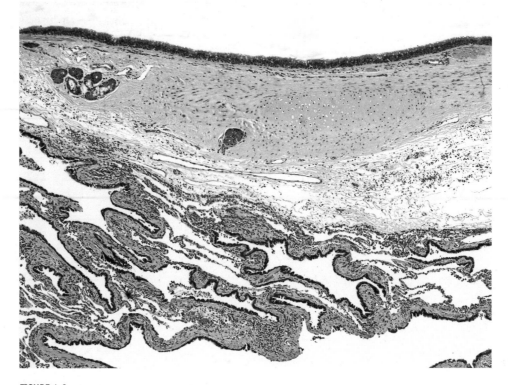

FIGURE 4-9

Bronchogenic cyst
Unlike the large cyst CCAM, an intrapulmonary bronchogenic cyst is self-contained and unilocular, without connection to the adjacent parenchyma. The lesion recapitulates a normal bronchus, including presence of cartilage plates and submucosal glands. In this case, the underlying parenchyma shows secondary changes due to airway obstruction.

pleuropulmonary blastoma (PPB) is an important differential of large cyst CCAM and should be considered and excluded in each case. Unlike CCAM (Stocker type 1), the low-grade cystic form of PPB is largely lined by alveolar epithelium with sometimes small foci of respiratory, but never mucigenic, epithelium. All have at least focal areas of interstitial hypercellularity and sometimes atypical cartilage, blastemal, and myogenic differentiation. Most examples of peripheral cystic CCAM (Stocker type 4) are thought to represent low-grade pleuropulmonary blastomas.

DISORDERS WITH ABNORMAL BRONCHIAL CONNECTION: BRONCHIAL ATRESIA, INTRALOBAR SEQUESTRATION, AND EXTRALOBAR SEQUESTRATION

CLINICAL AND PATHOLOGIC FEATURES

Bronchial atresia (BA) may occur at any level in the bronchial tree, resulting in lobar, segmental, or subsegmental distribution (Figures 4-10, 4-11). Isolated bronchial atresia typically presents in older children or adolescents with dyspnea, recurrent pneumonia, wheezing, or as an incidental finding on a chest x-ray. It is most often segmental and commonly involves the left upper lobe, but also occurs in the right upper or lower lobes. The widespread use of in utero ultrasound has resulted in early identification and surgical excision, making these lesions now more common in infants.

Although often isolated, bronchial atresia also may be associated with abnormal systemic arterial supply, in which case it is called a pulmonary sequestration. Venous drainage is most often by the ipsilateral pulmonary vein, but also may be aberrant to a systemic vein. Sequestrations have been subclassified as intralobar or extralobar depending on their relationship to the adjacent lung. Extralobar sequestration (ELS) is the more common, often identified in utero as a large mass that may become smaller relative to the normally connected lung as gestation advances. It appears as a separate, usually small, pyramidal portion of accessory lung tissue, with its own pleural investment and is unattached to the adjacent lung (Figures 4-12, 4-13). It may be seen in ectopic locations, including within the mediastinum, diaphragm, retroperitoneum, and abdomen. Intralobar sequestration (ILS) refers to a portion of lung contained within the confines of the visceral pleura of a lobe, but without normal

CCAM, LARGE CYST TYPE —FACT SHEET

Definition

▸ Focal developmental malformation of the lung usually forming a single large, often multiloculated, cystic structure

Incidence

▸ Uncommon, but commonest of the cystic maldevelopments

Morbidity and Mortality

▸ Variable, from asymptomatic to large, space-occupying lesions producing compression and rarely hypoplasia of the remaining lung
▸ Surgical excision is usually curative

Gender Distribution

▸ Slight male predominance

Clinical Features

▸ Increasing respiratory distress usually in the first week, but sometimes delayed

Radiologic Features

▸ In utero—hyperlucent region
▸ Post-natally—single, often multilocular, air-filled cystic lesion, enlarging, often with mediastinal shift
▸ Cannot be separated radiologically from low-grade cystic pleuropulmonary blastoma or intrapulmonary lymphangioma

Prognosis and Treatment

▸ Surgical excision
▸ Rarely, prolonged respiratory insufficiency with large lesions that have induced pulmonary hypoplasia
▸ Rarely, late development of bronchioalveolar carcinoma

CCAM, LARGE CYST TYPE—PATHOLOGIC FEATURES

Gross Findings

▸ Large cyst (>2 cm diameter), usually single and affecting only one lobe. May have septation or multiloculation
▸ Any lobe may be involved, lower lobe somewhat more commonly, and the left lung slightly more than the right

Microscopic Findings

▸ Respiratory epithelial lining with smooth muscle in wall and absent cartilage
▸ Connection of cyst cavity with adjacent parenchyma via smaller alveolar duct-like structures
▸ Focal mucigenic epithelium in some

Differential Diagnosis

▸ Bronchogenic cyst, pneumatocele, lymphangioma, lymphatic cyst, low-grade cystic pleuropulmonary blastoma (type I)

bronchial or arterial connections (Figures 4-14, 4-15). Because the alveolar parenchyma of this region communicates via collateral ventilation with adjacent normal parenchyma, intralobar sequestrations are susceptible to secondary infection and may present later in childhood or early adult life with recurrent pneumonia.

DIFFERENTIAL DIAGNOSIS

The differential diagnosis of bronchial atresia includes bronchogenic cyst, which is distinguished from the mucocele of bronchial atresia by the lack of direct connection to adjacent airways with mucus stasis. Congenital lobar overinflation (emphysema) is often caused by bronchomalacia, intrinsic narrowing due to webs or stenosis, or, less often, extrinsic compression of an airway. Unlike bronchial atresia, it typically does not have significant mucus stasis. The differential diagnosis of extralobar

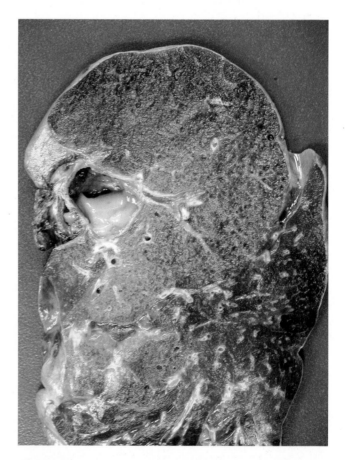

FIGURE 4-10

Bronchial atresia

Bronchial atresia results in a cystic mucus-filled central airway (mucocele), often producing a bulge or palpable mass lesion near the hilum. The parenchyma within the distribution of the atretic bronchus is hyperinflated and often shows dilated, mucus-filled branching airways. If the atretic bronchus is large, it may form a nodular focus of cartilage at the hilum of the lobe.

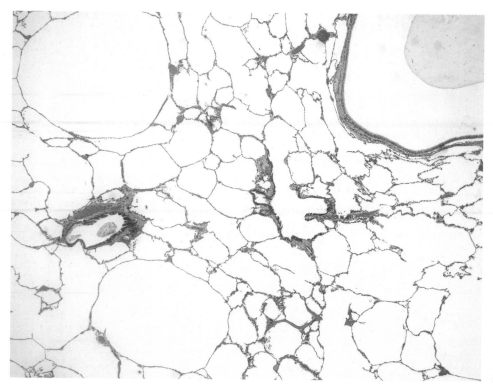

FIGURE 4-11

Bronchial atresia

Dilated distal airways are filled with mucus (top right). The surrounding alveoli show variable enlargement and rounded contours, with impaired development.

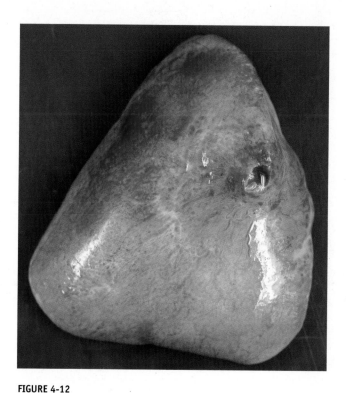

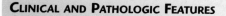

FIGURE 4-12

Extralobar Sequestration

Extralobar sequestrations are typically small triangular or pyramidal structures invested on all sides by smooth pleura. A vascular pole at the hilum contains a thick-walled systemic artery and one or more draining veins, but no evidence of a bronchus.

sequestration radiographically includes CCAM and other mass lesions, but is a pathologically distinctive lesion. The differential diagnosis of intralobar sequestration includes acute and organizing pneumonia (if infected) and large cyst CCAM (type I), particularly as approximately 25% of large cyst type CCAMs have a systemic arterial supply and, less frequently, abnormal venous connection. Both of these have normal bronchial connection of the involved lung.

PRIMARY PULMONARY LYMPHATIC DISORDERS

CLINICAL AND PATHOLOGIC FEATURES

Primary developmental disorders of lymphatics include lymphangiectasia, lymphangiomatosis, lymphangioma, and lymphatic dysplasia syndrome. Although the product of developmental errors, these conditions have a variable presentation and course. They can also be confused both clinically and on imaging studies with other primary pulmonary conditions, as they produce respiratory symptomatology and have an interstitial pattern on imaging studies. These lymphatic

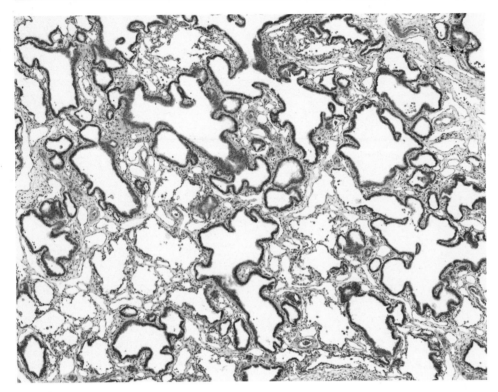

FIGURE 4-13

Extralobar sequestration
Microscopically, many of these lesions show parenchymal microcystic maldevelopment due to airway obstruction, resulting in increased branching bronchiolar profiles and simplified alveoli, also described as Stocker type 2 CCAM.

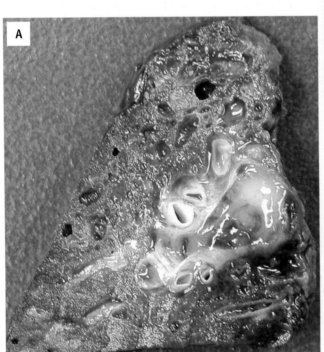

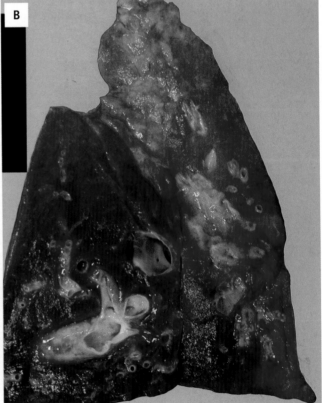

FIGURE 4-14

Intralobar sequestration
The gross appearance of intralobar sequestration is dependent upon the age at presentation, presence or absence of concurrent infection, and hemodynamic alterations. Like bronchial atresia, the gross appearance of intralobar sequestration reflects proximal bronchial obstruction, often with ectatic mucus-filled airways and small parenchymal cysts which may be filled with purulent material if infected **(A)**. Arteriovenous shunting may produce pronounced congestion, in this case defining the limits of the sequestered lung from the surrounding normal parenchyma **(B)**.

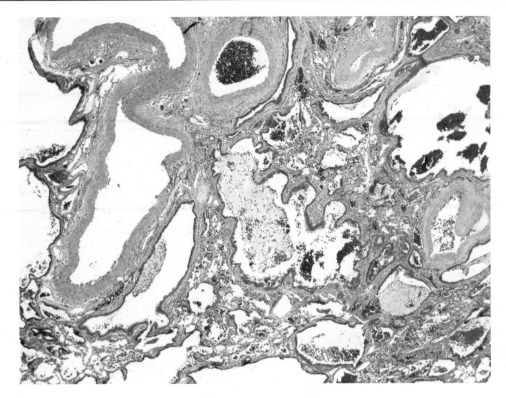

FIGURE 4-15

Intralobar sequestration
Similar to isolated bronchial atresia, there is mucus stasis in the airways. A dilated thick-walled systemic artery accompanies the ectatic airways near the hilum.

disorders are usually sporadic. However, primary pulmonary lymphangiectasis (Figures 4-16, 4-17) can be a component of chromosomal disorders (Turner syndrome, Down syndrome) and other genetic disorders (Noonan syndrome, Ehlers-Danlos syndrome), or can be found in association with cardiovascular malformations, both with and without pulmonary venous obstruction. Severely affected infants are often stillborn. Pulmonary lymphangiectasis occurs in two forms: primary (malformation of lymphatics isolated to lungs and sometimes the mediastinum) and secondary (following injury to the lymphatic system from surgery, radiation, infection, or trauma). At times, pulmonary lymphangiectasis is a component of a more generalized lymphatic disorder with involvement of extrathoracic sites. Lymphatic dysplasia syndrome refers to a group of quite varied disorders in which there is not always pulmonary involvement. These include primary lymphedema syndromes, congenital and idiopathic chylothorax, and the yellow nail syndrome. While pulmonary lymphangioma refers to a focal mass lesion, lymphangiomatosis is a diffuse proliferation of lymphatics expanding the pleura and interlobular septa (Figure 4-18).

PRIMARY CILIARY DYSKINESIA

CLINICAL FEATURES

Primary ciliary dyskinesia is usually a familial disorder with an autosomal recessive pattern of inheritance. Clinical manifestations typically include chronic sinusitis and otitis media, recurrent pneumonia, and male infertility. Situs inversus (Kartagener's syndrome) occurs in approximately half of cases. Presentation is usually in childhood, although some cases are not detected until adulthood, particularly when associated with male infertility. Absent or poorly coordinated ciliary motion results from a variety of defects of the ciliary apparatus.

PATHOLOGIC FEATURES

Poor clearance of secretions and recurrent infection result in bronchiectasis and progressive lung disease (Figure 4-19). Diagnostic evaluation for primary ciliary

DISORDERS WITH ABNORMAL BRONCHIAL CONNECTION —FACT SHEET

Definition

» A group of related disorders unified by the presence of complete bronchial obstruction and its secondary consequences

Incidence

» Uncommon

Age Distribution

» Neonates and infants (ELS)
» Neonates, infants, older children, adolescents, and young adults, depending on diagnostic modality (BA, ILS)

Clinical Features

» Asymptomatic finding on prenatal or postnatal chest imaging (ELS)
» May be associated with diaphragmatic defect or other developmental abnormality
» Asymptomatic, dyspnea, wheezing, recurrent pneumonia (BA)
» Asymptomatic, recurrent pneumonia (ILS)

Radiologic Features

» Absent bronchial connection in all
» May have hilar density caused by mucocele (BA)
» Systemic arterial supply (ILS, ELS) from thoracic or abdominal aorta, celiac, splenic, intercostal, or subclavian arteries. Single or multiple vessels
» Systemic venous drainage—more common in ELS, rare in ILS

Prognosis and Treatment

» Generally good prognosis
» Surgical resection is the predominant treatment modality

DISORDERS WITH ABNORMAL BRONCHIAL CONNECTION—PATHOLOGIC FEATURES

Gross Findings

» Location is most often the left upper lobe (BA), left lower lung field (ELS), or left lower lobe (ILS)

BA/ILS

» Enlarged lobe with atretic bronchus, cystically-dilated and mucus-filled bronchus (mucocele) distal to atresia, and dilatation of more distal airways
» Parenchymal overexpansion and sometimes microcystic change
» Hilar dome (mucocele) for lobar BA
» Segmental and subsegmental BA show regional parenchymal changes
» Affected region may be outlined by pleural pseudofissures

ILS

» Thick-walled systemic artery enters transpleurally separate from the hilum

ELS

» Pleurally enclosed portion of lung parenchyma with vessels but no airway in the pedicle
» Microcystic parenchyma or more solid appearance on cut surface

Microscopic Findings

BA/ILS

» Cystic dilation of airways and mucus stasis
» Distal obstructive parenchymal changes with airspace enlargement (pulmonary hyperplasia) and decreased density of airways and vessels
» May have superimposed acute and chronic inflammation with supervening infection

ILS

» Systemic artery rapidly anastomoses with pulmonary arteries and may show hypertensive changes when long-standing

ELS

» Central dilated bronchus and parenchymal maldevelopment with pulmonary hyperplasia
» Many show microcystic parenchymal maldevelopment (approximately 50%) of CCAM type 2 morphology
» Markedly dilated lymphatics occasionally, postulated to be due to torsion
» Rhabdomyomatous dysplasia rarely

dyskinesia includes direct examination of ciliary movement and ultrastructural examination of cilia. Light microscopic examination of unstained wet preparations using fresh ciliary brushings and/or biopsies is commonly used as a screening tool. Lack of coordinated and rhythmic movement of cilia may reflect primary ciliary dyskinesia, but may also be secondary to other factors including presence of squamous metaplasia or inflammation. Repeat biopsy after resolution of inflammation may be necessary in this circumstance. Ultrastructural analysis of cilia oriented in cross-section is used to detect variable structural abnormalities in the ciliary apparatus, including absent or short dynein arms, lack of radial spokes, compound cilia or abnormal ciliary orientation, and other microtubular abnormalities (Figure 4-20).

CYSTIC FIBROSIS

CLINICAL FEATURES

Cystic fibrosis is a systemic disease with an often prominent pulmonary component. It is the most common cause of chronic lung disease in children and accounts for the highest proportion of lung transplants performed in the pediatric age group. The severity of lung disease

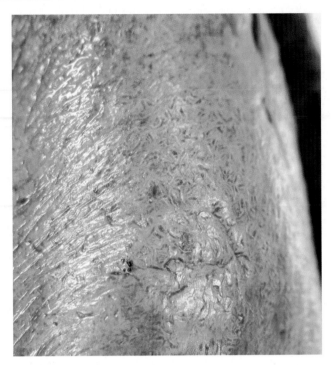

FIGURE 4-16

Lymphangiectasis
The pleura appears slightly thickened and opaque with a complex network of linear lymphatic markings.

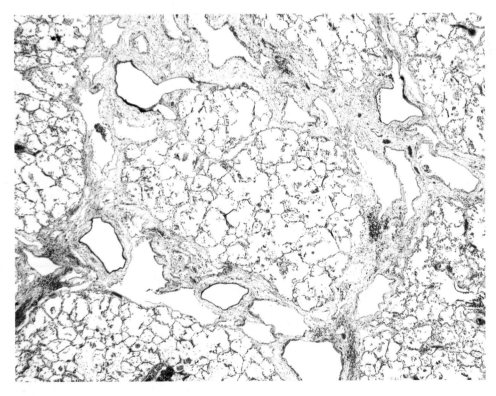

FIGURE 4-17

Lymphangiectasis
Primary pulmonary lymphangiectasis shows marked dilation of the lymphatic spaces in the interlobular septa. (Movat pentachrome)

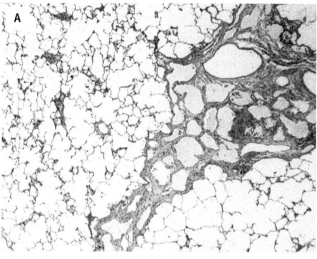 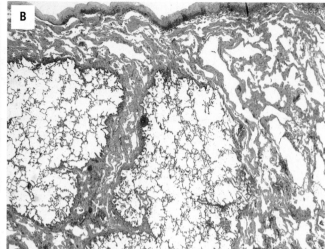

FIGURE 4-18

Lymphangiomatosis

The lymphatics are both dilated and proliferated within the pleura and interlobular septa. They may form numerous rounded spaces in some cases **(A)**, and more complex anastomosing channels in other cases **(B)**. Compact spindled kaposiform areas containing hemorrhage and hemosiderin may also be seen.

LYMPHATIC DISORDERS —FACT SHEET

Definition
➤ A group of developmental abnormalities of the lymphatic system
➤ Primary lymphangiectasis is likely due to failure of regression of interstitial tissue with subsequent lymphatic dilatation
➤ Lymphangioma is due to failure of lymphatic channels to connect properly during development
➤ Lymphangiomatosis is due to progressive non-tumoral proliferation of lymphatic channels in normal locations
➤ Congenital chylothorax is due to a deficiency in peripheral lymphatic channels or incompetent valves with reflux from the thoracic duct

Incidence
➤ Rare

Morbidity and Mortality
➤ Primary lymphangiectasis—stillborn, or fatal early in life
➤ Lymphangiomas—incidental
➤ Lymphangiomatosis—progressive, ultimately fatal
➤ Congenital chylothorax—significant morbidity from pleural effusion and often fatal

Gender and Age Distribution
➤ Primary lymphangiectasis—neonate; M>F
➤ Lymphangioma—early childhood, 90% before age 2 years; M=F
➤ Lymphangiomatosis—school-age children and adolescents; M=F
➤ Congenital chylothorax—neonate; M>F

Clinical Features
➤ Primary lymphangiectasis—severe respiratory failure; later onset when associated with cardiovascular maldevelopment; associated with Turner, Down, Noonan, and Ehlers-Danlos

Continued on next page...

LYMPHATIC DISORDERS—PATHOLOGIC FEATURES

Gross Findings
➤ Primary lymphangiectasis—bosselated pleural surface with dilated linear lymphatic markings
➤ Lymphangioma—mass lesion, may collapse when excised
➤ Lymphangiomatosis—diffuse pleural and septal widening without mass lesions
➤ Congenital chylothorax—cloudy pleural effusion

Microscopic Findings
➤ Primary lymphangiectasis—markedly dilated and tortuous lymphatics in normal numbers and locations without other vascular changes
➤ Lymphangioma—focal proliferation of lymphatic channels and associated connective tissue
➤ Lymphangiomatosis—diffuse proliferation of lymphatics in normal locations. Often dilated but smaller and more numerous than in lymphangiectasia; smooth muscle proliferation; some with Kaposiform spindle cell proliferation
➤ Congenital chylothorax—lymphocyte-rich effusion without organisms, protein- and lipid-rich

Immunohistochemical Features
➤ D2-40 specifically highlights lymphatic endothelium

Differential Diagnosis
➤ Primary lymphangiectasis—secondary lymphatic dilation; pulmonary interstitial emphysema
➤ Lymphangioma—hemangioma, other mass lesion
➤ Lymphangiomatosis—lymphangioleiomyomatosis; secondary lymphangiectasis; organizing pleural effusion; pulmonary interstitial emphysema
➤ Congenital chylothorax—other effusions and chylothorax of other etiologies

- Lymphangioma—incidental finding; mass lesion
- Lymphangiomatosis—early resembles asthma, later progressive restrictive disease; 75% with thoracic bony lesions
- Congenital chylothorax—autosomal recessive, early onset respiratory distress and chylous pleural effusion

Radiologic Features

- Primary lymphangiectasis—localized or diffuse interstitial infiltrates, pleural effusion
- Lymphangioma—intrapulmonary mass lesion; cystic with thin septa
- Lymphangiomatosis—bilateral interstitial infiltrates, pleural and/or pericardial effusion
- Congenital chylothorax—bilateral pleural effusion

Prognosis and Treatment

- Primary lymphangiectasis—poor prognosis, often fatal if early presentation; low-fat, high-protein diet
- Lymphangioma—good prognosis; excision
- Lymphangiomatosis—ultimately fatal; low-fat, high-protein diet, fluid drainage, pleurodesis
- Congenital chylothorax—variable prognosis related to degree of lung hypoplasia and associated low-fat, high-protein diet, fluid drainage, pleurodesis, replace losses of immune components

is highly variable between individual patients, but typically results in progressive decline in respiratory function due to airway obstruction, bronchiectasis, and recurrent infection. This autosomal recessive disorder is caused by homozygous or compound heterozygous mutations in the cystic fibrosis transmembrane regulator (CFTR) gene on chromosome 7. The mutations result in loss of function of a chloride transport channel with impaired removal of chloride ions from the respiratory epithelial cell and decreased sodium and water content in the luminal mucus. The resulting thick inspissated airway mucus causes chronic airway-centered infection with bacterial colonization (especially with mucoid strains of *Pseudomonas aeruginosa*, *Burkholderia cepacia*, *Staphylococcus aureus*, and *Haemophilus influenzae*). The airways may also be colonized by yeast and fungal organisms (20%), especially *Candida* or *Aspergillus*, which in some cases manifests as allergic bronchopulmonary fungal disease (10%). Colonization by non-tuberculous mycobacteria may also occur. Pulmonary complications include pneumothorax, hemoptysis, pulmonary hypertension, and right ventricular hypertrophy (cor pulmonale). Inspissation of ductal

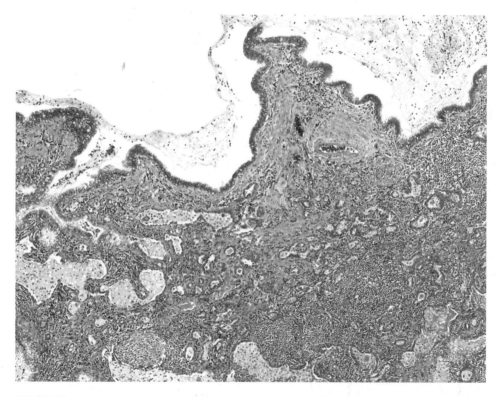

FIGURE 4-19

Primary ciliary dyskinesia

Prominent bronchiectasis with resolving pneumonia are the most prominent features in this lobectomy from an 18-year-old girl with primary ciliary dyskinesia due to absent outer dynein arms. The cilia are morphologically unremarkable by light microscopy.

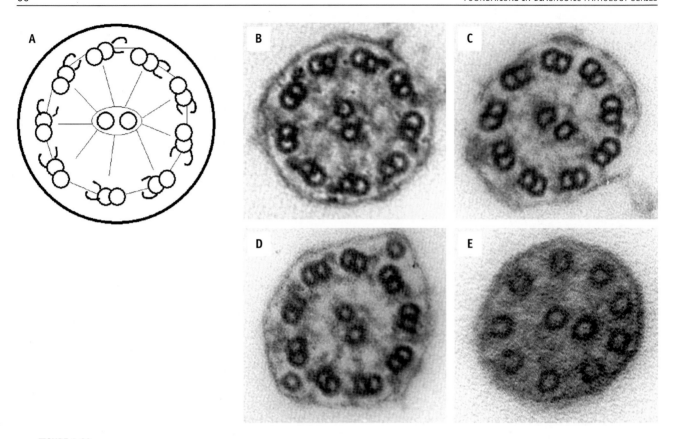

FIGURE 4-20

Ciliary dyskinesia

The normal ciliary skeleton is composed of 9 peripheral microtubule doublets, each with outer and inner dynein arms, and 2 central microtubules (**A,** diagram of normal cilia). A variety of ultrastructural abnormalities has been described in primary and secondary ciliary dyskinesia, most notably absent or shortened inner (**B**) and/or outer (**C**) dynein arms. Other abnormalities may include absent or reduced radial spokes, absent central microtubules, and aberrant peripheral microtubule position (**D**) and number (**E**). Abnormalities of dynein arms and central microtubules are associated with primary ciliary dyskinesia.

secretions in other exocrine organs causes end-organ damage, particularly pancreatic dysfunction (fat malabsorption, malnutrition, diabetes). Other manifestations include meconium ileus in the neonate, focal biliary cirrhosis with long-standing disease, and infertility in males. Although genetic testing is available for the common mutations in CFTR, the sweat test remains the mainstay of diagnosis. Sweat from patients with cystic fibrosis contains elevated levels of both sodium and chloride. Sweat is obtained by quantitative pilocarpine iontophoresis, and the chloride concentration is measured. Collection errors may affect results, and an abnormal result should always be confirmed.

PATHOLOGIC FEATURES

The lungs in cystic fibrosis show progressive changes, beginning with stasis of secretions leading to impaired airway clearance, supervening infection, sequestration of bacteria in abnormal mucus, local inflammation, and immunologic alterations leading to recurrent injury to airway walls with eventual destruction of smooth muscle and cartilage. Partial replacement of airway mucosa by granulation tissue and vascular changes from chronic infection favor the development of hemoptysis. Bronchiectasis is the pathologic hallmark of cystic fibrosis

PRIMARY CILIARY DYSKINESIA —FACT SHEET

Definition

» Primary structural disorder of ciliary apparatus resulting in abnormal ciliary motility

Incidence and Location

» Rare; 1:15,000 Caucasian
» Worldwide distribution

Morbidity and Mortality

» Impaired ciliary function results in situs inversus from abnormal embryonic patterning, and post-natally in poor airway clearance, severe otitis media, and sinusitis
» Abnormal sperm motility leads to male infertility
» Most morbidity is related to the respiratory system effects

Gender, Race, and Age Distribution

» M=F; no racial predilection
» Usual onset in early childhood

Clinical Features

» Chronic sinusitis, otitis media, recurrent upper and lower respiratory infections in early childhood, male infertility
» Familial predilection (autosomal recessive)

Prognosis and Treatment

Postural drainage, chest physiotherapy, maintenance of adequate hydration, mucolytics, and appropriate use of antibiotics for secondary infection

PRIMARY CILIARY DYSKINESIA—PATHOLOGIC FEATURES

Gross Findings

» Bronchiectasis with or without bronchopneumonia

Microscopic Findings

» Normal cilia by light microscopy
» Chronic airway injury with bronchiectasis and chronic active inflammation

Ancillary Studies

» Absent or dyscoordinated ciliary motion on direct wet preparation
» Abnormal ciliary beat frequency
» Abnormal ciliary structure by electron microscopy in most cases (e.g., absent inner or outer dynein arms)

Differential Diagnosis

» Bronchiectasis due to cystic fibrosis, immunodeficiency, and other etiologies

and is related to mucus plugging and secondary infection (Figures 4-21, 4-22).

PROGNOSIS AND THERAPY

There have been marked improvements in the management of cystic fibrosis, resulting in a marked increase in the mean survival, well into adulthood. Surgical intervention is now unusual, limited to rare lobectomies for more localized disease and lung transplantation. Hemoptysis is managed by embolization of the affected region.

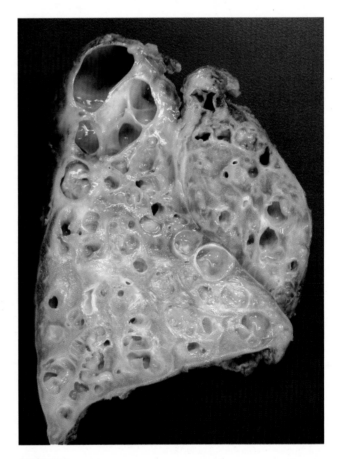

FIGURE 4-21

Cystic fibrosis

Bronchiectasis with tenacious mucopurulent secretions is the hallmark of cystic fibrosis, though there is individual variation in the degree of bronchiectasis and lobar distribution. The ectatic airways are thickened and fibrotic, and may show adjacent regions of parenchymal consolidation. Areas of preserved lung are generally pale and hyperinflated due to air-trapping.

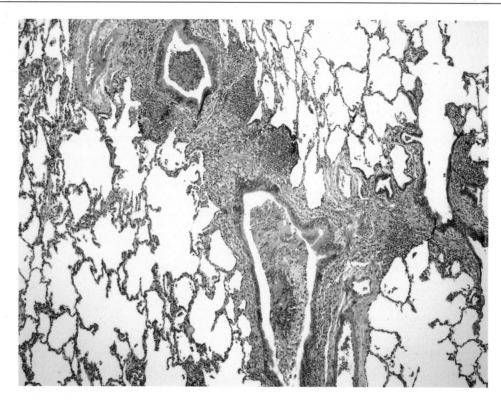

FIGURE 4-22

Cystic fibrosis
Dilated airways are accompanied by a dense, mixed inflammatory infiltrate of the airway wall with intraluminal eosinophilic inspissated secretions admixed with abundant neutrophils, bacteria, and karyorrhectic debris.

SUGGESTED READINGS

Diffuse Developmental Disorders

1. Boggs S, Harris MC, Hoffman DJ, et al. Misalignment of pulmonary veins with alveolar capillary dysplasia: affected siblings and variable phenotypic expression. *J Pediatr.* 1994;124:125-8.
2. Chambers HM. Congenital acinar aplasia: an extreme form of pulmonary maldevelopment. *Pathology.* 1991;23:69-71.
3. Janney CG, Askin FB, Kuhn C. Congenital alveolar capillary dysplasia: an unusual cause of respiratory distress in the newborn. *Am J Clin Pathol.* 1981;76:722-7.
4. Langston C. Misalignment of pulmonary veins and alveolar capillary dysplasia. *Pediatr Pathol.* 1991;11:163-70.
5. McMahon HE. Congenital alveolar dysplasia. *Am J Pathol.* 1948;24:919-30.
6. Rabah R, Poulik JM. Congenital alveolar capillary dysplasia with misalignment of pulmonary veins associated with hypoplastic left heart syndrome. *Pediatr Devel Pathol.* 2001;4:167-74.
7. Rutledge JC, Jensen P. Acinar dysplasia: a new form of pulmonary maldevelopment. *Hum Pathol.* 1986;17:1290-3.
8. Sen P, Thakur N, Stockton DW, Langston C, Bejjani BA. Expanding the phenotype of alveolar capillary dysplasia. *J Pediatr.,* 2004;145:646-51.

Surfactant Dysfunction Disorders

9. Cole FS, Hamvas A, Nogee LM. Genetic disorders of neonatal respiratory function. *Pediatr Res.* 2001;50:157-62.
10. DeMello DE, Nogee LM, Heymans S, et al. Molecular and phenotypic variability in the congenital alveolar proteinosis syndrome associated with inherited surfactant protein B deficiency. *J Pediatr.* 1994;124:43-50.
11. Fisher M, Roggli V, Merten D, et al. Coexisting endogenous lipoid pneumonia, cholesterol granulomas, and pulmonary alveolar proteinosis in a pediatric population. *Pediatr Pathol.* 1992;12:365-83.

12. Katzenstein A-LA, Gordon LP, Oliphant M, et al. Chronic pneumonitis of infancy. *Am J Surg Pathol.* 1995;19:439-47.
13. Nogee LM, deMello DE, Dehner LP, et al. Pulmonary surfactant protein B deficiency in congenital pulmonary alveolar proteinosis. *N Engl J Med.* 1993;328:406-10.
14. Nogee LM, Dunbar AE, Wert SE, et al. A mutation in the surfactant protein C gene associated with familial interstitial lung disease. *N Engl J Med.* 2001;344:573-9.
15. Shulenin S, Nogee LM, Annilo T, Wert SE, Whitsett JA, Dean M. ABCA3 gene mutations in newborns with fatal surfactant deficiency. *N Engl J Med.* 2004;350:1296-1303.

Congenital Cystic Adenomatoid Malformation, Large Cyst Type

16. Langston C. New concepts in the pathology of congenital lung malformations. *Semin Pediatr Surg.* 2003;12:17-37.
17. Stocker JT, Madewell JE, Drake RM. Congenital cystic adenomatoid malformation of the lung: classification and morphologic spectrum. *Hum Pathol.* 1977;8:151-71.

Disorders with Abnormal Bronchial Connection

18. Conran RM, Stocker JR. Extralobar sequestration with frequently associated congenital cystic adenomatoid malformation, type 2: report of 50 cases. *Pediatr Dev Pathol.* 1999;2:454-63.
19. Langston C. New concepts in pathology of congenital lung malformations. *Semin Pediatr Surg.* 2003;12:17-37.
20. Riedlinger WF, Vargas SO, Jennings RW, et al. Bronchial atresia is common to extralobar sequestration, introlobar sequestration, congenital cystic adenomatoid malformation, and lobar emphysema. *Pediatr Dev Pathol* 2006;9;361-73.

Lymphatic Disorders

21. Faul JL, Berry GJ, Colby TV, et al. Thoracic lymphangiomas, lymphangiectasis, lymphangiomatosis, and lymphatic dysplasia syndrome. *Am J Respir Crit Care Med*. 2000;161:1037-46.
22. Tazelaar HD, Kerr D, Yousem SA, et al. Diffuse pulmonary lymphangiomatosis. *Hum Pathol*. 1993;24:1313-22.

Primary Ciliary Dyskinesia

23. Hicks MJ. Chapter 235: Ciliary Dyskinesia. In: McMillan JA, Feigin RD, DeAngelis C, Jones MD, eds. *Oski's Pediatrics,* 4th ed. Philadelphia: Lippincott Williams and Wilkins, 2006;1423-4.
24. Holzmann D, Ott PM, Felix H. Diagnostic approach to primary ciliary dyskinesia: a review. *Eur J Pediatr*. 2000;159:95-8.
25. Meeks M, Bush A. Primary ciliary dyskinesia (PCD). *Pediatr Pulm*. 2000;29:307-16.

Cystic Fibrosis

26. Oppenheimer EH, Esterly JR. Pathology of cystic fibrosis: review of the literature and comparison with 146 autopsied cases. In: Rosenberg HS, Bolande RP, eds. *Perspective in Pediatric Pathology*, vol 2. Chicago: Year Book, 1975.
27. Orenstein DM, Winnie GB, Altman H. Cystic fibrosis: a 2002 update. *J Pediatr*. 2002;140:156-64.
28. Tomashefski JF Jr, Dahms B, Abramowsky CA. The pathology of cystic fibrosis. In: Davis PB, ed. *Cystic Fibrosis*. New York: Marcel Dekker; 1994:435-89.

5

Acquired Non-Neoplastic Neonatal and Pediatric Disorders

Gail H. Deutsch

- Introduction
- Growth Abnormalities
- Pulmonary Interstitial Glycogenosis
- Neuroendocrine Cell Hyperplasia of Infancy
- Persistent Pulmonary Hypertension of the Newborn
- Complications of Prematurity and its Therapy

INTRODUCTION

Acquired non-neoplastic neonatal and pediatric lung disorders comprise a heterogeneous group of conditions that can be divided into two broad categories, entities with a known etiology and those of unknown or poorly understood etiology. The well-characterized disorders include those that reflect altered lung growth and development or a poor transition from intrauterine to extrauterine life, including persistent pulmonary hypertension of the newborn, hyaline membrane disease, and bronchopulmonary dysplasia. Those classified as poorly understood include two idiopathic lung diseases unique to infants and very young children, pulmonary interstitial glycogenosis and neuroendocrine cell hyperplasia of infancy.

GROWTH ABNORMALITIES

Abnormalities of lung growth, specifically pulmonary hypoplasia and pulmonary hyperplasia, largely reflect the influence of a developmental process or malformation that alters lung maturation. Distension of the lung with liquid and fetal respiratory movements is required for normal fetal lung growth, so any mechanism that interferes with these processes can result in a prenatal growth disorder. Prenatal onset pulmonary hypoplasia ranges from mild to severe, depending on the mechanism of

hypoplasia and timing of the insult in relation to the stage of lung development (Table 5-1). Early insults that take place before 16 weeks' gestation (renal anomalies, congenital diaphragmatic hernia) may interfere with airway branching as well as acinar development, while later events (premature rupture of membranes) will exclusively impact acinar development. Since lung maturation continues well into the postnatal period, with most alveolarization occurring within 5 to 6 months of term birth, postnatal events can impact lung growth as well. Postnatal onset growth abnormalities are commonly associated with premature birth (see below, complications of prematurity and its therapy) and Down syndrome, and not infrequently seen in patients with congenital heart disease.

Like pulmonary hypoplasia, pulmonary hyperplasia, or excessive growth of the parenchyma, is a secondary phenomenon. During development it appears to be a response to airway obstruction, which blocks the outflow of fetal fluid, leading to increased alveolar growth. Pulmonary hyperplasia has also been referred to as polyalveolar lobe and Type 3 cystic adenomatoid malformation. The pathogenesis and clinical characteristics of this entity are related to congenital lobar overinflation/emphysema.

CLINICAL FEATURES

The majority of cases of pulmonary hypoplasia are secondary to congenital anomalies or pregnancy complications that inhibit lung development. Table 5-1 summarizes the most important conditions associated with prenatal pulmonary hypoplasia. The clinical profile and time of presentation are variable depending on the extent of hypoplasia and other anomalies.

Pulmonary hyperplasia is most frequently seen in a setting of airway obstruction. When all lobes are affected, this malformation is typically associated with a developmental upper airway obstruction such as tracheal or laryngeal atresia. Obstructive lesions causing focal hyperplasia include bronchial atresia and stenosis. Extrinsic airway compression from a bronchogenic cyst or vascular anomaly could also result in a hyperplastic or overinflated lung lobe. Affected neonates usually present with dyspnea in early life.

TABLE 5-1

Conditions and Anomalies Associated with Pulmonary Hypoplasia

Condition	Anomalies
Oligohydramnios	Bilateral renal agenesis or dysplasia, bladder outlet obstruction
	Prolonged premature rupture of membranes
Restriction of thoracic space	Diaphragmatic hernia
	Pleural effusions (usually due to hydrops fetalis)
	Thoracic deformity due to skeletal dysplasia syndromes
	Intrathoracic masses (congenital cystic adenomatoid malformation, thoracic neuroblastoma)
Decreased fetal breathing	Central nervous system lesions
	Neuromuscular diseases (myotonic dystrophy, spinal muscular atrophy)
	Arthrogryposis multiplex congenita
	Maternal depressant drugs
Congenital heart disease with poor pulmonary blood flow	Tetralogy of Fallot
	Hypoplastic right heart
	Pulmonary artery hypoplasia

RADIOLOGIC FEATURES

Radiographic identification of late onset pulmonary hypoplasia is often difficult. Secondary findings include spontaneous pneumothorax and pneumomediastinum. Pulmonary hypoplasia in Down syndrome may appear as peripheral cystic disease (Figure 5-1).

In pulmonary hyperplasia, chest radiographs demonstrate progressive hyperinflation or hyperlucency of a lobe. Marked overinflation may lead to compression of the adjacent lung and mediastinum (Figure 5-2).

PATHOLOGIC FEATURES

GROSS FINDINGS

Grossly, pulmonary hypoplasia is best defined by the ratio of lung weight to body weight, with an expected ratio of 0.012 for infants of 28 weeks' gestation or more and 0.015 for those of earlier gestation.

In pulmonary hyperplasia, lungs are large, bulky, and often pale, with normal lobation. It may affect all or some lobes.

MICROSCOPIC FINDINGS

To define pulmonary hypoplasia, specific criteria have been devised that are based on reduced lung weight, lung volume, DNA content, and radial alveolar count. The simplest method is the radial alveolar count, which is the number of alveoli transected by a perpendicular line drawn from the center of a respiratory bronchiole to the nearest septal division or pleural margin. The radial count in a full-term infant should average 5 alveolar spaces. In pulmonary hypoplasia there is a reduction of alveolar spaces for gestation age, which is often accompanied by

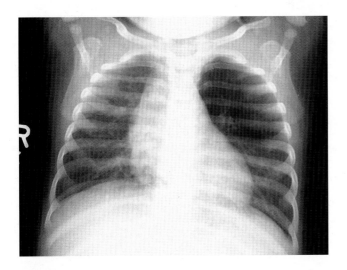

FIGURE 5-1

Pulmonary hyperplasia

Chest radiograph shows hyperlucency and hyperexpansion of the left upper lobe. (Courtesy of Dr. Alan Brody, Cincinnati, Ohio.)

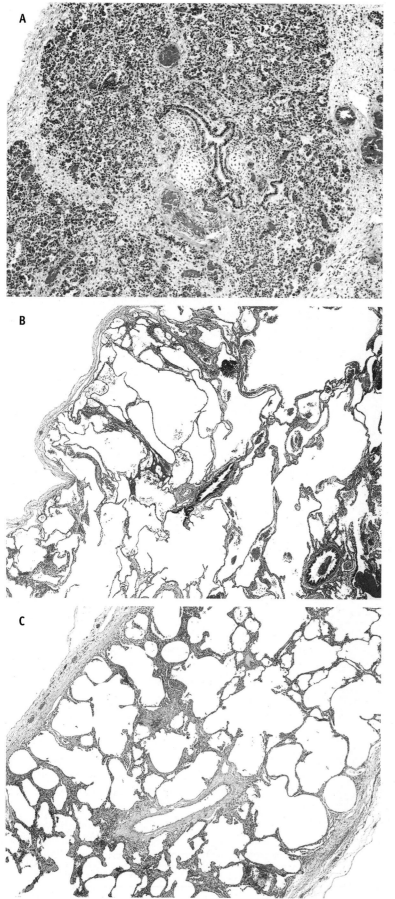

FIGURE 5-2

Pulmonary hypoplasia

(A) There is a prominence of cartilaginous bronchi and interstitial thickening in the lung of a term infant with bilateral renal dysplasia. The surrounding air spaces show collapse and marked congestion. (B) The lung of an infant with oligohydramnios, biopsied at 2.5 months, has markedly enlarged and simplified air spaces; compare with the size of a bronchiole. (C) In Down syndrome, the lung shows air space enlargement that is accentuated in the subpleural regions, but is also evident throughout the lobule.

prominence of the bronchovascular structures and a widened interstitium. Widened alveolar ducts, enlarged airspaces, and dilatation of the subpleural alveoli that may resemble cysts characterize deficient alveolarization of postnatal onset (Figure 5-3).

Pulmonary hyperplasia, diffuse or focal, is characterized by a striking increase in alveoli in relation to airways, which can be confirmed by the radial alveolar count. Alveoli are often abnormally enlarged and simplified, and there may be a decrease or absence of interlobular septae (Figure 5-4).

DIFFERENTIAL DIAGNOSIS

Due to the presence of alveolar enlargement, pulmonary hypoplasia is often misinterpreted as emphysematous change or remodeling after lung injury. However, unlike these processes, there is no evidence of a destructive process in a growth abnormality, including inflammation, type II cell hyperplasia, and significant fibrosis. Nonetheless, without proper orientation and handling, it may be difficult to recognize.

Pulmonary hyperplasia should be distinguished from congenital lobar overinflation, in which the volume increase is due to alveolar enlargement versus absolute increase in alveoli. Radial alveolar counts can be helpful for differentiating between the two processes.

PROGNOSIS AND THERAPY

Since prenatal onset pulmonary hypoplasia is frequently associated with severe and irreversible lesions, it carries a poor prognosis. Survivors are at risk for the complications frequently seen in infants with prematurity, including pneumothoraces, pulmonary interstitial emphysema, and persistent pulmonary hypertension. In entities such as diaphragmatic hernia, right-sided hypoplasia has a worse prognosis than left-sided, due to loss of bigger lung mass, more severe mediastinal shift and greater vessel displacement.

Pulmonary hyperplasia may be associated with in utero death due to compression of venous return to the heart and/or esophageal compression, resulting in polyhydramnios and fetal hydrops. The therapy for infants with lobar distension causing severe mediastinal shift and normal lung compression is surgical removal of the affected lobe or segment.

PULMONARY INTERSTITIAL GLYCOGENOSIS

Pulmonary interstitial glycogenosis (PIG), also known as cellular interstitial pneumonitis, and histiocytoid pneumonia, is a poorly understood entity seen exclusively in

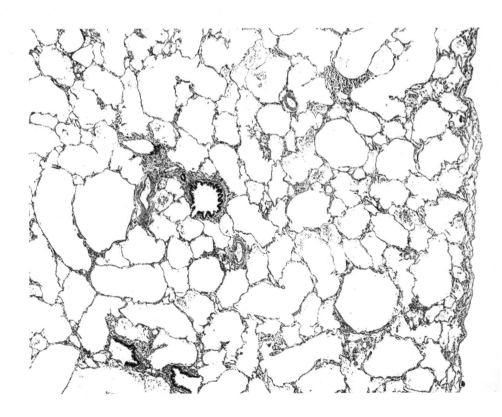

FIGURE 5-3

Pulmonary hyperplasia
Numerous, enlarged, and simplified air spaces are seen in the lung parenchyma distal to a focus of bronchial obstruction.

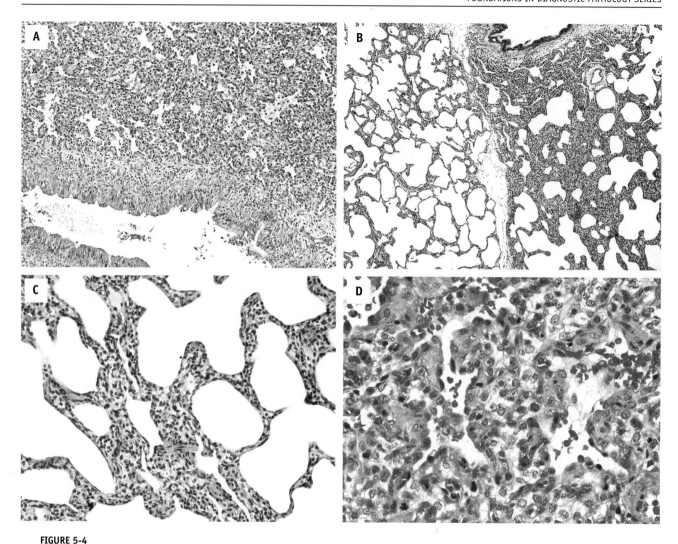

FIGURE 5-4

Pulmonary interstitial glycogenosis

The interstitial widening and increased cellularity seen in this condition can be diffuse **(A)** or patchy **(B)**, the latter typically associated with a growth disorder, such as bronchopulmonary dysplasia. Whether focal **(C)** or diffuse **(D)**, higher magnification demonstrates round to oval nuclei with vacuolated cytoplasm and indistinct cell borders.

infants less than 6 months of age. The hallmark histologic feature of PIG is a variable proliferation of glycogen-laden mesenchymal cells within the alveolar septae. PIG may be an isolated disorder or a component of another preexisting pulmonary condition, most commonly a growth abnormality such as bronchopulmonary dysplasia. There is debate concerning the underlying etiology of this condition. Some authors propose that accumulation of immature mesenchymal cells within the interstitium may represent a selective delay or aberration in the maturation of pulmonary mesenchymal cells, while others suggest that this accumulation is a nonspecific feature of several conditions that transiently alter lung growth and development in the neonatal period.

CLINICAL FEATURES

Infants generally present in the first few weeks of life, not uncommonly in the first few days, with tachypnea and hypoxemia. Deteriorating respiratory function occurs after an initial period of well-being, and patients frequently require mechanical ventilation and prolonged supplemental oxygen. Although these infants may be symptomatic for prolonged periods of time (up to 18 months after diagnosis), the overall clinical course is marked by general improvement, and mortality is rare if the patient does not have preexisting lung disease due to prematurity.

GROWTH ABNORMALITIES —FACT SHEET

Definition

▸ Pulmonary hypoplasia is the incomplete development of the lung, resulting in reduced numbers and complexity of acini

▸ Pulmonary hyperplasia, typically associated with an airway obstruction, is characterized by a marked increase in alveolar number

Incidence

Pulmonary Hypoplasia

▸ Estimated 10 per 10,000 live births

Morbidity and Mortality

Pulmonary Hypoplasia

▸ High mortality, ranging from 55-100%, depending on the mechanism of hypoplasia

▸ Increased mortality if severe oligohydramnios is present for more than 2 weeks

▸ Patients are at increased risk for pneumothorax, persistent pulmonary hypertension, and bronchopulmonary dysplasia

Pulmonary Hyperplasia

▸ May be fatal if associated with mediastinal shift and compression of unaffected lobes

Age Distribution

Pulmonary Hypoplasia and Pulmonary Hyperplasia

▸ Most present in the neonatal period

Clinical Features

Pulmonary Hypoplasia

▸ Typically associated with pregnancy complications or coexisting malformations

▸ Compression deformities may be present from prolonged oligohydramnios (contractures, Potter facies, arthrogryposes)

▸ In severe cases, neonates present with respiratory distress and difficulty in ventilation; they frequently get pneumothoraces and pulmonary interstitial emphysema

▸ Mild cases or those of postnatal onset may present later in life with dyspnea and cyanosis on exertion or a history of repeated respiratory infections

Pulmonary Hyperplasia

▸ When all lobes are affected, associated with tracheal or laryngeal atresia

▸ Focal lesions such as bronchial stenosis or atresia will cause subtotal involvement

▸ Most patients present with respiratory distress within the first 6 months of life

Radiologic Features

Pulmonary Hypoplasia

▸ Chest radiographic findings vary, depending on the mechanism and severity of hypoplasia

▸ Chest CT may show loss of lung volume and abnormal or absent normal airway branching

Pulmonary Hyperplasia

▸ Chest radiographs initially demonstrate an opacified lobe, commonly an upper lobe, which progresses to overinflation and hyperlucency

Continued

GROWTH ABNORMALITIES—PATHOLOGIC FEATURES

Gross Findings

Pulmonary Hypoplasia

▸ With early prenatal arrest, the lungs are notably small, and lung weight is often less than 40% of expected

▸ Postnatal arrest, as in Down syndrome, may manifest as peripheral cysts

Pulmonary Hyperplasia

▸ Diffuse or focal lobar overinflation

Microscopic Findings

Pulmonary Hypoplasia

▸ In prenatal arrest, there are fewer alveoli than expected for gestational age, with close approximation of the bronchi to the pleural surface

▸ Postnatal arrest is characterized by air space enlargement accentuated in subpleural and lobular areas with patchy overexpansion and collapse

Pulmonary Hyperplasia

▸ Absolute increase in the number of alveoli, which are mildly enlarged

Differential Diagnosis

Pulmonary Hypoplasia

▸ Remodeling after lung injury

Pulmonary Hyperplasia

▸ Congenital lobar overinflation/emphysema

PATHOLOGIC FEATURES

Lung biopsy shows a variable expansion of the interalveolar septae by spindle-shaped cells (Figure 5-4). A patchy distribution is typically seen in the presence of a growth abnormality. Inflammation, reactive changes, and fibrosis are absent. PAS stain demonstrates patchy PAS-positive diastase-labile material within the cytoplasm of these interstitial cells, consistent with glycogen. As the preservation of glycogen is influenced by the use of aqueous fixatives (i.e., 10 % formalin) this finding may be difficult to demonstrate on routine sections.

ANCILLARY STUDIES

ULTRASTRUCTURAL FEATURES

Ultrastructural examination shows interstitial mesenchymal cells with few cytoplasmic organelles and focally abundant monoparticulate glycogen; poor preservation of glycogen may manifest by empty-appearing cells

(Figure 5-5). Treating ultrathin sections with tannic acid enhances visualization of glycogen.

IMMUNOHISTOCHEMISTRY

The accumulated cells within the alveolar septae uniformly stain positive for vimentin (Figure 5-6). In normal conditions, one can see vimentin-positive cells around vessels, but not in alveolar walls.

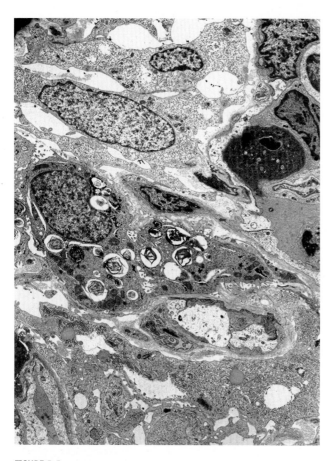

FIGURE 5-5

Pulmonary interstitial glycogenosis
Electron microscopic examination shows increased structural cells, with cytoplasmic glycogen and occasional lipid droplets. (Courtesy of Dr. Claire Langston, Houston, Texas.)

DIFFERENTIAL DIAGNOSIS

Because pulmonary interstitial glycogenosis carries a favorable prognosis, it is critical to distinguish it from other pediatric interstitial lung diseases that are associated with high morbidity and mortality. PIG/infantile cellular interstitial pneumonitis has sometimes been confused with chronic pneumonitis of infancy. Microscopically, the presence of uniform, prominent type II cells, some degree of PAS-positive material within air spaces, accumulation of macrophages, and occasional cholesterol clefts favors the diagnosis of chronic pneumonitis of infancy. Lung disease is not usually a prominent feature of storage diseases, but significant pulmonary involvement with accumulation of stored material can be seen in both air spaces and the interstitium in Gaucher disease, Niemann-Pick disease, Fabry's disease, Hermansky-Pudlak syndrome, infantile GM1 gangliosidosis, Krabbe disease, Pompe disease, and Farber's disease. Unlike PIG, the accumulating cells are histiocytes and should stain for macrophage markers.

PROGNOSIS AND THERAPY

Short-term pulse corticosteroids have been shown to be beneficial in patients with or without preexisting lung disease. A good response has also been reported with chloroquine. In infants without complications of prematurity, long-term follow-up has demonstrated a favorable outcome including normal growth and development and no significant residual pulmonary symptoms.

NEUROENDOCRINE CELL HYPERPLASIA OF INFANCY

Neuroendocrine cell hyperplasia of infancy (NEHI) is another poorly understood process that produces significant pulmonary symptomatology in infants and young children. In the literature, it has also been termed persistent tachypnea of infancy and chronic idiopathic bronchiolitis of infancy. Hyperplasia of neuroendocrine cells, as demonstrated by bombesin immunohistochemistry, is a consistent finding along with the distinctive clinical presentation and radiographic picture. It is currently unclear whether the pulmonary neuroendocrine cells are markers for this entity or involved in pathogenesis of the disorder. Based on the role of pulmonary neuroendocrine cells and bombesin in oxygen sensing as well as airway and arterial tone, it is hypothesized that neuroendocrine cells contribute to the disease process by creating a significant ventilation/perfusion

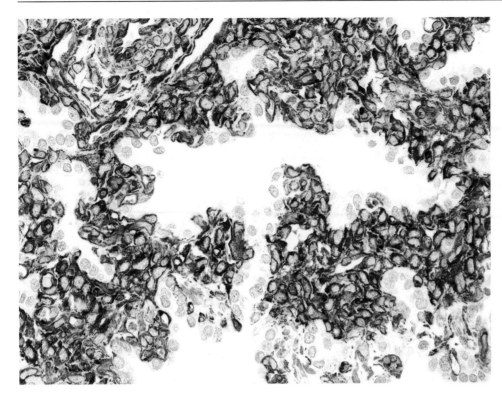

FIGURE 5-6

Pulmonary interstitial glycogenosis
The accumulated cells in the interstitium are strongly vimentin-positive.

mismatch within the lung. The stimulus for neuroendocrine cell hyperplasia is unknown, although many patients have a history of a respiratory illness preceding their clinical presentation.

CLINICAL FEATURES

At presentation, patients are extremely ill with tachypnea, hypoxia, and retractions. The onset of symptoms typically occurs at less than 1 year of age, although age at lung biopsy is often later. Familial cases with affected siblings have been identified, suggesting that there may be a genetic predisposition.

RADIOLOGIC FEATURES

Chest radiograph shows hyperexpansion and increased interstitial markings. High-resolution CT demonstrates scattered ground-glass opacities, reflective of air-trapping (Figure 5-7).

PATHOLOGIC FEATURES

Despite the apparent severity of the disease based on clinical symptoms, lung biopsies appear free of any diagnostic disease process, although most show minor and nonspecific abnormalities involving the distal airways (Figure 5-8). A mild periairway lymphocytic infiltrate is often seen but not prominent.

ANCILLARY STUDIES

Bombesin has been shown to be the most sensitive immunostain for detecting increased neuroendocrine cells in this disorder (Figure 5-9). Serotonin has also been shown to be effective. Neuron-specific enolase, calcitonin, synaptophysin, and chromogranin are much less reliable in demonstrating this increase. Immunohistochemical assessment of this disorder requires an adequate biopsy with at least 10-15 evaluable airways.

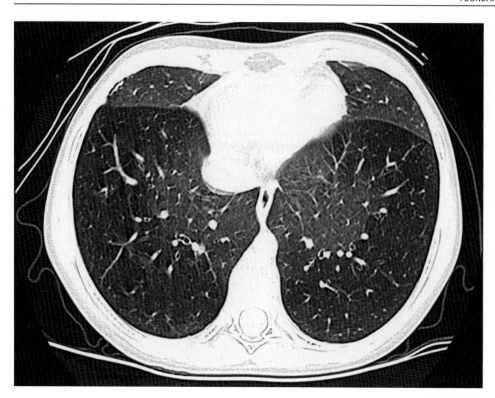

FIGURE 5-7

Neuroendocrine cell hyperplasia of infancy
The characteristic CT appearance of this disorder is hyperinflation with geographic ground-glass opacity. (Courtesy of Dr. Alan Brody, Cincinnati, Ohio.)

PULMONARY INTERSTITIAL GLYCOGENOSIS—FACT SHEET

Definition

» Idiopathic neonatal interstitial lung disease characterized by expansion of the interstitium by glycogen-laden mesenchymal cells

Incidence

» Rare, although recognition of the disorder is leading to identification of more cases

Mortality

» Mortality is rare and related to complications of prematurity

Gender and Age Distribution

» Preterm and term infants can be affected, and most become symptomatic in the first few weeks of life
» Unusual to see after 6 months of age
» May have a male predominance

Clinical Features

» Tachypnea and hypoxia

Radiologic Features

» Diffuse interstitial infiltrates with hyperinflation

Prognosis and Therapy

» If no underlying lung disorder, favorable outcome
» Short-term pulse corticosteroids and chloroquine have been shown to be beneficial

---

PULMONARY INTERSTITIAL GLYCOGENOSIS—PATHOLOGIC FEATURES

Microscopic Findings

» Variable proliferation of spindle-shaped cells in the interstitium
» Cells have indistinct cell borders, bland oval nuclei, and pale cytoplasm containing PAS-positive diastase-labile material that may be difficult to demonstrate
» Patchy distribution
» Often associated with a growth abnormality
» Associated inflammation, fibrosis, and accumulation of alveolar proteinaceous material should be absent

Ultrastructural Features

» Interstitial mesenchymal cells with few organelles
» Cells focally contain abundant monoparticulate glycogen
» Some cells may contain droeplets of neutral lipid

Immunohistochemical Features

» Cells always positive for vimentin, focally for smooth muscle actin
» Cells negative for desmin, leukocyte common antigen, CD68, and lysozyme

Differential Diagnosis

» Chronic pneumonitis of infancy
» Storage diseases

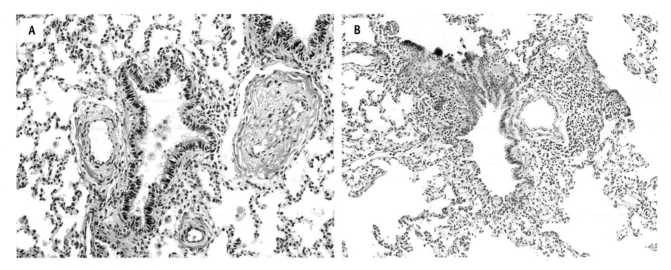

FIGURE 5-8

Neuroendocrine cell hyperplasia of infancy
(A) The lung biopsy shows minimal changes, including a mild increase in free alveolar macrophages and increased clear cells in the bronchiolar epithelium. **(B)** Mild hyperplasia of airway smooth muscle and periairway lymphocytic inflammation may be seen.

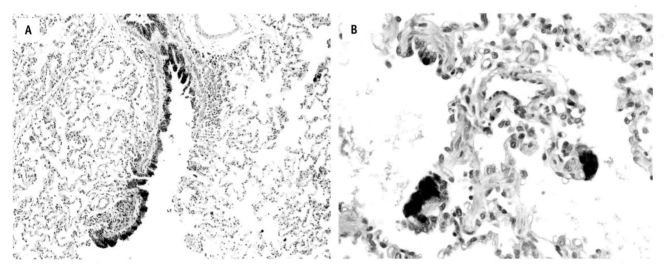

FIGURE 5-9

Neuroendocrine cell hyperplasia of infancy
Immunostain for bombesin reveals an increase in immunopositive cells within bronchioles **(A)** and highlights the neuroepithelial bodies within the lobular parenchyma **(B)**.

DIFFERENTIAL DIAGNOSIS

Neuroendocrine cell number is altered in several pediatric conditions including bronchopulmonary dysplasia, chronic bronchiolitis, cystic fibrosis, asthma, mechanical ventilation, and sudden infant death syndrome. Unlike most of these conditions, the lung biopsy in NEHI should be free of diagnostic abnormalities characteristic of a known pulmonary process, such as architectural disruption (seen in bronchopulmonary dysplasia) or changes of chronic lung injury (seen in chronic bronchiolitis, cystic fibrosis, asthma, or mechanical ventilation), including significant inflammation and prominent airway damage. Furthermore, unlike asthmatics, NEHI patients do not routinely wheeze or cough, and the process does not reverse with bronchodilators. Hence, correlation of the histology with the clinical presentation and radiographic findings is essential.

PROGNOSIS AND THERAPY

Although patients may be symptomatic and often require supplemental oxygen for months to years, their clinical condition improves over time. Symptoms are not reversible with bronchodilators, corticosteroids, hydroxychloroquine, and azathioprine. There have been no deaths reported, and no patients have progressed to respiratory failure or required lung transplantation. Patients may remain symptomatic with respiratory infections or exercise.

PERSISTENT PULMONARY HYPERTENSION OF THE NEWBORN

Persistent pulmonary hypertension of the newborn (PPHN), also referred to as "persistent fetal circulation," is a clinical syndrome characterized by maintenance of high pulmonary vascular resistance after birth. It is a significant cause of morbidity and mortality in the neonate and may be produced by a wide variety of disorders. In fetal life, pulmonary blood flow is low due to high pulmonary vascular resistance and shunts (foramen ovale, ductus arteriosus) that permit blood to bypass the pulmonary vascular bed. At birth, the pulmonary vascular resistance falls dramatically due to lung inflation and oxygenation. In PPHN this normal transition fails and pulmonary vascular resistance remains high. This results in right-to-left shunting at the foramen ovale and hypoxemia.

NEUROENDOCRINE CELL HYPERPLASIA OF INFANCY—FACT SHEET

Definition
- Idiopathic pediatric interstitial lung disease typified by a striking discrepancy between the severity of clinical symptoms and paucity of findings on lung biopsy, with the exception of neuroendocrine cell hyperplasia

Incidence
- Unknown, although more cases are being identified as recognition of the disorder increases

Morbidity and Mortality
- No deaths reported
- No progression to respiratory failure or lung transplantation

Gender and Age Distribution
- Infants (usually term) and young children, most presenting under 1 year of age
- May have a male predominance

Clinical Features
- Persistent tachypnea, hypoxemia, retractions
- Inspiratory crackles on exam
- Often diagnosed with failure to thrive, gastrointestinal reflux
- Symptoms may be preceded by a respiratory illness
- Infant pulmonary function tests demonstrate air-trapping with minimal airflow obstruction

Radiologic Features
- Scattered interstitial infiltrates and hyperinflation on chest radiograph
- Segmental ground-glass opacities on high-resolution CT

Prognosis and Therapy
- Good prognosis, with most patients achieving normal lung function, growth and development
- Patients often require long-term supplemental oxygen, with gradual improvement of symptoms
- May have persistent hyperinflation as well as intermittent pulmonary symptoms with viral infections or exercise
- No consistent response to corticosteroids, bronchodilators, and other agents

---

NEUROENDOCRINE CELL HYPERPLASIA OF INFANCY—PATHOLOGIC FEATURES

MIcroscopic Findings
- No morphologically specific disease process including extensive inflammation, reactive injury, architectural distortion, or fibrosis
- Minor and nonspecific changes including:
  - Mildly increased airway smooth muscle
  - Mildly increased numbers of alveolar macrophages
  - Occasional mild periairway lymphocytic infiltrates
  - Increased number of "clear cells" within bronchioles

Immunohistochemical Features
- Consistent increase in bombesin-immunoreactive cells within bronchioles
- At least 2/3 of airways contain immunopositive cells, present in small clusters (need 10-15 airways to evaluate)
- More than 10% of airway cells should be immunopositive in some bronchioles
- Size and number of neuroepithelial bodies in the lobules may be increased

Differential Diagnosis
- Neuroendocrine cells can be increased in chronic lung injury including:
  - Bronchopulmonary dysplasia
  - Chronic bronchiolitis
  - Asthma
  - Cystic fibrosis

CLINICAL FEATURES

Affected infants are term or post-term and present with cyanosis and respiratory distress at or shortly after birth. They have evidence of a right-to-left shunt with elevated pulmonary artery pressure. There are many known etiologies of PPHN, which may be classified as primary or secondary (Table 5-2). Primary PPHN is related to a reduction in the pulmonary vascular cross-sectional area, as in the case of pulmonary hypoplasia or alveolar capillary dysplasia with misalignment of the pulmonary veins. Secondary PPHN commonly occurs in the setting of congenital heart disease or severe acquired pulmonary disease (e.g., meconium aspiration, *Group B Streptococci* pneumonia), which results in clinically significant pulmonary vasoconstriction. The idiopathic form of PPHN is presumably related to prolonged, moderately severe decreased fetal perfusion or oxygenation. Premature closure of the ductus arteriosus, often related to the use of nonsteroidal anti-inflammatory agents late in pregnancy, is hypothesized to result in increased muscularization of pulmonary arteries due to increased pulmonary blood flow in utero. Fetal thrombotic syndromes may also result in this picture.

RADIOLOGIC FEATURES

Chest radiographic findings vary depending on the etiology. In idiopathic PPHN the lung fields are often hyperlucent, indicative of decreased blood flow.

PATHOLOGIC FEATURES

Microscopically, persistent pulmonary hypertension of the newborn is characterized by excessive muscularization of the small pulmonary arteries and abnormal extension of smooth muscle into normally nonmuscularized intra-acinar vessels (Figure 5-10). Extension of arterial smooth muscle into intra-acinar vessels is normally a postnatal phenomenon that does not begin until 6 months of age and is completed in adolescence. In addition to muscularization, there is often an increase in the adventitia around these vessels, thought to be a response to local hypoxia.

ANCILLARY STUDIES

Smooth muscle actin can be helpful in delineating the abnormally muscularized intra-acinar vessels (Figure 5-11).

DIFFERENTIAL DIAGNOSIS

Excessive muscularization of the small pulmonary arteries is a component of many hypoxic neonatal lung diseases, from disorders of lung growth and vascular patterning to congenital abnormalities of surfactant metabolism (e.g., chronic pneumonitis of infancy). It is important to define pathologically as well as clinically the potential cause of vascular remodeling.

TABLE 5-2
Causes of Persistent Pulmonary Hypertension of the Newborn*

Developmental deficit in cross-sectional area of the pulmonary vascular bed (primary)	Pulmonary hypoplasia, diffuse or unilateral
	Developmental aberration of lung growth/vascular patterning (acinar dysgenesis, congenital alveolar dysplasia, and alveolar capillary dysplasia with misalignment of the pulmonary veins)
Failure of postnatal decrease in pulmonary vascular resistance (secondary)	Large ventricular septal defect
	Hypoxic infant lung disease (severe pneumonia, respiratory distress syndrome)
Excessive prenatal muscularization of the distal pulmonary vasculature (secondary)	Associated with meconium aspiration
	Associated with cardiac malformations resulting in increased pulmonary arterial blood flow (hypoplastic left heart)
	Idiopathic

*Modified from suggested reading 13.

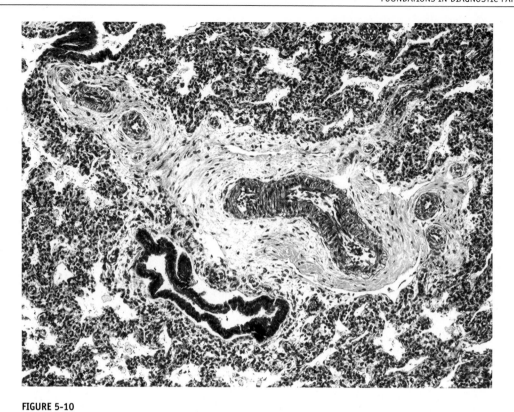

FIGURE 5-10

Persistent pulmonary hypertension of the newborn
Pentachrome stain delineates the medial thickening of this small pulmonary artery and the increased adventitia around this vessel.

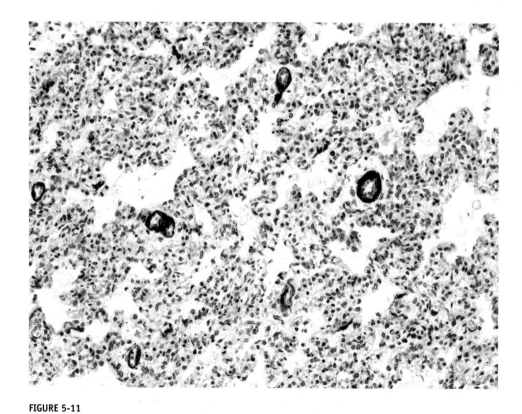

FIGURE 5-11

Persistent pulmonary hypertension of the newborn
Neomuscularization of normally nonmuscularized vessels in the distal alveolar parenchyma is highlighted by this smooth muscle actin stain.

PROGNOSIS AND THERAPY

Prognosis and therapy is determined by the underlying etiology of the condition. It is essential to evaluate a neonate with PPHN for cardiac disease, as this may be readily correctable. The primary therapy is supplemental oxygen with mechanical ventilation in infants who have significant respiratory distress and CO_2 retention. ECMO is needed for those in whom less invasive therapy is not effective. Nitric oxide, a selective pulmonary vasodilator, has been shown to be beneficial in infants without severe parenchymal disease or underlying developmental abnormalities of the lung. There remains a high mortality rate in infants with structurally abnormal lungs, as in congenital diaphragmatic hernia and alveolar capillary dysplasia with misalignment of the pulmonary veins.

COMPLICATIONS OF PREMATURITY AND ITS THERAPY

Complications of prematurity and its therapy, including hyaline membrane disease (HMD), bronchopulmonary dysplasia (BPD), and pulmonary interstitial emphysema (PIE), reflect a poor transition from intrauterine to extrauterine life, which requires replacement of intra-alveolar fluid with air and surfactant production to maintain adequate surface tension in the alveolus. These pulmonary disorders are the leading cause of morbidity and mortality in the preterm neonate, whose lungs are often morphologically and functionally immature. Term infants are also at risk for these complications in the setting of fetal asphyxia, infection, and other entities that result in acute and chronic lung injury.

PERSISTENT PULMONARY HYPERTENSION OF THE NEWBORN—FACT SHEET

Definition
- Syndrome associated with persistent postnatal elevation of pulmonary vascular resistance, characteristic of the fetal circulation
- Primary and secondary forms of PPHN exist

Incidence
- Estimated prevalence 1.9 per 1000 live births

Mortality
- Good survival in secondary PPHN
- High mortality (60%) in patients with primary PPHN

Gender and Age Distribution
- Term or post-term infants
- Slight male predominance

Clinical Features
- Onset of symptoms (cyanosis, respiratory distress) at or shortly after birth
- Pulmonary hypertension
- Right-to-left shunt, at ductus arteriosus or foramen ovale

Prognosis and Therapy
- Supplemental oxygen is needed, as well as high frequency oscillatory ventilation (HFOV) or ECMO in patients with significant respiratory distress and CO_2 retention
- Nitric oxide may also be helpful

PERSISTENT PULMONARY HYPERTENSION OF THE NEWBORN—PATHOLOGIC FEATURES

Microscopic Findings
- Muscularization of small pulmonary arteries with reduction of luminal diameters
- Neomuscularization of precapillary intra-acinar vessels
- Thickening of connective tissue sheaths around vessels

Immunohistochemical Features
- Smooth muscle actin highlights the smooth muscle hyperplasia of small vessels

Differential Diagnosis
- Evaluate for potentially associated conditions including:
  - Pulmonary hypoplasia
  - Alveolar capillary dysplasia with misalignment of pulmonary veins

Hyaline membrane disease, the pathologic correlate of respiratory distress syndrome (RDS) of the newborn, is largely an acute lung disease of the premature infant caused by inadequate amounts of surfactant. Decreased surfactant results in insufficient surface tension in the alveolus during expiration, leading to atelectasis, decreased gas exchange, and severe hypoxia and acidosis.

Chronic neonatal lung disease (CNLD), which encompasses bronchopulmonary dysplasia (BPD), is a disorder of lung injury and repair, classically attributed to prolonged positive pressure, mechanical ventilation, and oxygen toxicity resulting in interference with alveolar and vascular development.

Pulmonary interstitial emphysema (PIE) and persistent pulmonary interstitial emphysema (PPIE) are acquired conditions that may complicate any pulmonary disorder in which there is airway plugging or a requirement for mechanical ventilation. Air gains access to the interstitium of the lung via rupture of small bronchioles or alveoli, dissecting along connective tissue sheaths of the bronchovascular bundles, interlobular septa, and visceral pleura.

CLINICAL FEATURES

The incidence and severity of HMD are inversely proportional to gestational age and birth weight. It predominantly occurs in infants younger than 32 weeks' gestational age and in those weighing less than 1200 g. It is the most common cause of respiratory failure during the first day of life and the leading cause of mortality in infants. In addition to prematurity, predisposing factors include maternal diabetes, cesarean delivery without preceding labor, fetal asphyxia, prior affected infants, and being the second born of twins.

The diagnosis of BPD is based on persistent oxygen requirement at 36 weeks postmenstrual age or greater than 28 days post-delivery. While most cases of BPD follow HMD, some follow other forms of acute lung injury or disorders that require treatment with high concentrations of oxygen and mechanical ventilation, including pneumonia/sepsis, meconium aspiration, pulmonary hypoplasia and congenital heart disease. The incidence of BPD is increasing as the survival of extremely premature infants improves, but its clinical presentation is milder with current therapeutic practices. In contrast to classic BPD, in which postnatal inflammation and fibrosis due to barotrauma and oxygen toxicity played more of a role, "new BPD" is more related to extreme prematurity and failure of postnatal alveolarization.

PIE often occurs in conjunction with RDS, but other predisposing factors include meconium aspiration, perinatal asphyxia, and neonatal sepsis. Positive pressure ventilation and reduced lung compliance are significant predisposing factors. PIE can be acute (less than 1 week duration) or persistent (PPIE). By compressing adjacent functional lung tissue and vascular structures, its presence can further compromise an already critically ill infant by impeding oxygenation, ventilation, and blood flow.

RADIOLOGIC FEATURES

In infants with RDS, the typical radiographic appearance is one of decreased pulmonary expansion, with ground-glass opacification of the lungs and air bronchograms (Figure 5-12). Granular opacities represent the atelectatic terminal air spaces.

Before the advent of surfactant replacement therapy, chest radiographs of infants with classic BPD demonstrated coarse reticular lung opacities, cystic lucencies, and areas of atelectasis and hyperinflation. In the era of surfactant replacement, radiographic abnormalities are more subtle and include diffuse lung haziness, interstitial opacities, and areas of cystic change (Figure 5-13).

The radiographic appearance of PIE is small, cyst-like radiolucencies that may coalesce in subpleural locations to form pseudocysts (Figure 5-14).

PATHOLOGIC FEATURES

GROSS FINDINGS

In HMD, the lungs are dark red, firm, and congested. On cut section, they are relatively airless with marked atelectasis (Figure 5-15).

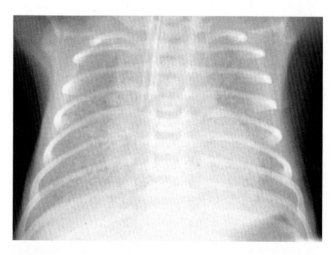

FIGURE 5-12

Hyaline membrane disease

Chest radiograph in a one-day-old premature infant with RDS demonstrates diffuse, granular parenchymal opacities. (Courtesy of Dr. Alan Brody, Cincinnati, Ohio.)

With advanced BPD, alternating areas of expansion, atelectasis, and scarring give the pleural surface a lobulated appearance (Figure 5-16). Dilated spaces due to chronic interstitial air are evident on sectioning. The trachea and mainstem bronchi may show diffuse or focal areas of mucosal edema, ulceration, granulation tissue, and scarring, depending on the duration and frequency of intubation and ventilation. In contrast, the gross appearance of the lung in "new BPD" is largely unremarkable, with evenly aerated parenchyma.

The extent of PIE can vary, with single or numerous cysts and involvement of one or multiple lung lobes (Figure 5-17).

MICROSCOPIC FINDINGS

The presence of hyaline membranes is the most common histologic finding in premature infants with clinically severe RDS. Hyaline membranes consist of cellular debris, fibrin, amniotic fluid, and transudate fluid.

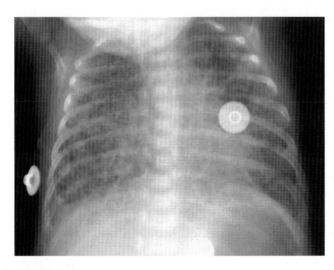

FIGURE 5-13

Bronchopulmonary dysplasia
Chest radiograph shows classic BPD with bilateral, coarse reticular opacities and "bubble-like" lucencies. (Courtesy of Dr. Alan Brody, Cincinnati, Ohio.)

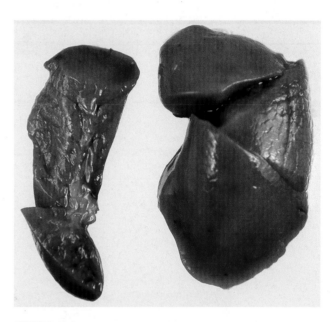

FIGURE 5-15

Hyaline membrane disease
Marked congestion and atelectasis impart a "liver-like" appearance to the lungs.

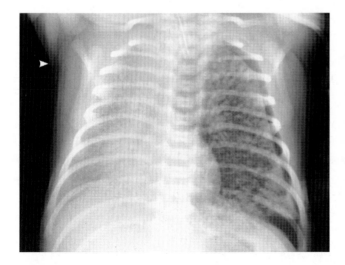

FIGURE 5-14

Pulmonary interstitial emphysema
This radiograph demonstrates the characteristic changes of PIE on the left side (linear and cyst-like radiolucencies), which is complicated by a pneumothorax. (Courtesy of Dr. Alan Brody, Cincinnati, Ohio.)

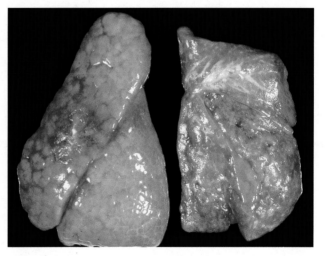

FIGURE 5-16

Bronchopulmonary dysplasia
In classic bronchopulmonary dysplasia, the pleural surface is distorted by alternating areas of expansion and collapse in the underlying parenchyma.

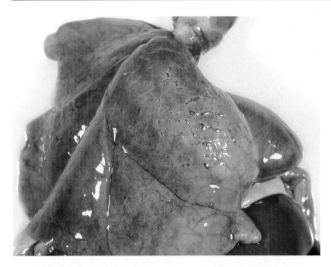

FIGURE 5-17

Pulmonary interstitial emphysema
Air collections in the subpleural and interlobular regions appear as linear cysts or bubbles.

They may be stained bright yellow if the infant has unconjugated hyperbilirubinemia (Figure 5-18). Hyaline membranes appear within 3 to 4 hours after the development of symptoms and are most prominent at approximately 12 hours. The surrounding lung shows alveolar collapse, congestion, hemorrhage, epithelial desquamation, and lymphatic dilatation. Since most infants are premature, there is underlying lung immaturity, which correlates with gestational age. If the process does not resolve, progression to BPD with both air space and interstitial fibroblastic proliferation may be seen as early as 36 hours after birth.

Classic BPD shows an evolution of injury and repair that can be divided into acute, subacute, and chronic or late-stage phases (Figure 5-19). The progression of the pathologic changes is shown in Table 5-3. The acute phase is characterized by severe epithelial injury in the airways and terminal air spaces, which may lead to occlusion of bronchiolar lumens by necrotic debris. Reparative

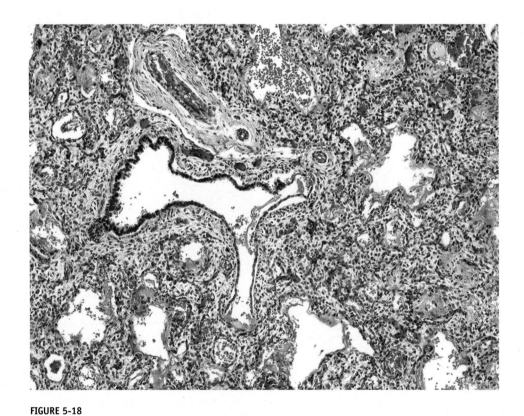

FIGURE 5-18

Hyaline membrane disease
Dilated distal airways are lined by hyaline membranes, many stained yellow in a premature infant with hyperbilirubinemia. There is congestion and collapse of the surrounding parenchyma.

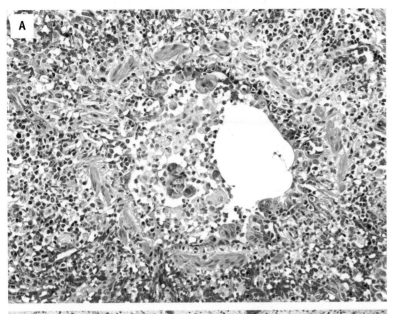

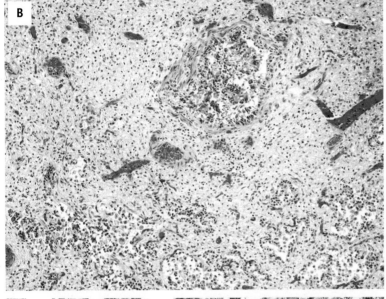

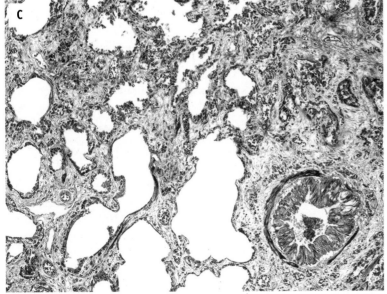

FIGURE 5-19

Classic bronchopulmonary dysplasia
(A) In the early phases there is bronchiolar necrosis with filling of the lumen by sloughed epithelium and inflammatory cells. **(B)** Periairway fibrosis and prominence of alveolar type 2 cells is seen in the subacute phase. **(C)** Late-stage "healed" bronchopulmonary dysplasia is characterized by interstitial fibrosis and honeycomb change (Trichrome stain).

TABLE 5-3

Phases of Classic Bronchopulmonary Dysplasia

Acute exudative phase (0-4 days)	Hyaline membranes
	Epithelial necrosis in the airways
	Bronchiolar plugging by necrotic debris
	Lymphatic dilatation
Subacute phase (<1 month)	Squamous metaplasia
	Variable bronchiolar obliteration and bronchiolectasis
	Periairway fibrosis
	Bronchiolar smooth muscle hyperplasia with extension into the lobule
	Type 2 cell hyperplasia
	Increasing interstitial fibrosis
Chronic phase (>1 month)	Foci of enlarged alveoli
	Interstitial fibrosis
	Medial hypertrophy of pulmonary arteries

changes in the subacute phase may lead to bronchiolar obliteration, bronchiolectasis and tracheal stenosis. Lobular remodeling with nonuniform inflation of the lung and a combination of enlarged alveoli and interstitial fibrosis typifies the chronic stage. At all stages, pulmonary interstitial air may be present. Morphometric studies done on lungs with BPD show a decrease in alveolar number coupled with larger than normal air spaces.

In the post-surfactant era, the lungs of infants with BPD, termed "new" BPD, show less fibrosis and more uniform inflation (Figure 5-20). However, alveoli remain simplified and enlarged, reflecting an interference with postnatal septation. Only the occasional case of "classic" acute BPD is still seen.

In PIE, elongated or round air-filled spaces of variable size and shape are present beneath the pleura and distending interlobular septa and bronchovascular bundles (Figure 5-21). They may be associated with hemorrhage and parenchymal distortion. With time (PPIE), the prolonged presence of air elicits a foreign-body response with giant cells and histiocytes.

DIFFERENTIAL DIAGNOSIS

Although characteristic of HMD, hyaline membranes are a nonspecific finding with a number of causes, which should be considered especially in the term and post-term infant with RDS. Hyaline membranes can be seen with meconium aspiration, neonatal pneumonia, pulmonary edema and hemorrhage and with various irritants to the terminal airways and alveoli.

Furthermore, the early stages of BPD and those related to therapeutic intervention cannot be easily separated from HMD. The air-filled spaces in PIE may be so large as to resemble a cystic malformation; however, the cystic spaces in PIE are limited to the interstitial tissues without parenchymal involvement (albeit significant parenchymal compression can be present). Diffuse pulmonary lymphangiectasia may also resemble PIE; immunostains to label the endothelium or lymphatics (e.g., CD31, D2-40) will be helpful in these circumstances.

PROGNOSIS AND THERAPY

The long-term survival and outcome of patients with RDS, BPD, and PIE has significantly improved with the use of exogenous surfactant therapy, improved ventilatory strategies, and supportive measures. Prophylactic surfactant in high-risk infants (less than 30 weeks' gestation) has resulted in a significant decrease in the incidence of HMD and improved survival without the development of BPD. In addition, antenatal administration of corticosteroids to mothers with threatened premature delivery is beneficial, by means of accelerating the maturity of the surfactant system. Although there has been a significant decrease in the incidence of central nervous system injury and BPD with current therapeutic modalities, the incidence of other morbidities such as necrotizing enterocolitis, patent ductus arteriosus (PDA), and late-onset sepsis has not substantially changed.

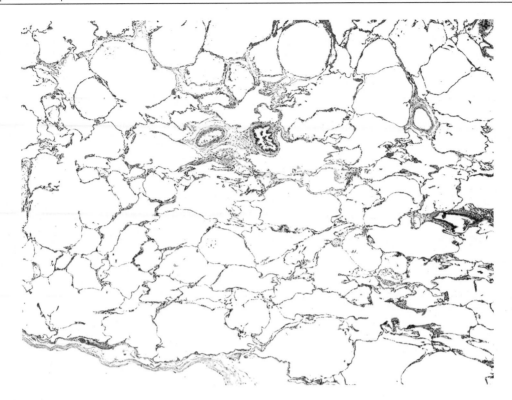

FIGURE 5-20

"New" bronchopulmonary dysplasia

In comparison to classic bronchopulmonary dysplasia, there is no evidence of scarring or significant airway injury. There is prominent alveolar simplification and distension.

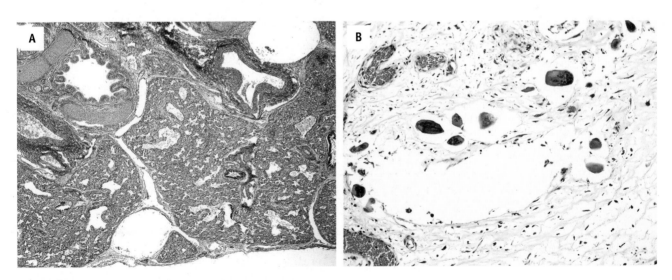

FIGURE 5-21

Pulmonary interstitial emphysema

(A) Air has dissected along the bronchovascular bundles and septae, and into the subpleural space. **(B)** In chronic or persistent pulmonary interstitial emphysema, the spaces are lined by foreign-body giant cells. (Courtesy of Dr. Megan Dishop, Houston, Texas.)

COMPLICATIONS OF PREMATURITY AND ITS THERAPY—FACT SHEET

Definition

- HMD is the result of a deficiency in surfactant related to pulmonary immaturity or injury to the pulmonary epithelium
- BPD and CNLD, which develop in infants who require prolonged support for neonatal respiratory disease, reflect ongoing injury and repair of the immature lung
- PIE and PPIE refer to collections of air inside the connective tissue of the lung, secondary to alveolar and terminal bronchiolar rupture

Incidence

Hyaline Membrane Disease

- 1% of live births
- The incidence increases from 5% at 35-36 weeks to 65% at 29-30 weeks' gestation

Bronchopulmonary Dysplasia

- Approximately 30% in infants with birth weights below 1000 g
- Infrequent in infants over 30 weeks' gestational age and above 1200 g

Pulmonary Interstitial Emphysema

- Limited information, but estimated 10% of preterm infants (< 30 weeks) with RDS
- Incidence increases with decreasing birth weight

Morbidity and Mortality

Hyaline Membrane Disease

- HMD and its complications account for approximately 20% of all neonatal deaths
- Morbidity and mortality are related to pulmonary disease, complications of hypoxemia (e.g., intraventricular hemorrhage, congestive heart failure due to left-to-right shunt through patent ductus arteriosus), or complications of assisted ventilation (e.g., PIE, pneumothorax)

Bronchopulmonary Dysplasia

- Infants remain at high risk during the first few years of life for increased susceptibility and symptomatology during respiratory infections, cardiac dysfunction, apneic spells, and late sudden unexpected death

Pulmonary Interstitial Emphysema

- Subpleural blebs can rupture into the pleural space to produce a pneumothorax, or can extend centrally to cause pneumomediastinum, pneumopericardium, pneumoperitoneum, or subcutaneous emphysema

Gender, Race, and Age Distribution

Hyaline Membrane Disease

- Premature infants
- Male predominance (M:F 5 2:1)
- Incidence higher among Caucasians

Bronchopulmonary Dysplasia

- Frequently premature infants

Pulmonary Interstitial Emphysema

- More frequent in infants with extreme prematurity

Clinical Features

Hyaline Membrane Disease

- Onset of symptoms occurs at or within the first few hours after birth

Continued

COMPLICATIONS OF PREMATURITY AND ITS THERAPY—PATHOLOGIC FEATURES

Gross Findings

Hyaline Membrane Disease

- "Liver-like" solid, congested lungs with marked atelectasis

Classic Bronchopulmonary Dysplasia

- Cobblestone appearance of pleural surface due to scarring and alternating hyperinflation and collapse of the underlying parenchyma

Pulmonary Interstitial Emphysema

- Air blebs (ranging from 0.1-0.5 cm) located beneath the pleura and interlobular septa
- May occur as an isolated lesion, multiple cysts localized to one portion of the lung, or diffuse involvement of both lungs
- Cysts in the localized form of PPIE tend to be larger (up to 5 cm) than cysts associated with more diffuse involvement

Microscopic Findings

Hyaline Membrane Disease

- Dilated terminal and respiratory bronchioles and alveolar ducts lined by acellular eosinophilic hyaline membranes
- Membranes can be stained bright yellow in the setting of unconjugated hyperbilirubinemia
- Alveolar collapse and congestion, epithelial desquamation of the airways
- Hyaline membranes are frequently absent in infants who die at less than 4 hours of age
- Fibroblastic organization (BPD) may be seen within 36 hours after birth

Bronchopulmonary Dysplasia

- Classic BPD is characterized by airway injury, inflammation and parenchymal fibrosis
- New BPD is typified by large, simplified alveoli with absence of scarring or significant airway injury

Pulmonary Interstitial Emphysema

- Air-filled cysts confined to the interlobular septa and around bronchovascular bundles
- Loose connective tissue and compressed parenchyma surround the cysts
- In PPIE, the cysts contain multinucleated foreign body giant cells

Differential Diagnosis

Hyaline Membrane Disease

- Meconium aspiration
- Pulmonary infection
- Pulmonary edema and hemorrhage

Bronchopulmonary Dysplasia

- Hyaline membrane disease

Pulmonary Interstitial Emphysema

- Cystic malformation
- Pulmonary lymphangiectasia

COMPLICATIONS OF PREMATURITY AND ITS THERAPY—FACT SHEET—Cont'd

» Tachypnea, retractions, expiratory grunting, progressive cyanosis, hypoxemia

» Prematurity is the most important predisposing factor, and other predisposing factors include maternal diabetes, cesarean delivery, fetal asphyxia, and multiple gestation

Bronchopulmonary Dysplasia

» Persistent oxygen requirement at 36 weeks' postmenstrual age or greater than 28 days postdelivery

» Tachypnea, cough, wheezing, and rhonchi; symptoms may persist for months

» Frequent history of prolonged oxygen therapy and mechanical ventilation

» May follow history of respiratory distress syndrome, acute lung injury

Pulmonary Interstitial Emphysema

» Frequently occurs in premature infants on ventilators for respiratory distress

» Often occurs in conjunction with respiratory distress syndrome

» Hypotension and difficulty in oxygenation and ventilation may suggest its presence

---

Radiologic Features

Hyaline Membrane Disease

» Diffuse, bilateral, ground-glass opacities with air bronchograms

Bronchopulmonary Dysplasia

» Classic BPD is typified by hyperexpansion, cystic lucencies, and areas of opacification

Pulmonary Interstitial Emphysema

» Often unilateral hyperinflation that causes a mediastinal shift

» Distinct rounded and linear lucencies distributed uniformly in the affected lung

Prognosis and Therapy

Hyaline Membrane Disease

» Prognosis correlates inversely with birth weight

» CNLD occurs in 20% of patients who survive HMD

» Infants receive exogenous surfactant therapy, oxygen, and mechanical ventilation

Bronchopulmonary Dysplasia

» Early complications include pulmonary air leak, patent ductus arteriosus, systemic hypertension, poor growth, and gastroesophageal reflux and aspiration

» Late complications include tracheal stenosis, bronchial hyperreactivity, small airway disease, and chronic airflow obstruction in adult life

» May require ventilation and/or supplemental oxygen for months to years

Pulmonary Interstitial Emphysema

» Complications include air leak, massive air embolism, chronic neonatal lung disease, and chronic lobar emphysema

» Lateral decubitus positioning, selective bronchial intubation and occlusion, and high frequency ventilation have been used with variable success

» Lobectomy reserved for severe localized lobar emphysema

SUGGESTED READINGS

Growth Abnormalities

1. Cooney TP, Wentworth PJ, Thurlbeck WM. Diminished radial count is found only postnatally in Down's syndrome. *Pediatr Pulmonol.* 1988;5:204-9.

2. Mani H, Suarez E, Stocker JT. The morphologic spectrum of infantile lobar emphysema: a study of 33 cases. *Paediatr Respir Rev.* 2004;5(Suppl A): S313-20.

3. Congenital anomalies and pediatric disorders. In: Travis WD, Colby TV, Koss MN, et al. *Atlas of Nontumor Pathology-Non-Neoplastic Disorders of the Lower Respiratory Tract.* Washington, DC: American Registry of Pathology and AFIP. 2002:473-538.

4. Thibeault DW, Haney B. Lung volume, pulmonary vasculature, and factors affecting survival in congenital diaphragmatic hernia. *Pediatrics.* 1998;101:289-95.

5. Winn HN, Chen M, Amon E. Neonatal pulmonary hypoplasia and perinatal mortality in patients with midtrimester rupture of amniotic membranes: a critical analysis. *Am J Obstet Gynecol.* 2000;182:1638-44.

Pulmonary Interstitial Glycogenosis

6. Canakis A, Cutz E, Manson D, O'Brodovich H. Pulmonary interstitial glycogenosis: a new variant of neonatal interstitial lung disease. *Am J Respir Crit Care Med.* 2002;165:1557-65.

7. Case Records of the Massachusetts General Hospital. Weekly clinicopathological exercises. Case 40-1999. A four-month-old girl with chronic cyanosis and diffuse pulmonary infiltrates. *N Engl J Med.* 1999;341:2075-83.

8. Langston C. Pediatric lung biopsy. In: Cagle P, ed. *Diagnostic Pulmonary Pathology.* New York: Marcel Dekker. 2000;1:19-47.

9. Schroeder SA, Shannon DC, Mark, EJ. Cellular interstitial pneumonitis in infants: a clinicopathologic study. *Chest.* 1992;101:1065-9.

Neuroendocrine Cell Hyperplasia of Infancy

10. Deterding R, Hay T, Langston C, Fan L. Persistent tachypnea of infancy (PTI). *Am J Respir Crit Care Med.* 1997;155:715.

11. Deterding RR, Pye C, Fan LL, Langston C. Persistent tachypnea of infancy is associated with neuroendocrine cell hyperplasia. *Pediatr Pulmonol.* 2005;40:157-65.

12. Hull J, Chow CW, Robertson CF. Chronic idiopathic bronchiolitis of infancy. *Arch Dis Child.* 1997;77:512-5.

13. Langston C. Pulmonary disorders in the neonate, infant and child. In: Churg AM, Myers JL, Tazelaar HD, Wright JL, eds. *Thurlbeck's Pathology of the Lung.* 3rd ed. New York: Thieme; 2005:119-72.

Persistent Pulmonary Hypertension of the Newborn

14. Konduri GG. New approaches for persistent pulmonary hypertension of newborn. *Clin Perinatol.* 2004;31:591-611.

15. Murphy JD, Rabinovitch M, Goldstein JD, Reid LM. The structural basis of PPHN. *Clin Perinatol.* 1984;11:525-49.

16. Walsh-Sukys ML, Tyson JE, Wright LL, et al. Persistent pulmonary hypertension in the newborn in the era before nitric oxide: practice variation and outcomes. *Pediatrics.* 2000. 105:12-20.

Complications of Prematurity and Its Therapy

17. American Thoracic Society. Statement on the care of the child with chronic lung disease of infancy and childhood. *Am J Respir Crit Care Med.* 2003;68:356-96.

18. Coalson JJ. Pathology of new bronchopulmonary dysplasia. *Semin Neonatol.* 2003;8:73-81.

19. Fanaroff AA, Hack M, Walsh MC. The NICHD neonatal research network: changes in practice and outcomes during the first 15 years. *Semin Perinatol.* 2003;281-7.

20. Margraf LR, Tomashefski JF Jr, Bruce MC, Dahms BB. Morphometric analysis of the lung in bronchopulmonary dysplasia. *Am Rev Respir Dis.* 1991;143:391-400.

21. Northway W Jr, Rosan R, Porter D. Pulmonary disease following respiratory therapy of hyaline-membrane disease: bronchopulmonary dysplasia. *N Engl J Med.* 1967;276:357-68.

22. Wilson JM, Mark EJ. Case 30-1997. A preterm newborn female triplet with diffuse cystic changes in the left lung. *N Engl J Med.* 1997;337:916-24.

6

Lung Neoplasms in Infants and Children

Michael H. Covinsky

- Introduction
- Inflammatory Myofibroblastic Tumor
- Pleuropulmonary Blastoma
- Epstein-Barr Virus-Associated Smooth Muscle Tumor

INTRODUCTION

Primary lung neoplasms in children are uncommon, and occur less frequently than congenital malformations and metastatic malignancies. Table 6-1 lists the histologic types of primary pulmonary neoplasms arising in the pediatric population, many of which resemble their counterparts arising in adults. This chapter focuses on neoplasms that occur primarily or uniquely in the pediatric population.

INFLAMMATORY MYOFIBROBLASTIC TUMOR

Inflammatory myofibroblastic tumors (IMTs) comprise over 80% of benign pediatric pulmonary neoplasms. Other names for this entity have included inflammatory pseudotumor, plasma cell granuloma, and pulmonary fibroxanthoma. Although there has been debate regarding the neoplastic vs. reactive nature of this process, IMT is now generally believed to represent a neoplastic disorder of cells demonstrating myofibroblastic characteristics.

CLINICAL AND RADIOLOGIC FEATURES

Although IMTs are most commonly seen in the second decade of life, they can occur in infants. Symptoms include fever, cough, chest pain, and hemoptysis, but many cases are asymptomatic. Imaging studies show a usually solitary nodule, and calcifications are present in 25%-33% of cases.

PATHOLOGIC FEATURES

GROSS FINDINGS

IMTs are tan-white or grey masses usually located in the periphery of the lung. They can appear deceptively well-circumscribed. Cut surfaces are white and firm and may be gritty in lesions with calcifications.

MICROSCOPIC FINDINGS

IMTs can have a wide variety of microscopic appearances both within an individual tumor and between tumors. Most lesions consist of proliferations of slender spindle-shaped cells and fibrosis, accompanied by variably intense mononuclear inflammatory cell infiltrates comprised primarily of plasma cells and lymphocytes (Figures 6-1 to 6-3). Either the myofibroblastic component or the inflammatory component may predominate. At one end of the histologic spectrum, lesions can resemble a fibrous histiocytoma, with short interlacing fascicles of spindle cells that can show storiform patterns and whorls. Alternatively, the lymphoplasmacytic infiltrate may predominate (Figure 6-4), with conspicuous lymphoid aggregates with germinal centers. There may be a dense scar at the center of the lesion and organizing pneumonia may be found at the periphery of the lesion. Other features may include intra-alveolar lymphohistiocytic inflammation, granulomatous inflammation, multinucleated giant cells, and abscesses. Foci of calcification, myxomatous changes, osseous metaplasia and intralesional vascular invasion may be present.

ANCILLARY STUDIES

IMMUNOHISTOCHEMISTRY

Immunohistochemical stains for vimentin, smooth muscle actin, and muscle-specific actin are generally positive. Anaplastic lymphoma kinase (ALK-1) is expressed in approximately 40% of cases, and the tumor may express p80. Cytokeratin, desmin and CD68 can be

---

TABLE 6-1

Pediatric Pulmonary Neoplasms

Inflammatory myofibroblastic tumor*

Carcinoid*

Pleuropulmonary blastoma

Salivary gland-type neoplasms

    Mucoepidermoid carcinoma

    Adenoid cystic carcinoma

    Acinic cell carcinoma

Conventional types of lung carcinoma

    Adenocarcinoma

    Squamous cell carcinoma

    Small cell carcinoma

    Large cell carcinoma

    Basaloid carcinoma

Sarcomas

    Fibrosarcoma

    Rhabdomyosarcoma

    Leiomyosarcoma

    Undifferentiated

Epstein Barr virus-associated smooth muscle tumors

Hamartoma

Granular cell tumor

Leiomyoma

Bronchial chondroma

Teratoma

---

*Most common neoplasms arising in the pediatric population.

focally positive, and stains for S100, myoglobin, epithelial membrane antigen, and p53 are negative.

CYTOGENETICS

Translocations involving the ALK locus at 2p23 are found in many lesions, and translocation partners can include clathrin heavy chain (CLTC), tropomyosin-3 and -4 (TPM-3 and TPM-4), cysteinyl tRNA synthetase (CARS), and Ran-binding protein 2 (RANBP2).

ULTRASTRUCTURAL STUDIES

Electron microscopy reveals features of a fibroblastic or myofibroblastic phenotype. Spindle cells often contain thin filaments and occasional pinocytotic vesicles. Lipid droplets may be seen. The nuclei are irregular with abundant euchromatin and a rim of heterochromatin along the nuclear membrane.

DIFFERENTIAL DIAGNOSIS

Since IMTs can vary in their histology, the differential diagnosis for an individual tumor will depend upon its particular histologic appearance. Solitary fibrous tumors and desmoid tumors are important entities in the differential diagnosis, but can usually be distinguished histologically and with application of immunohistochemistry. Solitary fibrous tumors characteristically show a patternless pattern including spindle cells and collagen, may have myxoid or hemangiopericytomatous areas, usually show less inflammation, and are immunoreactive for CD34 and usually negative for muscle markers and ALK-1. Desmoid tumors also consist of cells with myofibroblastic characteristics and variable amounts of collagen, but usually show less inflammation than IMTs. Both IMTs and desmoid tumors express muscle markers, but desmoid tumors do not stain for ALK-1. Synovial sarcoma can be distinguished by the appearance of the spindle cells, lack of inflammatory cells, CD99 immunoreactivity and demonstration of the t(X;18) translocation. Malignant fibrous histiocytomas have frankly malignant characteristics including pleomorphism and anaplasia, necrosis, and high mitotic activity. Leiomyomas and leiomyosarcomas tend to show little inflammation, lack the histologic variegation seen in IMTs, and strongly express muscle markers. For neoplasms with a prominent component of dense scar tissue, mediastinal fibrosis (sclerosing mediastinitis) may be considered, but does not typically display the cellular proliferation of myofibroblasts characteristic of IMTs.

PROGNOSIS AND THERAPY

For most IMTs, surgical excision and there represents the primary therapeutic approach. The borders of this lesion can be infiltrative, in some cases making complete excision difficult, but failure to obtain a clear margin can lead to recurrence. Extension into the chest wall is associated with a worsened prognosis. There is also some evidence that oral corticosteroids may be of benefit in extrapulmonary IMTs, and there are case reports of successful combination chemotherapy of IMTs.

Mortality may result from involvement of the aorta, esophagus, or pulmonary vessels. Sarcomatous transformation is rare. There are no dependable histological predictors of aggressive behavior, although the presence of atypia and ganglion-like cells have been associated with an increased risk of recurrence or malignant progression. Aneuploidy and p53 expression also suggest an increased risk of aggressive behavior.

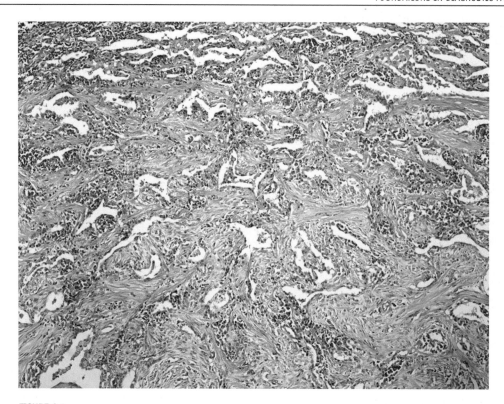

FIGURE 6-1

Inflammatory myofibroblastic tumor
This low-power view shows a background proliferation of spindle cells accompanied by a lymphoplasmacytic infiltrate. Compressed air spaces appear as angulated open spaces interspersed throughout the lesion.

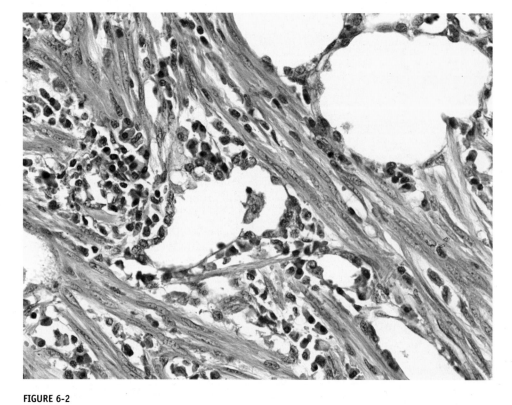

FIGURE 6-2

Inflammatory myofibroblastic tumor
Plasma cells are conspicuous amongst the cytologically bland spindle cells with elongated nuclei and fine chromatin. Residual air spaces are partially lined by reactive pneumocytes.

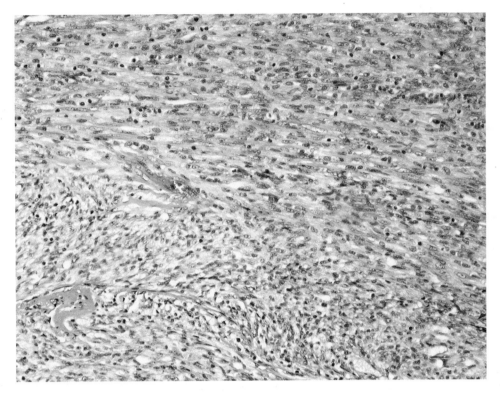

FIGURE 6-3

Inflammatory myofibroblastic tumor
This lesion has fewer inflammatory cells and consists primarily of bland spindle cells with a fascicular pattern.

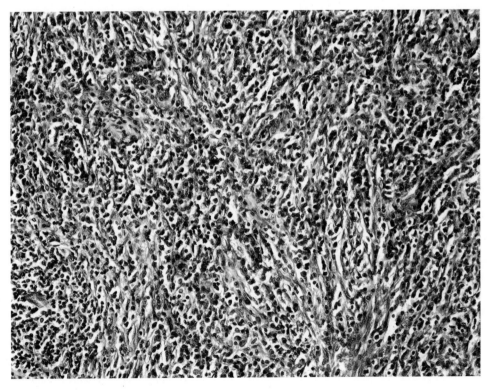

FIGURE 6-4

Inflammatory myofibroblastic tumor
A dense lymphoplasmacytic infiltrate obscures the myofibroblastic cells.

INFLAMMATORY MYOFIBROBLASTIC TUMOR—FACT SHEET

Definition

» A low-grade, locally aggressive tumor comprised of cells with myofibro-blastic/fibroblastic characteristics, associated with a variably intense mononuclear inflammatory cell infiltrate

Incidence

» Rare

Morbidity and Mortality

» Direct extension into other vital structures can cause death
» Metastases are rare
» Morbidity can arise from extension into the chest wall

Gender and Age Distribution

» Highest frequency in the second decade of life
» Can occur in infancy
» 10% occur in adults
» Slight female predominance (M:F 0.7)

Clinical Features

» Fever
» Chest pain
» Hemoptysis
» Cough

Radiologic Features

» Single round nodule
» Microcalcifications present in 1/4 to 1/3 of cases

Prognosis and Therapy

» Complete surgical excision is usually curative
» Incomplete resection can lead to recurrence
» Possible roles for corticosteroid therapy and chemotherapy

INFLAMMATORY MYOFIBROBLASTIC TUMOR—PATHOLOGIC FEATURES

Gross Findings

» Tan-white mass in the periphery of the lung
» Firm to gritty cut surface

Microscopic Findings

» Proliferation of slender spindle cells with accompanying fibrosis and inflammatory cell infiltrates, with variable balance between the components
» Inflammatory cell infiltrates typically include lymphocytes and plasma cells; lymphoid aggregates with germinal centers may be present
» Organizing pneumonia is common
» Scarring may be present

Immunohistochemical Features

» Generally positive for vimentin, smooth muscle actin, and muscle-specific actin
» ALK-1 positive in 30-40% of tumors

Cytogenetics

» Frequent abnormalities at the ALK-1 locus at 2p23

Ultrastructural Features

» Spindle cells frequently contain thin filaments and occasional pinocytotic vessels

Pathologic Differential Diagnosis

» Solitary fibrous tumor
» Desmoid tumor
» Organizing pneumonia
» Synovial sarcoma
» Malignant fibrous histiocytoma
» Leiomyoma
» Leiomyosarcoma
» Mediastinal fibrosis

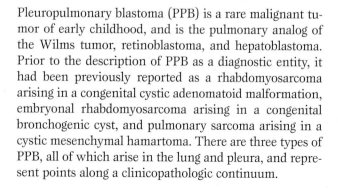

PLEUROPULMONARY BLASTOMA

Pleuropulmonary blastoma (PPB) is a rare malignant tumor of early childhood, and is the pulmonary analog of the Wilms tumor, retinoblastoma, and hepatoblastoma. Prior to the description of PPB as a diagnostic entity, it had been previously reported as a rhabdomyosarcoma arising in a congenital cystic adenomatoid malformation, embryonal rhabdomyosarcoma arising in a congenital bronchogenic cyst, and pulmonary sarcoma arising in a cystic mesenchymal hamartoma. There are three types of PPB, all of which arise in the lung and pleura, and represent points along a clinicopathologic continuum.

CLINICAL FEATURES

PPB is a rare lesion, with only 128 cases listed in the International Pleuropulmonary Blastoma Registry. It is usually diagnosed within the first four years of life, but can be diagnosed prenatally or present in older children or young adults. In approximately 25% of cases, evidence of a heritable tumor syndrome is found including a family history of childhood neoplasia or second tumors in the same patient. The additional tumors in these patients include thyroid malignancies, cystic nephromas and other nephroblastic lesions, medulloblastomas, ovarian teratomas, and second PPBs. Symptoms can include chest pain, fever, cough, and respiratory distress.

It is believed that type I PPBs can progress to type II and then type III PPBs. This is supported by the fact that the median age at diagnosis increases from 10 months for the type I PPB to 44 months for the type III PPB. Type I tumors can recur as type II and type III tumors, however type III tumors do not recur as type I or type II tumors. Since type I PPBs have a much better prognosis than type II and type III PPBs, it is important that pulmonary cystic lesions be excised as soon as clinically reasonable and thoroughly examined, with attention paid to surgical marginal status.

RADIOLOGIC FEATURES

Radiologic studies usually reveal air-filled cysts in the lung, unilocular or multilocular, and solid components may be present. Chest wall or mediastinal extension may be visible. Pneumothorax or pleural effusion may also be present.

PATHOLOGIC FEATURES

GROSS FINDINGS

Type I is purely cystic, type II is mixed cystic and solid, and type III is purely solid. The type I PPB shows thin-walled unilocular or multilocular cysts with no areas of thickening or nodularity. Type III is solid, usually white and gelatinous, with areas of hemorrhage and necrosis. Type II contains both solid and cystic components.

MICROSCOPIC FINDINGS

Cyst walls of type I PPBs are lined by non-neoplastic respiratory epithelia. Classically, a condensation of small, round immature mesenchymal cells is present beneath the epithelium (Figure 6-5), often resembling the cambium layer of a botryoid rhabdomyosarcoma. Anaplasia is rare. Rhabdomyoblast-like strap cells with prominent eosinophilic cytoplasm may be present, but can be quite focal. Nodules of immature cartilage may be observed (Figure 6-6). It is essential that cystic lesions be thoroughly, if not entirely, sampled, in order to facilitate detection of sarcomatous components.

The cystic areas of a type II PPB are similar to those of a type I PPB. If thickened areas of sarcomatous or blastematous overgrowth are found, this is sufficient for a diagnosis of type II PPB even in the absence of grossly visible solid areas. Type III PPBs and the solid portions of type II PPBs contain a mixture of cellular populations. Islands of immature blastematous cells are found alongside sarcomatous areas (Figure 6-7). The blastematous component is composed of small cells with round or oval nuclei, inconspicuous nucleoli, and scant cytoplasm. Mitotic figures are usually easy to find. The sarcomatous portion can be undifferentiated (Figure 6-8), but areas with rhabdomyoblastic differentiation can usually be found either with routine stains or with

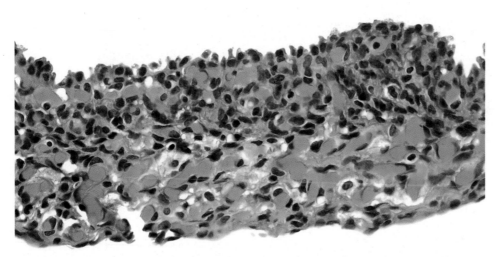

FIGURE 6-5

Pleuropulmonary blastoma

This type I PPB contains a hypercellular cyst wall with a condensation of small cells beneath a normal epithelium.

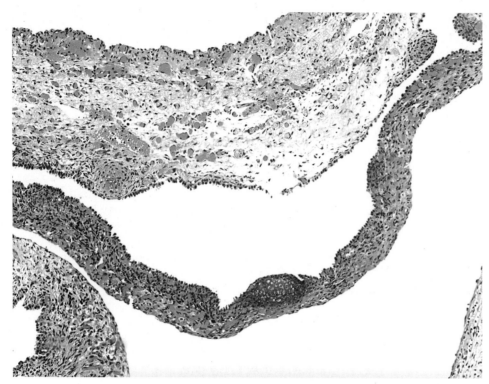

FIGURE 6-6

Pleuropulmonary blastoma
Small nodules of malignant cartilage are observed in this type I PPB.

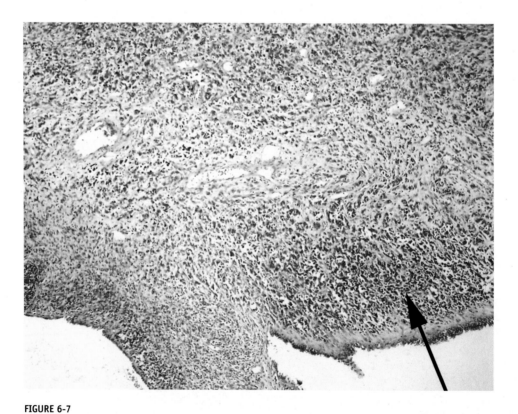

FIGURE 6-7

Pleuropulmonary blastoma
This type II PPB contains cystic (lower half) and solid (upper half) areas. Note the cambium layer (arrow) beneath the epithelial lining. (Courtesy of Dr. Megan Dishop, Texas Children's Hospital, Baylor College of Medicine, Houston, Texas.)

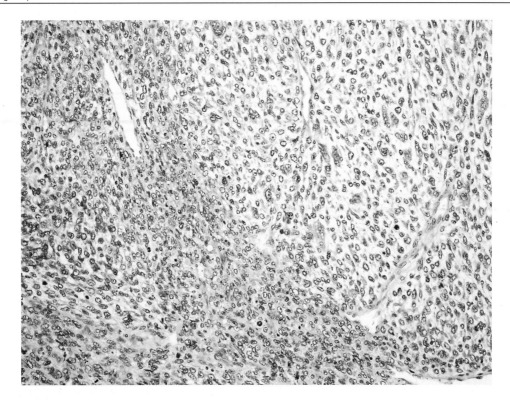

FIGURE 6-8

Pleuropulmonary blastoma

This type III PPB contains frankly malignant cells with frequent mitotic figures, including bizarre mitotic figures. (Courtesy of Dr. Megan Dishop, Texas Children's Hospital, Baylor College of Medicine, Houston, Texas.)

immunohistochemistry. Cartilaginous differentiation can often be found and usually manifests frankly malignant features. These differentiated areas can sometimes be the predominant population in these lesions. In contrast to type I lesions, anaplasia can usually be found in the undifferentiated or rhabdomyosarcomatous portions of type II and type III lesions.

Metastases generally have the appearance of a high-grade sarcoma and usually lack the cellular variability of the primary lesion. Rhabdomyoblastic or spindle cell sarcomatous patterns predominate. When there are multiple metastases, the appearances of the lesions are usually similar to one another.

ANCILLARY STUDIES

Immunohistochemistry can be helpful for supporting rhabdomyoblastic or cartilaginous differentiation. Sarcomatous areas will stain for vimentin, which is usually also weakly expressed by the blastematous cells. Muscle markers are expressed by rhabdomyoblasts and can sometimes be useful for highlighting these cells. S100 will stain cells with cartilaginous differentiation. Cytokeratin reactivity is confined to benign cyst lining cells and entrapped epithelia.

Electron microscopy can reveal abortive sarcomere development in rhabdomyoblasts with parallel thin and thick filaments and well to poorly formed Z bands. Blastematous areas and undifferentiated sarcomatous areas show no distinguishing characteristics.

Trisomy 2 and trisomy 8 have been detected in PPBs. Fluorescence in situ hybridization can demonstrate trisomy 8 in 50-70% of cases, and a positive result can help to confirm the malignant character of a histologically questionable case. This finding, however, does not differentiate between malignancies, and a negative result is noncontributory.

DIFFERENTIAL DIAGNOSIS

Because of the prognostic implications, it is important to differentiate between a type I and a type II PPB, using the criteria discussed above. More problematic is the distinction between PPB and congenital pulmonary adenomatoid malformation (CPAM). It has recently been suggested that type IV CPAM may be part of a spectrum with type I PPB. In fact, there is a documented case of a PPB arising in a patient with a previously diagnosed type IV CPAM. The type IV CPAM is also composed of thin walled cysts, but it should not have immature cartilaginous nodules, dense spindle cell proliferations, or subepithelial collections of spindled cells. A pathologist confronted with the possible diagnosis of a type IV CPAM should thoroughly sample the walls of the cyst or cysts and carefully search for the previously mentioned histologic features.

Synovial sarcoma can present as a cystic lesion, although it is often in patients older than those who typically present with type I PPB. Synovial sarcomas will contain spindle cells in interweaving bundles within the cyst walls. These spindle cells will usually be immunoreactive for cytokeratin, epithelial membrane antigen, and CD99. Molecular studies that demonstrate the t(X;18) translocation can also establish the diagnosis of synovial sarcoma. For type II and type III PPBs, the differential diagnosis also includes other primary and metastatic malignancies. Metastatic Wilms' tumor can be distinguished from a blastema-predominant PPB by a positive immunohistochemical stain for WT-1 in Wilms' tumor. Cytokeratin may be positive in Wilms' tumor if cells retain epithelial differentiation. Metastatic rhabdomyosarcoma will have a more uniform histology. Chondrosarcomas will lack blastematous areas. Congenital infantile fibrosarcoma is a low-grade lesion with a relatively uniform appearance of sheets and interlacing fascicles of spindle cells, also without a blastemal component. A t(12;15) translocation can be identified in some of these lesions. Adult-type pulmonary blastomas generally occur in young and middle-aged adults, but can occur in children or infants. They are biphasic tumors with malignant epithelial and stromal elements, in contrast to PPB, which lacks malignant epithelium. Heterologous elements may be present in the stromal component. Well differentiated fetal adenocarcinoma (WDFA) is also distinguished from PPB on the basis of malignant epithelium. These tumors are composed of malignant glands with a complex architecture that resembles fetal lung in the canalicular phase of development. Cells may contain cytoplasmic clearing due to glycogen.

PROGNOSIS AND THERAPY

For treatment of type I lesions, the current recommendation is complete excision followed by adjuvant chemotherapy with vincristine, actinomycin-D, and cyclophosphamide. Complete resection is also attempted for type II and type III lesions, followed by multi-agent chemotherapy. Neo-adjuvant chemotherapy may be used for some patients. Prognosis is highly dependent on the type of PPB. In one series, the 5-year survival rate for type I lesions was 83%, and for types II and III, 42%. Complete resection is associated with a better prognosis than incomplete resection, and extrapulmonary involve-

ment at diagnosis is reportedly associated with a worse prognosis.

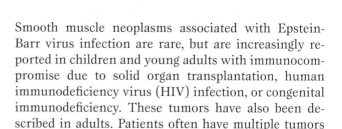

EPSTEIN-BARR VIRUS–ASSOCIATED SMOOTH MUSCLE TUMOR (EBV-SMT)

Smooth muscle neoplasms associated with Epstein-Barr virus infection are rare, but are increasingly reported in children and young adults with immunocompromise due to solid organ transplantation, human immunodeficiency virus (HIV) infection, or congenital immunodeficiency. These tumors have also been described in adults. Patients often have multiple tumors which are usually metachronous lesions, rather than metastases.

CLINICAL FEATURES

EBV-SMTs are found in patients with immunocompromise of various etiologies including transplantation-associated immunosuppression, HIV infection, severe combined immune deficiency, and ataxia-telangiectasia. Most tumors are diagnosed during childhood or early adulthood. Centrally located lesions can give rise to airway obstruction, while peripheral lesions can be asymptomatic. In addition to the lung, virtually any organ may be affected, and the most common sites of involvement are the liver and soft tissues. This lesion has been reported to occur in association with post-transplant lymphoproliferative disorder (PTLD).

PATHOLOGIC FEATURES

GROSS FINDINGS

These tumors are usually white, firm, and well circumscribed.

MICROSCOPIC FINDINGS

Tumors are well circumscribed with pushing borders, and are comprised of interlacing fascicles of spindle cells with eosinophilic cytoplasm and elongated blunted nuclei (Figure 6-9). There may be moderate nuclear atypia, necrosis and myxoid change. In 50% of tumors, there are nodules of primitive round cells. Mitotic activity is usually low but can range as high as 18 mitotic figures per 10 high-power fields. A T-cell-predominant lymphocytic infiltrate is often found within these tumors.

PLEUROPULMONARY BLASTOMA—FACT SHEET

Definition

➤➤ A sarcomatous tumor of infancy and childhood that is comprised of a spectrum of cystic and solid lesions arising in the lung or pleura

Incidence

➤➤ Rare

Mortality

➤➤ Survival is dependent upon type: five-year survival rates are 83% for type I and 42% for type II and type III

Gender and Age Distribution

➤➤ No gender predominance
➤➤ Median age: type I—10 months, type II—36 months, type III—44 months

Clinical Features

➤➤ Chest pain
➤➤ Fever
➤➤ Cough
➤➤ Respiratory distress
➤➤ Pneumothorax

Radiologic Features

➤➤ Unilocular or multilocular cysts with or without septal thickening or solid areas
➤➤ Pneumothorax may be present

Prognosis and Therapy

➤➤ Prognosis is dependent upon tumor type, completeness of resection, and presence or absence of extrapulmonary involvement at diagnosis
➤➤ Type I PPBs are treated with complete surgical excision, and adjuvant chemotherapy is usually given
➤➤ Type II and Type III PPBs are treated with complete surgical excision when possible, and adjuvant or neo-adjuvant chemotherapy
➤➤ Local recurrence is more common with types II and III PPBs (46%) than with type I PPBs (14%)
➤➤ Distant metastasis, especially to the brain, spinal cord, or bone, is not unusual in patients with type II or type III PPB

ANCILLARY STUDIES

To support the diagnosis, it is necessary to demonstrate the presence of Epstein-Barr virus. In situ hybridization studies for EBER-1 usually produce extensive nuclear staining (Figure 6-10). Immunohistochemical studies for EBV latent membrane protein-1 are frequently negative even when in situ hybridization is positive. Immunohistochemical stains for smooth muscle actin are typically strongly and diffusely positive. Desmin is expressed by approximately 50% of tumors. Ultrastructural studies reveal characteristics of smooth muscle cells: elongated spindled cells with oval or slightly indented nuclei, intracytoplasmic bundles of microfilaments with dense bodies, frequent submembranous

PLEUROPULMONARY BLASTOMA—PATHOLOGIC FEATURES

Gross Findings

➤➤ Location: 54% in the right hemithorax, 9% bilateral, 37% in the left hemithorax
➤➤ Type I PPB: thin-walled unilocular or multilocular cysts
➤➤ Type II PPB: solid and cystic components
➤➤ Type III PPB: tan-white solid tumor with areas of hemorrhage and necrosis

Microscopic Findings

Type I PPB:

➤➤ Cyst walls lined by benign epithelium and containing small primitive cells with or without rhabdomyoblastic differentiation, sometimes forming a cambium layer
➤➤ Strap cells may be present
➤➤ Nodules of immature cartilage may be present

Type II PPB:

➤➤ Thickened areas of sarcomatous or blastematous overgrowth within septae
➤➤ Solid component similar to that seen in type III PPB

Type III PPB:

➤➤ Mixture of sarcomatous and blastematous elements
➤➤ Blastema is composed of small cells with round nuclei, inconspicuous nucleoli, and scant cytoplasm
➤➤ Sarcomatous areas often contain rhabdomyosarcomatous and chondrosarcomatous areas as well as undifferentiated areas
➤➤ Mitotic activity is high
➤➤ Anaplasia and marked pleomorphism are usually present

Ultrastructural Features

➤➤ Sarcomere formation is seen within the rhabdomyosarcomatous component
➤➤ Granular matrix is seen within the chondrosarcomatous component

Immunohistochemical Features

➤➤ Immunohistochemical staining depends upon the components represented
➤➤ Rhabdomyoblastic areas stain with muscle markers
➤➤ Chondroid elements stain with S-100
➤➤ Blastema stains weakly for vimentin and smooth muscle actin
➤➤ Epithelium lining the cysts of type I PPB stains for cytokeratin

Pathologic Differential Diagnosis

Type I PPB:

➤➤ Type I or type IV congenital adenomatoid malformation

Type II PPB

➤➤ Cystic synovial sarcoma

Type II and Type III PPB

➤➤ Metastatic sarcomas
➤➤ Metastatic Wilms' tumor
➤➤ Synovial sarcoma
➤➤ Chondrosarcoma
➤➤ Undifferentiated sarcoma
➤➤ Congenital infantile fibrosarcoma

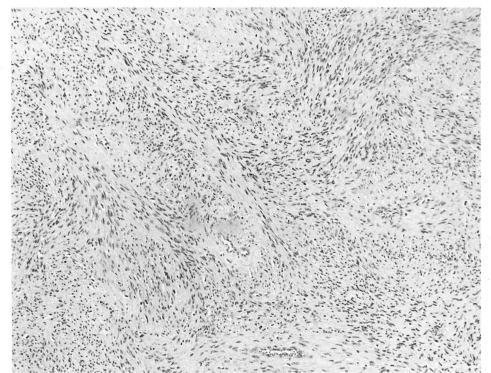

FIGURE 6-9

EBV-associated smooth muscle neoplasm
Intersecting fascicles of bland spindle cells with blunt-ended nuclei comprise this lesion.

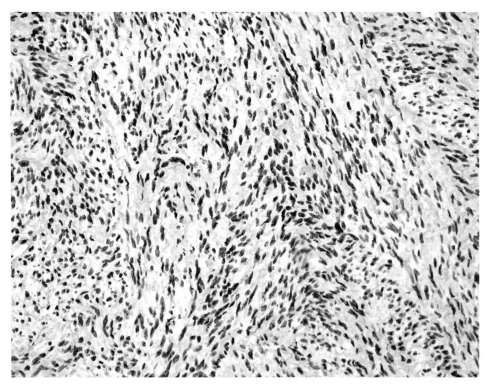

FIGURE 6-10

EBV-associated smooth muscle neoplasm
Chromogenic in situ hybridization for the Epstein-Barr virus coded RNA, EBER-1, demonstrates extensive strong nuclear signal.

EPSTEIN-BARR VIRUS-ASSOCIATED SMOOTH MUSCLE NEOPLASMS—FACT SHEET

Definition
- A proliferation of smooth muscle cells with evidence of Epstein-Barr virus infection, occurring in an immunocompromised patient

Incidence
- Rare

Mortality
- Mortality is usually the result of the underlying condition

Gender and Age Distribution
- EBV-SMTs usually arise in children or young adults, but can also occur in adults
- No gender predominance

Clinical Features
- Central lesions can present with airway obstruction
- Disease can be multifocal
- Rare association with PTLD

Prognosis and Therapy
- Prognosis is usually dependent on the underlying disease and comorbid conditions
- Rare fatal outcomes related to the tumor
- Therapy includes surgical excision and reduction of immunosuppression if the patient is receiving immunosuppressive medications

---

EPSTEIN-BARR VIRUS-ASSOCIATED SMOOTH MUSCLE NEOPLASMS—PATHOLOGIC FEATURES

Gross Findings
- White, well demarcated lesion

Microscopic Findings
- Fascicles of spindle cells with eosinophilic cytoplasm and blunt-ended nuclei
- Nodules of primitive round cells may be present
- Variable mitotic rate
- Necrosis or myxoid change may be present
- T-cell infiltrate is common

Ultrastructural Features
- Smooth muscle phenotype: elongated spindle cells, intracytoplasmic microfilament bundles with dense bodies, submembranous pinocytotic vesicles

Immunohistochemical Features
- Tumors are positive for smooth muscle actin
- 50% of tumors are positive for desmin

In Situ Hybridization
- In situ hybridization for EBER-1 is positive

Pathologic Differential Diagnosis
- Solitary fibrous tumor
- Inflammatory myofibroblastic tumor
- Schwannoma
- Sarcomas with differentiation other than smooth muscle

---

pinocytotic vesicles, and a surrounding basement membrane. The presence of intracytoplasmic viral particles is an inconsistent feature.

DIFFERENTIAL DIAGNOSIS

The clinical setting of immunocompromise should provide an important clue to the appropriate classification of this lesion, when considered in context of the histology and immunohistochemical staining results. Other entities that may be considered, however, are solitary fibrous tumor, inflammatory myofibroblastic tumor, schwannoma, and sarcomas of non-smooth muscle types. Solitary fibrous tumors usually show a patternless pattern, and may show more fibrosis, myxoid change, and hemangiopericytomatous features. Also, these tumors are CD34-positive and usually negative for muscle markers. Inflammatory myofibroblastic tumors usually demonstrate a more prominent lymphoplasmacytic infiltrate and include spindle cells with myofibroblastic characteristics. Schwannomas usually consist of spindle cells with wavy nuclear contours that express S100, show variable cellularity, and may show myxoid change. Epstein-Barr virus is not found in tumor cells.

Features of individual sarcomas are discussed in another chapter.

PROGNOSIS AND THERAPY

Prognosis depends primarily on the underlying disease and the nature of organ involvement by the EBV-SMT. A fatal outcome was reported in one patient with a high tumor burden. Therapy includes surgical excision for solitary or small numbers of tumors, and reduction of immunosuppression if the patient is receiving immunosuppressive medications.

SUGGESTED READINGS

General Information

1. Cohen MC, Kaschula RO. Primary pulmonary tumors in childhood: a review of 31 years' experience and the literature. *Pediatr Pulmonol.* 1992;14:222-32.
2. Corrin B, Nicholson AG. Tumours. In Corrin B, ed. *Pathology of the Lungs.* 2nd ed. New York: Churchill Livingstone; 2006:583-641.
3. Lal DR, Clark I, Shalkow J, et al. Primary epithelial lung malignancies in the pediatric population. *Pediatr Blood Cancer.* 2005;45:683-6.

4. Stocker JT. The respiratory tract. In: Stocker JT, Dehner LP, eds. *Pediatric Pathology*, 2nd ed. Philadelphia: Lippincott, Williams, and Williams; 2001:491-501.

Inflammatory Myofibroblastic Tumor

5. Coffin CM, Dehner LP, Meis-Kindblom JM. Inflammatory myofibroblastic tumor, inflammatory fibrosarcoma, and related lesions: an historical review with differential diagnostic considerations. *Semin Diagn Pathol*. 1998;15:102-10.
6. Fisher C. Myofibroblastic malignancies. *Adv Anat Pathol*. 2004;11(4):190-201.
7. Hussong JW, Brown M, Perkins SL, Dehner LP, Coffin CM. Comparison of DNA ploidy, histologic, and immunohistochemical findings with clinical outcome in inflammatory myofibroblastic tumors. *Mod Pathol*. 1999:12:279-86.

Pleuropulmonary Blastoma

8. Dehner LP. Pleuropulmonary blastoma is the pulmonary blastoma of childhood. *Semin Diagn Pathol*. 1994:11:144-51.
9. Indolfi P, Bisogno G, Casale F, et al. Prognostic factors in pleuropulmonary blastoma. *Pediatr Blood Cancer*. 2007;48:318-23.

10. Priest JR, Hill DA, Williams GM, Moertel et al. International Pleuropulmonary Blastoma Registry. Type I pleuropulmonary blastoma: a report from the International Pleuropulmonary Blastoma Registry. *J Clin Oncol*. 2006;24:4492-8.
11. Priest JR, McDermott MB, Bhatia S, Watterson J, Manivel JC, Dehner LP. Pleuropulmonary blastoma: a clinicopathologic study of 50 cases. *Cancer*. 1997;80:147-61.
12. Available at: www.ppbregistry.org.

Epstein-Barr Virus—Associated Smooth Muscle Tumor

13. Deyrup AT, Lee VK, Hill CE, et al. Epstein-Barr virus-associated smooth muscle tumors are distinctive mesenchymal tumors reflecting multiple infection events: a clinicopathologic and molecular analysis of 29 tumors from 19 patients. *Am J Surg Pathol*. 2006;30:75-82.
14. Monforte-Munoz H, Kapoor N, Saavedra JA. Epstein-Barr virus-associated leiomyomatosis and post-transplant lymphoproliferative disorder in a child with severe combined immunodeficiency: case report and review of the literature. *Pediatr Dev Pathol*. 2003;6:449-57.
15. Weiss SW. Smooth muscle tumors of soft tissue. *Adv Anat Pathol*. 2002;9:351-9.

7

Vascular Diseases

Carlyne D. Cool

INTRODUCTION

Pulmonary vascular diseases encompass a wide range of disorders of the lung. Abnormalities of the pulmonary vasculature not only cause lung disease, but can also result from secondary involvement by nonvascular pulmonary diseases. Many of the primary vascular diseases of the lung are severe, have no adequate available therapy, and pose dilemmas to both the clinician and pathologist. Diseases of the pulmonary vasculature can affect all compartments of the pulmonary vascular tree, including arteries, arterioles, capillaries, and veins. Patients who have these diseases typically present with insidious symptoms, including dyspnea upon exertion, fatigue, syncope, and lower extremity edema. Most patients with pulmonary vascular disease will not undergo lung biopsies, as the risk of the procedure may outweigh any benefits to the patient; thus many cases are diagnosed either clinically or post-mortem. However, it is important to understand and be able to evaluate the pulmonary vessels as some of these entities can be easily overlooked in biopsy specimens. This chapter deals with the most common of the vascular diseases (edema, congestive vasculopathy, and thromboembolism), as well as those entities rarely seen (idiopathic pulmonary arterial hypertension, veno-occlusive disease, pulmonary capillary hemangiomatosis, lymphangiomatosis, and arteriovenous malformation).

EDEMA

Congestion and edema of the lungs is common in heart failure and in areas of inflammation of the lung. Pulmonary edema is the leakage of fluid from the vascular compartment into the interstitium and alveoli of the lung. There are four major causes of pulmonary edema: (1) increased capillary hydrostatic pressure, (2) increased capillary permeability, (3) decreased plasma oncotic pressure, and (4) lymphatic obstruction. Recall that the fluid fluxes in the lung are governed by the Starling equation: the net fluid movement is dependent on the interrelationship between the capillary and interstitial hydrostatic and oncotic pressures. If the net fluid movement is positive, then fluid will leave the capillaries. If negative, fluid will tend to enter the capillaries.

CLINICAL FEATURES

Pulmonary edema may be found at any age. The most common cause of pulmonary edema, though, is cardiogenic. Cardiogenic pulmonary edema is caused by elevated pulmonary capillary hydrostatic pressure, which leads to a transudate of fluid into the interstitium and alveoli. Both left atrial outflow impairment and left ventricular dysfunction can lead to cardiogenic pulmonary edema. Permeability pulmonary edema, on the other hand, results from injury to the capillary endothelial cells. Intravascular hydrostatic pressures are normal, but the endothelial cells lose their integrity and no longer provide a semipermeable membrane. Most of these patients suffer from acute respiratory distress syndrome (ARDS).

Patients with pulmonary edema, if acute in onset, develop breathlessness, anxiety, and feelings of drowning. In those patients with a more gradual onset of symptoms, the most common complaints include dyspnea

99

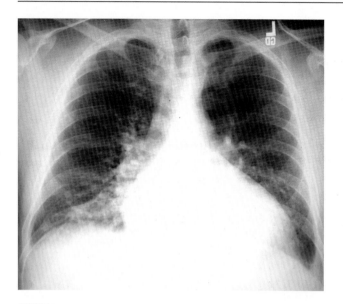

FIGURE 7-1

Pulmonary edema: chest x-ray findings
Chest radiograph illustrates the blunting of the costophrenic angles by pleural effusions as well as the bilateral infiltrates characterized by ill-defined opacities.

RADIOLOGIC FEATURES

Chest x-rays usually show classic features and thus are very helpful in distinguishing pulmonary edema from other causes of dyspnea. Alveolar edema is characterized by bilateral infiltrates in a butterfly pattern along with pleural effusions (Figure 7-1). Other helpful features include loss of sharp definition of pulmonary vasculature, haziness of hilar shadows, and thickening of interlobular septa (Kerley B lines). However, it may take up to 12 hours to develop these classic chest x-ray signs.

PATHOLOGIC FEATURES

GROSS FINDINGS

The gross appearance can take two forms in pulmonary edema, depending on the acuity of the process. In acute pulmonary edema, the lungs are heavy, become dark blue-red, and exude a frothy pink material from the airways and the cut lung surfaces. The Kerley B lines that are visible on chest x-ray correspond to widened, edematous interlobular septa. In the more chronic form of the disease, the lungs may become firm and take on a brown hue, the so-called "brown induration." The brown color is due to the numerous hemosiderin-laden macrophages ("heart failure cells") that accumulate within airspaces (Figure 7-2).

upon exertion, orthopnea, and paroxysmal nocturnal dyspnea. Cough may also be present. Patients with severe disease may present with pink, frothy sputum.

As the causes and severity of pulmonary edema are so varied, the morbidity and mortality of the disease is more related to the underlying etiology. However, the mortality may be as high as 20% in patients admitted to intensive care units.

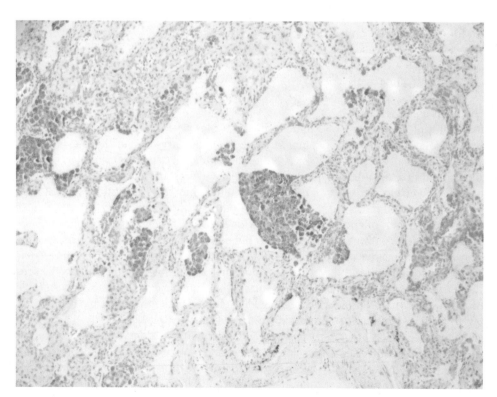

FIGURE 7-2

Pulmonary edema
Chronic leakage and uptake of hemosiderin by alveolar macrophages can lead to a grossly brown appearance of the lung due to the abundant golden-brown hemosiderin. The alveolar septa can become thickened due to this chronic hemorrhage.

MICROSCOPIC FINDINGS

Morphologically, pulmonary edema is recognized as a pink homogeneous fluid that fills the alveolar spaces (Figure 7-3). The capillaries are congested and dilated, and there may be leakage of blood into alveolar spaces. In the chronic forms, the leakage and breakdown of red blood cells leads to the formation of golden-brown granules of hemosiderin accumulating within macrophage cytoplasm (Figure 7-4). These macrophages may be called "heart failure cells" if associated with pulmonary congestion due to congestive heart failure. Additionally, in chronic, longstanding examples of pulmonary edema, there may be a mild associated thickening and fibrosis of the alveolar septa. Pulmonary veins are also commonly affected in chronic pulmonary edema. The histologic changes associated with chronic pulmonary venous hypertension are described in the next section.

DIFFERENTIAL DIAGNOSIS

The differential diagnosis of pulmonary edema chiefly includes diffuse alveolar damage (DAD), fibrin exudates, pulmonary alveolar proteinosis (PAP) and *Pneumocystis jiroveci* pneumonia (PJP). DAD is a disease characterized by hyaline membrane formation. The hyaline membranes diffusely line alveolar septa, but do not fill the alveoli. It may be difficult on occasion to differentiate the two, as DAD (clinically, ARDS) begins with pulmonary edema. Fibrin exudates can appear similar to pulmonary edema, but the fibrin exudates are denser and more eosinophilic, and other features of acute lung injury are often present. PAP can be difficult to distinguish from pulmonary edema. However, pulmonary edema lacks the granularity, acicular spaces and foam cells of PAP. PAS stains can also help distinguish PAP from pulmonary edema, as PAP contains PAS-positive, diastase-resistant material. PJP is associated with a frothy-appearing eosinophilic exudate that can be mistaken for pulmonary edema. PJP can be distinguished primarily by the more amphophilic appearance of the alveolar material as well as by the frothy, foamy appearance. Silver stains, of course, will highlight the *Pneumocystis*.

PROGNOSIS AND THERAPY

The prognosis of pulmonary edema is entirely dependent on the etiology. Many patients can be treated adequately with pharmacotherapy. The drugs used to treat pulmonary edema depend on the cause of the pulmonary edema. Cardiogenic pulmonary edema is treated with various drugs including preload reducers, afterload reducers, catecholamines, and phosphodiesterase inhibitors. Some patients may require surgical

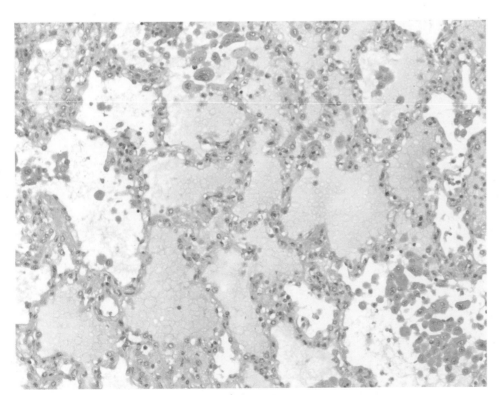

FIGURE 7-3
Pulmonary edema
The alveolar spaces are filled with pink, homogeneous material characteristic of pulmonary edema.

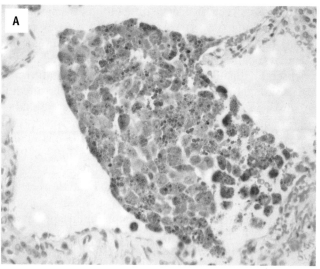

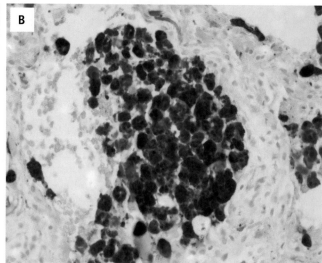

FIGURE 7-4

Pulmonary edema
(A) This is a high-power view of the golden-brown, chunky hemosiderin granules within air space macrophages. **(B)** An iron stain highlights the intense deposition of hemosiderin that can be seen in longstanding heart failure.

intervention with intra-aortic balloon pump insertion in order to obtain hemodynamic stabilization prior to definitive therapy. Patients with permeability pulmonary edema often require ventilatory support during the course of their disease.

CONGESTIVE VASCULOPATHY AND CHRONIC PASSIVE CONGESTION

Congestive vasculopathy and chronic passive congestion are the result of longstanding edema and congestion, often due to elevated left atrial pressure with consequent

EDEMA—FACT SHEET

Definition
▸▸ Leakage of fluid from the vascular compartment into the interstitium and alveoli of the lung, most often due to cardiogenic or permeability factors

Incidence
▸▸ Any age
▸▸ Common with heart failure and ARDS

Mortality
▸▸ Related to the underlying etiology
▸▸ 20% mortality in ICU patients

Clinical Features
▸▸ Acute: Breathlessness, anxiety, feelings of drowning
▸▸ Chronic: Dyspnea on exertion, orthopnea, paroxysmal nocturnal dyspnea, cough

Radiologic Features
▸▸ Butterfly pattern of bilateral infiltrates
▸▸ Pleural effusions
▸▸ Kerley B lines
▸▸ Loss of normal sharp definition of pulmonary vasculature

Prognosis and Therapy
▸▸ Prognosis is dependent on etiology
▸▸ Most cardiogenic patients are treated with drug therapy
▸▸ Ventilatory support is required for permeability pulmonary edema due to ARDS

EDEMA—PATHOLOGIC FEATURES

Gross Findings
▸▸ Acute: heavy lungs with frothy exudate and dark blue-red appearance
▸▸ Chronic: firm, brown appearance ("brown induration")

Microscopic Findings
▸▸ Acute: pink homogenous fluid fills air spaces, capillaries are congested, leakage of blood into air spaces
▸▸ Chronic: hemosiderin-laden macrophages within air spaces, alveolar septal thickening and fibrosis, changes of pulmonary venous hypertension

Pathologic Differential Diagnosis
▸▸ Diffuse alveolar damage
▸▸ Fibrin exudates
▸▸ Pulmonary alveolar proteinosis
▸▸ *Pneumocystis jiroveci* pneumonia

elevated pulmonary venous pressure. Over time, chronic passive congestion leads to fibrosis of the alveolar septa along with hemosiderin deposition, the so-called "brown induration" described above. Not only are the septa affected, but the pulmonary veins, arteries, and arterioles can also become remodeled.

CLINICAL FEATURES

Patients with a history of chronic congestive heart failure and/or recurring pulmonary edema may develop pulmonary venous hypertension. Pulmonary venous hypertension is the most common cause of pulmonary hypertension in clinical practice. These patients may develop orthopnea and paroxysmal nocturnal dyspnea prior to the development of exertional dyspnea. The clinical picture may become complicated because some of these patients remodel their pulmonary veins and arteries in response to the elevated left-sided pressures, leading to further elevations in pulmonary artery pressures and eventually right-sided heart failure.

RADIOLOGIC FEATURES

The radiographic picture of pulmonary venous hypertension is characterized by a change in the apparent size of major vessels in the upper lobes as compared to the lower lobes. Normally, when patients are upright, the upper lobe vessels are smaller than the lower vessels. With pulmonary venous hypertension, the upper lobe vessels became at least as large as, if not larger than, the lower lobe vessels. This can be a subtle finding. Other radiographic features can include cardiomegaly (since most congestive vasculopathies are due to left ventricular failure) and the findings of pulmonary edema described above. If mitral stenosis is present, then the chest x-ray shows prominence of the left atrial appendage.

PATHOLOGIC FEATURES

GROSS FINDINGS

The gross findings in congestive vasculopathy are typified by the "brown induration" of the lung due to chronic hemosiderin deposition.

MICROSCOPIC FINDINGS

As the pressure changes are relayed to the pulmonary veins, arteries, and arterioles, all can show changes of vascular remodeling. The pulmonary veins become thick-

ened by smooth muscle hypertrophy of the media. Additionally, elastic tissue stains demonstrate the acquisition of an external elastic lamina such that veins now resemble arteries (Figure 7-5). Venous adventitia often become fibrotic. Lymphatics within the interlobular septa often become dilated (Figure 7-6). The increased venous pressures translate to increased arterial/arteriolar pressures. Thus, the pulmonary arteries become hypertrophied by both medial and intimal expansion. The medial hypertrophy can become quite pronounced (Figure 7-7) and the intimal fibrosis is often eccentric rather than circumferential (Figure 7-8). The arterioles may become muscularized. Other changes in the lung include hemosiderin-laden macrophages within air spaces. In fact, this may become so severe in diseases such as mitral stenosis that the changes may mimic a bland alveolar hemorrhage syndrome. If the hemosiderin load is large, there may be encrustation of elastic fibers by iron and calcium deposits with resultant engulfment by foreign-body type giant cells. This appearance can also be seen in other causes of chronic pulmonary hemosiderosis (e.g., idiopathic pulmonary hemosiderosis) and has been termed "endogenous pneumoconiosis" (Figure 7-9). Iron and von Kossa stains will highlight this feature. Additional histologic findings may include septal thickening due to chronic edema and congestion.

DIFFERENTIAL DIAGNOSIS

If hemosiderosis is severe, particular attention should be paid to the vessels, as severe pulmonary venous hypertension can mimic alveolar hemorrhage syndromes. The only distinguishing feature may be the markedly abnormal vessels found in pulmonary venous hypertension. Pulmonary arterial hypertension does not affect the venous system, thus careful attention will distinguish the two. Additionally, plexiform lesions and arteritis are not features of pulmonary venous hypertension. Pulmonary veno-occlusive disease (PVOD) can be particularly difficult to distinguish from congestive vasculopathy associated with chronic passive congestion, especially in the adult population. Occlusion of veins in interlobular septa is a helpful distinguishing feature in PVOD.

PROGNOSIS AND THERAPY

The underlying etiology must be treated in order to affect the pulmonary venous hypertension. However, the pulmonary vascular findings may persist even after the clinical cause of the venous hypertension is resolved. There have been rare reports of complete regression of the histologic lesions.

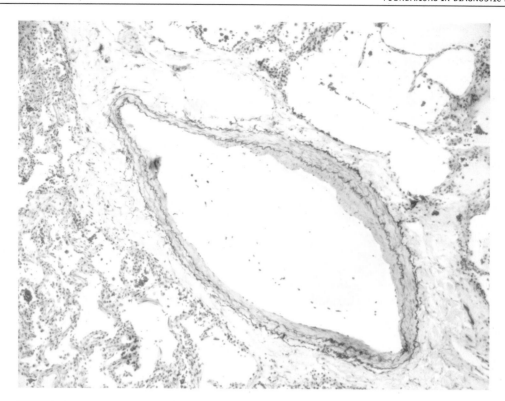

FIGURE 7-5

Pulmonary venous hypertension: arterialization of interlobular vein
A vein within the interlobular septum displays arterialization of its wall, with an additional elastic lamina, medial hypertrophy and mild intimal fibrosis. These changes are best appreciated with elastic tissue stains, such as this Movat or pentachrome stain. Note the absence of an accompanying airway, which would be seen with a true artery.

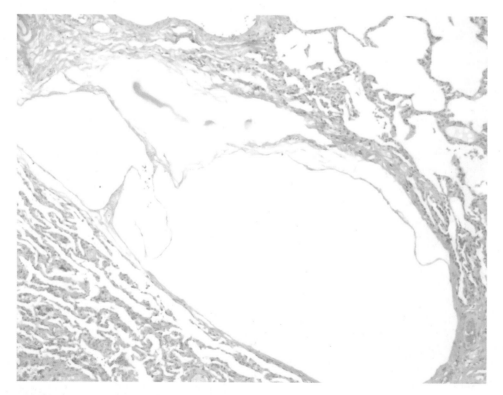

FIGURE 7-6

Pulmonary venous hypertension: dilated lymphatic
As a consequence of venous hypertension, lymphatics become dilated, as illustrated here. This lymph channel is located within an interlobular septum.

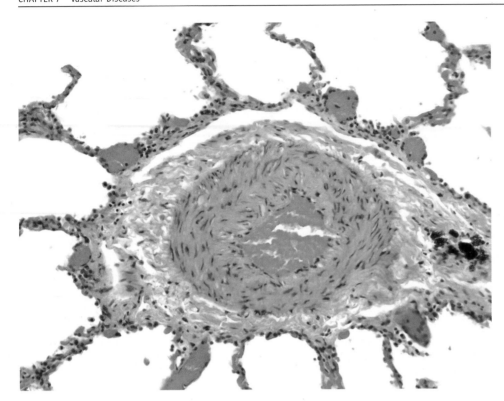

FIGURE 7-7

Pulmonary venous hypertension: medial hypertrophy of pulmonary artery
Pulmonary arteries can be secondarily affected by venous hypertension such that their medial layer becomes hypertrophied.

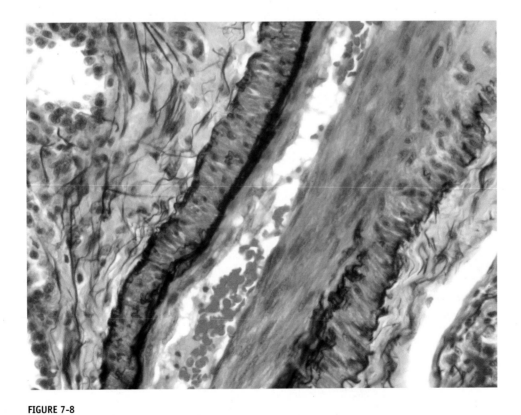

FIGURE 7-8

Pulmonary venous hypertension: eccentric intimal fibrosis of pulmonary artery
In contrast to other causes of hypertension, pulmonary venous hypertension leads to an eccentric, rather than concentric, intimal changes in pulmonary arteries. This is a high-power view of a Movat-stained section, illustrating an artery with one side showing minimal intimal change, while the other side shows more marked intimal hyperplasia along with focal loss of the internal elastic lamina. The aqua color indicates myofibroblastic change as well.

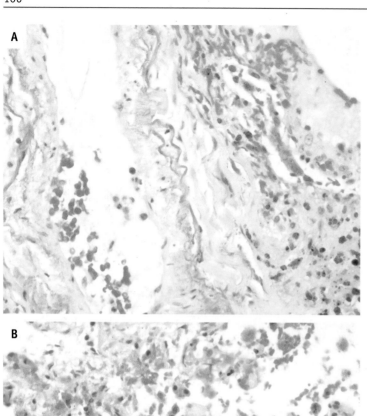

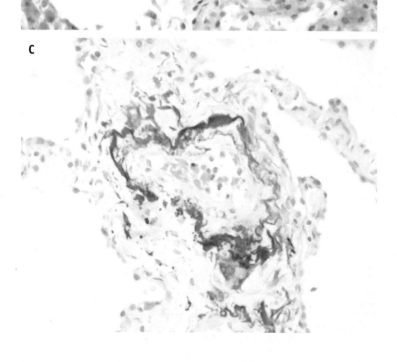

FIGURE 7-9

Pulmonary venous hypertension: chronic pulmonary hemosiderosis

(A) This H & E stain illustrates the encrustation of the vascular elastic fibers by calcium and iron deposits. The coated fibers take on a gray hue. Adjacent hemosiderin granules and vascular congestion are present. **(B)** In the center of this image, a multinucleated giant cell is seen engulfing some of the coated elastic fibers. This has given rise to the term "endogenous pneumoconiosis." **(C)** Iron staining highlights the iron composition of the encrusted elastic fibers. Von Kossa stains can also be used to highlight the calcium composition.

CONGESTIVE VASCULOPATHY AND CHRONIC PASSIVE CONGESTION—FACT SHEET

Definition
» End result of longstanding edema and congestion due to various etiologies, including chronic congestive heart failure and recurring pulmonary edema. Leads to pulmonary venous hypertension.

Incidence
» Any age
» Occurs most commonly in patients with chronic congestive heart failure and/or recurring pulmonary edema
» Mitral stenosis is another common cause

Mortality
» Related to the underlying etiology

Clinical Features
» Orthopnea and paroxysmal nocturnal dyspnea
» Eventually, exertional dyspnea

Radiologic Features
» Increase in size of the major vessels in the upper lobes
» Cardiomegaly
» Pulmonary edema pattern
» Enlarged left atrial appendage (if mitral stenosis is present)

Prognosis and Therapy
» Prognosis is dependent on etiology
» Pulmonary vascular changes may persist even after clinical resolution of the underlying etiology

---

CONGESTIVE VASCULOPATHY AND CHRONIC PASSIVE CONGESTION— PATHOLOGIC FEATURES

Gross Findings
» "Brown induration" of chronic congestion and edema

Microscopic Findings
Pulmonary Veins
» Medial hypertrophy
» Arterialization (acquisition of an external elastic lamina)
» Adventitial fibrosis

Pulmonary Lymphatics
» Dilatation

Pulmonary Arteries
» Medial hypertrophy
» Intimal fibrosis, often eccentric

Pulmonary Arterioles
» Muscularization

Alveolar Parenchyma
» Edema
» Alveolar septal thickening
» Hemosiderin-laden macrophages within air spaces
» Possible endogenous pneumoconiosis

Pathologic Differential Diagnosis
» Alveolar hemorrhage syndromes
» Pulmonary arterial hypertension
» Pulmonary veno-occlusive disease

THROMBOEMBOLISM

Pulmonary embolism is perhaps the most common cause of pulmonary vascular disease and likely the most clinically significant as well. Pulmonary emboli have been documented in up to half of all autopsied patients. Pulmonary embolism is a major contributing cause of death in up to 10% of patients dying in a hospital setting.

CLINICAL FEATURES

Thrombosis can occur in a number of disease settings. Hypercoagulability, injury, and inactivity can all lead to peripheral venous thrombosis and subsequent embolism to the pulmonary vasculature. Although occlusions of pulmonary arteries are almost always embolic in origin (greater than 95% arise from thrombi within lower leg veins), in situ thrombosis of small pulmonary arteries may occasionally lead to pulmonary hypertension. It should be cautioned that in situ thrombosis can occur in response to diffuse alveolar damage, and should not be interpreted as recurrent thromboembolic disease. Acute pulmonary thromboembolism rarely causes pulmonary hypertension except in massive cases, such as saddle embolism. Recurrent pulmonary thromboembolism, a subtle and difficult entity to diagnose, however, can often lead to sustained pulmonary hypertension. Diagnosis typically is made via spiral CT scan, ventilation-perfusion scan, or pulmonary angiography. However, occasionally such cases are diagnosed by a fortuitous lung biopsy.

Additionally, emboli of foreign or endogenous material, such as intravenous drug particles, tumor or fat emboli, and ova/parasites, may lead to pulmonary artery obstruction. Sickle cell disease can result in recurrent microvascular obstruction, leading to the development of pulmonary hypertension. Pulmonary hypertension is among the most common cause of death in patients with sickle cell disease. These patients often present with progressive dyspnea.

RADIOLOGIC FEATURES

Radiologic features of thromboembolism include enlargement of central pulmonary arteries, patchy areas of decreased vascularity (mosaic oligemia), and right-sided heart enlargement. Ventilation-perfusion scan is sensitive, but not specific, in diagnosing thromboembolic pulmonary hypertension. Spiral CT scans with contrast enhancement are the current procedure of choice for evaluating patients with suspected chronic thromboembolic pulmonary disease.

PATHOLOGIC FEATURES

GROSS FINDINGS

The gross features depend upon the age of the clot. Early on, the clot consists predominantly of fibrin and blood and is loosely adherent to the vessel wall. However, with time the clot becomes adherent to the wall and fibrous tissue develops. A clot in a large vessel can become recanalized, and the organized embolus then takes on the appearance of a fibrous intravascular web.

MICROSCOPIC FINDINGS

The microscopic appearance of a clot also depends upon its age. Within the first three days, there is little reaction between the embolus, which consists mainly of fibrin and blood, and the vascular endothelium (Figure 7-10). By the end of the first week, endothelial cells grow over the surface of the clot and migrate into the embolus itself. During the second week, fibroblasts and capillaries form. If resolution of the clot does not occur, then organization results. Organization begins with development of collagen fibers during the third and fourth weeks. A completely organized clot may show an eccentric intimal plaque within the pulmonary artery (Figure 7-11), or there may be recanalization of the vessel, resulting in multiple, round, well formed, vascular channels (Figure 7-12). Bridging fibrous webs may form in larger vessels (Figure 7-13). If there is poor blood supply to the region, infarction may occur (Figure 7-14). Often, a spectrum of recent, organizing, and organized thromboemboli is evident in the lung.

A variety of normal tissues can also embolize to the lung, with little or no functional consequence to the lung. Megakaryocytes from the bone marrow often lodge in pulmonary capillaries. In addition, bone marrow (Figure 7-15), adipose tissue, particles of skin, or hair can all become dislodged by trauma and embolize to the lungs. Air and gas can enter the circulation during surgery, trauma, or injection, or as the result of Caisson disease (decompression sickness). Gas emboli are seen as vacuoles in histologic preparations, and are indistinguishable from lipid emboli. Oil red O stain can be used to distinguish lipid from other vacuolated-appearing emboli, if fresh or frozen tissue is available. All these forms of tissue emboli are usually of little consequence to the pulmonary circulation.

Tumor emboli, on the other hand, can occasionally be extensive and lead to symptomatic and sustained

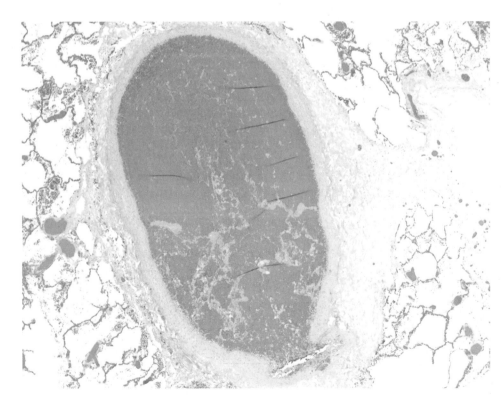

FIGURE 7-10

Thromboembolism
A recent embolus, characterized by intraluminal blood and fibrin.

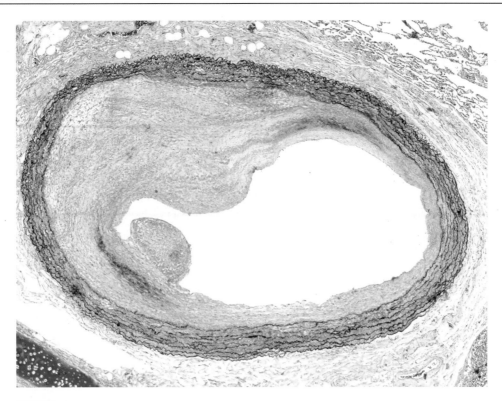

FIGURE 7-11

Thromboembolism: organizing clot

Movat stain of a large artery, showing prominent eccentric intimal fibrosis. On occasion, the intimal fibrosis may obliterate the lumen.

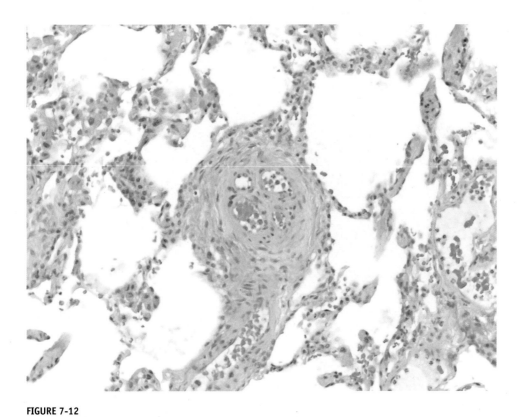

FIGURE 7-12

Thromboembolism: recanalized vessel

This small pulmonary artery shows recanalization, which is characterized by a punched-out, "cookie cutter" appearance of the lumen.

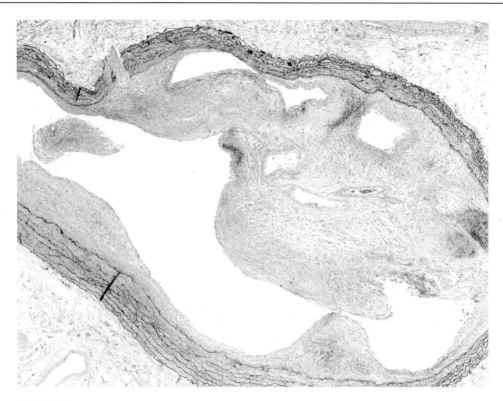

FIGURE 7-13

Thromboembolism: organizing clot
Movat stain of a larger artery showing an example of the bridging, fibrous intraluminal webs that can form over time. These may be visible on gross examination.

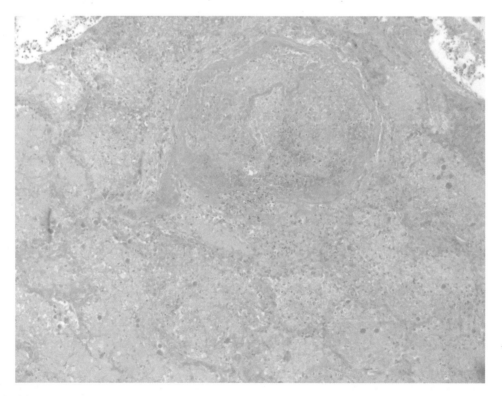

FIGURE 7-14

Thromboembolism: infarcted lung
If a clot is in a medium or large pulmonary artery, and there is insufficient blood supply to a region, then infarction results. The infarct is usually subpleural and wedge-shaped grossly, and on microscopic examination appears as a region of avascular, dead alveolar walls, as illustrated in this image.

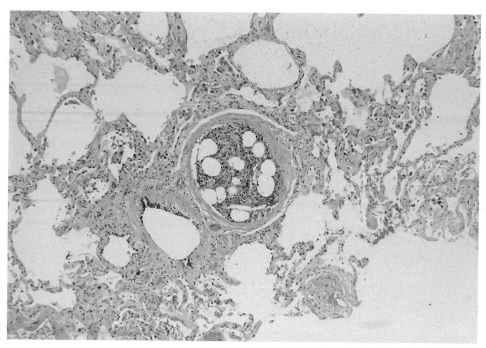

FIGURE 7-15

Thromboembolism: bone marrow embolus
Bone marrow emboli are usually incidental findings at autopsy, but can also be seen in surgical lung specimens. They may result from bony trauma or rib manipulation. There is almost never any clinical significance to these findings.

pulmonary hypertension. Tumors that commonly embolize to the lung include carcinomas of the liver, stomach, and breast.

Foreign body embolism can be encountered in therapeutic procedures such as catheterization studies in which cotton gauze fibers are inadvertently introduced into the circulation (Figure 7-16). Cotton fibers can cause granulomatous inflammation with rupture of the arterial wall. Talc, starch, and microcrystalline cellulose are often introduced through the use of intravenous drugs, and can occlude a substantial number of pulmonary arteries leading to pulmonary hypertension (Figure 7-17). Examination under polarized light is used to identify foreign particles in the lung. Sickled red blood cells can be seen in pulmonary vessels of patients who die from pulmonary hypertension secondary to sickle cell disease (Figure 7-18).

DIFFERENTIAL DIAGNOSIS

The most difficult lesion to distinguish from a recanalized pulmonary artery is the plexiform lesion seen in severe pulmonary arterial hypertension. However, the secondary lumens of the recanalized vessel are rounded, punched-out-appearing, and are lined by a single layer

of endothelial cells. By contrast, the plexiform lesion often shows irregular, slit-like secondary lumens surrounded by proliferating endothelial and smooth muscle cells (Figure 7-19).

PROGNOSIS AND THERAPY

Treatment regimens in many of these patients include anticoagulants. In larger vessels, pulmonary thromboendarterectomy may provide dramatic relief. However, the vascular changes in smaller vessels are often irreversible and may lead to pulmonary hypertension, cor pulmonale, and sudden death.

PULMONARY HYPERTENSION

Pulmonary hypertension has undergone a number of re-classifications in the last few decades. In 1958, Heath and Edwards published the pathology of hypertensive pulmonary vascular disease, giving a description of six grades of structural changes in the pulmonary arteries

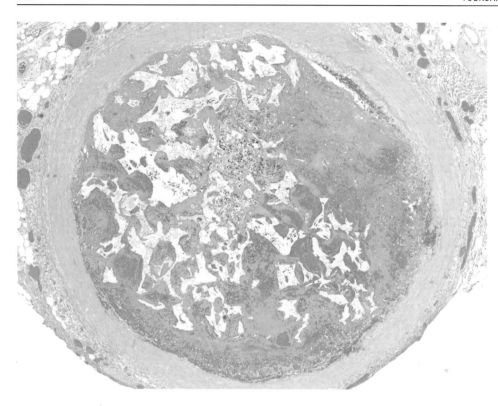

FIGURE 7-16

Thromboembolism: foreign material embolus
This pulmonary artery is occluded by cotton gauze fibers.

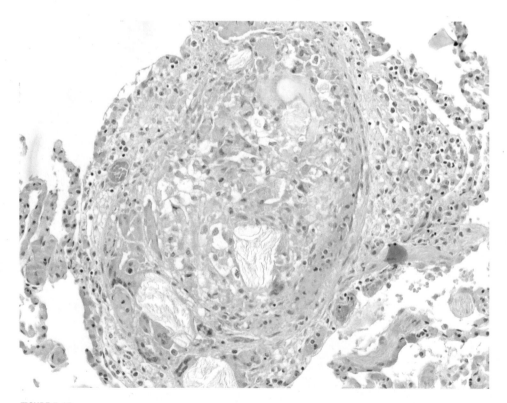

FIGURE 7-17

Thromboembolism: foreign material embolus
This pulmonary artery shows occlusion by foreign material that, when polarized, is doubly refractile, consistent with insoluble filler material found in oral preparations. There is often an associated giant cell reaction in the walls of the pulmonary arteries.

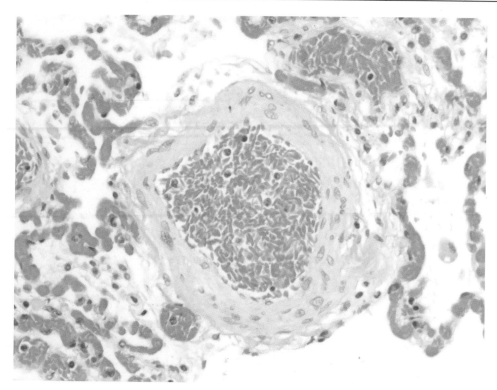

FIGURE 7-18

Pulmonary hypertension associated with sickle cell disease
This vessel shows occlusion by numerous sickled red blood cells, a common finding in sickle patients who die with pulmonary hypertension.

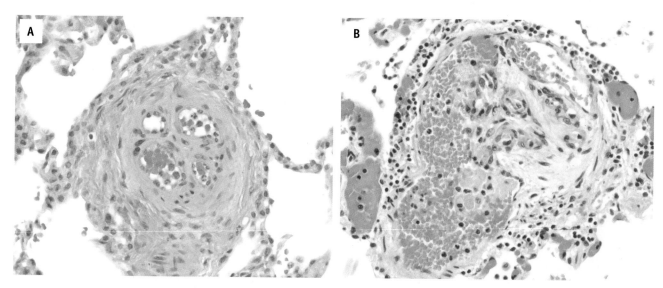

FIGURE 7-19

Comparison of recanalized pulmonary artery with plexiform lesion
(A) is a high-power view of the recanalized vessel in Figure 7-12 above. For comparison, **(B)** illustrates, at the same high power, the irregular lumens that are seen in plexiform arteriopathy.

with special reference to congenital cardiac septal defects (Table 7-1). However, over the years, this grading system has been used to classify other forms of pulmonary hypertension, including idiopathic pulmonary arterial hypertension (IPAH). In 1998, the World Health Organization (WHO) adopted a revised classification for pulmonary hypertension that combined clinical history, epidemiology, and pathology, in an attempt to provide meaningful diagnostic and prognostic information. At the 2003 World Health Organization Third World Conference on Pulmonary Hypertension, revisions were once again made not only to address shortcomings in the previous classification scheme, but also to address recent advances in pathogenetic mechanisms (Table 7-2).

THROMBOEMBOLISM—FACT SHEET

Definition

▸▸ Occlusion of pulmonary arteries which is usually embolic (most emboli arise from deep venous thrombi), and less often thrombotic in origin

Incidence

▸▸ Any age
▸▸ Common in hospitalized patients

Mortality

▸▸ Major contributor to death in 10% of patients dying in a hospital setting

Clinical Features

▸▸ Most frequently asymptomatic
▸▸ Sudden death is unusual
▸▸ Can cause acute or chronic pulmonary hypertension and right-sided heart failure with its associated symptoms

Radiologic Features

▸▸ Enlargement of central pulmonary arteries
▸▸ Patchy decreased vascularity (mosaic oligemia)
▸▸ Right-sided heart enlargement
▸▸ Ventilation-perfusion scans sensitive, but not specific
▸▸ Spiral CT with contrast best for chronic thromboembolic disease

Prognosis and Therapy

▸▸ May develop pulmonary hypertension, cor pulmonale, and sudden death
▸▸ Anticoagulants are the standard approach to prevention
▸▸ Pulmonary thromboendarterectomy can be performed for large vessel clots

THROMBOEMBOLISM—PATHOLOGIC FEATURES

Gross Findings

▸▸ Early: fibrin and blood loosely adherent to vessel wall
▸▸ Late: fibrous intravascular webs visible in larger arteries

Microscopic Findings

▸▸ Early (72 hours): fibrin and blood within arteries
▸▸ Mid (one week): endothelial cells cover the clot and grow into the embolus
▸▸ Mid (second week): fibroblasts and capillaries form within the embolus
▸▸ Late (third to fourth week): collagen fibers form, recanalization begins
▸▸ Depending on size of vessel and blood supply, infarcts may occur
▸▸ Non-blood clots can embolize to the pulmonary arteries, including megakaryocytes, bone marrow, adipose tissue, skin, hair, air, and gas. Most are incidental findings
▸▸ Tumor emboli can cause pulmonary hypertension
▸▸ Foreign body emboli can cause pulmonary hypertension

Pathologic Differential Diagnosis

▸▸ Plexiform lesions of pulmonary arterial hypertension

TABLE 7-1

Heath and Edwards Grading Scheme for Hypertensive Pulmonary Vascular Disease

Grade	Structural Change
Grade I:	Medial hypertrophy of arteries and muscularization of arterioles
Grade II:	Intimal proliferation develops in arteries
Grade III:	Intimal concentric laminar fibrosis becomes prominent in muscular arteries
Grade IV:	Dilatation of small arteries occurs with development of plexiform lesions
Grade V:	Plexiform and angiomatoid lesions become prominent; hemosiderin deposition present
Grade VI:	Necrotizing arteritis develops

From Heath D, Edwards JE. The pathology of hypertensive pulmonary vascular disease: a description of six grades of structural changes in the pulmonary arteries with special reference to congenital cardiac septal defects. *Circulation*. 1958;18:533-547.

TABLE 7-2

2003 Revised Nomenclature and Classification of Pulmonary Hypertension

I. Pulmonary arterial hypertension (PAH)

  A. Idiopathic (IPAH)

  B. Familial (FPAH)

  C. Associated with:

    1. Collagen vascular disease

    2. Congenital systemic to pulmonary shunts (large, small, repaired, or nonrepaired)

    3. Portal hypertension

    4. HIV infection

    5. Drugs and toxins

    6. Other (glycogen storage disease, Gaucher's disease, hereditary hemorrhagic telangiectasia, hemoglobinopathies, myeloproliferative disorders, splenectomy)

  D. Associated with significant venous or capillary involvement

    1. Pulmonary veno-occlusive disease

    2. Pulmonary capillary hemangiomatosis

II. Pulmonary venous hypertension

  A. Left-sided atrial or ventricular heart disease

  B. Left-sided valvular heart disease

III. Pulmonary hypertension associated with hypoxemia

  A. Chronic obstructive pulmonary disease

  B. Interstitial lung disease

  C. Sleep-disordered breathing

  D. Alveolar hypoventilation disorders

  E. Chronic exposure to high altitude

IV. Pulmonary hypertension due to chronic thrombotic and/or embolic disease

  A. Thromboembolic obstruction of proximal pulmonary arteries

  B. Thromboembolic obstruction of distal pulmonary arteries

  C. Pulmonary embolism (tumor, parasites, foreign material)

V. Miscellaneous: sarcoidosis, histiocytosis X, lymphangiomatosis, compression of pulmonary vessels (adenopathy, tumor, fibrosing mediastinitis)

Reprinted from Simonneau G, Galiè N, Rubin LJ, et al. Clinical classification of pulmonary hypertension. *J Am Coll Cardiol.* 2004;43 (12 Suppl S):5S-12S, with permission from Elsevier.

CLINICAL FEATURES

Pulmonary arterial hypertension (PAH) is defined clinically as a mean resting pulmonary artery pressure greater than 25 mm Hg, or pulmonary artery pressure greater than 30 mm Hg during exercise. Mild elevations in pulmonary artery pressure are usually asymptomatic, and most cases are diagnosed only when the pulmonary artery pressure exceeds 60 mm Hg. Symptoms of pulmonary hypertension include dyspnea, fatigue, syncope, lower extremity edema, and atypical chest pain.

The cases that are spontaneous, and seemingly idiopathic, as well as familial forms of the disease are considered "idiopathic (primary) pulmonary arterial hypertension," whereas those cases attributable to collagen vascular diseases, congenital shunts, portal hypertension, HIV, drug-exposure, and persistent pulmonary hypertension of the newborn are now categorized as "associated pulmonary arterial hypertension."

Idiopathic cases are more common in young females (mean age 36.4 years, male: female 1.0:1.7), but can occur at any age. The overall incidence is not known, but is estimated to be 1 to 2 per million.

Familial pulmonary arterial hypertension is rare (less than 6% of primary cases). The disease presents at an earlier age as compared to spontaneous cases, and appears to have an autosomal dominant inheritance pattern with incomplete penetrance. Germ-line mutations in BMPR2 (chromosome 2q31-32), a gene that encodes a receptor in the transforming growth factor beta (TGFβ) super-family, have been identified in patients with familial PAH. Only 10-20% of family members develop the disease. Despite the autosomal dominant inheritance, the disease shows a female predominance, similar to the spontaneous form of the disease.

All forms of collagen vascular disease have been seen in association with PAH. However, there is a wide range of risk based on the clinical classification of collagen vascular disease. CREST, a limited form of systemic sclerosis, has a very high incidence of pulmonary hypertension, with up to 30% of patients affected and over 50% with evidence of pulmonary hypertension at autopsy. Similar incidences have been reported in patients with mixed connective tissue disease. Systemic lupus erythematosus has a somewhat lower risk, with approximately 5-10% of individuals affected. Sjögren's disease, rheumatoid arthritis, and polymyositis/dermatomyositis rarely develop associated pulmonary hypertension.

Portal hypertension, most commonly in the setting of liver disease, can be associated with pulmonary hypertension. Porto-pulmonary hypertension (PPHTN) is seen in 2-5% of patients with liver disease, and may be even higher among patients who have undergone liver transplantation. The risk of pulmonary hypertension is associated with the duration, not the degree, of portal hypertension. Typically, pulmonary hypertension develops 4 to 7 years after the initial diagnosis of portal hypertension.

HIV appears to be a potent risk factor for the development of pulmonary hypertension, with an incidence of approximately 0.5% in the HIV-positive population. This represents at least a 2,000-fold increase in risk as compared with the general population.

Drug exposures may also be a risk factor in the development of pulmonary hypertension. Aminorex, fenfluramine, and dexfenfluramine have been associated with a 23-fold increase in the relative risk for pulmonary hypertension, purportedly affecting approximately 1 out of every 20,000 users of diet combination Fen-Phen. Other agents thought to be associated with pulmonary hypertension include toxic rapeseed oil, amphetamines, meta-amphetamines, cocaine, and L-tryptophan.

RADIOLOGIC FEATURES

The assessment of pulmonary arterial hypertension on chest x-ray is difficult and somewhat subjective. The central pulmonary arteries are enlarged, whereas the peripheral pulmonary arteries show rapid tapering ("peripheral pruning"). CT scans are better for assessing the size of the main pulmonary artery. Anything larger than 29 mm is abnormal. However, it should be remembered that there is poor correlation between the diameter of the central pulmonary arteries and the severity of the pulmonary arterial hypertension.

PATHOLOGIC FEATURES

GROSS FINDINGS

The gross findings of pulmonary arterial hypertension can be subtle, but the medium to small pulmonary arteries are often quite pronounced with a thickened, rigid, pipe-like appearance. Atheroscopic plaques can be seen in the large pulmonary arteries. In patients dying with right heart failure, there is usually right ventricular hypertrophy.

MICROSCOPIC FINDINGS

While many cases of pulmonary hypertension are diagnosed without lung biopsy, pathology can play a critical role in the diagnosis of patients with atypical clinical presentations. A common change in pulmonary arterial hypertension is medial hypertrophy of arterial walls (Figure 7-20). In children, muscularization of arterioles may be the only histologic finding in pulmonary hypertension, although this appears rarely to be the case in adults. There is often good correlation between the thickness of the medial smooth muscle and the measured pulmonary artery pressure. In contrast, intimal hyperplasia, while a common finding in pulmonary hypertension, has poor correlation with the severity of disease. Intimal hyperplasia is seen in two distinctive forms. Cellular intimal hyperplasia, a relatively nonspecific finding, is loose and lacking in collagen deposition (Figure 7-21). Concentric laminar intimal hyperplasia, on the other hand, has dense depositions of collagen and elastin, and is a finding rarely seen except in primary/idiopathic pulmonary arterial hypertension and some collagen vascular diseases (Figure 7-22). Occasionally, dilation creates vessels with large lumens and very thin walls that are reminiscent of pulmonary veins (Figure 7-23).

Plexiform lesions are the hallmark angioproliferative lesion of primary pulmonary hypertension, and are characterized by abnormal proliferation of endothelial cells, forming multiple irregular lumens in a glomeruloid plexus (Figure 7-24). Unlike the rigid round lumens of a recanalized thrombus, the plexiform lesion tends to form asymmetrical and slit-like channels within the vessel (Figure 7-19). Plexiform lesions may be very sparse in a case, requiring examination of multiple sections, or may be widespread. Some cases show only plexiform lesions and no evidence of medial hypertrophy. Plexiform lesions, though not pathognomic, are characteristic of the sporadic and familial forms of severe PAH. Fibrinoid necrosis and arteritis have been described, but are rarely seen

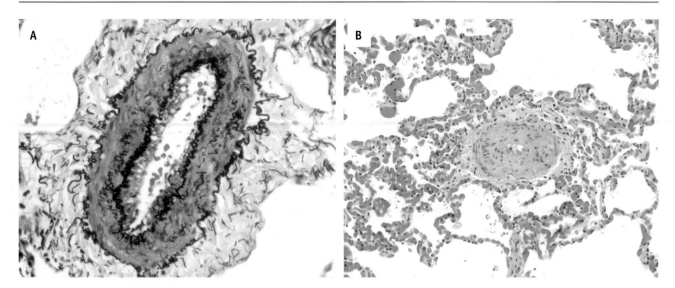

FIGURE 7-20

Pulmonary arterial hypertension: medial hypertrophy

(A) This Movat stain of a medium-sized pulmonary artery shows a thickened media between the internal and external elastic laminae. The intima also shows mild hyperplastic changes. **(B)** This smaller pulmonary artery shows significant medial hypertrophy, a common finding in severe pulmonary arterial hypertension. Note the mild intimal hyperplasia, a relatively nonspecific finding.

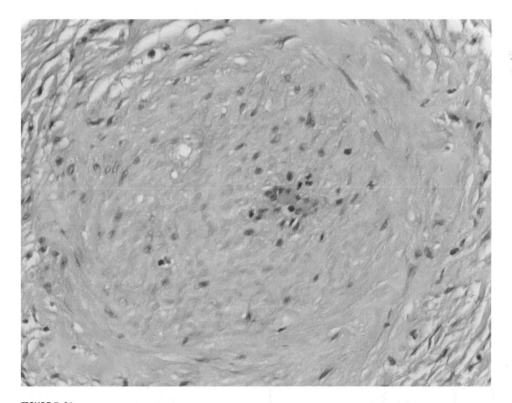

FIGURE 7-21

Severe pulmonary arterial hypertension: cellular intimal hyperplasia

This pulmonary artery shows near total obliteration of the lumen by a loose proliferation of intimal cells. Myxoid changes are noted.

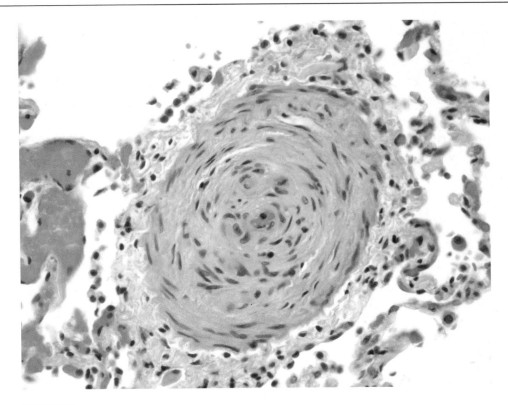

FIGURE 7-22

Severe pulmonary arterial hypertension: concentric laminar fibrosis

In contrast to the loose, myxoid intimal proliferation seen in Figure 7-21, concentric laminar fibrosis has a more "onionskin" appearance to the intima. This can be especially pronounced in cases of severe pulmonary arterial hypertension associated with collagen vascular diseases, especially CREST.

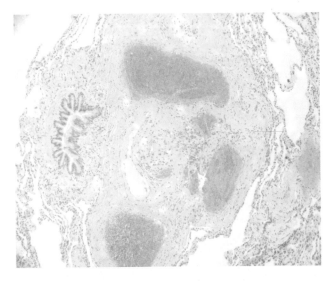

FIGURE 7-23

Severe pulmonary arterial hypertension: dilatation lesion

The pulmonary artery can be recognized by its location next to the airway (bronchiole). This pulmonary artery is markedly abnormal. The central portion of the lesion consists of a plexus of abnormal cells creating new lumens within the artery. Almost surrounding this plexus are markedly dilated channels filled with blood, the so-called dilatation lesions.

in treated patients. Thromboembolic lesions are now rarely seen in patients with severe pulmonary hypertension because these patients are usually effectively treated with anticoagulants.

In cases of PAH associated with collagen vascular disease, the vascular adventitia may be markedly thickened with collagen (Figure 7-25). In addition, these cases may show other features of collagen vascular disease, such as constrictive bronchiolitis and lymphoid aggregates with germinal centers.

DIFFERENTIAL DIAGNOSIS

The plexiform lesion is a unique vascular lesion. However, as described in the thromboembolism section, occasionally, recanalized vessels can be confused with plexiform lesions. In these cases, immunohistochemical stains for endothelial cells may help in the differentiation, as plexiform lesions often show a proliferation of endothelial cells within the lumen, while recanalized vessels show endothelial cell monolayer formation.

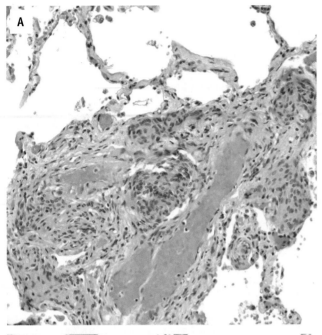

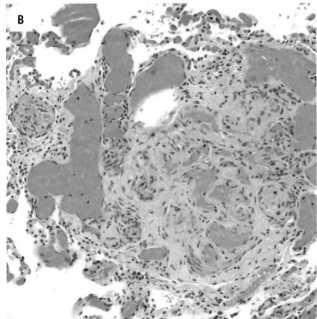

FIGURE 7-24

Severe pulmonary arterial hypertension: plexiform lesions
(A) shows a proliferation of the abnormal cells that comprise the plexiform lesions. This view shows why some, including this author, believe that these lesions are angioproliferative, neoplastic proliferations. **(B)** shows another example of a less cellular plexiform lesion. **(C)** demonstrates the strong immunoreactivity for Factor VIII-related antigen (von Willebrand factor) that can be seen in the cellular versions of the plexiform lesion.

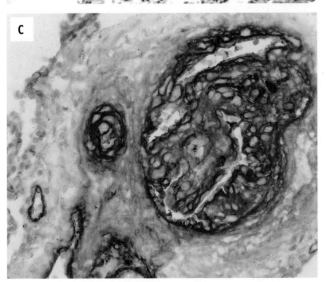

PROGNOSIS AND THERAPY

Since the symptoms of early pulmonary arterial hypertension are subtle and nonspecific, the disease is typically diagnosed late in its course. The natural history is one of relentless progression to right-sided heart failure, with a median survival of 2.8 years between diagnosis and death. Current treatment regimens have improved the survival considerably. Oxygen is used to treat patients with dyspnea and prevent further vasoconstriction from hypoxia. Patients have also been shown to derive benefit from long-term

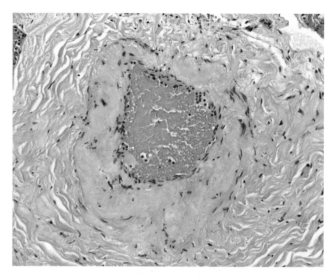

FIGURE 7-25

Severe pulmonary arterial hypertension: adventitial changes
There can be marked perivascular collagen deposition in the adventitia of vessels in patients with collagen vascular disease-associated pulmonary hypertension. This histologic feature is usually most prominent in the vessels of CREST/scleroderma patients.

PULMONARY ARTERIAL HYPERTENSION—FACT SHEET

Definition

▸ Pulmonary hypertension is subclassified into pulmonary arterial hypertension, pulmonary venous hypertension, pulmonary hypertension associated with hypoxemia, pulmonary hypertension due to chronic thrombotic and/or embolic disease, and miscellaneous
▸ Pulmonary arterial hypertension is defined as a mean resting pulmonary artery pressure greater than 25 mm Hg (greater than 30 mm Hg during exercise)

Incidence

▸ IPAH is rare (estimated annual incidence of 1 to 2 per million persons)
▸ Familial PAH is even rarer
▸ Secondary/associated cases are more common (up to 30% of patients with CREST, up to 5% of patients are with portal hypertension, 0.5% of HIV+ patients)

Mortality

▸ Untreated patients have a median survival of 2.8 years
▸ Treatment can increase survival in some patients

Gender, Race, and Age Distribution

▸ Idiopathic PAHS is more common in females (M:F = 1.0:1.7)
▸ Mean age of 36.4, but can occur at any age
▸ Individuals of all races are affected

Clinical Features

▸ Asymptomatic with mild elevations in pulmonary arterial pressures
▸ Increasing pulmonary arterial pressures lead to dyspnea, fatigue, syncope, lower extremity edema, and atypical chest pain
▸ Familial form is autosomal dominant

Radiologic Features

▸ Enlargement of central pulmonary arteries
▸ Rapid tapering of peripheral pulmonary arteries ("peripheral pruning")
▸ CT scan—29 mm main pulmonary artery

Prognosis and Therapy

▸ Poor prognosis, even with treatment
▸ Oxygen therapy, warfarin, oral vasodilators, and intravenous prostacyclin increase life expectancy; lung transplantation may be necessary
▸ Prognosis with lung transplantation—1 year, 73% survival; 5 year, 45% survival

---

PULMONARY ARTERIAL HYPERTENSION—PATHOLOGIC FEATURES

Gross Findings

▸ May show prominence and rigidity of pulmonary arteries and atherosclerosis of large pulmonary arteries
▸ Right heart enlargement and hypertrophy

Microscopic Findings

Pulmonary Arteries

▸ Plexiform lesions
▸ Medial hypertrophy
▸ Cellular intimal hyperplasia
▸ Concentric intimal fibrosis
▸ Dilatation lesions
▸ Rarely, fibrinoid necrosis

Pulmonary Arterioles

▸ Muscularization

Alveolar Parenchyma

▸ Usually normal, except in some cases of collagen vascular disease with other co-existing pathology

Pathologic Differential Diagnosis

▸ Recanalized vessels in chronic thromboembolic disease may mimic plexiform lesions
▸ Other causes of pulmonary hypertension may result in similar vascular changes.
▸ Plexiform lesions are unique to severe pulmonary arterial hypertension

anticoagulation. While oral vasodilators, such as calcium channel blockers, can provide long-term benefit, only 20% of patients with severe PAH respond to calcium channel blockers. Perhaps the most important advance in the treatment of severe IPAH has been the use of the prostacyclins, such as epoprostenol. Prostacyclins are potent, short-acting vasodilators and inhibitors of platelet aggregation that have improved exercise tolerance, quality of life, and long-term survival in patients. Despite the advancement in the medical management of severe PAH, many patients ultimately require lung transplantation. Lung transplant recipients with IPAH have a reported 1-year survival of 73% and a 5-year survival of 45%.

PULMONARY VENO-OCCLUSIVE DISEASE

CLINICAL FEATURES

Pulmonary veno-occlusive disease (PVOD) is a rare cause of pulmonary hypertension, with an estimated annual incidence of 0.1 to 0.2 cases per million persons. The disease may present at any age, but typically is seen in children and young adults. Adult cases show a male predominance (male: female = 2:1), whereas childhood cases show no gender predilection. The disease typically presents with symptoms of exertional dyspnea and fatigue. As the disease progresses, there are increasing symptoms of right-sided heart failure including exertional syncope, chest pain, cyanosis, and hepatosplenic congestion. Since these symptoms are also typical of severe PAH, there can be significant diagnostic confusion.

It appears that PVOD is a common pattern of injury from a wide variety of etiologies. Chemical and pharmaceutical exposures have been associated with the development of PVOD in a number of cases. Drugs with the highest association with PVOD include bleomycin, mitomycin, and carmustine. Additionally, some have suggested a greater risk in the setting of bone marrow transplantation. PVOD has also been associated with viral infections, toxins, radiation, autoimmune diseases, and pregnancy.

RADIOLOGIC FEATURES

Similar to severe IPAH, PVOD shows enlarged central pulmonary arteries on chest x-ray. Additional findings include interstitial pulmonary edema and, often, small bilateral pleural effusions. The radiographic findings are subtle and not often diagnostic.

PATHOLOGIC FEATURES

GROSS FINDINGS

The gross findings are not specific, but patchy congestion and a brown appearance from hemosiderin deposition are common.

MICROSCOPIC FINDINGS

PVOD is a disease affecting small veins and venules, with occasional involvement of the larger veins of the hilum. The process is primarily characterized by intimal fibrosis within pulmonary veins traversing the interlobular septa (Figure 7-26). The fibrosis is variably dense, and can appear very loose and edematous. The vein lumen is narrowed or occluded (Figure 7-27), and may show localized thrombosis or evidence of recanalization. Over time, veins may become arterialized with additional elastin fiber and smooth muscle, creating distinct internal and external laminae, and may be confused with pulmonary arteries if the anatomic location is not properly identified (Figure 7-5). Lymphatics are often dilated. Arteries and arterioles may show mild medial hypertrophy. Arterial thrombosis may also be seen in PVOD, a feature not shared with other forms of pulmonary venous hypertension. Plexiform lesions are not present. The surrounding lung parenchyma is edematous, and chronic hemorrhage is common. If the hemorrhage is longstanding, endogenous pneumoconiosis may develop (Figure 7-28). Foci of interstitial fibrosis may be seen. Some areas may show alveolar capillary proliferation in a pulmonary capillary hemangiomatosis-like pattern. In fact, some

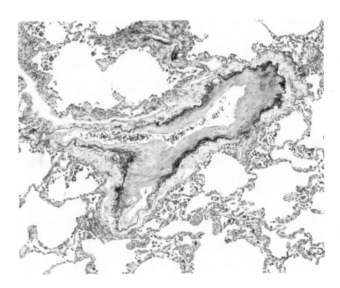

FIGURE 7-26
Pulmonary veno-occlusive disease
This elastic tissue stain highlights the intimal fibrosis of a pulmonary vein in an interlobular septum.

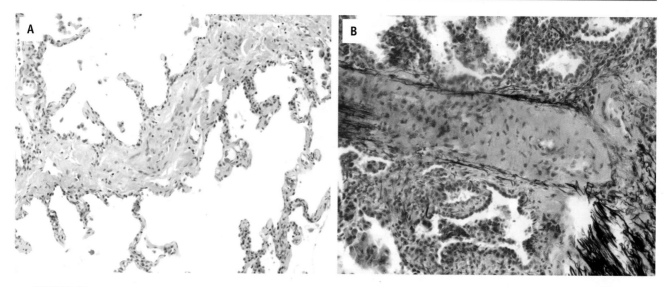

FIGURE 7-27

Pulmonary veno-occlusive disease
(A) Another example of PVOD illustrating the difficulty of identifying occluded veins on H & E stain. The vein, which is in the interlobular septum, is nearly occluded by fibrous tissue. **(B)** A Movat stain highlights the lumenal fibrous tissue. An elastic tissue stain can also often aid in identifying veins. The location of the vessel is also helpful in distinguishing veins from arteries, as some veins can become arterialized in PVOD.

believe that pulmonary capillary hemangiomatosis is a pattern of PVOD and not a distinct entity.

DIFFERENTIAL DIAGNOSIS

PVOD is a difficult entity to diagnose and is likely under-diagnosed. The pattern of lung involvement is so mixed that PVOD can easily be confused with entities

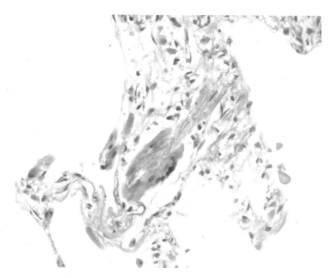

FIGURE 7-28

Pulmonary veno-occlusive disease: "endogenous pneumoconiosis"
A giant cell engulfs coated elastic fibers.

such as pulmonary capillary hemangiomatosis, chronic interstitial pneumonia, idiopathic pulmonary hemosiderosis, chronic passive congestion, lymphangiomatosis, and IPAH. Pulmonary capillary hemangiomatosis, although it may be a pattern of PVOD, lacks the venous changes of PVOD. Some cases of PVOD may have enough interstitial involvement that the vascular changes are overlooked and the interstitial component is over-diagnosed; thus, careful attention to vessels is needed. Both idiopathic pulmonary hemorrhage syndromes and chronic passive congestion lack the scarred veins of the interlobular septa that are classic for PVOD. As PVOD can cause lymphatic dilatation, lymphangiomatosis may be considered in the differential diagnosis, but elastic tissue stains will identify the abnormal veins. The arterial involvement in some cases of PVOD may raise the question of PAH; however, PVOD lacks plexiform lesions and the concentric laminar intimal fibrosis that are characteristic of severe PAH.

PROGNOSIS AND THERAPY

PVOD has a poor prognosis, with most patients dying within 2 years of diagnosis, unless lung transplantation is performed. Although various treatments have been tried, including vasodilators, anticoagulants, and immunosuppressive agents, success has been limited.

PULMONARY VENO-OCCLUSIVE DISEASE—FACT SHEET

Definition

» An occlusive disorder of the pulmonary veins associated with some drugs, bone marrow transplantation, viral infections, toxins, radiation, autoimmune diseases, and pregnancy

Incidence

» Rare (estimated annual incidence of 0.1 to 0.2 cases per million persons)

Mortality

» Most patients die within two years

Gender and Age Distribution

» Adults: M:F = 2:1
» Children: No gender predilection

Clinical Features

» Exertional dyspnea and fatigue
» With advancing disease, syncope, chest pain, cyanosis, and hepatosplenic congestion

Radiologic Features

» Enlarged central pulmonary arteries
» Interstitial pulmonary edema
» Small bilateral pleural effusions

Prognosis and Therapy

» Poor prognosis
» Only effective treatment is lung transplantation

PULMONARY VENO-OCCLUSIVE DISEASE—PATHOLOGIC FEATURES

Gross Findings

» Nonspecific, but may see patchy congestion and brown discoloration

Microscopic Findings

Pulmonary Veins and Venules

» Intimal fibrosis and occlusion of veins traversing interlobular septa
» Arterialization, including medial hypertrophy and acquisition of external elastic lamina

Pulmonary Lymphatics

» Often dilated

Pulmonary Arteries

» Mild medial hypertrophy
» Thrombosis

Pulmonary Arterioles

» Occasionally, muscularization

Pulmonary Parenchyma

» Edema and chronic hemorrhage
» Possibly, endogenous pneumoconiosis
» Occasionally, foci of interstitial fibrosis
» May have pulmonary capillary hemangio matosis-like areas

Pathologic Differential Diagnosis

» Pulmonary capillary hemangiomatosis
» Chronic interstitial pneumonias
» Idiopathic pulmonary hemosiderosis
» Chronic passive congestion
» Lymphangiomatosis
» Idiopathic pulmonary arterial hypertension

PULMONARY CAPILLARY HEMANGIOMATOSIS

Pulmonary capillary hemangiomatosis (PCH) is a locally aggressive vascular proliferation that is a rare cause of pulmonary hypertension.

CLINICAL FEATURES

PCH occurs in congenital, familial, and sporadic forms. Congenital PCH often occurs in association with other developmental abnormalities. The familial form has an autosomal recessive inheritance pattern, and is very rare, with only a single documented affected family. The more common spontaneous form of the disease, although de-

scribed in patients 6 to 71 years of age, typically presents in the 20-40 year age group with symptoms that mimic classic PAH. In fact, these cases are often initially diagnosed as IPAH or PVOD. However, the presence of hemoptysis or pleural effusions often raises the possibility of PCH. When clinically suspected, the lesion is typically diagnosed via pulmonary angiography. Biopsy can result in massive hemorrhage, and therefore the histologic findings are rarely seen except at autopsy.

RADIOLOGIC FEATURES

Similar to severe PAH and PVOD, chest x-rays show enlarged central pulmonary arteries. However, there are often multiple, bilateral, small, poorly defined nodular opacities on the CT scan that represent the scattered areas of capillary proliferation. Ventilation-perfusion scans may show matched defects.

PATHOLOGIC FEATURES

GROSS FINDINGS

The gross findings can be quite striking in PCH. There are nodular areas of red congestion that correspond to the CT scan images.

MICROSCOPIC FINDINGS

Microscopically, PCH is characterized by interstitial proliferations of small, capillary-sized vascular channels, often in a vaguely lobular and patchy distribution (Figure 7-29). There can be prominent vascular proliferations around bronchovascular bundles (Figure 7-30), as well as throughout the alveolar septa and pleura. Venous infiltration is associated with intimal fibrosis and secondary veno-occlusive disease. The alveolar septa are expanded, creating possible confusion with interstitial fibrosis. On high power, though, the expansion is by at least 2 layers of capillary-like, endothelial-lined vessels (Figure 7-31). The endothelial cells lining the capillary-like spaces are cytologically bland and stain with the usual endothelial markers, such as CD31, CD34, and Factor VIII-related antigen. Frequently, there are increased numbers of hemosiderin-laden macrophages in airspaces. True inter-stitial fibrosis with collagen deposition may be seen in cases with significant hemosiderosis.

DIFFERENTIAL DIAGNOSIS

The primary difficulty is differentiating PVOD from PCH. However, one should see widespread venous occlusion in PVOD versus rare veno-occlusive changes in PCH. Congestion (Figure 7-32) can lead to a prominence of alveolar capillaries, but the true proliferation of capillary-like vessels in PCH is not present in PVOD. Additionally, in PVOD, congestion is more diffuse, while it is patchy and nodular in PCH, showing intervening areas of normal, thin, and delicate septa. Patchy atelectasis can cause a low-power appearance similar to PCH, but high-power examination does not show the true proliferation of capillary-like vessels of PCH.

PROGNOSIS AND THERAPY

Overall, the prognosis of the disease is poor, with a median survival of 3 years from the time of diagnosis. The prostacyclins that are used to treat severe PAH are contraindicated in PCH because of the potential development of massive pulmonary edema. Lung transplantation remains the only effective therapy.

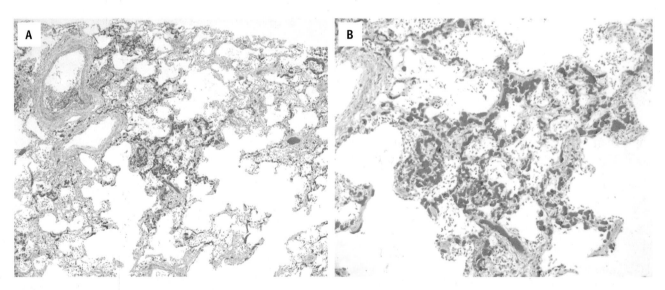

FIGURE 7-29

Pulmonary capillary hemangiomatosis

(A) This lower-power view shows the typical patchy, "congested" appearance of PCH. However, unlike typical congestion, this is a randomly distributed process throughout the lung parenchyma. **(B)** A higher power view of a lobular-appearing area of congestion. The alveolar septa are no longer lined by a single layer of capillaries, but are now expanded by multiple layers of capillary-sized vessels.

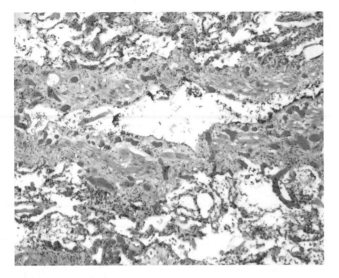

FIGURE 7-30

Pulmonary capillary hemangiomatosis
In this case of PCH, the abnormal proliferation of capillary-like vessels infiltrates a bronchiolar wall. Note that some of the alveolar septa adjacent to the bronchiole remain thin and delicate, without evidence of capillary proliferation.

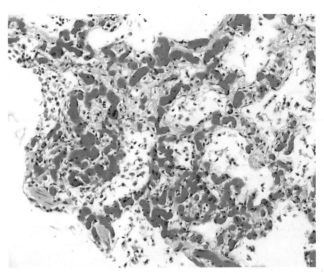

FIGURE 7-31

Pulmonary capillary hemangiomatosis
A high-power view highlights the multiple irregular capillary-like vessels that expand the alveolar septa.

PULMONARY CAPILLARY HEMANGIOMATOSIS—FACT SHEET

Definition
- Rare disease characterized by capillary-like vascular proliferations within the alveolar septa

Incidence
- Rare

Mortality
- Median survival of 3 years

Gender and Age Distribution
- No gender predilection
- Most common in 20- to 40-year age group

Clinical Features
- Congenital form is often associated with other developmental abnormalities
- Familial form is autosomal recessive
- Symptoms mimic classic PAH

Radiologic Features
- Enlarged central pulmonary arteries
- Multiple, bilateral, small, poorly defined nodules on CT scan
- Ventilation-perfusion scans show matched defects

Prognosis and Therapy
- Poor prognosis
- Only effective treatment is lung transplantation

LYMPHANGIOMATOSIS

Disorders of the lymphatics are rare in the lung, but the lymphatics play an important role in circulation, and their disruption can lead to serious pulmonary disease. The scarcity of lymphatic disorders often leads to misdiagnosis.

PULMONARY CAPILLARY HEMANGIOMATOSIS—PATHOLOGIC FEATURES

Gross Findings
- Patchy, nodular areas of congestion

Microscopic Findings
- Multifocal proliferations of capillary-like vessels within the alveolar septa
- May have prominent involvement of bronchovascular bundles and pleura
- Secondary pulmonary venous changes of intimal fibrosis and venous occlusion
- Abundant hemosiderin-laden macrophages are common
- Interstitial fibrosis may be seen if there is significant hemosiderosis

Pathologic Differential Diagnosis
- Pulmonary veno-occlusive disease
- Congestion
- Patchy atelectasis

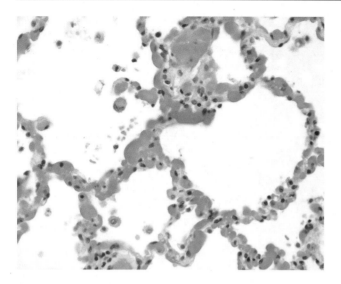

FIGURE 7-32
Congestion
In comparison to PCH, normal congested capillaries within the alveolar septa are a single layer in thickness.

CLINICAL FEATURES

Diffuse pulmonary lymphangiomatosis is rare. It is characterized by an abnormal number of anastomosing lymphatic spaces within the lymphatic routes of the lung (pleura, septa, and bronchovascular bundles). Lymphangiomatosis has been described in patients from birth to 80 years of age, but most patients present in childhood or early adulthood with respiratory distress, dyspnea, and/or wheezing. Males and females are equally affected. Chylous pleural and pericardial effusions are common. Many patients develop hemoptysis.

RADIOLOGIC FEATURES

Chest x-ray often shows bilateral interstitial infiltrates as well as pleural and/or pericardial effusions. CT scans demonstrate thickening of interlobular septa and bronchovascular bundles. There may be extensive involvement of mediastinal fat and perihilar regions.

PATHOLOGIC FEATURES

MICROSCOPIC FINDINGS

The histology is characterized by proliferation of thin-walled lymphatic channels along the lymphatic routes of the lung. Many of the channels are anastomosing; they may be irregular in shape and more numerous than normal (Figure 7-33). Mature smooth muscle may be present in the channel walls. The cells lining the lymphatic spaces are bland. If there is lymphangiomatous involvement of the airway submucosa, hemoptysis may result. Thus, hemosiderin-laden macrophages may be observed in adjacent lung parenchyma.

DIFFERENTIAL DIAGNOSIS

Diffuse pulmonary lymphangiomatosis may be difficult to distinguish from lymphangiectasia. However, lymphangiectasia is a dilatation of normal lymphatics, while lymphangiomatosis is a proliferation of abnormal anastomosing lymphatic spaces. Additionally, lymphangiomatosis may

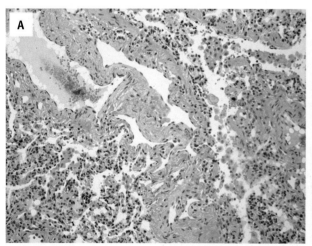
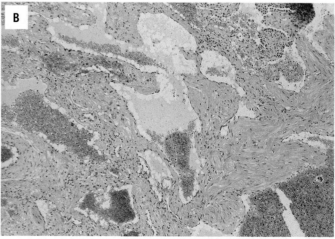

FIGURE 7-33
Lymphangiomatosis
(A) In this example of lymphangiomatosis, the interlobular septa show a proliferation of lymphatic spaces with some mature smooth muscle within their walls. **(B)** Abnormal anastomosing lymphatic channels highlight this disease. In this case, there is associated fibrosis. Both red blood cells and lymphatic fluid fill the abnormal spaces.

on occasion need to be distinguished from lymphangioleiomyomatosis (LAM). LAM is a proliferative smooth muscle process in the lung that occurs primarily in premenopausal women. The LAM cells are abnormal proliferations of smooth muscle cells that are HMB45-positive. Additionally, LAM lungs usually show prominent cystic changes, which are absent in lymphangiomatosis. The alveolar parenchyma is usually well preserved in lymphangiomatosis.

PROGNOSIS AND THERAPY

Diffuse pulmonary lymphangiomatosis is usually slowly progressive, but some patients may survive for years. Eventually, there is compression of adjacent structures by the proliferating lymphatic channels. Therapy is primarily palliative, aimed at controlling the recurrent chylous effusions.

ARTERIOVENOUS MALFORMATIONS

CLINICAL FEATURES

Most pulmonary arteriovenous malformations (AVMs) are congenital in origin and result when the blood vessels of the lung do not develop normally. There have been reports of acquired lesions, purportedly related to infections, neoplasma, or trauma. AVMs may be single or multiple. They are more common in the lower lobe. Many patients have hereditary hemorrhagic telangiectasia (Osler-Weber-Rendu disease). Patients with hereditary hemorrhagic telangiectasia (HHT) frequently have abnormal blood vessel development in the body, including the lungs, brain, nasal passages, liver, and gastrointestinal organs. Women are slightly more frequently affected than men. Patients with pulmonary AVM present with dyspnea (due to right-to-left shunting), cyanosis, and hemoptysis. Some patients are asymptomatic. Other clinical signs include clubbing and a murmur over the site of the malformation.

RADIOLOGIC FEATURES

Chest x-rays show one or more nodules or masses. CT imaging can often identify AVMs by the presence of a feeding artery and a draining vein. Pulmonary angiography can be used to define the size, number, and locations of the fistulae.

ARTERIOVENOUS MALFORMATION—FACT SHEET

Definition

➤ A tangled network of vessels that can be acquired, but is usually congenital

Incidence

➤ Rare, however may be present in up to 30% of patients with hereditary hemorrhagic telangiectasia

Morbidity and Mortality

➤ May develop paradoxical emboli
➤ Low mortality (0-15%), but morbidity may be significant and includes stroke, brain abscess, massive hemoptysis, infective endocarditis, and congestive heart failure

Gender and Age Distribution

➤ Slightly more common in women
➤ 10% identified in infancy or childhood, but increasing incidence with age

Clinical Features

➤ May be asymptomatic
➤ Patients with hereditary hemorrhagic telangiectasia and pulmonary AVMs have more symptomatology than those without hereditary hemorrhagic telangiectasia
➤ Dyspnea, cyanosis, hemoptysis
➤ Clubbing
➤ Murmur over the site of the malformation

Radiologic Features

➤ Nodules or masses
➤ CT imaging may identify feeding artery and draining vein
➤ Pulmonary angiography defines size, number, and location of fistulae

Prognosis and Therapy

➤ Prognosis worse in patients with hereditary hemorrhagic telangiectasia
➤ Asymptomatic patients may need no treatment
➤ Surgery and coil embolization may be performed in some patients

---

PATHOLOGIC FEATURES

GROSS FINDINGS

AVMs appear as single or multiple nodules consisting of tangled networks of dilated, wormlike channels that vary in size. Thrombi may be present.

MICROSCOPIC FINDINGS

AVMs consist of networks of anastomosing vessels of various sizes. The walls of the vessel are thickened to varying degrees. Often, they contain blood clots. The overlying visceral pleura may become thickened if the AVM abuts it.

ARTERIOVENOUS MALFORMATION—PATHOLOGIC FEATURES

Gross Findings

➤ Single or multiple nodules of tangled, dilated, wormlike channels of varying size. May have thrombosis

Pathologic Microscopic Findings

➤ Multiple or single plexiform mass of dilated, anastomosing vascular channels with little connective tissue stroma

---

PROGNOSIS AND THERAPY

Asymptomatic patients may need no treatment. However, most patients require either surgery to remove the abnormal vascular malformation or coil embolization of the AVM. Recurrent AVMs can be treated repeatedly with coil embolization. Some patients may develop paradoxical embolism, i.e., emboli from the lungs to the arms, legs, or brain.

DRUG-RELATED VASCULAR DISEASES

Drug-related vascular diseases are discussed in Chapter 19.

SUGGESTED READINGS

Edema

1. Andersson B, Waagstein F. Spectrum and outcome of congestive heart failure in a hospitalized population. *Am Heart J*. 1993;126:632-40.
2. Fraser RS, Muller NL, Pare PD. Pulmonary hypertension. In: *Fraser and Pare's Diagnosis of Diseases of the Chest*, 4th ed. Philadelphia: WB Saunders; 1999:1879-1945.
3. Lesur O, Berthiaume Y, Blaise G, et al. Acute respiratory distress syndrome: 30 years later. *Can Respir J*. 1999;6:71-86.
4. Ravin CE. Pulmonary vascularity: radiographic considerations. *J Thorac Imaging*. 1988;3:1-13.
5. Robbins, S.L. *Pathologic Basis of Disease*, 5 ed. Philadelphia, W.B. Saunders Co; 1994.
6. Wagenvoort CA, Mooi WJ. *Biopsy Pathology of the Pulmonary Vasculature*. London: Chapman and Hill; 1989.
7. Wagenvoort CA, Wagenvoort N. *Pathology of Pulmonary Hypertension*. New York: Wiley; 1977.

Thromboembolism

8. Augur WR, Fedullo PF, Moser KM. Chronic major-vessel thromboembolic pulmonary artery obstruction: appearance at angiography. *Radiology*. 1992;182:393-8.
9. Moser KM, Auguer WA, Fedulla PF: Chronic major vessel thromboembolic pulmonary hypertension. *Circulation*. 1990;81:1735-43.
10. Moser KM, Bloor CM. Pulmonary vascular lesions occurring in patients with chronic major vessel thromboembolic pulmonary hypertension. *Chest*. 1993;13:685-92.
11. Vichinsky E. Pulmonary hypertension in sickle cell disease. *New Engl J Med*. 2004;350:857-9.

12. Woodruff WW III, Hoeck BE, Chitwood WR Jr, Lyerly HK, Sabiston DC Jr, Chen JT. Radiographic findings in pulmonary hypertension from unresolved embolism. *AJR Am J Roentgenol*. 1985;144:681-6.

13. Yi ES, Kim H, Ahn H, et al. Distribution of obstructive intimal lesions and their cellular phenotypes in chronic pulmonary hypertension. A morphometric and immunohistochemical study. *Am J Respir Crit Care Med*. 2000;162:1577-86.

Pulmonary Hypertension

14. Bjornsson J, Edwards WD. Primary pulmonary hypertension: a histopathologic study of 80 cases. *Mayo Clin Proc*. 1985;60:16-25.

15. Cool CD, Stewart JS, Werahera P, et al. Three-dimensional reconstruction of pulmonary arteries in plexiform pulmonary hypertension using cell-specific markers: evidence for a dynamic and heterogeneous process of pulmonary endothelial cell growth. *Am J Pathol*. 1999;155:411-9.

16. D'Alonzo GE, Barst RJ, Ayres SM, et al. Survival in patients with primary pulmonary hypertension. Results from a national prospective registry. *Ann Intern Med*. 1991;115:34334-9.

17. Edwards WD. Pathology of pulmonary hypertension. *Cardiovasc Clin*. 1988;18:321-59.

18. Heath D, Edwards JE. The pathology of hypertensive pulmonary vascular disease: a description of six grades of structural changes in the pulmonary arteries with special reference to congenital cardiac septal defects. *Circulation*. 1958;18:533-47.

19. Hadengue A, Benhayoun MK, Lebrec D, et al. Pulmonary hypertension complicating portal hypertension: prevalence and relation to splanchnic hemodynamics. *Gastroenterology*. 1991;100:520-8.

20. Hoeper MM. Pulmonary hypertension in collagen vascular disease. *Eur Respir J*. 2002;19:571-6.

21. Lane KB, Machado RD, Pauciulo MW, et al. Heterozygous germline mutations in a TGF-beta receptor, BMPR2, are the cause of familial primary pulmonary hypertension. *Nat Genet*. 2000;26:81-4.

22. McLaughlin VV, Genthner DE, Panella MM, Rich S. Reduction in pulmonary vascular resistance with long-term epoprostenol (prostacyclin) therapy in primary pulmonary hypertension, *N Engl J Med*. 1998;338:273-7.

23. Rich, ed. Primary pulmonary hypertension. Executive summary from the world symposium, World Health Organization; September 6-10, 1998. Evian, France. Available at: www.who.int/ncd/cvd/pph.html. Accessed 1999.

24. Simonneau G, Galiè N, Rubin LJ, et al. Clinical classification of pulmonary hypertension. *J Am Coll Cardiol*. 2004;43(12 Suppl S):5S-12S.

25. Speich R, Jenni R, Opravil M, Pfab M, Russi EW. Primary pulmonary hypertension in HIV infection. *Chest*. 1991;100:1268–71.

Pulmonary Veno-Occlusive Disease

26. Carrington CB, Liebow AA. Pulmonary veno-occlusive disease. *Hum Pathol*. 1970;1:322-4.

27. Chawla SK, Kittle CF, Faber LP, Jensik RJ. Pulmonary venoocclusive disease. *Ann Thorac Surg*. 1976;22:249-53.

28. Mandel J, Mark EJ, Hales C. Pulmonary veno-occlusive disease. *Am J Respir Crit Care Med*. 2000;162:1964-73.

29. Palmer SM, Robinson LJ, Wang A, Gossage JR, Bashore T, Tapson VF. Massive pulmonary edema and death after prostacyclin infusion in a patient with pulmonary veno-occlusive disease. *Chest*. 1998;113:237-40.

30. Salzman D, Adkins DR, Craig F, Freytes C, LeMaistre CF. Malignancy-associated pulmonary veno-occlusive disease: report of a case following autologous bone marrow transplantation and review. *Bone Marrow Transplant*. 1996;18:755-60.

31. Veeraraghavan S, Koss MN, Sharma OP. Pulmonary veno-occlusive disease. *Curr Opin Pulm Med*. 1999;5:310-3.

32. Wagenvoort CA, Wagenvoort N, Takahashi T. Pulmonary veno-occlusive disease: involvement of pulmonary arteries and review of the literature. *Hum Pathol*. 1985;16:1033-41.

Pulmonary Capillary Hemangiomatosis

33. Almagro P, Julia J, Sanjaume M, et al. Pulmonary capillary hemangiomatosis associated with primary pulmonary hypertension. *Medicine*. 2002;81:417-24.

34. Faber CN, Yousem SA, Dauber JH, Griffith BP, Hardesty RL, Paradis IL. Pulmonary capillary hemangiomatosis: a report of three cases and a review of the literature. *Am Rev Respir Dis*. 1989;140:808-13.

35. Langleben D, Heneghan JM, Batten AP, et al. Familial pulmonary capillary hemangiomatosis resulting in primary pulmonary hypertension. *Ann Intern Med*. 1988;109:106-9.

36. Tron V, Magee F, Wright JL, Colby T, Churg A. Pulmonary capillary hemangiomatosis. *Hum Pathol*. 1986;17:1144-9.

37. Wagenvoort CA, Beetstra A, Spijker J. Capillary haemangiomatosis of the lung. *Histopathology*. 1978;2:401-6.

Lymphangiomatosis

38. Faul JL, Berry GJ, Colby TV, et al. Thoracic lymphangiomas, lymphangiectasis, lymphangiomatosis, and lymphatic dysplasia syndrome. *Am J Resp Crit Care Med*. 2000;161:1037-46.

39. Hillerdal G. Chylothorax and pseudochylothorax. *Eur Respir J*. 1997;10:1157-62.

40. Hilliard RI, McKendry JB, Phillips MJ. Congenital abnormalities of the lymphatic system: a new clinical classification. *Pediatrics*. 199;86:988-94.

41. Tazelaar HD, Kerr D, Yousem SA, Saldan MJ, Langston C, Colby TV. Diffuse pulmonary lymphangiomatosis. *Hum Pathol*. 1993;24:1313-22.

Pulmonary Arteriovenous Malformation

42. Burke CM, Safai C, Nelson DP, Raffin TA. Pulmonary arteriovenous malformation: a critical update. *Am Rev Respir Dis*. 1986;134:334-9.

43. Coley SC, Jackson JE. Pulmonary arteriovenous malformations. *Clin Radiol*. 1998;53: 396-404.

44. Langston C, Askin FB. Pulmonary disorders in the neonate, infant, and child. In: Thurlbeck WM, Churg AM, eds. *Pathology of the Lung*, 2nd ed. New York: Thieme; 1995;151-194.

45. Pick A, Deschamps C, Stanson AW. Pulmonary arteriovenous fistula: presentation, diagnosis, and treatment. *World J Surg*. 1999;23:1118-22.

8 Vasculitides and Other Causes of Pulmonary Hemorrhage

Andre L. Moreira • *William D. Travis*

- Introduction
- Wegener's Granulomatosis
- Churg-Strauss Syndrome
- Microscopic Polyangiitis
- Necrotizing Sarcoid Granulomatosis
- Antibasement Membrane Antibody Disease (Goodpasture's Syndrome)
- Idiopathic Pulmonary Hemosiderosis
- Behçet's Disease
- Other Uncommon Pulmonary Vasculitides
  Collagen Vascular Disease-Associated Vasculitis
  Polyarteritis Nodosa
  Henoch-Schönlein Purpura
  Vasculitis Associated with Cryoglobulinemia
  Takayasu's Arteritis
  Giant Cell Arteritis

The diagnosis and classification of pulmonary vasculitis is a challenging topic, because all types of pulmonary vasculitis are, in fact, pulmonary manifestations of systemic diseases. Extrapulmonary involvement is, in some cases, a significant source of morbidity and mortality. To further complicate matters, there is considerable overlap in the histological patterns of manifestations from different systemic vasculitis syndromes, as well as secondary inflammatory processes that affect blood vessels as seen in infectious granulomatous diseases and sarcoidosis.

To the pathologist, the difficulty in the interpretation of a surgical biopsy for the diagnosis of pulmonary vasculitis is contributed to by the fact that careful correlation between clinical, radiographic, and pathological features, rather than histological interpretation alone, is necessary to reach the correct diagnosis. In many cases, the biopsy is obtained early in the process when not all the classical criteria are present in the specimen or the

biopsy is taken after some course of treatment, which can modify the histological appearance of lesions. In these two circumstances, a strong clinical suspicion can help lead to the correct diagnosis. In addition, the rarity of pulmonary vasculitis syndromes prevents most pathologists from acquiring critical experience with the subtle criteria that are helpful in the distinction of these pathologic entities.

There are three major idiopathic vasculitis syndromes that commonly affect the lungs: Wegener's granulomatosis, Churg-Strauss syndrome, and microscopic polyangiitis. Their pathologic, clinical, and radiographic features will be the focus of this chapter. Other less common vasculitides and secondary conditions that affect the pulmonary blood vessels will be discussed briefly, mainly as they relate to the differential diagnosis of the three main syndromes named above.

WEGENER'S GRANULOMATOSIS

Wegener's granulomatosis (WG) is a systemic process characterized by necrotizing granulomatous vasculitis that primarily affects the upper and lower respiratory tract and the kidney. The pathogenesis of WG has not been fully elucidated, but there is evidence for an immunologically mediated process involving a T helper 1-like reaction. The presence of anti-neutrophil cytoplasmic antibodies in the serum from patients suffering from this condition raises the possibility of an autoimmune process. The pathogenesis is characterized by endothelial cell injury leading to activation of inflammatory mediators and accumulation of inflammatory cells (monocytes, neutrophils, eosinophils) producing vasculitis and other inflammatory lesions.

CLINICAL FEATURES

Wegener's granulomatosis is a rare condition that seems to have a peak incidence between the fourth and sixth decades of life with a slight male predominance.

130

The disease most frequently affects the upper and lower respiratory tracts and the kidneys, although it can affect any part of the body. The classical clinical triad of WG includes sinusitis, pneumonia, and glomerulonephritis. Most patients will complain of epistaxis and lower respiratory tract symptoms such as cough, chest pain, or dyspnea. In many patients, the clinical presentation will also include hypertension and edema, which are indications of renal involvement.

Laboratory tests are not specific and show results consistent with a chronic process, such as normochromic normocytic anemia, elevated sedimentation rates, and elevated C reactive protein. Urinalysis frequently reveals microhematuria and proteinuria.

The laboratory diagnosis of vasculitis has been revolutionized by the advent of the anti-neutrophil cytoplasmic antibody (ANCA) test, discussed more thoroughly in a later chapter. The two most common patterns of ANCA reactivity are based on the immunofluorescence patterns of cytoplasmic staining (c-ANCA) or perinuclear staining (p-ANCA). Proteinase 3 is the usual target antigen in c-ANCA reactivity, and myeloperoxidase is the usual target antigen in p-ANCA reactivity. In WG, c-ANCA is found in approximately 90% of cases. However, c-ANCA is not specific for WG. Cases of WG with a positive p-ANCA or even negative ANCA tests have been described. The latter is more commonly seen in indolent or previously treated disease, or in limited disease. The interpretation of an ANCA test should take into consideration the clinical context of a given patient, and the test should not be considered as an absolute parameter for the diagnosis of WG.

RADIOLOGIC FEATURES

Most patients affected by WG present with multiple bilateral opacities easily seen on computed tomography (CT) scan of the chest, with well marginated nodules. The lower lobes are involved most frequently. The nodules can present with spiculated margins mimicking a neoplasm, and very often show cavitation with thick walls. Careful examination of the CT scan can reveal an association with a feeding vessel. Lesions can wax and wane over time.

In some patients, pulmonary hemorrhage can be the only manifestation seen, and will appear radiographically as diffuse infiltrates or air space opacities. Another common finding in WG is the presence of a wedge-shaped peripheral opacity mimicking a pulmonary infarct. Rarely, the disease manifests as a solitary cavitary nodule. The diagnosis of WG in this setting should be made with caution because most solitary cavitary nodules are infectious in etiology. A strong clinical suspicion, as well as histological support, is necessary to establish the diagnosis of WG in this context.

PATHOLOGIC FEATURES

The histological manifestations of WG are varied but are composed of three main elements that are very helpful in the histological diagnosis of this entity. They include vasculitis, necrosis, and inflammatory background.

The vasculitis involves medium-sized and small veins and arteries. Capillaritis is also frequently present. In general, vasculitis is best appreciated in the parenchyma away from the other inflammatory lesions. The vasculitis is often focal with eccentric involvement of the vessel wall (Figure 8-1), or it can be limited to the endothelium and subendothelial spaces (Figure 8-2). The inflammatory cells that produce the vasculitis can include lymphocytes, macrophages, plasma cells, and occasionally eosinophils. A granulomatous reaction is often present within the vessel wall, and in some cases it can obscure and destroy the vessel. An elastic stain can be helpful for identification of the vessel wall within the granulomatous inflammation (Figure 8-3).

In WG, granulomas are generally poorly formed or may show palisading histiocytes (Figure 8-4). Well-formed sarcoid-like granulomas are uncommon in WG, and their presence should alert one to the possibility of other diagnoses. In these cases, an infectious process or necrotizing sarcoidosis should be considered in the differential diagnosis. In contrast to an infectious or sarcoid granuloma, the lesions in WG do not have a clear demarcation from the adjacent uninvolved pulmonary parenchyma, which is an important criterion for the differential diagnosis of these pathological entities. In WG, there is always an inflammatory overflow that extends beyond the area of granuloma (Figure 8-5).

The necrosis in WG is very often described as geographic and basophilic (Figures 8-5 and 8-6) It is considered geographic because it is irregular and is not confined to the center of the granulomatous process; in fact, it is thought to represent progressive collagenous necrosis and not infarct-like necrosis. The necrosis is considered basophilic because, contrary to the caseating necrosis of infectious granulomatous diseases, the area of necrosis in WG is rich in cellular debris and neutrophils, which imparts a "dirty" appearance.

Small foci of collagen necrosis can be seen around involved blood vessels or within the pulmonary parenchyma. The necrosis is characterized by a small collection of neutrophils (microabscess) around an area of dense eosinophilic collagen fibers (Figure 8-7).

Another helpful characteristic of the inflammatory infiltrate in WG is the presence of scattered multinucleated giant cells (Figure 8-8). They can be seen within the vasculitic process or within the background inflammatory infiltrate.

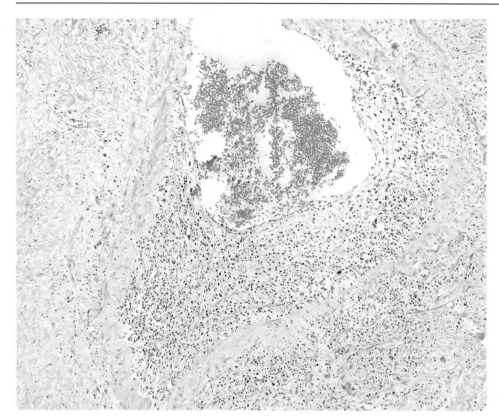

FIGURE 8-1

Wegener's granulomatosis: vasculitis

The inflammatory process is very often eccentric with partial involvement of the vessel wall. Note the thickened intima and transmural involvement of this medium-sized blood vessel.

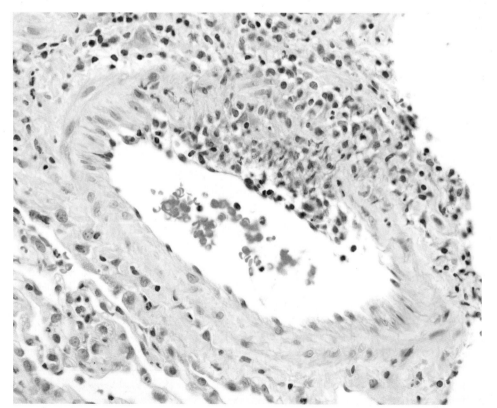

FIGURE 8-2

Wegener's granulomatosis: vasculitis

This is focal subendothelial involvement of a small blood vessel by a mixed inflammatory infiltrate.

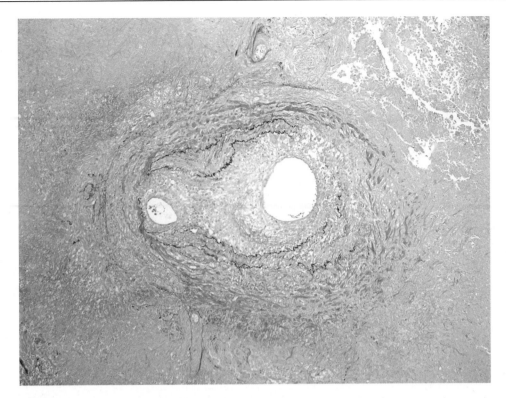

FIGURE 8-3
Wegener's granulomatosis: vasculitis (elastic stain)
Note that the inflammatory infiltrate is centered on a blood vessel, and there is destruction of elastic fibers.

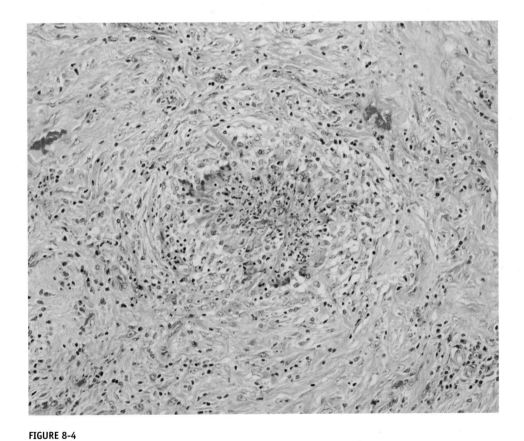

FIGURE 8-4
Wegener's granulomatosis: granuloma
The granuloma shows palisading histiocytes with no distinct border separating it from the surrounding parenchyma.
Note the presence of neutrophils in the necrotic center.

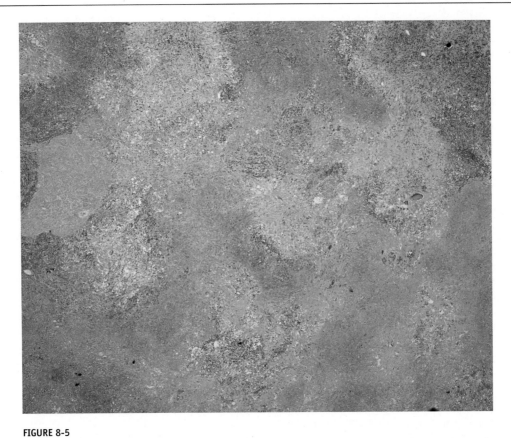

FIGURE 8-5

Wegener's granulomatosis: inflammation and necrosis
Note the poorly formed granulomas, the lack of circumscription to the inflammatory infiltrate, and the presence of basophilic geographic necrosis.

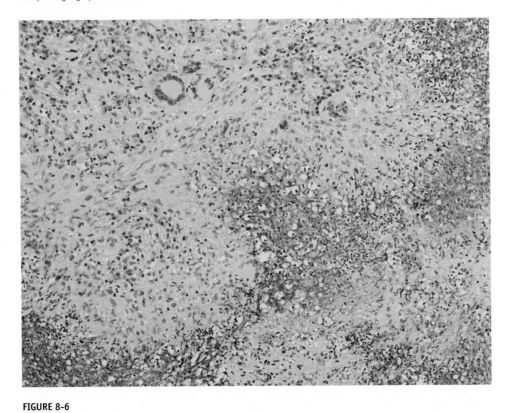

FIGURE 8-6

Wegener's granulomatosis: inflammation and necrosis
Note the palisading histocytes and geographic necrosis that is irregular and not in the center of the granulomatous reaction. Multinucleated giant cells are seen. The necrotic material is composed of cell debris and neutrophils.

Within the inflammatory background, areas of organizing pneumonia and hemosiderin-laden macrophages can also be found. The latter is an indication of chronic hemorrhage due to the vasculitic process (Figure 8-9). Bronchitis, bronchiolitis, and endogenous lipoid pneumonia can be observed.

The lung biopsy findings from patients with WG may not show the classical histological findings, especially if the biopsy is taken very early in the course of the disease or following treatment. Interstitial fibrosis sometimes with scattered giant cells, or bronchial and bronchiolar scarring or cicatricial vascular changes can be seen in biopsies of patients who received treatment.

DIFFERENTIAL DIAGNOSIS

Lymphomatoid granulomatosis (LYG) is an important consideration in the differential diagnosis of WG. The two entities have similar clinical and demographic features. Histologically, LYG is characterized by angiitis (vasculitis), poorly formed granulomatous inflammation, and a polymorphic lymphoid population. The difference between LYG and WG is in the cellular composition of the infiltrate. The former is composed of a mixture of small and large atypical lymphocytes, whereas in WG the infiltrate is composed of a mixture of acute and chronic inflammatory cells. Also, in WG, the inflammation causes necrosis of the vascular wall, whereas in LYG, the lymphocytes infiltrate the walls of the blood vessels. Immunostains for lymphoid markers usually reveal a T-cell rich B-cell lymphoma phenotype in LYG, discussed more extensively in another chapter.

Churg-Strauss syndrome and microscopic polyangiitis differ from WG in their clinical and laboratory features, as well as their histology. These disorders are discussed later in this chapter. Bronchocentric granulomatosis (BCG) also enters into the differential diagnosis of WG, since WG may have a bronchocentric pattern of lung involvement, and BCG may show secondary involvement of blood vessels. Systemic involvement is seen in WG, however, and a positive ANCA test also favors WG.

Necrotizing sarcoid granulomatosis is characterized by confluent areas of non-necrotizing granulomatous inflammation with extensive coagulative necrosis. Contrary to WG, the granulomas in this disease are well formed (sarcoid-like), there is a clear demarcation

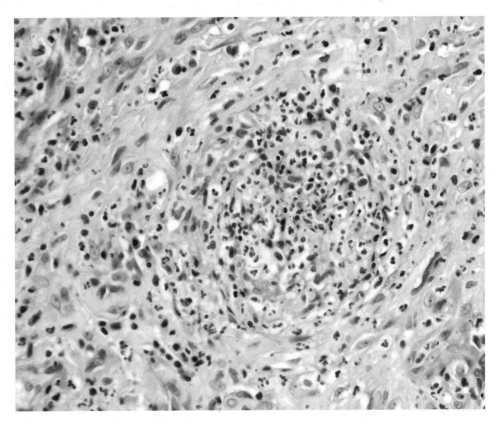

FIGURE 8-7

Wegener's granulomatosis: microabscess
Small collection of neutrophils and eosinophils around an area of eosinophilic collagen fibers.

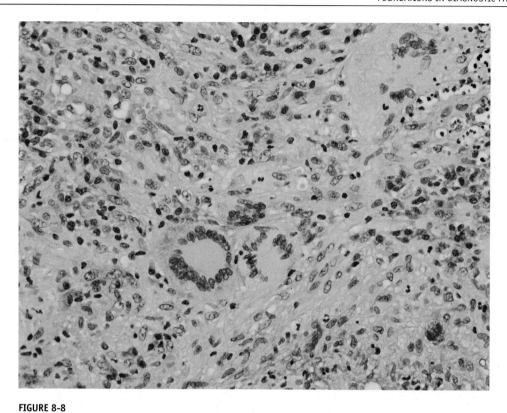

FIGURE 8-8

Wegener's granulomatosis: multinucleated giant cells
These cells can be seen in association with the granulomatous inflammation or within the background inflammatory infiltrate. Note that some of these multinucleated giant cells can have a bizarre appearance (upper right corner).

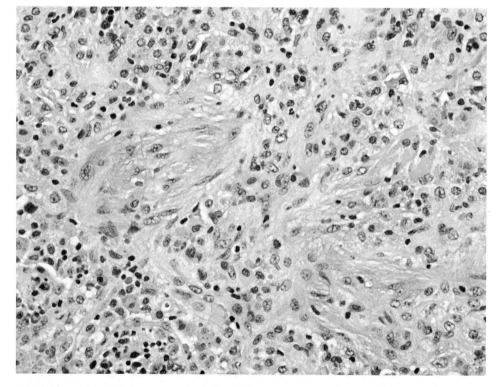

FIGURE 8-9

Wegener's granulomatosis: organizing pneumonia
Fibroblastic plugs fill alveolar spaces and hemosiderin-laden macrophages are seen in the inflamed and fibrotic tissue. The presence of hemosiderin-laden macrophages is a consequence of earlier hemorrhage due to capillaritis.

between granulomatous and normal pulmonary parenchyma, and the ANCA test is negative.

The differential diagnosis of WG and infectious granulomatous inflammation has been already discussed. An important point to keep in mind, however, is that whenever a granulomatous inflammatory process is identified in a biopsy, special stains to rule out the presence of microorganisms must be performed, even if WG is considered clinically and histologically.

Rheumatoid nodules usually occur in patients with a known diagnosis of rheumatoid arthritis, and lack the geographic necrosis and microabscess formation seen in WG.

Other causes of diffuse pulmonary hemorrhage with small vessel vasculitis (capillaritis) may also be considered in the differential diagnosis, if these findings are observed. These include drug-induced vasculitis, collagen vascular disease-associated vasculitis, cryoglobulinemia, antiphospholipid antibody syndrome, and other rarer processes. These processes lack the other inflammatory lesions of WG, and often have other associated laboratory abnormalities that can help to suggest the correct etiology.

WEGENER'S GRANULOMATOSIS—FACT SHEET

Definition

▸ Systemic necrotizing granulomatous vasculitis of unknown etiology

Incidence

▸ Rare (estimated incidence in the USA is 0.3 per million persons)
▸ Most common systemic vasculitis to involve the lung (90% of cases show pulmonary involvement)

Mortality

▸ Fatal disease if untreated
▸ Most patients die of renal or pulmonary insufficiency

Gender, Race, and Age Distribution

▸ Peak incidence is between the fourth and sixth decades (mean age, 50 years)
▸ Rare in children
▸ Slight male predominance
▸ No racial predilection

Clinical Features

▸ Classical triad includes sinusitis, pneumonia, and glomerulonephritis
▸ Most common signs and symptoms: epistaxis (sinusitis), cough, chest pain, dyspnea (pneumonia), hypertension and edema (glomerulonephritis), arthralgias, fever, cutaneous lesions, and weight loss
▸ 90% of patients have a positive c-ANCA test result

Radiologic Features

▸ Multifocal pulmonary nodular opacities that wax and wane and can be associated with a feeding vessel
▸ More frequent in the lower lobes
▸ Cavitation occurs in approximately 25 to 50% of cases
▸ Diffuse air space disease may be seen, corresponding to pulmonary hemorrhage
▸ A solitary nodule is rare

Prognosis and Therapy

▸ Treatment includes immunosuppressive drugs (corticosteroids and cyclophosphamide are the most commonly used drugs)
▸ 90% of affected patients respond to treatment
▸ 75% of patients have a complete remission
▸ Relapse rate is approximately 50%

WEGENER'S GRANULOMATOSIS—PATHOLOGIC FEATURES

Gross Findings

▸ Lung can be dark red due to pulmonary hemorrhage
▸ Solid nodular zones of consolidation with punctuate or geographic necrosis are often seen

Microscopic Findings

▸ Classical triad includes vasculitis, necrosis, and inflammatory background
▸ Vasculitis usually involves medium- and small-sized vessels
▸ Poorly formed granulomas and/or mixed inflammatory cell infiltrates permeate blood vessel walls
▸ Capillaritis (neutrophilic infiltrate within the alveolar wall) is often seen and accompanied by hemorrhage
▸ Necrosis is geographic and basophilic and contains neutrophils
▸ The inflammatory background is extensive and composed of macrophages, plasma cells, lymphocytes, neutrophils, and multinucleated giant cells
▸ Other abnormalities can include bronchitis, bronchiolitis, endogenous lipoid pneumonia, and organizing pneumonia
▸ There is a continuum between the areas of granulomatous reaction and the inflammatory background and there is no sharp demarcation between normal and affected lung
▸ Post-treatment changes include: interstitial fibrosis with scattered giant cells, bronchial/bronchiolar scarring, and cicatricial vascular changes

Ancillary Tests

▸ Elastic stain will highlight the angiocentric nature of the lesions
▸ Special stains to rule out microorganisms must be done with any granulomatous inflammation; no microorganisms are seen in WG

Pathologic Differential Diagnosis

▸ Lymphomatoid granulomatosis
▸ Churg-Strauss syndrome
▸ Microscopic polyangiitis
▸ Necrotizing sarcoid granulomatosis
▸ Infectious granulomatous inflammation
▸ Rheumatoid nodules
▸ Bronchocentric granulomatosis
▸ Other pulmonary hemorrhage syndromes

PROGNOSIS AND THERAPY

The use of corticosteroid and other immunosuppressive drugs such cyclophosphamide has revolutionized the natural course of WG. Before the advent of these drugs, WG was a fatal disease, with 90% of affected patients dying within 2 years of diagnosis. With therapy, approximately 90% of patients respond to treatment. 75% of these patients experience complete remission of the disease within a year of therapy. Even with a good response to therapy, most patients sustain sequelae of the disease or treatment, however. The relapse rate is high; for approximately 50% of affected patients, a second course of treatment is required.

The addition of trimethoprim-sulfamethoxazole to the treatment regimen has been suggested to reduce the relapse rate of patients in remission.

CHURG-STRAUSS SYNDROME

Churg-Strauss Syndrome (CSS) is a systemic disorder characterized by asthma, peripheral eosinophilia, and systemic vasculitis. CSS is basically a clinical entity, and its diagnosis is established in most cases based on clinical and laboratory findings. The parameters for the clinical diagnosis of CSS are: (1) asthma or history of allergy; (2) peripheral eosinophilia greater than 10% of white blood cell count; (3) neuropathy; (4) non-fixed radiographic pulmonary infiltrates; (5) sinusitis; and (6) a biopsy containing extravascular eosinophils. The combination of any four of these parameters is sufficient for the clinical diagnosis of CSS.

CLINICAL FEATURES

Although the true incidence of CSS is unclear, it most commonly affects patients between the third and fifth decades of life. It is usually seen in patients with asthma, some of whom have inadequate use of corticosteroids or a history of corticosteroid tapering. CSS progresses through three clinical phases: prodromic, vasculitic, and post-vasculitic. In the prodromic phase, the patient experiences peripheral blood eosinophilia and infiltration of eosinophils in the tissues. In the lung, this phase is characterized by the presence of eosinophilic pneumonia, with infiltrates of eosinophils in alveolar spaces. Another common site for eosinophilic tissue infiltration is the gastrointestinal tract. The vasculitic phase is characterized by systemic signs and symptoms such as neuropathy and cutaneous leukocytoclastic vasculitis. The post-vasculitic phase is often characterized by neuropathy. Cardiac in-

volvement is seen in approximately 47% of patients with CSS, a striking difference from other systemic vasculitides that involve the lung. The cardiac involvement can manifest as cardiac failure, pericarditis, and myocardial infarction. Contrary to Wegener's granulomatosis, renal involvement in CSS is less frequent and less severe.

There is no laboratory test that is specific for CSS. Apart from peripheral blood and bronchoalveolar lavage fluid eosinophilia, patients show nonspecific laboratory abnormalities such as chronic normocytic-normochromic anemia and elevated sedimentation rate. The ANCA test is often positive in the vasculitic phase, and will usually show the p-ANCA pattern (70% of the cases), although a c-ANCA pattern has also been demonstrated.

RADIOLOGIC FEATURES

The radiologic findings in CSS are nonspecific. The disease can manifest with multifocal parenchymal consolidation or nodules that wax and wane or change location. The consolidation is generally in the periphery of the lung, but can be widespread.

PATHOLOGIC FEATURES

The histopathological findings in biopsies of patients with CSS depend on the phase of the disease. In the prodromic phase, eosinophilic pneumonia is the most common finding (Figure 8-10). Extravasation of eosinophils in other anatomic sites or eosinophilic bronchitis can also be seen.

In the vasculitic phase, besides eosinophilic pneumonia, eosinophilic granulomas (allergic granulomas) and eosinophilic vasculitis can be seen. The granulomas are extravascular and consist of a necrotic center with eosinophils surrounded by palisading histiocytes (Figure 8-11). Multinucleated giant cells can be present. The vasculitis involves arteries, veins, and capillaries (Figure 8-12). The inflammatory infiltrate can include lymphocytes, neutrophils, plasma cells, and epithelioid macrophages, in addition to eosinophils. Diffuse pulmonary hemorrhage can occur in association with eosinophilic capillaritis.

Eosinophils are very sensitive to corticosteroid therapy. Therefore, in patients who have been treated with corticosteroids, the characteristic eosinophils can be absent or reduced in numbers, and may appear fragmented. These degenerative changes can make histologic interpretation more difficult, and it is possible to be misled into interpreting degenerated eosinophils as neutrophils. However, the larger size of the nuclear lobes in eosinophils as compared to neutrophils is a helpful clue, as well as the more eosinophilic appearance of the background as compared to the more basophilic

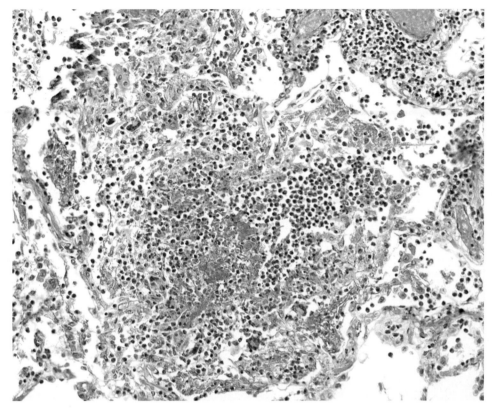

FIGURE 8-10

Churg-Strauss syndrome: eosino-philic pneumonia
Inflammatory infiltrate composed pre-dominantly of eosinophils in alveolar spaces.

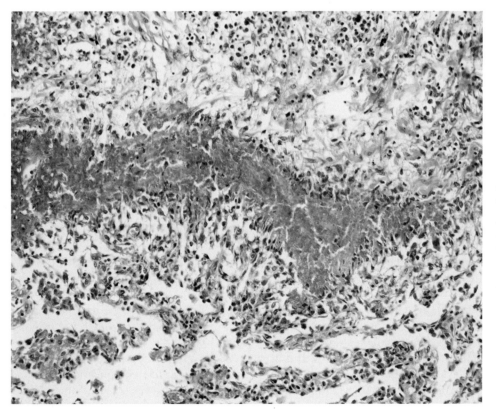

FIGURE 8-11

Churg-Strauss syndrome: allergic granuloma
Parenchymal granuloma with palisad-ing histiocytes and necrotic center composed predominantly of necrotic eosinophils.

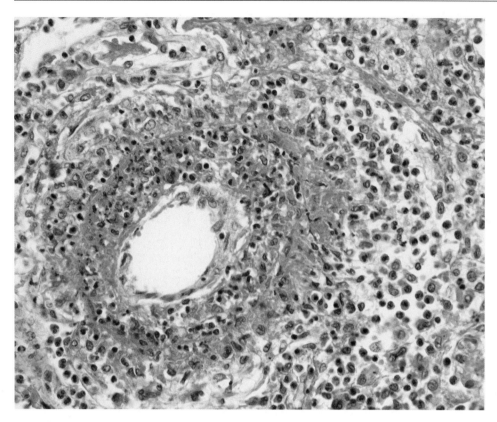

FIGURE 8-12

Churg-Strauss syndrome: vasculitis
Small-vessel vasculitis with fibrinoid necrosis and eosinophilic infiltrate.

appearance of the necrotic/inflammatory background with degenerating neutrophils.

DIFFERENTIAL DIAGNOSIS

The differential diagnosis of CSS includes other vasculitides and other pathological entities characterized by the presence of eosinophils.

CSS is distinguished from Wegener's granulomatosis by the clinical presentation, histopathology, and usual presence of c-ANCA (as opposed to p-ANCA in most patients with CSS). Although eosinophils can be seen in WG, they are not the predominant cells that compose the inflammatory infiltrate, and the range of histologic findings differs as discussed above. The ANCA test, although not specific, can be helpful in the differentiation between the two entities. Clinically, CSS is characterized by a spectrum of manifestations that differ from those of WG, and most patients have peripheral blood eosinophilia. In contrast, renal involvement is much more common in WG.

Eosinophilic pneumonia caused by other entities such as parasitic infections or drugs, must be differentiated

from CSS. Clinical information indicating a systemic process is helpful for making the correct diagnosis, since eosinophilic pneumonia can be an early manifestation of CSS (prodromic phase). Observation of vasculitis is also helpful for supporting a diagnosis of CSS.

Allergic bronchopulmonary fungal disease (ABPFD) can show eosinophilic pneumonia and bronchocentric granulomas. Unlike CSS, in ABPFD signs and symptoms of systemic vasculitis are absent.

PROGNOSIS AND THERAPY

Patients with CSS can usually be treated successfully with corticosteroids. Other immunosuppressive agents such as cyclophosphamide can also be used to prevent irreversible organ injury in patients who do not respond to corticosteroids.

If untreated, CSS is a fatal disease. Most patients who die of the disease have cardiac complications such as myocardial infarction and cardiac insufficiency. Other less common causes of death include renal failure, cerebral hemorrhage, respiratory failure, and gastrointestinal perforation.

CHURG-STRAUSS SYNDROME-FACT SHEET

Definition
»» Systemic disorder characterized by asthma, peripheral blood eosinophilia, and systemic vasculitis

Incidence
»» Occurs almost exclusively in patients with asthma or allergic rhinitis
»» The true incidence of CSS is unclear

Morbidity and Mortality
»» Cardiac involvement is the most common cause of death
»» Early recognition of the syndrome with early treatment is important to prevent irreversible organ injury

Age Distribution
»» Peak incidence is between the fourth and fifth decades of life

Clinical Features
»» The diagnosis is clinical and must include at least four of the following parameters: asthma, peripheral blood eosinophilia (10% of WBC), neuropathy, radiographic pulmonary infiltrate, sinusitis, and evidence of extravasated eosinophils in tissues
»» Common organs involved include the lungs, heart, central nervous system, kidney, gastrointestinal tract, and skin; renal involvement is less common than in Wegener's granulomatosis and microscopic polyangiitis
»» Three clinical phases: prodromic, vasculitic, and post-vasculitic
»» Symptoms depend upon the organ system(s) involved and the phase of the disease
»» Patients usually show a positive p-ANCA test result (70%)

Radiologic Features
»» Multifocal parenchymal consolidation that changes in location and appearance
»» Very often the consolidation shows a peripheral distribution
»» Cavitation is rare

Prognosis and Therapy
»» Generally has a good prognosis, but cardiac and severe gastrointestinal involvement are associated with a poor prognosis
»» Most patients with CSS show a good response to corticosteroids.
»» Cyclophosphamide is added in cases refractory to corticosteroids or with involvement of more than one organ system
»» The relapse rate is approximately 30%

CHURG-STRAUSS SYNDROME—PATHOLOGIC FEATURES

Gross Findings
»» Peripheral patchy nodular consolidations
»» Cavitation is extremely rare

Microscopic Findings
»» Microscopic findings depend on the phase of the disease
»» Eosinophilic pneumonia, gastroenteritis, or lymphadenitis are typical of the prodromic phase
»» Asthmatic bronchitis is usually present
»» Granulomas with palisading borders, multinucleated giant cells and necrotic centers containing eosinophils are frequent
»» Vasculitis with fibrinoid necrosis, containing eosinophils, that affects small arteries, venules, and capillaries, is typical
»» Diffuse pulmonary hemorrhage with small vessel vasculitis (capillaritis) can be seen
»» Samples obtained after corticosteroid therapy may lack well preserved eosinophils

Ancillary Tests
»» Bronchoalveolar lavage fluid contains eosinophils
»» Pleural fluid often contains eosinophils
»» Special stains to rule out microorganisms must be done in settings of granulomatous inflammation; no microorganisms are seen in CSS

Pathologic Differential Diagnosis
»» Eosinophilic pneumonia associated with drugs, infections, etc (see chapter 17).
»» Allergic bronchopulmonary fungal disease
»» Wegener's granulomatosis
»» Microscopic polyangiitis

MICROSCOPIC POLYANGIITIS

Microscopic polyangiitis (MPA) is a systemic vasculitis that involves small vessels (arterioles, venules, and capillaries). In the lung, the disease is manifested by diffuse pulmonary hemorrhage and small vessel vasculitis (capillaritis).

CLINICAL FEATURES

Microscopic polyangiitis has an incidence of 1 in 100,000 individuals, with a slight female to male predominance (1.5:1). It affects individuals most frequently in the fourth and fifth decades of life. In most patients, there is a rapid progression, but a more indolent form of the disease with onset of symptoms over a period of a year has also been reported. The most common clinical manifestation is glomerulonephritis, followed by other nonspecific systemic symptoms such as fever, weight loss, myalgias, and arthralgias. MPA is the most common cause of a pulmonary-renal syndrome, which is characterized by pulmonary hemorrhage and glomerulonephritis. The lung is involved in approximately 50% of the cases, followed by other sites such as ear and upper respiratory tract (30%), and skin (approximately 20%). Similar to other vasculitis syndromes, a positive ANCA test is found in MPA, with a p-ANCA pattern in approximately 80% of cases. Bronchoalveolar lavage fluid shows acute inflammation and hemosiderin-laden macrophages, non-specific findings in pulmonary hemorrhage syndromes.

RADIOLOGIC FEATURES

Microscopic polyangiitis has a pattern of diffuse pulmonary hemorrhage characterized radiographically by bilateral alveolar opacities without nodules that predominantly involve the lower lobes of the lungs.

PATHOLOGIC FEATURES

Biopsies typically show neutrophilic small vessel vasculitis (capillaritis) in a background of pulmonary hemorrhage (Figure 8-13). Neutrophilic capillaritis is characterized by patchy foci of acute inflammation focussed on the alveolar wall, which is distended and thickened by the neutrophilic infiltrate (Figure 8-14). Extravasation of neutrophils into the alveolar space can be seen in severe cases, resembling acute pneumonia. In these cases, recognition that the process is centered on the alveolar wall and the presence of pulmonary hemorrhage helps in reaching the correct diagnosis.

In alveoli, fibrin, hyaline membranes and plugs of fibroblastic tissue (organizing pneumonia) can also be seen (Figure 8-15). The presence of hemosiderin deposits is an indication of chronic hemorrhage that characterizes the disease.

DIFFERENTIAL DIAGNOSIS

In most cases, MPA can be separated histologically from Wegener's granulomatosis (WG) by the lack of granulomatous inflammation in MPA. However, granulomatous inflammation may not be seen in WG due to sampling error or if the tissue is obtained in an early phase of the disease or after treatment. In these cases, clinical correlation is very important for making the correct diagnosis. The ANCA test, although not specific, may provide some diagnostic aid, since c-ANCA is more frequently seen in WG, whereas a p-ANCA pattern is more often found in MPA.

Goodpasture's syndrome also falls into the differential diagnosis, with manifestations of pulmonary hemorrhage and glomerulonephritis, but patients have antibodies to the glomerular basement membrane that are demonstrable serologically or by immuno-fluorescence. Polyarteritis nodosa rarely affects the lungs but can occasionally enter into the differential diagnosis of MPA. However, contrary to MPA, which affects arterioles,

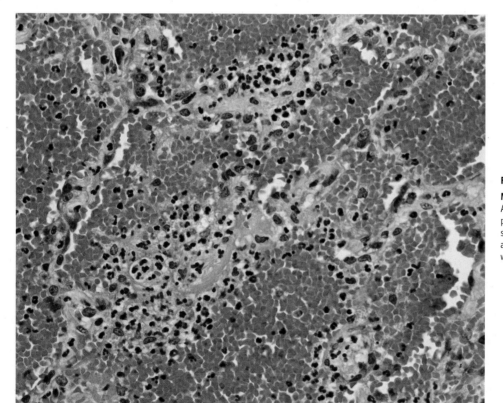

FIGURE 8-13

Microscopic polyangiitis: capillaritis
Alveolar capillaritis in a background of pulmonary hemorrhage. The alveolar septa are permeated by neutrophils and there is necrosis of capillary walls.

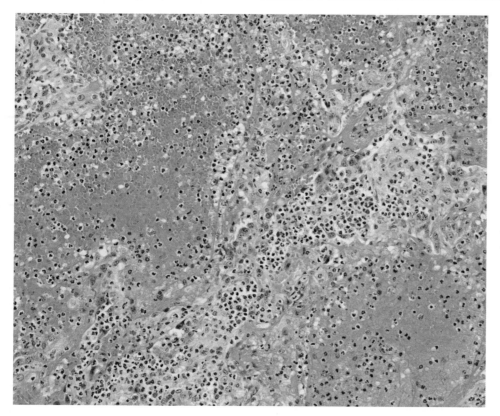

FIGURE 8-14

Microscopic polyangiitis: capillaritis
Foci of acute inflammation with clusters of neutrophils distending the alveolar wall. Note the hemorrhagic background and type II pneumocyte hyperplasia.

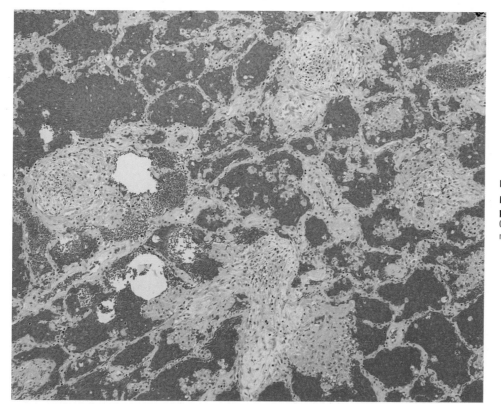

FIGURE 8-15

Microscopic polyangiitis: organizing pneumonia
Organization and hemosiderin-laden macrophages can also be seen in MPA.

venules, and capillaries, polyarteritis nodosa preferentially involves bronchial arteries. Polyarteritis nodosa can also be associated with a positive p-ANCA test.

MPA must also be separated from other vasculitides that affect small vessels. These include a heterogeneous group of vasculitis syndromes that can be caused by hypersensitivity reactions to drugs, collagen vascular diseases such as lupus and Henoch-Schönlein purpura, cryoglobulinemic vasculitis, serum sickness disease, and others. In contrast to some of these pathologic entities, MPA vasculitis shows minimal or absent immune complex deposition. These other entities are discussed in more detail later in this chapter.

PROGNOSIS AND THERAPY

Similar to WG, patients affected by MPA are treated with corticosteroids and cyclophosphamide. With this regimen, complete recovery is seen in approximately 70% of the patients. Relapses are frequent and affect about 40% of patients. In patients with complete remission of the disease, persistently abnormal pulmonary function tests have been observed.

NECROTIZING SARCOID GRANULOMATOSIS

Necrotizing sarcoid granulomatosis (NSG), originally described in 1973 by A.A. Liebow, is a disease that primarily affects the lungs. Although the histological features are similar to sarcoidosis, it remains unclear whether it represents a variant of that disease or is, in fact, a separate entity. Most currently view it primarily as a vasculitis.

MICROSCOPIC POLYANGIITIS—FACT SHEET

Definition
- Necrotizing vasculitis that affects small vessels (arterioles, venules, and capillaries) with few or no immune complex deposits

Incidence
- Rare (estimated incidence in the USA is 0.1 per million persons)

Morbidity and Mortality
- Causes of death include multiorgan system vasculitis and complications of treatment with immunosuppressive drugs
- Approximately 25% of patients have persistent pulmonary abnormalities after complete recovery

Gender, Race, and Age Distribution
- Peak incidence is between the fourth and sixth decades (mean age 56 years)
- Slight female predominance (1.5:1)
- No racial predilection

Clinical Features
- Affects predominantly the lungs and kidneys, and is the most common cause of pulmonary-renal syndrome
- 50% of cases show pulmonary involvement
- Most patients have a rapid onset of symptoms
- Most common clinical manifestation is glomerulonephritis
- Most common pulmonary finding is alveolar hemorrhage
- Systemic symptoms include arthralgias, myalgias, fever, weight loss, dyspnea, hemoptysis, cough, and chest pain
- 80% of the patients have a positive p-ANCA test result

Radiologic Findings
- Bilateral alveolar opacities (pulmonary hemorrhage) without nodules
- The lower lobes are affected more frequently

Prognosis and Therapy
- Treatment includes immunosuppressive drugs (corticosteroids and cyclophosphamide are the most commonly used drugs)
- Complete recovery is seen in approximately 70% of patients
- Relapse rate is approximately 40%

MICROSCOPIC POLYANGIITIS—PATHOLOGIC FEATURES

Gross Findings
- Lungs are dark due to pulmonary hemorrhage

Microscopic Findings
- Neutrophilic capillaritis in a background of hemorrhage
- Neutrophilic infiltrate may extend into the alveolar space, mimicking acute pneumonia
- Fibrin deposition, hyaline membranes, hemosiderin-laden macrophages, and organizing pneumonia may be present
- No granulomatous inflammation

Ancillary Test
- Bronchoalveolar lavage may show numerous hemosiderin-laden macrophages

Pathologic Differential Diagnosis
- Wegener's granulomatosis
- Goodpasture's syndrome
- Polyarteritis nodosa
- Other small-vessel vasculitides (Henoch-Schönlein purpura, cryoglobulinemia, lupus, and others)

CLINICAL FEATURES

The primary symptoms of NSG are respiratory and include cough, chest pain, fever and shortness of breath. Approximately 20 % of patients have no symptoms and present with changes on imaging studies. Unlike sarcoidosis, extra-pulmonary manifestations such as kidney or upper airway involvement are rare. Women are more commonly affected than men by a 2.2:1 ratio and the mean age of onset of this disease is 49 years (range, 11-75 years). Pulmonary function tests may show a number of abnormalities including decreased forced vital capacity and decreased arterial oxygen saturation. Laboratory findings usually include an elevated erythrocyte sedimentation rate (ESR). Unlike sarcoidosis, however, angiotensin-converting enzyme (ACE) levels are not commonly elevated in patients with NSG.

RADIOLOGIC FEATURES

Chest imaging studies usually reveal unilateral, localized disease with nodules or nodular infiltrates, more often in the lower lobes. However, bilateral lung involvement can occur, as can cavitation of both nodules and infiltrates. Pleural effusions may also be seen. Unlike sarcoidosis, hilar adenopathy is unusual, found in less than 10 % of patients.

PATHOLOGIC FEATURES

GROSS FINDINGS

Nodular lesions are typical of lung involvement by NSG. These lesions may show necrosis, but not to the extent that can be seen in Wegener's granulomatosis (WG).

MICROSCOPIC FINDINGS

Histologically, there is a confluence of non-necrotizing granulomas, which may surround a central area of necrosis (Figure 8-16). The distribution of the granulomas resembles that of sarcoidosis, generally following lymphatic routes (Figure 8-17). The necrosis present in the center of the mass usually has an infarct-like appearance (Figure 8-18). The vasculitis can affect both veins and arteries and consists of a lymphocytic infiltrate, giant cells or a combination of the two (Figure 8-19). Secondary features include organizing pneumonia and desquamative interstitial pneumonia-like collections of alveolar macrophages, which may contain hemosiderin.

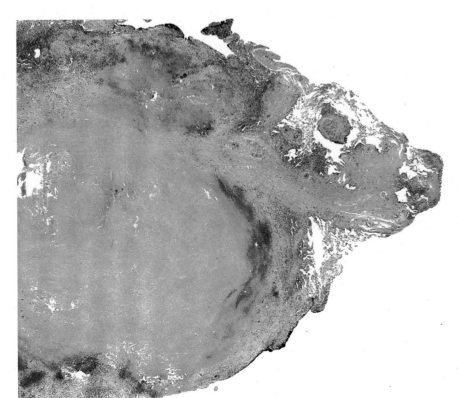

FIGURE 8-16

Necrotizing sarcoid granulomatosis

This mass includes an area of central necrosis and surrounding non-necrotizing granulomas and inflammation.

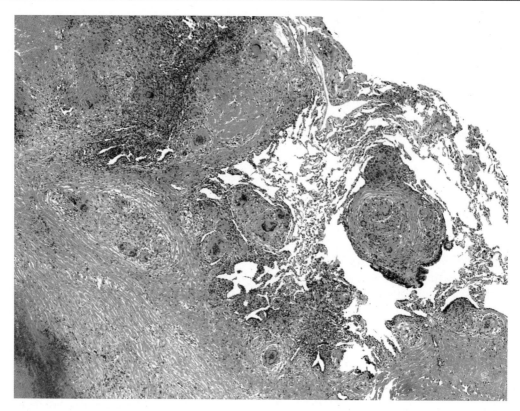

FIGURE 8-17
Necrotizing sarcoid granulomatosis
Non-necrotizing granulomas are visible in the surrounding lung.

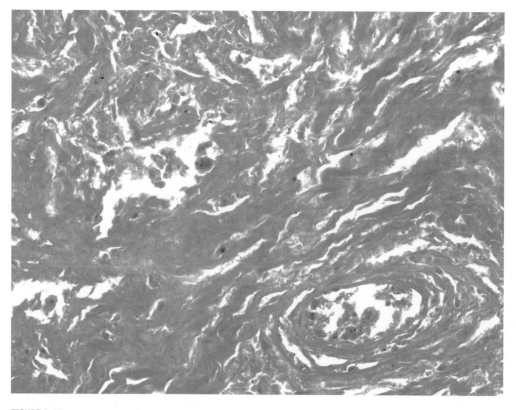

FIGURE 8-18
Necrotizing sarcoid granulomatosis
Necrosis in the center of the mass has infarct-like features with an eosinophilic appearance, unlike the basophilic appearance of WG.

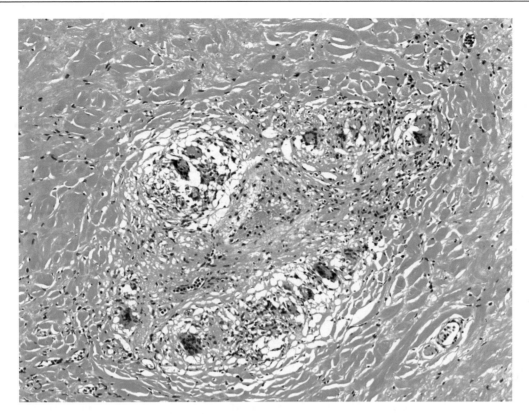

FIGURE 8-19
Necrotizing sarcoid granulomatosis
The vasculitis involves a small pulmonary artery and consists of giant cells.

NECROTIZING SARCOID GRANULOMATOSIS—FACT SHEET

Definition
- Disorder characterized by confluent sarcoidal granulomas with areas of necrosis and vasculitis

Gender and Age Distribution
- Female to male ratio of 2.2:1
- Average age is 49 years; range, 11-75 years

Clinical Features
- Cough, fever, dyspnea
- 20% of patients are asymptomatic at presentation

Radiologic Features
- Most commonly localized and unilateral
- Nodules and nodular infiltrates

Prognosis and Therapy
- No deaths due to disease have been reported
- Responds well to corticosteroids
- Surgical excision is curative for cavitating lesions

NECROTIZING SARCOID GRANULOMATOSIS—PATHOLOGIC FEATURES

Gross Findings
- Nodules with necrosis

Microscopic Findings
- Confluent masses of sarcoidal granulomas with central infarct-like necrosis
- Vasculitis involving pulmonary arteries and veins, consisting of lymphocytes, granulomas and giant cells

Ancillary Tests
- Elastic stains can help to define vascular destruction

Pathologic Differential Diagnosis
- Sarcoidosis
- Wegener's granulomatosis
- Mycobacterial and fungal infections

DIFFERENTIAL DIAGNOSIS

The major entities in the differential diagnosis for NSG are sarcoidosis, WG and granulomatous infections. Sarcoidosis usually does not demonstrate the extensive necrosis that is seen in NSG, and the extra-pulmonary involvement and hilar adenopathy that are frequent features of sarcoidosis are not seen in NSG. Well-formed, sarcoidal granulomas are not a feature of WG, and the necrosis in WG usually has a more basophilic appearance than the necrosis seen in NSG. Mycobacterial and fungal infections can elicit both necrotizing and nonnecrotizing granulomatous inflammation, and can therefore resemble NSG, so it is important to perform tissue organismal stains and microbiological cultures to exclude these diagnostic considerations before interpreting a case as NSG.

PROGNOSIS AND THERAPY

The prognosis for NSG is similar to that of sarcoidosis, with no deaths due to disease reported. NSG patients similarly respond well to corticosteroids. In cases with cavitation, surgical resection is curative.

ANTIBASEMENT MEMBRANE ANTIBODY DISEASE (GOODPASTURE'S SYNDROME)

Antibasement membrane antibody (ABMA) disease or Goodpasture's syndrome is a disease that affects both the lung and the kidneys, in which antibodies directed against the type IV collagen of both organs cause glomerulonephritis and pulmonary hemorrhage.

CLINICAL FEATURES

The disease is more common in men than women and has a bimodal age distribution with peaks at 30 and 60 years of age, and an average age at presentation of 35 years. The clinical presentation reflects the development of pulmonary hemorrhage and proliferative glomerulonephritis; most patients will have both features, and fewer patients will have disease restricted to the kidney or lung. Pulmonary symptoms include hemoptysis, cough and dyspnea, with rhonchi or crackles on auscultation. Systemic symptoms including fever, weight loss and arthralgias. Laboratory findings in this patient population include ABMAs in over 90% of patients and

antineutrophil cytoplasmic antibodies (ANCAs) in one-third of patients. Urinalysis reveals hematuria, granular casts and proteinuria.

RADIOLOGIC FEATURES

Chest imaging studies usually reveal bilateral consolidation, although the infiltrates may disappear and normal chest X-rays can be found in patients between periods of disease activity.

PATHOLOGIC FEATURES

GROSS FINDINGS

Lungs with ABMA disease have a dense, firm and red appearance without mass lesions or nodules.

MICROSCOPIC FINDINGS

Histologically, diffuse pulmonary hemorrhage is characteristic, with alveolar red blood cells, hemosiderin-laden macrophages, and with time, iron deposition on the elastic fibers in the alveolar septa. There may be a small vessel vasculitis and, if present, it may be accompanied by fibrin thrombi. The alveolar septa can be thickened with type 2 pneumocyte hyperplasia and organizing fibrosis (Figure 8-20). Hyaline membranes can be present in active disease. Immunofluorescence (IF) and ultrastructural analysis reveal linear deposition of IgG and complement along the capillaries in the alveolar septae and glomeruli (Figure 8-21; see chapter 39).

DIFFERENTIAL DIAGNOSIS

The differential diagnosis includes other causes of pulmonary small vessel vasculitis, and non-immunologic causes of pulmonary hemorrhage. The linear pattern of antibody deposition as seen by IF is specific to ABMA disease and helps to distinguish it from these other entities.

PROGNOSIS AND THERAPY

The most effective therapy for ABMA disease remains plasmapheresis to remove the circulating antibodies, and treatment with corticosteroids and, in some cases, cytotoxic drugs such as cyclophosphamide. Renal

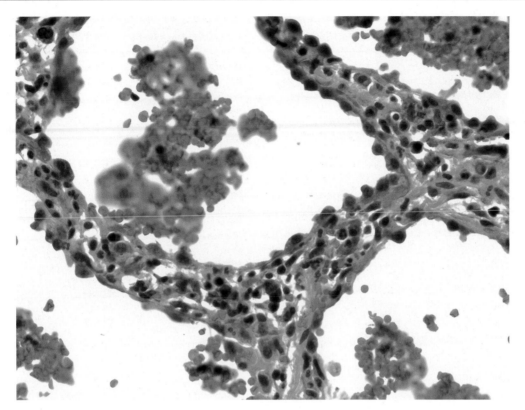

FIGURE 8-20

Antibasement membrane antibody disease
Interstitial thickening with type 2 pneumocyte hyperplasia is noted.

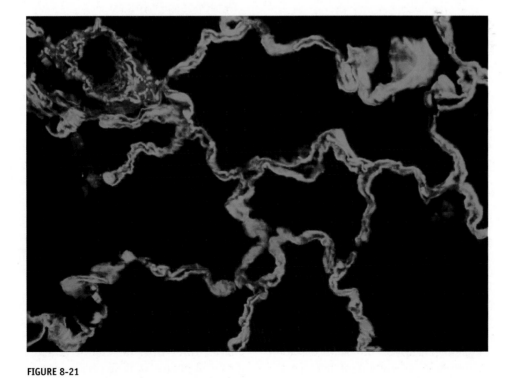

FIGURE 8-21

Anti basement membrane antibody disease
Immunofluoresence staining of a lung biopsy from a patient with Goodpasture's syndrome shows linear IgG staining along alveolar septa.

transplantation extends survival for patients who develop end stage kidney disease.

IDIOPATHIC PULMONARY HEMOSIDEROSIS

Idiopathic pulmonary hemosiderosis (IPH) is a rare disease that causes diffuse pulmonary hemorrhage, hemoptysis and anemia. Unlike ABMA disease, it is localized to the lungs.

CLINICAL FEATURES

This disorder is characterized by hemoptysis and anemia. Over 80% of cases occur in children, most in the first decade of life. Of the 20% of cases with adult onset, most are diagnosed before the age of 30 years. There is an equal distribution between males and females and familiar clustering has been reported, suggesting a possible genetic component. The acute clinical presentation is that of cough, dyspnea and fulminant hemoptysis, which can lead to respiratory failure. In the more chronic phase of the disease, fatigue, chronic cough and asymptomatic microcytic anemia predominate. In addition, failure to thrive, emaciation and pallor may be present. Pulmonary fibrosis can develop and, if so, physical examination may reveal bilateral crackles and clubbing.

RADIOLOGIC FEATURES

Findings on chest imaging vary with the phase of disease. In the acute phase, diffuse, ground-glass infiltrates are present, predominantly in the lower lobes. These resolve over time and reticulonodular infiltrates appear with fibrosis.

PATHOLOGIC FEATURES

GROSS FINDINGS

The gross appearance of IPH is one of brown induration secondary to the hemosiderin deposition.

MICROSCOPIC FINDINGS

Evidence of alveolar hemorrhage is present, including alveolar red blood cells and hemosiderin-laden macrophages. Interstitial thickening develops with time due to type 2 pneumocyte hyperplasia and collagen deposition (Figure 8-22). Ultrastructural analysis and immunofluorescence reveal no evidence of immunoglobulin deposits.

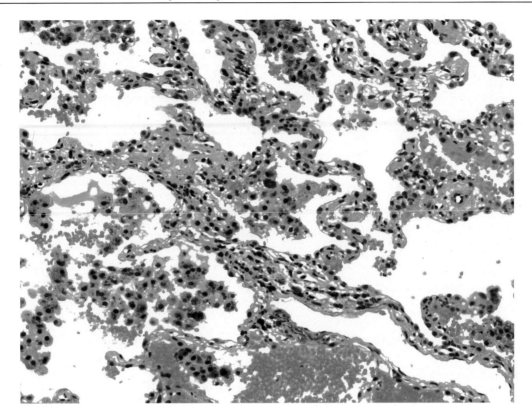

FIGURE 8-22
Idiopathic pulmonary hemosiderosis
There is hemosiderin deposition in the interstitium and within alveolar macrophages in areas of mild fibrosis.

IDIOPATHIC PULMONARY HEMOSIDEROSIS—FACT SHEET

Definition
▸ A rare disease that causes diffuse pulmonary hemorrhage and anemia

Gender and Age Distribution
▸ Equal distribution between male and females
▸ 80% of cases present during the first decade of life
▸ 100% of cases present before 30 years of age

Clinical Features
▸ Hemoptysis, dyspnea and iron deficiency anemia
▸ Chronic cases have pallor, fatigue, and emaciation
▸ Pulmonary fibrosis may be present and, if so, clubbing may be seen

Radiologic Features
▸ Diffuse, bilateral consolidation

Prognosis and Therapy
▸ Variable response to corticosteroids
▸ Median survival of 3-5 years

IDIOPATHIC PULMONARY HEMOSIDEROSIS—PATHOLOGIC FEATURES

Gross Findings
▸ Dense, firm brown lungs (brown induration)

Microscopic Findings
▸ Hemorrhage diffusely involving alveolar spaces
▸ Hemosiderin-laden macrophages
▸ Interstitial thickening with type 2 pneumocyte hyperplasia and fibrosis
▸ Minimal inflammation

Ancillary Tests
▸ Negative IF, ANCA and anti-basement membrane antibody tests

Pathologic Differential Diagnosis
▸ Immunologic and non-immunologic causes of pulmonary hemorrhage

BEHÇET'S DISEASE—FACT SHEET

Definition

▸ Chronic, systemic inflammatory disease, which presents with the clinical triad of relapsing uveitis, oral and genital ulcers

Location

▸ More common in East Asia and Mediterranean basin

Mortality

▸ In patients with pulmonary arterial aneurysms, less than 30% 2-year survival

Gender and Age Distribution

▸ Pulmonary involvement is more common in young males

Clinical Features

▸ Relapsing uveitis, oral and genital ulcers

Radiologic Features

▸ Hilar enlargement and lobulated opacities

Prognosis and Therapy

▸ Corticosteroids to reduce vasculitis
▸ Anticoagulation for thrombosis
▸ Surgical removal of lobe or lung for massive hemoptysis

DIFFERENTIAL DIAGNOSIS

The differential diagnosis includes ABMA disease, ANCA-associated vasculitides, and other immunologic and non-immunologic causes of pulmonary hemorrhage. IPH does not display small vessel vasculitis or immunoglobulin deposits by IF or electron microscopy. Also, IPH is predominantly found in a younger population than either ABMA disease or causes of pulmonary small vessel vasculitis.

PROGNOSIS AND THERAPY

Corticosteroids are the main therapy, although the response is variable. The long term prognosis is poor with a mean survival of 3 to 5 years.

BEHÇET'S DISEASE

Behçet's disease is a chronic, systemic inflammatory disease, which presents with the clinical triad of relapsing uveitis, oral and genital ulcers. Additional sites may

BEHÇET'S DISEASE—PATHOLOGIC FEATURES

Gross Findings

▸ Pulmonary arterial aneurysms with thrombosis in pulmonary trunk, main pulmonary artery and proximal branches

Microscopic Findings

▸ Lymphocytic and necrotizing vasculitis of pulmonary arteries (all sizes), veins and capillaries
▸ Eccentric intimal fibrosis with acute, organizing and recanalized thrombi
▸ Periadventitial fibrosis with collateral vessels

Pathologic Differential Diagnosis

▸ Thrombotic arteriopathy

be involved, the most common including the gastrointestinal tract and the central nervous system.

CLINICAL FEATURES

The disease, usually found in young men, is particularly common in eastern Asia and the Mediterranean basin. Pulmonary involvement is found in less than 5% of patients, most commonly as pulmonary artery aneurysms. Hemoptysis is the most common clinical symptom, usually caused by rupture of an aneurysm. This may be life threatening or fatal. Other pulmonary symptoms include cough, dyspnea and chest pain.

RADIOLOGIC FEATURES

Radiologic features include hilar enlargement or lobulated masses on chest radiographs secondary to pulmonary artery aneurysms. These are located in the main, segmental or lobar pulmonary arteries. Chest CT scans and magnetic resonance imaging can define saccular or fusiform dilatations in the proximal arteries. Parenchymal changes may be seen, but are nonspecific.

PATHOLOGIC FEATURES

MICROSCOPIC FINDINGS

The vasculitis is characterized by a perivascular inflammatory infiltrate that may be neutrophilic, mononuclear or mixed, involving arteries and veins of all sizes and capillaries. Elastic destruction in the vessel wall can be seen by elastic stains and thrombus formation is common, leading to narrowing and occlusion of vessels. Pulmonary infarction and arteriobronchial fistulas can occur and collateral vessels are commonly found in the periadventitial fibrosis surrounding the large affected vessels.

DIFFERENTIAL DIAGNOSIS

Because of the eccentric intimal fibrosis that is seen in this disease, pulmonary thrombotic arteriopathy can be mistaken for Behçet's disease.

PROGNOSIS AND THERAPY

Corticosteroids are used to control the vasculitis and anticoagulation is necessary to prevent thrombosis. Progression of the disease may require treatment with cyclophosphamide or azathioprine. Surgical resection (lobectomy or pneumonectomy) may be performed in cases of massive hemoptysis. The disease generally has a chronic course, characterized by exacerbations and remissions. It is most severe in young patients and 30% of patients with pulmonary arterial aneurysms die within 2 years.

OTHER UNCOMMON PULMONARY VASCULITIDIES

COLLAGEN VASCULAR DISEASE-ASSOCIATED VASCULITIS

Pulmonary involvement by collagen vascular diseases can manifest as vasculitis. This can take the form of small vessel vasculitis, or, less commonly, involvement of medium-sized arteries. The collagen vascular diseases most commonly associated with pulmonary vasculitis and hemorrhage are systemic lupus erythematosus (SLE) and rheumatoid arthritis.

POLYARTERITIS NODOSA

Polyarteritis nodosa (PAN) is a systemic vasculitis of medium-sized and small arteries that can involve the lung. Although there is considerable overlap in the histologic features of this entity with microscopic polyangiitis, PAN characteristically involves the bronchial arteries, usually sparing the pulmonary circulation.

HENOCH-SCHÖNLEIN PURPURA

Henoch-Schonlein purpura is a small vessel vasculitis that most commonly presents with gastrointestinal and renal involvement and palpable purpura of the skin. Rarely, the lung is involved and in these cases, patients present with hemoptysis due to pulmonary hemorrhage secondary to small vessel vasculitis.

VASCULITIS ASSOCIATED WITH CRYOGLOBULINEMIA

Cryoglobulinemia may occur in patients with lymphoproliferative disorders, infections or collagen vascular diseases. Pulmonary involvement is common, usually as an interstitial lung disease. Leukocytoclastic vasculitis of medium-sized arteries and small vessel vasculitis with pulmonary hemorrhage have been reported.

TAKAYASU'S ARTERITIS

Takayasu's arteritis is a giant cell arteritis usually found in women less than 40 years of age, which involves large vessels, most commonly the aorta and its proximal branches. Pulmonary involvement usually takes the form of a lymphocytic or giant cell arteritis that leads to elastic destruction, fibrosis, narrowing and occlusion of the affected vessels. Many times, pulmonary involvement by Takayasu's arteritis is diagnosed by angiography demonstrating narrowing and/or occlusion of the proximal pulmonary arteries.

GIANT CELL ARTERITIS

Giant cell arteritis, most common to the temporal artery, rarely involves the lung. In reported cases, both the main pulmonary artery and the trunk can be affected by a giant cell infiltrate resulting in destruction of the elastic fibers and fibrinoid necrosis. This disorder can be distinguished from Takayasu's arteritis by its involvement of the cranial arteries and its presentation in older patients.

SUGGESTED READINGS

1. Semple D, Keogh J, Forni L, Venn R. Clinical review: vasculitis on the intensive care unit—part 1: diagnosis. *Crit Care*. 2005;9:92-7.
2. Travis WD, Colby TV, Koss MN, Rosado-de-Christenson M, Muller NL, King TE Jr. Pulmonary vasculitis. In: King DW, ed. *Nonneoplastic Disorders of the Lower Respiratory Tract*. Washington, DC: American Registry of Pathology; 2002:233-64.

Wegener's Granulomatosis

3. Mark EJ, Flieder DB, Matsubara O. Treated Wegener's granulomatosis: distinctive pathological fi ndings in the lungs of 20 patients and what they tell us about the natural history of the disease. *Hum Pathol.* 1997;28:450-8.
4. Seo P, Min YI, Holbrook JT, et al. Damage caused by Wegener's granulomatosis and its treatment: prospective data from the Wegener's Granulomatosis Etanercept Trial (WGET). *Arthritis Rheum.* 2005;52:2168-78.
5. Yi ES, Colby TV. Wegener's granulomatosis. *Semin Diagn Pathol.* 2001;18:34-46.

Churg-Strauss Syndrome

6. Churg A. Recent advances in the diagnosis of Churg-Strauss syndrome. *Mod Pathol.* 2001;14:1284-93.
7. Katzenstein AL. Diagnostic features and differential diagnosis of Churg-Strauss syndrome in the lung: a review. *Am J Clin Pathol.* 2000;114:767-72.
8. North I, Strek ME, Leff AR. Churg-Strauss syndrome. *Lancet.* 2003;361:587-94.

Necrotizing Sarcoid Granulomatosis

9. Ma Y, Gal A, Koss MN. The pathology of pulmonary sarcoidosis: update. *Semin Diagn Pathol.* 2007;24:150-61.
10. Popper HH, Klemen H, Colby TV, et al. Necrotizing sarcoid granulomatosis-is it different from nodular sarcoidosis? *Pneumologie.* 2003;57:268-71.
11. Rosen Y. Pathology of sarcoidosis. *Semin Respir Crit Care Med.* 2007;28:36-52.

Antibasement Membrane Antibody Disease (Goodpasture's Syndrome)

12. Ball JA, Young KR, Jr. Pulmonary manifestations of Goodpasture's syndrome. Antiglomerular basement membrane disease and related disorders. *Clin Chest Med.* 1998;19:777-91.
13. Collard HR, Schwarz MI. Diffuse alveolar hemorrhage. *Clin Chest Med.* 2004;25:583-92.
14. DeRemee RA. The spectrum of pulmonary vasculitis. *Monaldi Arch Chest Dis.* 1996;51:35-8.
15. Kelly PT, Haponik EF. Goodpasture syndrome: Molecular and clinical advances. *Medicine (Baltimore).* 1994;73:171-85.

Idiopathic Pulmonary Hemosiderosis

16. Ioachimescu OC, Sieber S, Kotch A. Idiopathic pulmonary haemosiderosis revisited. *Eur Respir J.* 2004;37:476-84.
17. Milman N, Pedersen FM. Idiopathic pulmonary haemosiderosis. Epidemiology, pathogenic aspects and diagnosis. *Respir Med.* 1998;92:902-7.
18. Nuesslein TG, Teig N, Rieger CH. pulmonary haemosiderosis in infants and children. *Paediatri Respir Rev.* 2006;7:45-8.

Behçet's Disease

19. Erkan F, Esen K, Tunaci A. Pulmonary complications of Behçet's disease. *Clin Chest Med.* 2002;23:493-503.
20. Erkan F, Gul A, Fasali E. Pulmonary manifestations of Behçet's disease. *Thorax.* 2001;56:572-8.
21. Hiller N, Lieberman S, Chajet-Shaul T, et al. Thoracic manifestations of Behçet disease at CT. *Radiographics.* 2004;24:801-8.
22. Uzun O, Akpolat T, Erkan L. Pulmonary vasculitis in Behçet disease: A cumulative analysis. *Chest.* 2005;127:2243-53.

9 Acute Lung Injury

Mary Beth Beasley

- Introduction
- Diffuse Alveolar Damage
- Organizing Pneumonia (Bronchiolitis Obliterans-Organizing Pneumonia, Cryptogenic Organizing Pneumonia)
- Acute Fibrinous and Organizing Pneumonia

INTRODUCTION

The term "acute lung injury pattern" was originally proposed by Katzenstein to encompass the entities of diffuse alveolar damage (DAD) and the entity previously referred to as bronchiolitis obliterans with organizing pneumonia (BOOP), now known as organizing pneumonia. This designation was designed to reflect the relatively acute onset of both entities as well as the uniformity of both processes reflective of injury resulting from a single point in time. "Acute lung injury" in this context differs from the clinical definition of acute lung injury as defined by the American-European consensus conference in 1994. While most cases of organizing pneumonia do not meet the clinical definition of acute lung injury, this entity will be included in this chapter, as it should be considered when presented with a biopsy from a patient with a disease process of relatively short onset.

DIFFUSE ALVEOLAR DAMAGE

CLINICAL PRESENTATION

Diffuse alveolar damage is the histologic pattern most frequently encountered in association with acute respiratory distress syndrome (ARDS), which characteristically presents with rapidly progressive respiratory fail-

ure, typically within 24 to 48 hours following exposure to an initiating event. Profound hypoxemia is typically present, with nearly all patients requiring mechanical ventilation.

RADIOLOGIC FINDINGS

Standard chest x-rays demonstrate air space consolidation that is initially patchy but rapidly progresses to diffuse involvement (Figure 9-1). CT scans may appear patchy in comparison to the standard chest X-rays, with disease typically being more pronounced in dependent regions. Linear opacities, corresponding to the evolution of fibrosis, appear as the disease progresses.

PATHOLOGIC FINDINGS

GROSS FINDINGS

In the acute phase, the lungs are dark red, heavy, and consolidated. As the disease progresses, the lungs often become more fibrotic and develop a firm, yellowish-gray cut surface.

MICROSCOPIC FINDINGS

DAD is typically divided into an acute (exudative) phase and an organizing (proliferative) phase. A fibrotic phase is also included by some authors. The findings are typically diffuse and temporally uniform.

One to two days following the initial pulmonary insult, capillary congestion and intra-alveolar edema may be observed by light microscopy. Eosinophilic hyaline membranes, composed of plasma proteins and cellular debris, begin to appear by day 2 and reach a peak by day 4 or 5 (Figures 9-2 through 9-4). The membranes are found along alveolar septa with accentuation along alveolar ducts. Inflammation is typically sparse. The proliferative phase is usually considered to commence within 5 to 7 days after initial injury. The hyaline membranes are phagocytized by macrophages or are transformed into

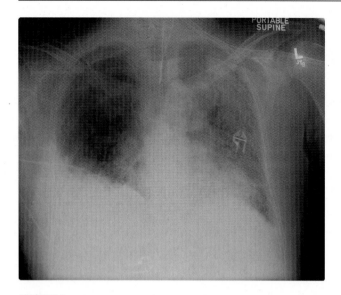

FIGURE 9-1

Diffuse alveolar damage

Air space consolidation may be patchy initially, but progresses quickly to diffuse involvement. (Radiograph courtesy of Dr. Stephen Zinck, Epic Imaging, Portland, Oregon.)

granulation tissue by proliferating myofibroblasts and are incorporated into the interstitium. The interstitium is expanded by loose, myxoid fibroblastic tissue that has a blue-gray appearance, as opposed to dense eosinophilic collagen fibrosis (Figure 9-5). Type 2 pneumocyte hyperplasia is typically quite pronounced, and the cells may

have atypical features (Figure 9-6). Squamous metaplasia may also be present (Figure 9-7). Thrombi may be seen in both phases and extensive vascular remodeling may be seen in the proliferative phase. Over time, patients develop varying degrees of collagenous fibrosis and airspace remodeling.

DIFFERENTIAL DIAGNOSIS

DAD can be difficult to diagnose on a small biopsy and may require a wedge biopsy for precise classification. DAD can be triggered by many agents, or it may be idiopathic in origin. Etiologic agents include infection, sepsis, trauma, aspiration, inhalational injury, drug reaction, metabolic disorders, and numerous other causes. Generally, the etiology is not apparent from the histology alone and must be determined based upon clinical and laboratory data. All cases of DAD should be routinely stained for fungi, particularly *Pneumocystis* as well as bacteria and mycobacteria. Other indicators of an infectious etiology such as granulomas and viral inclusions should also be sought. With immunocompromised patients, immunohistochemical staining for viruses including cytomegalovirus, herpes simplex viruses, and the respiratory viruses should be considered. Unusual agents such as rickettsiae, ehrlichiae, or uncommon viruses may also be in the differential diagnosis, depending upon the clinical circumstances.

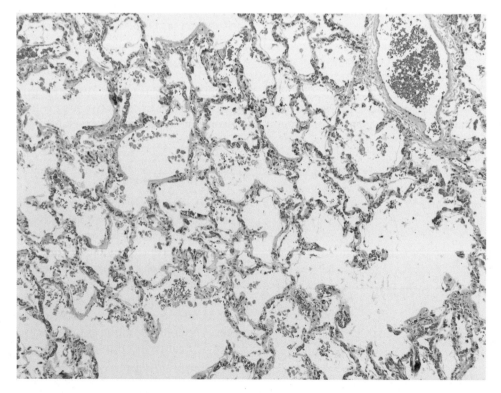

FIGURE 9-2

Diffuse alveolar damage, exudative phase

The process is temporally uniform. Alveolar septa are slightly widened and hyaline membrane formation is present.

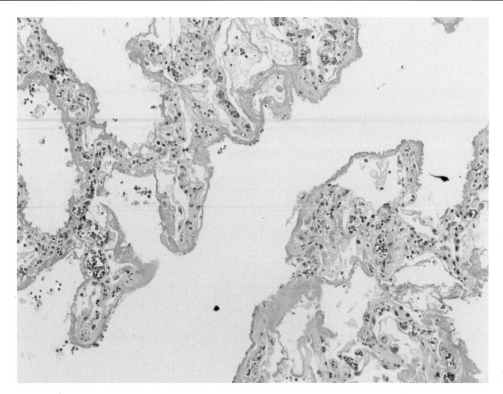

FIGURE 9-3

Diffuse alveolar damage, exudative phase
Hyaline membranes reach a peak by day 4 or 5 following initial injury and are found lining alveolar septa and alveolar ducts. Note that inflammation is relatively sparse.

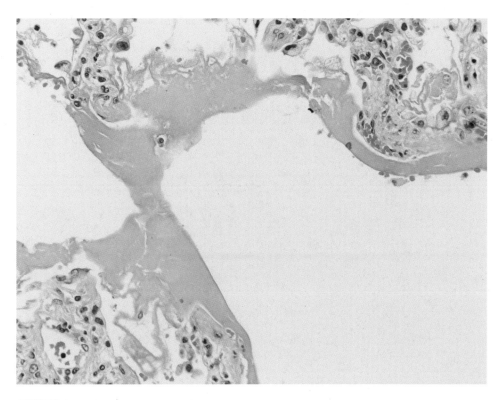

FIGURE 9-4

Diffuse alveolar damage, exudative phase
Hyaline membranes are composed of plasma proteins and cellular debris and have an eosinophilic refractile quality.

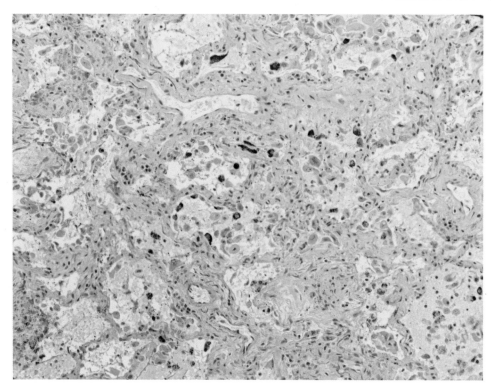

FIGURE 9-5

Diffuse alveolar damage, organizing phase

Approximately 5 to 7 days following initial injury, the alveolar septa are expanded by loose, myxoid-appearing fibroblastic tissue.

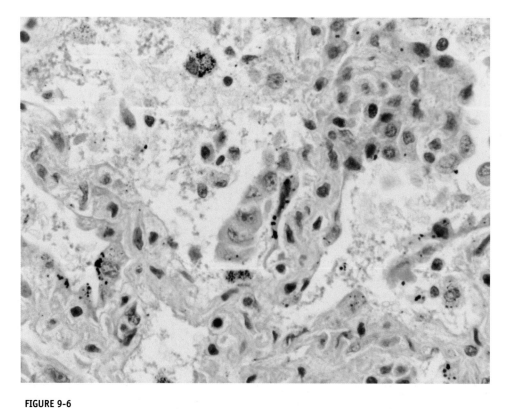

FIGURE 9-6

Diffuse alveolar damage, organizing phase

Type 2 pneumocyte hyperplasia is typically quite marked in organizing DAD, and the cells may have atypical cytologic features.

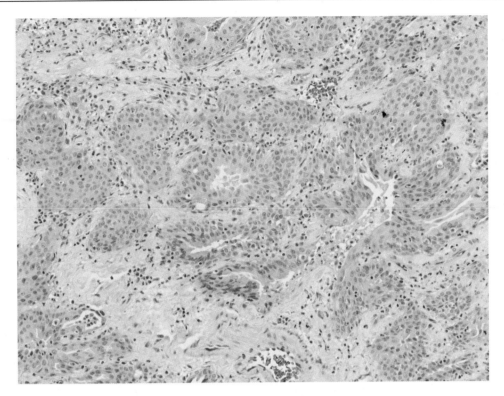

FIGURE 9-7
Diffuse alveolar damage, organizing phase
Squamous metaplasia may be present and, as in this case, quite pronounced.

If DAD is determined to be idiopathic in origin, the term "acute interstitial pneumonia (AIP)" is applied. Cases of AIP appear to correspond to the rapidly progressive idiopathic lung disease originally described by Hamman and Rich.

In addition to the above issues, the following entities may enter into the histologic differential diagnosis of DAD:

ACUTE EOSINOPHILIC PNEUMONIA (AEP)

AEP can present with acute respiratory distress and exhibit hyaline membranes similar to DAD, although prominent eosinophils are present and intra-alveolar fibrin and macrophages are also seen. AEP is exquisitely responsive to corticosteroid therapy and is therefore important to distinguish from DAD, given the therapeutic and prognostic implications.

NONSPECIFIC INTERSTITIAL PNEUMONIA (NSIP), FIBROSING VARIANT

Fibrotic NSIP is typically characterized by diffuse, densely collagenous fibrosis rather than the myxoid fibrosis of organizing DAD. Type 2 pneumocyte hyperplasia is generally not as pronounced. In some instances it

may be virtually impossible to separate fibrotic NSIP from DAD.

USUAL INTERSTITIAL PNEUMONIA (UIP)

In contrast to the diffuse, relatively uniform pattern seen in DAD, UIP is characterized by patchy fibrosis which is temporally heterogeneous. UIP may undergo what has been termed "accelerated decline," and in this situation hyaline membranes may be superimposed on otherwise typical features of UIP.

ORGANIZING PNEUMONIA/COP

OP is characterized by patchy intralumenal fibrosis as opposed to the predominantly interstitial fibrosis seen in DAD. Type 2 pneumocyte hyperplasia is not as pronounced, and hyaline membranes are not seen.

PROGNOSIS AND THERAPY

The mortality rate from DAD is generally reported as being between 40 to 60%, with some recent studies suggesting a slight decline with rates of 35%. Corticosteroid

---

DIFFUSE ALVEOLAR DAMAGE—FACT SHEET

Definition

» Temporally uniform acute lung injury pattern associated with the clinical presentation of acute respiratory distress syndrome
» Classically divided into acute and organizing phases histologically

Clinical Features

» Severe dyspnea, hypoxemia
» Rapidly progressive respiratory failure
» Mechanical ventilation required in essentially all cases

Radiologic Features

» Diffuse air space consolidation
» Progressive linear opacities with evolving fibrosis

Prognosis and Therapy

» 40-60% mortality rate, but more recent studies show some improvement

---

DIFFUSE ALVEOLAR DAMAGE—PATHOLOGIC FEATURES

Gross Findings

» Exudative phase: heavy, dark red, consolidated
» Proliferative phase: firm, yellow-gray, airless

Microscopic Findings

» Temporally uniform features reflective of an insult occurring at a single point in time

Exudative Phase

» Intra-alveolar edema
» Hyaline membranes (peak 4-5 days)
» Sparse inflammation
» Intravascular thrombi

Proliferative Phase

» Grayish-blue "myxoid" interstitial fibrosis
» Marked type 2 pneumocyte hyperplasia
» Variable squamous metaplasia
» Variable collagenous fibrosis and architectural remodeling

Pathologic Differential Diagnosis

» Organizing pneumonia
» Acute eosinophilic pneumonia
» Nonspecific interstitial pneumonia
» Usual interstitial pneumonia
» Acute fibrinous and organizing pneumonia
» Alveolar hemorrhage

---

regimens as well as nitric oxide, other vasodilators, and surfactant replacement therapies have met with mixed results but have been largely unsuccessful.

In patients who survive, radiographs will improve and pulmonary function typically returns to normal in 6 months to a year, although patients with significant fibrosis may retain some degree of restrictive deficit.

ORGANIZING PNEUMONIA (BRONCHIOLITIS OBLITERANS WITH ORGANIZING PNEUMONIA, CRYPTOGENIC ORGANIZING PNEUMONIA)

Organizing pneumonia (OP) refers to proliferations of fibroblastic tissue within small airways, alveolar ducts, and alveolar spaces. OP may occur as a nonspecific reaction to, or as a component of, a variety of processes, or it may occur as a specific pattern of patchy, bronchiolocentric lung disease ("OP pattern") as described below. This chapter will primarily address this specific "OP pattern" of disease. It should be noted that the term "OP pattern" is now the preferred term for the histologic pattern previously termed bronchiolitis obliterans with organizing pneumonia (BOOP) in the recent ATS/ERS consensus classification of idiopathic interstitial lung diseases.

When the OP pattern is present, it may be secondary to a variety of underlying etiologies (see below), or it may be idiopathic in origin. When the OP pattern occurs in an idiopathic setting, it is referred to clinically as cryptogenic organizing pneumonia (COP).

CLINICAL FINDINGS

The clinical syndrome of COP most commonly presents in the fifth and sixth decades with equal sex predilection. Patients typically present with a 2 to 3 month history of cough and dyspnea, although some cases may be more acute. Many patients report a history of an antecedent upper respiratory tract infection. Weight loss, fever, and chills may also be present. Inspiratory crackles are present on physical exam, and pulmonary function testing may show mild to moderate restrictive defects. Airflow obstruction is generally absent. Laboratory values may be normal or show nonspecific findings such as elevated erythrocyte sedimentation rate, C-reactive protein, or blood neutrophil count.

RADIOLOGIC FINDINGS

On standard chest x-rays, the OP pattern/COP typically exhibits patchy air space consolidation that is usually bilateral but may occasionally be unilateral. Small nodular opacities or a reticulonodular pattern may also occur. On CT scan, patchy airspace consolidation is observed in a peribronchial distribution more frequently involving the lower lobes (Figure 9-8). Other findings may include air bronchograms, ground-glass opacities, and small nodules around bronchovascular bundles. Larger nodules may be present in a small number of cases. Pleural effusion is rare.

PATHOLOGIC FINDINGS

GROSS FINDINGS

Few published gross descriptions exist, and typically describe nonspecific, ill-defined, consolidated areas without significant fibrosis.

MICROSCOPIC FINDINGS

The OP pattern is a temporally uniform process typified by patchy areas of organizing fibroblastic tissue occurring predominantly within alveolar ducts and alveolar spaces (Figure 9-9). The fibroblastic tissue plugs are composed of loose, myxoid-appearing tissue which appears bluish-gray on H&E stains. The process is predominantly centered on and around bronchioles (Figure 9-10). The alveolar septa in the areas of involvement generally contain mild to moderate lymphocytic infiltrates. Type 2 pneumocyte hyperplasia may be evident, but is not typically pronounced (Figure 9-11). Organizing fibroblastic plugs within bronchiolar lumens are seen in most cases (Figure 9-12), but may be absent and are not required for diagnosis in the presence of

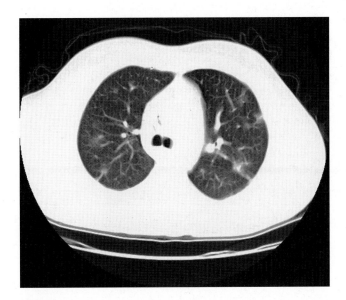

FIGURE 9-8

Chest CT demonstrating organizing pneumonia pattern
Patchy air space consolidation is present, which is accentuated peribronchially. (Radiograph courtesy of Dr. Stephen Zinck, Epic Imaging, Portland, Oregon.)

otherwise characteristic findings. Foamy macrophages may also be observed, secondary to airway obstruction (Figure 9-13). The lung parenchyma in between the areas of involvement is usually essentially normal. Significant fibrosis or architectural remodeling should not be present. Neutrophils and eosinophils should be essentially absent, and no granulomas should be seen.

DIFFERENTIAL DIAGNOSIS

The diagnosis of OP pattern should be made only when the specific pattern described above is present, and it is imperative to communicate to the clinician when one is referring to this specific pattern of disease rather than organizing pneumonia occurring in a different setting.

A precise diagnosis of OP pattern generally requires a wedge biopsy specimen and can be difficult to establish on a small or transbronchial biopsy. Furthermore, as previously mentioned, in addition to COP, organizing pneumonia can occur in a variety of other settings. In some of these settings, particularly infections, additional histologic, microbiologic, or serologic evaluation is indicated. For example, OP can occur as a component of hypersensitivity pneumonitis, Wegener's granulomatosis, or eosinophilic pneumonia. Additionally, OP may occur as a nonspecific reaction adjacent to an unrelated process such as a neoplasm, granuloma, or abscess. The OP pattern has been reported in association with a variety of chronic infections (bacterial, fungal, and viral) and special stains for microorganisms should be performed in all cases. The OP pattern may occur in association with collagen vascular diseases, especially rheumatoid arthritis and Sjögren's syndrome, more so than systemic lupus. Numerous therapeutic agents have caused OP as a side effect, and the OP pattern has also been rarely reported in association with inflammatory bowel disease, hematopoietic disorders, and hepatitis C. Further, OP may occur as a localized process presenting as a mass lesion, a condition termed "localized organizing pneumonia." For these reasons, the finding of OP requires careful clinical and radiographic correlation.

In addition to the above diagnostic issues, the following entities may enter the histologic differential diagnosis of the OP pattern:

DIFFUSE ALVEOLAR DAMAGE (DAD)

In contrast to OP, DAD typically presents with a more fulminant clinical course requiring mechanical ventilation. Histologically, DAD is diffuse rather than patchy, and, in the acute phase, hyaline membranes are present. In organizing DAD, the organizing fibroblastic tissue tends to be more interstitial rather than intralumenal, and type 2 pneumocyte hyperplasia is much more pronounced.

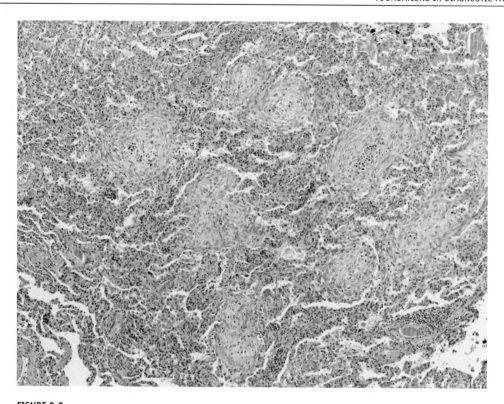

FIGURE 9-9

Organizing pneumonia pattern
Intra-alveolar organizing fibroblastic tissue is present in a patchy distribution. The alveolar septa contain mild chronic inflammatory infiltrates but significant fibrosis is absent.

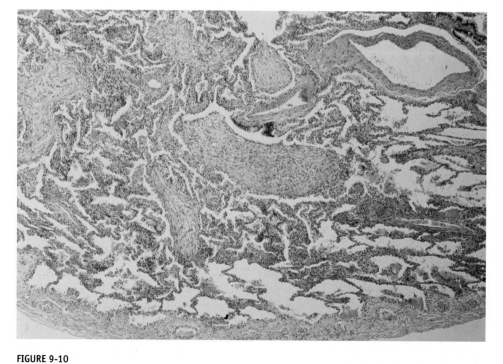

FIGURE 9-10

Organizing pneumonia pattern
Patchy organizing pneumonia is centered on bronchioles. An intralumenal fibroblastic plug is also present within a central bronchiole.

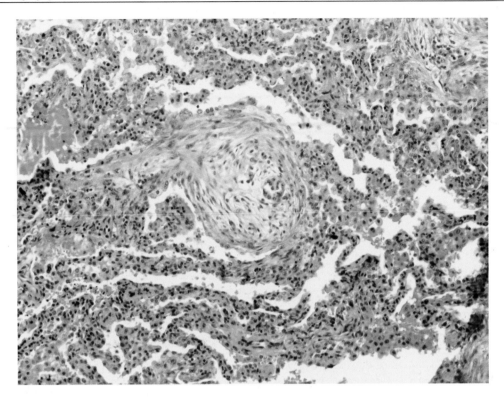

FIGURE 9-11

Organizing pneumonia pattern
The organizing fibroblastic tissue has a blue, myxoid appearance and is located within air spaces as opposed to the interstitium. Note lack of interstitial fibrosis and significant type 2 pneumocyte hyperplasia.

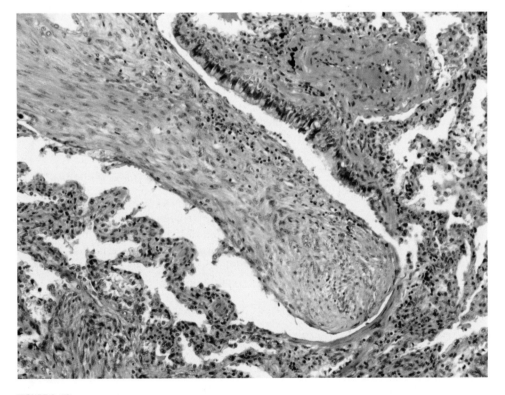

FIGURE 9-12

Bronchiolar involvement in organizing pneumonia
This intralumenal plug of fibroblastic tissue fills a bronchiolar lumen, as indicated by the respiratory mucosa.

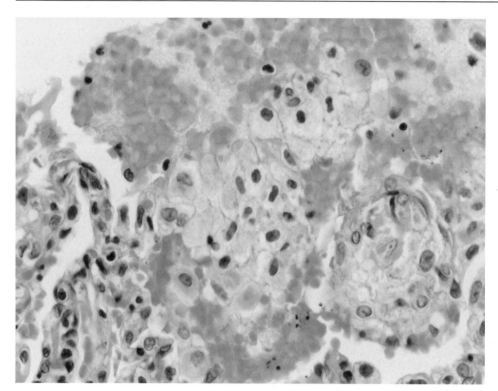

FIGURE 9-13

Intra-alveolar foamy macrophages in organizing pneumonia
This finding is frequently encountered in OP and is related to airway obstruction.

HYPERSENSITIVITY PNEUMONITIS (HSP)

OP may occur as a component of HSP, but is not the dominant finding. Additionally, granulomas are often present and significant fibrosis may be found, neither of which should be found in the OP pattern. Interstitial pneumonia, usually non-specific, and chronic bronchiolitis are other important features of HSP.

EOSINOPHILIC PNEUMONIA (EP)

OP may be present in cases of chronic EP. Eosinophils, intra-alveolar fibrin, and macrophage accumulation are typically also present and distinguish EP from the OP pattern. Peripheral blood eosinophilia is typically encountered in chronic EP and is not found in patients with OP/COP.

ACUTE FIBRINOUS AND ORGANIZING PNEUMONIA (AFOP)

AFOP may contain areas of OP, but the dominant finding is intra-alveolar fibrin balls, which should not be present to a significant degree in the OP pattern. The organizing fibroblastic tissue in AFOP may additionally have central cores of residual fibrin.

SO-CALLED "BOOP VARIANT" OF WEGENER'S GRANULOMATOSIS (WG)

OP may occasionally be a prominent finding in cases of WG. Other features of WG such as prominent neutrophils, areas of necrosis, giant cells, and vasculitis are usually present and point to the correct diagnosis.

NONSPECIFIC INTERSTITIAL PNEUMONIA (NSIP)

Focal areas of OP may be present in cases of NSIP, particularly the cellular subtype. However, OP is not the dominant finding in NSIP, and the background interstitial chronic inflammation is diffuse rather than patchy. The diffuse fibrosis present in fibrotic NSIP should readily distinguish this entity from OP.

PROGNOSIS AND THERAPY

The treatment of choice for COP is corticosteroid therapy, which usually leads to rapid and complete recovery in most cases. Occasional patients may relapse but recover with an additional course of corticosteroids.

ORGANIZING PNEUMONIA/COP—FACT SHEET

Definition

▸ A specific pattern of patchy, bronchiolocentric intra-alveolar organizing fibroblastic tissue with or without associated bronchiolar involvement

Gender and Age Distribution

▸ Fifth and sixth decades are most frequent
▸ M = F

Clinical Features

▸ 2- to 3-month history of cough and dyspnea with or without associated weight loss or fever
▸ Many patients report antecedent flu-like illness
▸ May be idiopathic or secondary to an underlying etiology

Radiologic Features

▸ Bilateral patchy air space consolidation/ground-glass opacities with or without small nodules around bronchovascular bundles

Prognosis and Therapy

▸ Excellent: essentially all patients respond to corticosteroid therapy

---

ORGANIZING PNEUMONIA/COP—PATHOLOGIC FEATURES

Microscopic Findings

▸ Intra-alveolar organizing fibroblastic tissue in a patchy, bronchiolocentric distribution
▸ Fibroblastic tissue in bronchioles
▸ Mild to moderate chronic interstitial inflammation in affected areas
▸ Intervening lung tissue is relatively normal
▸ Lung architecture is preserved; fibrosis is essentially absent

Pathologic Differential Diagnosis

▸ Diffuse alveolar damage
▸ Hypersensitivity pneumonia
▸ Eosinophilic pneumonia
▸ Usual interstitial pneumonia
▸ Nonspecific interstitial pneumonia
▸ Acute fibrinous and organizing pneumonia
▸ BOOP-like variant of Wegener's granulomatosis

Previously reported cases of BOOP/COP with a poor prognosis most likely represent other disease entities using current guidelines.

ACUTE FIBRINOUS AND ORGANIZING PNEUMONIA

Acute fibrinous and organizing pneumonia (AFOP) is a recently described histologic pattern associated with an acute or subacute clinical presentation that does not meet the strict histologic criteria for either OP/COP or DAD. Initial evaluation suggests that it may represent a variant of DAD. In contrast to OP and DAD, AFOP is characterized by the presence of organizing fibrin balls within alveolar spaces without associated hyaline membrane formation (Figure 9-14). A patchy distribution is typical, although some cases may appear more diffuse. Variable amounts of organizing intra-alveolar fibroblastic tissue may be present, which may contain fibrin cores. The alveolar septa in affected areas contain variable chronic inflammation, but fibrosis is essentially absent.

In the initial study of AFOP, patients presented with an average of 19 days of symptoms most commonly consisting of dyspnea and cough. A distinctive radiographic presentation was not found, but the most frequent finding was bilateral basilar infiltrates.

Diagnostic issues are similar to those encountered in DAD and OP. As with OP, organizing intra-alveolar fibrin may occur as the specific pattern of AFOP or as a nonspecific reaction at the periphery of an unrelated process such as a neoplasm or abscess. Therefore, the finding of intra-alveolar fibrin must be interpreted with caution on a small biopsy specimen. Like the other forms of acute lung injury, AFOP may be idiopathic, or it may occur secondary to a variety of etiologies, particularly infections, collagen vascular diseases, and drug reactions, which should be excluded clinically. Special stains for microorganisms should be performed in all cases.

The main histologic differential diagnoses for AFOP are OP, the exudative phase of DAD and eosinophilic pneumonia (EP). OP may occasionally have foci of fibrin, but it is not the dominant finding as is seen in AFOP. DAD may also have areas of organizing fibrin, which may be prominent, but hyaline membranes are still generally found, and type 2 pneumocyte hyperplasia is more pronounced. EP also typically has fairly pronounced intra-alveolar fibrin and variable organizing pneumonia. The main distinguishing feature of EP is the presence of abundant eosinophils. Macrophages are also generally present in EP and are not a prominent finding in AFOP. Of note, eosinophils disappear quickly with corticosteroid administration, and a partially treated EP should also be considered clinically if a biopsy is obtained subsequent to initiation of corticosteroid therapy. Peripheral blood eosinophilia has not been

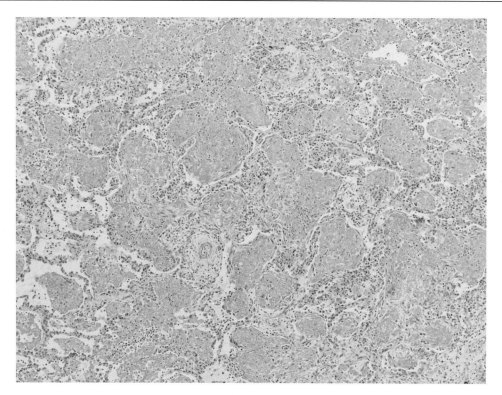

FIGURE 9-14

Acute fibrinous and organizing pneumonia
AFOP is characterized by the presence of intra-alveolar fibrin balls without formation of classic hyaline membranes. The process is typically patchy, but may be relatively diffuse.

found in cases of AFOP, but has not been extensively evaluated.

In the initial AFOP study, patients fell into one of two clinical patterns of disease. Slightly over half of patients presented with a fulminant illness progressing rapidly to death, with the remaining patients experiencing an indolent course with eventual recovery. No clinical or histologic features correlated with the eventual outcome, and an optimal therapy was not elucidated. As the mortality rate was found to be similar to that seen with DAD, at this point AFOP is probably best considered a variant of DAD, although further study is needed to clarify the relationship of AFOP to OP and EP, and to provide an explanation for the less fulminant course seen in a significant number of patients.

SUGGESTED READINGS

1. American Thoracic Society/European Respiratory Society international multidisciplinary consensus classification of the idiopathic interstitial pneumonias. *Am J Respir Crit Care Med*. 2002;165:277-304.
2. Beasley, MB. Acute lung injury. In: Cagle P, Fraire A, and Tomashefski J, eds. *Dail and Hammar's Pulmonary Pathology*, 3rd ed. New York: Springer-Verlag; In press.
3. Beasley MB, Franks TJ, Galvin JR, Gochuico B, Travis WD. Acute fibrinous and organizing pneumonia: a histological pattern of lung injury and possible variant of diffuse alveolar damage. *Arch Pathol Lab Med*. 2002;126:1064-70.
4. Bernard GR, Artigas A, Brigham KL, et al. The American-European Consensus Conference on ARDS. Definitions, mechanisms, relevant outcomes, and clinical trial coordination. *Am J Respir Crit Care Med*. 1994;149:818-24.
5. Cordier JF. Organising pneumonia. *Thorax*. 2000;55:318-28.
6. Epler GR, Colby TV, McLoud TC, Carrington CB, Gaensler EA. Bronchiolitis obliterans organizing pneumonia. *N Engl J Med*. 1985;312:152-8.
7. Hamman L, Rich A. Acute diffuse interstitial fibrosis of the lung. *Bull Johns Hopkins Hosp*. 1944;74:177.
8. Hasleton PS, Roberts TE. Adult respiratory distress syndrome: an update. *Histopathology*. 1999;34:285-94.
9. Katzenstein AL, Bloor CM, Leibow AA. Diffuse alveolar damage: the role of oxygen, shock, and related factors. A review. *Am J Pathol*. 1976;85:209-28.
10. Katzenstein AL. Acute lung injury patterns: diffuse alveolar damage and bronchiolitis-obliterans-organizing pneumonia. In Katzenstein AL, ed. *Katzenstein and Askin's Surgical Pathology of Non-neoplastic Lung Disease*. 3rd ed. Philadelphia: W.B. Saunders; 1997:14-47.
11. Tomashefski JF, Jr. Pulmonary pathology of acute respiratory distress syndrome. *Clin Chest Med*. 2000;21:435-66.
12. Travis WD, Colby T, Koss MN, Rosado de Christiansen ML, Muller NL, King TE Jr. Idiopathic interstitial pneumonia and other diffuse parenchymal lung disease. In *Non-neoplastic Disorders of the Lower Respiratory Tract*. Washington, D.C.: Armed Forces Institute of Pathology; 2004; 89-105.
13. Ware LB, Matthay MA. The acute respiratory distress syndrome. *N Engl J Med*. 2000;342:1334-49.

10 Bacterial Diseases

Carol F. Farver

INTRODUCTION

Bacterial infections in the lung can be classified in many different ways, i.e., pathogenesis, epidemiology, anatomic distribution (lobar or bronchopneumonia), time course, or etiologic agent. In practice, a combination of these approaches is needed to classify bacterial pneumonias. Indeed, the clinician and pathologist usually require clinical, pathologic, and microbiologic information to diagnosis most pneumonias. Therefore, for the purposes of this chapter, we will discuss each group of organisms and highlight the anatomic patterns it can cause and its distinguishing clinical and microbiologic features.

COMMON BACTERIAL PNEUMONIAS

Many organisms can cause pneumonia; however, the vast majority of respiratory illness is the result of infection by nine groups of organisms: *Streptococcus pneumoniae*, *Staphylococcus* sp, *Streptococcus* sp, *Legionella*, *Haemophilus influenzae*, *Pseudomonas aeruginosa*, anaerobic bacteria, Nocardia, and Actinomyces.

STREPTOCOCCUS PNEUMONIAE

INTRODUCTION

Streptococcus pneumoniae is also known as pneumococcus, a term coined soon after its discovery because of its association with pulmonary infections, and *Dip-*
lococcus pneumoniae, because it has paired cocci in tissue and liquid culture. It is a leading cause of meningitis, otitis media, bacteremia, and pneumonia in the United States.

CLINICAL FEATURES

Pneumonia due to *S. pneumoniae* is the most common cause of community-acquired pneumonia. It usually develops in infants or the elderly, in the setting of overcrowded environments or in individuals with an increased risk of aspiration such as alcoholics. Suppressed immune responses including damage to the mucociliary tree (smokers), defective immunoglobulin response, neutropenia, or defects in the complement cascade are also risk factors for this type of pneumonia.

The symptoms are characterized by sudden onset of chills, pleuritic chest pain, high fever, and cough productive of "rusty-colored" sputum. Tachycardia, tachypnea, and dyspnea are frequently seen. Laboratory values typically reveal a leukocytosis with a shift toward immature forms and, in severe cases, leukopenia.

RADIOLOGIC FEATURES

A typical chest x-ray shows patchy infiltrates that involve more than one lung segment and may progress to complete lobar consolidation, cavity formation, and pleural effusions.

PATHOLOGIC FEATURES

GROSS FINDINGS

Pneumococcal pneumonia is the most common cause of lobar pneumonia that progresses from a red hepatization phase to a grey hepatization phase (Figure 10-1). Fibrinous pleuritis and pleural effusions are common, and are the pathologic features responsible for the pleuritic pain that are usually experienced by these patients.

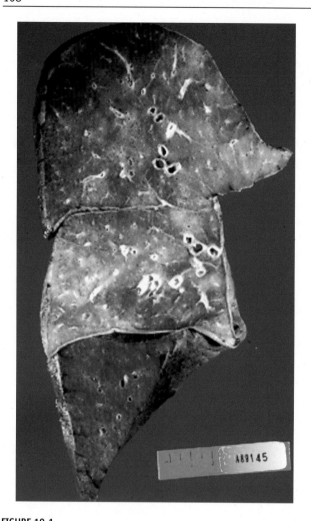

FIGURE 10-1

Lobar pneumococcal pneumonia
Localized red hepatization involving a segment of the lower left lung. (Courtesy of Dr. Joseph Tomashefski, MetroHealth Medical Center, Cleveland, Ohio.)

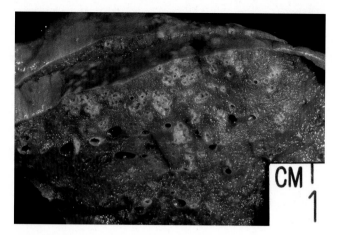

FIGURE 10-2

Lobular pneumococcal pneumonia
The early disease shows a red congested area with localized yellow foci of neutrophilic debris centered on the bronchioles.

undergo fibrosis, resulting in a firm lobe of lung encased within a fibrous capsule.

ANCILLARY STUDIES

MICROBIOLOGY

The organism is fragile and requires immediate plating for successful cultures. In culture, the organisms commonly grow in chains. Blood cultures are the best way to establish a diagnosis. Sputum cultures are sensitive, but may be difficult to interpret given the multiple organisms that may be present. Gram-positive lancet-shaped diplococci are seen within the neutrophils in smear preparations.

DIFFERENTIAL DIAGNOSIS

The differential diagnosis includes other predominantly non-necrotizing bacterial pneumonias due to *H. influenzae* and *Klebsiella pneumoniae*, and some viral pneumonias, especially influenza.

PROGNOSIS AND THERAPY

Penicillin is considered the drug of choice for *S. pneumoniae* pneumonia. However, because this infection has the potential to advance rapidly, usually initial treatment is started before microbiologic confirmation and consists of additional antibiotics including cephalosporins, doxycycline, macrolides, clindamycin, and fluoroquinolones.

The consolidation is more common in the posterior and lower segments of the lobe and more commonly seen in the lower lobes. The bronchi may exude a frothy fluid indicative of the marked congestion of the lung. Necrosis and cavitation are rare. Empyemas occur in approximately 2% of patients.

MICROSCOPIC FINDINGS

In the early stages of the disease, the infection has a lobular distribution (Figure 10-2). The alveoli show increased fluid with intra-alveolar fibrin, neutrophils, mononuclear cells and erythrocytes, congested and distended alveolar capillaries, and hyaline membranes within alveolar ducts (Figure 10-3). During this phase, the gram-positive organisms are abundant within neutrophils and macrophages. The fibrinous exudate present in the alveoli may also be found within the large airways. As the disease progresses, the intra-alveolar exudates will begin to organize and the pleuritis may

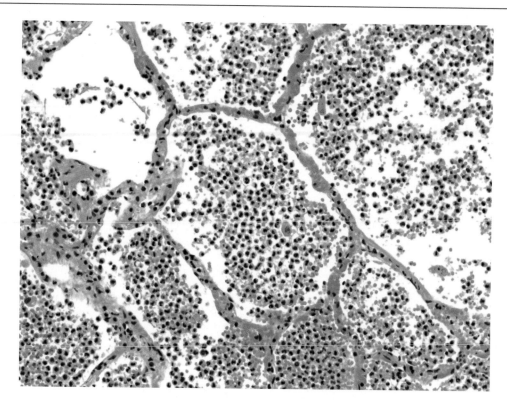

FIGURE 10-3

Acute pneumococcal bronchopneumonia
Alveoli with congested capillaries in alveolar walls. Intra-alveolar fibrin, neutrophils, and mononuclear cells are present.

Antibiotic resistance, an increasing problem, is found in approximately 30% of isolates. With prompt treatment, most individuals begin to recover within 1 to 2 days. Radiographic resolution is usually complete by 2 to 3 weeks.

Pneumococcal vaccine can prevent bacteremia in individuals at high risk for developing complications from this pneumonia. These include the young and the old, individuals with chronic obstructive pulmonary disease, diabetes, cardiovascular disease, alcoholism, asplenia, renal insufficiency, and immunosuppression of various types.

STAPHYLOCOCCUS SPECIES

INTRODUCTION

Pneumonia due to *Staphylococcus* species accounts for approximately 10% of all of pneumonias. *S. aureus*, the most common organisms isolated, is a gram-positive coccus that usually grows in clusters. *S. epidermidis* and *S. saprophyticus* may cause pneumonia, but are not common pathogens in the lungs. *Staphylococcus* sp gives off multiple toxins that may cause both localized tissue in-

jury in the form of abscesses and systemic tissue injury as is seen in toxic shock syndrome.

CLINICAL FEATURES

Pneumonia due to *Staphylococcus* species is usually the result of hematogenous spread from other sources, though it may also occur by spreading from upper airways infection or aspiration of oral secretions. It is two times more common as a nosocomial infection than as a community-acquired one. It is a common pathogen in patients with influenza or cystic fibrosis, in the immunocompromised, and in the very young and the very old. The clinical course is characterized by a high fever, chills, cough productive of purulent bloody sputum, and dyspnea.

RADIOLOGIC FEATURES

Staphylococcal pneumonia usually manifests as patchy, bilateral, lower-lobe infiltrates that may progress to complete consolidation. Early infection is based around the bronchioles as an early necrotizing pneumonia.

STREPTOCOCCUS PNEUMONIAE—FACT SHEET

Definition

▸ Also called Pneumococcus (*Diplococcus pneumoniae*), *S. pneumoniae* causes meningitis, otitis media, bacteremia, and pneumonia

Incidence

▸ Leading cause of community-acquired bacterial pneumonia
▸ Patients with immunoglobulin deficiencies, aspiration, splenectomy, and sickle cell disease at increased risk

Age Distribution

▸ More common in infants and elderly

Clinical Features

▸ Sudden onset of chills, pleuritic chest pain, high fever, "rust-colored" sputum
▸ Laboratory values show leukocytosis or leukopenia

Radiologic Features

▸ Infiltrates may involve any lobe
▸ Posterior and lower segments of lower lobes are the most common sites
▸ Patchy infiltrates that progress to lobar consolidation
▸ Cavities are rare; pleural effusions may be present

Prognosis and Therapy

▸ Penicillin is the drug of choice, though resistance is found in 30% of isolates
▸ Vaccine can prevent bacteremia in patients at risk for developing complications from the pneumonia
▸ Excellent prognosis with most individuals recovering in 1 to 2 days

Cavity formation may occur. Over half of patients have pleural effusions, and a majority of these will progress to empyema.

PATHOLOGIC FEATURES

GROSS FINDINGS

During the acute infection, the lungs are congested with a purple/red color and a minimal pleural reaction (Figure 10-4). Pleural effusions are common and usually of a serosanguineous quality. Airways and cut surfaces may contain bloody fluid, and a thick, exudative bronchitis with pseudomembrane formation has been seen. Progression of the disease usually results in a necrotizing, peribronchiolar pattern that develops into multiple, thin-walled cavities (pneumatoceles) from 1-5 cm in diameter with thick, yellow/green pus (Figure 10-5). These are especially common in children.

STREPTOCOCCUS PNEUMONIAE—PATHOLOGIC FEATURES

Gross Findings

▸ Lobar consolidation that progresses from red to grey hepatization phase
▸ Fibrinous pleuritis
▸ Pleural effusions may progress to empyemas (2% of patients)

Microscopic Findings

▸ Intra-alveolar fibrinous exudates with abundant neutrophils
▸ Marked capillary congestion
▸ Variable hemorrhage
▸ May see hyaline membranes

Microbiology

▸ Gram-positive cocci in pairs
▸ Sputum smear is more sensitive than cultures for diagnosis

Pathologic Differential Diagnosis

▸ Other non-necrotizing pneumonias such as *H. influenzae* and *K. pneumoniae*

MICROSCOPIC FINDINGS

Staphylococcal pneumonia can be acquired hematogenously or as a bronchopneumonia (Figure 10-6) that may arise out of an acute, necrotizing tracheobronchitis which spreads distally to involve the alveoli. This acute, exudative infiltrate usually expands to fill large areas of the surrounding lung and commonly develops into a necrotizing pneumonia with cavitation and abscess formation (Figure 10-7). Within the phagocytes of the infiltrates, gram-positive cocci are abundant, usually in grape-like clusters. Though pleuritis is uncommon, extension of these cavities to the pleural surface and empyema formation are common.

ANCILLARY STUDIES

MICROBIOLOGY

Staphylococci are gram-positive, catalase-producing anaerobes that grow well in culture. They are easy to culture from most body fluids and in smear preparations appear as irregular, grape-like clusters, but can be seen as singles or in pairs.

DIFFERENTIAL DIAGNOSIS

The differential diagnosis includes other cavitating pneumonias. These include bacterial pneumonias such as Pseudomonas pneumonia, fungal pneumonias, and mycobacterial pneumonias.

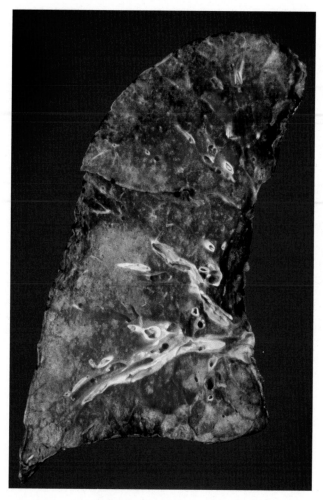

FIGURE 10-4

Acute bronchopneumonia due to staphylococcal pneumonia
Section of the lung reveals purple/red color in the area of infection that is progressing from the peribronchiolar areas and coalescing into large patches through the lung. (Courtesy of Dr. Joseph Tomashefski, MetroHealth Medical Center, Cleveland, Ohio.)

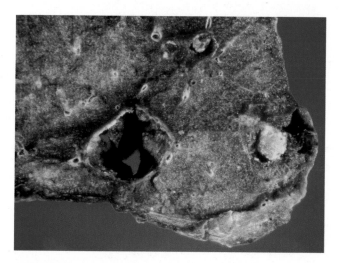

FIGURE 10-5

Staphylococcal pneumonia with cavitation
An abscess with yellow pus (right) is present in lung. These abscesses undergo healing and become thin-walled cavities (pneumatoceles) (center). (Courtesy of Dr. Joseph Tomashefski, MetroHealth Medical Center, Cleveland, Ohio.)

PROGNOSIS AND THERAPY

Staphylococcal pneumonia requires immediate treatment with penicillins or cephalosporin. Methicillin-resistant *Staphylococcus* is a growing problem and requires vancomycin as an alternative antibiotic. The mortality from *Staphylococcus* can be significant, usually 25-30%, and may be as high as 80% in the setting of complications such as bacteremia, cavitation, and empyema.

STREPTOCOCCUS SPECIES

INTRODUCTION

Streptococcus species refer to the gram-positive streptococci that are not pneumococci. There are now approximately 50 species of Streptococci, however, only five cause disease in humans. These include: Group A—beta-hemolytic, *S. pyogenes*; Group B—beta hemolytic, *S. agalactiae*; Group C—beta-hemolytic; Group D—*Enterococcus*; and, Group F—alpha-hemolytic, *S. viridans*. These account for approximately 1% of adult pneumonias, and most are due to Group A, beta-hemolytic streptococcus. Group B streptococci are a major cause of neonatal pneumonia.

CLINICAL FEATURES

Group A *Streptococcus* pneumonia is similar to *S. aureus* pneumonia in that it may result from either spread from a soft tissue or skin source or result from contamination from nasopharynx organisms and commonly follow a viral pneumonia. Epidemics have been reported in military recruits and after influenza. The clinical course is similar to *S. aureus*, with a fulminant onset with high fevers, chills, tachypnea, blood-streaked sputum, pleuritic chest pain, and, in severe cases of early shock, tachycardia.

RADIOLOGIC FEATURES

The initial radiographs may be normal, lagging behind the clinical symptoms, but quickly deteriorate to include bilateral diffuse infiltrates (usually lower lobe), empyema, and pneumatoceles. Lower lobe collapse can be seen as the disease progresses.

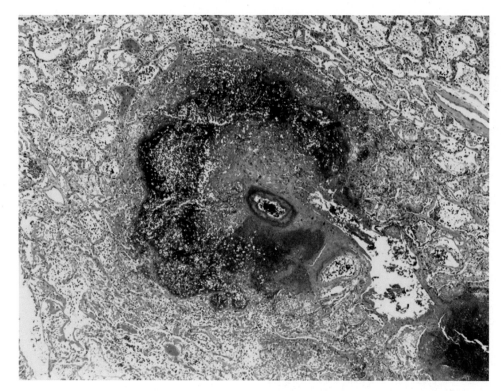

FIGURE 10-6

Acute staphylococcal bronchopneumonia
Acute inflammation with necrosis and basophilic neutrophilic debris develops around bronchioles in early acute bronchopneumonia due to *Staphylococcus aureus*.

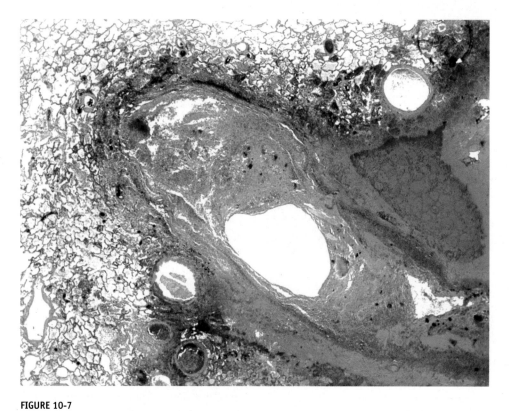

FIGURE 10-7

Acute staphylococcal pneumonia with early necrosis
The peribronchiolar necrosis expands to include large areas of the adjacent lung. These areas eventually form large cavities.

STAPHYLOCOCCUS SPECIES—FACT SHEET

Definition

» Bacteria produce toxins and cause localized tissue injury in the form of abscesses or systemic disease such as toxic shock syndrome

Incidence

» More common as nosocomial infections
» 10% of all pneumonias
» Common in patients with influenza, cystic fibrosis, and immunocompromise

Mortality

» 25-30% mortality and may be as high as 80% with complications such as bacteremia, cavitation, or empyema

Age Distribution

» More common in the very young and the very old

Clinical Features

» Pneumonia caused by hematogenous spread from other sites or acquired through the airways
» Twice as common as a nosocomial infection than as a community-acquired infection

Radiologic Features

» Patchy, bilateral, lower-lobe infiltrates
» May progress to complete consolidation
» Cavitation may occur
» Pleural effusions in over half of patients

Therapy

» Immediate treatment with penicillins or cephalosporins
» Methicillin resistance is growing problem, which requires vancomycin

STAPHYLOCOCCUS SPECIES—PATHOLOGIC FEATURES

Gross Findings

» Red/purple lungs with bloody fluid and exudative bronchitis
» Disease progression results in thin-walled cavities with thick yellow/green pus
» Extension of cavities to pleural surface and empyema formation is common

Microscopic Findings

» Bronchopneumonia pattern with dense neutrophil infiltrate, fibrin, and macrophages
» Necrosis with abscess formation and cavitation is typical

Microbiology

» Gram-positive cocci in grape-like clusters
» Easy to culture from most body fluids

Pathologic Differential Diagnosis

» Cavitating pneumonias such as *Pseudomonas* pneumonia, fungal pneumonias, and mycobacterial pneumonias

PATHOLOGIC FEATURES

GROSS FINDINGS

The anatomic distribution of the infection ranges from localized lobular to lobar pneumonia (Figure 10-8). The lungs in the acute phase are red and edematous with pleural effusions. Hemorrhagic fluid fills both the airways and the lung tissue. With progression of the disease, the congested areas develop a tan/yellow color as the inflammation begins to organize, and a fibrinous pleuritis and empyema develop in the overwhelming majority of the cases. Cavitation and pneumatocele formation commonly occur.

MICROSCOPIC FINDINGS

The histologic changes early in the disease center on the bronchioles and consist of a marked acute inflammatory infiltrate with abundant neutrophils. As bacterial

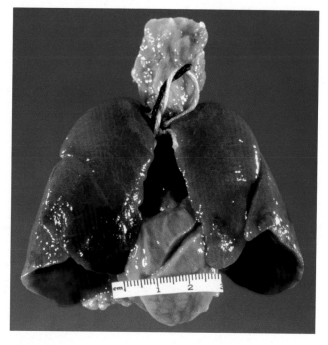

FIGURE 10-8

Group A streptococcal lobar pneumonia in neonatal lungs
The lungs are red and edematous. Hemorrhagic fluid fills both lungs, producing a dark red/purple color. (Photo courtesy of Dr. Beverly Dahms, Case Western Reserve University, Cleveland, Ohio.)

enzymes lyse these cells, neutrophilic debris is left behind, giving the histology a "dirty" appearance (Figure 10-9). Using a Gram stain, the organisms are visible within phagocytes as gram-positive cocci in chains. Organization of the infiltrate occurs, but tissue necrosis and eventual abscess formation is common.

ANCILLARY STUDIES

MICROBIOLOGY

Streptococcus species are gram-positive organisms measuring approximately 2 μm, which grow readily in culture. They are classified according to their hemolytic reaction on blood agar.

DIFFERENTIAL DIAGNOSIS

The clinical and pathologic features of this pneumonia must be distinguished from other necrotizing bacterial pneumonias, including those caused by *S. pneumoniae, S. aureus,* and *Pseudomonas* sp.

PROGNOSIS AND THERAPY

Group A pneumonia in adults and Group B pneumonia in neonates are usually treated successfully with penicillin or vancomycin. However, Group A pneumonia is often seen as a component of systemic Group A streptococcal infections, including toxic shock syndrome, or as a secondary infection in patients with influenza. In these settings, the pneumonia has a high mortality rate despite antibiotic treatment.

HEMOPHILUS INFLUENZAE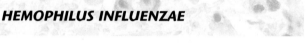

INTRODUCTION

H. influenzae, found in the upper respiratory tract, causes pneumonia either through hematogenous spread or by aspiration into chronically inflamed lungs. Six serotypes (A-F) are defined based on their capsular antigens. Both children and adults are susceptible to these pulmonary infections, usually by type B, an encapsulated strain.

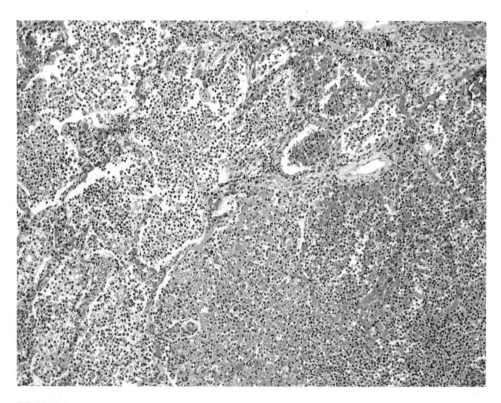

FIGURE 10-9

Group A streptococcal pneumonia

A marked, acute inflammatory infiltrate with an abundance of neutrophils fills the alveolar spaces. Lysis of these cells by bacterial enzymes produces a "dirty" appearance (lower right).

STREPTOCOCCUS SPECIES—FACT SHEET

Definition
- Refers to streptococci that are not pneumococci
- Approximately 50 species are present; 5 cause disease in humans

Incidence
- Account for 1% of adult pneumonias, most due to Group A—beta-hemolytic *Streptococcus*
- Group B streptococcus is a major course of neonatal pneumonia

Mortality
- Both Group A pneumonia in adults and Group B pneumonia in neonates have an excellent prognosis with antimicrobial treatment
- In the setting of systemic Group A streptococcal infections, there is a high mortality rate

Age Distribution
- Adults and neonates

Clinical Features
- Rapid onset of symptoms
- High fever, chills, tachypnea, blood-streaked sputum, pleuritic chest pain
- Typically occurs in winter and early spring
- Epidemics have occurred in military recruits and after influenza

Radiologic Features
- Bilateral diffuse infiltrates
- Usually lower lobe
- Empyema and pneumatoceles are common
- Lower lobe collapse may be seen with disease progression

Therapy
- Usually treated successfully with penicillin or vancomycin

STREPTOCOCCUS SPECIES—PATHOLOGIC FEATURES

Gross Findings
- Red, edematous, fluid-filled lung with pleural effusions
- Hemorrhagic fluid fills both the airways and lung tissue
- Yellow/tan color develops with progressive consolidation
- Pneumatocele and empyema are common

Microscopic Findings
- Abundant centrilobular neutrophilic infiltrate (bronchioles, alveoli)
- "Dirty" necrosis with progression
- Tissue necrosis and eventual abscess formation is common

Microbiology
- Gram-positive cocci usually found in chains
- Organisms classified according to their hemolytic reaction on blood agar

Pathologic Differential Diagnosis
- Other necrotizing pneumonias such as *S. aureus* and *Pseudomonas* sp.

These organisms are also responsible for a spectrum of other infections including meningitis, epiglottitis, otitis, and arthritis.

CLINICAL FEATURES

H. influenzae pneumonia is found predominantly in children. In adults, it is most commonly found in the elderly with underlying chronic lung disease such as chronic bronchitis, bronchiectasis or cystic fibrosis, with HIV infection, or in alcoholics. Epiglottitis is a common manifestation of this infection in children. The pneumonia is usually preceded by a viral or mycoplasmal infection that disrupts the airway mucosa, predisposing it to infections by these colonizing organisms. Symptoms of *H. influenzae* pneumonia are fever, a cough productive of purulent sputum, and myalgias. Most commonly found as a community-acquired pneumonia, its role as a nosocomial infection is increasing, especially in younger patients.

RADIOLOGIC FEATURES

H. influenzae pneumonia is usually localized, causing a lobar or segmental consolidation. In patients with hematogenous spread, a diffuse miliary pattern may be present. Cavitation or empyemas can be seen but are not common.

PATHOLOGIC FEATURES

GROSS FINDINGS

The pneumonia is usually a necrotizing pneumonia with a lobar pattern. Cavitation or pneumatoceles, when present, usually arise out of the lobar pattern and are more common in children.

MICROSCOPIC FINDINGS

The infiltrate is rich in neutrophils with fibroblastic proliferation and organization in the peripheral areas. A pleural effusion may be present with a fibrinous pleuritis.

ANCILLARY STUDIES

MICROBIOLOGY

H. influenzae is a gram-negative coccobacillus that is somewhat difficult to culture. Organisms can be seen in Gram-stained sputum. Most pneumonias are caused by the encapsulated type B, with type F the second most common strain isolated. Nontypeable (nonencapsulated) strains have been found in community and hospital-acquired pneumonia.

DIFFERENTIAL DIAGNOSIS

Streptococcal pneumonia or staphylococcal pneumonia and pneumonias caused by *K. pneumoniae* may mimic this predominantly non-necrotizing pneumonia.

PROGNOSIS AND THERAPY

Patients usually survive this pneumonia when treated promptly with antimicrobials. Due to increasing bacterial resistance, the treatment of choice is third-generation cephalosporin antibiotics. Mortality may be higher with bacteremia. A vaccine to *H. influenzae* type B (HIB vaccine) has been shown to be effective in preventing infections in children.

PSEUDOMONAS AERUGINOSA

INTRODUCTION

Pseudomonas aeruginosa is a gram-negative bacillus that is found throughout the environment, especially in warm water reservoirs. Human colonization is relatively low outside of the hospital, documented usually at rates of less than 10%. With hospitalization, that rate increases substantially to approximately 50% of all hospitalized patients. It may enter the body through a variety of routes, including the pharynx, the abdomen, and the urinary tract, usually due to disruption of the epithelial surfaces in these areas by cuts, burns, or therapeutic devices such as mechanical ventilators or intravascular catheters. Infection of the lower respiratory tract occurs through microaspiration of colonized secretions from the oropharynx, inoculation by an endotracheal tube, or hematogenous spread from an extrapulmonary infected site.

CLINICAL FEATURES

Pneumonia due to *Pseudomonas aeruginosa* is most commonly seen as a nosocomial infection in intensive care units, burn units, in patients with chronic obstructive pulmonary disease or with cystic fibrosis, and in patients who have undergone a prolonged hospitalization. The presentation is usually fulminant with marked dyspnea and respiratory failure and may progress to gram-negative sepsis. The diagnosis is usually made by cultures of either tracheobronchial aspirates or bronchoscopically retrieved specimens. Blood cultures and pleural fluids are rarely positive.

RADIOLOGIC FEATURES

Radiographic patterns of *Pseudomonas* pneumonia include uni- or multifocal opacities, usually in the lower lobes. Cavities are present in less than 10% of cases and pleural effusions are unusual.

PATHOLOGIC FEATURES

GROSS FINDINGS

Pseudomonas pneumonia due to aspiration from upper airway sources is characterized first by necrotizing bronchocentric pneumonia, which eventually progresses to confluent areas with abscess formation. *Pseudomonas* pneumonia due to hematogenous spread is characterized by areas of necrosis that are usually surrounded by a red halo of congestion and hemorrhage (Figure 10-10), which go on to form cavities (Figure 10-11).

MICROSCOPIC FINDINGS

Pseudomonas pneumonia begins as a bronchocentric, neutrophilic alveolitis that rapidly progresses to formation of microabscesses and, eventually, large abscesses. A necrotizing vasculitis can be seen, with abundant organisms present within vessel walls (Figure 10-12). Hemorrhagic infarction and thrombi may be seen.

ANCILLARY STUDIES

MICROBIOLOGY

Pseudomonas aeruginosa are gram-negative, motile, nonfermenting, obligate aerobic rods that have minimal growth requirements in culture. Identification is usually based on the colony morphology, which is round with a fluorescent greenish color. Mucoid strains are prevalent in cystic fibrosis patients. Most organisms are easily identified in tissue by either a Gram or Brown and Hopps stain within the areas of necrosis.

DIFFERENTIAL DIAGNOSIS

The differential diagnosis includes other types of fulminant, necrotizing pneumonia, most notably *Staphylococcus* pneumonia or *Klebsiella* pneumonia. Opportunistic organisms to consider may include *E. coli*.

PROGNOSIS AND THERAPY

Mortality depends upon co-existing risk factors, but is usually in the range of 20-50% for hospitalized patients. Rapid treatment is necessary and usually includes a combination of aminoglycosides (amikacin), β−lactams,

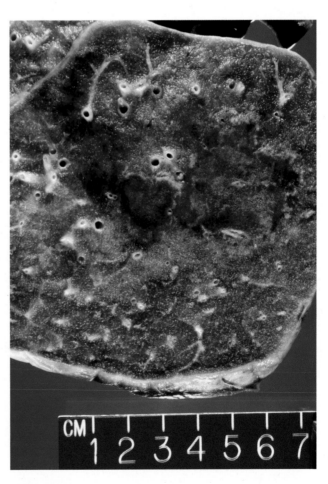

FIGURE 10-10

Early *Pseudomonas* pneumonia with necrotizing bronchocentric pattern
Yellow areas of necrosis are surrounded by a red halo of hemorrhage.

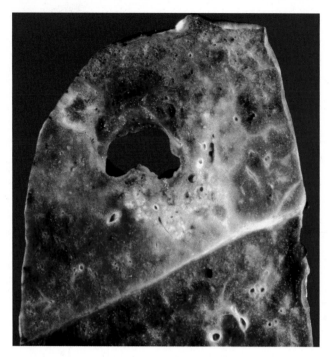

FIGURE 10-11

Cavitary *Pseudomonas* pneumonia
A healed cavity with a thin, fibrous wall, the result of of *Pseudomonas* pneumonia. (Courtesy of Dr. Joseph Tomashefski, MetroHealth Medical Center, Cleveland, Ohio.)

and quinolones (ciprofloxacin). Antibiotic resistance is present in 10-20% of patients.

LEGIONELLA SPECIES

INTRODUCTION

Legionella are gram-negative bacilli found predominantly in aquatic habitats such as lakes, rivers, ponds, and also in artificial reservoirs such as evaporator pans, cooling towers, humidifiers, and other water outlets. These man-made water reservoirs are the main source of bacteria that cause human infections. It has been estimated that approximately 50% of air conditioners contain *Legionella* bacilli. *Legionella pneumophila* has 15 serogroups, 3 of which cause the overwhelming majority of human infections. It is responsible for 10% of community-acquired pneumonias.

CLINICAL FEATURES

L. pneumophila causes two forms of clinical disease: legionnaires' disease, named after the outbreak of pneumonia caused by the bacillus at a 1976 American Legion convention in Philadelphia when the organism was first

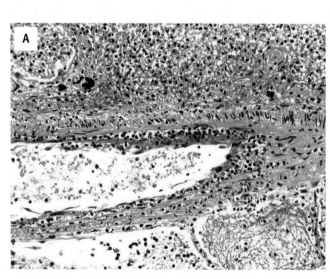

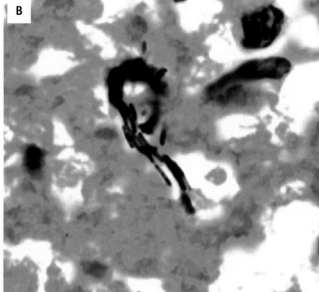

FIGURE 10-12

Necrotizing vasculitis of *Pseudomonas* pneumonia
An acute inflammatory infiltrate involves a medium-size artery, producing a transmural necrosis **(A)**; present within the areas of necrosis around the vessel are abundant organisms (B-Gram stain).

PSEUDOMONAS AERUGINOSA—FACT SHEET

Definition

▸ Pneumonia caused by *P. aeruginosa,* usually a result of micro-aspiration of colonized oropharyngeal material

Incidence

▸ 10% of pneumonias developing outside of the hospital; 50% of pneumonias developing in hospitalized patients
▸ Increased risk for patients with burns, chronic obstructive pulmonary disease, or cystic fibrosis, or those who have undergone prolonged hospitalization

Mortality

▸ Mortality of 20-50%, depending upon risk factors

Gender and Age Distribution

▸ Elderly and debilitated patients with underlying chronic lung disease

Clinical Features

▸ Clinical symptoms are usually fulminant with marked dyspnea and respiratory failure
▸ Progression to sepsis is common

Radiologic Features

▸ Unifocal or multifocal opacities, usually in the lower lobes
▸ Cavities present in less than 10% of cases

Therapy

▸ Antimicrobial therapy with combination of aminoglycosides, β-lactam, and quinolones
▸ Antibiotic resistance is present in 10-20%

PSEUDOMONAS AERUGINOSA—PATHOLOGIC FEATURES

Gross Findings

▸ Confluent consolidation progressing to abscess formation
▸ Necrosis surrounded by red halo of congestion and hemorrhage

Microscopic Findings

▸ Bronchocentric, neutrophilic alveolitis
▸ Microabscesses and larger abscesses
▸ Necrotizing vasculitis with abundant organisms
▸ Hemorrhagic infarction and thrombi are commonly seen

Microbiology

▸ Gram-negative, obligate aerobic rods that are easily identified in tissue by Gram stain

Pathologic Differential Diagnosis

▸ Fulminant, necrotizing pneumonia such as staphylococcal pneumonia, *Klebsiella* pneumonia, or pneumonia due to *E. coli*

---

isolated, and Pontiac fever (non-pneumonic legionellosis), a self-limiting flu-like disease with nonspecific symptoms. *Legionella* pneumonia is a severe, progressive pulmonary infection with eventual extrapulmonary complications, which include nausea, vomiting, diarrhea, and renal insufficiency. Chills and rigors are common, and a nonproductive or mucoid cough is usually present. Shortness of breath and pleuritic chest pain are common presenting symptoms. The pneumonia is more common in men than women.

RADIOLOGIC FEATURES

Early in the disease, the chest imaging studies usually show unilateral, lower lobe infiltrates, which progress very quickly to involve multiple lobes, even after antibiotic treatment has been started. Pleural effusions are quite common and loculated effusions, empyemas, and other pleural complications can occur, particularly in the immunocompromised patient. Cavitation is rare.

PATHOLOGIC FEATURES

GROSS FINDINGS

Lungs involved by *Legionella* pneumonia are firm, red, congested with a rubbery texture, and appear distended with fluid upon opening the thoracic cavity.

MICROSCOPIC FINDINGS

Legionella pneumonia has a dramatic microscopic appearance with a marked fibrinopurulent exudate and a cellular infiltrate of monocytes, macrophages, and neutrophils (Figure 10-13). This cellular exudate appears to carpet the alveolar spaces, and bacteria are easily seen in these areas. At the periphery of the acute pneumonia, there may be hyaline membranes and a fibrinoserous exudate. Abscesses, if present, are small.

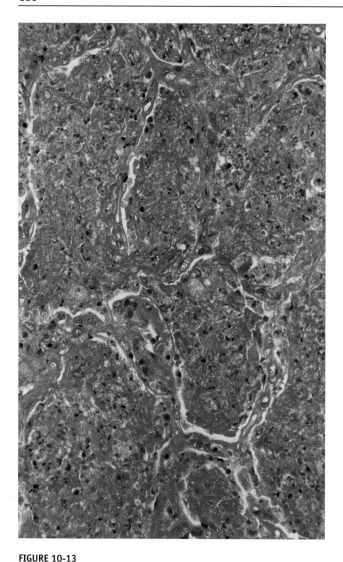

FIGURE 10-13

Legionella pneumonia
A fibrinopurulent exudate with monocytes, macrophages, and neutrophils fills the alveolar spaces.

ANCILLARY STUDIES

MICROBIOLOGY

Legionella is easily cultured from sputum, transtracheal aspirates, pleural effusions, and bronchoscopic specimens. This gram-negative bacillus grows easily on supplemented buffered charcoal yeast extract or a modified Mueller-Hinton agar. The most sensitive tissue organismic stains are the silver impregnation stains such as a Steiner, Warthin-Starry, or Dieterle; the bacilli are difficult to see on Gram and Brown and Hopps bacterial stains (Figure 10-14). Direct fluorescent antibody tests are commonly used, can be applied to deparaffinized, formalin-fixed tissue slides, and can have a sensitivity of up to 80%. Urinary antigens remain the most useful test to detect *L. pneumophila*, with a sensitivity of 90%.

DIFFERENTIAL DIAGNOSIS

The differential diagnosis includes other predominantly non-necrotizing bacterial pneumonias caused by *S. pneumoniae, H. influenzae,* and *Klebsiella pneumoniae,* and some viral pneumonias, especially influenza.

PROGNOSIS AND THERAPY

The new macrolides (azithromycin) and quinolones (ciprofloxacin and levofloxacin) are the most effective antibiotics for the treatment of Legionnaires' disease. Erythromycin is also effective but may have more side effects, including gastrointestinal symptoms. Clinical improvement is usually seen within 24 to 48 hours with most constitutional symptoms gone within 3 to 5 days. Mortality is reported in 5-25% of cases, with most deaths associated with delay of administration of appropriate antibiotics.

NOCARDIA

INTRODUCTION

Nocardiosis of the lung is caused by species of *Nocardia,* most commonly *Nocardia asteroides.* Pulmonary disease usually results from inhalation of the mycelial form of this gram-positive rod from its source in soil or organic matter. It is more commonly found in warmer climates, including the southern United States.

CLINICAL FEATURES

Nocardiosis usually occurs in adults and affects men twice as often as women. Normal hosts may be infected, but nocardiosis is much more common in immunocompromised patients. It is a common infection in patients with pulmonary alveolar proteinosis, chronic lung diseases, and mycobacterial and other granulomatous diseases. It takes the form of either a localized mycetoma or airway colonizer (healthy host) or invasive disease (immunocompromised host).

Nocardiosis usually presents as an indolent infection with symptoms present from 1 to several weeks before presentation. Cough is common and usually productive of thick, purulent sputum. Fever and weight loss occur as the disease progresses. Immunocompromised patients usually have a more acute course with fever, chills, dyspnea, and

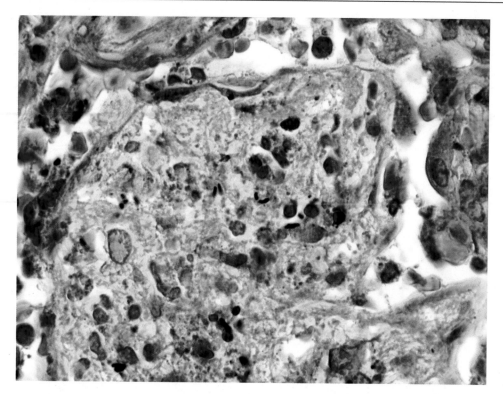

FIGURE 10-14

Legionella **pneumonia: identification of bacteria in tissue**
Legionella are gram-negative bacilli that are most easily seen in tissue using silver impregnation stains such as this Dieterle stain.

hemoptysis. Systemic involvement is not uncommon, particularly in the central nervous system and soft tissues.

RADIOLOGIC FEATURES

Chest imaging studies usually show bilateral infiltrates, which progress to consolidation, abscesses, and pleural involvement. Thin-walled cavities can be seen with abscess formation.

PATHOLOGIC FEATURES

GROSS FINDINGS

Suppurative necrosis and abscess formation is the usual gross picture of nocardiosis in the lung. The abscesses may be multiple and linked by sinus tracts filled with greenish, thick pus.

MICROSCOPIC FINDINGS

Neutrophils, macrophages, and necrotic debris are present in the middle of the abscesses, and epithelioid histiocytes and giant cells are sometimes seen around

the periphery. The organisms, which consist of long, filamentous gram-negative bacilli, can be seen randomly oriented in these areas of necrosis. As the abscess ages, these organisms may fragment into pleomorphic coccobacillary forms that can be seen within the phagocytes in the lesions. In the areas surrounding the abscesses, a fibrinopurulent acute pneumonia is present. Extension of both the acute pneumonia and the necrosis to the pleural surface is common, causing empyema to be present in a majority of cases.

ANCILLARY STUDIES

MICROBIOLOGY

Culturing these organisms may be difficult. Blood cultures are usually the most successful and may take 1 to 2 weeks for definitive results. Direct microscopic examination of tissue specimens is quicker and easier to make the diagnosis. *Nocardia* sp is a gram-negative bacillus approximately 1 micron wide that branches at right angles (Figure 10-15). In areas of necrosis, the organisms may be numerous and, because of their branching, are said to resemble Chinese characters. They are not usually seen on H and E staining, but are well visualized on Gram, Gomori methenamine, and partially

LEGIONELLA SPECIES—FACT SHEET

Definition

▸ Pneumonia caused by *L. pneumophila*

Incidence

▸ Responsible for less than 10% of community-acquired pneumonias

Mortality

▸ 5-25% mortality rate

Gender and Age Distribution

▸ More common in adults, though children and neonates can be affected
▸ 2-3:1 male to female ratio

Clinical Features

▸ Chills and rigors are common
▸ Shortness of breath, pleuritic chest pain, and nonproductive or mucoid cough
▸ Accompanying nausea, vomiting, diarrhea, and renal insufficiency

Radiologic Features

▸ Early disease is usually unilateral, lower lobe infiltrates
▸ Fast progression to multiple lobes
▸ Pleural effusions are common

Therapy

▸ Macrolides (azithromycin) and quinolones (ciprofloxacin and levofloxacin) are most effective

LEGIONELLA SPECIES—PATHOLOGIC FEATURES

Gross Findings

▸ Firm, red, congested lungs with a rubbery texture, which appear distended with fluid

Microscopic Findings

▸ Marked fibrinopurulent exudates with a necrotic cellular infiltrate of monocytes, macrophages, and neutrophils
▸ Exudate appears to "carpet" the alveolar space
▸ Periphery of the pneumonia may have hyaline membranes and a fibrinoserous exudate

Microbiology

▸ Gram-negative bacillus best seen on silver-impregnated stains (Steiner, Warthin-Starry, Dieterle)
▸ Easily cultured from sputum, transtracheal aspirates, pleural effusions, and bronchoscopic specimens

Pathologic Differential Diagnosis

▸ Non-necrotizing hemorrhagic *pneumonias* caused by *S. pneumoniae*, *H. influenzae*, or *K. pneumoniae*
▸ Some viral pneumonias such as influenza

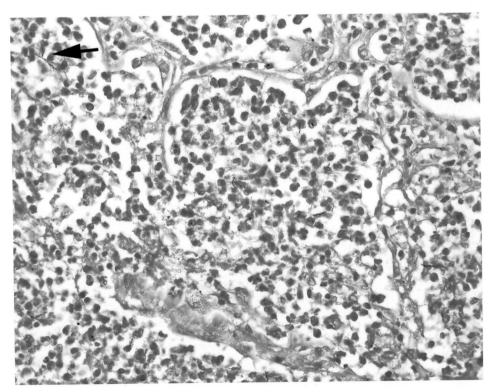

FIGURE 10-15

Nocardia: **identification of bacteria in tissue**

Nocardia is a gram-negative bacillus that branches at right angles (arrow). It can be seen in tissue using a Gram, Gomori methenamine silver, or partial acid-fast stain such as the Fite (shown here).

NOCARDIA—FACT SHEET

Definition

▸ Pneumonia caused by *Nocardia* sp., most commonly *Nocardia asteroides*
▸ Usually results from inhalation of soil or organic matter

Incidence

▸ Rare cause of pneumonia; usually found in immunocompromised patients
▸ Risk factors include pulmonary alveolar proteinosis, chronic lung diseases, and mycobacterial or other granulomatous diseases

Mortality

▸ 5% mortality with treatment

Gender and Age Distribution

▸ More common in adults than children
▸ 2:1 male to female ratio

Clinical Features

▸ Indolent infection, developing over one–several weeks
▸ Cough is productive of thick, purulent sputum
▸ Fever and weight loss may occur with disease progression
▸ Other systemic involvement may develop

Radiologic Features

▸ Bilateral infiltrates that progress to consolidation
▸ Abscesses (thin-walled cavities) and pleural involvement are common

Therapy

▸ Sulfonamides
▸ Surgery may be required to drain empyemas or abscesses

NOCARDIA—PATHOLOGIC FEATURES

Gross Findings

▸ Suppurative necrosis with abscess formation
▸ Multiple abscesses and sinus tracts with green, thick pus

Microscopic Findings

▸ Necrosis with neutrophils, macrophages, and necrotic debris
▸ Histiocytes may rim abscesses and multinucleated giant cells can be seen
▸ Fibrinopurulent acute pneumonia adjacent to abscesses
▸ Organisms may be numerous in areas of necrosis and resemble "Chinese characters"
▸ Organisms are best visualized on Gram, Gomori methenamine, and partially decolorized acid-fast stains (Fite)

Microbiology

▸ Long, filamentous, gram-negative bacilli branching at right angles
▸ Organisms may fragment into pleomorphic, coccobacillary forms within phagocytes
▸ May be difficult to culture; blood cultures are most successful

Pathologic Differential Diagnosis

▸ Other fulminant, necrotizing pneumonias such as staphylococcal pneumonia or *Klebsiella* pneumonia
▸ Microscopically may resemble *Actinomyces*, but does not form sulfur granules and is acid fast (Fite)-positive, unlike *Actinomyces*

---

decolorized acid fast stains such as Fite. With these stains, they appear beaded.

DIFFERENTIAL DIAGNOSIS

The differential diagnosis includes other forms of fulminant, necrotizing pneumonia, most notably staphylococcal pneumonia, and pneumonias due to *E. coli* or fungal pneumonias. Microscopically, the differential diagnosis includes *Actinomyces,* an organism that also appears filamentous but forms sulfur granules that are not seen with *Nocardia* sp. *Actinomyces,* however, does not stain with an acid fast stain. Mycobacteria, when numerous, can resemble *Nocardia*; however, they are usually shorter and do not branch.

PROGNOSIS AND THERAPY

Sulfonamides are the drugs of choice for the effective treatment of nocardiosis. Mortality is reported as less than 5% when therapy is not delayed. Surgery may be required to drain empyemas and abscesses, if formed.

ACTINOMYCES

INTRODUCTION

Actinomyces are endogenous commensals of the mouth, throat, GI tract, and vagina. They are gram-positive, branching, filamentous bacilli that are weakly pathogenic and usually infect previously traumatized or injured tissue. The main pathogenic species are *A. israelii, A. naeslundii, A. viscosus,* and *Arachnia propionica.* There are three major forms of actinomycosis: cervicofacial ("lumpy jaw"), thoracic, and abdomino-pelvic.

CLINICAL FEATURES

Pulmonary actinomycosis represents approximately 20% of all *Actinomyces* infections. The most common mode of introduction to the lung is through aspiration of colonizing bacteria in the oral cavity, usually in patients with poor dental hygiene, recent dental procedures, or those who have disorders that impair swallowing or consciousness, such as alcoholism or neurologic conditions. Clinically, it is characterized by a gradual onset of symptoms that include cough with sputum production, fever, and weight loss. These symptoms may be minimal even in extensive disease. Empyema and mediastinal involvement may occur, and thoracocutaneous fistula tracts have been reported.

RADIOLOGIC FEATURES

Chest X-rays are characterized by dense infiltrates, usually in the upper lobes, which can mimic lung cancer. Cavities are present in one-half of cases, but are usually small. Spread to adjacent bones, including ribs and vertebrae, can happen and produce a marked periosteal reaction known as wavy periostitis.

PATHOLOGIC FEATURES

GROSS FINDINGS

Lesions of actinomycosis grossly appear as yellow-gray and firm, and commonly cause overlying pleural fibrosis and adhesions. Invasion of the infection into the adjacent chest wall may occur with sinus tracts to the surface of the skin, which can show "sulfur granules" (see below). Small yellow abscesses are most common, but occasionally, a single, large abscess is seen.

MICROSCOPIC FINDINGS

The histologic picture is that of an abscess with actinomycotic "sulfur granules" in the center that appear as aggregates of filamentous, beaded bacteria with a radial orientation and eosinophilic material on the filaments (Figure 10-16). The eosinophilic material deposited on the bacteria is referred to as the Splendore-Hoeppli effect and can be seen in actinomycosis and other infections including those caused by fungi. Granules range in size up to 3000 microns, and grossly appear as yellow flecks. On the periphery of the abscess is inflamed granulation tissue. Giant cells may be seen in this area, but well formed granulomas are not part of the histologic picture.

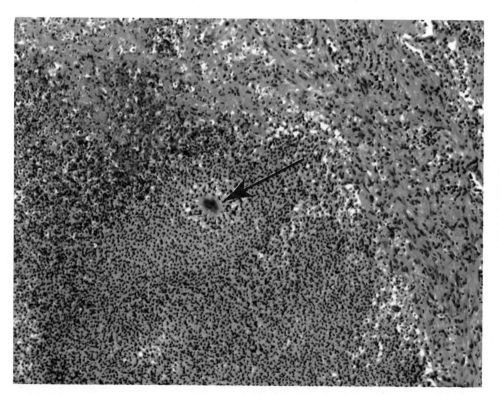

FIGURE 10-16

Actinomycosis

This pneumonia shows abscess formation with an aggregate of organisms (arrow highlighting sulfur granule) present in the center of the abscess.

ANCILLARY STUDIES

MICROBIOLOGY

Aggregates of the filamentous bacteria are easily appreciated on H & E stain, and are also highlighted by Gomori methenamine silver and Gram (Brown-Hopps or Brown-Brenn) stains (Figure 10-17). The bacterial filaments are gram-positive, 0.2-0.5 μm thick, branched, and slender, and extend into the peripheral rays. Staining with Gram stain may be weak and irregular, producing a beaded or even a gram-negative appearance.

DIFFERENTIAL DIAGNOSIS

The pathologic differential diagnosis includes other infections that can cause a Splendore-Hoeppli effect. These include botryomycosis, nocardiosis, and some fungal infections. Botryomycosis is usually a mixture of non-filamentous gram-positive and gram-negative organisms. Nocardiosis can be distinguished with a Fite stain. Fungal organisms, unlike *Actinomyces*, demonstrate thick, hyphal forms, readily distinguishable from the branching filaments found in the lesions of actinomycosis.

PROGNOSIS AND THERAPY

Penicillin in high doses is the treatment of choice for pulmonary actinomycosis. Successful therapy usually includes a six-week course of antibiotics followed by a six-month course of tetracycline to prohibit recurrence. Surgical excision of abscesses or fistula tracts may also be needed. Because of the indolent clinical features, diagnosis may be delayed. However, after diagnosis, chances of a cure are excellent with antibiotic administration.

SEQUELAE OF ASPIRATION

INTRODUCTION

Lung infections caused by aspiration are usually due to bacteria that normally live in the oropharyngeal region or stomach. These include anaerobic bacteria such as *Bacteroides* and *Actinomyces* species, streptococci and fusobacteria, as well as some aerobes such as *Enterobacter* and *Proteus*. Usually the infection is a mixed population of these organisms.

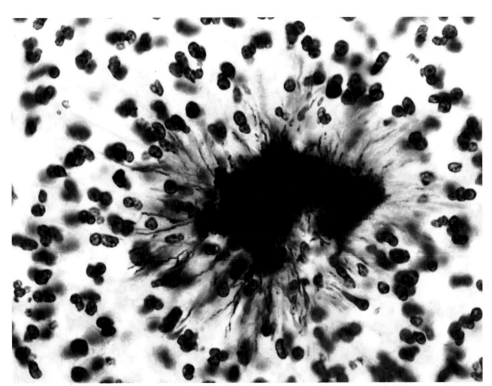

FIGURE 10-17
Actinomyces
The filamentous bacteria extend into peripheral rays (Gram stain).

ACTINOMYCES—FACT SHEET

Definition

» Pneumonia and abscesses caused by *Actinomyces*
» Usually introduced to the lungs via aspiration from the oropharynx

Incidence and Location

» Pulmonary infection accounts for 20% of all *Actinomyces* infections
» Rare infection in the United States
» Increased risk associated with poor dental hygiene, recent dental procedure, disorders of swallowing or consciousness
» Can be seen in immunocompromised hosts where disseminated infection may occur

Age Distribution

» Adults

Clinical Features

» Gradual onset of symptoms
» Productive cough

Radiologic Features

» Dense infiltrates, usually in the upper lobes
» May mimic lung cancer
» Cavities are present in one-half of cases
» Spread to adjacent bones may produce "wavy periostitis"

Prognosis and Therapy

» Six-week course of penicillin in high doses
» Long-term tetracycline to prohibit recurrence
» Surgical excision of abscesses or fistula tracts
» Excellent prognosis with long term antimicrobial therapy

ACTINOMYCES—PATHOLOGIC FEATURES

Gross Findings

» Yellow-grey, firm nodules
» Small yellow abscesses
» Fibrinous pleuritis and adhesions

Microscopic Findings

» Suppurative necrosis with sulfur granules containing filamentous, beaded bacteria in radial orientation (Splendore-Hoeppli effect)
» Periphery may include giant cells

Microbiology

» Gram-positive filamentous bacteria best seen on Brown-Hopps or Brown-Brenn stains

Pathologic Differential Diagnosis

» Other infections that cause Splendore-Hoeppli effect
  » Botryomycosis
  » Nocardiosis
  » Fungi

---

segment of the upper lobe, and the apical segment of the lower lobe. Also, because of the anatomically less acute angle of the right lung, aspiration is more common in the right lung than in the left lung. Clinically, fever, purulent sputum, and marked leukocytosis are common findings.

PATHOLOGIC FEATURES

GROSS FINDINGS

Aspiration pneumonia usually results in areas of necrotizing pneumonia with abscess formation with a characteristic malodorous smell. The consolidation is usually quite marked compared to other bacteria pneumonias. Chronic aspiration may result in peribronchial fibrosis and bronchiectasis (Figure 10-18).

MICROSCOPIC FINDINGS

Aspiration pneumonia causes a bronchopneumonia pattern of injury with alveoli filled with abundant neutrophils and fibrinopurulent exudates, and prominent suppurative necrosis (abscesses). Particles of food (plant matter, skeletal muscle) provoke a giant cell reaction. Aspiration of oral contents may be visualized using an immunohistochemical stain for cytokeratin, which highlights the aspirated squamous epithelium (Figure 10-19). Aspirated lipid material, such as mineral oil, can produce spaces in tissue where the droplets leached out during processing, with accompanying foamy macrophages (exogenous lipid pneumonia).

CLINICAL FEATURES

Risk factors for developing aspiration pneumonia include the following: 1) Loss of consciousness (during normal sleep or associated with central nervous system injury), 2) Impaired swallowing mechanics (myopathies or head and neck surgery), 3) abnormal esophageal motility (achalasia, esophageal strictures, scleroderma), and 4) gastro esophageal reflux.

RADIOLOGIC FEATURES

Chest X-rays usually reveal infiltrates with or without cavities in the parts of the lungs that were dependent at the time of aspiration. The regions most often involved are the basal segments of the lower lobes, the posterior

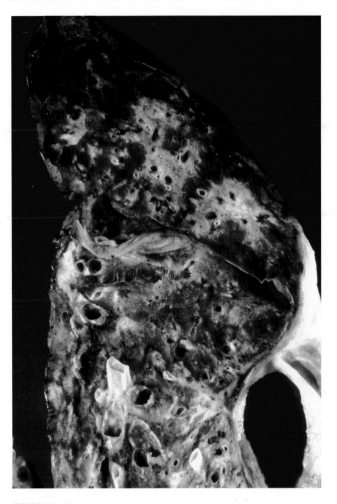

FIGURE 10-18

Chronic aspiration pneumonia
Bronchectasis and peribronchial fibrosis present in a lobectomy specimen. (Courtesy of Dr. Joseph Tomashefski, MetroHealth Medical Center, Cleveland, Ohio.)

ANCILLARY STUDIES

MICROBIOLOGY

Because the organisms responsible for this pneumonia are part of the normal flora of the upper respiratory tract, interpretation of microbiologic cultures is difficult. Therefore, blood and pleural or empyema fluid cultures may be more reliable. Transtracheal aspiration specimens are especially useful when pleural fluid is not available. Mixed bacterial infections are common with both anaerobes and aerobes. The most common isolates are *Bacteroides* and *Fusobacterium* species.

DIFFERENTIAL DIAGNOSIS

The pathologic differential diagnosis includes necrotizing pneumonias due to *Pseudomonas*, *Staphylococcus*, and other abscess-forming bacteria. The presence of food particles is diagnostically helpful. The anatomic location of the pneumonia is an important radiologic clue.

PROGNOSIS AND THERAPY

Combination antimicrobial therapy directed at the cultured bacteria is effective. However, mortality is as high as 30-50% with gastric acid aspiration, which can cause diffuse alveolar damage.

UNCOMMON BACTERIAL INFECTIONS

BURKHOLDERIA PSEUDOMALLEI

INTRODUCTION

Pulmonary melioidosis is caused by the gram-negative bacterium *Burkholderia pseudomallei*. It occurs predominantly in Southeast Asia, Asia, and northern Australia and usually follows percutaneous inoculation or inhalation of the bacterium that is present in soil and water. Its occurrence is associated with increased rainfall and has the capability of epidemic spread in non-endemic areas.

CLINICAL FEATURES

Pulmonary melioidosis presents either as an acute fulminant pneumonia or as an indolent cavitary disease. The clinical picture in the acute form of the disease is that of high fever, dyspnea, purulent sputum, and hemoptysis. Many patients ultimately develop sepsis with secondary hematogenous spread to the lung. The more chronic form of the disease has minimal symptoms, usually including fever, cough, and weight loss. Though some patients have no risk factors for this pneumonia, the majority of fatal cases have diabetes, alcoholism, or chronic renal disease. At least 10% of cases present with a chronic respiratory illness (>2 months) mimicking tuberculosis. Melioidosis and colonization with *B. pseudomallei* have been documented in cystic fibrosis patients visiting or resident in endemic areas.

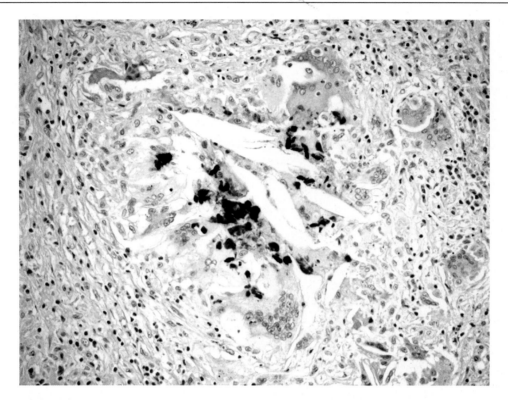

FIGURE 10-19

Aspiration pneumonia
In a background of pneumonia, aspirated cytokeratinaceous debris can be seen with a giant cell reaction (immunohisto-chemical study: pancytokeratin).

RADIOLOGIC FEATURES

Most commonly, chest imaging reveals upper lobe infil-trates and/or cavities that can mimic tuberculosis. In patients with the chronic form of the disease, apical cavities and scarring may be seen.

PATHOLOGIC FEATURES

GROSS FINDINGS

The lungs commonly have multiple, long-standing suppurative abscesses. Early disease begins as infil-trates, either unilobar or bilobar, in the upper lobes. Nodular lesions then coalesce to form cavities.

MICROSCOPIC FINDINGS

The histologic pattern of pulmonary melioidosis is that of either an acute necrotizing pneumonia with a prominent neutrophilic and exudative picture or a gran-ulomatous picture with ill-formed granulomas with palisading histiocytes and areas of necrosis.

ANCILLARY STUDIES

MICROBIOLOGY

Diagnosis is by culture of *B. pseudomallei* from blood, sputum, throat swab, or other samples. The organism, an aerobic gram-negative bacillus, grows readily in culture.

DIFFERENTIAL DIAGNOSIS

The main pathologic differential diagnosis is that of other necrotizing pneumonias caused by *Staphylococcus aureus*, *Klebsiella pneumoniae* and *Pseudomonas aerugi-nosa*. A history of travel to an endemic area and isolation of the organism in culture allow for rapid diagnosis.

PROGNOSIS AND THERAPY

Despite the introduction of ceftazidime- and carbapenem-based intravenous treatments, melioidosis is still associ-ated with significant mortality attributable to sepsis and its complications. Prolonged antibiotic therapy is required

---

ASPIRATION PNEUMONIA—FACT SHEET

Definition

» Pneumonia caused by aspiration of bacteria that normally live in the oropharyngeal area or stomach

» Common bacteria include *Bacteroides* sp, *Fusobacterium* sp

Incidence

» Common in patients with these risk factors:
  » Loss of consciousness
  » Impaired swallowing mechanics
  » Abnormal esophageal motility
  » Gastroesophageal reflux

Mortality

» 30-50% mortality with gastric aspiration

Age Distribution

» More common in adults

Clinical Features

» Cough productive of malodorous sputum
» Fever

Radiologic Features

» Infiltrates with or without cavities in the dependent parts of the lung
» Basal segments of lower lobes and posterior segment of upper lobe are most common

Therapy

» Antimicrobials directed at cultured organisms

ASPIRATION PNEUMONIA—PATHOLOGIC FEATURES

Gross Findings

» Abscesses with malodorous smelling material and consolidation of in dependent areas of lung

Microscopic Findings

» Bronchopneumonia with abundant neutrophils and fibrinopurulent exudates
» Abscesses
» Particles of food (plant matter, skeletal muscle) with giant cell reaction

Microbiology

» Infection is due to organisms of the upper respiratory tract
  » Anaerobic and aerobic
  » Mixed infections are common
» Interpretation of microbiological cultures may be difficult; best specimens are:
  » Transtracheal aspiration
  » Blood
  » Pleural or empyema fluid

Pathologic Differential Diagnosis

» Necrotizing pneumonias caused by *Pseudomonas*, *Staphylococcus*, or other abscess-forming bacteria

---

for eradication, and there is a high relapse rate. In non-endemic areas, reactivation is common months to years after the initial exposure to the organism.

MALAKOPLAKIA (R. EQUI)

INTRODUCTION

Malakoplakia, a term derived from the Greek "malakos" (soft) and "plax" (plaque) to describe the gross appearance, is an uncommon proliferation of histiocytes in response to infection. It is more commonly seen in the urinary, genital, and gastrointestinal tract. Gupta et al. reported the first case of pulmonary malakoplakia in

1972. To date, the cases of pulmonary malakoplakia reported are associated with *Rhodococcus equi* infection and occur in HIV-infected patients or patients with other immunocompromising conditions.

CLINICAL FEATURES

Immunocompromised patients (AIDS and non-AIDS) with malakoplakia usually present with unilobar, upper lobe pneumonia, which progresses slowly over several weeks. Symptoms at onset are cough, dyspnea, and low-grade fever. With progression, multilobar pneumonia, and eventually cavitation may occur. Empyema is common, and extra-pulmonary spread is seen in 7% of cases.

RADIOLOGIC FEATURES

Chest imaging usually reveals upper lobe dense consolidations or infiltrates, most commonly unilateral, but sometimes multifocal. If cavitation occurs, there may be a thick, fibrous capsule that can resemble postprimary tuberculosis.

BURKHOLDERIA PSEUDOMALLEI—FACT SHEET

Definition

▸ Pulmonary melioidosis is pneumonia caused by *Burkholderia pseudomallei*

Incidence and Location

▸ Occurs primarily in Southeast Asia, Asia, and northern Australia
▸ Associated with increased rainfall
▸ Capable of epidemic spread

Morbidity and Mortality

▸ Significant mortality due to sepsis
▸ Reactivation is common months to years after initial exposure

Age Distribution

▸ Found predominantly in adults

Clinical Features

▸ Two forms:
  ▸ Acute: high fever, dyspnea, purulent sputum, and hemoptysis
  ▸ Indolent cavitary: fever, cough, weight loss

Radiologic Features

▸ Upper lobe infiltrates with cavities
▸ Mimics tuberculosis

Therapy

▸ Prolonged antibiotic therapy with ceftazidime and carbapenems

---

BURKHOLDERIA PSEUDOMALLEI—PATHOLOGIC FEATURES

Gross Findings

▸ Early disease has areas of consolidation, unilobar or bilobar, primarily in upper lobes
▸ Multiple, long-standing abscesses

Microscopic Findings

▸ Acute necrotizing pneumonia with prominent neutrophilic and exudative picture
▸ Ill-formed granulomas with palisading histiocytes

Microbiology

▸ Aerobic gram-negative bacillus
▸ Grows rapidly in culture

Pathologic Differential Diagnosis

▸ Necrotizing pneumonias such as those caused by *Staphylococcus aureus*, *Klebsiella pneumoniae,* and *Pseudomonas aeruginosa*

PATHOLOGIC FEATURES

GROSS FINDINGS

Pulmonary malakoplakia associated with *R. equi* most commonly occurs as a single lesion, usually in the upper lobes. The gross lesions are yellow and round, and can have a distinctive gross appearance of tumefaction, similar to that of a neoplasm.

MICROSCOPIC FINDINGS

Histologically, there is a proliferation of histiocytes with abundant granular eosinophilic cytoplasm that contains Michaelis-Gutmann bodies (Figure 10-20A). These bodies are visible by light microscopy as basophilic structures with targetoid-like concentric laminations (Figure 10-20B). These inclusions can be highlighted with periodic-acid-Schiff and Von Kossa stains and frequently are iron-positive.

ANCILLARY STUDIES

MICROBIOLOGY

R. equi is a gram-positive pleomorphic coccobacillus that is weakly acid fast on Fite or Kinyoun stain. It is most commonly found in soil with animal feces, especially that of barnyard animals, and is acquired through inhalation.

ULTRASTRUCTURAL EXAMINATION

Ultrastructurally, Michaelis-Gutmann bodies have a characteristic electron-dense center with a less dense peripheral halo. Fragments of bacterial organisms can be found in these bodies and may form the nidus for calcification.

DIFFERENTIAL DIAGNOSIS

The differential diagnosis for the pathologist is to separate pulmonary malakoplakia secondary to *R. equi* infection from other histiocytic-predominant lesions in the lung. In the HIV-infected patient, this includes mycobacterial infections, both tuberculous and non-tuberculous, as well as other granulomatous infections caused by *Histoplasma*, *Cryptococcus,* and, occasionally, *Pneumocystis jiroveci*. Special stains are particularly helpful for demonstrating organisms, and should include silver stains

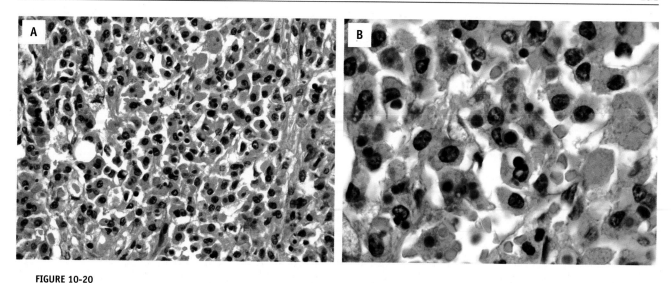

FIGURE 10-20

Pulmonary malakoplakia

This lesion is characterized by histiocytes with abundant eosinophilic cytoplasm **(A)**; numerous Michaelis-Gutmann bodies are present as basophilic structures with targetoid-like concentric laminations **(B)**.

(Histoplasma, Cryptococcus, Pneumocystis) and acid fast stains (mycobacteria), though *Rhodococcus equi* may be partially acid fast. Another infectious histiocytic lesions to consider in both HIV- and non-HIV-infected patients is Whipple's disease.

Noninfectious causes of histiocytic-rich lesions in the lung include storage diseases such as Niemann-Pick and Gaucher's disease, both of which have PAS-negative histiocytes and characteristic ultrastructural features. Amiodarone treatment may also cause foamy histiocytes within the lung. A clinical history of amiodarone exposure is extremely helpful. Other lesions that may be considered in this differential diagnosis include obstructive pneumonia and exogenous lipid pneumonia. Special stains for the *R. equi* will help to eliminate these entities.

PROGNOSIS AND THERAPY

R. equi pulmonary infections respond to erythromycin, vancomycin, and clindamycin. Rifampin is used commonly in combination with erythromycin. The prognosis is good with early medical intervention; however, long courses of parenteral antibiotics are usually required (2 to 6 months), and recurrence is common. Surgical excision of abscesses may be required in more severe cases.

BOTRYOMYCOSIS

INTRODUCTION

Botryomycosis is an uncommon bacterial disease of pyogenic bacteria, characterized by the microscopic formation of eosinophilic granules. It is sporadic and found worldwide. Multiple anatomic sites may be affected. When the lung is involved, it is usually a primary infection. Secondary, hematogenous spread may occur.

CLINICAL FEATURES

Pulmonary symptoms for botryomycosis are nonspecific and include dyspnea, shortness of breath, and pleuritic chest pain.

RADIOLOGIC FEATURES

The typical lesion is an infiltrate in the upper lobe. A mass or cavitating lesion may be seen, and spread to hilar lymph nodes causing adenopathy is common.

MALAKOPLAKIA—FACT SHEET

Definition

➤ Pneumonia with a prominent proliferation of histiocytes in response to bacteria (*R. equi*)

Incidence

➤ Rare
➤ Found in immunocompromised patients

Age Distribution

➤ Adults

Clinical Features

➤ Cough, dyspnea, and low-grade fever

Radiologic Features

➤ Upper lobe dense consolidations
➤ Usually unilateral, but may be multifocal
➤ Can cause cavitation with thick-walled capsule

Prognosis and Therapy

➤ Long term antimicrobial therapy including erythromycin, vancomycin, and clindamycin
➤ Good prognosis with early treatment

MALAKOPLAKIA—PATHOLOGIC FEATURES

Gross Findings

➤ Most commonly single, upper lobe lesion
➤ Yellow, round, with tumefaction

Microscopic Findings

➤ Histiocytes with abundant granular eosinophilic cytoplasm with Michaelis-Gutmann bodies
➤ Michaelis-Gutmann bodies are best seen with PAS, von Kossa, or iron stains

Microbiology

➤ *R. equi* is a gram-positive pleomorphic coccobacillus that is weakly acid fast
➤ *R. equi* is found in soil and animal feces, especially barnyard animals

Pathologic Differential Diagnosis

➤ Histiocytic lesions of the lung
 ➤ *Mycobacterium avium* complex
 ➤ Tuberculosis
 ➤ Fungal infections
 ➤ Whipple's disease
 ➤ Storage diseases: Niemann-Pick, Gaucher disease
 ➤ Amiodarone effect

PATHOLOGIC FEATURES

GROSS FINDINGS

The lungs are usually involved by multiple firm, yellow-green nodules with granules that are visible as yellow flecks. A suppurative bronchiectasis is commonly seen.

MICROSCOPIC FINDINGS

The histologic picture is that of bacterial colonies of mixed organisms found in the middle of abscesses. The bacteria are similar to those present in aspiration pneumonia, and the colony size varies. The colonies accumulate eosinophilic "clubbing" material referred to as a Splendore-Hoeppli reaction that is usually surrounded by lymphocytes and plasma cells, sometimes with a foreign body giant cell reaction. Bronchiectasis may be present. Granulation tissue and fibrosis may be seen in the abscess walls, and sinus tracts may occur.

ANCILLARY STUDIES

MICROBIOLOGY

The diagnosis of botryomycosis can be made when microscopic inspection and culture of the granules reveal gram-positive cocci or gram-negative bacilli. The organisms most commonly cultured include *Staphylococcus aureus*, *Escherichia coli*, and *Pseudomonas aeruginosa*. A Gram stain usually highlights the bacterial colonies and the eosinophilic material. A periodic acid Schiff (PAS) stain usually stains the inner part of the "clubbing" material.

DIFFERENTIAL DIAGNOSIS

Pulmonary botryomycosis can resemble actinomycosis, tuberculosis, or invasive carcinoma by causing a mass lesion with constitutional symptoms. The eosinophilic granules of botryomycosis can be confused with *Actinomyces*. Gram staining and cultures are needed for a definitive distinction.

PROGNOSIS AND THERAPY

The prognosis is excellent when the infection is treated promptly, but successful treatment often requires a combination of both surgical debridement and long-term intravenous antimicrobial therapy.

TROPHERYMA WHIPPELII

INTRODUCTION

The organism *Tropheryma whippelii* is responsible for Whipple's disease, the bacterial infection first described by George H. Whipple as an intestinal lipodystrophy in 1907. The characteristic feature of the disease is the presence of foamy macrophages that contain PAS-positive rod-shaped bacteria.

CLINICAL FEATURES

Whipple's disease most commonly affects the gastrointestinal tract and lymph nodes, but lung involvement is present in 35-60% of cases. There is a male-to-female ratio of 8:1 and mean age of onset around 50 years. Patients with pulmonary involvement by Whipple's disease usually have a nonproductive chronic cough, dyspnea, and pleuritic chest pain. The disease can mimic other interstitial lung diseases, especially sarcoidosis.

RADIOLOGIC FEATURES

The chest imaging studies of Whipple's disease usually show pleural effusions with diffuse or focal pulmonary infiltrates.

PATHOLOGIC FEATURES

GROSS FINDINGS

Gross features of pulmonary Whipple's disease are nonspecific, with scattered white/tan firm areas of consolidation, usually around the bronchovascular areas, similar to those of sarcoidosis.

MICROSCOPIC FINDINGS

The characteristic picture of Whipple's disease is that of foamy macrophages filled with bacteria and bacterial breakdown products that stain positive with PAS and silver stains. The distribution of these macrophages is usually around the bronchovascular areas.

ANCILLARY STUDIES

MICROBIOLOGY/MOLECULAR BIOLOGY

T. whippelii cannot be cultured; however, new tests using amplification of rRNA by polymerase chain reaction are being used in many laboratories to identify the organism.

HISTOCHEMISTRY

Confirmation of Whipple's disease is based on demonstration of diastase-resistant, non-acid-fast, PAS-positive inclusions in macrophages within the lesion.

ULTRASTRUCTURAL STUDIES

Electron microscopy is used to confirm the presence of the bacteria. These bacteria have a trilamellar membrane and a cell wall structure found in many gram-positive bacteria. The presence of these organisms within phagocytes, in combination with positive PAS staining, confirms the diagnosis.

DIFFERENTIAL DIAGNOSIS

Non-tuberculous mycobacteria, especially the Mycobacteria avium complex (MAC), usually presents in the lung of immunocompromised hosts as foamy macrophages, similar to those found in Whipple's disease. Acid-fast staining highlights these mycobacteria and should not stain *T. whippelii*. In addition, some systemic fungal infections in immunocompromised hosts, such as *Histoplasma*, may have similar macrophage infiltrates containing multiple yeast forms. The morphology of these yeasts on silver stains will help to distinguish fungal diseases from the rod-shaped bacteria of Whipple's disease.

PROGNOSIS AND THERAPY

Treatment of Whipple's disease involves long-term antimicrobial therapy. This usually includes trimethoprim-sulfamethoxazole for 1 year, sometimes preceded by

---

BOTRYOMYCOSIS—FACT SHEET

Definition
- Pneumonia due to pyogenic bacteria, characterized by microscopic formation of eosinophilic granules

Incidence and Location
- Sporadic, worldwide

Age Distribution
- Adults

Clinical Features
- Dyspnea
- Shortness of breath
- Pleuritic chest pain

Radiologic Features
- Upper lobe infiltrate
- Mass or cavitating lesion
- Spread to hilar lymph nodes and adenopathy is common

Prognosis and Therapy
- Long-term antimicrobials
- Surgical debridement if cavitation and abscess formation occurs
- Excellent prognosis

BOTRYOMYCOSIS—PATHOLOGIC FEATURES

Gross Findings
- Multiple, firm, yellow-green nodules with granules that are visible as yellow flecks
- Suppurative bronchiectasis is common

Microscopic Findings
- Abscess cavities with bacterial colonies of mixed organisms
- Colonies demonstrate eosinophilic "clubbing"—Splendore-Hoeppli reaction
- Foreign body giant cell reaction to granules can be seen

Microbiology
- Gram-positive cocci or gram-negative bacilli
- Most common organisms are *Staphylococcus aureus, E. coli, Pseudomonas aeruginosa*
- Gram stain highlights bacteria and eosinophilic material
- PAS stains inner part of "clubbing" material

Pathologic Differential Diagnosis
- Actinomycosis
- Tuberculosis

---

two weeks of parenteral penicillin or streptomycin. With treatment, the prognosis is excellent and relapse is uncommon.

BIOTERRORISM AGENTS

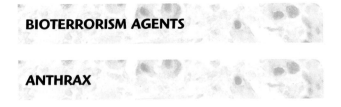

ANTHRAX

INTRODUCTION

Anthrax is a disease caused by *Bacillus anthracis.* It is primarily a disease of herbivores, but can cause infections in humans by direct contact with endospores, resulting in cutaneous anthrax and inhalation anthrax. Historically, it was referred to as "Woolsorters' Disease" because people who worked with sheep were prone to these infections. Cutaneous anthrax is rarely fatal, while inhalational (pulmonary) anthrax has a high mortality rate.

CLINICAL FEATURES

Inhalational anthrax begins with a brief prodrome resembling a viral respiratory illness followed by development of hypoxia and dyspnea. The disease progresses very quickly to septicemia, where abundant organisms can be seen in the circulating blood. Chills, fever, and a strident cough are symptoms of fulminant disease. Death occurs within 2 to 3 days.

RADIOLOGIC FEATURES

The characteristic x-ray for inhalational anthrax reveals mediastinal widening, lung infiltrates, and pleural effusions.

PATHOLOGIC FEATURES

GROSS FINDINGS

Lungs infected with *B. anthracis* are red, congested, and heavy, and massive hemorrhagic pleural effusions are present. Cavitation or abscess formation in the lungs is not seen. Hemorrhage is also present in the mediastinum, tracheobronchial lymph nodes, and mucosa of the cartilaginous airways.

TROPHERYMA WHIPPELII—FACT SHEET

Definition

▸ Whipple's disease is caused by *Tropheryma whippelii*
▸ Invasion of lung causes interstitial lung disease

Incidence

▸ Rare
▸ Lung involvement in 35-60% of cases

Gender and Age Distribution

▸ Adults with mean onset at 50 years
▸ Male-to-female ratio of 8:1

Clinical Features

▸ Nonproductive chronic cough, dyspnea, and pleuritic chest pain

Radiologic Features

▸ Diffuse or focal infiltrates
▸ Pleural effusions

Prognosis and Therapy

▸ Combination of surgical debridement and long-term intravenous antimicrobial therapy
▸ Excellent prognosis with long term treatment

TROPHERYMA WHIPPELII—PATHOLOGIC FEATURES

Gross Findings

▸ Scattered white/tan firm areas of consolidation, usually involving bronchovascular areas

Microscopic Findings

▸ Foamy macrophages filled with bacteria and bacterial breakdown products
▸ Bacteria stain positive with PAS and silver stains
▸ Distribution is usually around bronchovascular areas

Microbiology

▸ *T. whippelii* cannot be cultured
▸ Molecular tests using amplification of rRNA by PCR are useful for diagnosis
▸ Electron microscopy confirms the presence of bacteria
  ▸ Trilamellar membrane with cell wall structure of gram-positive bacteria

Pathologic Differential Diagnosis

▸ Non-tuberculous mycobacteria, especially *Mycobacterium avium* complex
▸ Some fungal diseases, such as histoplasmosis

MICROSCOPIC FINDINGS

The histologic picture of pulmonary anthrax is marked edema and hemorrhage involving the lungs, pleura, and mediastinum. There is usually a large serosanguineous pleural effusion. Within the alveolar spaces, there is fibrin and a macrophage infiltrate (Figure 10-21). There are scattered lymphocytes and lymphocytolysis; however, a neutrophilic infiltrate is not a prominent part of the histologic picture. There will be a prominent vasculitis involving many small vessels in the lung, and a Gram stain will show abundant organisms in the alveolar spaces and within the vessels.

ANCILLARY STUDIES

MICROBIOLOGY

Bacillus anthracis is a long gram-positive bacillus that measures 3-5 microns in length, with a "boxcar" type morphology. Endospores are formed by the bacilli and inhaled into the lungs to cause the disease. Spread to humans is by exposure to dead infected animals. Diagnosis is usually made by blood cultures.

DIFFERENTIAL DIAGNOSIS

The differential diagnosis for inhalational anthrax includes other hemorrhagic pneumonias with fulminant courses. These include *Legionella* pneumonia and pneumococcal pneumonia. However, both have a more prolonged clinical course. Viral hemorrhagic pneumonias may also be considered clinically.

PROGNOSIS AND THERAPY

B. anthracis is susceptible to penicillin. However, the organism produces virulent toxins, which causes it to progress despite antibiotic therapy. Death comes in 2 to 3 days after inhaling anthrax endospores in the majority of patients.

TULAREMIA

INTRODUCTION

Tularemia is an infection caused by *Francisella tularensis*, which can be acquired from a wide variety of domestic and wild animals and spread to humans. The

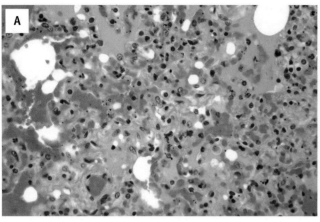
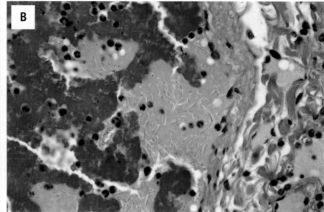

FIGURE 10-21

Pulmonary anthrax

Marked edema and hemorrhage with fibrin and macrophages involve the alveolar spaces **(A)**; scattered lymphocytes may be present, but neutrophils are not part of the histologic picture **(B).** (Courtesy of Dr. Joseph Tomashefski, MetroHealth Medical Center, Cleveland, Ohio.)

ANTHRAX—FACT SHEET

Definition

›› Pneumonia caused by *Bacillus anthracis*
›› Caused by direct contact with endospores

Incidence

›› Rare

Mortality

›› Fatal within 2 to 3 days

Gender, Race, and Age Distribution

›› Anyone exposed to endospores

Clinical Features

›› Prodrome resembling viral illness
›› Hypoxia and dyspnea
›› Quick progression to septicemia
›› Chills, fever, and strident cough

Radiologic Features

›› Mediastinal widening, diffuse bilateral lung infiltrates, and pleural effusions

Therapy

›› Penicillin

ANTHRAX—PATHOLOGIC FEATURES

Gross Findings

›› Red, congested, and heavy lungs

Microscopic Findings

›› Edema and hemorrhage
›› Alveolar spaces containing fibrin and macrophage infiltrates; neutrophils are absent
›› Prominent vasculitis

Microbiology

›› Gram-positive bacillus, 3-5 μ with "boxcar"-type morphology
›› Endospores are formed from the bacilli and inhaled into lungs
›› Spread to humans by exposure to dead infected animals

Pathologic Differential Diagnosis

›› Hemorrhagic pneumonias such as *Legionella* pneumonia, pneumococcal pneumonia, viral hemorrhagic pneumonias

CLINICAL FEATURES

The onset of symptoms for tularemia pneumonia is abrupt with severe chills, dyspnea, a nonproductive cough with pleuritic pain, and profuse sweating.

RADIOLOGIC FEATURES

Radiographs of tularemia pneumonia are varied. They can be unrevealing early in the disease, with a gradual development of nodular infiltrates, pleural effusions,

most common reservoirs are rabbits, hares, and ticks. Pneumonia is a common symptom of tularemia, usually a result of hematogenous spread from a skin ulcer from a tick bite or exposure of an open wound to an infected animal. In endemic areas, pneumonia may be a primary manifestation of the disease.

or adenopathy. Empyemas and bronchopleural fistulas can occur. Cavitation is present in 20% of cases.

PATHOLOGIC FEATURES

GROSS FINDINGS

The lungs show consolidation or grey/tan nodules with yellow necrosis and cavitation (Figure 10-22).

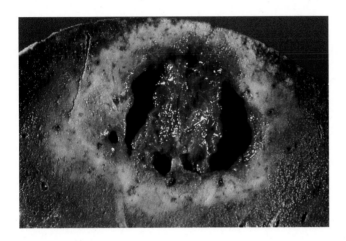

FIGURE 10-22
Tularemia pneumonia
A gray-tan nodule with a yellow central necrosis is present in a lung involved by tularemia pneumonia. (Courtesy of Dr. Joseph Tomashefski, MetroHealth Medical Center, Cleveland, Ohio.)

MICROSCOPIC FINDINGS

Acute tularemia pneumonia has a similar appearance to *Legionella* pneumonia with a marked fibrinous exudate in alveolar spaces and degenerating macrophages and neutrophils. There is extensive necrosis of the alveolar septa with vasculitis and thrombosis (Figure 10-23).

ANCILLARY STUDIES

MICROBIOLOGY

There are five subspecies of *F. tularensis*, but Type A is responsible for 70-90% of the cases in humans. It is a gram-negative coccobacillus found in mud, water, and decaying animal carcasses. It is most common in the temperate zones of the northern hemisphere. The diagnosis is made by cultures of sputum, bronchial fluid, or pleural fluid.

DIFFERENTIAL DIAGNOSIS

Legionella pneumonia is similar both clinically and pathologically to tularemia. However, *Legionella* organisms are larger on organism stains such as Dieterle.

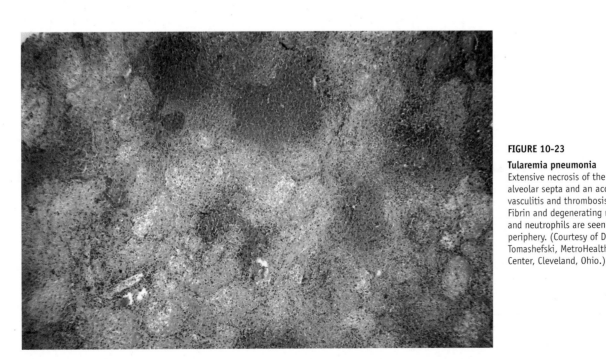

FIGURE 10-23
Tularemia pneumonia
Extensive necrosis of the alveolar septa and an accompanying vasculitis and thrombosis are seen. Fibrin and degenerating macrophages and neutrophils are seen in the periphery. (Courtesy of Dr. Joseph Tomashefski, MetroHealth Medical Center, Cleveland, Ohio.)

TULAREMIA—FACT SHEET

Definition

» Pneumonia caused by *Francisella tularensis*
» Acquired from a variety of domestic and wild animals (rabbits, hares, ticks)
» Pneumonia develops from hematogenous spread from a skin ulcer

Incidence and Location

» <200 cases per year in the United States
» Most common in the temperate zones of the northern hemisphere

Mortality

» 1-5% mortality

Clinical Features

» Abrupt onset of chills, dyspnea, non-productive cough
» Pleuritic pain
» Profuse sweating

Radiologic Features

» Early in disease, chest x-ray may be negative
» Gradual development of nodular infiltrates, pleural effusions, and adenopathy

Therapy

» Streptomycin

TULAREMIA—PATHOLOGIC FEATURES

Gross Findings

» Grey/tan nodules with yellow necrosis and early cavitation

Microscopic Findings

» Marked fibrinous exudates in alveolar spaces
» Infiltrates of degenerating macrophages and neutrophils
» Extensive necrosis of the alveolar septa with vasculitis and thrombosis

Microbiology

» Five subspecies
» Type A is responsible for 70-90% of human cases
» Gram-negative coccobacillus
» Diagnosis is made by cultures of sputum, bronchial fluid, or pleural fluid

Pathologic Differential Diagnosis

» *Legionella* pneumonia

PROGNOSIS AND THERAPY

Streptomycin is a very effective therapy for tularemia pneumonia. A two-week course of parenteral antibiotics is required to eradicate the disease. The mortality rate for diagnosed tularemia is 1-5%.

YERSINIA PESTIS

INTRODUCTION

Yersinia pestis, a gram-negative bacterium transmitted to humans by fleas, is the organism responsible for pneumonic plague. This disease, endemic to areas of wild rodents, is known for causing pandemics throughout history that have resulted in over 200 million deaths. Small outbreaks continue in modern times, mostly in Africa, Asia, and South America. In the United States, the western states have had sporadic cases, a result of direct contact with plague-infected animals, not from flea bites. Primary pneumonic plague, the result of inhalation of *Y. pestis,* is rare. Most plague pneumonias are secondary, a result of hematogenous spread from bubonic (lymph nodes) or septicemic plague.

CLINICAL FEATURES

Symptoms of pneumonic plague usually include fever, lymphadenopathy, cough, hemoptysis, and chest pain. Gastrointestinal symptoms are common, including vomiting, diarrhea, and abdominal pain. The clinical course can be rapid and fatal, with up to 90% mortality within 24 hours of presentation. The disease is highly contagious, with an incubation time ranging from 1 to 5 days.

RADIOLOGIC FEATURES

Chest radiographs are nonspecific, showing patchy bronchopneumonia, cavitation, and multilobar consolidation, usually a result of air space disease due to alveolar hemorrhage.

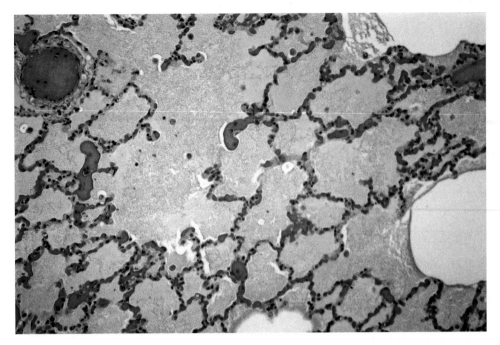

FIGURE 10-24
Yersinia **pneumonia**
A hemorrhagic exudate involves the alveolar spaces. Congested capillaries are present in the alveolar walls. (Courtesy of Dr. Joseph Tomashefski, MetroHealth Medical Center, Cleveland, Ohio.)

PATHOLOGIC FEATURES

GROSS FINDINGS

Lungs involved by primary pneumonic pneumonia have a lobular pneumonia that progresses to a widespread lobar pneumonia very quickly. The lungs are edematous and purple/red, and may contain scattered necrotic nodules. A fibrinopurulent pleuritis is common.

MICROSCOPIC FINDINGS

The histology of pneumonic pneumonia starts as peribronchiolar inflammation with numerous organisms and a marked exudate that is predominantly hemorrhagic without fibrin (Figure 10-24). Vasculitis with perivascular edema is a common finding (Figure 10-25). With progression, these areas grow to involve the entire lung and undergo necrosis and hemorrhage. Neutrophils are sparse (Figure 10-26).

ANCILLARY STUDIES

MICROBIOLOGY

Blood cultures, serologies, and nucleic acid amplification are the current tests used to establish the diagnosis of *Y. pestis*. Also, the organism can be identified in the peripheral blood by Gram stain. The organisms appear as bipolar bacilli in macrophages in large numbers and can be seen in tissue sections using Gram, Giemsa, or silver stains such as Warthin-Starry.

DIFFERENTIAL DIAGNOSIS

The pathologic differential diagnosis includes other causes of rapidly progressing hemorrhagic pneumonias such as *Legionella* pneumonia or pneumococcal pneumonia.

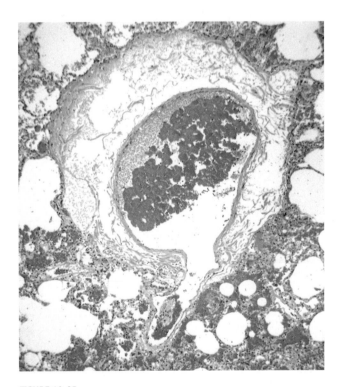

FIGURE 10-25
Yersinia **pneumonia**
Marked perivascular edema is a common feature. (Courtesy of Dr. Joseph Tomashefski, MetroHealth Medical Center, Cleveland, Ohio.)

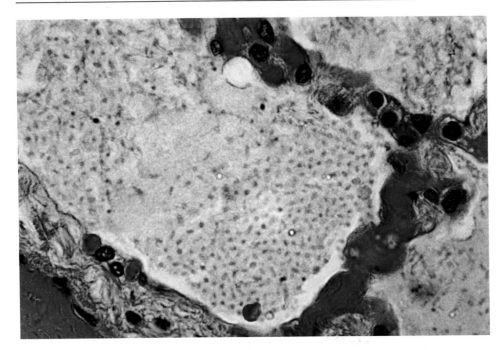

FIGURE 10-26

***Yersinia* pneumonia**
Abundant bacteria may be seen on H and E stain in the alveolar spaces. (Courtesy of Dr. Joseph Tomashefski, MetroHealth Medical Center, Cleveland, Ohio.)

YERSINIA PESTIS—FACT SHEET

Definition
- ▸ Pneumonic plague is due to infection of the lungs by *Yersinia pestis*
- ▸ Bacteria are usually transmitted to humans by fleas
- ▸ Most plague pneumonias are secondary to hematogenous spread from lymph nodes or septicemia

Incidence and Location
- ▸ Rare
- ▸ Highly contagious
- ▸ Small outbreaks mostly in Africa, Asia, and South America
- ▸ Sporadic cases in the USA

Mortality
- ▸ 60-90% mortality within 24 hours of presentation

Clinical Features
- ▸ Fever, lymphadenopathy, cough, hemoptysis, and chest pain
- ▸ Gastrointestinal symptoms including vomiting, diarrhea, and abdominal pain are common

Radiologic Features
- ▸ Patchy infiltrates progress to multilobar consolidation

Therapy
- ▸ Streptomycin, tetracycline, and chloramphenicol
- ▸ Contain spread of organism

YERSINIA PESTIS—PATHOLOGIC FEATURES

Gross Findings
- ▸ Lobular pneumonia that rapidly progresses to lobar pneumonia
- ▸ Edematous, purple, red lungs that may contain necrotic nodules
- ▸ Fibrinopurulent pleuritis

Microscopic Findings
- ▸ Starts as peribronchiolar inflammation
- ▸ Marked hemorrhagic exudates
- ▸ Neutrophils are sparse
- ▸ Abundant organisms

Microbiology
- ▸ Gram-negative bacillus, seen best on silver stain (Steiner, Warthin-Starry, Dieterle)

Pathologic Differential Diagnosis
- ▸ Other rapidly progressing hemorrhagic pneumonias such as *Legionella* pneumonia, pneumococcal pneumonia

PROGNOSIS AND THERAPY

Antimicrobial therapies of streptomycin, tetracycline, and chloramphenicol, if given early, can be effective. Isolation is important to prevent spread, given the contagious nature of the infection. Unfortunately, even with early treatment, the mortality is high, ranging from 60-90% within days.

SUGGESTED READINGS

General References

1. Donowitz GR, Mandell GL. Acute pneumonia. In: Mandell GL, Bennett JE, Dolin R, eds. *Principles and Practice of Infectious Diseases*, 5th ed. New York: Churchill Livingstone; 2000:717-42.
2. Rello J, Rodriguez R, Jubert P, Alvarez B. Severe community-acquired pneumonia in the elderly: epidemiology and prognosis: study group for severe community-acquired pneumonia. *Clin Infect Dis*. 1996;23:723-8.
3. Winn WC Jr, Allen SD, Janda WM, et al. *Koneman's Color Atlas and Textbook of Diagnostic Microbiology*. 6 ed. Philadelphia: J.B. Lippincott; 2006.

Streptococcus Pneumoniae

4. Johnston RB Jr. The host response to invasion by *Streptococcus pneumoniae*: protection and the pathogenesis of tissue damage. *Rev Infect Dis*. 1981;3:282-8.
5. Kadioglu A, Andrew PW. The innate immune response to pneumococcal lung infection: the untold story. *Trends Immunol*. 2004;25:143-9.
6. Kerem E, Bar Ziv Y, Rudenski B, Katz S, Kleid D, Branski D. Bacteremic necrotizing pneumococcal pneumonia in children. *Am J Respir Crit Care Med*. 1994;149:242-4.
7. Musher DM. Infections caused by *Streptococcus pneumoniae*: clinical spectrum, pathogenesis, immunity, and treatment. *Clin Infect Dis*. 1992;14:801-7.
8. Ort S, Ryan JL, Barden G, D'Esopo N. Pneumococcal pneumonia in hospitalized patients: clinical and radiological presentations. *JAMA*. 1983;249:214-8.
9. Watanakunakorn C, Bailey TA. Adult bacteremic pneumococcal pneumonia in a community teaching hospital, 1992-1996: A detailed analysis of 108 cases. *Arch Intern Med*. 1997;157:1965-71.
10. Winn WC Jr, Chandler FW. Bacterial infections. In: Dail DH, Hammar SP, eds. *Pulmonary Pathology*. 2nd ed. New York: Springer-Verlag; 1994: 255-330.

Staphylococcus Species

11. Kaye MG, Fox MJ, Bartlett JG, Braman SS, Glassroth J. The clinical spectrum of *Staphylococcus aureus* pulmonary infection. *Chest*. 1990;97: 788-92.
12. Kissane JM. Staphylococcal infections. In: Connor DH, Chandler FW, Manz HJ, et al., eds. *Pathology of Infectious Diseases*. Stamford: Appleton & Lange; 1997:805-16.
13. Musher DM, McKenzie SO. Infections due to *Staphylococcus aureus*. Medicine 1977;56:383-409.
14. Rello J, Quintana E, Ausina V, Puzo C, Net A, Prats G. Risk factors for *Staphylococcus aureus* nosocomial pneumonia in critically ill patients. *Am Rev Respir Dis*. 1990;142:1320-4.
15. Robertson L, Caley JP, Moore J. Importance of *Staphylococcus aureus* in pneumonia in the 1957 epidemic of influenza A. *Lancet*. 1958;2:233-6.

Streptococcus Species

16. Farley MM. Group B streptococcal disease in nonpregnant adults. *Clin Infect Dis*. 2001;33:556-61.

17. Farley MM, Harvey RC, Stull T, et al. A population-based assessment of invasive disease due to group B *Streptococcus* in nonpregnant adults. *N Engl J Med*. 1993;328:1807-11.
18. Kissane JM. Streptococcal infections and infections by streptococcus-like organisms. In: Connor DH, Chandler FW, Manz HJ, et al., eds. *Pathology of Infectious Diseases*. Stamford: Appleton & Lange; 1997:817-32.
19. Lerner PI, Gopalakrishna KV, Wolinsky E, et al. Group B *Streptococcus* bacteremia in adults: analysis of 32 cases and review of the literature. *Medicine*. 1977;56:457-73.
20. Mulla ZD. Group A streptococcal pneumonia. *Arch Intern Med*. 2003;163:2101-02.
21. Munoz P, Llancaqueo A, Rodriguez-Creixems M, Pelaez T, Martin L, Bouza E. Group B *streptococcus* bacteremia in nonpregnant adults. *Arch Intern Med*. 1997;157:213-6.
22. Outbreak of group A streptococcal pneumonia among Marine Corps recruits—California, November 1-December 20, 2002. *MMWR Morb Mortal Wkly Rep*. 2003;52:106-9.
23. Sarkar TK, Murarka RS, Gilardi GL. Primary streptococcus viridans pneumonia. *Chest*. 1989;96:831-4.
24. Shlaes DM, Lerner PI, Wolinsky E, Gopalakrishna KV. Infections due to Lancefield group F and related streptococci *(S. milleri, S. anginosus)*. *Medicine*. 1981;60:197-207.

Haemophilus Influenzae

25. Jorgensen JH. Update on mechanisms and prevalence of antimicrobial resistance in *Haemophilus influenzae*. *Clin Infect Dis*. 1992;14:1119-23.
26. Marley EF, Campos JM. *Haemophilus influenzae* infection. In: Connor DH, Chandler FW, Manz HJ, et al., eds. *Pathology of Infectious Diseases*. Stamford: Appleton & Lange; 1997:579-82.
27. Moxon ER, Wilson R. The role of *Haemophilus influenzae* in the pathogenesis of pneumonia. *Rev Infect Dis*. 1991;13:S518-27.
28. Musher DM, Kubitschek KR, Crennan J, Baughn RE. Pneumonia and acute febrile tracheobronchitis due to *Haemophilus influenzae*. *Ann Intern Med*. 1983;99:444-50.
29. Peltola H. Worldwide *Haemophilus influenzae* type B disease at the beginning of the 21st century: global analysis of the disease burden 25 years after the use of the polysaccharide vaccine and a decade after the advent of conjugates. *Clin Microbiol Rev*. 2000;13:302-17.
30. Takala AK, Meurman O, Kleemola M, et al. Preceding respiratory infection predisposing for primary and secondary invasive *Haemophilus influenzae* type B disease. *Pediatr Infect Dis J*. 1993;12:189-95.

Pseudomonas Aeruginosa

31. Bodey GP, Bolivar R, Fainstein V, Jadeja L. Infections caused by *Pseudomonas aeruginosa*. I. 1983;5:279-313.
32. Crnich CJ, Gordon B, Andes D. Hot tub-associated necrotizing pneumonia due to *Pseudomonas aeruginosa*. *Clin Infect Dis*. 2003;36:e55-7.
33. Fetzer AE, Werner AS, Hagstrom JW. Pathologic features of pseudomonal pneumonia. *Am Rev Respir Dis*. 1967;96:1121-30.
34. Hatchette TF, Gupta R, Marrie TJ. *Pseudomonas aeruginosa* community-acquired pneumonia in previously healthy adults: case report and review of the literature. *Clin Infect Dis*. 2000;31:1349-56.
35. Hoogwerf BJ, Khan MY. Community-acquired bacteremic *Pseudomonas* pneumonia in a healthy adult. *Am Rev Respir Dis*. 1981;123:132-4.
36. Pollack M. *Pseudomonas* species. In: Mandell GL, Bennett JE, Dolin R, eds. *Mandell, Douglas, and Bennett's Principles and Practice of Infectious Diseases*. New York: Churchill Livingstone, 2000. 2310-35.
37. Talon D, Mulin B, Rouget C, Bailly P, Thouverez M, Viel JF. Risks and routes for ventilator-associated pneumonia with *Pseudomonas aeruginosa*. *Am J Respir Crit Care Med*. 1998;157:978-84.

Legionella Species

38. Dondero TJ Jr., Rendtorff RC, Mallison GF, et al. An outbreak of Legionnaires' disease associated with a contaminated air-conditioning cooling tower. *N Engl J Med*. 1980;302:365-70.
39. Fraser DW, Tsai TR, Orenstein W, et al. Legionnaires' disease: description of an epidemic of pneumonia. *N Engl J Med*. 1977;297:1189-97.
40. Hernandez FJ, Kirby BD, Stanley TM, Edelstein PH. Legionnaires' disease: postmortem pathologic findings of 20 cases. *Am J Clin Pathol*. 1980;73:488-95.

41. Winn WC Jr. Legionnaires' disease: historical perspective. *Clin Microbiol Rev*. 1988;1:60-81.

42. Winn WC Jr, Glavin FL, Perl DP, Craighead JE. Macroscopic pathology of the lungs in Legionnaires' disease. *Ann Intern Med*. 1979;90:548-51.

43. Winn WC Jr, Glavin FL, Perl DP, et al. The pathology of Legionnaires' disease: fourteen fatal cases from the 1977 outbreak in Vermont. *Arch Pathol Lab Med*. 1978;102:344-50.

Nocardia

44. Beaman BL, Beaman L. Nocardia species: host-parasite relationships. *Clin Microbiol Rev*. 1994;7:213-64.

45. Burbank B, Morrione TG, Cutler SS. Pulmonary alveolar proteinosis and nocardiosis. *Am J Med*. 1960;28:1002-7.

46. Carlsen ET, Hill RB, Rowlands DT. Nocardiosis and pulmonary alveolar proteinosis. *Ann Intern Med*. 1964;60:275-81.

47. Curry WA. Human nocardiosis: a clinical review with selected case reports. *Arch Intern Med*. 1980;140:818-26.

48. Simpson GL, Stinson EB, Egger MJ, Remington JS. Nocardial infections in the immunocompromised host: a detailed study in a defined population. *Rev Infect Dis*. 1981;3:492-507.

49. Smego RAJ, Gallis HA. The clinical spectrum of *Nocardia brasiliensis* infection in the United States. *Rev Infect Dis*. 1984;6:164-80.

Actinomyces

50. Baron EJ, Angevine JM, Sundstrom W. Actinomycotic pulmonary abscess in an immunosuppressed patient. *Am J Clin Pathol*. 1979;72: 637-9.

51. Brown JR. Human actinomycosis: a study of 181 subjects. *Hum Pathol*. 1973;4:319-30.

52. Coelha Filho JC. Pulmonary cavities colonized by actinomycetes: report of six cases. *Rev Inst Med Trop Sao Paulo*. 1990;32:636-66.

53. Dicpinigaitis PV, Bleiweiss IJ, Krellenstein DJ, Halton KP, Teirstein AS. Primary endobronchial actinomycosis in association with foreign body aspiration. *Chest*. 1992;101:283-5.

54. Wright EP, Holmberg K, Houston J. Pulmonary actinomycosis simulating a bronchial neoplasm. *J Infect*. 1983;6:179-81.

Sequelae of Aspiration

55. Bartlett JG, Gorbach SL, Finegold SM. The bacteriology of aspiration pneumonia. *Am J Med*. 1974;56:202-7.

Burkholderia Pseudomallei

56. Everett ED, Nelson RA. Pulmonary melioidosis: observations in thirty-nine cases. *Am Rev Respir Dis*. 1975;112:331-40.

57. McCormick JB, Sexton DJ, McMuray JG, Carey E, Hayes P, Feldman RA. Human-to-human transmission of *Pseudomonas pseudomallei*. *Ann Intern Med*. 1973;83:512-3.

58. Piggott JA, Hochholzer L. Human melioidosis: a histopathologic study of acute and chronic melioidosis. *Arch Pathol*. 1970;90:101-11.

59. Wong KT, Puthucheary SD, Vadivelu J. The histopathology of human melioidosis. *Histopathology*. 1995;26:51-5.

Malakoplakia (R. equi)

60. Colby TV, Hunt S, Pelzmann K, Carrington CB. Malakoplakia of the lung: a report of two cases. *Respiration*. 1980;39:295-9.

61. Emmons W, Reichwein B, Winslow DL. *Rhodococcus equi* infection in the patient with AIDS: literature review and report of an unusual case. *Rev Infect Dis*. 1991;13:91-6.

62. Hamrock D, Azmi FH, O'Donnell E, Gunning WT, Philips ER, Zaher A. Infection by *Rhodococcus equi* in a patient with AIDS: histological appearance mimicking Whipple's disease and *Mycobacterium avium-intracellulare* infection. *J Clin Pathol*. 1999;52:68-71.

63. Harvey RL, Sunstrum JC. *Rhodococcus equi* infection in patients with and without human immunodeficiency virus infection. *Rev Infect Dis*. 1991;13:139-45.

64. Hodder RV, St George-Hyslop P, Chalvardjian A, Bear RA, Thomas P. Pulmonary malakoplakia. *Thorax*. 1984;39:70-1.

65. Kwon KY, Colby TV. *Rhodococcus equi* pneumonia and pulmonary malakoplakia in acquired immunodeficiency syndrome: pathologic features. *Arch Pathol Lab Med*. 1994;118:744-8.

66. Prescott JF. *Rhodococcus equi*: an animal and human pathogen. *Clin Microbiol Rev*. 1991;4:20-34.

67. Weingarten JS, Huang DY, Jackman JD, Jr. *Rhodococcus equi* pneumonia. An unusual early manifestation of the acquired immunodeficiency syndrome (AIDS). *Chest*. 1988;94:195-6.

68. Yuoh G, Hove MG, Wen J, Haque AK. Pulmonary malakoplakia in acquired immunodeficiency syndrome: an ultrastructural study of morphogenesis of Michaelis-Gutmann bodies. *Mod Pathol*. 1996;9:476-83.

Botryomycosis

69. Greenblatt M, Heredia R, Rubenstein L, Alpert S. Bacterial pseudomycosis ("botryomycosis"). *Am J Clin Pathol*. 1964;41:188-93.

70. Paz HL, Little BJ, Winkelstein JA. Primary pulmonary botryomycosis: a manifestation of chronic granulomatous disease. *Chest*. 1992;101:1160-2.

71. Speir WA, Mitchener JW, Galloway RF. Primary pulmonary botryomycosis. *Chest*. 1971;60:92-3.

Tropheryma Whippelii

72. Bentley SD, Maiwald M, Murphy LD, et al. Sequencing and analysis of the genome of the Whipple's disease bacterium *Tropheryma whippelii*. *Lancet*. 2003;361:637-44.

73. Durand DV, Lecomte C, Cathebras P, Rousset H, Godeau P. Whipple disease: clinical review of 52 cases. The SNFMI Research Group on Whipple Disease. Société Nationale Française de Médecine Interne. *Medicine*. 1997. 76:170-84.

74. Dutly F, Altwebb M. Whipple's disease and *Tropheryma whippelii*. *Clin Microbiol Rev*. 2001;14:561-83.

75. Kelly CA, Egan M, Rawlinson J. Whipple's disease presenting with lung involvement. *Thorax*. 1996;51:343-5.

76. Mahnel R, Marth T. Progress, problems and perspectives in diagnosis and treatment of Whipple's disease. *Clin Exp Med*. 2004;4:39-43.

77. Maizel H, Ruffin JM, Dobbins WO III. Whipple's disease: a review of 19 patients from one hospital and a review of the literature since 1950. *Medicine*. 1993;72:343-55.

78. Raoult D, Birg ML, La Scola B, et al. Cultivation of the bacillus of Whipple's disease. *N Engl J Med*. 2000;342:620-5.

79. Relman DA, Schmidt TM, MacDermott RP, Falkow S. Identification of the uncultured bacillus of Whipple's disease. *N Engl J Med*. 1992;327: 293-301.

80. Symmons DP, Shepherd AN, Boardman PL, Bacon PA. Pulmonary manifestations of Whipple's disease. *Q J Med*. 1985;56:497-504.

81. Winberg CD, Rose ME, Rappaport H. Whipple's disease of the lung. *Am J Med*. 1978;65:873-80.

Anthrax

82. Guarner J, Jernigan JA, Shieh WJ, et al. Pathology and pathogenesis of bioterrorism-related inhalational anthrax. *Am J Pathol*. 2003;163: 701-9.

83. Jernigan DB, Raghunathan PL, Bell BP, et al. Investigation of bioterrorism-related anthrax, United States, 2001. epidemiologic findings. *Emerg Infect Dis*. 2002;8:1019-28.

84. Jernigan JA, Stephens DS, Ashford DA, et al. Bioterrorism-related inhalational anthrax: the first 10 cases reported in the United States. *Emerg Infect Dis*. 2001;7:933-44.

85. Kaya A, Tasyaran MA, Erol S, Ozkurt Z, Ozkan B. Anthrax in adults and children: a review of 132 cases in Turkey. *Eur J Clin Microbiol Infect Dis*. 2002;21:258-61.

Francisella Tularensis

86. Bell JH. Woolsorters' disease. *Lancet*. 1880;1:909-11.

87. Ellis J, Oyston PC, Green M, Titball RW. Tularemia. *Clin Microbiol Rev*. 2002;15:631-46.

88. Evans ME, Gregory DW, Schaffner W, McGee ZA. Tularemia: a 30-year experience with 88 cases. *Medicine (Baltimore)*. 1985;64:251-69.

89. Gill V, Cunha BA. Tularemia pneumonia. *Semin Respir Infect*. 1997;12: 61-7.

90. Pullen RL, Stuart BM. Tularemia analysis of 225 cases. *JAMA*. 1945;129: 495-500.

91. Sunderrajan EV, Hutton J, Marienfeld RD. Adult respiratory distress syndrome secondary to tularemia pneumonia. *Arch Intern Med*. 1985;145: 1435-7.

92. Taylor JP, Istre GR, McChesney TC, et al. Epidemiologic characteristics of human tularemia in the southwest-central states, 1981-1987. *Am J Epidemiol*. 1991;133:1032-8.

Yersinia Pestis

93. CDC. Pneumonic plague—Arizona, 1992. *MMWR Morb Mortal Wkly Rep*. 1992;41:737-9.

94. Krishma G, Chitkara K. Pneumonia plague. *Semin Respir Infect*. 2003;18:159-67.

95. Smith JH, Reisner BS. Plague. In: Connor DH, Chandler FW, Manz HJ, Schwartz DA, Lack EE, eds. *Pathology of Infectious Diseases*. Stamford: Appleton & Lange; 1997:729-38.

11 Mycobacterial Diseases

Jaishree Jagirdar

- Tuberculosis
- Non-Tuberculous Mycobacterial Infections

TUBERCULOSIS

INTRODUCTION

Tuberculosis (TB), caused by *Mycobacterium tuberculosis hominis* (MTB), is responsible for 2 million deaths annually worldwide and is a major cause of death in individuals infected with the human immunodeficiency virus (HIV). MTB was discovered by Louis Pasteur in 1887. Much has been learned about MTB since this time; the entire genome has been sequenced, information has been uncovered regarding virulence and latency, and molecular methodologies have revolutionized rapid diagnosis of the infection. The treatment has shifted from fresh air in the sanatorium in 1903 to pharmacogenetically targeted therapy in 2007. About a third of the world's population is infected with MTB, and approximately 10% of this group will develop mycobacterial disease at some point during their lives. In the immunocompromised HIV-infected host, however, the annual incidence of active disease development is 10%. This contributed to the rising prevalence of TB seen in the 1980s, during the height of the HIV epidemic. In the early 1990s, multidrug-resistant TB began to emerge as another challenge to the treatment of the disease. The spectrum of disease morphology also changed to include not only the well formed necrotizing granulomas in the immunocompetent host, but also poorly formed granulomas and less organized macrophage infiltrates in the immunocompromised host.

Classically, TB has been divided into primary and secondary (postprimary) forms of disease. Primary TB is defined as an infection caused by MTB in a previously uninfected host. It is usually clinically silent and discovered incidentally via a positive purified protein derivative (PPD) test or on a chest radiograph. These infections induce a granulomatous response in the lung as well as in other bodily sites that are seeded with the organisms. Over time, these infected foci usually become surrounded by fibrous rims and calcify, but organisms are believed to remain dormant in the foci and contribute to the persistence of reactivity with PPD. These foci remain latent in most individuals, but can reactivate to produce postprimary TB in about 10% of infected people, sometimes after there is a compromise to host immunity. In a smaller number of individuals, the primary foci do not involute, but instead can grow, cavitate, and disseminate (progressive primary TB). Progressive primary TB is more likely in immunocompromised people than in those with intact immune functions. Chronic pulmonary TB, also known as secondary or postprimary TB, refers to TB developing in a previously sensitized individual, usually due to reactivation of a latent infection or less commonly via reinfection from an external source. Lesions are most often found in one or both apices of the lungs. They present as areas of consolidation that can enlarge, cavitate, and disseminate in the lungs or systemically. The spectrum of associated pathology is described below.

CLINICAL FEATURES

The MTB infection rate in foreign-born persons in the United States is 8.7 times that of people born in the U.S. Hispanics, African-Americans, and Asians have MTB rates that are 7.3, 8.3, and 19.6 times higher than Caucasians, respectively. Males are more likely to be infected than females. Today, MTB is most commonly diagnosed in the elderly and in people with HIV infection. In the U.S., the incidence of MTB has declined in children, unlike in other countries with higher incidences, and exposure to MTB often occurs for the first time in young adults. The risk of active disease is increased with coexisting diabetes, alcoholism, congenital heart disease, chronic lung disease, immunocompromise, or other debilitating illnesses. Transmission usually occurs via inhalation of organism-bearing particles (droplet nuclei and dust-associated particles) released by a patient with an airway-communicating lesion, by coughing, sneezing, or speaking. A history of prolonged contact with the infected individual is often present. Rarely, infections can be acquired through an open skin wound or mucous membrane.

Patients typically develop vague symptoms of cough, fever, anorexia, fatigue, chest pain, and night sweats. Purulent sputum may be present, and hemoptysis is seen in 7-33% of patients with tuberculosis. Clubbing may be observed and is indicative of severe pulmonary disease. Headache can occur with central nervous system involvement. The most prominent chronic constitutional symptom is wasting; hence MTB was called "phthisis" or "consumption." Some patients are asymptomatic.

RADIOLOGIC FEATURES

Radiologic techniques more commonly detect lesions of chronic pulmonary TB than primary TB. Reactivation TB lesions are located in the apicoposterior aspects of the lungs in 84% of patients. About 10% of cases occur in the superior segments of the lower lobes. Lesions can be solid or cavitary; cavities tend to be thick-walled and may demonstrate air-fluid levels. Some lesions are slightly spiculated and may present as solitary coin lesions mimicking carcinoma. Consolidation may also be seen. Mediastinal and hilar adenopathy and associated pleural effusions may be evident and often reflect immune compromise. Pulmonary nodules and hilar lymph nodes may be calcified. CT findings of central low attenuation in lymph nodes may reflect active disease.

The Ghon focus is the focus of primary pulmonary infection with MTB, and may be visible as a 1.0-1.5 cm. focus of consolidation, most commonly in the lower part of an upper lobe or the upper part of a lower lobe adjacent to the pleura (regions that receive the greatest flow of air). Enlarged, infected tracheobronchial lymph nodes may accompany this pulmonary focus; the combination may be referred to as the "Ghon complex." The foci of primary infection may not be visible on chest radiograph.

PATHOLOGIC FEATURES

GROSS FINDINGS

Grossly, adult TB usually presents as a necrotizing consolidative process in one or both lung apices (Figure 11-1). The necrosis is described as "caseous," referring to the chalky or cheese-like appearance of the necrotic

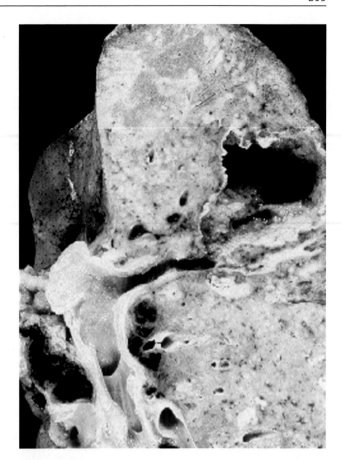

FIGURE 11-1
Chronic pulmonary tuberculosis
This lung displays a large cavity which empties into an airway, apical consolidation, and necrotic nodules. (Courtesy of Dani S. Zander, MD, Penn State Milton S. Hershey Medical Center, Hershey, PA.)

material. There may be cavitation with erosion into bronchi, which can lead to intrabronchial spread of the infection to other lobes of lung and promote aerogenous spread of the infection to other individuals. Cavities are usually located in the upper lobes, often measure between 3 and 10 cm, have thick walls, and contain variable amounts of caseous material (Figure 11-2). Chronic cavities have thicker, more fibrotic walls than expanding recent ones. Obliterated or aneurysmal pulmonary arteries can be seen traversing the cavity.

Other presentations of TB also occur. TB can appear as a circumscribed nodule (Figure 11-3), mass or masses (tuberculomas), and these lesions are occasionally resected due to concern about carcinoma. Some of the nodules represent foci of primary TB. These are usually solitary 1.0-1.5 cm. nodules with central necrosis, calcification, and/or fibrosis, frequently in the mid-zones of the lung, and often accompanied by enlarged, infected tracheobronchial lymph nodes. In miliary TB, innumerable 1-3 mm. nodules (granulomas) are distributed throughout the lungs and other systemic sites (Figure 11-4). In

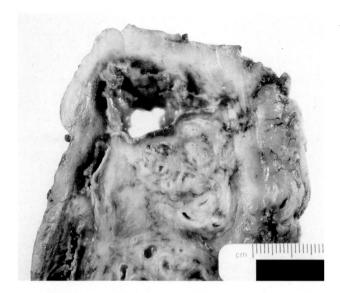

FIGURE 11-2
Chronic pulmonary tuberculosis
This shrunken lung has advanced fibrosis and an apical cavity. Note the pleural fibrosis and fatty infiltration.

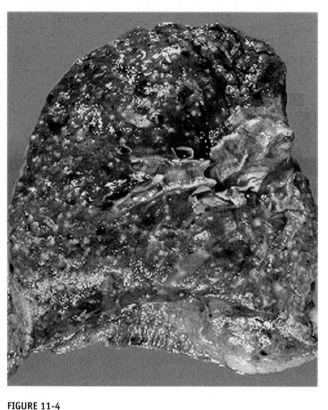

FIGURE 11-4
Miliary tuberculosis
The lung displays numerous 1-2 mm granulomas throughout. (Courtesy of Dani S. Zander, MD, Penn State Milton S. Hershey Medical Center, Hershey, PA.)

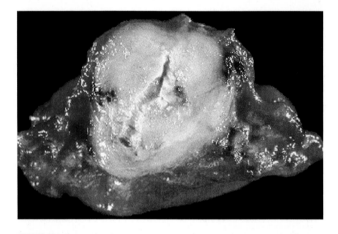

FIGURE 11-3
Tuberculosis
This granuloma presented as a coin lesion. It has a soft necrotic center. (Courtesy of Dani S. Zander, MD, Penn State Milton S. Hershey Medical Center, Hershey, PA.)

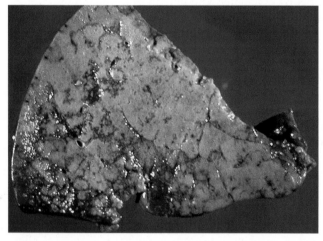

FIGURE 11-5
Tuberculous pneumonia
The majority of this lobe is consolidated, resembling a bacterial pneumonia. (Courtesy of Dani S. Zander, MD, Penn State Milton S. Hershey Medical Center, Hershey, PA.)

tuberculous pneumonia, parenchymal consolidation can be extensive, and the gross and radiographic features can resemble bacterial pneumonia (Figure 11-5). Pleural TB can manifest with thickened, shaggy pleura, sometimes showing discrete granulomas and associated with a pleural effusion (Figure 11-6). Although involvement of any bodily site can occur, the meninges and bones represent more common sites of involvement, and display granulomatous and necrotizing changes similar to those observed in the lung.

MICROSCOPIC FINDINGS

The granuloma is the hallmark of the usual host response to MTB. A granuloma consists of a discrete cluster of epithelioid macrophages which may be accompanied by Langhans-type giant cells, and it is often

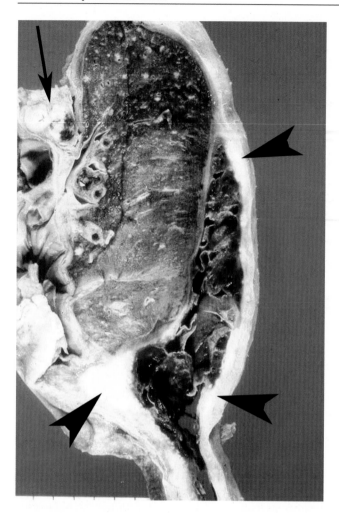

FIGURE 11-6

Pleural tuberculosis and tuberculous lymphadenitis
The pleural cavity contains necrotic exudate (arrowheads) infected with MTB, and hemorrhagic material, and hilar lymph nodes are largely replaced by granulomatous inflammation (arrow). (Courtesy of Dani S. Zander, MD, Penn State Milton S. Hershey Medical Center, Hershey, PA.)

sites that are seeded by the MTB. Non-necrotizing granulomas can accompany the necrotizing granulomas or represent the predominant host response to the infection. Over time, the granulomas will usually become fibrotic and calcified. However, if healing does not occur in the primary phase, the infection can progress (progressive primary TB), with enlarging areas of granulomatous inflammation and cavitation. Lesions of chronic pulmonary TB are also characteristically granulomatous. These foci can also undergo fibrosis and calcification, or they can progress with formation of cavities (cavitary fibrocaseous TB), tracheobronchial spread, miliary spread through the vasculature or lymphatics, pleural involvement, or spread to virtually any site.

COMPLICATIONS OF PULMONARY TUBERCULOSIS

Although the granulomatous reaction is essentially an attempt to contain the tuberculous infection, granulomas, especially when large and cavitary, can lead to complications. Erosion of a granuloma into a pulmonary artery can lead to significant and sometimes fatal bleeding (Rasmussen's aneurysm). Erosion through pleura can lead to formation of a bronchopleural fistula and pleural tuberculous empyema. A cavity can become colonized by aspergilli and develop a fungus ball (aspergilloma) (Figure 11-8). Rare scar carcinomas develop in association with scars caused by chronic tuberculous infections. Amyloidosis is another very rare complication of chronic infection.

STAINING CHARACTERISTICS OF MYCOBACTERIA

Acid fast stains or other procedures discussed below are necessary for demonstrating the bacilli, which are not visible in hematoxylin-eosin-stained preparations. Acid-fast stains include the Ziehl-Neelsen stain (Figure 11-9), the Kinyoun stain, and the Fite stain. Most practitioners choose either the Ziehl-Neelsen or the Kinyoun stain, neither of which will stain *Nocardia* (unlike the Fite stain). Owing to their waxy cell wall components, the bacilli of TB are acid fast; that is, they retain the red dye, carbol fuchsin, after rinsing with acid solvents. Oftentimes, the bacilli have a beaded appearance. Detection of one or more mycobacteria in an area of granulomatous inflammation is highly specific and indicative of infection. Unfortunately, however, over 100 mycobacteria per milliliter of tissue are usually necessary before the organisms can be visualized by light microscopy, so a negative stain does not exclude a diagnosis of TB. It must also be remembered that mycobacteria cannot be speciated based upon morphologic features; other techniques (culture, molecular assays) must be used to determine the mycobacterial species. Staining of mycobacteria is inconsistent with Gram stain. In some cases, mycobacteria can be stained by Gomori methenamine silver stain or periodic acid–Schiff stain. Other stains that are useful and more

surrounded by lymphocytes (Figure 11-7). Granulomas can be necrotizing (caseating) or non-necrotizing. Acid-fast staining often demonstrates the bacilli of MTB in the necrotic areas or in the giant cells, and sometimes in the epithelioid macrophages as well. Small numbers of neutrophils may also be present. With conditions that impair cell-mediated immunity, granulomas may be less well formed or even absent, and the host response can take the form of less-organized macrophage infiltrates and zones of necrosis. In these cases, acid fast bacilli are often more numerous and easier to identify.

Primary pulmonary infection by MTB results in a small patch of pneumonia that converts to necrotizing (caseous) granulomatous inflammation after the infected individual develops type IV hypersensitivity to the MTB. Similar granulomatous lesions appear in the draining hilar lymph nodes as well as in other bodily

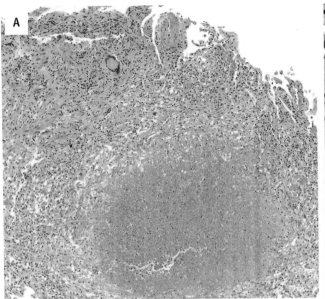

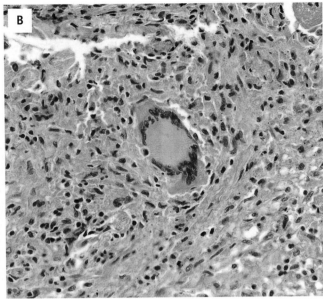

FIGURE 11-7

Necrotizing granuloma

(A) The necrotic center is surrounded by epithelioid histiocytes and then by a rim of lymphocytes. **(B)** This higher power view highlights a Langhans giant cell in a background of epithelioid histiocytes.

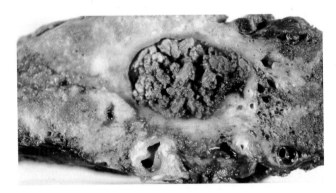

FIGURE 11-8

Aspergilloma (fungus ball) in tuberculous cavity

An aggregate of *Aspergillus* fills this chronic cavity.

sensitive, but perhaps not as specific, are the auramine-O (Figure 11-10) and the rhodamine stains.

ANCILLARY STUDIES

IMMUNOHISTOCHEMISTRY

With the availability of antibodies to mycobacteria, it is possible to detect mycobacteria in tissues using immunohistochemistry. Humphrey and Weiner tested rabbit polyclonal antibodies and found a slightly improved detection rate of mycobacteria in caseous lesions as compared to the traditional Ziehl-Neelsen stain. Their antibody weakly cross-reacted with atypical mycobacteria, but was found to be highly specific for mycobacterial infections. Other authors, using monoclonal antibodies against different mycobacterial antigens (28, 35, and 65 kDa), were able to improve upon the false-negative results obtained by traditional staining methods. Recently, Mustafa et al. reported increased sensitivity using an antibody to the MTB antigen MPT64, but a few of their negative controls were immunoreactive.

ULTRASTRUCTURAL STUDIES

With the electron microscope, epithelioid cells show highly ruffled interdigitating cell membranes and well developed endoplasmic reticulum, and may contain thick-walled mycobacteria and large Golgi complexes.

CYTOLOGIC DIAGNOSIS

Fine needle aspiration (FNA) in patients with suspected mycobacterial infection is valuable as a screening procedure, particularly in superficial, easily accessible locations such as cervical and submandibular regions. Three different patterns are observed: epithelioid granulomas without necrosis, epithelioid granulomas with

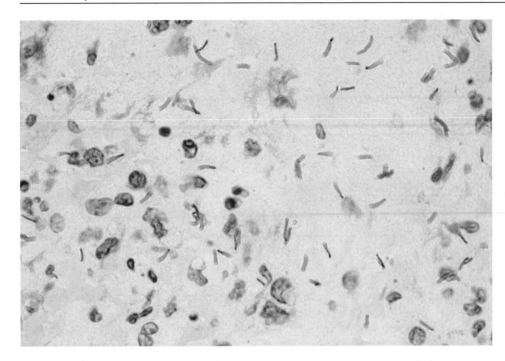

FIGURE 11-9

Mycobacterium tuberculosis
(Ziehl-Neelsen stain)
Numerous red mycobacteria are visible
in an untreated case of TB in a patient
with HIV.

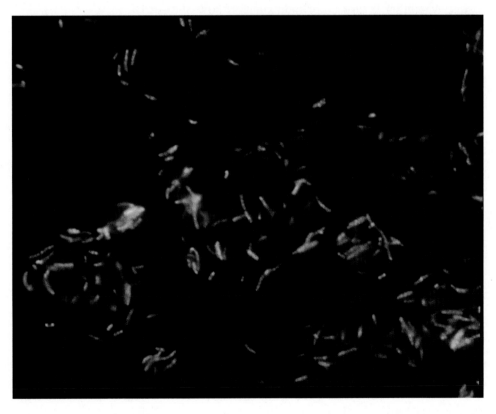

FIGURE 11-10

Mycobacterium tuberculosis
(Auramine stain)
Examination under the immunofluorescence microscope shows numerous
bacilli.

necrosis, and necrosis alone. Acid fast bacilli are seen most readily in patients with necrosis alone (77%). Finfer and colleagues found that when caseous or grossly purulent material was aspirated in the proper clinical setting, it was highly specific. Lau and coauthors reported that FNA has a specificity of 93% and a sensitivity of 77% for diagnosis of TB. On average, the chance of detecting acid fast bacilli in these specimens appears to be between 40% and 56%. Cases of TB have also been diagnosed in transbronchial needle aspiration specimens.

DIFFERENTIAL DIAGNOSIS

The differential diagnosis includes other granulomatous and necrotizing conditions. Infections with non-tuberculous mycobacteria, fungi, and *Nocardia,* as well as Wegener's granulomatosis and sarcoidosis, are important entities that can resemble TB. Sarcoidal lesions following alpha-interferon therapy, hypersensitivity pneumonia, malakoplakia, and silicotic nodules may also be considered. MTB cannot be morphologically distinguished from non-tuberculous mycobacteria; differentiation requires culture or molecular techniques. Fungal infections, especially histoplasmosis, can have very similar histology and patient presentation, but methenamine silver staining and culture can usually identify fungi in the lesions. *Nocardia asteroides* is a branching filamentous bacterium that is acid fast when stained with the Fite stain, but will not be visible with Ziehl-Neelsen or Kinyoun stains; it can also be seen with silver and Gram stains. Wegener's granulomatosis manifests a spectrum of histologic changes including geographic necrosis, in which the necrotic areas can have granulomatous-appearing rims. Vasculitis is also frequently present, but can also be observed occasionally in TB. In Wegener's granulomatosis, cultures of the lesions will not yield mycobacteria and should be performed. Assessment of antinuclear cytoplasmic antibody status is also very helpful in evaluating individuals for Wegener's granulomatosis. Additional information regarding the spectrum of pathologic and clinical presentations in patients with Wegener's granulomatosis can be found in the chapter dealing with this disorder. Sarcoidal granulomas tend to be small, compact, and well formed, and often have a distinctive onion skin cuffing of collagen around the epithelioid cells (Figure 11-11). They are usually non-necrotizing, or if they do have necrosis, it is punctate. Sarcoidal granulomas, however, can occur in a setting of TB, and diagnosis of sarcoidosis requires not only demonstration of the correct histology, but exclusion of TB and other granulomatous infections. Silicotic nodules usually have central zones of dense collagen in association with variable quantities of black pigment, and polarizable silicates implying mixed-dust exposure (Figure 11-12). The presence of necrosis in silicotic nodules is suggestive of superimposed mycobacterial infection, which does occur in approximately 30% of cases.

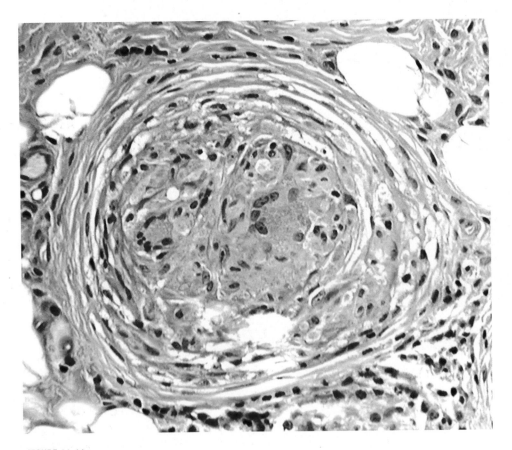

FIGURE 11-11

Sarcoidosis
This compact non-necrotizing granuloma shows distinct onion skinning around the aggregate of epithelioid macrophages.

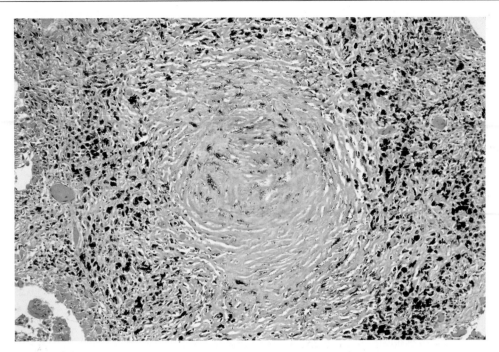

FIGURE 11-12

Silicotic nodule

The nodule consists of dense eosinophilic collagen surrounded by macrophages containing anthracotic material.

PROGNOSIS AND THERAPY

In the absence of therapy, there is a 49% mortality rate over 5 years. For most individuals with TB, however, the prognosis is excellent, provided treatment guidelines are followed carefully and the infection is not with a multidrug-resistant strain. Infections with the latter are associated with a poorer prognosis. The principles of therapy hinge upon making a rapid diagnosis and instituting treatment promptly so that the patient is rapidly rendered noninfectious. Until the 1940s, no effective antimicrobial agents were available, but the discovery of Streptomycin changed things. Although streptomycin was effective against TB, it became apparent that monotherapy would not work due to rapid development of drug resistance. Soon after, PAS (para-aminosalicylic) and INH (isoniazid) were discovered. The concept of multidrug therapy emerged as a major advance that reduced the development of drug resistance and relapse. Unfortunately, however, infected patients needed long-term treatment, usually between 18 and 24 months, before cure was achieved. This hurdle was overcome with the introduction of rifampin in 1966, and later pyrazinamide (PZA). Today, drug therapy decisions are made primarily based on disease presentation and drug sensitivities. Patients are usually rendered non-

infectious within 2 months and cured by 6 months of multidrug therapy consisting of INH, rifampin, and streptomycin or PZA plus ethambutol. The relapse rate is generally low. Multidrug resistance is a vexing issue, however, and requires individualized treatment.

NON-TUBERCULOUS MYCOBACTERIAL INFECTIONS

INTRODUCTION

Non-tuberculous mycobacteria (NTM) is the term used to distinguish environmental mycobacteria from the mycobacteria that cause leprosy (*Mycobacterium leprae*), and tuberculosis (*Mycobacterium tuberculosis hominis*). *M. avium* and *M. intracellulare* are closely related members of the group that are usually considered together as *Mycobacterium avium* complex (MAC) or *Mycobacterium avium intracellulare;* these agents are most commonly responsible for infections with NTM. However, other mycobacteria such as *Mycobacterium abscessus, Mycobacterium fortuitum, Mycobacterium gordonae, Mycobacterium kansasii, Mycobacterium*

TUBERCULOSIS—FACT SHEET

Definition

» Infection caused by *Mycobacterium tuberculosis hominis* (MTB)

Incidence and Location

» About one-third of people throughout the world are infected with MTB
» Tuberculous disease develops in approximately 10% of infected individuals
» Infection is most commonly diagnosed in the elderly and people with HIV infection

Morbidity and Mortality

» Mortality is extremely uncommon in treated patients
» Morbidity depends upon the severity and distribution of lesions in individuals with active disease

Gender, Race, and Age Distribution

» Males are more often affected than females
» Incidence is higher in foreign-born individuals than in individuals born in the United States
» Hispanics, African-Americans, and Asians have higher infection rates than Caucasians
» Primary infection is more common in young adults in the U.S.

Clinical Features

» Typical symptoms include cough, fever, anorexia, fatigue, weight loss, chest pain, and night sweats
» Purulent sputum, hemoptysis, and clubbing may be present
» Some patients are asymptomatic

Radiologic Features

» Chronic pulmonary TB is detected more often than primary TB
» Chronic pulmonary TB:
  » Lesions are characteristically located in the apicoposterior aspects of the lungs, and can be nodular, cavitary, or infiltrates
  » Mediastinal and hilar lymphadenopathy, with or without calcification, and pleural effusions may be evident
» Primary pulmonary TB:
  » 1.0-1.5 cm, focus of consolidation most commonly in the lower part of an upper lobe or the upper part of a lower lobe adjacent to the pleura
  » Enlarged, infected tracheobronchial lymph nodes may be seen
  » The focus of primary infection may not be visible on chest radiograph

Prognosis and Therapy

» Excellent prognosis for most patients, provided treatment guidelines are adhered to and infections are not due to multidrug-resistant strains
» Poorer prognosis with multidrug-resistant organisms
» Drug therapy decisions are made primarily based upon disease presentation and drug sensitivities

TUBERCULOSIS—PATHOLOGIC FEATURES

Gross Findings

» Most common presentation is as a necrotizing consolidative process in one or both lung apices
» Caseous necrosis is often observed
» Cavities, usually located in the upper lobes and often measuring between 3 and 10 cm, may be present
» Enlarged, infected tracheobronchial or mediastinal lymph nodes can be seen
» Other findings can include:
  » Circumscribed nodule, mass, or masses (tuberculoma)
  » Miliary TB: innumerable 1-3 mm nodules (granulomas) distributed throughout the lungs and other systemic sites
  » Primary TB: solitary 1.0-1.5 cm nodule with central necrosis, calcification, and/or fibrosis, most often in the lower part of an upper lobe or the upper part of a lower lobe, usually subpleural
  » Pleural TB: thickened pleura, sometimes showing discrete granulomas, with effusion
  » Bronchopleural fistula

Microscopic Findings

» Necrotizing (caseating) and non-necrotizing granulomas
» With chronicity and healing, granulomas undergo fibrosis and calcification
» With immunocompromise, less-organized macrophage infiltrates and necrotic areas can be seen
» Mycobacteria can often be demonstrated with an acid fast stain
» A negative acid fast stain does not rule out TB

Immunohistochemical Features

» Some reports of benefits of immunohistochemical stains for detection of MTB

Ultrastructural Findings

» Epithelioid cells show highly ruffled interdigitating cell membranes and well developed endoplasmic reticula, and may contain thick-walled mycobacteria and large Golgi complexes

Cytologic Diagnosis

» Fine needle aspiration and transbronchial needle aspiration can be very helpful for diagnosis

Pathologic Differential Diagnosis

» Infections with non-tuberculous mycobacteria, fungi, and *Nocardia*
» Wegener's granulomatosis
» Sarcoidosis
» Sarcoidal lesions following α-interferon therapy
» Hypersensitivity pneumonitis
» Malakoplakia
» Silicotic nodule

malmoense, and *Mycobacterium xenopi* can cause disease as well. NTM are found primarily in water, soil, dust, animals, and food, and survive chlorination, ozonization, and filtration. These agents do not normally cause disease in healthy humans, and there is no evidence of person-to-person transmission. With impairment of host defenses or disruption of skin or mucosal barriers, however, they can become pathogenic. Infections with NTM occur in diverse settings such as cystic fibrosis, immunosuppression associated with transplantation, other forms of iatrogenic immunosuppression, immune reconstitution inflammatory syndrome, fibronodular bronchiectasis, and exogenous lipoid pneumonia. These agents most commonly cause skin and soft tissue infections, lymphadenitis, and lung disease. Disseminated infection may occur in patients with the acquired immune deficiency syndrome (AIDS), and in patients with interleukin (IL)-12 and interferon (IFN)-γ receptor abnormalities. As the rate of MTB has declined, there seems to have been an apparent increase in infections with NTM. This could, at least in part, however, be due to more diligent searching for these organisms and better detection techniques. BACTEC liquid culture systems and the development of nucleic acid amplification and DNA probes allow more rapid diagnosis of mycobacterial disease and more rapid differentiation of NTM from MTB. High-performance liquid chromatography, polymerase chain reaction, and restriction fragment length polymorphism analysis have also helped to identify new NTM species.

CLINICAL FEATURES

Typically, patients develop cough and sputum production, shortness of breath, hemoptysis, and systemic symptoms such as fatigue, lassitude, weight loss, fever, and night sweats, much like patients with MTB. Some culture-positive patients, however, are asymptomatic, and in this setting it can be difficult to assess whether a positive culture result reflects colonization of the respiratory tract by the organisms or active infection. NTM is seen most commonly in males and is typically associated with other predisposing diseases, such as chronic obstructive pulmonary disease or HIV. The American Thoracic Society (ATS) has developed guidelines for diagnosing infection due to NTM in both HIV-seropositive and HIV-seronegative individuals. The ATS criteria include the presence of symptoms, pertinent radiologic findings as stated below, and microbiologic evidence of infection (3 positive sputum cultures, or 2 positive cultures and a positive smear). If the above criteria are not met, and other diseases can be excluded, a transbronchial biopsy showing granulomas or acid-fast bacilli may be sufficient to render a diagnosis in a suspected case of NTM.

Infections with NTM can be associated with previous TB, pneumoconioses, cystic fibrosis (usually MAC, occasionally *M. abscessus*), bronchiectasis (MAC and *M. abscessus*), transplantation (MAC and *M. abscessus* in lung transplant patients) and pulmonary alveolar proteinosis. In the HIV setting, infections usually develop when the CD4 count drops below 100/microliter, whereas MTB can occur at any time during an HIV infection. MAC is the most common non-tuberculous mycobacterial infection in HIV-infected patients, and dissemination is common. Immune reconstitution syndrome (IRIS) can also develop with the use of anti-HIV therapy. As the immune system begins to mount a response to the MAC, there is worsening of symptoms and radiologic findings. Some patients require corticosteroids to treat IRIS.

Patients with "hot tub lung" (HTL) are typically young, immunocompetent women in their 40s. Patients often have significant indoor hot tub exposure for several months or years. Household showers have also been implicated in some cases. Signs and symptoms include cough, dyspnea, chest tightness, fatigue, and hypoxia. Catheter-related infections can be caused by MAC, and anti-tumor necrosis factor antagonists used for rheumatoid arthritis and Crohn's disease are associated with infections with NTM. Patients who take mineral oil for constipation are at risk for developing *M. fortuitum* and *M. chelonei* infection, as well as exogenous lipoid pneumonia. An interesting presentation of pulmonary MAC infection, known as Lady Windermore Syndrome, has also been described, and occurs in otherwise healthy middle-aged women. In this condition, pulmonary consolidation is localized to the lingula and right middle lobe. In these women, it was felt that the infection was related to cough suppression by these ladies due to societal expectations for etiquette.

RADIOLOGIC FEATURES

The classic radiographic appearance of NTM infection is indistinguishable from that of pulmonary TB. Most patients have upper lobe disease, which may be cavitary, with associated pleural thickening. Plain radiographs can be normal, however, despite active pulmonary infection. Pleural effusions and adenopathy are uncommon. Radiographic findings of bronchiectasis and small nodules, predominantly located within the right middle lobe and lingula, are seen in some middle-aged and elderly females. In HTL, diffuse interstitial or nodular infiltrates are noted on chest radiographs. A high-resolution CT scan of the chest typically demonstrates ground-glass opacities and scattered nodules. Mosaic attenuation is common and reflects air-trapping consistent with bronchiolitis.

PATHOLOGIC FEATURES

GROSS FINDINGS

Cavitary lesions and solitary nodular lesions resembling those of MTB are often present. Multiple nodules may also be seen in association with bronchiectasis in the Lady Windermere Syndrome. In HTL, interstitial widening and small nodules may be visible.

MICROSCOPIC FINDINGS

The morphologic features in the classic fibro-cavitary lesions resemble those of TB, with granulomas representing the predominant host response. Granulomas can be necrotizing or non-necrotizing, well circumscribed or poorly formed, and variable numbers of neutrophils may be present (Figure 11-13). In some cases, neutrophilic infiltrates predominate or occur without granulomatous inflammation. Acid fast staining often reveals organisms in the granulomatous lesions or acutely inflamed areas. In Lady Windermere Syndrome, nonnecrotizing granulomas are usually identified. The granulomas are centered on airways with bronchiectasis. In HTL, centrilobular granulomas, usually non-necrotizing but sometimes focally necrotizing, and in association with organizing pneumonia and patchy interstitial pneumonitis, are present, overlapping with the findings of hypersensitivity pneumonia (Figure 11-14). Sputum cultures from patients with HTL are consistently positive for MAC, and cultures of the tub water often yield the organism. In HIV-positive patients with NTM infections, the granulomas are usually poorly formed and there are fewer giant cells. With CD4+ T-cell counts below 100, numerous acid fast bacilli may be seen (Figure 11-15). Occasionally, the lesions in this setting may form pseudotumors with spindle cells, resembling dermatofibromas (Figure 11-16). Cytologic diagnosis can be made using an acid fast stain. On a Diff Quik stain, acid fast bacilli can be seen as negative images when they are numerous (Figure 11-17).

DIFFERENTIAL DIAGNOSIS

The differential diagnostic considerations are essentially the same as for TB.

PROGNOSIS AND THERAPY

The most common therapy employed for MAC infection is a three-drug regimen of either clarithromycin or azithromycin, with ethambutol, and rifampin or rifabutin for 12 months after sputum conversion. This regimen results in sputum conversion in approximately 90% of those who tolerate the regimen. Drug intolerance is common, and relapse may occur after apparently successful therapy. HTL will usually respond to discontinuation of exposure to the contaminated water or treatment with corticosteroids.

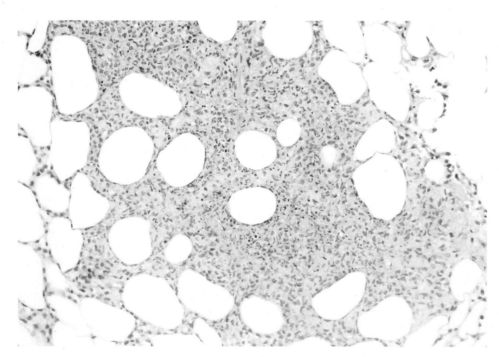

FIGURE 11-13

Mycobacterium avium **complex**
This poorly organized collection of epithelioid histiocytes and neutrophils represents the host response to MAC infection in an HIV-infected patient with low CD4+ T-cell counts.

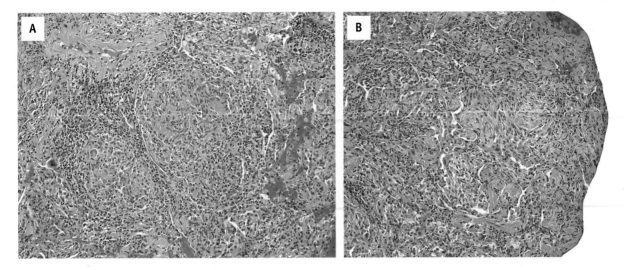

FIGURE 11-14
Hot tub lung
(A) Two granulomas are present, with punctate necrosis in the granuloma on the right. **(B)** Organizing pneumonia accompanied the granulomas in this case. (Courtesy of Dani S. Zander, MD, Penn State Milton S. Hershey Medical Center, Hershey, PA.)

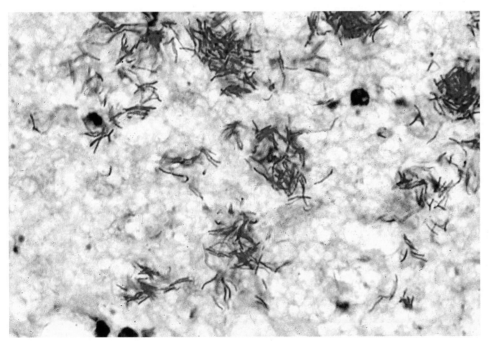

FIGURE 11-15

***Mycobacterium avium* complex**
Numerous acid fast organisms are visible in this sample from an HIV-infected patient. (Courtesy of Dani S. Zander, MD, Penn State Milton S. Hershey Medical Center, Hershey, PA.)

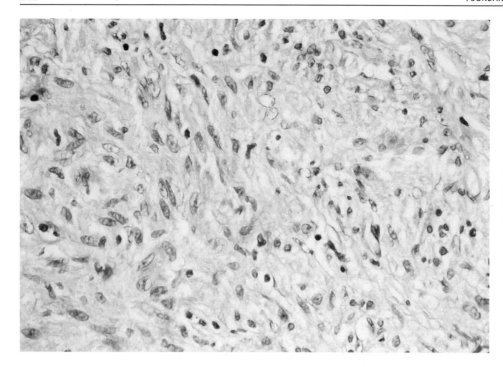

FIGURE 11-16
Spindle cell pseudotumor due to
***Mycobacterium avium* complex.**
The histology resembles a dermatofibroma.

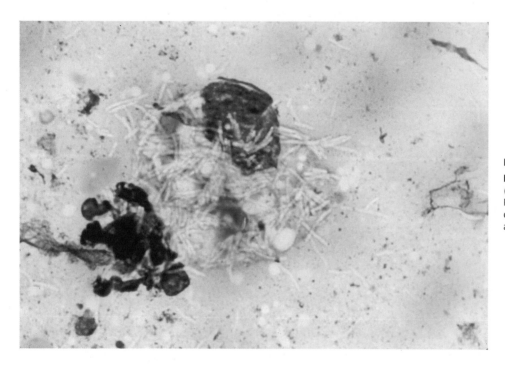

FIGURE 11-17
Non-tuberculous mycobacteria
(Diff Quik stain)
Fine needle aspiration yielded a foam cell with mycobacteria evident as negative images.

NONTUBERCULOSIS MYCOBACTERIAL INFECTIONS—FACT SHEET

Definition

» Infection caused by a species of mycobacteria other than *Mycobacterium leprae* and *Mycobacterium tuberculosis hominis*

Incidence and Location

» Prevalence appears to be on the rise
» Worldwide distribution
» Incidence is higher in HIV-positive individuals
» Other associations include cystic fibrosis, immunosuppression associated with transplantation, other forms of iatrogenic immunosuppression

Morbidity and Mortality

» Mortality is uncommon due to NTM.
» Morbidity depends upon the severity and distribution of lesions in individuals with active disease and on the immune status of the patient

Gender and Age Distribution

» Males tend to develop more cavitary lesions
» In Lady Windermere Syndrome, middle-aged females are most often affected
» "Hot tub lung" typically occurs in young women and men who use hot tubs with water contaminated by NTM

Clinical Features

» Typical symptoms include cough, fever, anorexia, fatigue, weight loss, chest pain, and night sweats
» Some patients are asymptomatic

Radiologic Features

» Lesions can be nodular, multinodular, cavitary, or diffusely infiltrative
» Bronchiectasis can be observed
» Mediastinal and hilar lymphadenopathy, with or without calcification, and pleural effusions may be evident, but are not common as in MTB

Prognosis and Therapy

» Prognosis for most patients is good provided treatment guidelines are followed
» Drug resistance is more common than in MTB, and prognosis is poorer with multidrug-resistant organisms and immunocompromise
» For hot tub lung, the prognosis is excellent with discontinuation of patient exposure to contaminated water; corticosteroids can be given for more severe cases and usually produce improvement

NONTUBERCULOSIS MYCOBACTERIAL INFECTIONS—PATHOLOGIC FEATURES

Gross Findings

» Cavitary and nodular lesions resembling MTB
» Multiple nodules may be seen in association with bronchiectasis in the right middle lobe or lingula, in the Lady Windermere Syndrome
» In hot tub lung, interstitial widening and small nodules may be present.

Microscopic Findings

» Granulomatous inflammation, with or without necrosis, is the predominant host response
» Neutrophils can be present in varying numbers, and in some cases can represent the predominant response

Pathologic Differential Diagnosis

» Infections with non-tuberculous mycobacteria, fungi, and *Nocardia*
» Wegener's granulomatosis
» Sarcoidosis
» Sarcoidal lesions following α-interferon therapy
» Hypersensitivity pneumonitis
» Malakoplakia
» Silicotic nodule

7. Dannenberg Am Jr. Pathogenesis of tuberculosis. In AP Fishman, ed. *Pulmonary Disease and Disorders*. New York: McGraw-Hill; 1980: 1264-81.
8. Finfer M, Perchick A, Burstein DE. Fine needle aspiration biopsy diagnosis of tuberculous lymphadenitis in patients with and without the acquired immune deficiency syndrome. *Acta Cytol*. 1991;35:325-32.
9. Flance IJ. Scar cancer of the lung. *JAMA*. 1991;266:2003-4.
10. Goldberg HJ, Fiedler D, Webb A, Jagirdar J, Hoyumpa AM, Peters J. Sarcoidosis after treatment with interferon-alpha: a case series and review of the literature. *Respir Med*. 2006:100;2063-8.
11. Guy E, Rocha MP, Faith R, et al. Pathogenicity of multi-drug resistant *M. tuberculosis* in the guinea pig. *Am Rev Respir Dis*. 1994;149:A614.
12. Heimbeck J. Incidence of tuberculosis in young adult women with special reference to employment. *Br J Tuberc Dis Chest*. 1938;32:154-66.
13. Hill AR, Premkumar S, Burstein S, et al. Disseminated tuberculosis in the acquired immunodeficiency syndrome era. *Am Rev Respir Dis*. 1991;144:1164-70.
14. Humphrey DM, Weiner MH. Mycobacterial antigen detection by immunohistochemistry in pulmonary tuberculosis. *Hum Pathol*. 1987;18:701-8.
15. Jagirdar J, Zagzag D. Pathology and insights into the pathogenesis of tuberculosis. In Rom WN, Garay SM, eds. *Tuberculosis*. 2nd ed. Philadelphia: Lippincott Williams and Wilkins; 2004:323-44.
16. Laennec RTH. *Deflauscultation Mediate*. Paris: Brosson, 1918.
17. Lau SK, Wei WI, Hsu C, et al. Efficacy of fine needle aspiration cytology in the diagnosis of tuberculous cervical lymphadenopathy. *J Laryngol Otol*. 1990;104:24-7.
18. Madri JA, Carter D. Scar cancers of the lung; origin and significance. *Hum Pathol*. 1984;15:625-31.
19. Mankiewicz E. Bacteriophage types of mycobacteria. *Can J Public Health*. 1972;63:111:307-12.
20. McGuinness G, Naidich DP, Jagirdar J, et al. High resolution CT finding in miliary lung disease. *J Comput Assist Tomogr*. 1992;16:384-90.
21. Medlar EM. The behavior of pulmonary tuberculous lesions: a pathological study. *Monograph*. 1955.
22. Mustafa T, Wiker HG, Mfinanga SGM, Mørkve O, Sviland L. Immunohistochemistry using a mycobacterium tuberculosis complex specific antibody for improved diagnosis of tuberculous lymphadenitis. *Mod Pathol*. 2006:19;1606-14.
23. Pennington JE. Aspergillus lung disease. *Med Clin North Am*. 1980;64:475-90.
24. Stead WW. Pathogenesis of a first episode of chronic pulmonary tuberculosis in man: recrudescence of residuals of the primary infection or exogenous reinfection? *Am Rev Respir Dis*. 1967;95:729-45.

SUGGESTED READINGS

Tuberculosis

1. Arora B, Arora DR. Fine needle aspiration cytology in diagnosis of tuberculous lymphadenitis. *Indian J Med Res*. 1990;91:189-92.
2. Barbolini G, Biseti A, Colizzi V, et al. Immunohistologic analysis of mycobacterial antigens by monoclonal antibodies in tuberculosis and mycobacteriosis. *Hum Pathol*. 1989;20:1078-83.
3. Chandrasekhar S, Ratnam S. Studies on cell-wall deficient non-acid-fast variants of M. tuberculosis. *Tuberc Lung Dis*. 1992;73:273-9.
4. Chauduri MR. Primary pulmonary scar carcinomas. *Indian J Med Res*. 1973;61:858-69.
5. Dacosta NA, Kinare SG. Association of lung carcinoma and tuberculosis. *J Postgrad Med*. 1991;37:185-9.
6. Daniels M, Ridehaligh F, Springett VH, et al. *Tuberculosis in Young Adults: Report of the Prophit Tuberculosis Survey 1935-1944*, 1st ed. London: Lewis; 1948.

25. Stead WW. Pathogenesis of the sporadic cases of tuberculosis. *N Engl J Med*. 1967;277:1008-12.

26. Stead WW. The pathogenesis of pulmonary tuberculosis among older persons. *Am Rev Respir Dis*. 1965;91:811-22.

27. Wear DJ, Hadfield TL, Connor DH, et al. Letters to the editor. *Arch Pathol Lab Med*. 1985;109:701-2.

Non-Tuberculous Mycobacteria

28. Brandwein M, Choi HS, Strauchen J, Stoler M, Jagirdar J. Spindle cell reaction to nontuberculous mycobacteriosis in AIDS mimicking a spindle cell neoplasm: Evidence for dual histiocytic and fibroblast-like characteristics of spindle cells. *Virchows Arch A Pathol Anat Histopathol*. 1990;416:281-6.

29. Bruijnesteijn Van Coppenraet ES, Lindeboom JA, Prins JM, Peeters MF, Claas EC, Kuijper EJ. Real-time PCR assay using fine-needle aspirates and tissue biopsy specimens for rapid diagnosis of mycobacterial lymphadenitis in children. *J Clin Microbiol*. 2004;42:2644-50.

30. Ellison E, Lapuerta P, Martin SE. Fine needle aspiration diagnosis of mycobacterial lymphadenitis: Sensitivity and predictive value in the United States. *Acta Cytol*. 1999;43:153-7.

31. Ellison E, Lapuerta P, Martin SE. Fine needle aspiration (FNA) in HIV+ patients: results from a series of 655 aspirates. *Cytopathology*. 1998;9:222-9.

32. Field SK, Cowie RL. Lung disease due to the more common nontuberculous mycobacteria. *Chest*. 2006;129:1653-72.

33. Hilborn Ed, Covert TC, Yakrus MA, et al. Persistence of nontuberculous mycobacteria in a drinking water system after addition of filtration treatment. *Appl Environ Microbiol*. 2006;72:5864-9.

34. Kobashi Y, Fukuda M, Yoshida K, Miyashita N, Okay M. Pulmonary mycobacterium intracellulare disease with a solitary pulmonary nodule detected at the onset of pneumothorax. *J Infect Chemother*. 2006;12:203-6.

35. Kommareddi S, Abramowsky C, Swinehart GL, et al. Nontuberculous mycobacterial infections: comparison of the fluorescent auramine-O and Ziehl-Neelsen techniques in tissue diagnosis. *Hum Pathol*. 1984;15:1085-9.

36. Levin DL. Radiology of pulmonary *Mycobacterium* avium-intracellulare complex. *Clin Chest Med*. 2002;23:603-12.

37. Ridaura-Sanz C, Lopez-Corella E, Salazar-Flores M. Exogenous lipoid pneumonia superinfected with acid-fast bacilli in infants: a report of nine cases. *Fetal Pediatr Pathol*. 2006;25:107-17.

38. Waninger KN, Young Jr. Hot tub lung: is it on your list of respiratory ailments? *J Fam Pract*. 2006;55:694-6.

12 Fungal Diseases

Abida K. Haque

INTRODUCTION

Fungi are unicellular or multicellular organisms that have chitinous cell walls and reproduce either asexually, sexually, or both ways. Fungal cells are larger and more complex than bacteria, with their cell walls containing polysaccharides, proteins, sugars, and antigens. Pulmonary fungal infections follow inhalation of aerosolized fungi from the environment. The infections can remain either localized to the lungs, or can disseminate to produce systemic disease in immunocompromised individuals. Common fungal infections included in this chapter are histoplasmosis, coccidioidosis, candidiasis, aspergillosis, cryptococcosis, phaeohyphomycosis, and zygomycosis. Uncommon fungal infections presented at the end of the chapter include the following: pseudallescheriasis, fusariosis, trichosporonosis, penicilliosis, paracoccidioidomycosis, and geotrichosis. Protothecosis, adiaspiromycosis, malasseziosis, and rhinosporidiosis are other uncommon fungal infections that occur in the lung, but are not discussed in this chapter.

COMMON FUNGAL INFECTIONS

HISTOPLASMOSIS

Histoplasmosis is a respiratory infection caused by inhalation of infectious conidia or mycelia of *Histoplasma capsulatum* var. *capsulatum*. In the United States, the Mississippi and Ohio River valleys are highly endemic areas. The avian and chiropteran habitats such as chicken coops, roosting shelters, caves, and attics favor the growth and multiplication of histoplasma in soil enriched with fecal material.

CLINICAL FEATURES

Almost 75% of infections are asymptomatic and self-limited, and heal without treatment. The remaining 25% of patients may develop symptomatic disease manifested as: 1) acute pulmonary disease; 2) disseminated disease; 3) chronic pulmonary disease, and 4) fibrosing mediastinitis.

Acute pulmonary disease clinically manifests as fever with cough and chest pain, approximately 1 to 4 weeks after exposure. Symptoms can resolve in a few days to two weeks, but may persist up to several months. Disseminated histoplasmosis is seen in patients with impaired cell-mediated immunity with development of severe systemic symptoms including weight loss, malaise, hepatosplenomegaly, purpura, and oropharyngeal and intestinal ulcerations. The mortality without antifungal therapy can be as high as 80%. Chronic pulmonary histoplasmosis is primarily a disease of adults with symptoms similar to other chronic progressive pulmonary infections such as tuberculosis.

Fibrosing mediastinitis is a histologically benign disorder caused by proliferation of collagen within the mediastinum as a result of histoplasmosis; however, cases secondary to tuberculosis, zygomycosis, and Langerhans cell histiocytosis are also reported. Most of the patients are young and present with respiratory symptoms. The disease is slowly progressive, and may result in extensive fibrosis with entrapment and invasion of structures adjacent to the mediastinal lymph nodes including the heart, great vessels, and esophagus.

RADIOLOGIC FEATURES

In the acute phase, chest radiographs may show hilar lymphadenopathy and a single small area of pulmonary infiltrate forming the primary complex. With disease evolution, chest radiographs may show patchy nodular pulmonary infiltrates and pleural effusion. Four radiologic patterns have been described in chronic pulmonary histoplasmosis: infiltrative, cavitary, fibrosis with emphysema, and residual solitary nodule or histoplasmoma.

PATHOLOGIC FEATURES

GROSS FINDINGS

In the acute pulmonary disease, patchy bronchopneumonia and hilar lymphadenopathy may be seen. In disseminated histoplasmosis, the lungs may show edema, congestion, and granulomas. Chronic pulmonary histoplasmosis may be seen as diffuse pulmonary infiltrates, frequently apical, but may be bilateral, associated with cavitary lesions, as seen in tuberculosis. Fibrosis may be severe and associated with bronchiectasis. Histoplasmoma, or the "coin" (lesion), may be confused with carcinoma, especially when it is noncalcified. However, histoplasmomas are often rounded, subpleural, and show a concentric calcification pattern, accompanied by enlarged and calcified hilar lymph nodes.

MICROSCOPIC FINDINGS

The characteristic histologic lesion of histoplasmosis is a granuloma, with or without central necrosis, surrounded by lymphocytes, macrophages, and multinucleated giant cells. The fungus is an oval, 2-5 micron yeast that does not have a capsule and shows narrow-necked budding (Figure 12-1). The yeast often occurs in clusters due to its intracellular proliferation in phagocytes. In hematoxylin-eosin-stained sections, the basophilic cytoplasm of the yeast is often retracted from the poorly stained cell wall, creating a false impression of an unstained capsule or a "halo" effect. Poorly formed pseudohyphae consisting of cells attached to each other and germ tubes are often seen in active lesions. The yeast stains strongly with methenamine silver (GMS) stain,

and may be seen in the central areas of old "coin" lesions. The histoplasmoma consists of a large central zone of caseous necrosis surrounded by a thick fibrous capsule that contains lymphoid aggregates and rare epithelioid and multinucleated giant cells. The central necrotic material may be calcified and may show osseous or myeloid metaplasia.

DIFFERENTIAL DIAGNOSIS

The differential diagnosis includes *Candida glabrata*, which is of similar size, but amphophilic and without "halo" effect on H & E stain. *Penicillium marneffei* is also of similar size and shape, but does not bud and divides by fission through the center and can form short hyphae-like or allantoid forms. Poorly encapsulated cryptococci may appear similar, but are round, have narrow point budding, are pleomorphic, and stain with mucicarmine. Microforms of *Blastomyces dermatitidis* should be considered but are multinucleated, with thick double-contoured walls, and have broad-based budding.

Leishmania amastigotes have dot-like intracellular basal bodies or kinetoplasts. However, these do not stain with GMS. *Toxoplasma gondii* also has a similar appearance, stains with H & E, but does not show budding and does not stain with GMS.

PROGNOSIS AND THERAPY

Acute histoplasmosis is usually a benign, self-limited illness that heals without antifungal therapy. However, the progressive pulmonary and disseminated infections require prompt and sometimes prolonged treatment with either amphotericin B or one of its lipid formulations, ketoconazole, itraconazole, or fluconazole. Newer antifungal agents such as triazole and posaconazole are also being used. Fibrosing mediastinitis may require antifungal therapy combined with corticosteroids.

BLASTOMYCOSIS

Blastomycosis is a systemic infection caused by the dimorphic fungus *Blastomyces dermatitidis*. The disease is endemic in the southeastern, south central, and midwestern United States; however, cases have been reported from northern states and Canada also. The natural habitat and precise ecologic niche of *B. dermatitidis* are not completely understood; however, it appears that the fungus exists as a wood saprophyte, and infection occurs via respiratory tract.

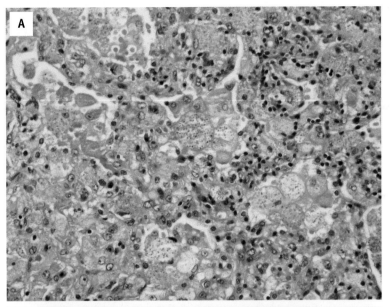

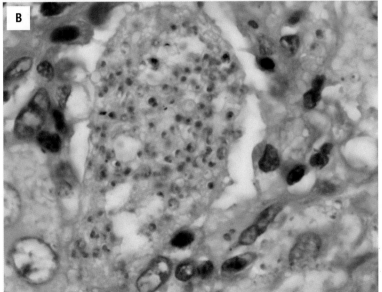

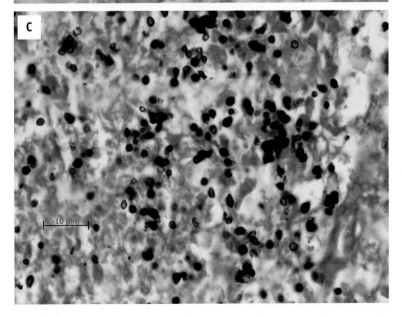

FIGURE 12-1

Histoplasmosis

(A) Lung section from a patient with AIDS shows alveolar macrophages filled with *Histoplasma capsulatum* organisms. **(B)** Higher magnification shows the small 2-4 micron organisms. **(C)** Silver stain (GMS) show small budding yeasts with buds connected by a narrow neck.

HISTOPLASMOSIS—FACT SHEET

Definition

➤ Respiratory infection caused by *Histoplasma capsulatum* var. *capsulatum*

Incidence and Location

➤ Endemic in midwest states of USA
➤ Common in avian and chiropteran habitats

Clinical and Radiologic Features

➤ Infections asymptomatic in almost 75%
➤ 25% develop symptomatic disease manifested as:
  ➤ Acute infection with pulmonary infiltrates and hilar lymphadenopathy
  ➤ Disseminated infection (in immunocompromised patients) with generalized symptoms, and high mortality
  ➤ Chronic infection with symptoms similar to other chronic pulmonary infections; radiologic patterns may show infiltrative, cavitary, fibrotic, and nodular lesions
  ➤ Fibrosing mediastinitis with slowly progressive collagen proliferation and entrapment of vital mediastinal structures

Prognosis

➤ Acute histoplasmosis is self-limited
➤ Mortality in immunocompromised patients with progressive and disseminated infections is high (up to 80% without treatment)

HISTOPLASMOSIS—PATHOLOGIC FEATURES

Gross Findings

➤ Acute infection has patchy bronchopneumonia and hilar adenopathy
➤ Disseminated infection shows edema, congestion, and granulomas
➤ Chronic infection has diffuse infiltrative lesions, apical bilateral cavitary lesions, bronchiectasis, or histoplasmomas or "coin lesions"

Microscopic Findings

➤ Granulomas with or without central necrosis surrounded by lymphocytes, macrophages, and multinucleated giant cells
➤ The fungus is oval, 2-5 microns, with narrow-based budding, often seen in the center of the granuloma; there may be a "halo effect" from retraction of the cell wall, and rarely pseudohyphae and germ tubes may be seen

Differential Diagnosis

➤ *Candida glabrata*
➤ *Penicillium marneffei*
➤ Poorly encapsulated cryptococci
➤ Microforms of *Blastomyces dermatitides*
➤ *Leishmania* amastigotes
➤ *Toxoplasma gondii*

CLINICAL FEATURES

The disease occurs most frequently in young males and presents either as acute or chronic infection. Pulmonary infection can either remain confined to the lungs or disseminate hematogenously to other organs, and may be fatal in severe progressive infections. Following inhalation of the infectious conidia, patients develop a nonspecific flu-like illness progressing to acute pneumonia, with high fever and pleuritic chest pain. Symptoms may persist for a few days to two weeks and often result in a self-limited infection. Rarely a more rapid clinical course with development of acute respiratory distress syndrome, pulmonary necrosis, and cavitation may be seen. Chronic blastomycosis presents with respiratory symptoms lasting weeks to months, associated with fever, chest pain, weight loss, and night sweats.

RADIOLOGIC FEATURES

Acute pulmonary blastomycosis manifests as patchy areas of consolidation, often bilateral, and less commonly associated with pleural effusion and cavitations. The posterior segments of lower lobes are most often involved, but middle and upper lobes may also be affected. A severe infection may result in lobar consolidation and formation of miliary infiltrates. Chronic blastomycosis is associated with linear pulmonary infiltrates, fibronodular densities with cavitations similar to chronic active tuberculosis, and mediastinal lymphadenopathy. Pleural involvement is common.

PATHOLOGIC FEATURES

GROSS FINDINGS

The lesions of blastomycosis may have a nodular pattern mimicking localized tumors, or a miliary pattern. Chronic pulmonary lesions show fibrosis, hyalinization of the nodules, and cavitation, similar to that seen in other granulomatous diseases. A primary pulmonary-lymph node complex is much less frequent than in histoplasmosis. Solitary residual fibrocaseous nodule "coin" lesions are rare, and calcification is even rarer.

MICROSCOPIC FINDINGS

Blastomyces dermatitidis is a dimorphic fungus that measures 8-15 microns in diameter with a thick cell wall and solitary blastoconidia attached by a broad-based septum (Figure 12-2). The lesions are characterized by abscess-like neutrophil collections, surrounded by epithelioid or palisading macrophages, and multinucleated giant cells. The fungus is found usually at the edge of the abscesses, and calcification is not common.

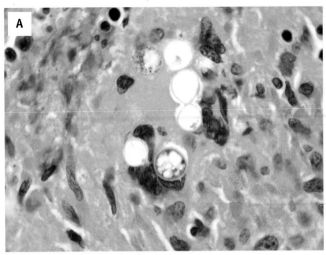
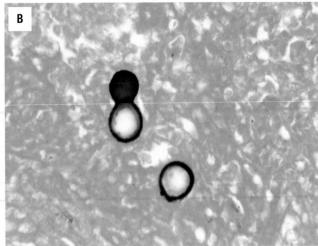

FIGURE 12-2

Blastomycosis

(A) Thick, double-contoured hyaline wall of *Blastomyces dermatitidis* is seen in this surgical biopsy from a patient with acute progressive blastomycosis. Multiple nuclei can be seen. **(B)** Silver stain (GMS) demonstrates the 8-15 micron in diameter yeasts, multinucleated, with broad-based budding. The double contour of the wall is usually not apparent in silver stains.

BLASTOMYCOSIS—FACT SHEET

Definition

» Systemic infection caused by the dimorphic fungus *Blastomyces dermatitidis*

Incidence and Location

» Endemic in southeastern, south central, and midwestern states of USA
» Natural habitat most likely wood

Clinical Features

» Self-limited illness, frequent in young males
» Acute infection with flu-like illness, pneumonia, high fever, and pleuritic chest pain
» Rarely acute respiratory distress syndrome and cavitary lesions
» Chronic infection with fever, weight loss, and night sweats

Radiologic Features

» Acute infection has bilateral patchy consolidation most often in the posterior segments of the lower lobes and pleural effusion
» Severe acute infection may cause lobar consolidation
» Chronic infection shows linear pulmonary infiltrates, fibronodular densities, and cavitation

Prognosis

» Acute primary infection is self-limited, but long-term follow-up is recommended to detect extrapulmonary infection

---

BLASTOMYCOSIS—PATHOLOGIC FEATURES

Gross Findings

» Nodular or miliary pattern with hyalinization, fibrosis, and cavitation of nodules
» Pulmonary-lymph node complex infrequent

Microscopic Findings

» Characteristic lesion is abscess-like neutrophil collection surrounded by palisading macrophages, lymphocytes, plasma cells, and multinucleated giant cells, with fungus at the edge of the abscess
» Fungus is 8-15 microns in diameter, has a thick cell wall and solitary blastoconidium attached by a broad septum

Differential Diagnosis

» *H. capsulatum* var. *duboisii*
» *Cryptococcus neoformans*
» *Coccidiosis immitis*

DIFFERENTIAL DIAGNOSIS

The differential diagnosis includes *Histoplasma capsulatum* var. *duboisii*, which has broad-based attachments. Small atypical forms of *B. dermatitidis* can be confused with *H. capsulatum,* however, microforms of blastomyces are always present as part of a continuum of small to large yeast forms. *Cryptococcus neoformans* is similar in size as blastomyces, but is mucicarmine-positive. *Coccidioides immitis* is distinguished by the presence of spherules with double walls.

PROGNOSIS AND THERAPY

Acute primary blastomycosis is often self-limited, and antifungal therapy is not required. However, long-term follow-up is necessary because patients may present with extrapulmonary lesions from months to years after resolution of the primary pulmonary infection. Itraconazole and amphotericin B are the drugs of choice.

CRYPTOCOCCOSIS

Cryptococcosis is a systemic infection caused by the yeast *Cryptococcus neoformans,* found in avian, particularly pigeon, excreta. The respiratory tract is the portal of entry for aerosolized cryptococci in human infections. Disseminated cryptococcosis is almost always seen in immunocompromised hosts.

CLINICAL FEATURES

Two clinical forms of cryptococcosis are seen: pulmonary and cerebro meningeal. The pulmonary disease may present in three different forms: 1) transient, asymptomatic colonization of tracheobronchial tree; 2) self-limited or progressive pulmonary disease with or without extrapulmonary dissemination; and 3) residual pulmonary nodule or "cryptococcoma". Colonization of the respiratory tract is seen in patients who have pre-existing lung disease, such as tuberculosis, chronic bronchitis, asthma, neoplasms, and allergic bronchopulmonary aspergillosis. An invasive infection is not seen in these patients. The majority of immunocompetent people with cryptococcosis have asymptomatic or self-limited pulmonary infections with formation of residual fibrocaseous nodules or cryptococcomas. These nodules are usually subpleural, rounded, 0.2 to 7.0 cm in diam-

eter, and show no calcification. Rarely, a primary pulmonary-lymph node complex may be formed. Progressive pulmonary infection may be asymptomatic or associated with low-grade fever, cough, pleuritic chest pain, and weight loss.

RADIOLOGIC FEATURES

Chest radiographs may show interstitial infiltrates, nodules that resemble neoplasms, segmental or lobular consolidation, and, less commonly, hilar lymphadenopathy, pleural effusion, and empyema. The upper lobes are reportedly more frequently involved. Fibrosis and calcification are uncommon. Diffuse interstitial, peribronchial, or miliary infiltrates can develop in profoundly immunodeficient patients.

PATHOLOGIC FEATURES

GROSS FINDINGS

The severe infection often seen in AIDS patients presents as diffuse miliary lesions or as areas of patchy consolidation with a mucoid appearance in freshly sectioned lungs. Sometimes cystic lesions composed of densely packed organisms may be seen in immunodeficient patients. In immunocompetent individuals, lesions remain localized and either resolve or become granulomatous with formation of nodules. The firm grayish-white fibrocaseous nodules, "cryptococcomas," show central necrosis and cavitation, and resemble lesions seen in histoplasmosis and coccidioidomycosis; however, these lesions rarely show calcifications. Smaller satellite nodules may also be present.

MICROSCOPIC FINDINGS

In H&E stained tissue sections, typical cryptococci appear as pleomorphic, eosinophilic, uninucleate, thin-walled, round yeast forms, 2-20 microns in diameter, surrounded by a wide, clear polysaccharide capsule (Figure 12-3). Budding is seen as a single blastoconidium attached to the parent cell by a narrow neck. Active lesions can contain large number of rapidly dividing cryptococci. The fungi stain with usual fungus stains as well as with mucin stains such as mucicarmine and alcian blue. *Cryptococcus* species are the only common pathogenic fungi that produce mucinous capsular material. The host response to *C. neoformans* depends on the immune status of the host, with immunodeficient patients developing profuse multiplying lakes of cryptococci with little surrounding host response. The cryptococci may appear to fill the alveolar spaces

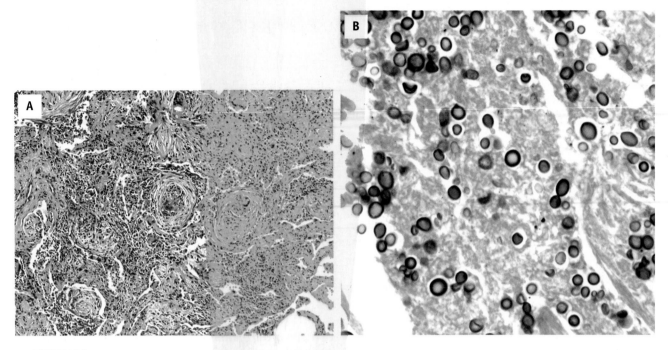

FIGURE 12-3

Cryptococcosis

(A) Lung from an immunocompromised patient containing areas of organizing pneumonia with giant cells, which contain multiple yeast forms. **(B)** An area of pulmonary necrosis with cryptococci, some with early budding (GMS stain).

CRYPTOCOCCOSIS—FACT SHEET

Definition

➤ Systemic infection caused by *Cryptococcus neoformans*, usually acquired from avian excreta

Clinical Features

➤ Acute pulmonary infection may be asymptomatic, transient colonization of respiratory tract, or self-limited pulmonary disease
➤ Residual "cryptococcomas" are subpleural small nodules without calcification
➤ Progressive infection, seen in immunocompromised patients, is either asymptomatic or has low-grade fever, cough, pleuritic pain, and weight loss

Radiologic Features

➤ Interstitial infiltrates, nodules, consolidation, pleural effusion, empyema, and hilar lymphadenopathy
➤ Upper lobes more often involved
➤ Fibrosis and calcification are uncommon

Prognosis

➤ Depends upon immune status, and the severity and extensiveness of the infection

---

CRYPTOCOCCOSIS—PATHOLOGIC FEATURES

Gross Findings

➤ Severe infection has diffuse miliary lesions or patchy consolidation with mucoid surface on cut section
➤ Cryptococcomas are nodules which show central necrosis and cavitation, but no calcifications

Microscopic Findings

➤ Immunocompromised host has profusely multiplying yeasts filling the alveoli, alveolar septa, and capillaries
➤ Immunocompetent hosts have a granulomatous response with caseation and fibrosis
➤ Pleomorphic, eosinophilic, uninucleate, thin-walled round yeast forms, 2-20 μm, surrounded by a wide, clear capsule and narrow-based budding
➤ Only pathogenic fungus that stains with mucin stains (mucicarmine, alcian blue)
➤ Capsule-deficient small *C. neoformans* stain black or brown with Fontana-Masson stain

Differential Diagnosis

➤ Capsule-deficient forms of *C. neoformans* need to be differentiated from:
  ➤ *H. capsulatum* var. *capsulatum*
  ➤ *B. dermatitidis* microforms
  ➤ *S. schenckii*
  ➤ *C. glabrata*
  ➤ *Candida* sp.
  ➤ Immature spherules of *C. immitis*

and the thickened alveolar septa and septal capillaries. Immunocompetent individuals and capsule-deficient strains of cryptococci may cause a granulomatous inflammatory response with caseation and fibrosis surrounding the small 2-4 micron in diameter capsule-deficient and distorted cryptococci. In these lesions, GMS or modified Fontana-Masson stain can be used to identify the poorly encapsulated cryptococci.

DIFFERENTIAL DIAGNOSIS

The capsule-deficient small *C. neoformans* should be differentiated from *H. capsulatum* var. *capsulatum*, microforms of *B. dermatitides, S. schenckii, C. glabrata* blastoconidia of *Candida* species, and immature spherules of *C. immitis*. A Fontana-Masson stain is helpful, since capsule-deficient cryptococci stain black or brown with this stain, however *S. schenckii* and *C. immitis* spherules may also stain positive.

PROGNOSIS AND THERAPY

Amphotericin B and 5-fluorocytosine is the treatment of choice for progressive pulmonary cryptococcosis and cerebromeningeal cryptococcosis. Maintenance suppressive therapy with fluconazole can be used.

CANDIDIASIS

Candidiasis is the most common opportunistic infection among immunocompromised patients, with approximately nine different species that are pathogenic in humans. *Candida albicans* is the most common. *C. albicans* is part of normal microflora of mouth and oropharynx, digestive tract, and vagina. Factors that impair host defense mechanisms predispose to invasive candidiasis. Broad-spectrum antibiotic and corticosteroid therapy, and neutropenia, are predisposing factors for development of candidiasis in immunocompromised patients.

CLINICAL FEATURES

The clinical features of pulmonary candidiasis resemble other opportunistic pulmonary infections. Common symptoms include persistent fever unresponsive to broad-spectrum antibiotic therapy and cough associated with dyspnea.

RADIOLOGIC FEATURES

The radiographic diagnosis of pulmonary candidiasis is neither specific nor sensitive and depends on the underlying disease associated with candidiasis. Patients may have patchy or diffuse bilateral air space consolidation, bilateral miliary nodules reflecting hematogenous spread of candidiasis, or pulmonary edema, hemorrhage, infarcts, or diffuse alveolar damage. In almost 50% of patients with pulmonary candidiasis, no radiographic abnormalities can be identified, most likely either due to agranulocytosis, small size of the lesions, or technically inferior films.

PATHOLOGIC FEATURES

GROSS FINDINGS

The gross features of pulmonary candidiasis are determined by the route of infection. Airway infection due to aspiration of *Candida* from the oropharynx or upper respiratory tract produces patchy, asymmetric areas of consolidation, especially in the lower lobes. Extensive pulmonary hemorrhage may be seen in about 50% of cases, associated with central small yellow abscesses. Hematogenous spread of candidiasis to the lungs from another focus results in bilateral, random, symmetrically distributed miliary or nodular lesions. These nodules, termed "target lesions," are round, well circumscribed, 2 to 4 mm in diameter, with a yellow granular center and peripheral hemorrhagic margins. Embolic pulmonary candidiasis is almost always associated with indwelling venous catheters and is especially seen in infants. The hemorrhagic infarcts may undergo liquefaction and cavitation. Pulmonary infarcts are highly unusual in adult patients with disseminated candidiasis.

MICROSCOPIC FINDINGS

The lesions of candidiasis show pale blue or lilac-colored oval yeast cells or blastoconidia, 3-5 microns in diameter, pseudohyphae 3-5 microns wide with periodic constrictions at the point where budding yeast cells are joined end-to-end, and occasionally true hyphae (Figure 12-4). All pathogenic *Candida* species have a similar appearance in histologic sections, and therefore cannot be speciated by their morphology. However, a predominance of well developed pseudohyphae is suggestive of *C. albicans, C. tropicalis,* or *C. krusei*. Small yeast cells without pseudohyphae suggest *C. parapsilosis* complex and *C. glabrata*.

The microscopic pattern and distribution of pulmonary lesions are determined by the route of infection. With endobronchial infection, the yeast cells and pseudohyphae proliferate within the small airways and extend

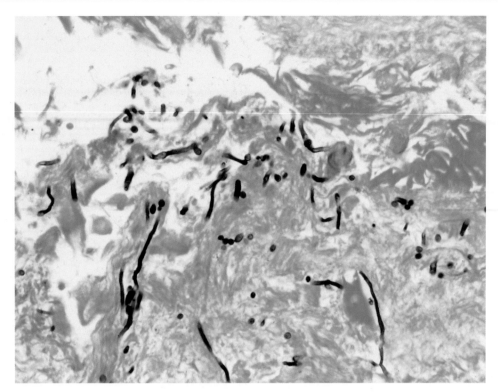

FIGURE 12-4
Candidiasis
Candida yeast forms, oval, 3-5 microns in diameter, are mixed with pseudohyphae of the same width showing constrictions at the points where the budding yeast cells are joined together.

from the airway lumens through their walls into the peribronchial alveolar spaces. Hematogenous infection produces angiocentric lesions with a central core of necrotic pulmonary parenchyma containing yeast cells, surrounded by a zone of neutrophils and a peripheral zone of parenchymal hemorrhage, the "target lesions." A necrotic vessel can usually be found within or at the edge of the "target lesions." With passage of time these lesions may enlarge and develop abscesses. The cellular reaction of invasive *Candida* infection is characteristically neutrophilic, with mixed yeast cells and pseudohyphae or hyphae present within the inflammation, and sometimes forming compact radiating microcolonies. In granulocytopenic hosts, the cellular reaction is minimal, and lesions are mainly characterized by coagulative necrosis and hemorrhage. Occasionally chronic eosinophilic pneumonia may be seen in patients who are sensitized to *Candida* species.

DIFFERENTIAL DIAGNOSIS

Candida species can easily be distinguished from most other yeast forms in histologic sections if both the budding yeast cells and filamentous elements (pseudo-

hyphae and hyphae) are present. *B. dermatitidis*, *C. neoformans*, *H. capsulatum*, and *S. schenckii* tissue forms consist of yeasts, and none of these fungi typically produce pseudohyphae or hyphae in sections. *Aspergillus*, *Fusarium*, and *Pseudallescheria* produce hyphae or pseudohyphae, and do not produce yeasts in tissues. *Trichosporon* species may be difficult to distinguish from *Candida* species in tissue sections, because both produce yeast cells, pseudohyphae, and hyphae. However, the yeast forms of *Trichosporon* species are slightly larger and more pleomorphic, and also produce arthroconidia. Dematiacious fungi may be confused with *Candida* species, but they have poorly pigmented cell walls.

PROGNOSIS AND THERAPY

Candida septicemia has a high mortality rate and needs treatment with azole compounds (miconazole, ketoconazole, fluconazole, and itraconazole). Amphotericin B in lipid vehicles and other azole compounds are under development. *C. glabrata* is often resistant to fluconazole and may need treatment with intravenous liposomal amphotericin B and intravenous caspofungin.

CANDIDIASIS—FACT SHEET

Definition
- Most common opportunistic infection in immunocompromised patients
- *Candida albicans* is a true endogenous pathogen

Clinical Features
- Fever, cough, and dyspnea

Radiologic Features
- Almost 50% have negative radiographs
- Patchy or diffuse bilateral consolidation, miliary nodules, pulmonary edema, hemorrhage, infarcts, or diffuse alveolar damage may be seen

Prognosis
- *Candida* septicemia has a high mortality rate

CANDIDIASIS—PATHOLOGIC FEATURES

Gross Findings
- Patchy consolidation with endobronchial infection
- Miliary or nodular lesions with hematogenous infection; the "target lesions" are 2-4 mm nodules with a yellow center and hemorrhagic periphery

Microscopic Findings
- Lesions contain pale-blue- or lilac-colored oval yeasts 3-5 microns in diameter with budding, pseudohyphae, and rarely true hyphae
- Target lesions have a necrotic center surrounded by a zone of neutrophils, and an outer zone of hemorrhage; a thrombosed/necrotic vessel may be seen at the periphery

Differential Diagnosis
- Yeast forms, without hyphae or pseudohyphae:
  - *B. dermatitidis*
  - *C. neoformans*
  - *H. capsulatum*
  - *S. schenckii*
  - *Trichosporon*
- Fungi with hyphae, but no yeast forms:
  - *Aspergillus*
  - *Fusarium*
  - *Pseudallescheria*

ASPERGILLOSIS

Aspergillosis remains a major cause of morbidity and mortality in immunosuppressed patients, particularly in those with hematologic diseases. *Aspergillus* species are common molds, ubiquitous within the environment in a world-wide distribution, isolated from soil, decaying vegetation, and organic debris. Although there are numerous *Aspergillus* species, only a few are human pathogens, including *A. fumigatus, A. flavus, A. niger,* and *A. terreus. A. fumigatus* is the most common agent of invasive pulmonary aspergillosis, and *A. niger* of intracavitary aspergilloma.

CLINICAL FEATURES

The spectrum of pulmonary aspergillosis includes: 1) allergic reactions in hypersensitive hosts, which includes eosinophilic pneumonia, allergic bronchopulmonary aspergillosis, mucoid impaction of proximal bronchi, bronchocentric granulomatosis, and perhaps some cases of necrotizing sarcoid granulomatosis; 2) colonization of pre-existing cavities in patients with normal immunity, with formation of aspergillomas; the clinical diagnosis of aspergilloma is suspected by the triad of hemoptysis, positive serology, and radiographic demonstration of an intracavitary mass; 3) localized airway-invasive infections; 4) chronic necrotizing pulmonary aspergillosis (CNPA), a progressive, locally destructive form of aspergillosis occuring in mildly compromised patients, occupying an intermediate position in the spectrum between colonizing and invasive forms of aspergillosis; predominant clinical symptoms include fever, productive cough, dyspnea, weight loss, malaise, and serum antibodies against *Aspergillus* antigens; 5) invasive pulmonary aspergillosis (IPA), a fulminant and highly lethal opportunistic infection of severely compromised patients who are profoundly granulocytopenic, have hematologic malignancies, or are receiving corticosteroids, cytotoxic agents, or broad-spectrum antibiotic therapy.

RADIOLOGIC FEATURES

Allergic aspergillosis and colonization of pre-existing cavities produce no specific radiographic findings. Aspergilloma or fungus ball can be seen on radiographs as a thick-walled cavity, usually 3-5 cm in diameter in the upper lobe or apex, that contains an opaque, rounded mass surrounded by a crescent of air (Monod's sign) with thickening of the adjacent pleura and positional movement of the fungus ball with decubitus films. Chest radiographs in CNPA may show pulmonary infiltrates and thick-walled cavities involving the upper lobes or superior segments of the lower lobes, often with pleural thickening. Less than half of these patients may develop fungus balls in these newly formed cavities. Chest radiographs in patients with IPA show a variety of abnormalities that include patchy, multifocal, diffuse, bilateral areas of consolidation or nodules, peripheral wedge-shaped, pleural-based infiltrates in an infarct pattern, and, rarely, bilateral miliary nodules. Follow-up films may show cavitation of the nodules and infarcts. However, up to one-third of patients may have negative chest radiographs.

PATHOLOGIC FEATURES

GROSS FINDINGS

In allergic bronchopulmonary aspergillosis (ABPA), bronchiectasis with mucoid impaction is usually seen, and is sometimes accompanied by peripheral consolidation. The intracavitary aspergilloma or fungus ball appears as a lobulated, yellowish-brown, friable mass that fills most of the cavity, but is usually unattached to the wall of the cavity. The cavities are usually round or oval, 1-7 cm or more in diameter, with a 1-5 mm-thick fibrous wall, and a smooth or shaggy inner surface that often communicates with the bronchial tree. The major findings in CNPA include a cavity that contains a well formed fungus ball with focal superficial invasion and limited destruction of surrounding lung parenchyma. The characteristic lesion of IPA is a nodular pulmonary infarct or "target lesion" that results from hyphal invasion of a peripheral pulmonary artery branch. The lesion can measure up to several centimeters in diameter, is centrally yellowish-gray and necrotic, with a hemorrhagic rim. An occluded necrotic artery can often be identified within or at the edge of the lesion.

MICROSCOPIC FINDINGS

The histologic diagnosis of *Aspergillus* infection depends on the identification of *Aspergillus* hyphae with their characteristic features of 3 to 6 micron width, uniform shape, regular septation, and parallel walls (Figure 12-5). The branches of the hyphae arise at acute angles from the parent hyphae with progressive and dichotomous branching (of same size as the parent hyphae). Often calcium oxalate crystals are deposited within aspergillomas, particularly those formed by *A. niger*.

The pathologic features of ABPA are discussed more extensively in another chapter, but include mucoid impaction of bronch, bronchocentric granulomatosis, eosinophilic pneumonia, and exudative bronchitis. Intracavitary aspergillomas have thick, vascularized, fibrous walls infiltrated by lymphocytes, plasma cells, histiocytes, and occasionally neutrophils and eosinophils. Occasionally, granulomas may be found in the walls of the cavities. Cavities formed by ectatic bronchi may be lined by respiratory or metaplastic epithelium.

The pathologic diagnosis of CNPA requires demonstration of invasion and destruction of noncavitary lung tissue in an appropriate clinical and radiologic setting. CNPA is distinguished from IPA by the limited extent of parenchymal invasion, and the absence of vascular invasion and infarction in the former.

IPA shows nodular pulmonary infarcts or target lesions composed of a central zone of ischemic necrosis, intermediate zone of fibrinous exudate that may contain degenerated neutrophils, and a peripheral zone of parenchymal hemorrhage. An occluded necrotic artery can often be identified within or at the edge of the lesion, with abundant hyphae extending through the vessel wall and invading the surrounding pulmonary tissue.

ANCILLARY STUDIES

Although visible with H&E stain, hyphal morphology is best demonstrated with silver or other fungal stains. The viable hyphae are basophilic on H&E stain, whereas necrotic hyphae are hyaline or eosinophilic.

DIFFERENTIAL DIAGNOSIS

Fusarium and *Pseudallescheria* have branched septate hyphae that closely resemble *Aspergillus* and require special studies for differential diagnosis, such as fluorescent antibodies or immunoperoxidase conjugates. *Absidia* and *Rhizopus* have broader hyphae with non-parallel walls, wide-angled branching, and few septa. *Candida* and *Trichosporon* have yeast cells, pseudohyphae, and hyphae with arthroconidia, which are absent in *Aspergillus*.

PROGNOSIS AND THERAPY

Amphotericin B is the drug of choice; however, itraconazole, posaconazole, and voriconazole and the less toxic lipid formulations of amphotericin are also effective against aspergilli. Surgical excision is advised for localized infection and for aspergillomas.

ZYGOMYCOSIS (MUCORMYCOSIS)

Zygomycosis, also referred to as mucormycosis, is an opportunistic infection caused by fungi in the class Zygomycetes (formerly Phycomycetes). The agents of zygomycosis include species within several genera including *Rhizopus, Absidia, Mucor, Rhizomucor, Saksenaea, Cunninghamella, Mortierella, Syncephalastrum,* and *Apophysomyces*. The *Rhizopus* and *Absidia* species

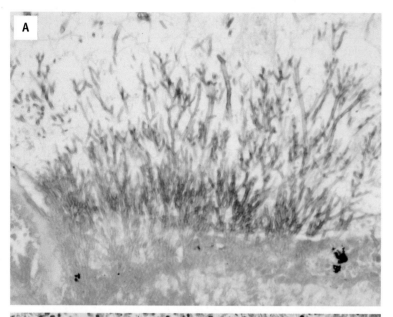

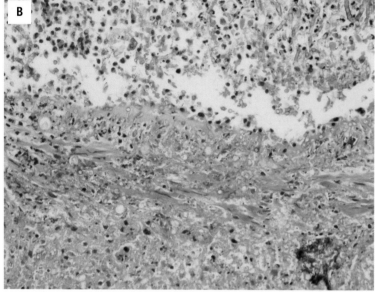

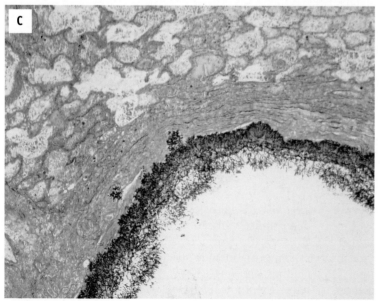

FIGURE 12-5

Aspergillosis
(A) Alveolar wall shows invasion by uniform, homogeneous hyphae, 3-6 microns, with parallel contours and regular septa. **(B)** Fungal cavity wall with acute infiltrate and hyphae present within necrotic debris. **(C)** The dichotomous branching pattern and the parallel walls of the *Aspergillus* hyphae are clearly seen with the silver stain (GMS).

ASPERGILLOSIS—FACT SHEET

Definition

» Infections caused by species of *Aspergillus*, which is a common mold that is ubiquitous in the environment, present in soil and organic debris

Clinical Features

» Symptoms vary depending on host factors and form of disease
» Spectrum of clinical presentations includes:
  » Allergic bronchopulmonary aspergillosis (ABPA), with manifestations of mucoid impaction, bronchocentric granulomatosis, and eosinophilic pneumonia
  » Aspergilloma (colonization of pre-existing cavity)
  » Localized airway-invasive infection
  » Chronic necrotizing pulmonary aspergillosis (CNPA)
  » Invasive pulmonary aspergillosis (IPA)

Radiologic Features

» ABPA: bronchiectasis, infiltrates
» Aspergilloma: opaque round mass surrounded by a crescent of air in a thick-walled cavity
» CNPA: pulmonary infiltrates and thick-walled cavities
» IPA: patchy nodules, infarcts with cavitation later

ASPERGILLOSIS—PATHOLOGIC FEATURES

Gross Findings

» ABPA: bronchiectasis with mucoid impaction of bronchi and/or parenchyma consolidation
» Aspergilloma: yellowish-brown friable mass fills a cavity with a fibrous wall
» CNPA: thick-walled cavities with surrounding consolidation
» IPA: nodular infarcts (target lesions) with yellowish necrotic centers and hemorrhagic rims, and larger wedge-shaped infarcts

Microscopic Findings

» Fungal hyphae 3-6 microns wide, uniform with regular septa, and parallel walls
» Hyphae branch dichotomously, at acute angles
» Conidial heads consist of a vesicle with 1 to 2 layers of phialides and attached conidia
» Splendore-Hoeppli effect may be seen
» Calcium oxalate crystals (common with *A. niger*)
» ABPA: bronchiectasis with mucoid impaction of bronchi, bronchocentric granulomas, eosinophilic pneumonia, and/or exudative bronchitis
» Aspergilloma: concentric layers of *Aspergillus* hyphae
» CNPA: limited invasion of lung parenchyma, without vascular invasion or infarction
» IPA: pulmonary infarcts with central zone of necrosis, intermediate zone of fibrinous exudate, and peripheral zone of hemorrhage and vascular invasion by fungal hyphae

Differential Diagnosis

» *Fusarium*
» *Pseudallescheria*
» *Absidia* and *Rhizopus*
» *Candida*
» *Trichosporon*

are the most frequently implicated fungi in human infections. These fungi are widely distributed in nature and can be isolated from soil and decaying organic material.

CLINICAL FEATURES

Pulmonary zygomycosis occurs most frequently in patients with hematologic malignancies, poorly controlled diabetes mellitus, renal failure, severe burns, other causes of immunocompromise, and/or treatment with corticosteroids. The clinical features of pulmonary zygomycosis are similar to those of invasive aspergillosis. Patients develop persistent fevers and new or progressive pulmonary infiltrates unresponsive to antibacterial therapy.

RADIOLOGIC FEATURES

Chest radiographs show patchy infiltrates and solitary or multiple areas of consolidation. Cavitation and pleural effusion are infrequent. A miliary or nodular pattern may also be seen in patients with hematogenous dissemination.

PATHOLOGIC FEATURES

GROSS FINDINGS

The characteristic feature is pulmonary infarction, which is usually hemorrhagic, perihilar or peripheral. Proximal infarcts are rounded or irregular in shape, whereas peripheral infarcts are typically wedge-shaped and accompanied by pleural invasion. Acute exudative bronchopneumonia may be seen in non-granulocytopenic patients, and cavities may develop in some infarcts. Abscesses are, however, uncommon and often signify secondary bacterial infection. Complications of infections include rupture of pulmonary arteries secondary to hyphal invasion, resulting in massive hemoptysis.

MICROSCOPIC FINDINGS

Pulmonary zygomycosis results from germination of inhaled sporangiospores, or aspiration of hyphae from a focus of infection in the upper respiratory tract, with proliferation of the fungi within the airways. The fungus is highly invasive and penetrates through the bronchial wall into the adjacent blood vessels, particularly the arteries, resulting in thrombosis and pulmonary infarction. The hyphae may be seen within the infarcted areas, as pleomorphic and broad (10 to 25 microns or more in width), with delicate thin walls and rare septa (Figure 12-6). The hyphae are often twisted, folded, or wrinkled because of their broad size, and show variation in caliber. The branching pattern is also irregular, and branches are often oriented at right angles to the parent hyphae. The fungus can be seen with H & E as well as silver stains. Occasionally thick-walled, round, or ovoid chlamydoconidia and sporangia may be found with the invasive hyphae.

DIFFERENTIAL DIAGNOSIS

Aspergillus is the main differential diagnosis, but the *Aspergillus* hyphae are narrower, more uniform, regularly septate, and have an orderly, progressive, dichotomous pattern of branching.

PROGNOSIS AND THERAPY

Pulmonary zygomycosis has a high mortality rate because of the underlying disease of the patient, difficulty in diagnosing the infection early, and rather ineffective

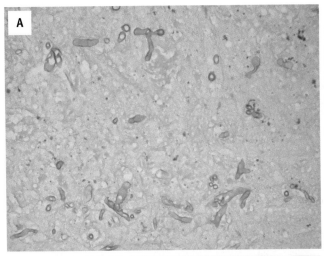

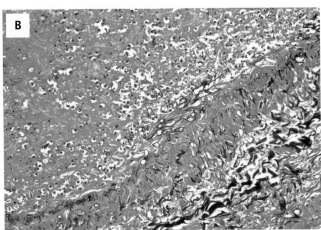

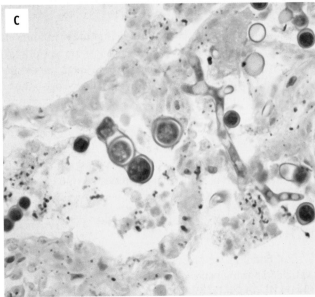

FIGURE 12-6

Zygomycosis
(A) Zygomycosis shows broad non-septate, empty-appearing fungal hyphae with right-angled branching pattern. **(B)** GMS stain demonstrates vascular invasion by the irregular broad hyphae of zygomycosis. **(C)** *Rhizopous macroconidia* with transverse septation.

ZYGOMYCOSIS (MUCORMYCOSIS)—FACT SHEET

Definition

» Infections caused by several species of zygomycetes; *Rhizopus* and *Absidia* are the most common human pathogens
» Widely distributed in soil and decaying organic material

Clinical Features

» Fever and hemoptysis due to rupture of pulmonary vessels from hyphal invasion
» Incidence is higher in patients with hematologic malignancies, transplants, diabetes meilitus, burns, renal failure, and corticosteroid therapy

Radiologic Features

» Patchy infiltrates and consolidations on chest radiographs
» Miliary pattern may be seen in patients with hematogenous dissemination

Prognosis

» High mortality rate

ZYGOMYCOSIS (MUCORMYCOSIS)—PATHOLOGIC FEATURES

Gross Findings

» Pulmonary infarction, perihilar (round) or peripheral (wedge-shaped)
» Acute exudative bronchopneumonia
» Abscesses rare, except with secondary bacterial infections
» Rupture of pulmonary arteries

Microscopic Findings

» Pleomorphic, broad hyphae, 10-25 μm or more in width, thin, delicate walls, rare septa, irregular and right-angled branching
» Hyphae are folded and wrinkled
» Chlamydoconidia and sporangia occasionally found
» Parenchyma and angioinvasion with thrombosis and infarction

Differential Diagnosis

» *Aspergillus*

responses to antifungal treatments. Amphotericin B is the drug of choice. Localized focus of infection may be amenable to surgical resection.

COCCIDIOIDOMYCOSIS

Coccidioidomycosis is caused by *Coccidioides immitis,* which is endemic to the semi-arid desert climate of the southwestern United States, and exists as septate, branched hyphae and arthroconidium in soil. Infection is acquired by inhalation of the arthroconidium, which is approximately 3-5 microns in size. Predisposing factors include corticosteroid therapy, chemotherapy, transplantation, AIDS, and pregnancy. The majority of cases resolve spontaneously, however, pregnant women have a higher risk of developing disseminated disease.

RADIOLOGIC FEATURES

Chest radiographs in patients with acute coccidioidomycosis infection may be normal in up to 20% of symptomatic patients, or show soft, hazy, patchy, or segmental pneumonic infiltrates. Less commonly, solitary or multiple nodules, cavitary lesions, hilar lymphadenopathy, and pleural effusions may occur. In patients with chronic pulmonary coccidioidomycosis, there are usually bi-apical fibronodular lesions with cavities and retraction of pulmonary parenchyma. Miliary coccidioidomycosis

has features similar to infection with miliary tuberculosis. Coccidioidoma appears as a solitary coin lesion, 1-4 cm in diameter in the upper lobes and mid-lung fields, with either cavitation or calcification. Fibrocavitary coccidioidomycosis demonstrates either thin-walled or thick-walled cavities, 2-4 cm in size, often solitary, and in the upper lung fields.

PATHOLOGIC FEATURES

GROSS FINDINGS

The pathologic features of primary pulmonary coccidioidomycosis are not well studied, since patients usually recover from the infection. However, pneumonic infiltrates and occasionally suppurative infection may be seen. Coccidioidal cavities in chronic infections develop from fibrocaseous nodules or represent bronchiectatic cavities, a result of necrotizing bronchitis. Cavities may contain coccidioidal fungus balls, whsich are often soft, grayish-brown, friable or pultaceous. The fibrocavitary lesions and coccidioidomas show discrete upper lobe nodules and cavities, 0.5 to 3.5 cm in diameter, and often subpleural.

MICROSCOPIC FINDINGS

The fibrocaseous nodules consist of granulomatous inflammation, surrounded by mixed cellular infiltrates. The diagnostic sporulating spherules (Figure 12-7) can be found in at least 50% of the nodules, along with hyphae and arthroconidia in about 15%. The spherules are abundant in active pulmonary and disseminated lesions, but are difficult to find in the residual inactive

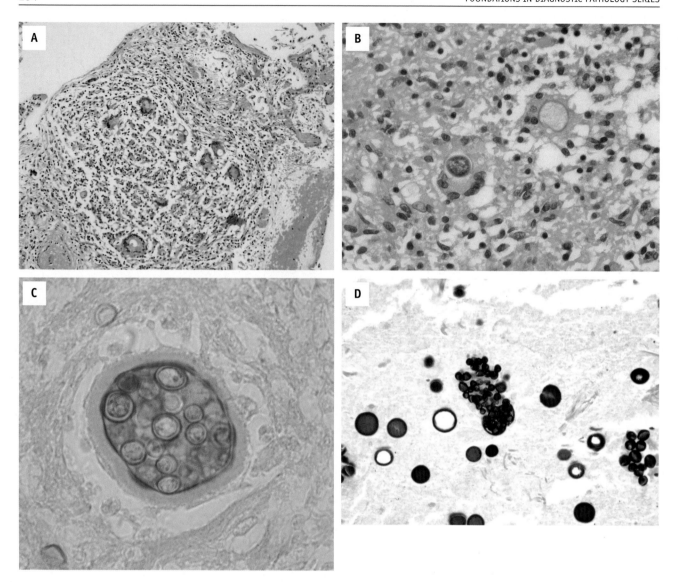

FIGURE 12-7

Coccidioidomycosis

(A) This granuloma includes multinucleated giant cells containing round, thick-walled fungi of different sizes, suggestive of coccidioidomycosis. **(B)** Spherules are seen on hematoxylin-eosin stain in an area of necrosis. **(C)** High magnification photomicrograph of a *Coccidiosis immitis* thick-walled fungal spherule containing endospores. **(D)** *Coccidioides immitis* spherule with partial rupture of the wall, releasing the endospores (GMS).

lesions. Their morphology is best demonstrated with a GMS stain. Different stages of maturation of spherules may be seen in active infection, and these may be surrounded by eosinophilic Splendore-Hoeppli material. The spherules are 30-100 microns in diameter and show internal septations and endospores, which are released into the infected tissue with rupture of the spherules. Each endospore then potentially develops into another spherule and repeats the cycle. Under certain circumstances, endospores can germinate within host tissue to produce hyphae and arthroconidia, which can then develop into spherules. The barrel-shaped arthroconidia are approximately 3-5 microns in size, and the septate branched hyphae are 2-4 microns in width.

DIFFERENTIAL DIAGNOSIS

Rhinosporidium seeberi is the main fungus that can be confused with *C. immitis*, since it is also large and replicates by endosporulation. *Rhinosporidium* endospores are distributed in a distinct zonal pattern within the sporangia, contain globular inclusions, and have carminophilic walls. Myospherulosis, a pseudomycosis of peripheral soft tissues, has parent bodies and spherules, may be confused with *C. immitis*. It is seen in the upper respiratory tract and middle ear. The spherules have an inherent brown pigment, but do not stain with GMS or PAS stains. Immature spherules of *C. immitis* may resemble the budding yeast cells of *B. dermatitidis*; however, the latter contain broad-based blastoconidia, bud pores, and multiple nuclei. Finally, the endospores of *C. immitis* may resemble *Histoplasma capsulatum* var. *capsulatum*,, but *C. immitis* are much larger in size than the yeast of *H. capsulatum* and do not show budding.

PROGNOSIS AND THERAPY

In most patients the infection is self-limited, and symptoms resolve within a few weeks without treatment. However, persistent coccidioidal pneumonia is diagnosed when symptoms persist beyond 6 to 8 weeks, requiring treatment with amphotericin B. Amphotericin B lipid-formulation may be advantageous. Azole therapy is generally inferior to amphotericin B in disseminated disease.

PHAEOHYPHOMYCOSIS

Phaeohyphomycosis comprises a heterogeneous group of subcutaneous and systemic infections caused by a wide variety of dematiaceous (naturally pigmented) opportunistic fungi that develop as black molds in culture and as dark-walled, brown, septate hyphae in tissues. Most of these fungi are common saprophytes of wood, soil, and decaying organic matter. Some of the common fungi in this group include *Alternaria, Anthopsis, Aureobasidium, Bipolaris, Chaetomium, Cladophialophora, Cladosporium, Curvularia, Exophiala, Ochroconis, Phialophora, Scedosporium, Scytalidium* and *Thermomyces.*

CLINICAL FEATURES

Two main clinical forms of these infections are recognized in humans: subcutaneous and systemic. The subcutaneous infection is much more common than pulmonary infection, and occurs when the fungi enter the body through a skin wound or traumatic implantation of a wood splinter. The lesion develops as a firm to fluctuant, painless, subcutaneous abscess that may enlarge up to 7.0 cm in diameter and is associated sometimes with lymphangitis and regional lymphadenopathy. The most common agent that produces pulmonary and systemic infection is *Cladophialophora bantianum.* Pulmonary infection may be associated with cough, chest pain, dyspnea, and hemoptysis, or may be asymptomatic. The fungus often reaches the brain via hematogenous dissemination from the primary pulmonary site, resulting in cerebral lesions that may be solitary or multiple encapsulated abscesses or generalized inflammatory infiltrates.

PATHOLOGIC FEATURES

MICROSCOPIC FINDINGS

Infection can present as a pulmonary fungus ball, granulomatous pulmonary disease, or allergic bronchopulmonary disease. The fungi appear as individual or small, loose aggregates of irregularly shaped, short or long septate and branched hyphae, 2-6 micron wide budding yeast cells, occasional pseudohyphae, and large thick-walled vesicles in the necrotic centers of granulomas (Figure 12-8). The brown pigmented cell walls of the hyphal and yeast structures are easily detected in H&E-stained sections, but GMS and PAS stains are usually needed for detailed morphologic studies. Fontana-Masson stain for melanin can be used to demonstrate the presence of melanin in the fungus cell wall.

DIFFERENTIAL DIAGNOSIS

Eumycotic mycetomas are the main differential diagnosis. These have large granules of interwoven mycelia, up to 3.0 mm in diameter, whereas phaeohyphomycosis never forms granules.

Chromoblastomycosis has dark brown muriform cells with thick walls and divides by septation into vertical and horizontal planes.

PROGNOSIS AND THERAPY

Azoles such as itraconazole and amphotericin B are treatments of choice for systemic and pulmonary phaeohyphomycosis.

PNEUMOCYSTOSIS

Pneumocystis pneumonia, or pneumocystosis, is one of the most common pulmonary infections in persons with impaired cell-mediated immunity and those infected with the human immunodeficiency virus, HIV-1. The organisms are ubiquitous and globally distributed, having been identified in virtually every mammalian species. The species that infects humans, *P. jiroveci,* is different from the one that infects other mammals, and there is no cross-species infection. The infection is acquired by inhalation, with primary exposure occurring early in

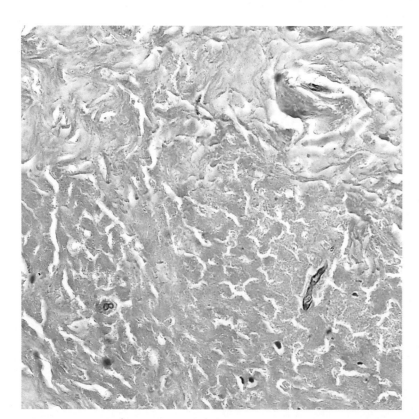

FIGURE 12-8
Phaeohyphomycosis
Brown hyphae are noted in a necrotic background.

life, so that most children have serum antibodies to *Pneumocystis* by age 2 or 3. Infection is presumed to be asymptomatic. The organisms remain latent within the host, and propagate when the host immune system becomes compromised.

CLINICAL FEATURES

There are two major clinical forms of *P. jiroveci* pneumonia (PJP), each with a different epidemiological pattern: 1) the infantile form designated plasma cell interstitial pneumonia, and 2) the adult form (*P. jiroveci* pneumonia in immunocompromised hosts). The plasma cell interstitial pneumonia historically occurred in institutional settings in underdeveloped countries, mainly affecting premature and malnourished children. The infants develop respiratory difficulty characterized by tachypnea, cyanosis, cough, and progressive respiratory failure, with diffuse pulmonary infiltrates or consolidation on chest radiographs.

The adult infection (also called the sporadic form) is a leading causes of fatal opportunistic infection in AIDS patients and other immunocompromised hosts. The infection indicates the existence of an underlying cellular immunodeficiency with impairment of CD4-positive (T-helper) lymphocyte function. The incidence of PJP has undergone a significant reduction with the institution of chemoprophylaxis in AIDS patients. The clinical and radiographic findings are not specific, and mimic those of other opportunistic infections. The onset of symptoms in AIDS patients is insidious, with development of fever, dyspnea, tachypnea, and nonproductive cough. Less frequently, there is weight loss, chest pain, night sweats, chills, fatigue, and malaise. In a small subset of HIV-positive patients the presentation is more acute, with fulminant onset of respiratory symptoms progressing to respiratory failure within 1 to 2 weeks.

The disease in non-AIDS patients often presents as an acute illness with an abrupt onset, and less commonly as a more indolent disease. Symptoms often start when corticosteroid therapy is tapered or discontinued, and are present for a short time, usually 1 to 2 weeks before a diagnosis of PJP is established.

RADIOLOGIC FEATURES

Typical radiographic findings in PJP include bilateral, diffuse, interstitial, and alveolar infiltrates, initially predominant in perihilar regions and lower lung fields, with progression to extensive areas of bilateral air-space consolidation. Atypical manifestations may be seen and include unilateral upper lobe infiltrates, nodular lesions, consolidation, cavitated masses or nodules, pneumatocele, pneumothorax, pneumomediastinum, atelectasis, bronchiectasis, lymphadenopathy, and pleural effusion. Classically, ground-glass perihilar interstitial infiltrates are seen in the early stages, with progression to involve all lung fields in untreated patients. The lung apices are relatively spared, but may be involved with the use of prophylactic inhaled pentamidine, presumably due to the relatively poor distribution of aerosolized pentamidine to these regions. As many as 10-20% of AIDS patients with PJP present initially with no detectable radiological abnormalities, however, high-resolution computed tomography in these cases may reveal ground-glass attenuation or cystic lesions.

PATHOLOGIC FEATURES

GROSS FINDINGS

The lungs are heavy with pale-gray or tan, granular, firm, consolidated cut surfaces. Occasionally, nodules or cavities may be seen.

MICROSCOPIC FINDINGS

Infantile PJP has intense plasmacytic and lymphocytic interstitial inflammation. Pathologic findings in adult type PJP may be divided into two major groups: typical and atypical forms. Typical pathologic features are seen in the lungs of patients who are not on prophylactic treatment or highly active antiretroviral therapy (HAART). Microscopically, a variety of patterns may be seen. The typical histopathologic pattern is characterized by a mild interstitial chronic inflammatory infiltrate and type II pneumocyte hyperplasia, associated with an eosinophilic, foamy exudate in alveolar spaces (Figure 12-9). Higher magnification of the exudate shows round basophilic dots which correspond to the nuclei of the sporozoites and trophozoites. The alveolar exudate is composed predominantly of abundant *P. jiroveci* trophozoites mixed with cysts, membranotubular extensions, surfactant, and cellular debris enmeshed in fibrin. The alveolar exudate may be focal or diffuse, depending on the severity of the infection. In progressive chronic infection, interstitial and intra-alveolar fibrosis may be seen. In acute progressive infection with respiratory failure, there is diffuse alveolar damage with hyaline membranes and reactive alveolar epithelial cell proliferation.

Atypical pathologic features include dense interstitial lymphocytic infiltrates, granulomas, multinucleated giant cells, and focal calcifications. The fibrocaseous nodular pattern of atypical PJP is characterized by confluent parenchymal necrosis with lysis of the alveolar septa, and formation of cavities, 1-6 cm, surrounded

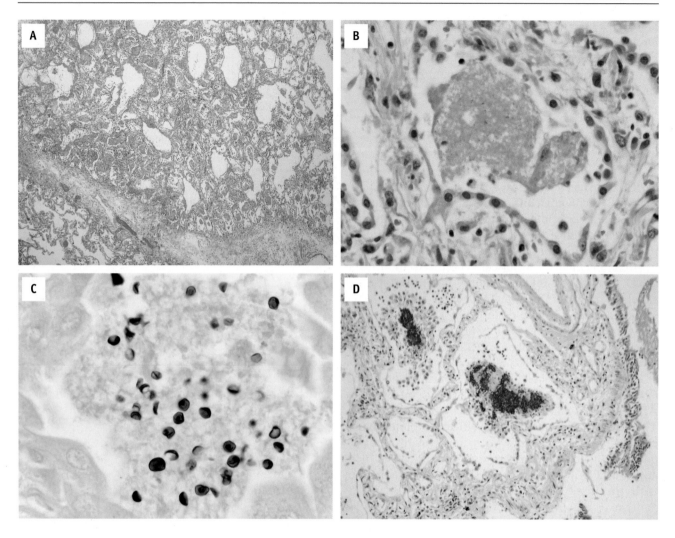

FIGURE 12-9

Pneumocystis jiroveci

(A) Lung section from a patient with AIDS shows eosinophilic alveolar exudates, mild alveolar wall fibrosis, and type II pneumocyte hyperplasia.
(B) Higher magnification of the alveolar exudates demonstrates the frothy appearance and the tiny blue dots characteristic of *Pneumocystis* infection.
(C) Silver stain (GMS) accentuates the cyst wall and the central "dot." A few collapsed forms of the cysts are also seen, the so-called boat-shaped or navicular forms. The trophozoites do not stain with GMS. **(D)** Immunostains are very useful in cases of treated pneumocystosis, to demonstrate the trophozoites.

by a zone of necrotic lung parenchyma. The necrotic lung parenchyma is often replaced by confluent masses of eosinophilic foamy material with abundant PJP cysts. Rarely, *Pneumocystis* vasculitis characterized by massive infiltration of blood vessel walls by the cysts may be seen. Cystic changes can occur in atypical PJP, either in the parenchyma or in the subpleural areas, with cysts ranging from microscopic to 1 cm in size. The walls of the cysts are formed by alveoli filled with *P. jiroveci* or by a thin layer of fibrous tissue and chronic inflammatory infiltrates. Microcalcifications are an important atypical feature and may be seen with or without foamy exudates. Several patterns of calcification may be seen, including a bubbly pattern with vacuolations, plate-like, elongated and conchoidal patterns. The calcifications often contain *P. jiroveci* on GMS stains and represent dystrophic calcifications of degenerated *P. jiroveci* organisms. Margins of cavitary lesions as well as subpleural areas may demonstrate microcalcifications.

ANCILLARY STUDIES

Special stains (GMS) demonstrate cysts that are round to oval and focally curved, disc-shaped or boat-shaped. The trophozoites cannot be seen on H&E stain, but can be demonstrated with Giemsa, Wright-Giemsa, and Diff-Quik stains. Immunohistochemical studies can be used to highlight the trophozoites in treated cases of pneumocystosis.

PNEUMOCYSTIS JIROVECI—FACT SHEET

Definition

▸ A common AIDS-defining infection with *P. jiroveci*, acquired by inhalation
▸ *P. jiroveci* is ubiquitous in the environment and causes asymptomatic infections in childhood

Clinical Features

▸ Infantile form or plasma cell interstitial pneumonia affects malnourished children, who develop respiratory difficulty and failure
▸ Adult form affects immunocompromised patients with impaired CD4-positive T-lymphocyte functions; usually, there is an insidious onset with respiratory and generalized symptoms of fever, dyspnea, tachypnea, cough, weight loss, fatigue, etc., and less frequently the presentation is that of ARDS
▸ Extrapulmonary pneumocystosis can develop with prophylactic pentamidine therapy

Radiologic Features

▸ Infantile form: diffuse pulmonary infiltrates or consolidation
▸ Adult form: ground-glass perihilar interstitial infiltrates in early stage, and diffuse, bilateral interstitial and alveolar infiltrates later

PNEUMOCYSTIS JIROVECI—PATHOLOGIC FEATURES

Gross Findings

▸ Pulmonary consolidation with tan, granular, cut surfaces
▸ Atypical findings include fibrocaseous nodules, cystic changes, vascular permeation and, rarely, lymphadenopathy

Microscopic Findings

▸ Mild chronic interstitial lymphoplasmacytic infiltrate, type II pneumocyte hyperplasia, eosinophilic foamy alveolar exudate
▸ Round, basophilic dots in the alveolar exudate
▸ GMS stain shows round to oval, curved-disc or boat-shaped cysts; trophozoites seen only by Giemsa and Diff-Quik stains
▸ Atypical features include dense interstitial lymphocytic infiltration, interstitial fibrosis, granulomas, and calcifications

Differential Diagnosis

▸ *H. capsulatum*
▸ *C. glabrata*
▸ *C. neoformans*
▸ *T. gondii*

PROGNOSIS AND THERAPY

Two standard drugs used to treat most patients with PJP are trimethoprim-sulfamethoxazole (TMP-SMX), and pentamidine isothionate. Early adjunctive therapy with corticosteroids can reduce the morbidity and mortality associated with moderate or severe PJP. Patients who are at high risk to develop PJP, specifically HIV-infected patients with CD4-positive T-lymphocyte counts of less than 200 cells per mm, and all AIDS patients who have already had one or more episodes of PJP, benefit from prophylactic therapy with TMP-SMX and aerosolized pentamidine. The latter, however, may predispose to extra-pulmonary pneumocystosis. It has been the introduction of combination antiretroviral therapy including HAART that has contributed to the reduced incidence of PJP. Other drugs under development include echinocandins, pneumocandins which inhibit beta-glucan synthesis, and sordarins which inhibit fungal protein synthesis.

DIFFERENTIAL DIAGNOSIS

H. capsulatum, *C. glabrata*, and *C. neoformans* are most difficult to distinguish from the cysts of *P. jiroveci*. The single or paired argyrophilic focus in the wall of the *P. jiroveci* cyst is never seen in the walls of other yeasts, however, and formation of blastoconidia by budding, a characteristic feature of yeasts, is never seen in PJP. *Cryptococcus neoformans* has a mucopolysaccharide mucicarmine-positive and Masson-Fontana (melanin) stain-positive capsule. The yeast forms of *C. glabrata* are accompanied by pseudohyphae and true hyphae, which are not seen with *Pneumocystis jiroveci*.

Tissue elements such as leukocytes, erythrocytes, and mucus vacuoles are all weakly argyrophilic and may complicate screening and diagnosis of slides that may be over-stained with GMS.

UNCOMMON FUNGAL INFECTIONS

PSEUDALLESCHERIASIS

Pseudallescheria boydii is a ubiquitously occurring fungus that rarely causes infection in immunocompetent hosts. It is a cosmopolitan saprophyte that can be isolated from moist soil, polluted water, and sewage. It is a common cause of fungal pneumonia after near-drowning and is associated with a high mortality. Pulmonary infection caused by *Pseudallescheria boydii* comprises two distinct clinicopathological entities: colonization of cavities in patients with underlying lung disease and invasive necrotizing pneumonia in immunocompromised patients.

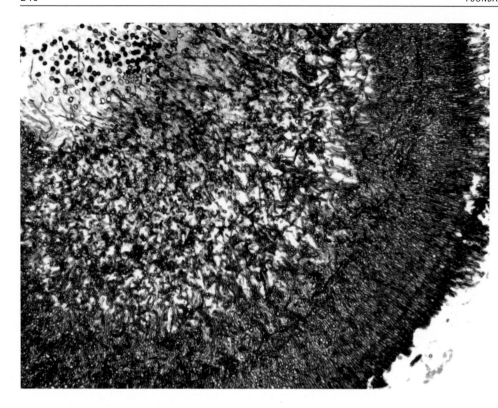

FIGURE 12-10
Pseudallescheria
Fungus ball consisting of aggregates of hyphae with concentric rings (GMS).

PATHOLOGIC FEATURES

The colonizing form of pseudallescheriasis develops as a soft, amorphous fungus ball in a cavity that may communicate with the bronchial tree. The wall of the cavity may consist of granulation tissue with suppurative or granulomatous inflammation, or rarely respiratory epithelium with squamous metaplasia. The invasive pulmonary infection is seen as a destructive, necrotizing pneumonia with abscess formation (Figure 12-10).

FUSARIOSIS

Fusariosis is an emerging infectious disease in immunocompromised patients that may present as a localized skin infection, mycetoma, or pneumonia. Localized and disseminated infections have been reported in patients with hematologic malignancies, burns, transplants, and aplastic anemia.

PATHOLOGIC FEATURES

Invasive and disseminated lesions of *Fusarium* consist of abscesses, infarcts secondary to vascular invasion and thrombosis, and granulomas. The hyphae of *Fusarium* are hyaline and septate, measure 3-7 microns in diameter, and are sparsely branched, with often perpendicular branching (Figure 12-11). Intercalated vesicles are occasionally found, but characteristic conidia are not produced in tissues. Disseminated infection is characterized by hyphal vascular invasion. Three major human pathogens are included within the genus *Fusarium*. These are *F. oxysporum*, *F. moniliforme*, and *F. solani*, and they are widely distributed in nature as soil saprophytes and plant pathogens. Disruption of the mucosa or cutaneous barrier appears to be a major factor in the pathogenesis of invasive fusariosis.

SPOROTRICHOSIS

Sporotrichosis is a chronic, localized, or rarely disseminated infection caused by the dimorphic fungus *Sporothrix schenckii*. The fungus grows as a saprophyte on plants, trees, wood timbers, sphagnum moss, and other plant material. Most infections are nonpulmonary, resulting from accidental cutaneous inoculation of the fungus. Primary pulmonary infections are rare and result from inhalation of conidia by immunosuppressed patients, alcoholics, or patients with AIDS.

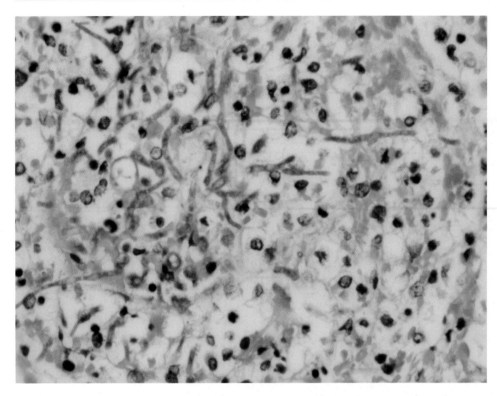

FIGURE 12-11

Fusarium

Septate hyphae of *Fusarium* species with haphazard branching pattern, including some branches arising perpendicular to the parent hyphae.

PATHOLOGIC FEATURES

Pulmonary lesions consist of large, often confluent, necrotizing and non-necrotizing granulomas that contain scattered or clustered yeast cells of *S. schenckii*. The granulomas may also be fibrotic, however calcification is rare. Because of their scarcity, *S. schenckii* cells are difficult to see in H & E-stained sections; however, they are often demonstrated with GMS or PAS stains. The fungi appear as round or oval cells, with some blastoconidia that appear elongated and cigar-shaped. The yeast cells and blastoconidia are 2-6 microns or more in diameter, and the yeast cells may be coated with eosinophilic, refractile, radially oriented Splendore-Hoeppli material to form asteroid bodies within microabscesses or granulomas. Rarely, *S. schenckii* can form hyphae in tissues and intracavitary fungus balls.

PARACOCCIDIOIDOMYCOSIS

Paracoccidioidomycosis (South American blastomycosis) is a chronic progressive fungal infection largely confined to Latin America and Mexico; however, cases have been diagnosed in the United States in patients who acquired the infection in endemic areas. The fungus has been isolated from wood fragments, soil, and thorns. Primary infection begins in the lungs and is followed by dissemination to upper respiratory tract, skin, lymph nodes, liver, spleen, adrenals, intestines, and other organs.

PATHOLOGIC FEATURES

Lungs with chronic progressive pulmonary paracoccidioidomycosis may have a cobblestone appearance resulting from advanced fibrosis and emphysema. In the interstitial form of the disease, linear streaks of fibrosis radiate peripherally from the hilum, accompanied by emphysema. The residual lesions usually consist of solitary granulomas; however, multifocal lesions consisting of miliary, interstitial, or tuberculoid granulomas with central caseous or suppurative necrosis may be seen. Acute bronchopneumona may be observed in patients with an acute or subacute clinical course, often in young patients treated with corticosteroids.

The yeast cells of *P. brasiliensis* can be identified in tissue sections with a silver stain (GMS). The cells vary in diameter from 3-30 microns, and may reach up to 60 microns, with thick walls measuring up to 1.0 micron

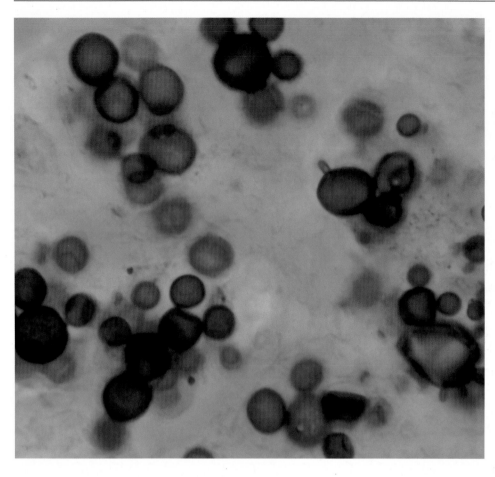

FIGURE 12-12
Paracoccidioides brasiliensis
Yeast forms with multiple oval buds attached to the parent cell by narrow necks.

(Figure 12-12). The specific histologic diagnosis can be made when typical multiple budding cells are identified. Two patterns of budding may be found, the large teardrop (blastoconidia attached to the parent cell by narrow necks), and smaller oval or tubular blastoconidia. Rarely, hyphae and pseudohyphae may be seen. Yeast cells with fractured walls, so-called mosaic forms, are almost constantly present in chronic pulmonary lesions. While still attached to the parent cell, the daughter cells form their own daughter blastoconidia, 1-3 microns in diameter, attached by narrow necks, with the entire mass of blastoconidia resembling a mariner's wheel. Such budding is often referred to as multiple budding and is characteristic of *P. brasiliensis* in culture and in tissues.

TRICHOSPORONOSIS

Trichosporonosis is a disseminated opportunistic fungal infection caused by multiple species of *Trichosporon*, including *T. asahii*, *T. asteroides*, *T. beigelii*, *T. inkin*, *T. mucoides*, and *T. ovoides*. These fungi are soil saprophytes, widely distributed in nature, and they cause infection primarily in immunocompromised hosts, par-

ticularly those with hematopoietic malignancies and patients who have received transplants.

PATHOLOGIC FEATURES

Pulmonary lesions appear as hemorrhagic, necrotizing bronchopneumonia or nodular infarcts. Histologically, radiating fungal colonies with little inflammatory response and widespread mycotic emboli within the hemorrhagic infarcts are seen. In tissue sections, *T. beigelii* appears as pleomorphic hyaline yeast-like cells, 3-8 microns in diameter, with septate hyphae, and arthroconidia. The arthroconidia are produced by fragmentation of the hyphae.

GEOTRICHOSIS

Geotrichosis is a rare, opportunistic fungal infection caused by *Geotrichum candidum*, a ubiquitous saprophyte seen in soil, decomposing organic matter, and contaminated foods and vegetables.

PATHOLOGIC FEATURES

In tissue sections *G. candidum* appears as hyaline, septate, infrequently branching hyphae, 3-6 microns wide, with nonparallel contours and acute angle branching. Rectangular to oval arthroconidia, 4-10 microns wide with rounded or squared ends, are produced by disarticulation of the hyphal segments. Occasionally, thick-walled spherical cells 12 microns or less in diameter and germ tubes may be seen, causing confusion with *Candida* species and *Trichosporon* species. The absence of blastoconidia or budding cells distinguishes *G. candidum* from these two other fungi.

PENICILLIOSIS

Penicillium marneffei is a dimorphic fungus and an emerging AIDS-related infection. *Penicillium* species are ubiquitous environmental saprophytes that rarely cause invasive infection in immunocompetent individuals. Only one species, *P. marneffei*, is known to cause invasive pulmonary disease.

PATHOLOGIC FEATURES

Three inflammatory patterns are described in penicilliosis: 1) granulomatous, 2) suppurative and necrotizing, and 3) anergic; the first two are seen in patients with intact immunity, and the third in patients who are immunocompromised. In H&E- and GMS-stained sections, the yeast cells are seen within histiocytes, and measure 2.5-5.0 microns in diameter. The fungus produces a single transverse septum that stains more intensely and is wider than the external cell wall. Intracellular forms of *P. marneffei* are more pleomorphic than those of *H. capsulatum* var. *capsulatum*. Additionally, short hyphal forms and elongated oval and curved forms, up to 20 microns in length with one or more septa and rounded ends are occasionally seen in necrotic foci and pulmonary cavities.

SUGGESTED READINGS

General

1. Alexander BD. Diagnosis of fungal infection: new technologies for the mycology laboratory. *Transpl Infect Dis*. 2002;4(Suppl 3):32-7.
2. Haque AK. Pathology of common pulmonary fungal infections. *J Thorac Imaging*. 1992;7:1-11.
3. Marchevsky A, Rosen JM, Chrystal G, et al. Pulmonary complications of the acquired immunodeficiency syndrome: a clinicopathologic study of 70 cases. *Hum Pathol*. 1984;16:659-70.
4. Saubolle MA. Fungal pneumonias. *Semin Respir Infect*. 2000;15:162-77.
5. Vartivarian SE, Anaissie EJ, Bodey GP. Emerging fungal pathogens in immunocompromised patients: classification, diagnosis and management. *Clin Infect Dis*. 1993;17:S487-91.
6. Walsh TJ, Groll A, Heimenz J, et al. Infections due to emerging and uncommon medically important fungal pathogens. *Clin Microbiol Infect*. 2004;10:48-66.

Histoplasmosis

7. Goodwin RA Jr, Des Prez RM. Histoplasmosis: state of the art. *Am Rev Respir Dis*. 1978;117:929-56.
8. Shore RN, Waltersdorff RL, Edelstein MV, et al. African histoplasmosis in the United States. *JAMA*. 1981;245:734.
9. Silverman FN. Roentgenographic aspects of histoplasmosis. In: Sweany HC, ed. *Histoplasmosis*. Springfield, Ill: Thomas; 1960:337-81.
10. Wheat LJ, Connolly-Stringfield PA, Baker RL, et al. Disseminated histoplasmosis in the acquired immune deficiency syndrome: clinical findings, diagnosis and treatment, and review of the literature. *Medicine (Baltimore)*. 1990;69:361-74.

Blastomycosis

11. Bradsher RW, Chapman SW, Pappas PG. Blastomycosis. *Infect Dis Clin North Am*. 2003;17:21-40.
12. Lemos LB, Guo M, Baliga M. Blastomycosis: organ involvement and etiologic diagnosis. A review of 123 patients from Mississippi. *Ann Diagn Pathol*. 2000;4:391-406.
13. Wallace J. Pulmonary blastomycosis. *Chest*. 2002;121:677-9.

Cryptococcosis

14. Chandler FW, Kaplan W, Ajello L. *Color Atlas and Text of the Histopathology of Mycotic Diseases*. Year Book Medical Publishers, Chicago, 1980;70-81.
15. Chandler FW, Watts JC. Cryptococcosis. In: Connor DH, Chandler FW, eds. *Pathology of Infectious Diseases*. Stamford, Conn: Appleton & Lange; 1997:989-97.
16. Clark RA, Greer D, Atkinson W, et al. Spectrum of *Cryptococcus neoformans* infection in 68 patients infected with human immunodeficiency virus. *Rev Infect Dis*. 1990;12:768-77.

Candidiasis

17. Cliff PR, Sandoe JA, Heritage J, et al. Retrospective survey of candidemia in hospitalized patients and molecular investigation of a suspected outbreak. *J Med Microbiol*. 2005;54:391-4.
18. Haron E, Vartivarian S, Annissie E, et al. Primary *Candida* pneumonia: experience at a large cancer center and review of the literature. *Medicine*. 1993;72:137-42.

Aspergillosis

19. Denning DW. Invasive aspergillosis. *Clin Infect Dis*. 1998;26:781-805.
20. Lemos LB, Jensen AB. Pathology of aspergillosis. In: Al-Doory Y, Wagner GE, eds. *Aspergillosis*. Springfield, Ill: Thomas; 1984:156-95.
21. Minamoto GY, Barlam TF, Vander Els NJ. Invasive aspergillosis in patients with AIDS. *Clin Infect Dis*. 1992;14:66-74.
22. Patterson TF, Kirkpatrick WF, White M, et al. Invasive aspergillosis: disease spectrum, treatment practices, and outcomes. 13 Aspergillus Study Group. *Medicine (Baltimore)*. 2000;79:250-60.
23. Yousem S. The histologic spectrum of necrotizing forms of pulmonary aspergillosis. *Hum Pathol*. 1997;28:650-6.
24. Zander DS. Allergic bronchopulmonary aspergillosis: an overview. *Arch Pathol Lab Med*. 2005;129:924-8.

Zygomycosis

25. Csomor J, Nikolova R, Sinko J, et al. Mucormycosis. *Orv Hetil*. 2004;145:2507-13.
26. Frater JL, Hall GS, Procop GW. Histologic features of zygomycosis: emphasis on perineural invasion and fungal morphology. *Arch Pathol Lab Med*. 2001;125:375-8.
27. Gonzales C. Zygomycosis. *Infect Dis Clin North Am*. 2002;16:895-914.

Coccidioidomycosis

28. Crum NF, Lederman ER, Stafford CM, et al. Coccidioidomycosis: a descriptive survey of a reemerging disease. Clinical characteristics and current controversies. *Medicine (Baltimore)*. 2004;83:149-75.
29. Galgiani JN. Coccidioidomycosis: a regional disease of national importance. *Ann Intern Med* .1999;130:293-300.
30. Kirkland TN, Fierer J. Coccidioidomycosis: a reemerging infectious disease. *Emerg Infect Dis*. 1996;2:192-9.
31. Singh VR, Smith DK, Lawrence J, et al. Coccidioidomycosis in patients infected with human immunodeficiency virus: review of 91 cases at a single institution. *Clin Infect Dis*. 1996;23:563-8.
32. Stevens, DA. Current concepts: Coccidioidomycosis. *N Engl J Med*. 1995;332:1077-82.

Phaeohyphomycosis

33. Borges MC Jr, Warren S, White W, et al. Pulmonary phaeohyphomycosis due to *Xylohypha bantiana*. *Arch Pathol Lab Med*. 1991;115:627-9.
34. Fader RC, McGinnis MR. Infections caused by dematiaceous fungi: chromoblastomycosis and Phaeohyphomycosis. *Infect Dis Clin North Am*. 1988;2:925-38.

Pneumocystosis

35. Stringer JR, Beard CB, Miller RF, Wakefield AE. A new name *(Pneumocystis jiroveci)* for pneumocystis from humans. *Emerg Infect Dis*. 2002;8:891-6.
36. Thomas CF Jr., Limper AH. Pneumocystis pneumonia. *N Engl J Med*. 2004;350:2487-98.
37. Travis WD, Pittaluga S, Lipschik GY, et al. Atypical pathologic manifestations of *Pneumocystis carinii* pneumonia in the acquired immune deficiency syndrome: review of 123 lung biopsies from 76 patients with emphasis on cysts, vascular invasion, vasculitis, and granulomas. *Am J Surg Pathol*. 1990;14:615-25.
38. Watts JC, Chandler FW. Pneumocystosis. In DH Connors, FW Chandler, et al. (eds). *Pathology of Infectious Diseases*. Stamford, CT: Appleton & Lange; 1997:1241-51.
39. Wazir JF, Ansari NA. Pneumocystic carinii infection: update and review. *Arch Pathol Lab Med*. 2004;128:1023-7.

Pseudallescheriasis

40. Kwon-Chung K, Bennett JE. Pseudallescheriasis and *Scedosporium* infection. In Kwon-Chung K, Bennett JE, eds. *Medical Mycology*. Philadelphia: Lea and Febiger; 1992:678-94.
41. Miller MA, Greenberger PA, American R, et al. Allergic bronchopulmonary mycosis caused by *Pseudallescheria boydii*. *Am Rev Respir Dis*. 1993;148:810-2.
42. Scherr GR, Evans SG, Kiyabu MT, Klatt EC. *Pseudallescheria boydii* infection in the acquired immunodeficiency syndrome. *Arch Pathol Lab Med*. 1992;116:535-6.

43. Vartivarian SE, Anaissie EJ, Bodey GP. Emerging fungal pathogens in immunocompromised patients: classification, diagnosis and management. *Clin Infect Dis*. 1993;17:S487-91.

Fusariosis

44. Anaissie E, Kantarjian H, Ro J, et al. The emerging role of *Fusarium* infections in patients with cancer. *Medicine (Baltimore)*. 1988;67:77-83.
45. Venditti M, Micozzi A, Gentile G, et al. Invasive *Fusarium solani* infections in patients with acute leukemia. *Rev Infect Dis*. 1988;10:653-60.
46. Wheeler MS, McGinnis MR, Schell WA, et al. *Fusarium* infection in burned patients. *Am J Clin Pathol*. 1981;75:304-11.

Sporotrichosis

47. England DM, Hochholzer L. Primary pulmonary sporotrichosis: report of eight cases. *Am J Surg Pathol*. 1985;9:193-204.

Paracoccidioidomycosis

48. Bethlem NM, Lemle A, Bethlem E, et al. Paracoccidioidomycosis. *Semin Respir Med*. 1991;12:81-97.
49. Brumer E, Castaneda E, Restrepo A. Paracoccidioidomycosis: an update. *Clin Microbiol*. 1993;6:89-117.

Trichosporonosis

50. Kimura M, Takahashi H, Satou T, et al. An autopsy case of disseminated trichosporonosis with candidiasis of the urinary tract. *Virchows Arch A Pathol Pathol Anat*. 1989;416:159-62.

Geotrichosis

51. Anaissie E, Bodey GP, Kantarjian H, et al. New spectrum of fungal infections in patients with cancer. *Rev Infect Dis*. 1989;11:369-78.
52. Jagirdar J, Geller SA, Bottone EJ. *Geotrichum candidum* as a tissue invasive human pathogen. *Hum Pathol*. 1981;12:668-71.

Penicilliosis

53. Cooper CR Jr, McGinnis MR. *Penicillium marneffei*, an emerging acquired immunodeficiency syndrome-related pathogen. *Arch Pathol Lab Med*. 1997;121:798-804.
54. McGinnis MR. *Penicillium marneffei*, dimorphic fungus of increasing importance. *Clin Microbiol Newsl*. 1994;4:29-31.

13 Viral Diseases

Sherif R. Zaki • Christopher D. Paddock

- Introduction
- Adenoviruses
- Hantaviruses
- Severe Acute Respiratory Syndrome (SARS) Coronavirus
- Cytomegalovirus
- Herpes Simplex Viruses
- Varicella Zoster Virus
- Influenza Viruses
- Measles
- Human Parainfluenza Viruses
- Respiratory Syncytial Virus
- Human Metapneumovirus
- Henipah Viruses
- Hemorrhagic Fever Viruses

INTRODUCTION

Influenza viruses remain the most frequently identified causes of viral infection in the lung. Nonetheless, the diversity of viral agents that cause pulmonary disease is extremely broad, and continues to expand (Table 13-1). Several newly recognized viral pathogens have been identified in the past two decades that are among the most feared and lethal of all emerging infections, including those caused by Hantaviruses, Nipah virus, and SARS coronavirus. Conversely, certain viral infections, particularly those that occur in vulnerable patient cohorts, have diminished during this same interval. For example, the U.S. incidence of varicella pneumonia has declined more than 65% since universal childhood vaccination for varicella was implemented in 1995, and advances in the clinical management of transplant recipients have reduced the incidence of cytomegalovirus pneumonia.

ADENOVIRUSES

Adenoviruses are represented by a ubiquitous and diverse group of at least 51 serotypes found naturally in the upper respiratory tracts and gastrointestinal systems of humans, other mammals, and birds. More than 50% of the known adenovirus serotypes are associated with human diseases. The others are rarely encountered and may or may not cause recognizable disease.

CLINICAL FEATURES

It is estimated that approximately 5-10% of all pneumonias in infants and young children are caused by adenoviruses. Most pediatric cases of adenovirus pneumonia occur between 6 months and 5 years of age, and serotypes 3, 7, and 21 are the most common causes of pneumonia in this patient cohort. Serotypes 3 and 7 are particularly pathogenic adenoviruses that can cause disseminated and often fatal disease in previously healthy children. In adults, pneumonia is generally associated with serotypes 3, 4, and 7. Periodic epidemics of adenovirus pneumonia in young adults have been identified, particularly among military recruits. In a manner similar to other pathogens, adenoviruses take advantage of impaired or destroyed immune systems to establish persistent and disseminated infections in immunocompromised hosts. Immunocompromised patients are also susceptible to a broader range of different adenovirus serotypes. Because some adenoviruses establish latency in lymphoid tissues and the kidneys of their host, it is believed that many, possibly most, cases of clinical disease caused by adenoviruses in immunocompromised patients are reactivated infections.

RADIOLOGIC FEATURES

Chest films typically show bilateral, multifocal, lobar, or segmental consolidations, bronchial wall thickening, hyperaeration, and lobar atelectasis. Pleural effusions and pneumatoceles are reported less frequently.

TABLE 13-1

Viral Infections in the Lung

Family/Agents	Virus
Adenoviridae	Adenovirus
Bunyaviridae	Hantavirus
Coronaviridae	SARS Coronavirus
Herpesviridae	Cytomegalovirus
	Herpes simplex
	Varicella zoster
Orthomyxoviridae	Influenza
Paramyxoviridae	Measles
	Parainfluenza
	Respiratory syncytial virus
	Human metapneumovirus
	Nipah
	Hendra
Viral hemorrhagic fevers	Arenaviruses, bunyaviruses, flaviviruses, and filoviruses

PATHOLOGIC FEATURES

GROSS FINDINGS

The lungs of patients with adenovirus pneumonia are heavy and edematous, and the bronchi are filled with mucoid, fibrinous, or purulent exudates. The mucosae of the large airways are generally hemorrhagic and congested. Necrotic and inflammatory foci in the pulmonary parenchyma are often represented by yellow palpable nodules.

MICROSCOPIC FINDINGS

The primary histopathologic findings include necrotizing bronchitis and bronchiolitis with extensively denuded epithelium, particularly in medium-sized (1-2 mm in diameter) intrapulmonary bronchi (Figure 13-1A). Affected airways may be occluded by homogeneous eosinophilic material, mixed inflammatory cells, detached epithelium, and cellular debris. The lamina propria of bronchi and bronchioles is typically congested and infiltrated by predominantly mononuclear inflammatory cell infiltrates. Bronchial serous and mucous glands are also often involved and show necrosis and mixed inflammatory infiltrates. As the infection progresses, there is involvement of the more distal pulmonary parenchyma, forming foci of bronchocentric necrosis with hemorrhage, neutrophilic and mononuclear cell infiltrates, and karyorrhexis.

These findings occur against a background of diffuse alveolar damage. Adenoviruses form intranuclear inclusions in respiratory epithelial cells of the trachea, bronchi, and bronchioles, in the acinar cells of bronchial glands, and in alveolar pneumocytes, and are generally most abundant at the viable edges of necrotic foci. On hematoxylin-eosin stain, early inclusions appear as small, dense, amphophilic structures surrounded by a cleared zone and peripherally marginated chromatin, similar to herpetic inclusions. As the cellular infection progresses, the inclusion becomes larger (as large as 14 microns in some cells) and more basophilic, and the margins of the nuclear membrane become blurred to form the characteristic "smudge cell" (Figure 13-1B).

ANCILLARY STUDIES

Various methods can be used to diagnose adenovirus infections, including antigen detection (fluorescence antibody assays and enzyme immunoassays), cell culture, electron microscopy, molecular assays, and serologic testing for group-specific or type-specific antibodies. Immunohistochemical (IHC) staining methods can detect adenovirus-infected cells in formalin-fixed, paraffin-embedded tissues using various commercially available adenovirus group-specific antibodies (Figure 13-1C). Electron microscopy of adenovirus-infected tissues reveals a paracrystalline array of virions represented by icosahedral capsids that measure 70 to 90 nm in diameter (Figure 13-1D). Most adenoviruses can be isolated in cell culture from bronchial washings, tracheal aspirates, or lung biopsy specimens during the early stage of the illness. Molecular assays, particularly gene amplification using polymerase chain reaction (PCR) and in situ hybridization (ISH) methods, have been developed to detect adenovirus nucleic acid in respiratory secretions and in formalin-fixed, paraffin-embedded tissues.

DIFFERENTIAL DIAGNOSIS

The differential diagnosis includes those agents that cause necrotizing bronchiolitis, pneumonia, and intranuclear viral inclusions, particularly herpes simplex viruses, varicella-zoster virus, and cytomegalovirus. Histologic clues to distinguish these agents from adenovirus include the presence (herpes simplex virus [HSV] and varicella zoster virus [VZV]) or absence (adenovirus) of multinucleated cells, cytoplasmic inclusions (CMV), or distinctive smudge cells (adenovirus); however, ancillary studies are generally required for confirmation.

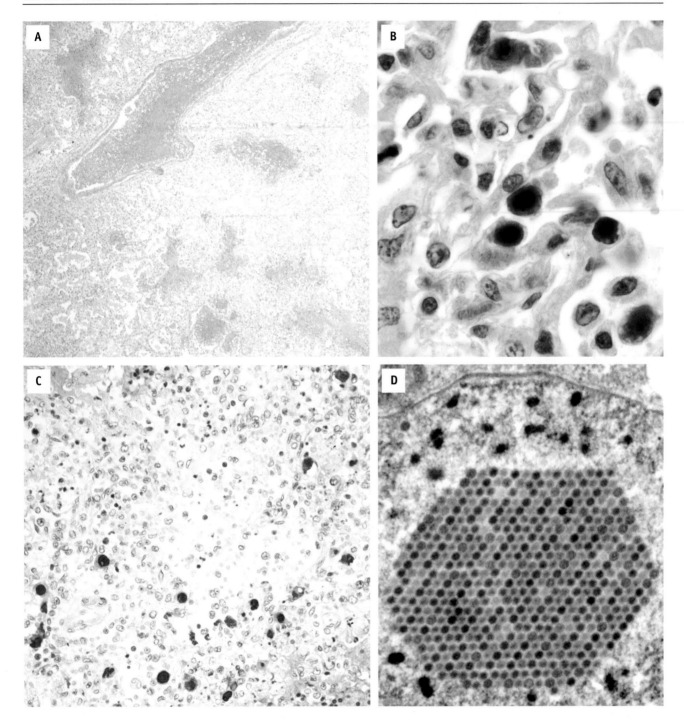

FIGURE 13-1

Adenovirus pneumonia
(A) Bronchioles and scattered alveoli containing necrotic debris comprised of surface epithelium, fibrin, and mixed inflammatory cells. **(B)** Large, basophilic, intranuclear inclusions in alveolar pneumocytes, forming characteristic "smudge cells" that can be observed in advanced adenovirus infections. **(C)** Immunohistochemical localization of adenovirus-infected cells in a patient with fatal adenovirus pneumonia (immunoalkaline phosphatase). **(D)** Paracrystalline arrays of 70-90 nm adenovirus particles in the nucleus of an infected pneumocyte.

PROGNOSIS AND THERAPY

In immunocompromised patients, the case fatality rate of adenoviral pneumonia approaches 60%, compared with an approximately 15% mortality in immu-nocompetent patients. There is no proven effective antiviral therapy for adenovirus infections. Most patients receive only supportive care for symptoms of the disease, which includes cessation of immune-suppressing drugs in those patients with iatrogenic immunosuppression.

HANTAVIRUSES

Hantaviral diseases in humans are caused by a group of closely related, trisegmented, negative-sense RNA viruses of the genus *Hantavirus*, of the family *Bunyaviridae.* Two classes of hantavirus-associated illnesses have been described: Hemorrhagic Fever Renal Syndrome, (HFRS) for disease in which the kidneys are primarily involved, and Hantavirus Pulmonary Syndrome (HPS), for disease in which the lungs are primarily affected.

CLINICAL FEATURES

The initial symptoms of HFRS and HPS are similar and resemble those seen in early phases of many other viral diseases. Fever, myalgia, headache, vomiting, weakness, and cough are common symptoms in early phases of both HFRS and HPS. Renal involvement is seen in all cases of HFRS, and the clinical presentation ranges from a mild illness with minimal renal dysfunction to a more severe form with acute renal failure and shock. Only HFRS patients who die during the later phases of renal failure typically show significant pulmonary edema. The clinical picture for HPS is quite different from that for HFRS. The initial prodrome is followed by rapidly progressive pulmonary edema, respiratory insufficiency, and shock. In fatal cases, the majority of deaths occur within 2 days of hospitalization. Hemorrhages and peripheral signs of vasomotor instability, such as flushing, conjunctival injection, and periorbital edema as seen in HFRS, are extremely rare.

RADIOLOGIC FEATURES

Chest radiographs may be normal early in the course of HPS, but evidence of interstitial edema can be observed in the majority of cases within 48 hours of hospitalization.

PATHOLOGIC FEATURES

GROSS FINDINGS

Large quantities of protein-rich, gelatinous retroperitoneal edema fluid are found in the hypotensive phase of severe HFRS, while all HPS patients have large bilateral pleural effusions and heavy, edematous lungs. In fatal Far Eastern HFRS, a distinctive triad of hemorrhagic necrosis of the junctional zone of the renal medulla, right atrium of the heart, and anterior pituitary can be seen. In patients with HPS, hemorrhages are exceedingly rare, and ischemic necrotic lesions, except those attributed to shock, are not seen.

MICROSCOPIC FINDINGS

Histologically, morphologic changes of the endothelium are uncommon but, when seen, consist of prominent and swollen endothelial cells. Vascular thrombi and endothelial cell necrosis are rare. In HFRS, the most severe and characteristic microscopic lesions involve the kidney; however, an interstitial pneumonitis can also be seen in some fatal cases. In contrast, the microscopic changes in HPS are principally seen in the lung and spleen. The lungs (Figure 13-2) show a mild to moderate interstitial pneumonitis characterized by variable degrees of edema and an interstitial mononuclear cell infiltrate composed of a mixture of small and enlarged mononuclear cells with the appearance of immunoblasts. Focal hyaline membranes composed of condensed proteinaceous intraalveolar edema fluid, fibrin, and variable numbers of inflammatory cells are observed. Typically, neutrophils are scanty and the alveolar pneumocytes are intact with no evidence of cellular debris, nuclear fragmentation, or hyperplasia. In fatal cases, with a prolonged survival interval, tissues show features more characteristic of the exudative and proliferative stages of diffuse alveolar damage (Figure 13-2B). Other characteristic microscopic findings in HPS cases include variable numbers of immunoblasts within the splenic red pulp and periarteriolar white pulp

(Figure 13-2E), lymph nodal paracortical zones, hepatic portal triads, and peripheral blood.

ANCILLARY STUDIES

Virus-specific diagnosis and confirmation can be achieved through serology, PCR for hantavirus RNA, or IHC for hantaviral antigens. Serologic testing can detect hantavirus-specific immunoglobulin M or rising titers of immunoglobulin G in patient sera and is considered the method of choice for laboratory confirmation of HPS. PCR detects viral RNA in blood and tissues and is extremely useful for diagnostic and epidemiologic purposes. Hantaviral RNA can also be detected in formalin-fixed, paraffin-embedded archival tissues by RT-PCR. IHC testing of formalin-fixed tissues is a sensitive method to confirm hantaviral infections, and viral antigens are found primarily within capillary endothelia throughout various tissues in both HPS and HFRS (Figure 13-2C). In HPS, marked accumulations of hantaviral antigens are found in the pulmonary microvasculature and in splenic and lymph nodal follicular dendritic cells. Electron microscopic studies of HPS lung tissue demonstrate infection of endothelial cells and macrophages. The virus or virus-like particles observed are infrequent and extremely difficult to identify in autopsy tissues; in contrast, typical endothelial granulofilamentous inclusions are seen more frequently (Figure 13-2D).

DIFFERENTIAL DIAGNOSIS

HPS should be suspected in cases of acute respiratory distress syndrome (ARDS) without a known precipitating cause among previously healthy individuals. The level of suspicion should be particularly high when patients have a known exposure to rodents in areas where *Peromyscus maniculatus* or other reservoirs of hantavirus are found. Physicians need to differentiate HPS from other common acute respiratory diseases, such as pneumococcal pneumonia, influenza virus, and unexplained ARDS. Diseases that need to be distinguished pathologically from HPS include a relatively large number of different viral, rickettsial, and bacterial infections, as well as various noninfectious disease processes.

PROGNOSIS AND THERAPY

Recovery in HFRS is usually complete, with no apparent long-term sequelae. Mortality rates for HFRS range from 1-15%, with shock and uremia being the main contributing causes of death, although pulmonary

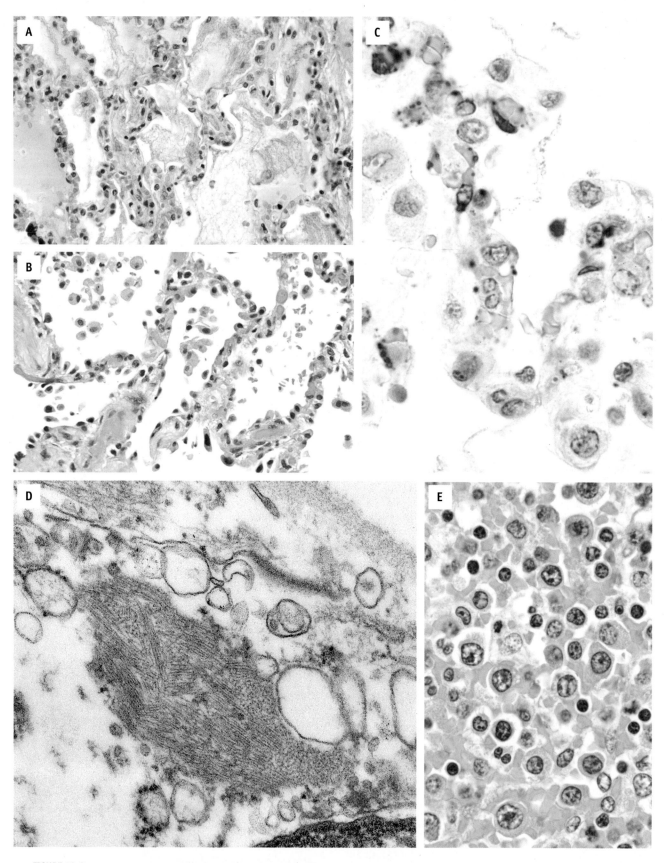

FIGURE 13-2

Hantavirus Pulmonary Syndrome (HPS)

(A) Mild mononuclear interstitial pneumonitis and edema in a typical case of HPS. (B) Type II pneumocyte hyperplasia as seen in patients with HPS who die after a prolonged clinical course. (C) Widespread immunostaining of hantaviral antigens in the pulmonary microvasculature of an HPS patient (immunoalkaline phosphatase). (D) Ultrastructural appearance of a typical granulofilamentous hantavirus inclusion within the pulmonary capillary endothelium. (E) Spleen from a fatal case in which immunoblasts are seen in the periarteriolar sheath. Note the prominent nucleoli and high nuclear-to-cytoplasmic ratio.

HANTAVIRUSES—FACT SHEET

Definition

» Hantaviral diseases are caused by closely related, trisegmented, negative-sense RNA viruses of the genus *Hantavirus*, of the family *Bunyaviridae*

» Two classes of hantavirus-associated illnesses have been described: Hemorrhagic Fever Renal Syndrome (HFRS) for disease in which the kidneys are primarily involved and Hantavirus Pulmonary Syndrome (HPS) for disease in which the lungs are primarily affected

Incidence and Location

» Zoonotic viruses maintained in nature by asymptomatic infection of rodents

» Transmission to humans is usually associated with exposure to rodents in and around the home, performing agricultural activities, cleaning animal sheds, sleeping on the ground, and with certain occupations

» Serotypes are distributed throughout the world

» HFRS is more common in Europe and Asia, while HPS is almost exclusively seen in the Americas

» Rare cause of pneumonia

Morbidity and Mortality

» In HFRS, mortality rates range from 1-15%

» In HPS, mortality rates may exceed 50%

» In survivors of HFRS, recovery is usually complete, with no long-term sequelae

Gender, Race, and Age Distribution

» No specific gender, race, or age distribution is generally seen

Clinical Features

» Prodrome of fever, myalgias, headache, vomiting, weakness, and cough is common in both HFRS and HPS

» Renal involvement is seen in all cases of HFRS, and the clinical presentation ranges from a mild illness with minimal renal dysfunction to a more severe form with acute renal failure and shock

» In HPS, the prodrome is followed by rapidly progressive pulmonary edema, respiratory insufficiency, and shock

Radiologic Features

» Interstitial edema without consolidation in the majority of cases within 48 hours of hospitalization

» Pleural effusions are very common

Prognosis and Therapy

» Supportive therapy, such as dialysis and circulatory and respiratory support

» Ribavirin is effective in treatment of HFRS but not HPS

HANTAVIRUSES—PATHOLOGIC FEATURES

Gross Findings

» Severe HFRS: gelatinous retroperitoneal collections, and a distinctive triad of hemorrhagic necrosis of the junctional zone of the renal medulla, right atrium of the heart, and anterior pituitary

» HPS: large bilateral pleural effusions and heavy edematous lungs

Microscopic Findings

» HFRS: the most severe and characteristic microscopic lesions involve the kidney

» HPS:

» Lungs—an interstitial pneumonitis is seen in most cases, characterized by edema and an interstitial mononuclear cell infiltrate, and sometimes focal hyaline membranes

» Extrapulmonary-immunoblasts in spleen, lymph nodes, and peripheral blood

Immunohistochemical Features

» IHC testing of formalin-fixed tissues is a sensitive method to confirm infection

» Hantaviral antigens are most commonly detected in endothelial cells of involved organs in HPS and HFRS

Ultrastructural Features

» Virus particles are 70-120 nm in diameter and generally appear spherical to oval in shape

» A lipid envelope containing glycoprotein spikes surrounds a core consisting of the genome nucleocapsids arranged in delicate tangles of filaments

» Granulofilamentous viral inclusions can be seen in endothelial cells

» Viral particles can be extremely difficult to visualize in tissues

Pathologic Differential Diagnosis

» Histopathologic and hematologic findings suggest the diagnosis in HPS and HFRS; however, laboratory confirmation is essential for confirmation of the diagnosis

» Differential diagnosis includes a large number of viral, rickettsial, bacterial infections, as well as non-infectious diseases

SEVERE ACUTE RESPIRATORY SYNDROME (SARS) CORONAVIRUS

The causative agent of SARS is an enveloped, positive-stranded RNA virus that is a member of the genus *Coronavirus*, of the family *Coronaviridae*. SARS was recognized during a global outbreak of severe pneumonia that began in late 2002 in Guangdong Province, China, and gained prominence in early 2003 as cases were identified in Asia, Europe, and in North and South America. Initial studies pointed to palm civets as a possible animal reservoir. However, it appears likely that the role of civets and other small mammals is as amplifier hosts within animal markets rather than as the natural reservoir of the virus. More recently, a novel SARS-like coronavirus was found in *Rhinolophus* bats in mainland

edema has been implicated in some patients. In HPS, mortality rates may exceed 50%, depending on serotype involved. Management of patients with HPS or HFRS is often complex and phase-specific. Supportive therapy, such as dialysis and circulatory and respiratory support, is the basis of treatment. Controlled studies suggest that ribavirin, a nucleoside analog, is effective in the treatment of hantaviral infection if administered early. Ribavirin has not proven effective in therapy of HPS.

China, suggesting that is the more likely species to be the natural reservoir from which the SARS coronavirus emerged.

CLINICAL FEATURES

The disease causes an influenza-like illness that typically presents with acute onset of fever, myalgia, malaise, and chills, with rhinorrhea and sore throat being less common features. A dry cough is common, but shortness of breath and tachypnea are prominent only later in the course of the disease. Watery diarrhea occurs in some patients, typically associated with clinical deterioration in the second week of illness. People of all ages can develop the illness and children tend to have a much milder clinical course than adults. Transmission is from person to person, and the estimated incubation period is 2 to 14 days.

RADIOLOGIC FEATURES

The radiologic features of SARS include the peripheral appearance of lung opacities, lower lobe predominance, and a mixture of ground-glass opacities, interstitial thickening, and bronchiectasis. Pneumomediastinum without preceding positive-pressure ventilation or intubation can be seen later in the disease. Multifocal peripheral subpleural ground-glass opacification or consolidation has been the most commonly observed CT feature at the time of diagnosis in patients with SARS.

PATHOLOGIC FEATURES

GROSS FINDINGS

In fatal cases of SARS, the lungs are usually heavy and edematous with varying degrees of red and gray hepatization. Multiple bilateral hemorrhagic infarcts are commonly seen in association with subpleural hemorrhages.

MICROSCOPIC FINDINGS

The main histopathologic pattern is diffuse alveolar damage (Figure 13-3A). Increased mononuclear cell infiltrates in the interstitium can be seen in some cases. Other findings identified in some patients include focal intra-alveolar hemorrhage, necrotic inflammatory debris in small airways, and organizing pneumonia. In addition, multinucleated syncytial cells may be seen in the alveolar spaces of some pa-

tients who die 14 days or more after onset of illness (Figure 13-3B).

ANCILLARY STUDIES

ISH and IHC studies of tissues from SARS patients have identified coronavirus in ciliated columnar epithelial cells in the trachea, bronchi, and bronchioles (Figure 13-3C) and in pneumocytes (Figure 13-3D,E) and occasional macrophages in some patients. Antigens are more readily identified in patients who die within the first 2 weeks of onset of illness. Electron microscopic examination can show coronavirus particles and nucleocapsid inclusions in cytoplasmic vesicles and along the cell membranes of pneumocytes, in phagosomes of macrophages, and associated with fibrin in alveolar spaces. Negative stains reveal particles averaging 80-100 nm in size with a characteristic crown-like fringe on the surface (Figure 13-3F).

DIFFERENTIAL DIAGNOSIS

The histopathologic findings seen in the lungs of patients who die from SARS are somewhat nonspecific and can also be seen in acute lung injury cases caused by infectious agents, trauma, drugs, or toxic chemicals. Multinucleated syncytial cells similar to those seen in some SARS patients can also be found in many viral infections, including measles, parainfluenza viruses, respiratory syncytial virus, and Nipah virus infections. An unequivocal diagnosis can be made only by laboratory tests such as viral culture, direct fluorescent antibody, serology, PCR, or IHC.

PROGNOSIS AND THERAPY

Patients with SARS can undergo complete recovery; however, the disease can progress to acute respiratory failure and death in about 5-10% of infected individuals. About 20-30% of all patients need observation in intensive care, and most of these require mechanical ventilation. The clinical management of patients with SARS includes respiratory support with intensive care support as needed. Ribavirin, lopinavir, and type I IFN show inhibition of SARS virus in tissue culture. However, their utility in SARS-infected patients is inconclusive, and they may actually be harmful. Similarly, studies of corticosteroid use are inconclusive and again these agents may possibly cause harm to the patient. Experimental and clinical trials are needed to evaluate the efficacy of various treatments.

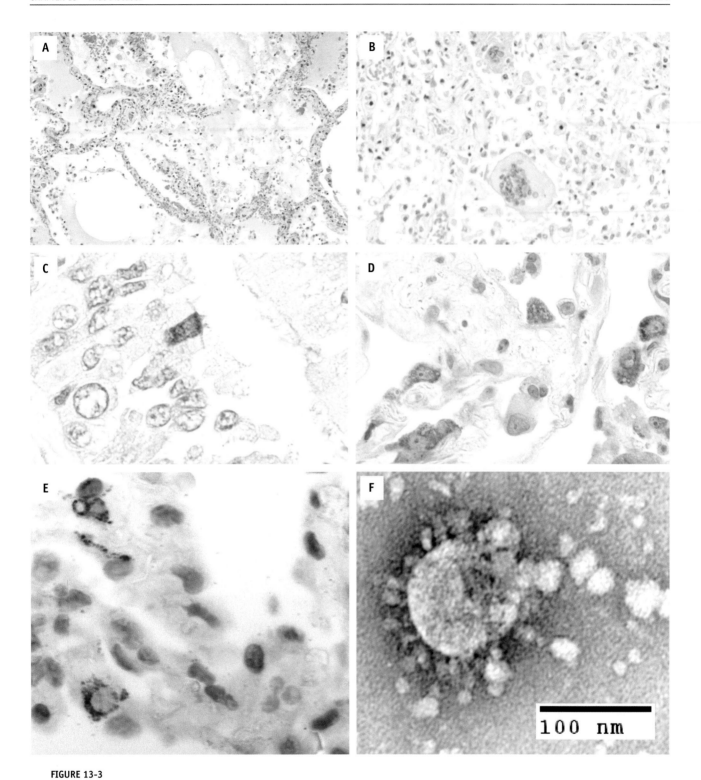

FIGURE 13-3

Severe Acute Respiratory Syndrome (SARS)

(A) Prominent edema, congestion and focal hemorrhage, and mild interstitial inflammation. **(B)** Multinucleated syncytial giant cells as seen in some cases of fatal SARS. Note the absence of discernible viral inclusions. **(C)** Ciliated upper airway epithelial cell containing viral antigens (immunoalkaline phosphatase). **(D)** Immunostaining of coronavirus antigens in alveolar pneumocytes (immunoalkaline phosphatase). **(E)** ISH showing infected pneumocytes and macrophages containing viral nucleic acids (digoxigenin-labeled probe followed by immunoalkaline phosphatase staining). **(F)** Electron micrograph showing 80-100 nm coronavirus particles, named for the characteristic crown-like fringe on their surfaces.

SARS CORONAVIRUS—FACT SHEET

Definition

- SARS coronavirus is an enveloped, positive-stranded RNA virus that is a member of the genus *Coronavirus*, of the family *Coronaviridae*

Incidence and Location

- First reported in Guangdong Province in Southern China in 2002, but rapidly spread to become a worldwide illness in 2003

Morbidity and Mortality

- SARS is fatal in about 5-10% of patients
- In patients who survive the illness, the recovery is usually complete
- Mortality and risk of complications are higher among elderly persons and persons of any age with certain underlying health conditions
- Children have a much milder clinical course than adults
- Secondary bacterial pneumonias with organisms may occur as a complication

Gender, Race, and Age distribution

- People of all ages are vulnerable to SARS
- No recognized gender or racial predilection

Clinical Features

- SARS coronavirus is spread person-to-person, primarily through the coughing and sneezing of infected persons
- Estimated incubation period is 2 to 14 days
- Uncomplicated SARS illness is an influenza-like illness characterized by an abrupt onset of fever, myalgia, headache, malaise, nonproductive cough, sore throat, and rhinitis

Radiologic Features

- Peripheral lung opacities with lower-lobe predominance, and a mixture of ground-glass opacities, interstitial thickening, and bronchiectasis
- CT at the time of diagnosis shows multifocal peripheral subpleural ground-glass opacities
- Pneumomediastinum can be seen later in the disease

Prognosis and Therapy

- Supportive respiratory and intensive care therapy
- Inconclusive studies regarding the efficacy of antivirals and corticosteroids
- Specific antibiotic therapy in cases with secondary bacterial infection
- Prevention of nosocomial transmission is an important strategy for management of cases in a hospital setting

---

SARS—PATHOLOGIC FEATURES

Gross Findings

- Lungs are usually heavy and edematous with varying degrees of red and gray hepatization
- Multiple bilateral pulmonary hemorrhagic infarcts and subpleural hemorrhages can be seen

Microscopic Findings

- Diffuse alveolar damage
- Hemorrhage
- Edema
- Multinucleated cells in about 10% of cases
- Viral inclusions cannot be identified by light microscopy

Immunohistochemical Features

- IHC reveals SARS-CoV antigens primarily in the respiratory epithelial cells of airways and pneumocytes, particularly in patients who die within the first two weeks of onset of the illness

Ultrastructural Features

- Virions form by alignment of the helical nucleocapsids along the membranes of the endoplasmic reticulum or Golgi complex and acquire an envelope by budding into the cisternae
- Cellular vesicles become filled with virions and progress to the cell surface for release of viral particles
- Negative stains reveal particles averaging 80-100 nm in size with a characteristic crown-like fringe on the surface

Pathologic Differential Diagnosis

- Other causes of diffuse alveolar damage, including many viral, rickettsial, and bacterial infections, as well as non-infectious diseases (trauma, drugs, and toxins)

CYTOMEGALOVIRUS

Cytomegalovirus (CMV), a large, double-stranded DNA virus, is a ubiquitous human pathogen, and in North America infects approximately 50-90% of the population. Like all herpesviruses, CMV remains with its host for life after primary infection and establishes latency in various cell types, including vascular endothelial cells, monocytes and macrophages, neutrophils, and renal and pulmonary epithelial cells. Activation of viral replication occurs in persons with severely compromised immunity.

CLINICAL FEATURES

Most CMV infections are inapparent, although cases of primary infection in otherwise healthy individuals can result in a self-limited mononucleosis syndrome resembling the illness caused by Epstein-Barr virus. Pulmonary involvement in CMV mononucleosis occurs in approximately 6% of these cases. Adults and children with advanced HIV disease and recipients of hematopoietic stem cell and lung transplants are particularly at risk for developing CMV pneumonia. Before the use of CMV screening and effective anti-viral prophylaxis regimens, 10-30% of all patients undergoing allogeneic bone marrow transplantation for leukemia, and 15-55% of solid organ transplants, developed CMV pneumonia with case fatality rates greater than 80% in some series. Neonates are also at risk. Symptomatology includes fever, cough, rales, and hypoxemia. Systemic dissemination and extrapulmonary involvement can occur in some patients.

RADIOLOGIC FEATURES

Pulmonary CMV disease typically appears as bilateral nodular or reticular opacities on chest radiographs. Pleural effusions are identified in approximately 10-30% of patients. Because some patients may be co-infected with other pulmonary pathogens, radiologic findings may be confusing. Some patients with documented infection have normal radiographs.

PATHOLOGIC FEATURES

GROSS FINDINGS

There are several general patterns of pulmonary CMV infection. The lungs are typically heavy and may appear diffusely consolidated, or show scattered nodular foci of hemorrhage and necrosis. Rarely, CMV infection of the lungs manifests as a single pulmonary nodule.

MICROSCOPIC FINDINGS

Multiple histopathologic patterns have been reported for CMV pneumonia. Extensive intra-alveolar hemorrhage with scattered cytomegalic cells and relatively scant inflammatory cell infiltrates may occur. In a similar manner, extensive involvement of the alveolar epithelium with minimal inflammation or overt evidence of parenchymal injury has also been described. Other patterns include multifocal or miliary lesions with mixed inflammatory cell infiltrates, hemorrhage, necrosis, and cytomegalic cells, or a diffuse, predominantly mononuclear cell infiltrate, interstitial pneumonitis with intra-alveolar edema and fibrin deposition, and diffusely distributed cytomegalic cells. The cytomegalic changes of CMV-infected cells are evident on standard hematoxylin-eosin staining and are virtually pathognomonic of active CMV infection. The cells are enlarged (25-40 microns) and contain amphophilic to deeply basophilic intranuclear and intracytoplasmic inclusions (Figure 13-4A,B). The single intranuclear inclusion is comprised of viral nucleoprotein and assembled capsids, and is a large (up to 20 microns), round-to-ovoid body with a smoothly contoured border that is generally surrounded by a clear halo that gives the inclusion a distinctive "owl's eye" appearance. Cytoplasmic inclusions are small (1-3 microns), granular bodies that appear after the intranuclear inclusion is well developed and are not uniformly present in all CMV-infected cells. These inclusions represent a mixture of virions and various cellular organelles, and increase in size and number as the infection progresses. Unlike the intranuclear inclusions, the cytoplasmic inclusions stain with periodic acid-Schiff stain and are deeply argyrophilic with methenamine silver stains.

ANCILLARY STUDIES

CMV pneumonia is defined by the presence of signs or symptoms of pulmonary disease combined with the detection of CMV in bronchoalveolar lavage fluid or lung tissue samples. Detection methods that support this definition include virus isolation, histopathologic observation of cytomegalic cells, ISH, or IHC stains (Figure 13-4C). Detection by PCR alone is considered too sensitive for the diagnosis of CMV pneumonia and is insufficient for this purpose. CMV is most often cultured in human diploid fibroblasts using a shell vial method to enhance infectivity and can usually yield diagnostic results within 48 hours.

DIFFERENTIAL DIAGNOSIS

Because the histopathologic features of CMV pneumonia are varied, the differential diagnosis depends on the predominant pattern of histologic pattern (hemorrhage, miliary inflammatory lesions, or diffuse interstitial pneumonitis). The cytopathologic changes of CMV-infected cells are generally sufficient to establish a diagnosis. CMV inclusions may on occasion, however, be confused with those of other herpesviruses, adenoviruses, or measles, but none of these pathogens collectively shows cytomegaly, a single large nuclear inclusion with a prominent halo, and multiple small cytoplasmic inclusions. Reactive pneumocytes can occasionally show enlarged nuclei, but the nuclei will be immunonegative with IHC for CMV.

PROGNOSIS AND THERAPY

Ganciclovir, foscarnet, and intravenous CMV immune globulin remain important lines of treatment for CMV pneumonia and have diminished mortality in immunosuppressed patients with this disease. Nonetheless, mortality attributable to CMV pneumonia is approximately 50%.

HERPES SIMPLEX VIRUSES

Human herpes simplex viruses (HSV) are large, enveloped, double-stranded DNA-viruses approximately 100-110 nm in diameter. Two serologic types are recognized, and each is most frequently associated with particular disease syndromes; however, either serotype may cause any of the clinical syndromes associated with either serotype. HSV-1 causes gingivostomatitis, pharyngitis, esophagitis, keratoconjunctivitis, and encephalitis, and is the serotype most commonly associated with adult

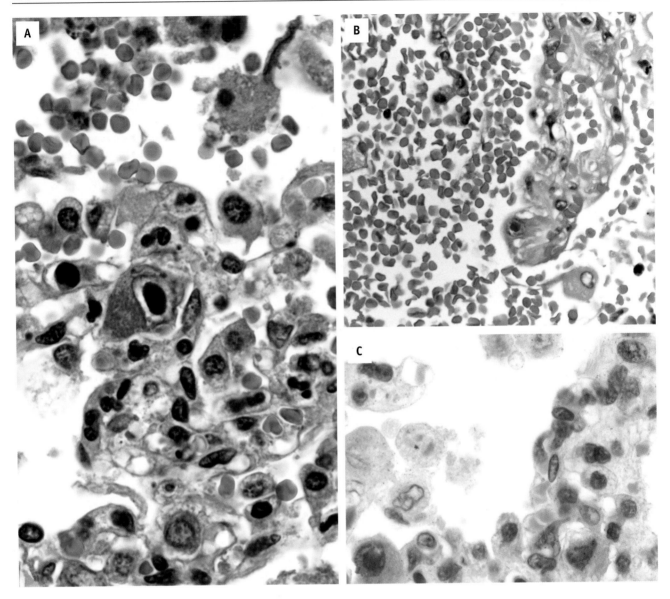

FIGURE 13-4

Cytomegalovirus pneumonia
(A) CMV-infected cell with large, basophilic "owl's eye" intranuclear inclusion and smaller, amphophilic cytoplasmic inclusions. **(B)** Alveolar hemorrhage with relatively little inflammation and CMV-infected pneumocytes. **(C)** Immunohistochemical localization of CMV-infected cells in the pulmonary parenchyma (immunoalkaline phosphatase).

HSV pneumonia. HSV-2 typically infects genital sites and is the serotype associated with approximately 80% of disseminated disease and pulmonary infections in newborn infants.

CLINICAL FEATURES

HSV, like all herpesviruses, has the ability to persist in an inactive state for varying periods of time and then recur spontaneously following undefined stimuli associated with physical or emotional stress, trauma to nerve roots or ganglia, fever, immunosuppression, or exposure to ultraviolet radiation. Tracheobronchitis and pneumonia

are the primary respiratory tract manifestations of HSV infection. In adults, infection of the respiratory tract with HSV may be associated with disseminated herpetic infection, but is more commonly identified as an isolated disease manifestation resulting from reactivation of latent herpetic infections in the oropharynx. Mucocutaneous herpetic infection generally precedes HSV pneumonia, and aspiration of virus-containing secretions into the lower respiratory tract is believed to be the most frequent cause of pulmonary infection with HSV; however, oral lesions may be absent in patients with herpetic laryngo-tracheitis and bronchopneumonia. Disease can also be associated with airway trauma caused by tracheal intubation or from hematogenous dissemination of HSV. Newborn infants, severely immunosuppressed or burned

CYTOMEGALOVIRUS PNEUMONIA—FACT SHEET

Definition

▸ Human CMV is a β-herpesvirus with the largest genome (230 kbp) of all the herpesviruses known to infect humans

Incidence and Location

▸ Common cause of pneumonia in immunocompromised patients
▸ Woldwide distribution
▸ CMV is a ubiquitous human pathogen, and in North America infects approximately 50-90% of the population
▸ Patients with advanced HIV disease and recipients of hematopoietic stem cell and lung transplants are particularly at risk of developing CMV pneumonia

Mortality

▸ Mortality attributable to CMV pneumonia is approximately 50%

Gender, Race, and Age Distribution

▸ Can develop in patients of any age
▸ No apparent gender or racial predilection

Clinical Features

▸ Fever, nonproductive cough, rales, and hypoxemia
▸ Disseminated infection may also cause adrenalitis, hepatitis, or encephalitis

Radiologic Features

▸ Common findings are bilateral nodular or reticular opacities
▸ Pleural effusions are identified in approximately 10-30% of patients
▸ Some patients with documented infection have normal radiographs

Therapy

▸ Ganciclovir, foscarnet, and intravenous CMV immune globulin remain important lines of treatment

CYTOMEGALOVIRUS PNEUMONIA—PATHOLOGIC FEATURES

Gross Findings

▸ Lungs are typically heavy and may appear diffusely consolidated or show scattered nodular foci of hemorrhage and necrosis
▸ Rarely, the infection manifests as a single pulmonary nodule

Microscopic Findings

▸ Multiple histopathologic patterns have been reported, including extensive intra-alveolar hemorrhage, diffuse interstitial pneumonitis, and miliary inflammatory foci with necrosis
▸ Virally induced cytopathic changes include cytomegaly (25-40 microns) and amphophilic to deeply basophilic intranuclear and intracytoplasmic inclusions in various cell types including macrophages, pneumocytes, glandular epithelium, endothelium, and fibroblasts
  ▸ The single intranuclear inclusion is a large (up to 20 microns), round to ovoid body with a smoothly contoured border that is generally surrounded by a clear halo
  ▸ Cytoplasmic inclusions are small (1-3 microns), stain with periodic acid-Schiff stain, and are deeply argyrophilic with methenamine silver stains

Immunohistochemical Features

▸ Commercially available antibodies can assist in the diagnosis of CMV

Ultrastructural Features

▸ Mature enveloped virions from 150- 200 nm

Pathologic Differential Diagnosis

▸ Herpes simplex viruses, varicella zoster virus, and adenoviruses
▸ Reactive pneumocytes

---

patients, and patients with severe trauma are at greatest risk of developing HSV pneumonia. Lower respiratory tract disease in neonates is most commonly associated with disseminated herpetic infections. Most cases of neonatal disease represent primary HSV infections and are acquired during parturition from HSV-infected mothers. The incidence of neonatal HSV infection is approximately 1 in 3,200 deliveries, and disseminated disease develops in approximately 25% of infected neonates. In disseminated infections, signs and symptoms appear a mean of 5 days after birth (range, 0 to 12 days), and approximately 40-50% of these patients develop pneumonia.

RADIOLOGIC FEATURES

Chest radiographs of patients with HSV pneumonia show ill-defined nodular or reticular densities of various sizes scattered in both lung fields. During the early stages of disease, these nodules measure 2-5 mm and are best seen in the periphery of the lungs. As the disease progresses, these lesions coalesce and enlarge to form more extensive segmental and subsegmental infiltrates. Computed tomography shows patchy ground-glass opacities with scattered areas of consolidation and nodular densities. Pleural effusions are common.

PATHOLOGIC FEATURES

GROSS FINDINGS

HSV tracheobronchitis appears as 5-15 mm ulcers covered by fibrinopurulent exudate on the mucous membranes. In HSV pneumonia acquired through the airways, the lungs are heavy and show nodular hemorrhagic foci that are generally distributed around bronchi and bronchioles. In hematogenously acquired HSV pneumonia, hemorrhagic foci usually have a random or miliary distribution.

MICROSCOPIC FINDINGS

Herpetic tracheobronchitis is an ulcerative process characterized by large areas of denuded mucosal epithelium and fibrinopurulent exudate containing necrotic cells. Despite extensive tissue damage, cells with intranuclear inclusions may be sparse and are found most often at the margins of the ulcerated epithelium or occasionally in the mucous glands below the ulcerated mucosa. In the lung, herpetic lesions show extensive necrosis and karyorrhectic debris, and are associated with hemorrhage and a sparse-to-moderate neutrophilic infiltrate (Figures 13-5A,B). Intranuclear inclusions are best appreciated in cells at the leading edge of necrotic foci. Inclusions appear either as homogeneous, amphophilic, and glassy (e.g., Cowdry type B inclusions), or as eosinophilic with a halo separating the inclusion from the nuclear membrane (e.g., Cowdry type A inclusions). Other changes associated with HSV, including multinucleation and nuclear molding, ground-glass nuclear chromatin, and ballooning degeneration of the cytoplasm, are more frequently associated with squamous epithelium and less often encountered in the lung.

ANCILLARY STUDIES

Virus isolation remains an important diagnostic method; however, because HSV can be isolated from oropharyngeal secretions and occasionally from the lower respiratory tract of patients who lack overt pulmonary disease, virologic cultures must be interpreted in the context of complementary clinical, radiographic, and histopathologic findings as much as possible. PCR methods that amplify HSV DNA from clinical specimens, including tissue and blood, can be particularly useful for distinguishing between HSV-1 and HSV-2 infections. Commercially available antibodies exist for IHC detection of HSV in tissues (Figure 13-5C). Electron microscopy can also be used to demonstrate encapsulated viral particles with a targetoid appearance arranged in a lattice-like pattern (Figure 13-5D).

DIFFERENTIAL DIAGNOSIS

HSV, varicella-zoster virus (VZV), adenoviruses, measles virus, and CMV can cause necrotizing hemorrhagic pneumonias, and each produce intranuclear inclusions that may be difficult to differentiate. The viral inclusions of HSV are identical to those of VZV; separation can be accomplished by IHC, molecular methods, or culture. Distinction from adenoviruses can be accomplished if smudge cells are identified (supporting the presence of adenovirus). HSV does not produce cytoplasmic inclusions, which should be seen in CMV and in measles.

PROGNOSIS AND THERAPY

Prior to the discovery and use of antiviral therapies, 85% of neonates with disseminated HSV disease died from the infection. With early diagnosis and high-dose acyclovir therapy, however, mortality has been reduced to approximately 30%. Foscarnet has been used effectively in some acyclovir-resistant patients.

VARICELLA ZOSTER VIRUS

Variclla zoster virus (VZV), is a human alpha-herpesvirus closely related to HSV. Primary infection causes varicella (chickenpox), and reactivation of latent virus causes herpes zoster (shingles). VZV is ubiquitous in human populations around the world, and humans are the only known host. During the prevaccine era in the United States, approximately 4 million cases, 4,000 to 9,000 hospitalizations, and 50 to 140 deaths were reported annually. VZV-related deaths have declined sharply in the United States, however, since universal childhood vaccination was implemented in 1995.

CLINICAL FEATURES

Primary infection with VZV occurs by inoculation of respiratory mucosa with infectious aerosols or by direct contact with skin lesions of patients with varicella or herpes zoster. After a primary viremia in the reticuloendothelial system, and secondary viremia in circulating mononuclear cells, the virus is disseminated to the skin, where it initiates a pruritic vesicular rash (chickenpox), and is disseminated back to mucosal sites in the lungs. The attack rate for previously uninfected household contacts exposed to varicella is approximately 90%. VZV also establishes latent infection within satellite cells and neurons of the trigeminal and dorsal root ganglia and can reactivate under various conditions to cause herpes zoster, a painful unilateral vesicular eruption distributed in a dermatomal distribution. Although chickenpox is usually a relatively benign infection in children, adult patients are approximately 25 times more likely than children to develop pneumonia. Pneumonia occurs in approximately 10-15% of adults primarily infected with VZV; however, the incidence of pneumonia in bone marrow transplant recipients and acute leukemia patients may be as high as 30-45%. The greatest risk of severe

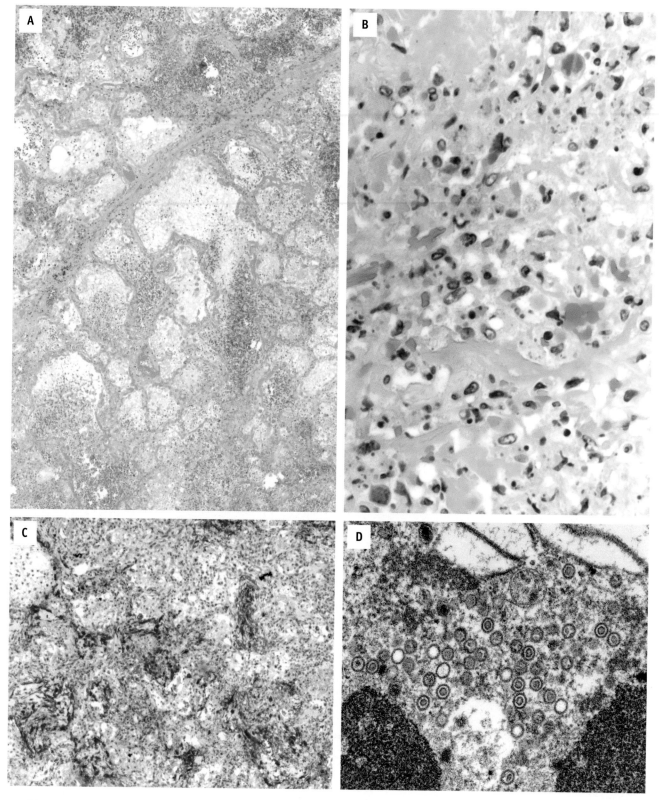

FIGURE 13-5

Herpes simplex virus pneumonia

(A) Extensive necrosis and hemorrhage associated with HSV pneumonia. **(B)** Glassy, amphophilic, intranuclear inclusions in HSV-infected cells at the margin of a necrotic focus in the lung. **(C)** Immunohistochemical localization of HSV in a patient with fatal HSV pneumonia (immunoalkaline phosphatase). **(D)** Ultrastructural view of HSV-infected cell showing complete enveloped virions in the cytoplasm. (Courtesy of Cynthia Goldsmith, Centers for Disease Control and Prevention, Atlanta, Georgia).

Definition

» Human herpes simplex viruses (HSV) are large, enveloped, double-stranded DNA-viruses that exist in two serologic types
  » HSV-1 is the serotype most commonly associated with adult HSV pneumonia
  » HSV-2 is the serotype associated with approximately 80% of disseminated disease and pulmonary infections in newborn infants

Incidence and Location

» Worldwide distribution
» Newborn infants, severely immunosuppressed or burned patients, and patients with severe trauma are at greatest risk of developing HSV pneumonia
» Most cases of neonatal disease represent primary HSV infections and are acquired during parturition from HSV-infected mothers; the incidence of neonatal HSV infection is approximately 1 in 3,200 deliveries

Mortality

» Prior to the discovery and use of antiviral therapies, 85% of neonates with disseminated HSV disease died from the infection
» With early diagnosis and high-dose acyclovir therapy, mortality has been reduced to approximately 30%

Gender, Race, and Age Distribution

» People of all ages are susceptible
» No recognized gender or racial predilection

Clinical Features

» In adults, infection of the respiratory tract with HSV may be associated with disseminated herpetic infection, but is more commonly identified as an isolated disease manifestation resulting from reactivation of latent herpetic infections in the oropharynx
» Disseminated disease develops in approximately 25% of infected neonates; approximately 40-50% of these patients develop pneumonia
» Infants with disseminated neonatal HSV infections first show signs and symptoms a mean of 5 days after birth (range, 0 to 12 days). As the disease progresses, the clinical picture often resembles bacterial sepsis, evolving rapidly to pneumonia, shock, and disseminated vascular coagulopathy

Radiologic Features

» Ill-defined nodular or reticular densities of various sizes scattered in both lung fields
» During the early stages of disease, these nodules measure 2-5 mm and are best seen in the periphery of the lungs; as the disease progresses, these lesions coalesce and enlarge to form more extensive segmental and subsegmental infiltrates
» Pleural effusions are commonly identified

Therapy

» Antiviral therapies include acyclovir, valacyclovir, and famcyclovir
» Foscarnet has been used effectively in some acyclovir-resistant patients

Gross Findings

» HSV tracheobronchitis: 5-15 mm ulcers covered by fibrinopurulent exudate on the mucous membranes of the large airways
» HSV pneumonia acquired through the airways: lungs are heavy and show nodular hemorrhagic foci that are generally distributed around bronchi and bronchioles
» Hematogenously acquired HSV pneumonia: hemorrhagic foci have a random or miliary distribution

Microscopic Findings

» HSV tracheobronchitis: large areas of denuded epithelium and exudate containing necrotic cells; cells with intranuclear inclusions may be sparse and are found most often at the margins of the ulcerated epithelium or occasionally in the mucous glands below the ulcerated mucosa
» HSV pneumonia: lesions show hemorrhage and necrosis with karyorrhectic debris; intranuclear inclusions are best appreciated in cells at the edge of necrotic foci
» Inclusions appear as homogeneous, amphophilic, and glassy or as eosinophilic with a halo separating the inclusion from the nuclear membrane
» Multinucleation and nuclear molding, ground-glass nuclear chromatin, and ballooning degeneration of the cytoplasm are more frequently associated with squamous epithelia and less often encountered in the lung

Immunohistochemical Features

» IHC testing of formalin-fixed tissues is a sensitive method to confirm HSV infections; antibodies reactive with both HSV-1 and HSV-2 are commercially available

Ultrastructural Features

» Virus particles are encapsulated and approximately 100-110 nm in diameter
» Individual particles demonstrate a targetoid appearance and are arranged in a lattice-like pattern

Pathologic Differential Diagnosis

» Varicella-zoster virus pneumonia
» Adenovirus pneumonia
» Measles pneumonia
» CMV pneumonia

disease and pneumonia occurs in those patients with chronic lung disease, immune-suppressing conditions, neonates, and pregnant women. The occurrence of pneumonia during herpes zoster is rare, and limited primarily to profoundly immunosuppressed patients, particularly bone marrow transplant recipients. VZV pneumonia develops 2 to 7 days following the onset of rash and is characterized by fever, cough, tachypnea, chest pain, and hemoptysis. Massive pulmonary hemorrhage and pulmonary infarcts are frequent terminal events. Hematopoietic cell transplant recipients may present with signs of visceral dissemination and pneumonia 1 to 4 days before the localized cutaneous eruption of herpes zoster appears, and lower respiratory tract disease has been described in the absence of skin lesions, particularly in neonates and bone marrow transplant recipients.

RADIOLOGIC FEATURES

The lungs show multifocal, bilateral, poorly defined nodular densities that measure 5-10 mm in greatest dimension. These opacities may coalesce to form more extensive areas of consolidation. Hilar adenopathy may also occur, but pleural effusions are uncommon. Some patients who survive VZV pneumonia show persistent parenchymal nodules that may mineralize and persist as small (2-3 mm) calcifications, predominantly in the lower zones of the lungs.

PATHOLOGIC FEATURES

GROSS FINDINGS

The lungs of patients with fatal VZV pneumonia are 2 to 3 times heavier than normal, firm, and plum-colored. There are often multiple necrotic and hemorrhagic lesions on the visceral and parietal pleura that resemble the pox lesions of skin. The trachea and bronchi are generally edematous and erythematous with occasional vesicles on the mucosal surfaces, and there may be lobular consolidation of the lungs as well as randomly distributed hemorrhagic lesions.

MICROSCOPIC FINDINGS

The lungs show interstitial pneumonitis and diffuse miliary foci of necrosis and hemorrhage in the pulmonary parenchyma involving alveolar walls, blood vessels, and bronchioles (Figure 13-6A,B). Other findings can include intra-alveolar collections of edema, fibrin, or hemorrhage, diffuse alveolar damage, and septal edema. Virally infected cells with intranuclear inclusions may be identified in respiratory epithelial cells of the trachea and bronchi, pneumocytes, interstitial fibroblasts, or capillary endothelium. Eosinophilic intranuclear inclusions and multinucleated syncytial cells may be difficult to locate but are best identified at the edges of necrotic foci. In cases of disseminated disease, similar necrotizing hemorrhagic lesions and occasional viral cytopathic changes in epithelial cells or fibroblasts may be observed in many other tissues and organs.

ANCILLARY STUDIES

Because pulmonary symptoms most often occur several days following the onset of the characteristic rash of varicella, a pathologic diagnosis is seldom required for a real-time diagnosis of VZV pneumonia. Antigen detection kits using fluorescein-conjugated VZV monoclonal antibodies can be helpful for rapid diagnosis of cutaneous VZV infection. Antibodies are also commercially available for IHC detection of VZV in tissue specimens (Figure 13-6C); however, relatively few laboratories are able to provide well-validated assays. Some commercial laboratories offer PCR amplification to detect viral nucleic acid in clinical specimens. Isolation of the virus in cell culture remains the reference standard for the diagnosis of VZV. Infectious VZV is usually recoverable from the clear fluid of cutaneous vesicles of varicella for approximately 3 days after the appearance of these lesions and for approximately 1 week from herpes zoster lesions. By using electron microscopy, VZV has an icosahedral nucleocapsid that is indistinguishable in appearance from other herpesviruses. The enveloped viral particle is pleomorphic to spherical in shape and 180-200 nm in diameter.

DIFFERENTIAL DIAGNOSIS

The histopathologic appearance of VZV pneumonia most closely resembles disease caused by HSV with respect to the general pattern of lung injury (e.g., multicentric, necrotizing, and hemorrhagic lesions) and to the appearance of the glassy intranuclear inclusions.

PROGNOSIS AND THERAPY

The U.S. incidence of varicella pneumonia declined markedly since universal childhood vaccination for varicella was implemented in 1995. Vaccine efficacy at preventing severe disease is approximately 97%. Untreated adult varicella pneumonia is fatal in approximately 10% of cases, but mortality is as high as 25% to 40% in certain high-risk cohorts, including pregnant women, transplant recipients, and neonates. Intravenous acyclovir is recommended for use in all patients for whom the risk of disseminated disease is particularly high or unpredictable, including patients with leukemia, bone marrow transplant recipients, and severely immune suppressed persons.

INFLUENZA VIRUSES

Influenza viruses belong to the *Orthomyxoviridae* family, and include the two important influenza viruses, types A and B, which are associated with significant human disease. All influenza viruses have a segmented, negative-sense RNA core surrounded by a lipid envelope. Influenza A viruses are further classified into subtypes

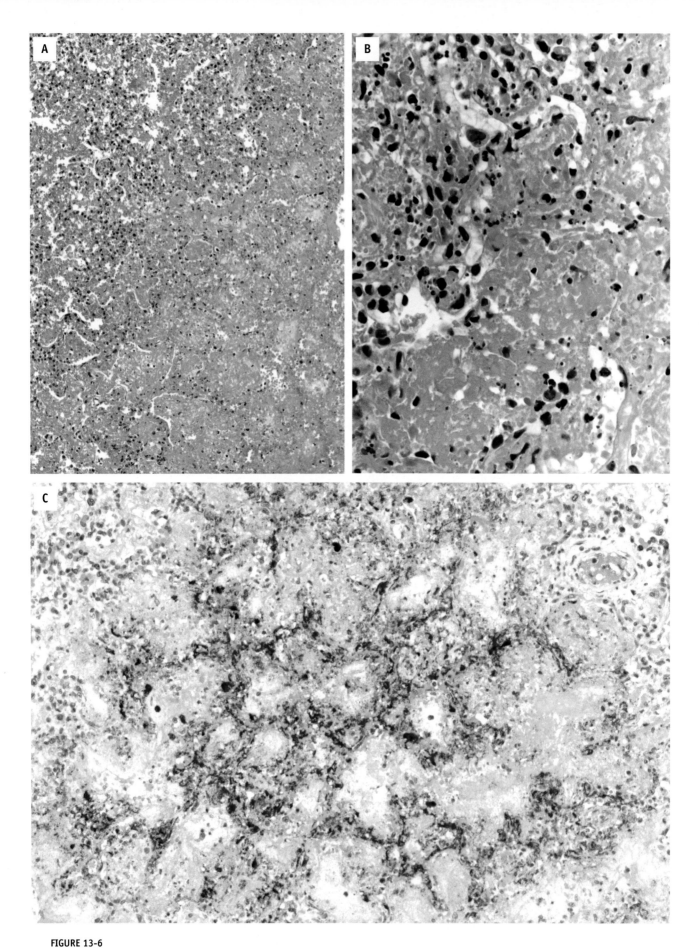

FIGURE 13-6

Varicella zoster virus pneumonia
(A) The periphery of a necrotic and hemorrhagic lesion in a case of fatal VZV pneumonia. (B) Eosinophilic intranuclear inclusions in VZV-infected cells at the edge of a necrotic focus. (C) Immunohistochemical staining of VZV antigens in a patient with fatal VZV pneumonia (immunoalkaline phosphatase).

VARICELLA ZOSTER VIRUS—FACT SHEET

Definition

▸▸ Primary infection causes varicella (chickenpox) and reactivation of latent virus causes herpes zoster (shingles)

Incidence and Location

▸▸ Ubiquitous worldwide pathogen, and humans are the only known host
▸▸ Highly contagious virus; the attack rate for previously uninfected household contacts exposed to varicella is approximately 90%
▸▸ The U.S. incidence of varicella pneumonia has dropped by two-thirds since universal childhood vaccination for varicella was implemented in 1995

Mortality

▸▸ Untreated adult varicella pneumonia is fatal in approximately 10% of cases
▸▸ Mortality is as high as 25-40% in certain high-risk cohorts, including pregnant women, transplant recipients, and neonates

Gender, Race, and Age Distribution

▸▸ Adult patients with varicella are approximately 25 times more likely than children to develop pneumonia; pneumonia occurs in approximately 10-15% of adults infected with VZV
▸▸ The greatest risk of severe disease and pneumonia occurs in those patients with chronic lung disease, immune-suppressing conditions, neonates, and pregnant women
▸▸ The incidence of pneumonia in bone marrow transplant recipients and acute leukemia patients infected with varicella may be as high as 30-45%
▸▸ No apparent gender or racial predilection

Clinical Features

▸▸ Primary infection occurs by inoculation of respiratory mucosa with infectious aerosols or by direct contact with skin lesions of patients with varicella or herpes zoster
▸▸ VZV pneumonia generally develops within 2 to 7 days following the onset of rash and may be characterized by fever, cough, tachypnea, chest pain, and hemoptysis

Radiologic Features

▸▸ Multifocal, bilateral, poorly defined nodular densities that measure 5-10 mm in greatest dimension, and may coalesce to form more extensive areas of consolidation
▸▸ Pleural effusions are uncommon
▸▸ Some survivors of VZV pneumonia show persistent parenchymal nodules that mineralize and persist as small (2-3 mm) calcifications, predominantly in the lower zones of the lungs

Prognosis and Therapy

▸▸ Intravenous acyclovir is recommended for use in all patients for whom the risk of disseminated disease is particularly likely or unpredictable, including patients with leukemia, bone marrow transplant recipients, and severely immune-suppressed persons

VARICELLA-ZOSTER VIRUS—PATHOLOGIC FEATURES

Gross Findings

▸▸ Trachea and bronchi are generally edematous and erythematous with occasional vesicles or ulcers on the mucosal surfaces
▸▸ The lungs are generally 2 to 3 times heavier than normal, firm, and "plum-colored"
▸▸ There are often multiple necrotic and hemorrhagic lesions on the pleura and in the lung parenchyma that resemble the pox lesions of skin

Microscopic Findings

▸▸ Interstitial pneumonitis and diffuse miliary foci of necrosis and hemorrhage in the pulmonary parenchyma
▸▸ Other findings may include alveolar collections of edema, fibrin, or hemorrhage, diffuse alveolar damage, and septal edema
▸▸ Virally infected cells with intranuclear inclusions may be identified in respiratory epithelial cells of the trachea and bronchi, pneumocytes, interstitial fibroblasts, or capillary endothelium
▸▸ Eosinophilic intranuclear inclusions and multinucleated syncytial cells may be difficult to locate but are best identified at the edges of necrotic foci
▸▸ In disseminated disease, similar necrotizing hemorrhagic lesions and occasional viral cytopathic changes are observed in other tissues and organs

Immunohistochemical Features

▸▸ IHC testing of formalin-fixed tissues is a sensitive method to confirm VZV infection and distinguish it from other viral infections, particularly HSV

Ultrastructural Features

▸▸ The enveloped viral particle is pleomorphic to spherical and 180-200 nm in diameter
▸▸ Viral particles are located within the nuclei of infected cells

Pathologic Differential Diagnosis

▸▸ HSV pneumonia (histology is identical)
▸▸ Adenovirus pneumonia
▸▸ Measles pneumonia
▸▸ CMV pneumonia

based on the antigenicity of their hemagglutinin (HA) and neuraminidase (NA) surface glycoproteins. Only one type of HA and one type of NA are recognized for influenza B. Influenza A occurs in both pandemic and interpandemic forms. The epidemiologic pattern of influenza in humans is related to two types of antigenic variation of its envelope glycoproteins, namely antigenic drift and antigenic shift. Fortunately, pandemics, defined as worldwide outbreaks of severe disease, occur infrequently and result from antigenic shift and emergence of new potentially pandemic influenza A viruses that possess a novel HA alone or in combination with a novel NA. Interpandemic influenza occurs virtually every year as a result of antigenic drift resulting from point mutations in the surface glycoproteins, and emergence of new strains related to those circulating in previous epidemics. This enables the virus to evade the immune system, leading to repeated outbreaks during interpandemic years.

CLINICAL FEATURES

Influenza viruses are spread person-to-person primarily through the coughing and sneezing of infected persons. The typical incubation period is 1 to 4 days. Adults can be infectious from the day before symptoms begin through approximately 5 days after illness onset. Children can be infectious for 10 or more days, and young children can shed virus for several days before their illness onset. Severely immunocompromised persons can shed virus for weeks or months. Respiratory illness caused by influenza is difficult to distinguish from illnesses caused by other respiratory pathogens on the basis of symptoms alone. Uncomplicated influenza illness is characterized by the abrupt onset of constitutional and respiratory signs and symptoms including fever, myalgia, headache, malaise, nonproductive cough, sore throat, and rhinitis. Among children, otitis media, nausea, and vomiting are also commonly reported. Influenza typically resolves after 3 to 7 days in most patients, although cough and malaise can persist for more than 2 weeks. Complications include secondary bacterial pneumonias, febrile seizures, and, uncommonly, encephalopathy, transverse myelitis, Reye's syndrome, myositis, myocarditis, and pericarditis. The risks for complications, hospitalizations, and deaths from influenza are higher among persons aged 65 years or older, young children, and persons of any age with certain underlying health conditions, than among healthy older children and younger adults.

RADIOLOGIC FEATURES

The main findings include unilateral or bilateral patchy consolidation of the lungs, which may progress to confluent lung disease. Pleural effusions are uncommon.

PATHOLOGIC FEATURES

GROSS FINDINGS

Lungs in influenza virus pneumonia, not associated with a bacterial infection, can have different degrees of hemorrhage and edema. Airways can be filled with varying amounts of exudate, and the mucosae of the trachea and large bronchi are hyperemic and swollen. Cross-sections of the lungs show a more or less granular appearance, in which the lower lobes are more affected than the upper lobes. The gross pathologic features in secondary infections depend largely on the specific microbial (usually bacterial)

pathogen involved. The mucosae of the large airways can demonstrate hyperemia, hemorrhages, or purulent necrotic debris. In the lungs, the extent of the pathologic process in the lower lobes is generally greater than the upper and may include consolidation, abscesses, hemorrhages, and empyema. Secondary inflammation in the regional lymph nodes may be present. Purulent mediastinitis and pericarditis may also be found in some cases.

MICROSCOPIC FINDINGS

The histopathologic features of non-fatal and fatal influenza include necrotizing bronchitis, diffuse alveolar damage, hemorrhage, edema, and thrombi. The pathology is more prominent in larger bronchi, and inflammation may vary in intensity (Figure 13-7A-C). Viral inclusions cannot be identified by light microscopy (Figure 13-7F). Secondary bacterial infections with organisms such as *Streptococcus pneumoniae,* group A Streptococcus, *Staphylococcus aureus*, and *Haemophilus influenzae* may occur as a complication in about 50-75% of fatal cases and make it difficult to recognize the pathologic changes associated with the primary viral infection. The histopathologic features in other organs may include myocarditis, cerebral edema, rhabdomyolysis, and hemophagocytosis (Figures 13-8A,B).

Recent studies suggest that, unlike human influenza viruses, avian virus H5N1 preferentially infects cells in the lower respiratory tract of humans, resulting in extensive damage of the lungs with minimal pathology in the upper respiratory tract (Figures 13-8C,D). This may explain why the H5N1 avian influenza virus is so lethal to humans but so difficult to spread from person to person. These studies show that the avian virus preferentially binds to the α-2,3 galactose receptors, which are found only in and around the alveoli. This is in contrast to the human influenza viruses which preferentially bind to the α-2,6 receptors, which are found throughout the respiratory tract from the nose to the lungs.

ANCILLARY STUDIES AND DIFFERENTIAL DIAGNOSIS

Because of the absence of any characteristic viral inclusions and because the overall pathologic features of influenza may resemble other viral, rickettsial, and certain bacterial infections, an unequivocal diagnosis can be made only by laboratory tests such as viral culture, direct fluorescent antibody and rapid antigen assays, serology, IHC, and ISH. IHC and ISH assays can demonstrate viral antigens and nucleic acids in epithelial cells of small airways (Figure 13-7D,E,G). Antigens are more readily identified in patients who die within 3 to 4 days of onset of illness..

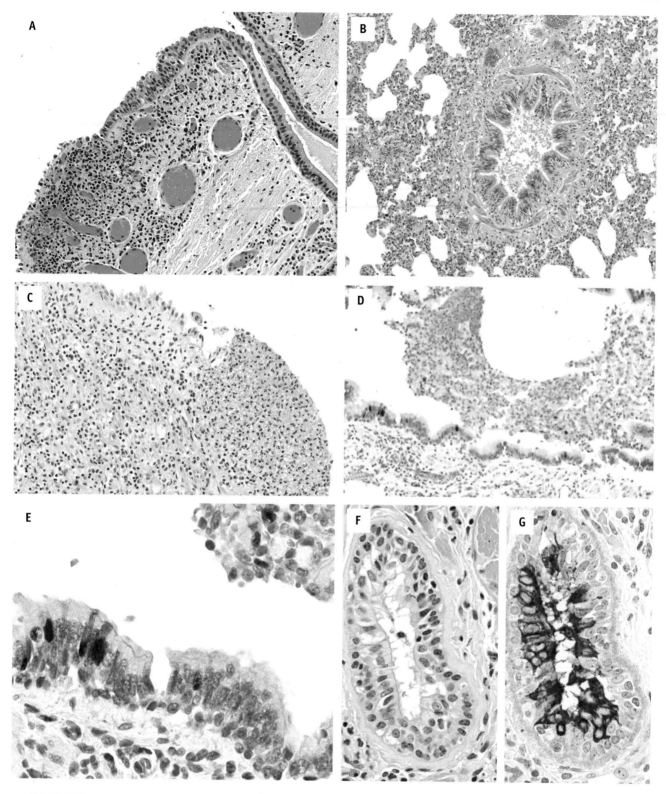

FIGURE 13-7

Influenza

(A) Trachea from a child with fatal influenza B showing congestion and predominantly mononuclear inflammatory cell infiltrates in the lamina propria and submucosa. **(B)** Bronchiole containing necrotic debris and surrounding congested lung parenchyma in a patient with fatal influenza B. **(C)** Ulcerated respiratory epithelium in a large airway of a patient with fatal influenza B. **(D, E)** Immunohistochemical staining of influenza B virus in the respiratory epithelium of an airway (immunoalkaline phosphatase). **(F, G)** Respiratory epithelial cells infected by influenza A, demonstrated with an immunohistochemical stain for hemagglutinin antigen **(G)** (immunoalkaline phosphatase).

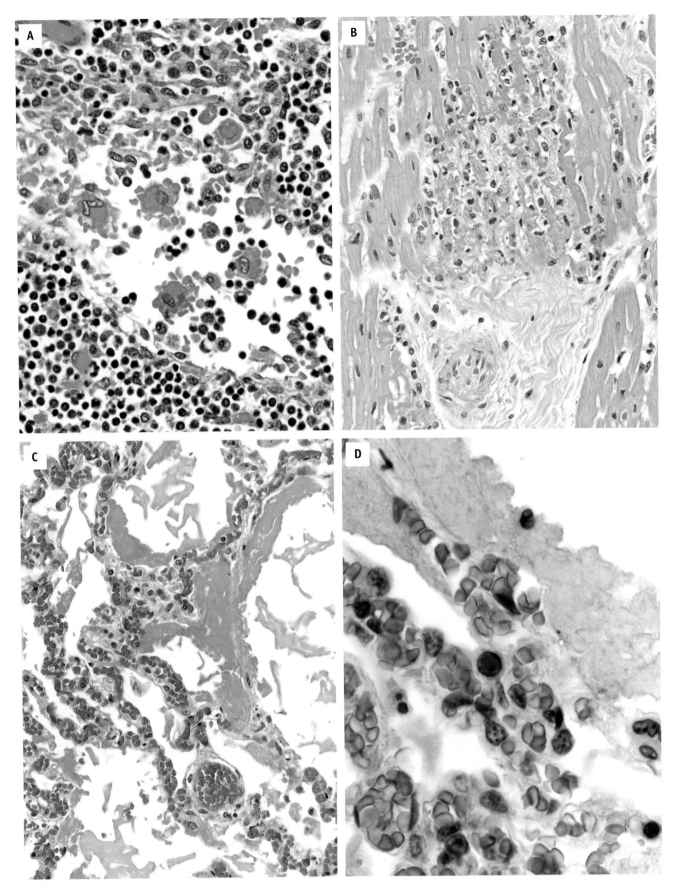

FIGURE 13-8

Influenza

(A) Hemophagocytosis in a peribronchial lymph node in a patient with fatal influenza B. **(B)** Focus of myocyte necrosis accompanied by a mixed inflammatory cell infiltrate in the heart of a patient with fatal influenza B. **(C)** Diffuse alveolar damage in a patient with fatal avian influenza (H5N1) showing hyaline membrane formation and congestion. **(D)** Influenza virus A (H5N1) antigens in the nucleus of a pneumocyte of a patient with fatal avian influenza (immunoalkaline phosphatase). Unlike other influenza viruses that cause disease in humans, H5N1 preferentially infects alveolar epithelial cells, and causes relatively minimal pathology in the upper respiratory tract.

PROGNOSIS AND THERAPY

Vaccination is an important strategy in the prevention of influenza virus infections. Influenza is seldom fatal in the immunocompetent host, and recovery is usually complete. Supportive management with bed rest, hydration, and antipyretics is the basis of treatment. Antiviral agents may be helpful early in the course of illness. NA, a major antigenic determinant of influenza viruses, catalyses the cleavage of glycosidic linkages to sialic acid and the release of progeny virions from infected cells. Accordingly, it has become an important target for drug inhibitors such as oseltamivir and zanamivir. The M2 surface component and channel of influenza A (not present in influenza B virus) regulates the internal pH of the virus and is blocked by the antiviral drug amantidine.

MEASLES

Measles (rubeola) is an infectious, acute febrile viral illness characterized by upper respiratory tract symptoms, fever, and a maculopapular rash. The causative agent, a member of the genus *Morbillivirus*, of the family *Paramyxoviridae,* is an enveloped virus that contains a negative sense, single-stranded RNA genome. Measles has a worldwide distribution. Although still a significant problem in underdeveloped countries, measles infection became uncommon in the United States after the development and widespread use of an effective measles vaccine. However, a recrudescence of measles infection occurred in several large U.S. urban centers in recent years, associated with reduced use of the vaccine among children and young adults.

CLINICAL FEATURES

Measles virus is highly contagious and is spread by aerosols and droplets from respiratory secretions of acute cases. Children are usually infected by 6 years of age, resulting in lifelong immunity, and almost all adults are immune either from vaccination or exposure. Clinical infection in children younger than 9 months of age is generally uncommon because of passive protection afforded the infant by the transfer of maternal antibodies, although occasional infections have occurred in this age group. A person with acute measles is infective from just before the onset of symptoms to the end of fever. After an incubation period of about 1 to 2 weeks, the prodromal phase of measles begins with fever, rhinorrhea, cough, and conjunctivitis. Koplik's spots, which are small, irregular red spots with a bluish-white speck

in the center, appear on the buccal mucosa in 50-90% of cases shortly before rash onset. An erythematous maculopapular rash begins on the face 3 to 4 days after prodromal symptoms and usually spreads to the trunk and extremities. The symptoms gradually resolve, with the rash lasting for approximately 6 days, fading in the same order as it appeared.

RADIOLOGIC FEATURES

Chest radiographs typically show fine reticular and ground-glass opacities as well as nodules and patchy consolidation. Bronchial thickening and peribronchial opacities may also be observed in some patients. Pleural effusions are rare.

PATHOLOGIC FEATURES

GROSS FINDINGS

In fatal cases, the lungs are heavy and show congestion, hemorrhage, and edema. The gross pathologic features in secondary infections depend largely on the specific microbial (usually bacterial) pathogen involved.

MICROSCOPIC FINDINGS

A focal or generalized interstitial pneumonitis, similar to that seen in many other viral infections, is seen in the lungs of measles patients. Histopathologic features include various degrees of peribronchial and interstitial mononuclear cell infiltrates, squamous metaplasia of bronchial endothelium, proliferation of type II pneumocytes, and intra-alveolar edema with or without mononuclear cell exudates and hyaline membranes. Secondary changes created by bacterial or viral superinfection or organizational changes, may alter the original pathology. The hallmark of the disease is the formation of multinucleated epithelial giant cells. These cells, which are often numerous, are formed by fusion of bronchiolar or alveolar lining cells (Figure 13-9A). These cells generally contain characteristic nuclear and cytoplasmic inclusions. The intranuclear inclusions are homogenous, eosinophilic, and surrounded by a slight indistinct halo (Figure 13-9B). The cytoplasmic inclusions are deeply eosinophilic and may form large masses with a "melted tallow" appearance (Figure 13-9B). These giant cells may undergo degenerative changes with progressive loss of cytoplasm, increasing basophilia, and shrinkage of nuclei. The presence of measles virus in these giant cells may be demonstrated by immunofluorescence, IHC, and ISH techniques (Figures 13-9C,D). These giant cells can also be seen in extrapulmonary tissues (Figure 13-9E).

INFLUENZA—FACT SHEET

Definition

»» Influenza viruses belong to the *Orthomyxoviridae* family and include the two important influenza virus types, A and B, which are associated with significant human disease

»» All influenza viruses have a segmented, negative-sense RNA core surrounded by a lipid envelope

»» Influenza A viruses are further classified into subtypes based on the antigenicity of their hemagglutinin (HA) and neuraminidase (NA) surface glycoproteins

»» There are 16 recognized HA subtypes and 9 NA subtypes of influenza A virus

»» Only one type of HA and one type of NA are recognized for influenza B

Incidence and Location

»» Worldwide distributions

»» Influenza A occurs in both pandemic and interpandemic forms

Morbidity and Mortality

»» Seldom fatal in the immunocompetent host, and recovery is usually complete

»» Mortality and risk for complications from influenza are higher among persons aged 65 years or older, young children, and persons of any age with certain underlying health conditions

»» Secondary bacterial pneumonias with organisms such as *Streptococcus pneumoniae*, group A streptococcus, *Staphylococcus aureus*, and *Haemophilus influenzae* may occur as a complication

Gender, Race, and Age Distribution

»» People of all ages are vulnerable to influenza pneumonia

»» No recognized gender or racial predilection

Clinical Features

»» Spread primarily through the coughing and sneezing of infected persons

»» Typical incubation period is 1 to 4 days

»» Uncomplicated influenza illness is characterized by the abrupt onset of fever, myalgia, headache, malaise, nonproductive cough, sore throat, and rhinitis

Radiologic Features

»» Unilateral or bilateral consolidation of the lungs

»» Rarely associated with pleural effusions

Therapy and Prevention

»» Vaccination is an important preventive strategy

»» Supportive therapy, such as bed rest, oral hydration, and antipyretics

»» Antivirals such as oseltamivir, zanamivir, and amantadine may be helpful early in the course of infection

»» Specific antibiotic therapy in cases with secondary bacterial infection

INFLUENZA—PATHOLOGIC FEATURES

Gross Findings

»» Airways show hyperemia, hemorrhage, and edema and may be filled with exudate

»» Cross-sections of the lungs have a granular appearance, in which the lower lobes are more affected than the upper lobes

»» Gross pathologic features in secondary infections depend largely on the specific microbial (usually bacterial) pathogen involved, and include consolidation, abscess formation, hemorrhage, and empyema

Microscopic Findings

»» Necrotizing bronchitis and tracheitis

»» Diffuse alveolar damage

»» Thrombi

»» Hemorrhage

»» Edema

»» Viral inclusions cannot be identified by light microscopy

Immunohistochemical Features

»» IHC is extremely valuable for confirming infection

»» Influenzaviral antigens are usually sparse and are primarily seen in the epithelial cells of larger airways

»» Antigens are more readily identified in patients who die within 3 to 4 days of onset of illness

Ultrastructural Features

»» Viral particles are pleomorphic (filamentous and spherical)

»» A 10-12 nm layer of HA (rod-shaped) and NA (mushroom-shaped) spikes project radially from the surfaces of the influenza A and B viruses

Pathologic Differential Diagnosis

»» A large number of viral, rickettsial, bacterial infections, as well as non-infectious diseases, may have similar histologic features

»» Unequivocal diagnosis can be made by laboratory tests such as viral culture, direct fluorescent antibody and rapid antigen assays, serology and IHC

fluorescence or by serologic methods using hemagglutination inhibition, neutralization, or enzyme immunoassay. Specimens for serologic testing consist of acute and convalescent-phase serum pairs. The presence of specific IgM antibody can be used to diagnose recent infection. IHC and ISH can be performed on tissue specimens. Ultrastructurally, measles virions are pleomorphic, generally spherical, enveloped particles from 120-250 nm in diameter, with a lipid envelope surrounding a helical nucleocapsid composed of RNA and protein.

ANCILLARY STUDIES

Laboratory confirmation is useful to avoid possible confusion with other rash-causing illnesses. Diagnostic laboratory procedures consist of either direct detection of the virus or viral antigens, usually by indirect immuno-

DIFFERENTIAL DIAGNOSIS

In typical cases, the diagnosis of measles can usually be made on the basis of clinical signs and symptoms. Other causes of a similar rash, but without other features of

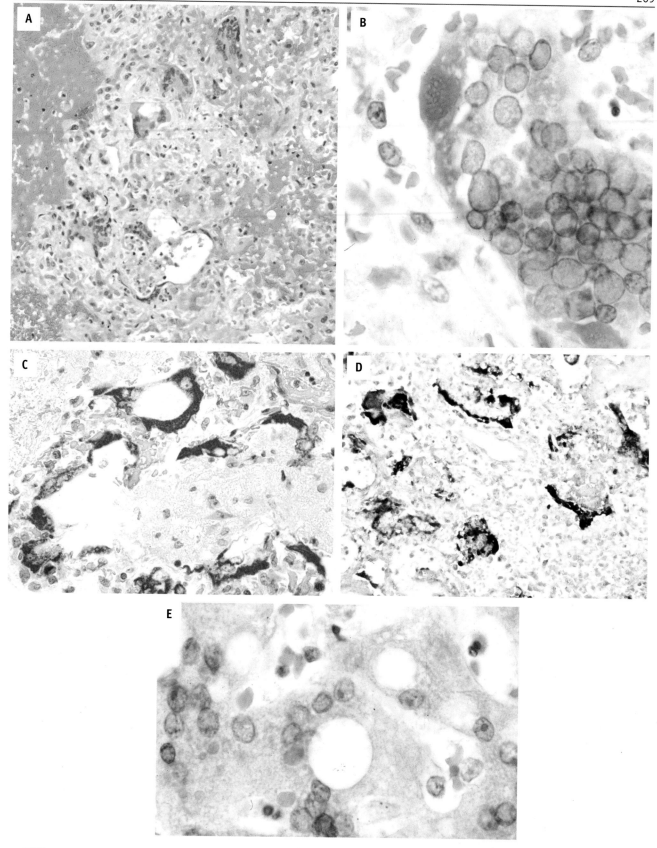

FIGURE 13-9

Measles pneumonia

(A) Multinucleated giant cells generally line the alveoli, although some are found lying free within alveolar spaces. **(B)** Multinucleated giant cell with eosinophilic cytoplasmic inclusions. The inclusions may be large and have a characteristic "melted tallow" appearance. Intranuclear inclusions are also seen, but are ill-defined, eosinophilic, and lack clear circumscription. **(C)** Viral antigens in the cytoplasm of giant cells, highlighted by immunohistochemistry (immunoalkaline phosphatase). **(D)** Numerous measles giant cells are seen by chromogenic in situ hybridization (digoxigenin-labeled probes followed by immunoalkaline phosphatase). **(E)** Multinucleated epithelial giant cells in the liver from a fatal case of measles.

measles, include rubella, dengue virus, enteroviruses, and drug reactions, especially to ampicillin. The histologic diagnosis is facilitated by the identification of the characteristic giant cells in a setting of interstitial pneumonitis. These giant cells are not seen in all cases of measles pneumonia, however, and their absence should not exclude the diagnosis. Furthermore, other viral pathogens, such as respiratory syncytial virus, parainfluenza, metapneumovirus, VZV, and the recently discovered Henipa viruses, may also give rise to pneumonias with giant cells and should be considered in the differential diagnosis. IHC or ISH testing can demonstrate viral antigens or nucleic acids in the majority of cases, assisting in the histologic diagnosis.

PROGNOSIS AND THERAPY

Supportive therapy, such as bed rest, oral hydration, and antipyretics usually produces rapid and complete recovery. Immune globulins can be useful if treatment is given early in the infection. Vaccination can also be helpful in the treatment regimen if given within 3 days of exposure. In a smaller number of patients, complications can arise as a result of continued and progressive virus replication, bacterial or viral superinfections, or abnormal host immune response. The most common complications are secondary bacterial pneumonia and otitis media. In these settings, specific antibiotic therapy is administered. Other complications include febrile convulsions, encephalitis, liver function abnormalities, chronic diarrhea, and sinusitis. Several pulmonary and central nervous system syndromes that are often fatal have been described. Death occurs in about 1 of every 1000 measles cases; however, the risk of death and other complications is substantially increased in infants, malnourished and immunocompromised individuals, persons with underlying illnesses, and non-immunized populations in underdeveloped countries.

HUMAN PARAINFLUENZA VIRUSES

Human parainfluenza viruses (HPIVs) are second only to respiratory syncytial virus (RSV) as a cause of lower respiratory tract disease in young children. HPIVs are negative-sense, nonsegmented, single-stranded, enveloped RNA viruses that possess fusion and hemagglutinin-neuraminidase glycoprotein "spikes" on their surface. The four serotypes of HPIV belong in the family *Paramyxoviridae*, subfamily *Paramyxovirinae*, and genera *Respirovirus* (HPIV-1 and -3) and *Rubulavirus* (HPIV-2 and -4).

CLINICAL FEATURES

HPIVs are spread from respiratory secretions through close contact with infected persons or contact with contaminated surfaces or objects. Infection can occur when infectious material contacts mucous membranes of the eyes, mouth, or nose, and possibly through the inhalation of droplets generated by a sneeze or cough. HPIVs are ubiquitous and infect most people during childhood. Serologic surveys have shown that 90-100% of children aged 5 years and older have antibodies to HPIV-3, and about 75% have antibodies to HPIV-1 and -2. The different HPIV serotypes differ in clinical presentations, with HPIV-1 and HPIV-2 most frequently associated with outbreaks of croup and HPIV-3 more often associated with bronchiolitis and pneumonia. HPIV-4 is infrequently detected, possibly because it is less likely to cause severe disease. The incubation period is generally from 1 to 7 days. The HPIVs can also cause repeated infections throughout life, usually manifested by an upper respiratory tract illness (e.g., cold and sore throat). Serious lower respiratory tract disease (e.g., pneumonia, bronchitis, and bronchiolitis) can also occur with repeat infection, especially among the elderly, and among patients with compromised immunity.

RADIOLOGIC FEATURES

The main findings associated with HPIV pneumonia include diffuse interstitial opacities, bronchial wall thickening, and peribronchial consolidation. Infection is rarely associated with pleural effusions.

PATHOLOGIC FEATURES

GROSS FINDINGS

In fatal cases, the lungs are typically heavy and display congestion, hemorrhage, and edema.

MICROSCOPIC FINDINGS

In patients with severe HPIV infection, multinucleated giant cells derived from the respiratory epithelium may be seen in association with an interstitial pneumonitis, diffuse alveolar damage, bronchiolitis, and organizing changes (Figure 13-10A,B). These giant cells, which may contain intracytoplasmic eosinophilic inclusions (Figure 13-10B), have also been reported in extrapulmonary tissues such as kidney, bladder, and pancreas.

Definition

▸ Measles virus is a single-stranded RNA virus and a member of the genus *Morbillivirus*, of the family *Paramyxoviridae*

Incidence and Location

▸ Highly communicable disease of worldwide distribution
▸ A significant problem in underdeveloped countries
▸ Uncommon infection in the United States after the widespread use of the vaccine

Morbidity and Mortality

▸ The most common complications are secondary bacterial pneumonia and otitis media
▸ Death occurs in about 1 of every 1,000 patients with measles
▸ The risk of death and other complications is substantially increased in infants, malnourished and immunocompromised individuals, persons with underlying illnesses, and non-immunized populations

Gender, Race, and Age Distribution

▸ Infection in children younger than 9 months of age is uncommon because of passive protection from immune mothers
▸ Children (non-vaccinated) are usually infected by 6 years of age
▸ Natural infection results in lifelong immunity and almost all adults are immune either due to exposure or vaccination
▸ No recognized gender or racial predilection

Clinical Features

▸ Typical incubation period is 1 to 2 weeks
▸ Brief prodrome characterized by fever, rhinorrhea, cough, and conjunctivitis
▸ Koplik's spots can be seen in the buccal mucosa shortly before rash onset
▸ An erythematous maculopapular rash begins on the face 3 to 4 days after prodromal symptoms and usually spreads to the trunk and extremities
▸ The rash lasts for approximately 6 days, fading in the same order as it appeared

Radiologic Features

▸ Fine reticular and ground-glass opacities in the lungs
▸ Nodules and patchy consolidation throughout the lungs may be seen
▸ Rarely associated with pleural effusions

Prognosis and Therapy

▸ Recovery is rapid and complete in most cases
▸ Supportive therapy is administered, such as bed rest, oral hydration, and antipyretics
▸ Immune globulins can be useful if treatment is given early in the infection
▸ Vaccination can also be helpful if given within 3 days of exposure

Gross Findings

▸ Lungs are typically heavy, congested, hemorrhagic, and edematous
▸ Gross findings in cases with secondary infections depend largely on the specific microbial (usually bacterial) pathogen involved, and may include consolidation, abscess formation, hemorrhage, and empyema

Microscopic Findings

▸ Interstitial pneumonitis with mononuclear cell infiltrates
▸ Diffuse alveolar damage
▸ Multinucleated giant cells with characteristic nuclear and cytoplasmic inclusions

Immunohistochemical Features

▸ Measles antigens can be detected in giant cells and alveolar lining cells

Ultrastructural Features

▸ Measles virions are pleomorphic, generally spherical, enveloped particles from 120-250 nm in diameter
▸ A lipid envelope surrounds a helical nucleocapsid composed of RNA and protein

Pathologic Differential Diagnosis

▸ Other viral pathogens that can cause giant cell pneumonia, such as respiratory syncytial virus, parainfluenza, metapneumovirus, VZV, and Henipa viruses
▸ Unequivocal diagnosis can be made by laboratory tests such as viral culture, direct fluorescent antibody and rapid antigen assays, serology, and IHC

ANCILLARY STUDIES

Diagnosis of infection with HPIVs can be made by virus isolation, direct detection of viral antigens by EIA or IFA in clinical specimens, detection of viral RNA by RT-PCR, demonstration of a rise in specific serum antibodies, or a combination of these approaches. HPIV infections of lung can be confirmed by IHC testing of formalin fixed tissues (Figure 13-10C); viral antigens can be detected in giant cells, pneumocytes, and respiratory epithelial cells. Ultrastructural studies demonstrate variably shaped virions of varying size (ranging from 150-300 nm), with a lipid envelope surrounding a helical nucleocapsid composed of RNA and protein.

DIFFERENTIAL DIAGNOSIS

Other viral causes of giant cell pneumonia, including measles and RSV, should be considered in the histopathologic differential diagnosis, and laboratory testing, including IHC, can be useful in determining the correct diagnosis.

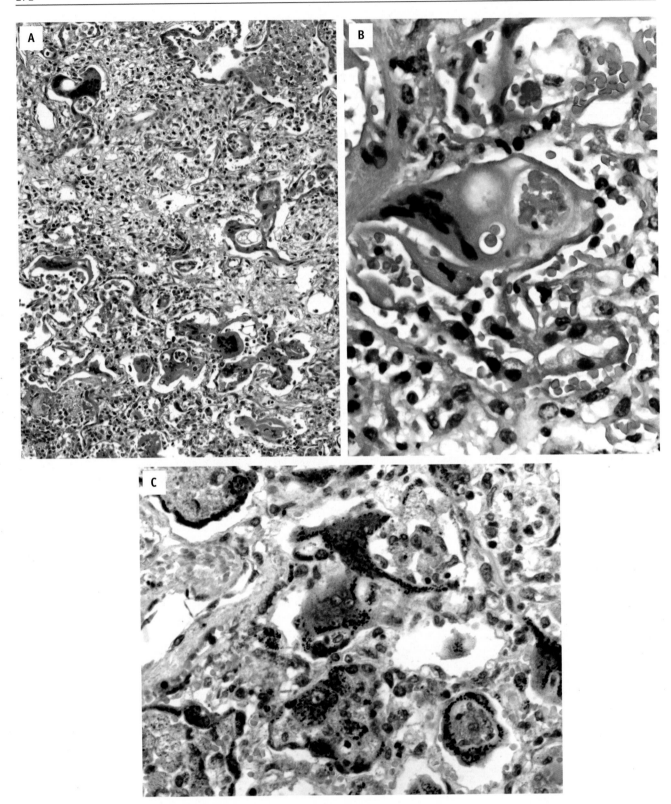

FIGURE 13-10

Parainfluenza virus pneumonia

 (A) Giant cell pneumonia showing numerous giant cells, interstitial pneumonitis, and hemorrhage. **(B)** Giant cell containing eosinophilic cytoplasmic inclusions. **(C)** Parainfluenza virus antigens in giant cells localized by IHC (immunoalkaline phosphatase).

PROGNOSIS AND THERAPY

Most HPIV infections cause a mild, self-limited illness. The highest rates of serious HPIV illnesses occur among young children. HPIV infections are also being increasingly recognized as an important cause of severe morbidity and mortality in immunocompromised adults. The mortality of bone marrow transplant patients with HPIV-3 infection has been reported to be as high as 60%. Supportive management with bed rest, oral hydration, and antipyretics is the basis of treatment. Aerosolized ribavirin has shown some efficacy in the treatment of severe cases of HPIV infection.

RESPIRATORY SYNCYTIAL VIRUS

RSV is a negative-sense, nonsegmented, single-stranded, enveloped RNA virus. RSV is a member of the family *Paramyxoviridae,* and can be further distinguished genetically and antigenically into two subgroups, A and B. The subgroup A strains are usually associated with more severe infections.

CLINICAL FEATURES

RSV is the most common cause of bronchiolitis and pneumonia among infants and children under 1 year of age. In temperate climates, RSV infections usually occur during annual community outbreaks, often lasting several months, during the late fall, winter, or early spring months. The timing and severity of outbreaks in a community vary from year to year. RSV spreads efficiently during the annual outbreaks, infecting as many as 50% of children in their first year of life. Most children will have serologic evidence of RSV infection by 2 years of age. Illness begins most frequently with fever, runny nose, cough, and sometimes wheezing. During their first RSV infection, between 25% and 40% of infants and young children have signs or symptoms of bronchiolitis or pneumonia, and 0.5-2% require hospitalization. The majority of children hospitalized for RSV infection are under 6 months of age, or are children with cyanotic congenital heart disease, cystic fibrosis, bronchopulmonary dysplasia, or immunosuppression. RSV can also cause repeated infections throughout life, and severe lower respiratory tract disease may occur at any age, especially among the elderly or among those with compromised cardiac, pulmonary, or immune systems.

RADIOLOGIC FEATURES

Children with RSV infection most commonly show multifocal air space consolidation and peribronchial thickening. In adults, disease is characterized by bilateral interstitial opacities and multifocal consolidations.

PATHOLOGIC FEATURES

GROSS FINDINGS

Large and small airways can contain necrotic debris and mucus, and may show ulceration. The lungs may be heavy and diffusely firm and may show areas of hyperexpansion or atelectasis.

MICROSCOPIC FINDINGS

The major histopathologic changes described in fatal RSV infections are necrotizing bronchiolitis and interstitial pneumonia. Bronchial lumens and airways are usually filled with necrotic debris and inflammatory cells. Airways show mixed or predominantly mononuclear infiltrates with hyperplastic epithelial changes (Figure 13-11A). These findings may be accompanied by diffuse alveolar damage (Figure 13-11E), and secondary bacterial superinfection. Giant cell pneumonia is seen in some cases (Figure 13-11C). The multinucleated giant cells represent epithelial cells in bronchi, bronchioles, and alveoli, and sometimes contain irregular, intracytoplasmic, eosinophilic inclusions surrounded by a clear halo (Figures 13-11C,D).

ANCILLARY STUDIES

Diagnosis of RSV infection can be made by virus isolation, direct detection of viral antigens in clinical specimens by EIA, IFA, or IHC (Figure 13-11B, F), detection of viral RNA by RT-PCR, or demonstration of a rise in RSV-specific serum antibodies. The virus is labile and attempts at culture isolation are often unsuccessful if there is delay or mishandling of the clinical specimen. Ultrastructural studies reveal virions of variable shape and size that range from 120 to 300 nm, with numerous 12-nm glycoprotein spikes.

DIFFERENTIAL DIAGNOSIS

Other viral causes of giant cell pneumonia should be considered in the histopathologic differential diagnosis, primarily parainfluenza viruses and measles viruses. Herpes

HUMAN PARAINFLUENZA VIRUSES—FACT SHEET

Definition

» The causative agents are negative-sense, nonsegmented, single-stranded, enveloped RNA viruses of the family *Paramyxoviridae*
» Four serotypes exist: HPIV-1 and 3 are included in the genus *Respirovirus*, and HPIV-2 and through HPIV-4 are included in the genus *Rubulavirus*

Incidence and Location

» Highly communicable disease of worldwide distribution
» Activity varies with serotype: HPIV-1 and 2 peak in the fall, HPIV-3 peaks in the spring and summer, and HPIV-4 is infrequently detected (less likely to cause severe illness)
» Common cause of upper respiratory illness, but an uncommon cause of lower respiratory tract disease

Morbidity and Mortality

» The highest rates of serious HPIV respiratory illnesses occur among young children
» HPIV infections are also an important cause of severe morbidity and mortality in immunocompromised adults

Gender, Race, and Age Distribution

» HPIVs infect most people by 5 years of age, and can cause repeated infections throughout life
» No recognized gender or racial predilection

Clinical Features

» Usually manifests as an upper respiratory illness (cold, sore throat, and croup) with a typical incubation period of 1 to 7 days
» Less commonly presents with symptoms of a lower respiratory illness (pneumonia, bronchitis, and bronchiolitis) in elderly or immunosuppressed patients

Radiologic Features

» Interstitial opacities, bronchial wall thickening, and peribronchial consolidation
» Rarely associated with pleural effusions

Prognosis and Therapy

» Recovery is rapid and complete in most cases
» Supportive management with bed rest, oral hydration, and antipyretics
» Aerosolized ribavirin can be used in immunosuppressed patients with severe illness

HUMAN PARAINFLUENZA VIRUSES—PATHOLOGIC FEATURES

Gross Findings

» Lungs can appear heavy, congested, hemorrhagic, and edematous

Microscopic Findings

» Interstitial pneumonitis with mononuclear cell infiltrates
» Diffuse alveolar damage
» Bronchiolitis
» Organizing pneumonia
» Multinucleated giant cells with characteristic cytoplasmic inclusions

Immunohistochemical Features

» HPIV antigens can be detected in giant cells and alveolar lining cells

Ultrastructural Features

» The virions are variable in shape and size, ranging from 150-300 nm
» A lipid envelope surrounds a helical nucleocapsid composed of RNA and protein
» The virus is morphologically indistinguishable from other members of the *Paramyxoviridae* family when viewed by negative contrast electron microscopy

Pathologic Differential Diagnosis

» Other viral pathogens that can cause giant cell pneumonia, such as measles, respiratory syncytial virus, metapneumovirus, VZV, and Henipa viruses
» Unequivocal diagnosis can be made by laboratory tests such as viral culture, direct fluorescent antibody and rapid antigen assays, serology, and IHC

---

simplex and varicella zoster viruses less commonly produce multinucleated giant cells in the lung.

PROGNOSIS AND THERAPY

Mortality in otherwise healthy children hospitalized for RSV pneumonia is less than 1%. However, the disease is fatal in as many as 15-40% of patients with immune suppression or underlying disease. Mortality is greatest in infants with congenital heart disease and pulmonary hypertension, where it approaches 70%. At present, the only antiviral drug with *in vitro* efficacy against RSV is ribavirin.

HUMAN METAPNEUMOVIRUS

Human metapneumovirus (HMPV), first identified in 2001 from clinical specimens obtained from patients with acute respiratory illnesses, is a negative-sense, non-segmented, single-stranded, enveloped RNA virus. HMPV has been categorized in the family *Paramyxoviridae*, subfamily *Pneumovirinae*, genus *Metapneumovirus*. HMPV can be further distinguished genetically and antigenically into two subgroups, A and B.

CLINICAL FEATURES

HMPV infection is ubiquitous and occurs during infancy and early childhood, with annual epidemic peaks occurring late in the winter and spring months in temperate

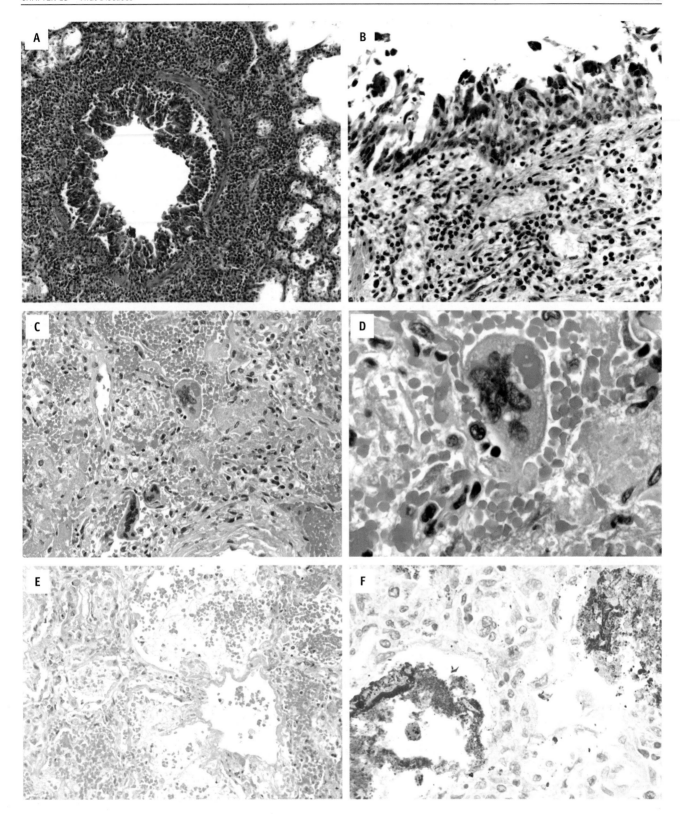

FIGURE 13-11

Respiratory syncytial virus pneumonia
(A) Bronchiolar and peribronchiolar inflammation in RSV infection. **(B)** RSV antigens in the lining epithelial cells of the same bronchiole, highlighted by IHC (immunoalkaline phosphatase). **(C)** Interstitial pneumonitis, hemorrhage, and giant cells in RSV pneumonia. **(D)** Giant cell with "melted tallow"-like inclusion similar to those of measles. **(E)** Diffuse alveolar damage in RSV pneumonia. **(F)** RSV antigens associated with hyaline membranes and necrotic debris (immunoalkaline phosphatase).

RESPIRATORY SYNCYTIAL VIRUS PNEUMONIA—FACT SHEET

Definition

» Respiratory syncytial virus (RSV) is a negative-sense, nonsegmented, single-stranded, enveloped RNA virus that is a member of the family *Paramyxoviridae*

Incidence and Location

» Worldwide distribution
» RSV spreads efficiently among children during annual outbreaks, infecting as many as 50% of children in their first year of life
» Most children will have serologic evidence of RSV infection by 2 years of age
» 0.5-2% of infants and young children infected with RSV are hospitalized
» Most children hospitalized for RSV infection are under 6 months of age or have cyanotic congenital heart disease, cystic fibrosis, bronchopulmonary dysplasia, or immunosuppression

Mortality

» Mortality in otherwise healthy children hospitalized for RSV pneumonia is less than 1%
» RSV pneumonia is fatal in as many as 15-40% of patients with immune suppression or underlying disease
» Mortality is greatest in infants with congenital heart disease associated with pulmonary hypertension, where it approaches 70%

Gender, Race, and Age Distribution

» RSV is the most common cause of bronchiolitis and pneumonia among infants and children under 1 year of age
» No recognized gender or racial predilection

Clinical Features

» Fever, runny nose, cough, sometimes wheezing
» During their first RSV infection, between 25% and 40% of infants and young children have signs or symptoms of bronchiolitis or pneumonia
» RSV can cause repeated infections throughout life, usually associated with moderate-to-severe cold-like symptoms
» Severe lower respiratory tract disease may occur at any age, especially among the elderly or among those with compromised cardiac, pulmonary, or immune systems

Radiologic Features

» Children most commonly show multifocal air space consolidation and peribronchial thickening
» Bilateral interstitial opacities and multifocal consolidations are usually seen in adults

Prognosis and Therapy

» Otherwise healthy children usually recover completely
» Higher mortality in specific patient groups (see above)
» The only antiviral drug with in vitro efficacy against RSV is ribavirin

RESPIRATORY SYNCYTIAL VIRUS PNEUMONIA—PATHOLOGIC FEATURES

Gross Findings

» Large and small airways can contain necrotic debris and mucus and may show ulceration
» The lungs may be heavy and firm, and show areas of hyperexpansion or atelectasis

Microscopic Findings

» Necrotizing bronchiolitis
» Interstitial pneumonia
» Hyperplastic airway epithelium
» Multinucleated giant cells (in some cases) in bronchi, bronchioles, and alveoli, that contain irregular, intracytoplasmic, eosinophilic inclusions surrounded by a clear halo

Immunohistochemical Features

» Viral antigens in multinucleated cells and respiratory epithelial cells

Ultrastructural Features

» The virion is variable in shape and size and ranges from 120 nm to 300 nm
» Particles show numerous 12-nm glycoprotein spikes

Pathologic Differential Diagnosis

» Other viral causes of giant cell pneumonia should be considered, primarily parainfluenza viruses and measles viruses
» Herpes simplex and varicella zoster viruses rarely produce multinucleated cytologic changes in the lung
» Confirmation of diagnosis is by clinical laboratory tests on IHC

spectrum of respiratory disease, most infections cause a mild, self-limited illness. The patient may be asymptomatic, or symptoms may range from mild upper respiratory tract illness to severe bronchiolitis and pneumonia. During their first HMPV infection, about 10-15% of infants and young children have signs or symptoms of bronchiolitis or pneumonia. About one-half of the cases of lower respiratory illness in children occur in the first 6 months of life, suggesting that young age is a major risk factor for severe disease. Underlying pulmonary disease, especially asthma, may increase the risk of hospitalization for HMPV pneumonia. Like RSV and the HPIVs, studies suggest that HMPV may also contribute to respiratory disease in elderly adults and the immunocompromised.

RADIOLOGIC FEATURES

Radiographic findings include interstitial infiltrates with focal consolidation commonly involving the lower lobes of the lung.

regions, often overlapping in part or in whole with the annual RSV epidemic. Seroprevalence studies reveal that 25% of all children aged 6 to 12 months have antibodies to HMPV; by age 5 years, 100% of patients have evidence of past infection. The incubation period is generally from 2 to 8 days. Although HMPV has been associated with a

PATHOLOGIC FEATURES

GROSS FINDINGS

In fatal cases, the lungs are typically heavy and display congestion, hemorrhage, and edema.

MICROSCOPIC FINDINGS

Histopathologic descriptions are few, and assessment of their validity is complicated by the uncertainty, in some cases, of the clinical significance of detecting this ubiquitous virus. Nonetheless, BAL specimens collected from patients within a few days of a positive HMPV assay show degenerative changes and cytoplasmic inclusions within epithelial cells, multinucleated giant cells, and histiocytes. The intracytoplasmic inclusions are ill-defined, eosinophilic

structures that measure 3-4 μm. Necrotizing bronchiolitis may be found on lung biopsy. Lung tissue later in the disease shows chronic airway inflammation, intra-alveolar foamy and hemosiderin-laden macrophages, acute and organizing lung injury, and organizing pneumonia (Figure 13-12A-C). In such cases, typical multinucleated giant cells or viral inclusions cannot be identified. ISH studies on a limited number of human cases suggest infection of alveolar and bronchial epithelial cells.

ANCILLARY STUDIES

HMPV is difficult to identify with commonly used viral diagnostic procedures. The virus replicates slowly in primary and tertiary monkey kidney cell lines, and cytopathic effects can be difficult to discern.

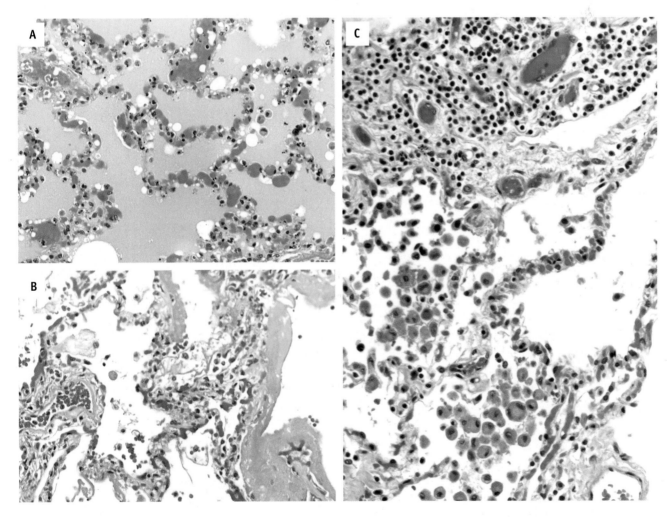

FIGURE 13-12

Human metapneumovirus pneumonia
(A) Severe pulmonary edema in fatal HMPV infection. **(B)** Diffuse alveolar damage in fatal HMPV infection. **(C)** Accumulation of alveolar macrophages in interstitial pneumonia associated with HMPV.

Antibodies to HMPV are not widely available; however, they can be used for identification of the virus by IFA. Most HMPV studies have been conducted using RT-PCR assays or by demonstration of a rise in HMPV-specific serum antibodies. The enveloped virion is variable in shape and size and ranges from 150 to 300 nm.

DIFFERENTIAL DIAGNOSIS

Other viral causes of giant cell pneumonia and diffuse alveolar damage, including measles, RSV, HPIV, measles, VZV, and HSV, may be considered, as well as noninfectious causes of diffuse alveolar damage. Laboratory testing, including IHC and ISH, can be useful in making this differentiation possible.

PROGNOSIS AND THERAPY

Supportive management with bed rest, oral hydration, and antipyretics is the basis of treatment, and usually leads to complete recovery. There are no licensed therapies or prophylactic treatments for HMPV at this time. Ribavirin and intravenous immunoglobulin, which have activity against RSV, were tested against HMPV *in vitro* and were found to have equivalent activity against HMPV and RSV.

HENIPA VIRUSES

Hendra and Nipah viruses belong to the recently designated genus *Henipavirus* within the family *Paramyxoviridae*, subfamily *Paramyxovirinae*, and are nonsegmented, negative-stranded RNA viruses. These zoonotic pathogens were first identified in Australia and Malaysia and have been associated with acute febrile encephalitis and respiratory tract disease.

CLINICAL FEATURES

Hendra was identified in 1994 when patients who came in close contact with sick horses developed an influenza-like illness with fever, myalgia, headache, lethargy, sore throat, nausea and vomiting. Two patients died with pneumonitis and multiorgan failure. The closely related Nipah virus was identified during an outbreak in Malaysia and Singapore during 1998-1999 that included more than 250 patients. The incubation period ranged from 2 days to 1 month, but in most cases lasted between 1 and 2 weeks. Patients presented with a severe acute encephalitic syndrome, but some also had significant pulmonary manifestations. In Bangladesh in 2001 and 2003, outbreaks of Nipah encephalitis occurred. Similar to the Malaysian outbreak, the most prominent symptoms were fever, headache, vomiting, and an altered level of consciousness. Respiratory illness was much more common in the Bangladesh cases, however, with 64% having cough and dyspnea. Epidemiologic and laboratory investigations identified fruit bats of the *Pteropus* genus as asymptomatic carriers of Hendra and Nipah viruses and possible animal reservoirs. Food-borne transmission has also been reported in an individual who consumed fruit contaminated by *Pteropus* bats.

RADIOLOGIC FEATURES

In patients with respiratory illness, chest radiographs reveal bilateral infiltrates consistent with ARDS.

PATHOLOGIC FEATURES

GROSS FINDINGS

In fatal infections, the lungs are heavy, congested, edematous, and hemorrhagic.

MICROSCOPIC FINDINGS

Histopathologic findings in fatal cases of Hendra and Nipah infections are similar, with varying degrees of central nervous system and respiratory tract involvement. Findings include a systemic vasculitis with extensive thrombosis, endothelial cell damage, necrosis, and syncytial giant cell formation in affected vessels (Figures 13-13A,B). Multinucleated giant cells with intranuclear inclusions can occasionally be seen in lung, spleen, lymph nodes, and kidneys. In the lung, vasculitis and fibrinoid necrosis can be seen in the majority of cases (Figure 13-13A). Multinucleated giant cells with intranuclear inclusions are usually noted in alveolar spaces adjacent to necrotic areas (Figure 13-13C).

ANCILLARY STUDIES AND DIFFERENTIAL DIAGNOSIS

The diagnosis of Nipah virus infection, suspected by patient history and clinical manifestations, can be supported by characteristic histopathological findings. The

HUMAN METAPNEUMOVIRUS (HMPV)—FACT SHEET

Definition

- Human metapneumovirus (HMPV) is a negative-sense, nonsegmented, single-stranded, enveloped RNA virus, that is a member of the family *Paramyxoviridae*, subfamily *Pneumovirinae*, genus *Metapneumovirus*
- HMPV can be distinguished genetically and antigenically into two subgroups, A and B

Incidence and Location

- Worldwide distribution
- About 25% of all children aged 6 to 12 months and all children by age 5 years will have serologic evidence of HMPV infection
- Annual epidemic peaks occur late in the winter and spring months in temperate regions, often overlapping in part or in whole with RSV epidemics
- About 4% of all infant hospitalizations for acute respiratory illness or fever are associated with HMPV; the majority of children hospitalized for HMPV infection are under 6 months of age or children with underlying pulmonary disease, especially asthma
- May also contribute to respiratory disease in elderly or immunocompromised adults

Mortality

- Mortality in otherwise healthy children hospitalized for HMPV pneumonia is less than 1%
- Disease may be fatal in as many as 30-40% of patients with immune suppression or underlying disease

Gender, Race, and Age Distribution

- Common cause of bronchiolitis and pneumonia among infants under 1 year of age
- No recognized gender or racial predilection

Clinical Features

- Most infections cause a mild, self-limited upper respiratory tract illness
- During their first HMPV infection, about 10-15% of outpatient infants and young children have signs or symptoms of bronchiolitis or pneumonia
- Severe lower respiratory tract disease (bronchiolitis, pneumonia) may occur at any age, especially among the elderly or among those with compromised cardiac, pulmonary, or immune systems

Radiologic Features

- Bilateral multifocal air space consolidation and interstitial infiltrates

Prognosis and Therapy

- With supportive care, most children recover from illness in 1 to 2 weeks
- No licensed therapies or prophylactic treatments for HMPV
- The only antiviral drug shown to have in vitro efficacy against HMPV is ribavirin

HUMAN METAPNEUMOVIRUS (HMPV)—PATHOLOGIC FEATURES

Gross Findings

- In fatal cases, the lungs are heavy and display congestion, hemorrhage, and edema

Microscopic Findings

- Histopathologic features have received relatively little study
- Necrotizing bronchiolitis that evolves to chronic bronchiolitis has been described, as well as interstitial pneumonitis, acute or organizing diffuse alveolar damage, and increased intra-alveolar macrophages
- Organizing DAD and chronic airway disease in patients who die later in the course of the illness
- BAL specimens may show multinucleated giant cells with cytoplasmic inclusions

Ultrastructural Features

- The virion is variable in shape and size, ranging from 150-300 nm, and is morphologically indistinguishable from other members of the *Paramyxoviridae* family when viewed by negative-stain electron microscopy

Pathologic Differential Diagnosis

- Other viral causes of giant cell pneumonia, necrotizing bronchiolitis, and interstitial pneumonitis and diffuse alveolar damage
- Non-infectious causes of diffuse alveolar damage

most unique histopathologic finding is the presence of syncytial and parenchymal multinucleated endothelial cells. However, this feature occurs in only about one-fourth of the cases and cannot be used as a sensitive criterion for the diagnosis of Henipa virus infections; furthermore, similar cells can also be seen in measles virus, RSV, HPIV, herpesviruses, and other infections. In addition to these viral infections, other non-infectious causes of diffuse alveolar damage may also be considered in the differential diagnosis. Unequivocal diagnosis can be made only by laboratory tests such as IHC, cell culture isolation, PCR, or serology. IHC can reveal widespread presence of Nipah virus antigens in endothelial and smooth muscle cells of blood vessels as well as in various parenchymal cells (Figures 13-13D–F). Ultrastructural studies can also demonstrate the pleomorphic viral particles which are composed of helical nucleocapsids enclosed within an envelope.

PROGNOSIS AND THERAPY

Only 3 persons are known to have been infected with Hendra virus, and 2 of them died. Death occurs in about 30-40% of patients infected with Nipah virus and is more frequent in patients with rapidly developing severe neurologic signs. Residual neurologic signs are common among survivors. Treatment is supportive, including mechanical ventilation for patients in a deep

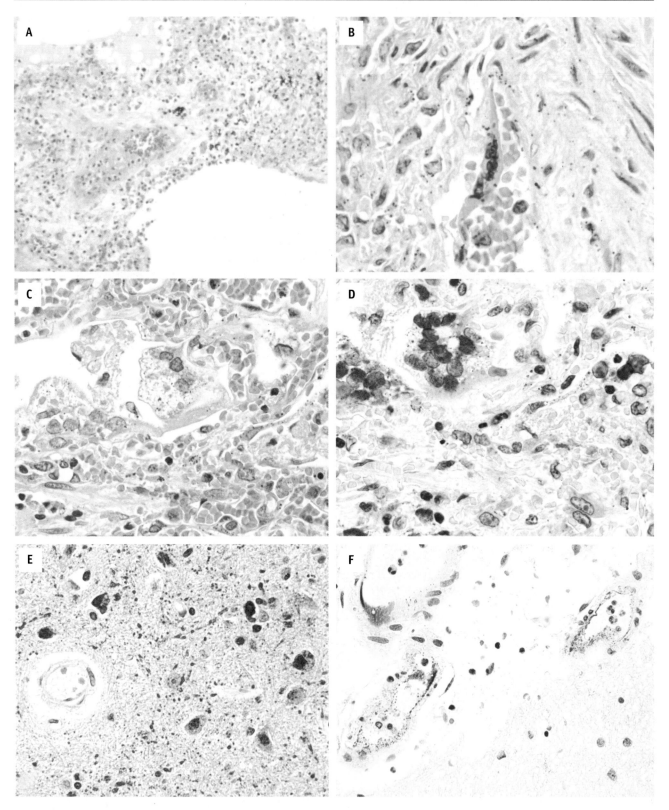

FIGURE 13-13

Nipah virus pneumonia

(A) Interstitial pneumonitis, edema, congestion, and focal thrombosis. **(B)** Pulmonary vessel showing a multinucleated endothelial syncytium. **(C)** Interstitial pneumonitis with intra-alveolar multinucleated giant cells with nuclear inclusions. **(D)** Viral nature of giant cells, in **C**, as evidenced by immunostaining for Nipah viral antigens (immunoalkaline phosphatase). **(E, F)** Immunostaining of Nipah viral antigens in neurons and vascular endothelium in the central nervous system (immunoalkaline phosphatase).

HENIPA VIRUSES—FACT SHEET

Definition

▸ Hendra and Nipah viruses are nonsegmented, negative-stranded RNA viruses, members of the family *Paramyxoviridae* and subfamily *Paramyxovirinae*

Incidence and Location

▸ Rare cases have occurred in Australia and Asia throughout the distribution of the animal reservoir, the fruit bat of the *Pteropus* genus
▸ Infection has occurred primarily in patients who have contact with sick horses and pigs
▸ Food-borne transmission has also been reported in an individual who consumed fruit contaminated by *Pteropus* bats

Morbidity and Mortality

▸ Death occurs in about 30-40% of Nipah cases associated with rapidly developing severe neurologic signs
▸ 2 of 3 of the known Hendra cases died with pneumonitis and multiorgan failure

Gender, Race, and Age Distribution

▸ Patient demographics depend largely on the mode of exposure, in most cases occupational
▸ No apparent gender or racial predilection

Clinical Features

▸ Acute febrile encephalitis and influenza-like illness

Radiologic Features

▸ Bilateral infiltrates consistent with the acute respiratory distress syndrome

Therapy

▸ Treatment is supportive, including mechanical ventilation when needed
▸ Equivocal data regarding the efficacy of ribavirin in treatment

---

HENIPA VIRUSES—PATHOLOGIC FEATURES

Gross Findings

▸ In fatal cases, the lungs are heavy and display congestion, hemorrhage, and edema

Microscopic Findings

▸ Histopathologic involvement of the central nervous system and respiratory system
▸ Vasculitis, thrombosis, endothelial cell damage, and syncytial cell formation
▸ Multinucleated giant cells with intranuclear and cytoplasmic inclusions in the brain, lung, and other organs
▸ Organizing diffuse alveolar damage in patients who die later in the course of the illness

Immunohistochemical Features

▸ Widespread presence of Henipa virus antigens can be seen by IHC in endothelial and smooth muscle cells of blood vessels, as well as in various parenchymal cells

Ultrastructural Features

▸ Pleomorphic viral particles composed of helical nucleocapsids enclosed within an envelope

Pathologic Differential Diagnosis

▸ Other viral causes of encephalitis, giant cell pneumonia, and diffuse alveolar damage, as well as noninfectious causes of diffuse alveolar damage

---

coma who are unable to maintain airways. Ribavirin was used in humans during the Nipah outbreak in Malaysia, with equivocal results.

HEMORRHAGIC FEVER VIRUSES

The combination of fever and hemorrhage can be caused by different viruses, rickettsiae, bacteria, protozoa, and fungi. However, the term "viral hemorrhagic fever" (VHF) is usually reserved for systemic infections characterized by fever and hemorrhage caused by a special group of viruses transmitted to humans by arthropods and rodents. VHFs are febrile illnesses characterized by abnormal vascular regulation and vascular damage and are caused by small, lipid-enveloped RNA viruses. This syndrome can be caused by RNA viruses belonging to four different families that differ in their genomic structure, replication strategy, and morphologic features (*Arenaviridae, Bunyaviridae, Flaviviridae,* and *Filoviridae*). Arenaviruses, bunyaviruses, and filoviruses are negative-stranded, whereas flaviviruses are positive-stranded RNA viruses. Hemorrhagic fever viruses are distributed worldwide, and the diseases they cause are traditionally named according to the location where they were first described. The oldest and best known is yellow fever virus; others include Lassa fever, lymphocytic choriomeningitis, Ebola, and dengue viruses. The distributions of the individual VHFs are related to the distributions of their specific arthropod and rodent vectors.

CLINICAL FEATURES

VHF is characterized clinically by its disproportionate effect on the vascular system. Typical manifestations are related to a loss of vascular regulation (vasodilatation and hypotension), vascular damage (leakage of protein into the urine, edema in soft tissues of the face and other loose connective tissues, and petechial hemorrhage in the skin and internal organs), and severe systemic derangement that presents as fever, myalgia, and asthenia proceeding to a state of prostration. Hemorrhage is common with most of these diseases and usually originates from mucosal surfaces. Patients with severe hemorrhagic fever generally develop shock, diffuse bleeding, and central nervous system dysfunction.

RADIOLOGIC FEATURES

In patients with respiratory illness, chest radiographs may reveal bilateral interstitial and alveolar edema and hemorrhage.

PATHOLOGIC FEATURES

GROSS FINDINGS

In fatal VHF, the lungs show congestion, hemorrhage, and edema. Pleural effusion may be found with certain infections.

MICROSCOPIC FINDINGS

At autopsy, common findings include widespread petechial hemorrhages and ecchymoses involving skin, mucous membranes, and internal organs. However, in many VHF patients manifestations of bleeding may be minimal or absent. Effusions, occasionally hemorrhagic, are also frequently seen. Widespread, focal, and sometimes massive necrosis is commonly observed in all organ systems and is often ischemic in nature. Necrosis is usually most prominent in the liver and lymphoid tissues. The most consistent microscopic feature is found in the liver and consists of multifocal hepatocellular necrosis with cytoplasmic eosinophilia,

Councilman bodies, nuclear pyknosis, and cytolysis (Figure 13-14D). Inflammatory cell infiltrates and necrotic areas are usually mild and, when present, consist of neutrophils and mononuclear cells. Commonly observed histopathologic changes in the lung include various degrees of hemorrhage, intra-alveolar edema, interstitial pneumonitis, and diffuse alveolar damage (Figure 13-14A,E,H).

ANCILLARY STUDIES AND DIFFERENTIAL DIAGNOSIS

The diagnosis of VHF should be suspected in patients with appropriate clinical manifestations returning from an endemic area, particularly if there is travel to rural areas during seasonal or epidemic disease activity. The diagnosis suspected by history and clinical manifestations can also be supported histopathologically. However, because of similar pathologic features seen in VHF and a variety of other viral, rickettsial, and bacterial infections, as well as noninfectious causes of hemorrhage, edema, and diffuse alveolar damage, unequivocal diagnosis can be made only by laboratory tests such as cell culture isolation, serology, PCR, and IHC (Figure 13-14B,F,G,I,J). Ultrastructural studies can also demonstrate the presence of virions. All viruses have a lipid envelope that is acquired by budding at either the cell surface or the internal membranes. The size and shape of these viruses vary from relatively small (35-50 nm), uniform, round particles, as seen with flaviviruses, to more pleomorphic, rod-shaped particles (measuring occasionally up to 15,000 nm) in the case of filoviruses (Figure 13-14C).

PROGNOSIS AND THERAPY

Case mortality ranges from about 15% with infections such as Lassa fever up to 90% with filovirus infections such as Ebola. Treatment depends on the particular agent and may include the use of passive antibodies, antiviral drugs such as ribavirin, or supportive therapy. Supportive therapy should include the reasonable measures that would be employed in any very ill patient with a fragile vascular bed. Volume replacement may be particularly important in some patients, especially with dengue hemorrhagic fever.

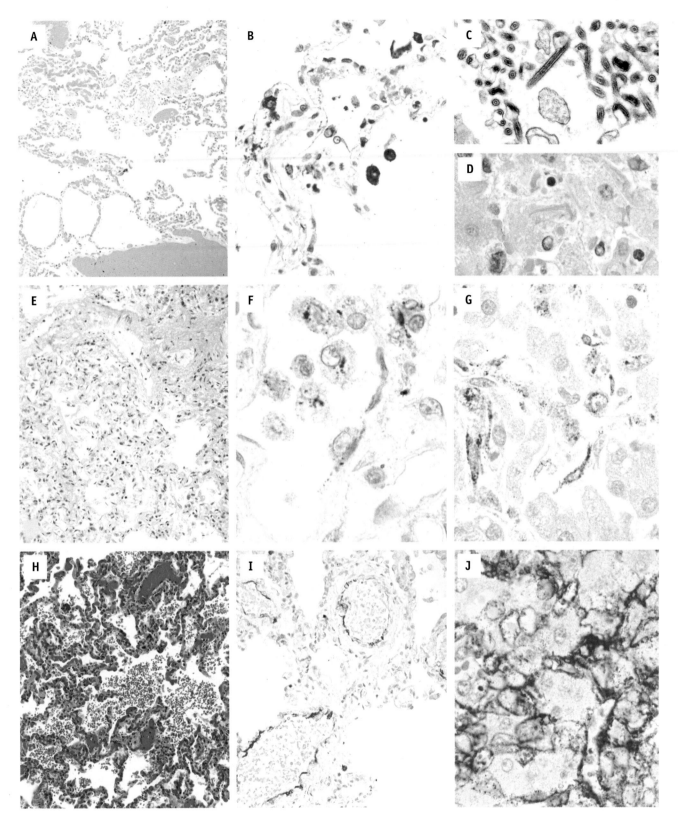

FIGURE 13-14

Viral hemorrhagic fevers

(A) Lung from a fatal Ebola case showing congestion and no significant inflammation. **(B)** Ebola viral antigens in alveolar macrophages, endothelial cells, fibroblasts, and other interstitial cells in the same patient seen in **A** (immunoalkaline phosphatase). **(C)** Ebola viral particles are seen within an intra-alveolar space by electron microscopy. **(D)** Numerous filamentous Ebola virus inclusions are seen within hepatocytes. **(E)** Mild interstitial pneumonitis in a fatal case of dengue hemorrhagic fever. **(F)** Dengue viral antigen-containing circulating mononuclear cells in a pulmonary vessel. Note also the viral antigens in a lining endothelial cell (immunoalkaline phosphatase). **(G)** Immunostaining of liver showing viral antigens predominantly within sinusoidal Kupffer cells. Note the absence of hepatocyte staining (immunoalkaline phosphatase). **(H)** Pulmonary congestion and absence of significant inflammatory response in a case of Lassa fever. **(I)** Lassa viral antigens in endothelial cells lining medium-sized vessels in the lung (immunoalkaline phosphatase). **(J)** IHC reveals Lassa virus antigens in the cytoplasm of hepatocytes and sinusoidal lining cells in association with areas of hepatocellular necrosis (immunoalkaline phosphatase).

VIRAL HEMORRHAGIC FEVERS—FACT SHEET

Definition

» Viral hemorrhagic fevers (VHFs) are systemic infections characterized by fever and hemorrhage, caused by a group of viruses transmitted to humans by arthropods and rodents

» Viruses belong to four different families that differ in their genomic structure, replication strategy, and morphologic features (*Arenaviridae, Bunyaviridae, Flaviviridae,* and *Filoviridae*)

» Arenaviruses, bunyaviruses, and filoviruses are negative-stranded, whereas flaviviruses are positive-stranded RNA viruses

Incidence and Location

» Rare diseases

» Hemorrhagic fever viruses are distributed worldwide, and the diseases they cause are traditionally named according to the location where they were first described

» The distributions of particular VHFs are related to the distributions of their specific arthropods and rodent vectors

Mortality

» Case mortality ranges from about 15% with infections such as Lassa fever up to 90% with filovirus infections such as Ebola

Gender, Race, and Age Distribution

» Patient demographics depend largely on the agent and mode of exposure

» People of all ages are vulnerable to VHFs

» No recognized gender or racial predilection

Clinical Features

» Fever, myalgia, asthenia, and prostration

» Loss of vascular regulation, shock, and central nervous system dysfunction

» Hemorrhage

Radiologic Features

» Bilateral interstitial or alveolar edema and infiltrates

Prognosis and Therapy

» Supportive therapy

» Passive antibodies

» Antivirals (ribavirin)

VIRAL HEMORRHAGIC FEVERS—PATHOLOGIC FEATURES

Gross Findings

» In fatal cases, the lungs display congestion, hemorrhage, and edema

» Widespread petechial hemorrhages and ecchymoses are present systemically

Microscopic Findings

» Histopathologic changes in the lung include varying degrees of hemorrhage, edema, interstitial pneumonitis, and diffuse alveolar damage

» Other systemic pathology as described in the text

Immunohistochemical Features

» Viral antigens can commonly be detected by IHC in the mononuclear phagocytic system and endothelium, as well as in parenchymal cells, depending on the particular VHF agent

Ultrastructural Features

» Features vary for the four families of viruses that cause VHF syndromes

» All viruses have a lipid envelope that is acquired by budding at either the cell surface or the internal membranes

» The sizes and shape of these viruses vary from relatively small (35-50 nm), uniform round particles, as seen with flaviviruses, to more pleomorphic, rod-shaped particles (occasionally measuring up to 15,000 nm) in the case of filoviruses

Pathologic Differential Diagnosis

» Other causes of hemorrhage, edema, and diffuse alveolar damage

» Unequivocal diagnosis can be made only by laboratory tests such as cell culture isolation, serology, PCR, and IHC

7. Mahy BWJ, Collier L, eds. *Microbiology and Microbial Infections: Virology.* 9 ed. London: Arnold; 1998.
8. Palmer EL, Martin ML. *Electron Microscopy in Viral Diagnosis.* Boca Raton, Florida: CRC Press, Inc.; 1988.

Adenoviruses

9. Becroft DM. Histopathology of fatal adenovirus infection of the respiratory tract in young children. *J Clin Pathol.* 1967;20:561-9.
10. Dudding BA, Wagner SC, Zeller JA, Gmelich JT, French GR, Top FH Jr. Fatal pneumonia associated with adenovirus type 7 in three military trainees. *N Engl J Med.* 1972;286:1289-92.
11. Hierholzer JC. Adenoviruses in the immunocompromised host. *Clin Microbiol Rev.* 1992;5:262-74.
12. Pham TT, Burchette JL Jr, Hale LP. Fatal disseminated adenovirus infections in immunocompromised patients. *Am J Clin Pathol.* 2003;120: 575-83.
13. Zahradnik JM. Adenovirus pneumonia. *Semin Respir Infect.* 1987;2: 104-11.

Hantaviruses

14. Duchin JS, Koster FT, Peters CJ, et al. Hantavirus pulmonary syndrome: a clinical description of 17 patients with a newly recognized disease. The Hantavirus Study Group. *N Engl J Med.* 1994;330:949-55.
15. Lukes RJ. The pathology of thirty-nine fatal cases of epidemic hemorrhagic fever. *Am J Med.* 1954;16:639-50.
16. Nolte KB, Feddersen RM, Foucar K, et al. Hantavirus pulmonary syndrome in the United States: a pathological description of a disease caused by a new agent. *Hum Pathol.* 1995;26:110-20.
17. Zaki SR, Greer PW, Coffield LM, et al. Hantavirus pulmonary syndrome. Pathogenesis of an emerging infectious disease. *Am J Pathol.* 1995;146:552-79.

SUGGESTED READINGS

General

1. Connor DH, Chandler FW, Schwartz DA, Manz HJ, Lack EE, eds. *Pathology of Infectious Disease,* 1st ed. Connecticut: Appleton & Lange; 1997.
2. Winn WC, Walker DH. Viral infections. In: Dail DH, Hammar SP, eds. *Pulmonary Pathology.* 2nd ed. New York: Springer-Verlag; 1994:429-64.
3. de Roux A, Marcos MA, Garcia E, et al. Viral community-acquired pneumonia in nonimmunocompromised adults. *Chest.* 2004;125: 1343-51.
4. Fields BN, Knipe DM, Howley PM, eds. *Fields Virology.* 4 ed. Philadelphia: Lippincott-Williams & Williams; 2001.
5. Infection unusual pneumonias. In: Katzenstein AL, ed. *Katzenstein and Askin's Surgical Pathology of Non-neoplastic Lung Diseases.* Philadelphia: Saunders Co.; 1997:247-85.
6. Travis WD, Colby TV, Koss MN, et al. Lung infections. In: King DW, ed. *Non-Neoplastic Disorders of the Lower Respiratory Tract.* Washington, DC: American Registry of Pathology and the Armed Forces Institute of Pathology; 2002.

18. Zaki SR, Khan AS, Goodman RA, et al. Retrospective diagnosis of hantavirus pulmonary syndrome, 1978-1993: implications for emerging infectious diseases. *Arch Pathol Lab Med*. 1996;120:134-9.

SARS Coronavirus

19. Chong PY, Chui P, Ling AE, et al. Analysis of deaths during the severe acute respiratory syndrome (SARS) epidemic in Singapore: challenges in determining a SARS diagnosis. *Arch Pathol Lab Med*. 2004;128:195-204.
20. Ding Y, Wang H, Shen H, et al. The clinical pathology of severe acute respiratory syndrome (SARS): a report from China. *J Pathol*. 2003;200:282-9.
21. Franks TJ, Chong PY, Chui P, et al. Lung pathology of severe acute respiratory syndrome (SARS): a study of 8 autopsy cases from Singapore. *Hum Pathol*. 2003;34:743-8.
22. Goldsmith CS, Tatti KM, Ksiazek TG, et al. Ultrastructural characterization of SARS coronavirus. *Emerg Infect Dis*. 2004;10:320-6.
23. Ksiazek TG, Erdman D, Goldsmith CS, et al. A novel coronavirus associated with severe acute respiratory syndrome. *N Engl J Med*. 2003;348:1953-66.
24. Nicholls JM, Poon LL, Lee KC, et al. Lung pathology of fatal severe acute respiratory syndrome. *Lancet*. 2003;361:1773-8.
25. Shieh WJ, Hsiao CH, Paddock CD, et al. Immunohistochemical, in situ hybridization, and ultrastructural localization of SARS-associated coronavirus in lung of a fatal case of severe acute respiratory syndrome in Taiwan. *Hum Pathol*. 2005;36:303-9.
26. To KF, Tong JH, Chan PK, et al. Tissue and cellular tropism of the coronavirus associated with severe acute respiratory syndrome: an in-situ hybridization study of fatal cases. *J Pathol*. 2004;202:157-63.

Cytomegalovirus

27. Beschorner WE, Hutchins GM, Burns WH, Saral R, Tutschka PJ, Santos GW. Cytomegalovirus pneumonia in bone marrow transplant recipients: miliary and diffuse patterns. *Am Rev Respir Dis*. 1980;122:107-14.
28. Herry I, Cadranel J, Antoine M, et al. Cytomegalovirus-induced alveolar hemorrhage in patients with AIDS: a new clinical entity? *Clin Infect Dis*. 1996;22:616-20.
29. Ison MG, Fishman JA. Cytomegalovirus pneumonia in transplant recipients. *Clin Chest Med*. 2005;26:691-705, viii.
30. Ljungman P, Griffiths P, Paya C. Definitions of cytomegalovirus infection and disease in transplant recipients. *Clin Infect Dis*. 2002;34:1094-7.
31. Wallace JM, Hannah J. Cytomegalovirus pneumonitis in patients with AIDS: findings in an autopsy series. *Chest*. 1987;92:198-203.

Herpes Simplex Viruses

32. Feldman S, Stokes DC. Varicella zoster and herpes simplex virus pneumonias. *Semin Respir Infect*. 1987;2:84-94.
33. Kimberlin DW. Neonatal herpes simplex infection. *Clin Microbiol Rev*. 2004;17:1-13.
34. Nash G. Necrotizing tracheobronchitis and bronchopneumonia consistent with herpetic infection. *Hum Pathol*. 1972;3:2832-91.
35. Ramsey PG, Fife KH, Hackman RC, Meyers JD, Corey L. Herpes simplex virus pneumonia: clinical, virologic, and pathologic features in 20 patients. *Ann Intern Med*. 1982;97:813-20.
36. Singer DB. Pathology of neonatal herpes simplex virus infection. *Perspect Pediatr Pathol*. 1981;6:243-78.

Varicella Zoster Virus

37. Feldman S. Varicella-zoster virus pneumonitis. *Chest*. 1994;106:22S-7S.
38. Harger JH, Ernest JM, Thurnau GR, et al. Risk factors and outcome of varicella-zoster virus pneumonia in pregnant women. *J Infect Dis*. 2002;185:422-7.
39. Mermelstein RH, Freireich AW. Varicella pneumonia. *Ann Intern Med*. 1961;55:456-63.
40. Triebwasser JH, Harris RE, Bryant RE, Rhoades ER. Varicella pneumonia in adults: report of seven cases and a review of literature. *Medicine (Baltimore)*. 1967;46:409-23.
41. Waring JJ, Neubuerger K, Geever EF. Severe forms of chickenpox in adults. *Arch Intern Med*, 1942;69:384-408.

Influenza Viruses

42. Guarner J, Paddock CD, Shieh WJ, et al. Histopathologic and immunohistochemical features of fatal influenza virus infections in children during the 2003-2004 season. *Clin Infect Dis*. 2006;43:132-40.
43. Guarner J, Shieh WJ, Dawson J, et al. Immunohistochemical and in situ hybridization studies of influenza A virus infection in human lungs. *Am J Clin Pathol*. 2000;114:227-33.
44. Hers JF, Masurel N, Mulder J. Bacteriology and histopathology of the respiratory tract and lungs in fatal Asian influenza. *Lancet*. 1958;2:1141-3.
45. Hers JFP. Changes in the respiratory mucosa resulting from infection with influenza virus B. *J Pathol Bacteriol*. 1957;73:565-8.
46. Martin CM, Kunin CM, Gottlieb LS, Barnes MW, Liu C, Finland M. Asian influenza A in Boston, 1957-1958: I. Observations in thirty-two influenza-associated fatal cases. *AMA Arch Intern Med*. 1959;103:515-31.
47. Nolte KB, Alakija P, Oty G, et al. Influenza A virus infection complicated by fatal myocarditis. *Am J Forensic Med Pathol*. 2000;21:375-9.
48. Shinya K, Ebina M, Yamada S, Ono M, Kasai N, Kawaoka Y. Avian flu: influenza virus receptors in the human airway. *Nature*. 2006;440:435-6.
49. Ungchusak K, Auewarakul P, Dowell SF, et al. Probable person-to-person transmission of avian influenza A (H5N1). *N Engl J Med*. 2005;352:333-40.
50. Van Riel D, Munster VJ, de Wit E, et al. H5N1 virus attachment to lower respiratory tract. *Science*. 2006;312:399.
51. Yeldandi AV, Colby TV. Pathologic features of lung biopsy specimens from influenza pneumonia cases. *Hum Pathol*. 1994;25:47-53.

Measles

52. Akhtar M, Young I. Measles giant cell pneumonia in an adult following long-term chemotherapy. *Arch Pathol*. 1973;96:145-8.
53. Archibald RW, Weller RO, Meadow SR. Measles pneumonia and the nature of the inclusion-bearing giant cells: a light- and electron-microscope study. *J Pathol*. 1971;103:27-34.
54. Breitfeld V, Hashida Y, Sherman FE, Odagiri K, Yunis EJ. Fatal measles infection in children with leukemia. *Lab Invest*. 1973;28:279-91.
55. Kipps A, Kaschula RO. Virus pneumonia following measles: a virological and histological study of autopsy material. *S Afr Med J*. 1976;50:1083-8.
56. Monafo WJ, Haslam DB, Roberts RL, Zaki SR, Bellini WJ, Coffin CM. Disseminated measles infection after vaccination in a child with a congenital immunodeficiency. *J Pediatr*. 1994;124:273-6.
57. Sata T, Kurata T, Aoyama Y, Sakaguchi M, Yamanouchi K, Takeda K. Analysis of viral antigens in giant cells of measles pneumonia by immunoperoxidase method. *Virchows Arch A Pathol Anat Histopathol*. 1986;410:133-8.
58. Sobonya RE, Hiller FC, Pingleton W, Watanabe I. Fatal measles (rubeola) pneumonia in adults. *Arch Pathol Lab Med*. 1978;102:366-71.

Parainfluenza

59. Akizuki S, Nasu N, Setoguchi M, Yoshida S, Higuchi Y, Yamamoto S. Parainfluenza virus pneumonitis in an adult. *Arch Pathol Lab Med*. 1991;115:824-6.
60. Butnor KJ, Sporn TA. Human parainfluenza virus giant cell pneumonia following cord blood transplant associated with pulmonary alveolar proteinosis. *Arch Pathol Lab Med*. 2003;127:235-8.
61. Jarvis WR, Middleton PJ, Gelfand EW. Parainfluenza pneumonia in severe combined immunodeficiency disease. *J Pediatr*. 1979;94:423-5.
62. Little BW, Tihen WS, Dickerman JD, Craighead JE. Giant cell pneumonia associated with parainfluenza virus type 3 infection. *Hum Pathol*. 1981;12:478-81.
63. Madden JF, Burchette JL Jr, Hale LP. Pathology of parainfluenza virus infection in patients with congenital immunodeficiency syndromes. *Hum Pathol*. 2004;35:594-603.
64. Weintrub PS, Sullender WM, Lombard C, Link MP, Arvin A. Giant cell pneumonia caused by parainfluenza type 3 in a patient with acute myelomonocytic leukemia. *Arch Pathol Lab Med*. 1987;111:569-70.
65. Wendt CH, Weisdorf DJ, Jordan MC, Balfour HH Jr, Hertz MI. Parainfluenza virus respiratory infection after bone marrow transplantation. *N Engl J Med*. 1992;326:921-6.

Respiratory Syncytial Virus

66. Delage G, Brochu P, Robillard L, Jasmin G, Joncas JH, Lapointe N. Giant cell pneumonia due to respiratory syncytial virus. Occurrence in severe combined immunodeficiency syndrome. *Arch Pathol Lab Med*. 1984;108: 623-5.
67. Englund JA, Sullivan CJ, Jordan MC, Dehner LP, Vercellotti GM, Balfour HH Jr. Respiratory syncytial virus infection in immunocompromised adults. *Ann Intern Med*. 1988;109:203-8.
68. Neilson KA, Yunis EJ. Demonstration of respiratory syncytial virus in an autopsy series. *Pediatr Pathol*. 1990;10:491-502.

Human Metapneumovirus

69. Cane PA, van den Hoogen BG, Chakrabarti S, Fegan CD, Osterhaus AD. Human metapneumovirus in a haematopoietic stem cell transplant recipient with fatal lower respiratory tract disease. *Bone Marrow Transplant*. 2003;31:309-10.
70. Kuiken T, van den Hoogen BG, van Riel DA, et al. Experimental human metapneumovirus infection of cynomolgus macaques *(Macaca fascicularis)* results in virus replication in ciliated epithelial cells and pneumocytes with associated lesions throughout the respiratory tract. *Am J Pathol*. 2004;164:1893-1900.
71. Sumino KC, Agapov E, Pierce RA, et al. Detection of severe human metapneumovirus infection by real-time polymerase chain reaction and histopathological assessment. *J Infect Dis*. 2005;192:1052-60.
72. van den Hoogen BG, de Jong JC, Groen J, et al. A newly discovered human pneumovirus isolated from young children with respiratory tract disease. *Nat Med*. 2001;7:719-24.

Henipah Viruses

73. Chua KB, Bellini WJ, Rota PA, et al. Nipah virus: a recently emergent deadly paramyxovirus. *Science*. 2000;288:1432-5.
74. Halpin K, Young PL, Field HE, Mackenzie JS. Isolation of Hendra virus from pteropid bats: a natural reservoir of Hendra virus. *J Gen Virol*. 2000;81:1927-32.
75. Hooper P, Zaki S, Daniels P, Middleton D. Comparative pathology of the diseases caused by Hendra and Nipah viruses. *Microbes Infect*. 2001;3:315-22.
76. Murray K, Selleck P, Hooper P, et al. A *Morbillivirus* that caused fatal disease in horses and humans. *Science*. 1995;268:94-7.
77. O'Sullivan JD, Allworth AM, Paterson DL, et al. Fatal encephalitis due to novel paramyxovirus transmitted from horses. *Lancet*. 1997;349: 93-5.
78. Paton NI, Leo YS, Zaki SR, et al. Outbreak of Nipah-virus infection among abattoir workers in Singapore. *Lancet*. 1999;354:1253-6.
79. Wong KT, Shieh WJ, Kumar S, et al. Nipah virus infection: pathology and pathogenesis of an emerging paramyxoviral zoonosis. *Am J Pathol*. 2002;161:2153-67.

Hemorrhagic Fever Viruses (Ebola, Dengue, Lassa)

80. Bhamarapravati N, Tuchinda P, Boonyapaknavik V. Pathology of Thailand haemorrhagic fever: a study of 100 autopsy cases. *Ann Trop Med Parasitol*. 1967;61:500-10.
81. Burke T. Dengue haemorrhagic fever: a pathological study. *Trans R Soc Trop Med Hyg*. 1968;62:682-92.
82. Burt FJ, Swanepoel R, Shieh WJ, et al. Immunohistochemical and in situ localization of Crimean-Congo hemorrhagic fever (CCHF) virus in human tissues and implications for CCHF pathogenesis. *Arch Pathol Lab Med*. 1997;121:839-46.
83. Walker DH, McCormick JB, Johnson KM, et al. Pathologic and virologic study of fatal Lassa fever in man. *Am J Pathol*. 1982;107:349-56.
84. Zaki SR, Peters CJ. Viral hemorrhagic fevers. In: Connor DH, Chandler FW, Schwartz DA, Manz HJ, Lack EE, eds. *Pathology of Infectious Diseases*. Stamford, CT: Appleton and Lange; 1997:347-64.

14 Human Parasitic Pulmonary Infections

Gary W. Procop • Ronald C. Neafie

INTRODUCTION

Parasitic infections remain an important cause of pulmonary disease throughout the world, although less frequently encountered in developed countries. The most common protozoal parasite-associated lung diseases throughout the world are caused by *Plasmodium falciparum* (falciparum malaria) and *Toxoplasma gondii* (toxoplasmosis). Helminths cause a variety of pulmonary diseases. The most common diseases caused by nematodes include the transient disease associated with transpulmonary migration, the aberrant migration of the larvae of zoonotic pathogens (i.e., visceral larva migrans), hypersensitivity reactions to parasite antigens, and infection by *Strongyloides stercoralis*, which includes the possibility of hyperinfection. Echinococcosis is the most important pulmonary disease caused by a cestode, but the recognition of pulmonary cysticercosis is also critical. *Paragonimus* is the most commonly recognized trematode that causes pulmonary disease, but schistosomes, because of their wide range of endemicity and the vast number of people infected, also are an important cause of pulmonary disease. The recognition of these infections is important, since specific antiparasitic chemotherapy and/or surgery are required to produce a cure.

In excised tissues, parasites may be dead, degenerated, incompletely sampled, or tangentially sectioned, posing a diagnostic dilemma for the pathologist. Under such conditions, a specific diagnosis based on parasite morphology can only be achieved when unique morphologic features of the organisms are present. The definitive identification of parasites in human tissue may not be possible in some instances. A thorough understanding of the parasites most likely to be encountered in the lungs and their morphologic features, however, helps to suggest the correct possibility. The definitive diagnosis is often achieved by using a combination of studies, which in addition to the morphologic findings, includes serology, a thorough history to evaluate the possibility of exposure (e.g., travel to an endemic area), and molecular diagnostics.

Greater than forty types of parasites can be found in the lungs of humans (Table 14-1). Two of these, *Paragonimus* and *Echinococcus* species, preferentially infect the lungs. The remainder are either lost in the wrong tissue or host or in transit to another anatomic site, or pulmonary involvement is part of disseminated disease. This review is not comprehensive and describes only the parasites that are most likely to be encountered by the practicing pathologist and clinician in North America. It focuses primarily upon pulmonary manifestations of these organisms. The reader who desires additional information is referred to the references at the end of this chapter.

PROTOZOAL CAUSES OF LUNG DISEASE

The majority (perhaps all) of the protozoal parasites that infect the lungs are not limited to this anatomic site, but are usually part of a disseminated, multiorgan infection.

TABLE 14-1

Parasites of the Human Lung

	Protozoa	Metazoa
More Common*	*Plasmodium falciparum* and *Toxoplasma gondii*	*Dirofilaria immitis, Strongyloides stercoralis, Toxocara* species, *Paragonimus* species, *Schistosoma* species, *Taenia solium, Echinococcus* species
Less Common*	*Entamoeba histolytica, Cryptosporidium* species, *Leishmania donovani, Trypanosoma cruzi, Acanthamoeba* species, and *Trichomonas tenax*	*Wuchereria bancrofti, Brugia malayi, Onchocerca volvulus, Capillaria aerophila, Mammomonogamus laryngeus, Ascaris lumbricoides, Ascaris suum, Mansonella perstans, Angiostrongylus cantonensis, Halicephalobus (Microema) deletrix, Metastrongylus elongates, Enterobius vermicularis, Lagochilascaris minor, Baylisascaris procyonis,* anisakids, *Gnathostoma spinigerum, Alaria* species, *Fasciola hepatica, Clinostomum complanatum, Spirometra* species, mites, fly larvae, *Armillifer* species, *Linguatula serrata* and *Limnatis nilotica*

*More common and less common do not refer to the overall prevalence of infection, but rather to the frequency of the parasite reported in histologic sections from the lung. For example, although *Ascaris* is one of the most common nematode infections in the world, it causes minimal pulmonary disease during pulmonary transmigration and therefore is infrequently encountered in histologic sections from the lung.

The following discussion is focused upon infections caused by *Plasmodium* species (*P. falciparum* [falciparum malaria] and *Toxoplasma gondii* [toxoplasmosis]), because of their wide distribution and the severity of the diseases they may cause.

FALCIPARUM MALARIA (*PLASMODIUM FALCIPARUM*)

Although malaria is far less common in North America than in previous centuries, it remains one of the most serious public health problems in the world. This disease kills approximately 2 million people each year, mostly children. Four species of *Plasmodium* are responsible for human disease: *P. falciparum, P. vivax, P. ovale,* and *P. malariae.* The most serious form is falciparum malaria, and is the type that most commonly causes pulmonary manifestations (i.e., malarial lung).

CLINICAL FEATURES

The presentation of soldiers with pulmonary malaria has been described as variable, with symptoms ranging from dry cough to acute respiratory distress similar to that encountered in patients with asthma. Pulmonary disease is usually associated with evidence of multisystem progression, such as brain involvement (i.e., cerebral ma-

laria) and kidney involvement (acute renal failure). Characteristically, the onset of malarial lung is abrupt and progresses rapidly from cough/dyspnea to severe hypoxia and respiratory arrest. The terminal event is usually preceded by breathing abnormalities, such as Cheyne-Stokes breathing, suggestive of brain stem dysfunction.

Acute pulmonary insufficiency, without cardiac decompensation or fluid overload, occurs in approximately 7% of nonimmune patients with falciparum malaria, and presents usually 2 to 3 days after the onset of fever and chills. Although initially the respiratory rate, blood pressure, and clinical examination may be normal, the clinical features of these patients change rapidly. The first clinical signs of pulmonary involvement may be circumoral cyanosis, dyspnea, and increased respiratory rate. The cyanosis spreads to the face and extremities. A spasmodic cough may develop, and there is a decrease in the hematocrit. Scattered rhonchi and rales may be heard in the basal aspects of the lungs, and foamy, blood-tinged sputum may be produced. Death usually occurs 24 hours after the recognition of malarial involvement of the lung. In addition to the malaria-induced lung injury, iatrogenic fluid overload and secondary bacterial pneumonias are perils for these patients.

RADIOLOGIC FEATURES

The chest radiograph is normal in the early phases of pulmonary involvement, with changes becoming discernible 6 to 24 hours after the onset of dyspnea. Signs of pulmonary edema appear, such as a generalized increase in the interstitial markings, and progress to fluffy infiltrations in both lungs. Evidence of a secondary bacterial pneumonia may also be detected.

PATHOLOGIC FEATURES

GROSS FINDINGS

The lungs of patients with pulmonary involvement by *P. falciparum* are congested, edematous, and heavy. Focal hemorrhages may be seen throughout, and pink foamy fluid fills the airways. A serosanguineous pleural effusion may be present. Areas of consolidation will be evident if secondary bacterial pneumonia is present.

MICROSCOPIC FINDINGS

Microscopically, there is severe pulmonary edema with capillary congestion and thickened alveolar septa. Hyaline membranes are present in approxi-

mately 50% of patients, but thrombosis and infarcts are absent. The edema fluid that fills the alveoli contains macrophages that, in turn, contain hemozoin pigment (Figure 14-1). The astute observer may note the presence of infected erythrocytes within the capillaries of the thickened alveolar septa. Evidence of disseminated intravascular coagulation is usually absent, but rarely has been described. Secondary bacterial pneumonia, usually bronchopneumonia, is often present.

ANCILLARY STUDIES

Rapid antigen detection assays are useful in the field, and are likely comparable to good microscopy. A variety of nucleic acid amplification methods have been described for the detection and differentiation of *Plasmodium* species, including real-time PCR assays that detect all four *Plasmodium* species and differentiate them based on post-amplification melt curve analysis (Figure 14-2).

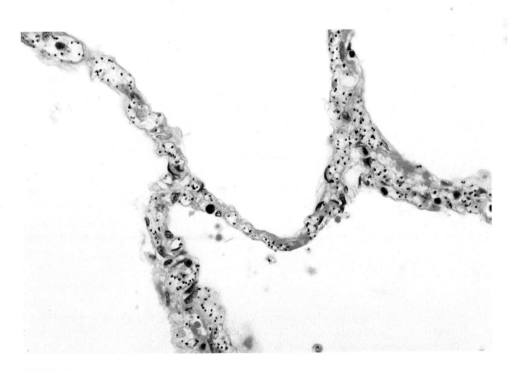

FIGURE 14-1

Plasmodium falciparum **infection**
The hemozoin pigment produced by *Plasmodium* species is readily detected in routinely stained sections. Prominent involvement of the pulmonary alveolar capillaries is demonstrated here.

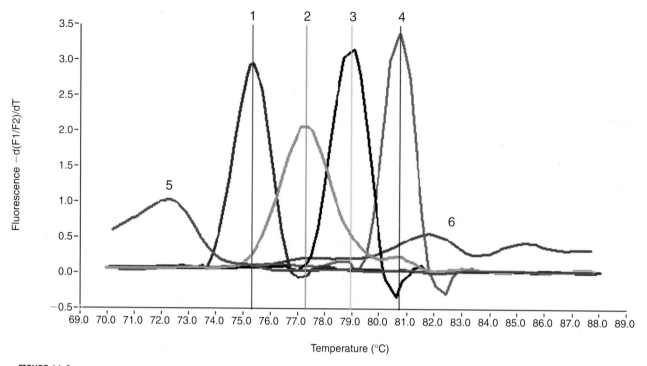

FIGURE 14-2

Post-amplification melt curve analysis
The four *Plasmodium* species that commonly cause human disease are differentiated using post-amplification melt curve analysis. 1 = *P. malariae*, 2 = *P. falciparum*, 3 = *P. ovale*, 4 = *P. vivax*, 5 = Primer dimers, 6 = Human DNA (negative control). (This image is compliments of Kathy Mangold and Dr. Karen L. Kaul, Evanston Northwestern Healthcare, Evanston, IL.)

DIFFERENTIAL DIAGNOSIS

The differential diagnosis of malaria is extensive and includes diseases such as typhoid fever, typhus, dengue, and the cyclic fevers caused by filarial worms, among others. Other differential diagnostic considerations for of the pulmonary manifestations in patients with falciparum malaria include secondary bacterial pneumonia and metabolic acidosis.

PROGNOSIS AND THERAPY

The severity of falciparum malaria depends on a variety of factors, such a previous infection (i.e., some degree of immunity), the host inflammatory response, and pregnancy, among others. The mortality for those who develop severe falciparum malaria is high, with a rate of 15-30% even with intensive care treatment. In contrast, the mortality of uncomplicated acute falciparum malaria is about 0.4%. There is a high mortality associated with development of malarial lung.

Pulmonary edema associated with severe falciparum malaria may present at any time during the course of illness, even when the patient is improving clinically and there is a resolution or reduction in the parasitemia. Pregnant women are at a particularly high risk. The mortality rate for patients with pulmonary edema who do not have ventilatory support is approximately 80%. However, even with ventilatory support the mortality rate of affected patients is higher than those without pulmonary involvement. Patients so affected often die within 3 to 8 days after onset of malaria, usually within 24 hours of the recognition of pulmonary involvement.

The prompt diagnosis and treatment of falciparum malaria may curtail the development of malarial lung. Successful treatment of malaria includes the administration of antimalarials and maintenance of optimal ventilation. The use of exchange transfusion is controversial, but may benefit some patients. Patients with complicating bacterial pneumonia should be treated with appropriate antibacterial agents.

FALCIPARUM MALARIA (MALARIAL LUNG)—FACT SHEET

Definition

- Four *Plasmodium* species, *P. falciparum*, *P. vivax*, *P. ovale*, and *P. malariae*, cause human malaria
- *Plasmodium falciparum* causes the most serious form of malaria and can cause pulmonary disease

Epidemiology

- Malaria, transmitted by the *Anopheles* mosquito, kills approximately 2 million people each year
- Disease is present in all hemispheres, but is more prevalent in a tropical and sub-tropical areas

Clinical Features

- Malarial lung presents approximately 2 to 3 days after the onset of fever and chills
- Pulmonary presentation is variable, but progression is usually rapid from cough/dyspnea to severe hypoxia and respiratory arrest
- Iatrogenic fluid overload and secondary bacterial pneumonia are also risks for these patients

Radiologic Features

- Radiographic changes manifest from 6 to 24 hours after the onset of dyspnea
- Chest radiographs show signs of pulmonary edema

Prognosis and Therapy

- The mortality rate for those with severe falciparum malaria is 15-30% even with intensive care treatment; pregnant women are at a particularly high risk
- Pulmonary edema in falciparum malaria is a poor prognostic sign, with 80% mortality without ventilatory support
- Death usually occurs within 3 to 8 days after the onset of malaria and usually within 24 hours of the recognition of pulmonary involvement
- Typical treatments for cardiogenic pulmonary edema are not helpful
- Successful treatment will include antimalarials, maintaining optimal ventilation, managing metabolic acidosis and hypovolemia while avoiding overhydration, and prompt treatment for secondary bacterial infections

---

FALCIPARUM MALARIA (MALARIAL LUNG)—PATHOLOGIC FEATURES

- Severe pulmonary edema, with capillary congestion and thickened alveolar septa
- Macrophages with hemozoin pigment and infected erythrocytes within the capillaries
- Diffuse alveolar damage occurs in 50% of patients

TOXOPLASMOSIS *(TOXOPLASMA GONDII)*

Toxoplasma gondii infection is highly prevalent throughout the world, and it is estimated that 50% of the world population is infected. Herein, we concentrate on the far less common pulmonary manifestations of toxoplasmosis.

CLINICAL FEATURES

People with an intact immune system who become infected respond to and contain the parasite. Such patients may be asymptomatic, develop a mononucleosis-like syndrome, or develop localized lymphadenopathy. Disseminated *Toxoplasma gondii* infections, which may have pulmonary involvement, occur in three clinical situations: 1) congenital toxoplasmosis, 2) in patients with AIDS, and 3) in patients with a non-HIV-associated immunosuppressive condition. In congenital toxoplasmosis, the infection is acquired during pregnancy and transmitted from the mother to the fetus. Congenital toxoplasmosis may be acute, subacute, or chronic. Acute severe disease results in death *in utero*. Parasitic infection with *T. gondii* is an important cause of morbidity and mortality for patients with advanced HIV infection or AIDS. Cerebral toxoplasmosis is most common in these patients, secondary to the reactivation of latent bradyzoite cysts. Patients with AIDS will less commonly (approximately 2%) have extracerebral toxoplasmosis, with a 0.5% prevalence of pulmonary toxoplasmosis. The non-AIDS immunocompromising conditions associated with toxoplasmosis are hematopoietic malignancy, transplantation (particularly stem cell/bone marrow transplantation), and conditions wherein high-dose or prolonged corticosteroid use is employed. Disseminated toxoplasmosis in these patients may have a prominent pulmonary component.

Pulmonary involvement occurs in more than 70% of patients with disseminated toxoplasmosis. A nonproductive cough and dyspnea are the most common symptoms, and fever is the most common sign. In some patients, the presenting or most significant features may be empyema or pleural effusion. Infection of lung tissue indicates dissemination of the parasite. There is a high likelihood of death in these patients from bronchopneumonia or meningoencephalitis.

RADIOLOGIC FEATURES

Chest radiographs lack both sensitivity and specificity; chest CT scanning is superior for more sensitive detection of findings. Radiographic patterns described in patients with pulmonary toxoplasmosis include bilateral diffuse pneumonia, miliary nodules, and interstitial and lobar infiltrates. CT scans may show ground-glass opacities and possibly superimposed septal thickening and intralobular linear opacities. Hilar and mediastinal lymphadenopathy is usually absent.

PATHOLOGIC FEATURES

GROSS FINDINGS

At autopsy, the lungs are heavily congested, with petechial hemorrhages and areas of consolidation and necrosis.

MICROSCOPIC FINDINGS

The proliferative form of *Toxoplasma* is the crescentic, subtly pyriform tachyzoite. It may be detected in cytologic preparations from sputa or bronchoalveolar lavage fluid. It is 4-8 microns in smear preparations, but in histologic sections it is approximately half this size. Tachyzoites, which are plentiful in fulminant disease, stain well with the routine hematoxylin-eosin stain, but can also be highlighted with the Giemsa or eosin-methylene blue stains. Oil immersion microscopy may be necessary because of the small size of these organisms. Tachyzoites can likely replicate in any nucleated cell, but are most frequently seen in the brain, heart, liver, intestine, lungs, and lymph nodes.

Coagulation necrosis and an alveolar fibrinous exudate are seen in the lungs, with chronic inflammation and edema. Many alveoli may be collapsed and contain cells packed with tachyzoites. Pseudocysts are prevalent in areas of necrosis. True cysts may also be observed (Figure 14-3). True cysts, which are present in chronic disease, may be differentiated from the pseudocysts of acute toxoplasmosis with histochemical stains.

The periodic acid–Schiff (PAS) and Gomori methenamine silver (GMS) stains highlight true cysts; the cyst wall is usually argyrophilic and bradyzoites are usually PAS-positive. In contrast, pseudocyst walls and tachyzoites stain weakly with those reagents, but are readily identified in hematoxylin and eosin stained sections in tissues from patients with fulminant disease.

ANCILLARY STUDIES

Serologic studies are useful for the diagnosis of toxoplasmosis. The presence of IgM antibody or a four-fold rise in the IgG antibody is indicative of acute infection. The presence of stable IgG antibody is indicative of prior infection, which means the patient likely has bradyzoite cysts dormant in his or her tissues and is at risk for reactivation toxoplasmosis in the event of profound immunosuppression.

Immunohistochemical staining has been described as likely superior to histochemical staining for the detection of rare organisms. However, because there are usually a large number of organisms present in dissemination disease, it is questionable whether immunohistochemistry is truly necessary to achieve the diagnosis. Nucleic acid amplification assays, such as the polymerase chain reaction (PCR), hold the greatest promise as a useful ancillary method of detection. PCR assays have been used to detect toxoplasmosis in amniotic fluid, cerebrospinal fluid, aqueous humor, blood, and bronchoalveolar lavage fluid.

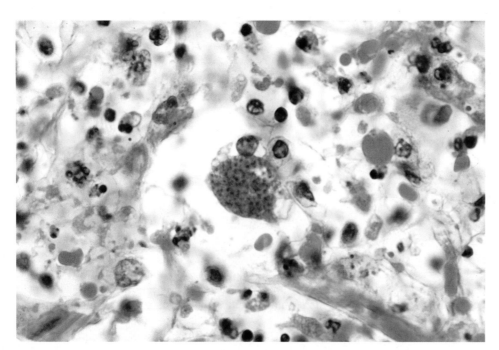

FIGURE 14-3

Toxoplasma gandii
A cyst filled with bradyzoites is present in this patient with pulmonary involvement by *T. gondii*.

TOXOPLASMOSIS—FACT SHEET

Definition

▸ Pulmonary toxoplasmosis, which is part of disseminated disease caused by *Toxoplasma gondii*, occurs with congenital toxoplasmosis and with infections of immunocompromised patients

Epidemiology

▸ *Toxoplasma gondii* infection is highly prevalent throughout the world
▸ Oocysts are passed in the feces of the definitive hosts, members of the family *Felidae* (i.e., cats), and are consumed by humans and other intermediate hosts wherein they asexually replicate and encyst

Clinical Features

▸ Infection of people with an intact immune system is subclinical, or consists of a mononucleosis-like syndrome with or without localized lymphadenopathy
▸ Disseminated infections occur in congenital disease, and in patients with AIDS and other types of immuncompromise
▸ Pulmonary involvement occurs in more than 70% of immunocompromised patients with disseminated toxoplasmosis, and the likelihood of death is high in this situation
▸ A nonproductive cough and dyspnea are the most common symptoms, and fever is the most common sign

Radiologic Features

▸ Radiographic findings include bilateral diffuse pneumonia, miliary nodules, and interstitial and lobar infiltrates
▸ CT scans may show ground-glass opacities and superimposed septal thickening and intralobular linear opacities

Prognosis and Therapy

▸ The prognosis is poor for patients with disseminated toxoplasmosis; the death rate is up to 92% in bone marrow transplant recipients who develop pulmonary toxoplasmosis
▸ The prophylaxis and treatment of choice is pyrimethamine/ sulfadoxine, but this therapy kills only the proliferating tachyzoites, not the quiescent cysts
▸ Prevention of primary toxoplasmosis includes avoiding contact with cat feces, good hand washing, washing of fruits and vegetables, and thorough cooking of meats before consumption

TOXOPLASMOSIS—PATHOLOGIC FEATURES

▸ The proliferative form of *Toxoplasma*, which is morphologically diagnostic, is the crescentic, subtly pyriform tachyzoite
▸ Pseudocysts and true cysts are also present
▸ Coagulation necrosis, an alveolar fibrinous exudate, interstitial chronic inflammation and edema are present

PROGNOSIS AND THERAPY

The prognosis is poor for patients with disseminated toxoplasmosis. A 92% death rate has been reported for bone marrow transplant recipients who develop pulmonary toxoplasmosis, with approximately half of the deaths occurring within 3 days after the onset of symptoms. The prophylaxis and treatment of choice is with pyrimethamine/sulfadoxine. This therapy kills the proliferating tachyzoites, but is not active against quiescent cysts. Therefore, the immunocompromised patient remains at risk for reactivation toxoplasmosis at any time.

Preventive measures to avoid contracting primary toxoplasmosis include avoidance of contact with cat feces, good hand-washing, thorough washing of fruits and vegetables, and complete cooking of meats before consumption. These measures are helpful in preventing congenital toxoplasmosis associated with a primary infection, but are not helpful in reducing reactivation toxoplasmosis associated with immunosuppression.

LESS COMMON PROTOZOAL CAUSES OF LUNG DISEASE

A variety of other protozoa have been identified as causes of human pulmonary infections, including *Cryptosporidium* species, *Entamoeba histolytica* (Figure 14-4), *Trypanosoma cruzi* and *Leishmania donovani*.

HELMINTHIC CAUSES OF LUNG DISEASE

NEMATODES

Ascaris lumbricoides and other roundworms, such as hookworms and filariae, infect millions of people throughout the world, but are a relatively rare cause of pulmonary disease. Part of the success of these parasites is that the migration, maturation, and subsequent

DIFFERENTIAL DIAGNOSIS

The differential diagnosis of congenital toxoplasmosis includes other infectious diseases known to cause intrauterine fetal demise, such as cytomegalovirus and herpes simplex virus. There are numerous causes of pneumonia in immunocompromised patients, including opportunistic pathogens such as *Pneumocystis jiroveci*, *Aspergillus*, zygomycetes, *Nocardia*, and multiple viruses, as well as agents causing pneumonia in healthy hosts.

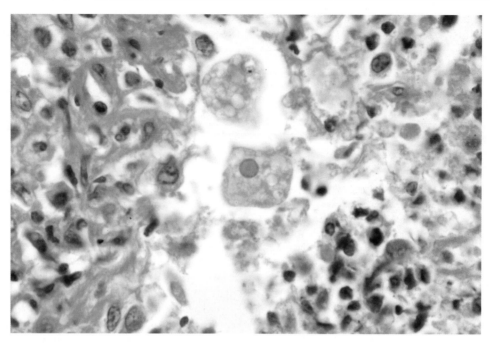

FIGURE 14-4

Entamoeba histolytica

The peripheral chromatin and tiny central karyosome of the trophozoite of *E. histolytica* is demonstrable in this patient with pulmonary involvement by this amoeba.

dwelling in the intestine usually causes minimal tissue damage (i.e., the most biologically successful parasites do not significantly harm the host). The significant conditions caused by nematodes, for the most part, may be separated into several categories: 1) hyperinfection of the immunocompromised host by *Strongyloides stercoralis*; 2) the aberrant migrations of animal nematodes (i.e., visceral larva migrans) and, more rarely, nematodes that normally infect humans; and 3) hypersensitivity reactions to parasite antigens.

STRONGYLOIDIASIS (STRONGYLOIDES STERCORALIS)

Strongyloidiasis refers to an infection with *Strongyloides stercoralis*, a geohelminth that has both a parasitic and a free-living life cycle. The areas of endemicity are widespread in tropical and subtropical regions, including the southeastern United States. The infective filariform larvae of this helminth, like the cercariae of schistosomes and the larvae of hookworms, have the ability to penetrate intact human skin. Following skin penetration, the larvae migrate to the lungs, where they penetrate the alveoli and enter the airways. The larvae are then swallowed, and mature into adult females in the distal stomach and small intestine. The parasitic female *S. stercoralis* is parthenogenetic, thus does not

require a male for reproduction. Unlike other intestinal helminths that produce eggs that are passed intact in the stool and embryonate in the soil, the eggs of *Strongyloides* release rhabditiform larvae within the intestinal tract that are then passed in the feces. Rhabditiform larvae may differentiate into either infective filariform larvae or mature into male and female adults. Male and female adults copulate, and the gravid female produces eggs; this is the free-living, nonparasitic cycle. Alternatively, the rhabditiform larvae may differentiate into the infective filariform larvae in the intestinal tract. This feature affords the parasite the opportunity to auto-infect the host, which may occur internally through the bowel wall or externally through the skin in the perianal region. This difference between *Strongyloides* and other intestinal geohelminths is important, since it is pivotal for the establishment of chronic strongyloidiasis and, in immunocompromised hosts, the commonly fatal hyperinfection.

CLINICAL FEATURES

The clinical manifestations of strongyloidiasis may be separated into acute disease, uncomplicated chronic disease, or complicated chronic disease, which includes the hyperinfection syndrome.

In acute disease, there is a transient, mild dermatitis that is pruritic and erythematous, which occurs after filariform larvae penetrate the skin and begin migration. About a week later, cough and sore throat may develop, followed by nonspecific abdominal complaints, such as diarrhea and a feeling of fullness.

Patients who have chronic strongyloidiasis may have nutritional deficits, but most often the infection is subclinical, remains undetected, and persists for years secondary to low-grade reinfection. Between 15 and 30% of patients with uncomplicated chronic strongyloidiasis are asymptomatic. The remainder have nonspecific findings similar to those described above. Gastrointestinal symptoms are most common at this stage, followed by pulmonary complaints that may include wheezing and dyspnea.

Complicated chronic strongyloidiasis manifests in the elderly and those with an immunocompromising condition or taking immunosuppressive medications. Although the reproductive activity of the worms in patients with chronic uncomplicated strongyloidiasis is regulated in some manner so that the host is not in danger from an enormous worm burden, the host-parasite regulatory mechanism is lost in patients with compromised immunity, and increasing autoinfection leads to life-threatening hyperinfection. In the gut of hyperinfected patients, numerous adult worms produce rhabditiform larvae that molt into filariform larvae that migrate through most organs, particularly the lungs. The severity of pulmonary symptoms correlates with the number of migrating larvae. Pulmonary symptoms consist of dyspnea, cough, hemoptysis, cyanosis, and respiratory distress. Eosinophilia may be present, but is often suppressed due to the effects of corticosteroids.

RADIOLOGIC FEATURES

The initial infection and the transient migration of *Strongyloides* larvae, and for that matter the transient transpulmonary migration of any human intestinal helminths (e.g., *Ascaris lumbricoides*), result in changes that range from normal to the transient pulmonary infiltrates of Löffler's Syndrome. Patients with uncomplicated chronic strongyloidiasis usually have normal chest radiographs. The radiologic findings associated with the *Strongyloides* hyperinfection include normal chest radiographs, nonsegmental patchy infiltrates, nodular infiltrates, or multiple infiltrates. Lung abscesses, nodules that mimic tuberculosis, diffuse infiltrates, and pleural effusions may also be seen.

PATHOLOGIC FEATURES

The morphologic diagnosis is usually made by the identification of larvae in sputum, bronchoalveolar lavage (BAL) fluid, or feces (Figure 14-5). The fortuitous demonstration of migrating larvae in either ascitic or cerebrospinal fluid also can provide the diagnosis. In hyperinfection, filariform larvae may appear in virtually any organ and must be differentiated from other parasites of humans such as *Ascaris, Necator,* and *Ancylostoma,* as well as zoonotic pathogens that cause visceral larva migrans (e.g., *Toxocara* or *Baylisascaris*). The invasive filariform larvae of *S. stercoralis* measure 400-700 microns in length X 12-20 microns in diameter.

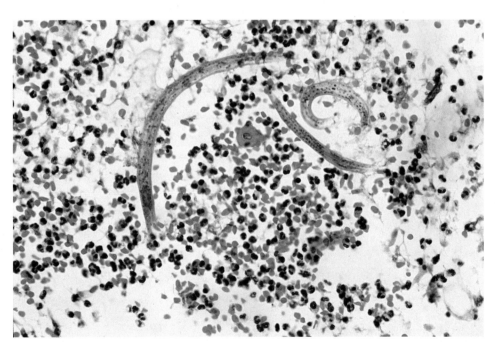

FIGURE 14-5

Strongyloides stercoralis
Filariform larvae are present in sputum admixed with acute inflammation and abundant eosinophils.

Larvae migrate to the pulmonary capillaries, where they penetrate alveoli, causing small hemorrhages that occasionally become severe (Figure 14-6). Infiltrates of polymorphonuclear leukocytes and monocytes follow. Tracts of tissue necrosis are left in the wake of the migrating larvae. More rarely, both cavities and abscesses of the lung have been associated with filariform larvae.

ANCILLARY STUDIES

A stool examination for the presence of the larvae of *Strongyloides* is often the first method attempted to make the diagnosis. If the larvae are present, the diagnosis is confirmed. However, the sensitivity of the stool examination varies from 27-73%. Similarly, the sensitivity of the duodenal fluid examination (i.e., the string test) varies from 39-76%. Therefore, serologic assays that usually measure parasite-specific IgG are commonly used diagnostic tests. The sensitivities of these assays range from 85-88% and the specificities range from 97-99%. Not surprisingly, there is some cross-reactivity with antibodies directed against other parasites, such as *Ascaris lumbricoides*. Although nucleic acid amplification assays for the detection of *S. stercoralis* have been described, these are not used in common practice.

DIFFERENTIAL DIAGNOSIS

The differential diagnosis for patients with eosinophilia includes other parasitic and nonparasitic disorders. The symptomatology of acute and uncomplicated chronic strongyloidiasis is also very nonspecific, so the differential diagnosis is broad. The possibility of a *Strongyloides* hyperinfection syndrome is usually considered in ill immunocompromised patients with appropriate symptomatology, however, given the severity and notoriety of this infection. Other disorders, such as sepsis, disseminated or invasive fungal infections, disseminated CMV, or post-transplant lymphoproliferative disorder, amongst many others, may be considered in an immunocompromised person who becomes severely ill.

PROGNOSIS AND THERAPY

There is no appreciable mortality associated with acute and uncomplicated chronic disease. Hyperinfection syndrome, however, is one of the most deadly infections of the transplant recipient. The mortality of *Strongyloides* hyperinfection in one series was noted to be 86%.

Thiabendazole is one of the most commonly used drugs for the treatment of strongyloidiasis. Albendazole

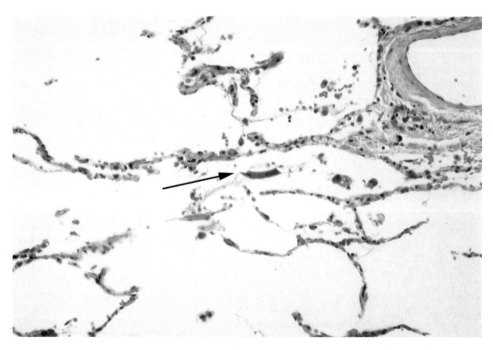

FIGURE 14-6

Strongyloides stercoralis
This tangentially sectioned portion of a filariform larva of *S. stercoralis* could easily be overlooked.

VISCERAL LARVA MIGRANS

Visceral larva migrans (VLM) is an infection by zoonotic helminth larvae that migrate aimlessly throughout the body because they are in an aberrant host. A variety of worms cause this disease, but the most common is *Toxocara canis*, the intestinal ascarid of dogs and other canids. Other causes include infections by *T. cati*, the intestinal ascarid of cats, and *Baylisascaris procyonis*, the raccoon roundworm. *Toxocara* is present in almost all young dogs, and infects cats at some time during their lives. A puppy in a household is a significant risk factor for VLM. The disease occurs worldwide, and is most often found in young children living in crowded dwellings where they are exposed to dog feces. Geophagia-pica is an obvious risk factor. Sandboxes and parks where dogs or other animals defecate are common areas where infection may occur. Dogs and cats become infected by ingesting embryonated eggs, after which larval migration and maturation resembles that of *Ascaris* in humans.

CLINICAL FEATURES

Humans acquire VLM by ingesting eggs of *Toxocara canis* or another zoonotic helminthic parasite. Alternatively, disease may also be contracted by consuming the larvae in the raw or undercooked meat of a paratenic host, such as a pig. Eggs that enter the stomach or small intestine release larvae that penetrate the mucosa and enter blood vessels. Larvae are carried to liver, lung, brain, eye, and other organs where they may migrate; they then become dormant but remain viable to possibly migrate again. Eventually they die.

Most patients infected by significant numbers of larvae have pulmonary symptoms, but severe pulmonary disease is rare. An example of a typical patient is a child with hypereosinophilia, pneumonitis, fever, hypergammaglobulinemia, and a history of potential exposure.

and ivermectin are other excellent therapeutic options. Hyperinfection requires hospitalization and prolonged courses of the antiparasitic agent, possibly with long-term suppressive therapy. In addition to specific antiparasitic therapy, immunosuppressive therapy should be discontinued or reduced as much as possible. Serum immunoglobulin levels may be used to follow therapy; a significant decline should be noted within 4 months following successful therapy.

Other common findings include pruritus, a rash, anorexia, weakness, pain in muscles and joints, fever, irritability, weight loss, and nocturnal sweats. Patients with pneumonia have manifestations that range from cough and mild wheezing to severe asthma-like symptoms and acute respiratory distress. Rales and rhonchi are found throughout the lungs. Unlike hyperinfection with strongyloidiasis, the sputum does not contain larvae.

RADIOLOGIC FEATURES

At least half of patients with VLM have a normal chest radiograph. Radiologic findings described in the remainder of the patients are variable, and include bilateral patchy infiltrates that may be migratory, or less commonly segmental or alveolar infiltrates.

PATHOLOGIC FEATURES

A biopsy is not usually needed to achieve the diagnosis. Diagnostic suspicions are usually confirmed with a positive serology in a child who eats dirt and has Löffler's syndrome. Eggs of *Ascaris* or *Trichuris* in the stool do not exclude the possibility of VLM, since these worms are commonly found in patients with VLM (i.e., there are shared risk factors for all geohelminth infections).

The morphologic diagnosis is made by identifying larvae in biopsy specimens or at autopsy. The *Toxocara canis* larvae are 400-500 × 18-21 μm and have minute, single lateral alae (Figure 14-7), whereas the larvae of *T. cati*, which have similar features (e.g., minute lateral alae) and length, but have a diameter of 15-17 μm. There is necrosis of tissues secondary to larval migration, and

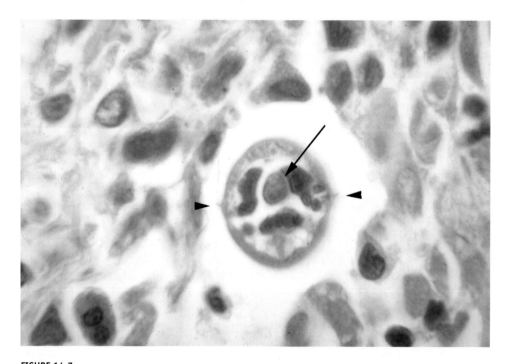

FIGURE 14-7

Toxocara canis
The migrating larva of *T. canis* has small lateral alae (arrowheads), which are useful for identification. A centrally located esophagus (long arrow) is surrounded by ganglionic cells in this anteriorly located section of the worm.

eosinophils dominate the early inflammatory response to larvae in lungs. Histiocytes eventually surround degenerating larvae, and eosinophilic granulomas are formed.

ANCILLARY STUDIES

Eosinophilia is the laboratory finding that may initially suggest the possibility of a parasitic infection. The degree of eosinophilia correlates with the degree of infection. There is also an increase in the total IgE levels and an elevation of parasite-specific immunoglobulins, which help establish the diagnosis.

DIFFERENTIAL DIAGNOSIS

The differential diagnosis includes Löffler's syndrome secondary to other causes, such as migrating human parasites like *Ascaris lumbricoides* (Figure 14-8),

Churg-Strauss syndrome, tropical pulmonary eosinophilia (TPE), idiopathic hypereosinophilic syndrome, and systemic vasculitides, among others. Many of these may readily be excluded based on lack of exposure (TPE, for example) and the profile of the patient.

PROGNOSIS AND THERAPY

Visceral larva migrans is rarely life-threatening, although the prognosis is guarded for patients with a heavy larval burden. The vast majority of infections are self-limited, and symptoms resolve without treatment. However, long-term morbidity such as blindness or seizures may persist. Albendazole is the drug of choice, although there is no therapy that has been proven effective. Other therapeutic alternatives are mebendazole, thiabendazole, and diethylcarbamazine (DEC). Concomitant corticosteroids may be necessary to attenuate an intense inflammatory response.

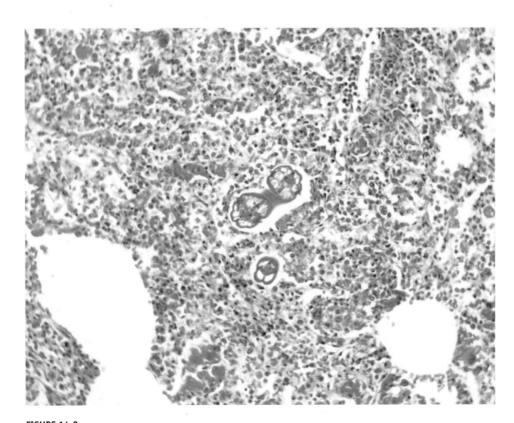

FIGURE 14-8

Ascaris lumbricoides
Löffler's or eosinophilic pneumonia in this instance was caused by the transpulmonary migration of the larvae of *Ascaris lumbricoides*.

VISCERAL LARVA MIGRANS—FACT SHEET

Definition

▸ Visceral larva migrans (VLM) is an infection by zoonotic helminth larvae that migrate aimlessly throughout the body because they are in an aberrant host

▸ *Toxocara cati*, the intestinal ascarid of dogs and other canids, is the most common cause; other causes include but are not limited to infections by *T. canis*, the intestinal ascarid of cats, and *Baylisascaris procyonis*, the raccoon roundworm

Epidemiology

▸ *Toxocara* is present in almost all puppies, and infects cats at some point during their lives

▸ Risk factors include crowded dwellings, exposure to dog feces, and geophagia-pica

▸ VLM occurs worldwide, with varying prevalence depending on location

Clinical Features

▸ The manifestations are determined by the extent of the infection and the organs most heavily involved

▸ Light infections may be asymptomatic, whereas heavy infections may result in severe morbidity, and rarely even death

▸ Death is usually secondary to lung and/or brain involvement. Severe morbidity results from ocular involvement

▸ Common findings include hypereosinophilia, pneumonitis, fever, hypergammaglobulinemia, a history of potential exposure, pruritus, a rash, anorexia, weakness, pain in muscles and joints, fever, irritability, weight loss, and nocturnal sweats; hepatomegaly is found secondary to an accumulation of the larvae in the liver

▸ Pulmonary manifestations range from cough and mild wheezing to severe asthma-like symptoms and acute respiratory distress; unlike *Strongyloides* hyperinfection, the sputum does not usually contain larvae

Radiologic Features

▸ At least half of patients with VLM have a normal chest radiograph, but others have bilateral patchy infiltrates that may be migratory or segmental alveolar infiltrates

Prognosis and Therapy

▸ Visceral larva migrans is rarely life-threatening and is usually self-limited, and symptoms resolve without treatment

▸ The prognosis is guarded for patients with a heavy larval burden, and long-term morbidity, such as blindness or seizures, may persist

▸ Albendazole and other anthelminthic drugs, such as mebendazole, thiabendazole, and diethylcarbamazine (DEC), have been used

▸ Anti- inflammatory and antiepileptic medications may also be necessary

---

VISCERAL LARVA MIGRANS—PATHOLOGIC FEATURES

▸ A positive serology in the appropriate clinical setting is usually sufficient; a biopsy is not usually needed to achieve the diagnosis

▸ *Toxocara canis* larvae are 400-500 μm × 18-21 μm with a minute, single lateral ala

▸ Associated histologic changes include necrosis of tissues secondary to larval migration, eosinophilic infiltrates, and eosinophilic granulomas or abscesses

---

PULMONARY DISEASES CAUSED BY FILARIAL WORMS

There are three types of human pulmonary disease caused by filarial worms. *Dirofilaria* granuloma results from the incomplete development of the dog heartworm, *Dirofilaria immitis*, in humans. Two filarial worms that naturally infect humans, *Wuchereria bancrofti* and *Brugia malayi*, rarely cause pulmonary disease during their aberrant migration through the lung. Tropical pulmonary eosinophilia (TPE) is the other important pulmonary disease caused by the immunologic response to the microfilariae produced by the adult filarial worms.

DIROFILARIASIS *(DIROFILARIA IMMITIS)*

Dirofilariasis refers to infection of humans with the dog heartworm, *Dirofilaria immitis,* which can also infect other animals such as the wolf, bear, and domestic cat. The microfilariae are transmitted from the animal host to the human by several types of mosquitoes in the genera *Aedes, Culex,* and *Anopheles.* This parasite infects dogs in temperate and tropical areas of the Western Hemisphere and Asia, where it is well known to veterinarians, but does not routinely occur in Europe or Africa. The geographic distribution of canine dirofilariasis for the rest of the world remains to be determined. It is most prevalent in the southern United States, particularly along the Gulf and Atlantic coasts and along the Mississippi river. The prevalence of infection in humans parallels the prevalence in dogs, which underscores the importance of zoonotic control. Other risk factors include the prevalence of the mosquito vectors and the participation in activities that expose humans to the mosquito vectors. Dog ownership, however, is not a risk factor for dirofilariasis.

Dirofilariasis occurs following the bite of an infected mosquito. The blood of infected dogs contains microfilariae, which are produced by the adult worm that resides in the right ventricle of the animal's heart. Microfilariae mature to the infective third-stage larvae within the mosquito and are transferred to either the human or animal host during a blood meal. The parasite then migrates through subcutaneous tissue, where it molts and enters the bloodstream to reach the heart. In a suitable host, the worm matures into an adult and the cycle is complete. Humans, however, are unsuitable hosts, and the worm dies before reaching maturity. It is subsequently swept into the pulmonary arterial circulation, where it lodges in a pulmonary artery and causes thrombosis, infarction, inflammation, and eventually a granulomatous reaction surrounded by a wall of fibrous tissue.

CLINICAL FEATURES

People of all ages may become infected, but this disease is rare in childhood. Reported patient ages range from 8 to 80 years old, with the average in the mid-fifties. The male to female ratio has been reported as 2:1 and 1:1 in two series. The majority of patients with dirofilariasis, from 51.4-62.4%, are asymptomatic. Patients with symptoms may complain of cough, chest pain, hemoptysis, low-grade fever, chills, and malaise. 5-10% of patients have peripheral eosinophilia.

In addition to the lung, *D. immitis* has also rarely been identified in subcutaneous abscesses, the abdominal cavity, the eyes, and the testes. Other *Dirofilaria* species, however, more commonly reside in the subcutaneous tissues and must be considered as possible etiologic agents when one is examining a specimen that contains a filarial worm in a subcutaneous location.

RADIOLOGIC FEATURES

Nodules caused by *D. immitis* are usually discovered by a routine chest radiograph. These are usually (approximately 90%) single, but rarely 2 or 3 nodules may be present. Calcification is rare. The nodules average 1.9 cm in diameter.

PATHOLOGIC FEATURES

GROSS FINDINGS

Nodules are tan and firm, characteristically small (0.8–4.5 cm; mean 1.9 cm), subpleural, spherical, and well circumscribed. In one study, 76% of the lesions were present in the right lung.

MICROSCOPIC FINDINGS

The adult *D. immitis* in the dog measures 0.7-2.0 mm in diameter, but the worms found in human lungs are immature and much smaller, measuring 100-359 μm

in diameter. They have a smooth, thick cuticle (5-25 μm) with the 3 distinct layers characteristic of the genus *Dirofilaria*. The thick, multilayered cuticle projects inwardly at the lateral chords, forming two prominent, opposing, internal longitudinal ridges. The somatic musculature is typically prominent, but the lateral chords are usually poorly preserved. Transverse sections reveal two large uteri and a much smaller intestine in female worms (Figure 14-9); a single reproductive tube and intestine is present in the males.

ANCILLARY STUDIES

Fine needle aspirates have rarely been reported to yield a definitive diagnosis, and are usually nondiagnostic due to sampling error. Although the use of immunofluorescence antibodies and PCR has been described, these techniques have not proven to be of practical value, nor are they widely used. Serologic studies have not proven useful.

DIFFERENTIAL DIAGNOSIS

Immature *Dirofilaria* in the lung should not be confused with larval nematodes that may occur in the lung, because *Dirofilaria* is much larger and contains reproductive organs. Adult nematodes with fully developed reproductive organs are rarely found in lungs, and include *Enterobius vermicularis*, *Wuchereria bancrofti*, *Brugia malayi*, and *Angiostrongylus cantonensis*. They are morphologically very distinct from *D. immitis*. The definitive identification of the worm based on internal structures may be difficult to impossible, given the advanced stage of worm degeneration in many of these specimens (Figure 14-10). However, a parasitic worm in a pulmonary artery, associated with a pulmonary infarct/granuloma, is probably *D. immitis*. Documenting the presence of the worm is necessary for diagnosis, which may necessitate submitting the entire lesion for histologic study. This should be done only after other diagnostic possibilities, such as tuberculosis, have been excluded, since in these instances culture and antimicrobial susceptibility testing should be performed.

PROGNOSIS AND THERAPY

The excision of the nodule is curative. Additional antiparasitic therapy is not needed.

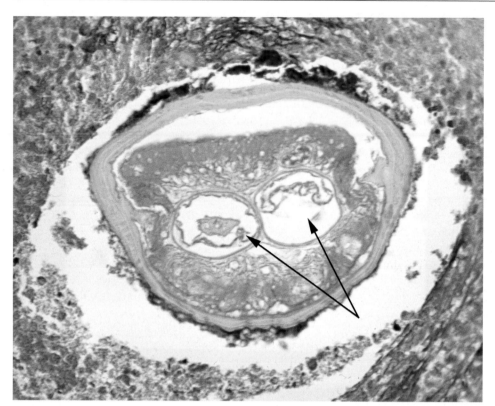

FIGURE 14-9

Dirofilaria immitis
Although degenerate, the multilayer cuticle, two uteri (arrows), and intestinal tract are evident in this immature female *D. immitis*. Note, however, that the uteri contain no microfilariae. Movat stain.

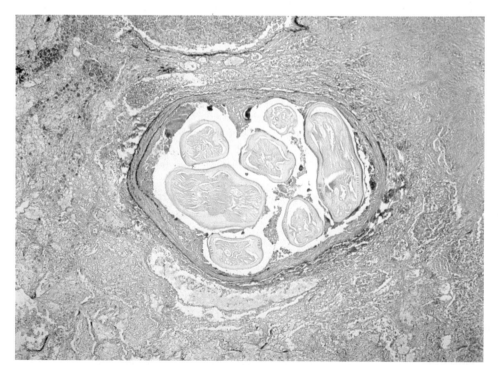

FIGURE 14-10

Dirofilaria immitis
A coiled immature male *D. immitis* is present in a pulmonary artery in an infarct.

individuals are more likely to develop TPE than people in endemic areas, and men are 4 times more likely than women to develop disease. Most affected individuals are in their second to fourth decades of life.

CLINICAL FEATURES

TPE is a hypersensitivity reaction to the microfilariae of *Wuchereria bancrofti* and *Brugia malayi*. Although this disease is caused by the microfilariae, these forms are notably absent from the blood smears of affected patients. This is because the microfilariae released by the adult filarial worm are rapidly cleared by the lung and other organs, such as the spleen. Pulmonary manifestations early in disease reflect hyperreactivity of the airways and include wheezing, dyspnea, and a paroxysmal cough that is worse at night. Fever, malaise, and weight loss are nonspecific features. Some patients develop nausea, vomiting, and/or diarrhea. Apparent spontaneous resolutions may occur, only to be followed by relapses. Late in the course of disease, patients develop pulmonary fibrosis.

Patients with adult filarial worms that have aberrantly migrated to the lung may be asymptomatic. Those with symptoms have reported chest pain and hemoptysis. All reported patients had visited endemic areas and developed symptomatology 2 to 3 years after returning to a nonendemic area.

RADIOLOGIC FEATURES

The most common reported finding is of bilateral reticulonodular infiltrates, miliary mottling, and increased bronchovascular markings. The parenchymal changes predominate in the middle and lower lung zones, whereas the increased vascular markings predominate in the bases. Less commonly, the chest radiograph demonstrates hilar adenopathy, pneumonitis, or pleural

TROPICAL PULMONARY EOSINOPHILIA AND ABERRANT FILARIA

Two filarial worms that naturally infect humans and cause tropical pulmonary eosinophilia (TPE) are considered here, *Wuchereria bancrofti* and *Brugia malayi*, the causes of bancroftian and brugian filariasis, respectively. The adult filarial worms of these genera do not usually cause lesions in the lungs, but occasionally become lost during migration and may be found in the lungs. Similarly, more rarely encountered animal filarial worms may occasionally be found in human tissues (e.g., zoonotic *Brugia* species).

Both *Wuchereria bancrofti* and *Brugia malayi* are found exclusively in tropical and subtropical areas. *Brugia malayi* is found in Southeast and East Asia, whereas *W. bancrofti* occurs in Asia, Africa, and Central and South America. However, infected patients could present in any part of the world, given the ease of travel. Approximately 3.3 billion people live in filarial endemic areas, and an estimated 78.6 million people are infected with these lymphatic filarial parasites. Although numerous people are infected, less than 1% of infected people develop tropical pulmonary eosinophilia, and only very rare instances of aberrant filarial worms in the lungs have been reported. Nonimmune

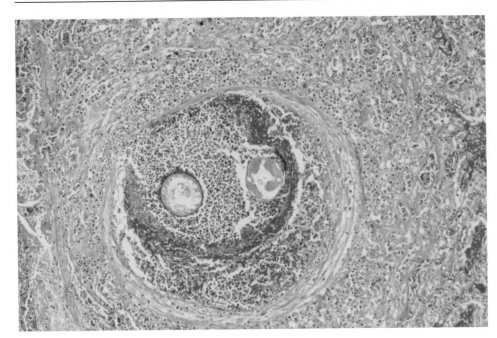

FIGURE 14-11
Wuchereria bancrofti
An adult male *W. bancrofti* in the pulmonary artery. Movat stain.

effusion. Sometimes, however, the chest radiograph may be entirely normal.

PATHOLOGIC FEATURES

The examination of tissues is usually not necessary for the diagnosis of TPE, but the histologic changes of this disease have been described. Early in the disease, there is an influx of eosinophils and histiocytes into the small airways and interstitium. These produce eosinophilic pneumonia, eosinophilic abscesses, and occasionally eosinophilic granulomas. The histopathologic demonstration of microfilariae in the lungs of patients with TPE is exceedingly rare, since microfilarial clearance has already occurred. If discovered, they are surrounded by eosinophils. Later in disease (6 months to 2 years), the infiltrate becomes more mixed, containing chronic inflammatory cells, as well as eosinophils and histiocytes. Interstitial fibrosis at this stage is minimal, but progressive. Finally (after more than 2 years), the infiltrate contains only rare eosinophils and is predominantly composed of chronic inflammatory cells and histiocytes. Fibrosis is the most striking finding at this stage.

The finding of aberrantly migrated adult filarial worms makes for more striking histopathology. When *Brugia malayi* and *W. bancrofti*, which are normally lymphatic-dwelling worms, aberrantly migrate in humans or animals, there is a propensity for deposition in a cardiopulmonary location. Pulmonary arteries, however, are an unnatural or inhospitable site for these worms, and those found in this location have been infertile. Adult *Wuchereria bancrofti* or *Brugia malayi* have been reported in the lungs of at least 6 patients. In each patient, the worms were associated with thrombosis of a small pulmonary artery and an associated infarct (Figure 14-11). Like *D. immitis*, the presence of these adult filarial worms in the pulmonary artery causes thrombosis, occlusion, infarction, and a surrounding granulomatous reaction. The pulmonary nodules formed range in diameter from 2 to 8 cm, the center of which is characterized by coagulation necrosis. The worm may extend beyond the thrombus and appear in histologic sections of artery surrounded by normal tissue. Worms in pulmonary arteries are tightly coiled. A single cross-section of artery usually contains several sections of the worm. In histopathologic sections, adult *W. bancrofti* and *B. malayi* are very similar, but may be distinguished by their diameters. It is difficult to assign a range of diameters for infertile female worms, but in the few patients reported, *B. malayi* was usually about 100 μm, whereas *W. bancrofti* was greater than 140 μm. The adult male *B. malayi* was less than 100 μm in diameter, whereas *W. bancrofti* was greater than 100 μm in diameter.

ANCILLARY STUDIES

Laboratory studies are necessary to confirm the diagnosis of TPE. Most patients have leukocytosis, which is primarily due to the significant eosinophilia. The eosinophils present in the peripheral smear are often degranulated and may reach levels of 70,000/mm^3 or higher. As noted earlier, the peripheral smear characteristically lacks the causative microfilariae. Extremely high levels of IgE are characteristic of this disease, as are elevated parasite-specific IgA, IgM, and IgG levels. Less-specific findings include an elevated erythrocyte sedimentation rate and low levels of alpha-1-antitrypsin. Although nonspecific, these markers are easily monitored and return to normal following appropriate therapy. Molecular diagnostic tools such as PCR have been used, as have blood antigen detection assays, but the utility of such assays remains to be determined.

DIFFERENTIAL DIAGNOSIS

The differential diagnosis of TPE includes other parasitic diseases, such as Löffler's syndrome and visceral larva migrans. Nonparasitic causes include allergic bronchopulmonary aspergillosis, Churg-Strauss syndrome, drug reactions, and vasculitides such as polyarteritis nodosa and Wegener's granulomatosis. The diagnosis of TPE in patients with an appropriate exposure history and typical pulmonary symptoms is made by demonstrating the presence of (1) persistent hypereosinophilia; (2) high titers of filarial antibody; (3) absence of microfilariae in peripheral blood; (4) elevated IgE; and (5) rapid relief of symptoms when treated with diethylcarbamazine (DEC).

The histologic lesions produced by aberrant adult *Wuchereria bancrofti* and *Brugia malayi* raise the possibility of *D. immitis*. The main concern raised by the radiologic findings is the possibility of carcinoma.

PROGNOSIS AND THERAPY

The prognosis of patients with TPE varies depending upon the time to diagnosis and the access to appropriate medical care. Approximately 95% of individuals treated early respond to DEC. This is in contrast to a response rate of only 60% for patients who have had disease for

---

TROPICAL PULMONARY EOSINOPHILIA AND ABERRANT ADULT FILARIA—FACT SHEET

Definition

▸ Tropical pulmonary eosinophilia (TPE) is a hypersensitivity reaction to the microfilariae of *Wuchereria bancrofti* and *Brugia malayi*
▸ Rarely, adult filarial worms aberrantly migrate to the lungs and cause disease

Epidemiology

▸ *Wuchereria bancrofti* and *Brugia malayi* are found exclusively in tropical and subtropical areas, and are transmitted through the bite of an infected mosquito
▸ Although over 3.3 billion people live in endemic areas, and an estimated 78.6 million people are infected, less than 1% of infected people develop TPE
▸ Nonimmune individuals are more likely to develop TPE than people in endemic areas
▸ Men are four times more likely than women to develop TPE

Clinical Features

▸ Early pulmonary manifestations reflect airway hyperreactivity and include wheezing, dyspnea, and a paroxysmal cough that is worse at night
▸ Fever, malaise, weight loss, nausea, vomiting, and/or diarrhea are nonspecific features
▸ Later, features of pulmonary fibrosis dominate
▸ Patients with aberrantly migrated adult filarial worms may be asymptomatic or have chest pain and hemoptysis

Radiologic Features

▸ Bilateral reticulonodular infiltrates, miliary mottling, and increased bronchovascular markings are the most common findings
▸ An adult filarial worm that has aberrantly migrated to the lung produces patchy or well-circumscribed pulmonary lesions that prompt surgical excision because of the possibility of malignancy

Prognosis and Therapy

▸ Prognosis of patients with TPE varies with time to diagnosis and access to therapy
▸ 95% of individuals treated early respond to diethylcarbamazine (DEC) treatment, in contrast to only 60% of patients who have had disease for 2-5 years
▸ Only supportive care can be provided for end-stage, chronic restrictive lung disease caused by TPE
▸ A bacterial endosymbiont (*Wolbachia* species) of filarial worms may be important in the pathogenesis of filariasis; treatment with doxycycline, which targets these bacteria, appears to result in a significant decrease in microfilaremia

---

TROPICAL PULMONARY EOSINOPHILIA AND ABERRANT ADULT FILARIA—PATHOLOGIC FEATURES

▸ Microfilariae are absent from the blood smears of affected patients
▸ Laboratory studies are necessary to confirm the diagnosis of TPE
▸ Hypereosinophilia, extremely high IgE levels, and elevated parasite-specific immunoglobulins are characteristics of this disease
▸ Early histopathologic changes include an influx of eosinophils and histiocytes, with the formation of eosinophilic pneumonia, eosinophilic abscesses, and occasionally eosinophilic granuloma; microfilariae in the lungs of patients with TPE are rare or more commonly absent
▸ Later in disease (6 months to 2 years), a mixed infiltrate is seen that consists of chronic inflammatory cells, as well as eosinophils and histiocytes, and early fibrosis
▸ Finally (after more than 2 years), the infiltrate contains only rare eosinophils and is predominantly composed of chronic inflammatory cells and histiocytes; fibrosis is the most striking finding at this stage
▸ Rare patients have an adult filarial worm in the pulmonary artery which causes thrombosis, infarction, and a surrounding granulomatous reaction, producing a 2-8 cm diameter nodule

2 to 5 years. Only supportive care can be provided for end-stage, chronic lung disease caused by TPE.

The drug of choice for the treatment of filariasis and TPE is DEC. Although the relapse rate of TPE following treatment is 10-20%, relapses resolve with another course of treatment. The excision of the adult filarial worm is curative for the associated pulmonary disease, but a course of DEC is warranted since other adults may be present in more typical locations. Recently, a bacterial endosymbiont (*Wolbachia* species) has been found to be associated with filarial worms and is possibly important for a certain degree of their pathogenesis, particularly disease associated with the microfilariae. Treatment with doxycycline, which targets these bacteria, appears to result in significant decreases in microfilaremia.

OTHER NEMATODES CAUSING LUNG DISEASE

A large number of other nematodes rarely cause pulmonary disease, incuding *Capillaria philippinensis*, *C. hepatica*, *C. aerophila*, *Mammomonogamus laryngeus*, *Trichinella spiralis*, *Metastrongylus elongatus*, *Halicephalobus deletrix*, *Enterobius vermicularis*, *Lagochilascaris minor*, *Anisakis* species, *Gnathostoma spinigerum*, and possibly others.

CESTODAL CAUSES OF LUNG DISEASE

Echinococcosis is arguably the most important pulmonary disease caused by cestodes, and is covered in detail below. Cysticercosis is another disease caused by a cestode, *T. solium*, which may have a pulmonary component. Although infrequently encountered, the number of people at risk is large, and, most importantly, the detection of pulmonary cysticercosis identifies a patient who almost certainly has lesions elsewhere which could be fatal without treatment.

ECHINOCOCCOSIS (ECHINOCOCCUS GRANULOSUS, E. MULTILOCULARIS)

Echinococcosis is one of the most important diseases caused by cestodes (i.e., tapeworms). It is easily acquired in endemic areas, pulmonary cysts are common, and it may be fatal. Cystic echinococcosis is caused by *E. granulosus*, alveolar echinococcosis is caused by *E. multilocularis*, and, far less commonly, polycystic echinococcosis is caused by *E. vogeli* and *E. oligarthrus*. *Echinococcus granulosus* is distributed worldwide, whereas *E. multilocularis* is endemic in the northern hemisphere.

Echinococcosis in humans is an infection with the larval-stage metacestode of tapeworms of the genus *Echinococcus*. It is also commonly known as hydatid disease, and hydatidosis. The adult tapeworms in this group live attached to the wall of the small intestine of carnivorous canids (wolf, dingo, dog, jackal, hyena), are very small (2-7 mm long), and cause no harm to the definitive host. Canids become infected when they eat the internal organs of intermediate hosts that contain a hydatid cyst. The intermediate hosts are primarily grazing ungulates (sheep, goats, cattle, horses, and pigs for *E. granulosus*; deer, elk, bison, moose, and antelope for *E. multilocularis*). Humans contract echinococcosis by consuming eggs from the feces of a definitive host, such as a dog. This is more often through dog contact than by the consumption of contaminated food or water. Humans are accidental, "dead-end hosts" when they ingest the eggs of *Echinococcus*, but the lesions formed are like those formed in the intermediate hosts, namely visceral cysts. Males are more likely to contract echinococcosis than females, and persons in rural locales are at higher risk than city dwellers.

Hydatid cysts may occur in any tissue or organ, but most often (70-90%) develop in the liver, followed by the lung (10-30%). Single organ involvement with a single cyst is most common, but 20-40% of people with a hydatid lung cyst will also have a liver cyst. Hydatid cysts of the lungs slightly predominate on the right side (60%) and in the lower lobes of the lungs (60%). Multiple pulmonary cysts are found in 30% of affected patients, and bilateral cysts are found in 20%. The lung is likely the most common site of infection in children. Pulmonary involvement with *E. multilocularis* is far less common than with *E. granulosus*, with only 8 of 96 (8%) patients in one series showing pulmonary disease.

CLINICAL FEATURES

The clinical manifestations of pulmonary hydatid disease may not appear for 5 to 10 years after the initial infection. Symptoms result from mass effect, rupture, or invasion of the vasculature. The pulmonary signs and symptoms are nonspecific and may include cough, chest pain, hemoptysis, dyspnea, fever, and allergic reactions. Invasion of the heart and inferior vena cava may result in embolization of cyst contents; in such instances, death occurs secondary to anaphylactic shock, massive embolism, or hemorrhage.

Cysts may rupture into either the airway or the pleural space. Between 29 and 33% of pulmonary hydatid cysts demonstrate evidence of rupture or secondary infection. The patient experiences *hydatid vomica* with the cyst rupture into an airway, which manifests as hemoptysis, cough, and the expectoration of the clear and salty cyst contents through the mouth and nose. The complications of bronchial fistulization and cyst rupture include asphyxia, anaphylactic shock, secondary hydatid spread, hemoptysis, retention of the cyst wall, and secondary infection. Rupture of the cyst into the pleural cavity is less frequent (3.5-6%).

The fragility of the cyst must be taken into account when diagnostic testing is considered. Although cyst rupture following exploratory puncture is relatively infrequent at approximately 5%, the consequences of rupture can be devastating.

RADIOLOGIC FEATURES

The role of radiology is paramount in the diagnosis of echinococcosis. The plain chest radiograph is usually sufficient for the identification of these lesions. The unruptured cyst appears as a simple, spherical, homogeneous opacity with clearly delineated or blurred borders. The blurring is associated with pericystic atelectasis, pneumonia, or allergic reaction. The presence of daughter cysts within the larger sphere is diagnostic. Penetrating air associated with cysts that have ruptured or are impending rupture can be seen as an air/fluid level or an onion-peel appearance, respectively. Following rupture, the residual cyst membrane may be seen folded upon itself, the "serpent sign." Alternatively, in a cyst with incomplete rupture, the collapsed membrane may be seen floating on the residual fluid to produce the "camalote," or "water lily sign." Finally, solid, residual membranes may be visualized in cysts that are completely evacuated; these will resolve into a scar. The rupture of a cyst into the pleural cavity produces the radiologic features of a hydrothorax, or if air is present a hydropneumothorax. Calcification of pulmonary hydatid cysts is uncommon, whereas calcification of liver hydatid cysts is frequently seen. Pulmonary disease may be a complication of liver involvement. Therefore, if a pulmonary hydatid cyst is discovered, radiologic imaging studies of the liver should be performed.

PATHOLOGIC FEATURES

An echinococcal cyst is mature by 5 to 6 months, and usually 10 cm or less, but some may be 20 cm in diameter. The cysts of *E. granulosus* and *E. multilocularis* are quite different, but both contain liquid and "hydatid sand," which is a mixture of protoscolices, hooklets, and debris. The cyst of *E. granulosus,* which is the type most likely to be encountered, is single and has a thick, acellular laminated membrane. The cyst is usually surrounded by a thick, fibrous capsule of host origin. Internal to the laminated membrane is the thin germinal membrane with nuclei and calcareous corpuscles, which gives rise to brood capsules and protoscolices. The gross examination of a cyst of *E. granulosus* reveals a white, fragile exocyst that consists of concentric sheets of hyaline (Figure 14-12). The inner aspect of the cyst wall, the endocyst, is transparent, fragile, and granular. The adjacent lung demonstrates tissue compression and may show dilated or stenotic bronchi and evidence of a bronchial-cystic fistula. The rupture of cysts into bronchi causes chronic suppuration and abscess formation. In rare instances, an entire lobe of the lung may be destroyed. In contrast, the cysts of *E. multilocularis* have only a thin laminated layer, which is surrounded by necrotic debris (i.e., there is no host-derived fibrous capsule). The larval mass of this species proliferates by budding of the germinal membrane, producing an alveolar-like pattern of microvesicles that are not contained by a fibrous capsule. These cysts have poorly defined borders and infiltrate in a manner reminiscent of a cancer.

The histopathologic demonstration of parasitic structures confirms the diagnosis (Figure 14-13).

Occasionally, hydatid cysts have been diagnosed by fine needle aspiration, usually when this diagnosis was not suspected. Needle aspiration is not recommended if this disease is suspected because patients with echinococcosis are in danger of anaphylactic shock and metastatic proliferation when the cyst is penetrated, even with a thin needle.

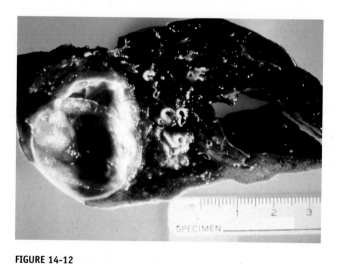

FIGURE 14-12

Echinococcus granulosus
This hydatid cyst of the lung is unilocular and well circumscribed.

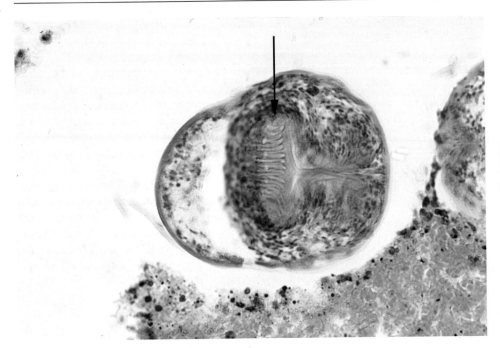

FIGURE 14-13
Echinococcus granulosis
The protoscolex demonstrates a prominent row of hooklets (arrow).

ANCILLARY STUDIES

A variety of immunodiagnostic assays are available to assist in the diagnosis of echinococcosis. The indirect immunofluorescence assay is reportedly greater than 95% sensitive in patients with hepatic cystic hydatidosis, whereas the sensitivity is poor for patients with pulmonary and bone hydatidosis. False-positive serologic reactions have occurred in patients with cysticercosis, likely due to cross-reactivity, and for unknown reasons in patients with malignancy. Positive serology supports the radiologic diagnosis. Patients who are successfully treated have been shown to be antibody-negative (< 1:128) within a year after therapy.

DIFFERENTIAL DIAGNOSIS

Hydatid cysts are occasionally mistaken for tuberculosis or carcinoma, although an accurate preoperative diagnosis is usually possible from the radiologic appearance. The differential diagnosis is essentially the radiologic differential, since the pathologic findings are pathognomonic. The association of a cyst with mediastinal structures can raise the possibility of an enlarged left auricle, an aortic aneurysm, or a mediastinal tumor. Pleural-associated cysts can be mistaken for loculated pleural effusions or pleurisy. Cysts that contain air can be mistaken for congenital cysts. Multiple cysts may have the appearance of metastatic disease.

PROGNOSIS AND THERAPY

The prognosis in pulmonary cystic hydatid disease is generally good, but complications may develop during treatment. The approach to therapy for a pulmonary hydatid cyst is different in many ways from the treatment of a liver hydatid cyst. Cysts in the liver resist medical treatment, whereas pulmonary cysts respond well to standard antiparasitic drugs. A combined surgical and medical approach is the standard for treatment of pulmonary echinococcal cysts. Medical treatment using a benzimidazole, such as mebendazole or albendazole, may be given preoperatively for easier removal of the cyst, postoperatively as adjuvant therapy, or as the sole method for the treatment of patients who can not tolerate surgery or who have disseminated disease. A variety of surgical approaches have been described.

Definition

- Echinococcosis is caused by infection with the larval metacestode stage of tapeworms of the genus *Echinococcus*
- *Echinococcus granulosus* (cystic echinococcosis) and *E. multilocularis* (alveolar echinococcosis) are the most common causes, with the former species predominating in the lung

Epidemiology

- The adult tapeworms are intestinal parasites of canids, which are the definitive hosts, whereas the natural intermediate hosts are primarily grazing ungulates
- *Echinococcus granulosus* is distributed worldwide, whereas *E. multilocularis* is in the Northern Hemisphere

Clinical Features

- Humans acquire echinococcosis by ingesting eggs and are accidental "dead-end intermediate hosts," but suitable for the development of the metacestode in visceral cysts
- 70-90% of hydatid cysts occur in the liver; the lung is the second most common site (10-30%)
- Single cysts predominate (70%), but 20-40% of people with a lung cyst will also have a liver cyst
- The lung is likely the most common site of infection in children
- Pulmonary hydatid disease, usually caused by *Echinococcus granulosus*, may not appear for as long as 5 to 10 years after infection; symptoms usually result from mass effect or secondary to rupture
- Most of the signs and symptoms of hydatid disease are nonspecific, such as cough, chest pain, hemoptysis, dyspnea, fever, and allergic reactions
- *Hydatid vomica*, which may occur with cyst rupture, refers to hemoptysis, cough, and the expectoration of the clear and salty cyst contents through the mouth and nose
- Complications include bronchial fistulization, secondary bacterial infection, and cyst rupture with hemoptysis, asphyxia, anaphylactic shock, and secondary hydatid spread

Radiologic Features

- The role of radiology is paramount in the diagnosis of echinococcosis
- The unruptured cyst appears as a simple, spherical, homogeneous opacity with clearly delineated or blurred borders
- Air/fluid level, residual fluid and cyst membrane, and residual cyst membrane alone may also be seen
- Calcification of pulmonary hydatid cysts is uncommon, whereas calcification of liver hydatid cysts is frequently seen
- Pulmonary disease may be a complication of liver involvement, so if a pulmonary hydatid cyst is discovered, radiologic imaging studies of the liver should be performed

Prognosis and Therapy

- The prognosis in pulmonary echinococcosis is generally good, but severe complications may arise
- Percutaneous aspiration of a pulmonary echinococcal cyst is not recommended
- The combination of surgical and medical treatment with mebendazole or albendazole is the standard for the treatment

- Most hydatid cysts are 10 cm or less, but some may be 20 cm in diameter
- The cyst of *E. granulosus* has two parasite-derived layers, the thick outer acellular laminated layer and the inner germinal layer. External to these is a host-derived fibrous capsule
- In contrast, the cysts of *E. multilocularis* have only a thin laminated layer, which is surrounded by necrotic debris (i.e., there is no host-derived fibrous capsule)
- Histopathologic demonstration of protoscolices, hooklets, and the cyst wall confirm the diagnosis
- Collapsed cysts of *E. granulosus* may resemble the cyst of *E. multilocularis* (i.e., the wall may be branching, sterile, and surrounded with necrotic debris)
- The lung adjacent to the hydatid cyst may be atelectatic or show bronchial stenosis, bronchiectasis, and inflammation with interstitial fibrosis

TREMATODAL CAUSES OF LUNG DISEASE

Trematodes belong to the phylum *Platyhelminthes*, the flatworms, and are commonly referred to as flukes. The two most important groups of trematodes that cause human lung disease are the *Paragonimus* species, or lung flukes, and the schistosomes, which are perhaps the most important helminthic parasite of humans overall. Schistosomiasis is second only to malaria as a parasitic cause of worldwide morbidity and mortality. As an agent of pulmonary disease schistosomiasis is minor, but demands attention given the prevalence of this disease.

PARAGONIMIASIS (PARAGONIMUS SPECIES)

Paragonimiasis results from an infection by a member of the genus *Paragonimus*, the lung fluke. The most common lung fluke that infects humans is *P. westermani*. *Paragonimus* species are the only helminthic parasite that naturally inhabits the lungs as an adult worm. These adult worms have also been described in a variety of ectopic sites that include the brain, liver, skeletal muscle, testes, and lymph nodes.

Paragonimiasis most frequently occurs in Asia, Africa, and South America. The adult, gravid *Paragonimus* fluke produces eggs while in the lungs. These may be expectorated or swallowed and passed with feces. After approximately two weeks in an appropriate aqueous environment, a ciliated miracidium emerges from the egg and infects a molluscan intermediate host. Asexual replication occurs within the mollusk during the next several weeks, resulting in the production of infective cercariae. These emerge into the water and penetrate the gills of a crustacean, most commonly a crab or crayfish. These larvae migrate to soft tissue where they encyst as metacercariae. The consumption of the metacercariae results in infection in a suitable host. After ingestion, the metacercariae emerge from the cyst, penetrate the wall of the stomach, migrate to and penetrate the diaphragm, and settle in the lungs where they mature into adult worms and the life cycle is completed. The adult worms cause chronic infections that may last for an extended time period.

CLINICAL FEATURES

Human paragonimiasis most commonly results from the consumption of raw or insufficiently cooked crabs or crayfish that contain infective metacercariae. The patient is often asymptomatic during the initial migration of the larvae. The clinical onset of paragonimiasis is variable, but often insidious, with the onset of symptoms varying from months to years. Patients present with hemoptysis and cough due to cyst rupture. The rusty hemoptysis is said to resemble "iron filings." Between 40% and 60% of patients have episodic pleuritic chest pain; a febrile episode occurs in two-thirds of the patients during some phase of the illness. Dyspnea, chronic bronchitis, and wheezing occur as the disease progresses. Rales and rhonchi may be heard in a minority (15-28%) of patients, but many have no abnormal findings on physical examination. A pleural effusion is reported in almost half of infected patients. The diagnostic triad of cough, hemoptysis, and eggs in sputa or feces seen in pulmonary paragonimiasis is not present in patients with pleural-based disease. The pleural effusion is an important sign of infection in these patients.

RADIOLOGIC FEATURES

Patients with paragonimiasis may have a completely normal chest radiograph. More commonly, however, some type of abnormality is present. The radiologic findings are variable, but the following lesions have been described. A pleural lesion of some type is present in up to 70% of these patients. These range from simple pleural thickening to hydropneumothorax. Approximately 60% of patients develop patchy, round, low-density air space consolidations. Single unilateral nodular/cavitating lesions are common, as is ipsilateral pleurisy. Other findings include transient diffuse pulmonary infiltrates and ring shadows resembling annular opacities, which correlate with the presence of a cyst. Multiple worms that encyst close to one another

may give a "soap-bubble" appearance in the chest radiograph. Rarely, single linear tracts may be seen and have been referred to as a "burrow sign." A pleural effusion alone may be seen in some patients with pleural-based paragonimiasis.

PATHOLOGIC FEATURES

GROSS FINDINGS

The average cyst is about 1.5 cm in diameter, and has a necrotic center.

MICROSCOPIC FINDINGS

The adult *P. westermani* is ovoid, plump, and measures 7-12 mm long × 4-6 mm wide (Figure 14-14). The tegument contains numerous tooth-like spines. This hermaphroditic worm contains two deeply lobed testes in the posterior third of the body, an ovary and a uterus. Worms that have been present for some time will usually be in a cyst. The cyst may communicate with a bronchiole or bronchus, and contains the adult worm, eggs, and necrotic debris.

An exudate of eosinophils and neutrophils may be seen associated with the worm or worms. Around the parasite, a collagenous capsule (i.e., a fibrous wall) develops that is initially thin, but becomes several millimeters thick with time. Associated bronchopneumonia is common if an airway communication is present.

Eggs that become lodged in parenchyma provoke a granulomatous response and ultimately fibrosis. The eggs of *P. westermani* are yellowish brown, ovoid, operculate, and measure 75-120 µm × 45-70 µm (Figure 14-15). The operculum is characteristically flattened. The morphology of the eggs from the various *Paragonimus* species has been described, and if eggs are abundant and well preserved, may be used for species-level identification. The eggs of *P. kellicotti*, the North American *Paragonimus* species, although similar to *P. westermani*, are broadest in the central aspect of the egg and lack the abopercular thickening present in the eggs of *P. westermani* (Figure 14-16). The eggs of *Paragonimus* species are birefringent when viewed using plane-polarized light. This feature is useful for differentiating the eggs of *Paragonimus* from the eggs of other parasites, such as the schistosomes, which may occasionally be found in the lungs. In addition to lacking birefringence, schistosome eggs also lack an operculum.

The detection of eggs in sputa or feces is the least invasive means to achieve the definitive diagnosis of paragonimiasis. The pleural effusion is exudative and demonstrates eosinophilia, but eggs are usually not present. Surgical excision of the thickened pleura may be necessary to morphologically diagnose patients with pleural paragonimiasis.

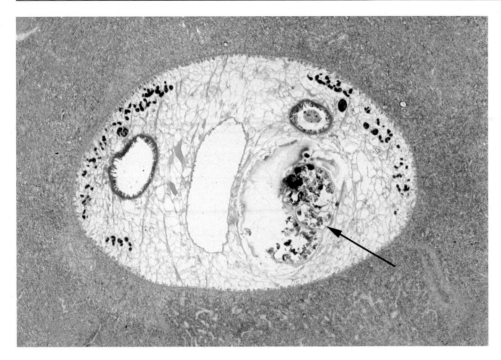

FIGURE 14-14
Paragonimus westermani
A rarely seen section through an adult worm. Note the presence of eggs in the uterus (arrow).

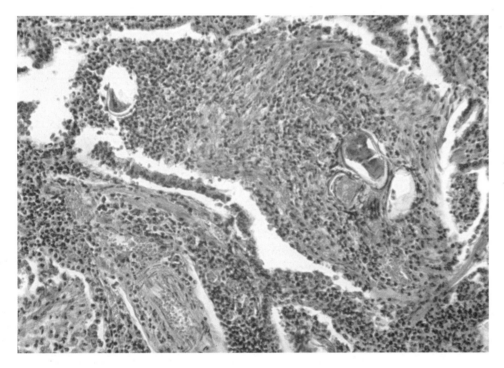

FIGURE 14-15
Paragonimus westermani
Distorted eggs of *P. westermani* lie in inflamed connective tissue in this bronchiole.

ANCILLARY STUDIES

Serologic studies are very useful for the assessment of patients suspected to have paragonimiasis. Approximately 98% of patients with paragonimiasis will have IgG antibodies in their serum and/or pleural fluid, if an effusion is present. Similarly, the sensitivity and specificity of an ELISA assay for *P. heterotremus*, an etiologic agent of paragonimiasis in Thailand, was reported as 100% and 96%, respectively. The specificity was less than 100% due to the cross-reactivity of serum from patients with fascioliasis. Approximately 80% of patients with paragonimiasis have eosinophilia or an elevated IgE level.

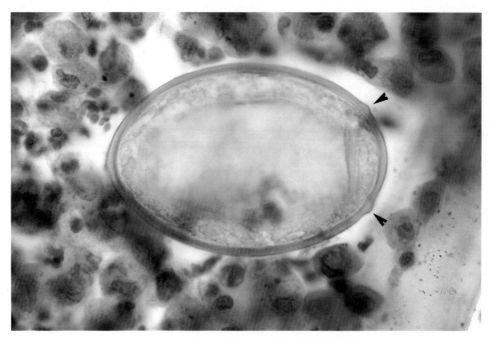

FIGURE 14-16

Paragonimus kellicotti
This golden brown egg of *P. kellicotti* has distinct opercular shoulders (arrowheads), is broadest centrally, and lacks the abopercular thickening of *P. westermani*. This patient contracted paragonimiasis in the Central United States after consuming undercooked crayfish. Papanicolaou stain.

PARAGONIMIASIS—FACT SHEET

Definition

➤ Paragonimiasis is an infection by a member of the genus *Paragonimus*, the lung fluke

Epidemiology

➤ *Paragonimus* species are the only adult helminths that naturally infect the lungs
➤ *Paragonimus westermani* is the most common species that infects humans, but many other species infect humans in Asia, Africa, and the Americas; *Paragonimus kellicotti* causes North American paragonimiasis
➤ The *Paragonimus* life cycle includes a carnivorous or omnivorous definitive host and two intermediate hosts, a mollusk and a crustacean. Paratenic hosts may also be involved

Clinical Features

➤ Human paragonimiasis usually results from the consumption of raw or insufficiently cooked crabs or crayfish that contain infective metacercariae
➤ The clinical onset of paragonimiasis is variable, but often insidious, with the onset of symptoms varying from months to years after infection; patients commonly develop cough and "iron filings" rusty hemoptysis
➤ 40-60% have episodic pleuritic chest pain, and two-thirds have a febrile episode during some phase of the illness; dyspnea, chronic bronchitis, and wheezing occur as the disease progresses
➤ A pleural effusion is reported in almost half of infected patients
➤ The diagnostic triad is cough, hemoptysis, and eggs in sputa or feces
➤ Ectopic paragonimiasis is caused by aberrant migration of the *Paragonimus* larvae or adults into other parts of the body
➤ Cerebral paragonimiasis is particularly life-threatening and may cause seizure, abnormal vision, and sensory/motor deficits

DIFFERENTIAL DIAGNOSIS

The differential diagnosis is usually based on the radiologic and clinical findings. Solid, mass-like areas may be confused with malignancy. Tuberculosis is the most common misdiagnosis of patients with pulmonary paragonimiasis, being made in 50-70% of patients. Therefore, laboratory findings should be used to establish the diagnosis of either tuberculosis or paragonimiasis in patients at risk for these diseases. If operculate eggs are found in the feces, the differential diagnosis includes *Clonorchis, Opisthorchis, Fasciolopsis, Fasciola,* and *Diphyllobothrium*. These eggs are differentiated from those of *Paragonimus* by size and other morphologic features.

PARAGONIMIASIS—PATHOLOGIC FEATURES

➤ The cyst contains worm(s), eggs, and necrotic debris
➤ Eggs elicit a granulomatous response and ultimately fibrosis, worms are associated with an exudate of eosinophils and neutrophils
➤ The eggs of *Paragonimus westermani* are yellowish-brown, ovoid, operculate, and 75-120 μm × 45-70 μm, and are birefringent when exposed to plane-polarized light
➤ The detection of eggs in sputa or feces is the least invasive means to achieve the definitive diagnosis of paragonimiasis

PARAGONIMIASIS—FACT SHEET—cont'd

Radiologic Features

» Some type of abnormality is usually present in the chest radiograph, but it may be completely normal

» 70% have a pleural lesion; approximately 60% of patients develop patchy, round, low-density air space consolidations

» Single unilateral nodular/cavitating lesions are common, as is ipsilateral pleurisy

» Transient diffuse pulmonary infiltrates and ring shadows resembling annular opacities, which correlate with the presence of a cyst, are other possible findings

» A pleural effusion alone may be seen for some patients with pleural-based paragonimiasis

Prognosis and Therapy

» The outcome of cerebral paragonimiasis is often fatal, even with aggressive treatment, whereas the prognosis of pulmonary paragonimiasis is good

» Praziquantel is the drug of choice for paragonimiasis and is uniformly effective against pulmonary paragonimiasis

PROGNOSIS AND THERAPY

The outcome of cerebral paragonimiasis is often fatal, even with aggressive treatment, whereas the prognosis of pulmonary paragonimiasis is good. Pulmonary paragonimiasis is rarely fatal, even without treatment. Praziquantel is the drug of choice for paragonimiasis and is uniformly effective against pulmonary paragonimiasis. Treatment with praziquantel has, however, caused patients to cough up living worms, a rather unpleasant side effect.

OTHER TREMATODES CAUSING LUNG DISEASE

Schistosomiasis is one of the most prevalent tropical diseases in the world, with an estimated 200 million people at risk for disease in the more than 70 countries where it is endemic. Pulmonary disease can be associated with acute infection as an immunologic reaction, or can be associated with chronic disease. Chronic pulmonary schistosomiasis develops when eggs are swept into the portal venous circulation and bypass hepatic capillaries because of the portovenous anastomoses that have been formed secondary to portal hypertension, which itself is part of the disease. The eggs lodge in pulmonary arterioles and provoke granulomatous endarteritis that can over time result in pulmonary hypertension and eventually cor pulmonale. Although *Schistosoma*-induced cor pulmonale is rare, it does occur in all schistosome-endemic areas of the world. It is most often reported in Egypt and Brazil associated with *S. mansoni* infections.

Numerous other trematodes may infect humans, and some of these may aberrantly migrate to the lung. For example, rare human pulmonary infections have been reported with *Opisthorchis viverrini*, a liver fluke that is found in northeastern Thailand; *Fasciola hepatica,* the liver fluke of sheep; and *Clinostomum complanatum*, a fluke that occurs in the esophagus and pharynx of herons and gulls.

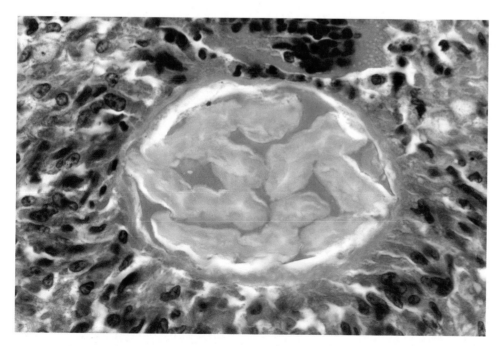

FIGURE 14-17
Lentil pneumonia
Starch grains, which may be seen in lentil pneumonia, may be mistaken for a parasite.

MIMICS OF PARASITES IN HUMAN TISSUES

When considering the possibility of a parasitic infection as a diagnosis, one should also consider the possibility of a mimic. Foreign material has been mistaken for parasites. Ciliocytophthoria has been mistaken for a parasite in cytologic preparations, a diagnosis that is especially tempting if a wet preparation is made and the suspect structures are found to be motile. The identification of parasites in tissue sections requires the demonstration of specific morphologic features. People who are unfamiliar with the morphologic features of parasites can mistake unusual structures in histologic sections for parasites.

We suggest the following to help the pathologist when he or she encounters a possible pulmonary parasite. First, try to determine if the structure present is actually a parasite. For helminthes, the identification of internal biologic structures, such as intestines, may help. Be skeptical of "parasites" in bizarre locations. Attempt to measure the maximum length and/or diameter, if possible. When the diagnosis is considered, check published, known dimensions, taking into account shrinkage that occurs during processing. Then, obtain the opinion of a valued colleague, and if the diagnoses do not agree, explore the reasons. Remember, a specific diagnosis may not be possible based on the material available. For example, lentil pneumonia, which is caused by aspiration of starch grains from legumes, results in lentil grains present in lung tissue with pyogranulomatous inflammation; these have been thought to resemble the eggs of helminthes (Figure 14-17). Periodic acid-Schiff vividly stains the walls and starch compartments of the grain.

SUGGESTED READINGS

General

1. Gutierrez Y. *Diagnostic Pathology of Parasitic Infections*. 2nd ed. New York, NY: Oxford University Press; 2000.
2. Orihel TC, Ash LR. *Parasites in Human Tissues*. Chicago, Ill: ASCP Press; 1995.
3. DH Connor, FW Chandler (eds.). *Pathology of Infectious Diseases*. Stamford, Conn: Appleton & Lange; 1997.
4. Meyers WM, ed. *Pathology of Infectious Diseases. Volume I: Helminthiases*. Washington DC: Armed Forces Institute of Pathology; 2000.

Falciparum Malaria (Malarial Lung)

5. Kemper CA. Pulmonary disease in selected protozoal infections. *Semin Respir Infect*. 1997;12:113-21.
6. Taylor WRJ, White NJ. Malaria and the lung. *Clin Chest Med*. 2002;23:457-68.
7. World Health Organization. Severe falciparum malaria. *Trans R Soc Trop Med Hyg*. 2000;94(Suppl 1):S1-90.

Toxoplasmosis *(Toxoplasma gondii)*

8. Campagna AC. Pulmonary toxoplasmosis. *Semin Respir Infect*. 1997;12:98-105.
9. Kemper CA. Pulmonary disease in selected protozoal infections. *Semin Respir Infect*. 1997;12:113-21.
10. Sing A, Leitritz L, Roggenkamp A, et al. Pulmonary toxoplasmosis in bone marrow transplant recipients: report of two cases and review. *Clin Infect Dis*. 1999;29:429-33.

Strongyloidiasis *(Strongyloides stercoralis)*

11. Loutfy MR, Wilson M, Keystone JS, Kain KC. Serology and eosinophil count in the diagnosis and management of strongyloidiasis in a non-endemic area. *Am J Trop Med Hyg*. 2002;66:749-52.
12. Schaeffer MW, Buell JF, Gupta M, Conway GD, Akhter SA, Wagoner LE. Strongyloides hyperinfection syndrome after heart transplantation: case report and review of the literature. *J Heart Lung Transplant*. 2004;23:905-11.
13. Wehner JH, Kirsch CM. Pulmonary manifestations of strongyloidiasis. *Semin Respir Infect*. 1997;12:122-9.

Visceral Larva Migrans

14. Chitkara RK, Sarinas PSA. Dirofilaria, visceral larva migrans, and tropical pulmonary eosinophilia. *Semin Respir Infect*. 1997;12:138-48.

Filarial Worms

15. Chitkara RK, Sarinas PSA. Dirofilaria, visceral larva migrans, and tropical pulmonary eosinophilia. *Semin Respir Infect*. 1997;12:138-48.
16. Shah MK, Human pulmonary dirofilariasis: review of the literature. *South Med J*. 1999;92:276-9.
17. Walther M, Muller R. Diagnosis of human filariases (except onchocerciasis). *Adv Parasitol*. 2003;53:149-93.

Tropical Pulmonary Eosinophilia and Aberrant Filaria

18. Chitkara RK, Sarinas PSA. Dirofilaria, visceral larva migrans, and tropical pulmonary eosinophilia. *Semin Respir Infect*. 1997;12:138-48.
19. Cooray JHL, Ismail MM. Re-examination of the diagnostic criteria of tropical pulmonary eosinophilia. *Respir Med*. 1999;93:655-9.
20. Ong RK, Doyle RL. Tropical pulmonary eosinophilia. *Chest*. 1998;113:1673-9.
21. Walther M, Muller R. Diagnosis of human filariases (except onchocerciasis). *Adv Parasitol*. 2003;53:149-93.

Echinococcosis *(Echinococcus granulosus, E. multilocularis)*

22. Biava MF, Dao A, Fortier B. Laboratory diagnosis of cystic hydatic disease. *World J Surg*. 2001;25:10-4.
23. Gottstein B, Reichen J. Hydatid lung disease (echinococcosis/hydatidosis). *Clin Chest Med*. 2002;23:397-408.
24. Morar R, Feldman C. Pulmonary echinococcosis. *Eur Respir J*. 2003;21:1069-77.
25. Ramos G, Orduna A, Garcia-Yuste M. Hydatid cyst of the lung: diagnosis and treatment. *World J Surg*. 2001;25:46-57.

Paragonimiasis *(Paragonimus species)*

26. Im JG, Chang KH, Reeder MM. Current diagnostic imaging of pulmonary and cerebral paragonimiasis, with pathological correlation. *Semin Roentgenol*. 1997;4:301-24.
27. Kagawa FT. Pulmonary paragonimiasis. *Semin Respir Infect*. 1997;12:149-58.
28. Nawa Y. Re-emergence of paragonimiasis. *Intern Med J*. 2000;39:353-4.
29. Maleewong W. Recent advances in the diagnosis of paragonimiasis. *Southeast Asian J Trop Med Public Health*. 1997;28:134-8.

15 Chlamydial, Mycoplasmal, Rickettsial, and Ehrlichial Diseases

David H. Walker

INTRODUCTION

The unusual bacterial pneumonias described in this chapter are caused by agents that are phylogenetically diverse and reside in a wide variety of locations ranging from extracellular *Mycoplasma* attached to respiratory epithelium to obligately intracellular organisms. The obligately intracellular agents range from *Rickettsia* and *Orientia*, living in the cytosol of endothelial cells, to *Chlamydia, Ehrlichia,* and *Anaplasma,* living in modified cytoplasmic vacuoles, to *Coxiella,* living in acidic cytoplasmic phagolysosomes of macrophages. Transmission varies from person-to-person communicability *(Mycoplasma, C. trachomatis, C. pneumoniae)* to vector-borne inoculation by ticks *(Rickettsia, Ehrlichia,* and *Anaplasma)*, lice or fleas *(Rickettsia)*, and mites *(Orientia* and *Rickettsia)*. The organisms themselves vary from gram-negative bacteria with cell walls containing lipopolysaccharide (LPS) and peptidoglycan *(Rickettsia)*, cell walls containing LPS but no peptidoglycan *(Chlamydia)*, cell walls containing neither LPS nor peptidoglycan *(Orientia, Ehrlichia,* and *Anaplasma)* to bacteria lacking a cell wall altogether *(Mycoplasma)*. Although generally having small genomes owing to selective genome reduction, these organisms are highly adapted to their individual ecologic niches. Their composition and interaction with the host, including the particular target cells in the lung, determine the pulmonary pathology that they cause.

For some of these diseases, such as *Mycoplasma* and chlamydial pneumonias and Q fever, fatality and biopsy are exceedingly rare. Clinical microbiology laboratories seldom undertake cultivation of these agents from respiratory samples, if even at all. Thus, recognizing the pathologic lesions and establishing an etiologic diagnosis is a challenge.

MYCOPLASMA PNEUMONIA

Mycoplasma pneumonia is among the most common lower respiratory infections worldwide. Its pathologic features reflect the secretion of peroxide by bacteria attached to the respiratory epithelium and the response of the host defenses (Figures 15-1 and 15-2).

CHLAMYDIAL PNEUMONIAS

The three species, *Chlamydia trachomatis, C. pneumoniae,* and *C. psittaci,* that cause pneumonia affect patients in different clinicoepidemiologic settings. *Chlamydia trachomatis* is usually a postnatal respiratory infection. *Chlamydia pneumoniae* is a frequent cause of community-acquired pneumonia. *Chlamydia psittaci* is a zoonotic pneumonia classically transmitted from infected birds.

The pathologic lesions of chlamydial pneumonias result from entry of the infectious, metabolically inert elementary body into respiratory epithelial cells, where conversion to the 10-100 times larger, metabolically active, replicating reticulate body occurs. After growth to substantial numbers, reticulate bodies change into elementary bodies that are released to infect other cells in the same or another person.

Chlamydia trachomatis infection of infants often occurs in association with infection by other agents of the maternal genital tract (e.g., cytomegalovirus), confounding the delineation of the pathologic lesions of pure chlamydial pneumonia of infants. Infiltration of the interstitium and bronchiolar walls by lymphocytes,

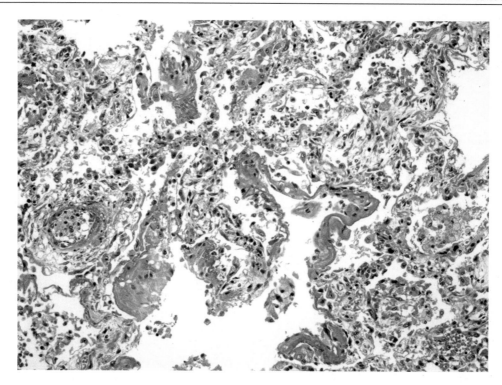

FIGURE 15-1
Mycoplasma **pneumonia**
Although *Mycoplasma* infections usually involve the attachment of the bacteria to the epithelium of the airways, in this case of severe pneumonia, the lung shows diffuse alveolar damage with abundant hyaline membranes. (Generously provided by Christopher Paddock, MD, Centers for Disease Control and Prevention.)

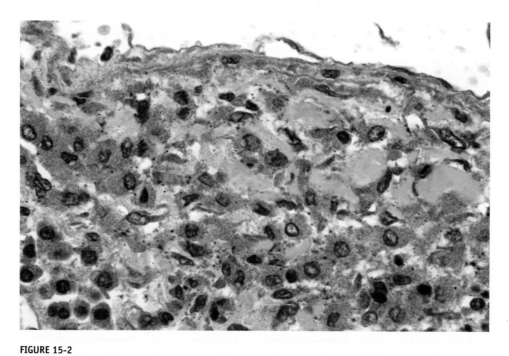

FIGURE 15-2
Mycoplasma **pneumonia**
Immunohistochemical demonstration of *M. pneumoniae* antigen in the lung. (Generously provided by Christopher Paddock, MD, Centers for Disease Control and Prevention.)

MYCOPLASMA PNEUMONIA—FACT SHEET

Definition

» Lower respiratory tract infection and inflammatory consolidation caused by *Mycoplasma pneumoniae*

Incidence

» One of the most common community-acquired pneumonias

Mortality

» A fatal outcome is rare

Age Distribution

» Highest incidence in 5-20 year olds
» 9% of community-acquired pneumonia isolates in patients younger than 5 years, 51% in 5-9 year olds, 74% in 9-15 year olds, and 3.3-18% in adults; in university students, 11% of clinically diagnosed pneumonias and 22% of radiologically confirmed pneumonias

Clinical Features

» Gradual onset of headache, malaise, fever, sore throat, and cough
» *Mycoplasma* tracheobronchitis occurs 30 times more frequently than pneumonia
» Similar incidence of productive cough, rales, and diarrhea as community-acquired pneumococcal or *Legionella* pneumonia, but with more frequent upper respiratory symptoms, normal leukocyte count, and younger age

Radiologic Features

» Bronchopneumonia usually involving a single lobe, subsegmental atelectasis, peribronchial thickening, and streaky interstitial densities
» High-resolution computerized tomography shows centrilobular consolidation, acinar shadows less than 1 cm diameter, air bronchograms and bronchiolograms, and thickening of the bronchovascular bundle

Prognosis and Therapy

» Usually self-limited
» The duration of illness, but not *Mycoplasma* carriage, is shortened by oral ambulatory treatment with doxycycline, erythromycin, clarithromycin, azithromycin, sparfloxacin, levofloxacin, gatifloxacin, or moxifloxacin for 14 to 21 days

MYCOPLASMA PNEUMONIA—PATHOLOGIC FEATURES

Gross Findings

» Because *Mycoplasma* pneumonia is rarely fatal, the gross pathologic lesions have not been described

Microscopic Findings

» Limited human autopsy and biopsy materials and similar observations in a hamster model show peribronchial, peribronchiolar, and interstitial infiltrates of macrophages, CD4 and CD8 T lymphocytes, B lymphocytes, and plasma cells
» Airway lumens contain mucus, fibrin, polymorphonuclear leukocytes, and detached respiratory epithelial cells, which frequently cause obstruction leading to segmental and subsegmental atelectasis
» In some cases, combinations of bronchiolitis obliterans, organizing pneumonia, and interstitial fibrosis occur rather than resolution

Immunohistochemical Features

» An immunohistochemical method for detection of *Mycoplasma pneumoniae* has been developed

Ultrastructural Findings

» Experimental studies of animals have demonstrated attachment of *M. pneumoniae* to the cell surface of respiratory epithelial cells between cilia by a specialized tip structure
» Cilia are shed, intercellular junctions are disrupted, and the respiratory epithelial cells detach from the basement membrane

Pathologic Differential Diagnosis

» Influenza A and B, parainfluenza 1-4 pneumonia, respiratory syncytial virus pneumonia and chlamydial pneumonias (*C. trachomatis, C. pneumoniae, C. psittaci*)

CHLAMYDIA TRACHOMATIS PNEUMONIA—FACT SHEET

Definition

▸▸ Lower respiratory tract infection and inflammatory consolidation caused by *Chlamydia trachomatis*

Incidence

▸▸ *Chlamydia trachomatis* is the etiologic agent of 25-36% of the cases of pneumonia requiring hospitalization in 1- to 3-month-old infants
▸▸ Of infants born to mothers harboring *C. trachomatis* genital infection, 17-22% develop chlamydial pneumonia

Morbidity and Mortality

▸▸ Usually a prolonged self-limited illness, *C. trachomatis* can cause severe pneumonia in low-birth-weight neonates

Age Distribution

▸▸ Infection is usually required intrapartum, with onset of symptoms at 4 to 12 weeks of age
▸▸ Pneumonia caused by *C. trachomatis* is rare in adults, even immunocompromised patients

Clinical Features

▸▸ Typical onset is characterized by afebrile, staccato cough, tachypnea, rales, hypoxemia, and mild peripheral eosinophilia
▸▸ Chlamydial conjunctivitis is present in only 50% at the presentation with pneumonia

Radiologic Features

▸▸ Chest radiographs reveal hyperexpansion and diffuse or patchy interstitial infiltrates

Prognosis and Therapy

▸▸ Rarely fatal
▸▸ Infants are treated with erythromycin (12.5 mg/kg 4 times daily for 2 weeks) or sulfisoxazole (37.5 mg/kg 4 times daily for 2 weeks)

CHLAMYDIA PNEUMONIAE PNEUMONIA—FACT SHEET

Definition

▸▸ Lower respiratory tract infection and inflammatory consolidation caused by *Chlamydia pneumoniae*

Incidence

▸▸ *C. pneumoniae* is the fourth most common cause of infectious pneumonia, responsible for 6-12% of cases
▸▸ Based on the detection of antibodies in half of the adult population, *C. pneumoniae* infection is likely nearly universal with frequent reinfections

Morbidity and Mortality

▸▸ Generally a mild or asymptomatic infection (90%), it is more severe in older patients
▸▸ Rarely fatal

Age Distribution

▸▸ Persons of all ages greater than 5 years may become infected

Clinical Features

▸▸ Infected children less than 11 years of age are more likely to develop bronchitis, otitis media, and rhinitis than asymptomatic infection, pneumonia, pharyngitis, laryngitis, tonsillitis, or croup
▸▸ Initially presenting with pharyngitis, infection gradually proceeds to cough and pneumonia over days to a week
▸▸ Adults manifest cough (61%) that is productive of sputum (44%), rales (61%), and fever (56%)

Radiologic Features

▸▸ Primary *C. pneumoniae* pneumonia in adults causes alveolar infiltrates on admission more frequently than interstitial infiltrates, but interstitial infiltrates occur more often with reinfection
▸▸ More than half of cases develop pleural effusions

Prognosis and Therapy

▸▸ Infection is self-limited
▸▸ Doxycycline (tetracycline), erythromycin, azithromycin, or clarithromycin is given for 14 days

sometimes forming germinal centers, plasma cells, eosinophils, and polymorphonuclear leukocytes and of alveoli by mononuclear cells and eosinophils causes a combination of interstitial pneumonia, alveolar pneumonia, and bronchiolitis. Obstruction of airways may lead to patchy distal atelectasis.

Experimental infection of mice and rabbits with *C. pneumoniae* causes infection of respiratory epithelial cells, early polymorphonuclear leukocyte response, and later interstitial and peribronchial, peribronchiolar, perivascular, and alveolar lymphocytes, macrophages, and plasma cells.

Psittacosis pneumonia is characterized by variable quantities of early infiltration of alveoli by polymorphonuclear leukocytes, red blood cells, and fibrin followed later by macrophages, lymphocytes, and plasma cells.

Definition

▸ Lower respiratory tract infection and inflammatory consolidation caused by *Chlamydia psittaci*

Incidence

▸ Although more than 813 cases of psittacosis were reported to the CDC from 1988 to 1998, only 10-24 cases were registered annually in 2001-2004

Mortality

▸ Although the case fatality rate was 15-20% in the pre-antibiotic era, it is less than 1% in appropriately treated cases

Age Distribution

▸ Predominantly an occupational or avocational disease (e.g., turkey processors, pet shop workers, and bird fanciers), psittacosis is mild and uncommon in childhood and commonly affects adults

Clinical Features

▸ In addition to classical psittacosis with pneumonia, some patients have subclinical, nonspecific febrile or typhoidal forms
▸ Typically abrupt onset of fever, headache, chills, malaise, and myalgia are followed by nonproductive cough
▸ Examination frequently reveals pharyngeal redness, rales, and hepatomegaly

Radiologic Features

▸ The chest radiograph is abnormal in three-quarters of patients and frequently reveals more extensive infiltrates than suggested by auscultation
▸ Consolidation may appear alveolar or interstitial, and small pleural effusions are common

Prognosis and Therapy

▸ The treatment of choice is doxycycline for 2 to 3 weeks (at least 10 days after defervescence)
▸ Erythromycin is an alternative, but may be less effective
▸ Subjective amelioration frequently occurs after 24 hours, and resolution of symptoms after 48 to 72 hours of treatment

Macrophages and lymphocytes also multifocally infiltrate alveolar septa.

Q FEVER PNEUMONIA

Coxiella burnetii is inhaled into the lungs, and only a few of these highly infectious bacteria are required to establish infection in alveolar macrophages. A high propor-

tion (60%) of infections are asymptomatic, and in a well investigated outbreak only 4.4% of patients were hospitalized with pneumonia. The pathologic lesions range from macrophage-rich pneumonia to poorly resolving pulmonary pseudotumor (Figures 15-3 and 15-4).

RICKETTSIAL PNEUMONIAS

Respiratory signs, symptoms, and life-threatening pulmonary inflammation and edema occur in patients with severe Rocky Mountain spotted fever (Figures 15-5 and 15-6), epidemic typhus, Mediterranean spotted fever, and murine typhus (Figure 15-7) because of extensive rickettsial infection of the pulmonary microcirculation.

SCRUB TYPHUS PNEUMONIA

A prevalent infection in indigenous populations, scrub typhus also occurred among US soldiers who entered regions infested by *O. tsutsugamushi*-infected chiggers during World War II and the Vietnam War and travelers whose itineraries include such exposures (Figures 15-8 and 15-9). The pulmonary lesions can be life-threatening.

EHRLICHIAL PNEUMONIA

Life-threatening respiratory failure is a component of a portion of cases of human monocytotropic ehrlichiosis (HME) (Figures 15-10 and 15-11). Patients with fatal HME are either immunocompetent patients who die with scant organisms likely because of immunopathologic mechanism(s) or immunocompromised patients who die with overwhelming infection and large ehrlichial loads.

Our knowledge of the pathology of HME is based on a small number of autopsies. Gross consolidation has been observed. Histopathology reveals interstitial pneumonia and diffuse alveolar damage with interstitial lymphocytes and macrophages. Immunohistochemical examination with anti-ehrlichial antibodies demonstrates *E. chaffeensis* in macrophages in the pulmonary interstitium. *Ehrlichia* have two distinct ultrastructural forms, a smaller form with an electron-opaque central condensation and a larger reticulate cell with dispersed electron-lucent protoplasm. They reside in a cytoplasmic vacuole that contains matrices and other structures of ehrlichial origin.

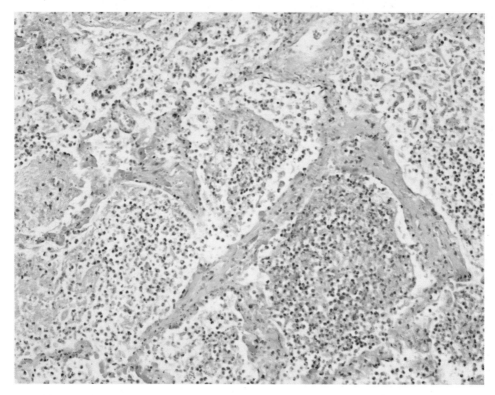

FIGURE 15-3
Q fever
Q fever pneumonia shows alveoli filled with a mixture of leukocytes and fibrin. (Generously provided by J. Stephen Dumler, MD, Johns Hopkins Medical Institutions.)

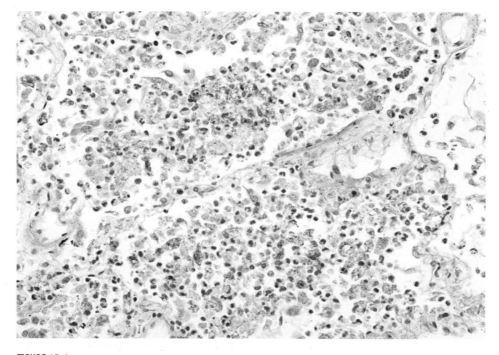

FIGURE 15-4
Q fever
Immunohistochemical demonstration of *Coxiella burnetii* in the cytoplasm of numerous macrophages in pulmonary alveoli. (Generously provided by J. Stephen Dumler, MD, Johns Hopkins Medical Institutions.)

Q FEVER PNEUMONIA—FACT SHEET

Definition

» Lower respiratory tract infection and inflammatory consolidation caused by *Coxiella burnetii*

Incidence

» Global seroprevalence studies indicate that *C. burnetii* infection is common
» Clinical diagnosis of Q fever with laboratory confirmation is rare in the US, but was documented to be the cause of 3-6% of cases of community-acquired pneumonia when careful studies were performed

Morbidity and Mortality

» Q fever is rarely fatal even when co-morbid conditions are present
» In the pre-antibiotic era a case-fatality rate of 1.5% was reported

Age Distribution

» Infection with *C. burnetii* can occur at any age

Clinical Features

» Patients with acute Q fever pneumonia manifest fever, fatigue, inspiratory rales, and severe headache
» In one series, only 28% complained of cough, which was nonproductive
» Myalgia, nausea, vomiting, diarrhea, or pleuritic chest pain may occur in some patients

Radiologic Features

» The chest radiograph of a patient with Q fever can have a variety of abnormalities: segmental or subsegmental consolidation, rounded opacity, atelectasis, pleural effusion, and hilar lymphadenopathy

Prognosis and Therapy

» Acute Q fever pneumonia resolves over a period of 10 days to 2 months, usually within 15 to 30 days
» The drug of choice is doxycycline for a course of 15 to 21 days
» There is evidence that some quinolones may also be effective

Q FEVER PNEUMONIA—PATHOLOGIC FEATURES

Gross Findings

» Focal consolidation

Microscopic Findings

» Bronchioloalveolitis
» Alveolar macrophages, lymphocytes, fibrin, red blood cells, and few polymorphonuclear leukocytes

Immunohistochemical Features

» Specific immunohistochemical method detects *C. burnetii* in the cytoplasm of alveolar macrophages

Ultrastructural Findings

» Small and large cell forms of *C. burnetii* in large phagolysosomes of alveolar macrophages

Pathologic Differential Diagnosis

» Any agent causing macrophage-rich pneumonia, including *Legionella pneumophila*

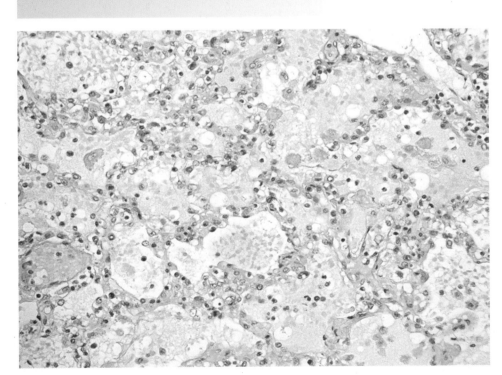

FIGURE 15-5

Fatal Rocky Moutain spotted fever
Lung from a three-year-old girl from Tennessee shows interstitial pneumonia and alveolar edema.

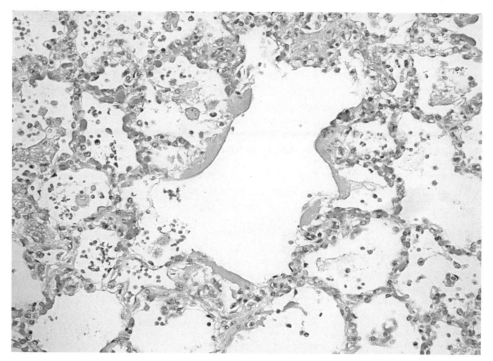

FIGURE 15-6
Fatal Rocky Mountain spotted fever
Diffuse alveolar damage with prominent hyaline membranes.

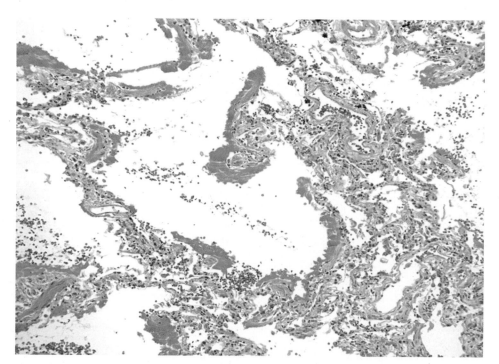

FIGURE 15-7
Fatal murine typhus
Lung from an 81-year-old woman from Texas with hyaline membranes.

RICKETTSIAL PNEUMONIAS—FACT SHEET

Definition

➤ Interstitial pneumonia in some cases associated with noncardiogenic pulmonary edema caused by *Rickettsia rickettsii, R. prowazekii, R. conorii,* or *R. typhi*

Incidence

➤ Respiratory signs, symptoms, and failure are associated with severe illness that affects patients with Rocky Mountain spotted fever (RMSF), epidemic louse-borne typhus, Mediterranean spotted fever (MSF), and murine typhus in descending order of the proportion of cases
➤ In 2005, 1766 cases of RMSF were reported in the U.S.
➤ Louse-borne typhus fever has occurred in recent years as outbreaks in zones of extreme poverty or social disruption by warfare involving several to 100,000 cases
➤ The incidences of MSF and murine typhus are poorly reported and are probably important in some parts of the world

Morbidity and Mortality

➤ Case fatality rates range downwards from 23% for RMSF in the pre-antibiotic era; current estimates are 4% for RMSF, epidemic typhus, and MSF and 1% for murine typhus
➤ Risk factors for a fatal outcome include older age, delay in antirickettsial treatment, and male gender

Age Distribution

➤ Rickettsioses can affect patients of any age; the highest incidence of RMSF occurs in childhood

Clinical Features

➤ Rickettsioses present with fever, headache, myalgia, and, for MSF, an eschar at the site of tick bite inoculation of rickettsiae
➤ Rash appears on day 3 to 5 or later and occurs in a high portion of lightly pigmented patients
➤ The occurrence of petechiae reflects the severity of illness; involvement of the palms and soles is present in RMSF and MSF
➤ The most severe cases manifest neurologic and respiratory involvement; cough occurs in a third or more of cases of RMSF, epidemic typhus, and murine typhus and 10% of cases of MSF
➤ A fatal outcome is frequently associated with development of the acute respiratory distress syndrome

Radiologic Features

➤ Approximately one-third of patients with RMSF have radiographic abnormalities, particularly those with severe disease and delayed treatment
➤ Diffuse interstitial infiltrate progresses to diffuse air space consolidation
➤ Diffuse infiltrates are a grave prognostic sign with a fatal outcome in 50% of cases
➤ Survivors' pulmonary infiltrates resolve within 5 days
➤ Pleural effusions are observed radiographically in approximately 10% of cases

Prognosis and Therapy

➤ Virtually all patients with rickettsial infection who are treated within 5 days of onset of illness recover without sequelae
➤ The treatment of choice except for pregnant or tetracycline-hypersensitive patients is doxycycline
➤ Chloramphenicol is an alternative, but with less favorable results

RICKETTSIAL PNEUMONIAS—PATHOLOGIC FEATURES

Gross Findings

➤ Diffuse consolidation in most fatal cases

Microscopic Findings

➤ Interstitial pneumonia and edema
➤ Alveolar edema, fibrin, macrophages, petechiae
➤ Interlobular septal edema
➤ Lymphohistiocytic vasculitis
➤ Diffuse alveolar damage

Immunohistochemical Findings

➤ Specific immunohistochemical methods identify numerous spotted fever group rickettsiae *(R. rickettsii, R. conorii)* or typhus group rickettsiae *(R. prowazekii, R. typhi)* in endothelial cells of alveolar septa, pulmonary arteries and pulmonary veins

Ultrastructural Findings

➤ Small ($0.3 \times 1 \ \mu m$) gram-negative bacteria free in the cytosol of endothelial cells surrounded by an electron-lucent halo presumed to be a rickettsial slime layer

Pathologic Differential Diagnosis

➤ Other bacterial and viral interstitial pneumonias

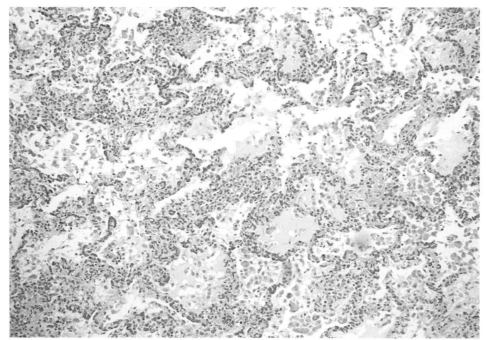

FIGURE 15-8

Fatal scrub typhus
Lung reveals severe interstitial pneumonia and pulmonary edema.

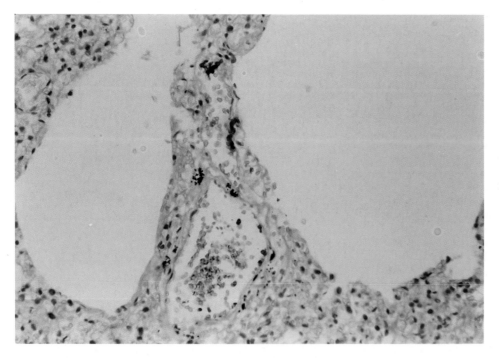

Figure 15-9

Fatal scrub typhus
Immunohistochemical demonstration of *Orientia tsutsugamushi* in endothelial cells of the pulmonary interstitium.

SCRUB TYPHUS PNEUMONIA—FACT SHEET

Definition

➤ Interstitial pneumonia caused by *Orientia tsutsugamushi*

Incidence

➤ In the region within the polygon encompassed by the Russian Far East, Korea, Japan, islands of the southwest Pacific Ocean, northern Australia, islands of the Indian Ocean, India, and Afghanistan, a huge rural population is at risk
➤ An incidence of 3.2-3.9% of the population being infected with *O. tsutsugamushi* monthly has been observed with a point seroprevalence of 50%

Mortality

➤ Case fatality rates ranged from less than 1% to 30% in the pre-antibiotic era
➤ Lethality is age-dependent with greatest severity in the elderly

Age Distribution

➤ Infection occurs in persons of all ages exposed to infected larval mites

Clinical Features

➤ An eschar develops at the site of feeding of the infected chigger in half of primary infections, followed by fever, regional lymphadenopathy, headache, and myalgia
➤ A rash may appear at the end of the first week of illness
➤ Cough and tachypnea occur frequently and may progress to dyspnea and acute respiratory distress syndrome

Radiological Features

➤ Radiographic pulmonary infiltrates are frequently present, varying from interstitial infiltrates to patchy infiltrates or frank consolidation

Prognosis and Therapy

➤ Patients generally become afebrile within 24 to 36 hours of treatment with doxycycline
➤ Chloramphenicol is effective, but less so than the tetracyclines
➤ Tetracycline- and chloramphenicol-resistant strains in northern Thailand have responded to treatment with rifampin or azithromycin
➤ Clarithromycin has been used during pregnancy

SCRUB TYPHUS PNEUMONIA—PATHOLOGIC FEATURES

Gross Findings

➤ Diffuse congestion, hemorrhages, and edema

Microscopic Findings

➤ Alveolar septal infiltration by macrophages and lymphocytes
➤ Alveolar edema and hemorrhage
➤ Diffuse alveolar damage with hyaline membranes

Immunohistochemical Findings

➤ *Orientia tsutsugamushi* is detected by a specific immunohistochemical method in endothelial cells and macrophages

Ultrastructural Findings

➤ Small (0.5 × 1.2 μm) gram-negative bacteria that reside free in the cytosol of endothelial cells and differ from *Rickettsia* in cell wall structure and absence of a surrounding electron-lucent zone

Pathologic Differential Diagnosis

➤ Other bacterial and viral interstitial pneumonias such as typhus and spotted fever

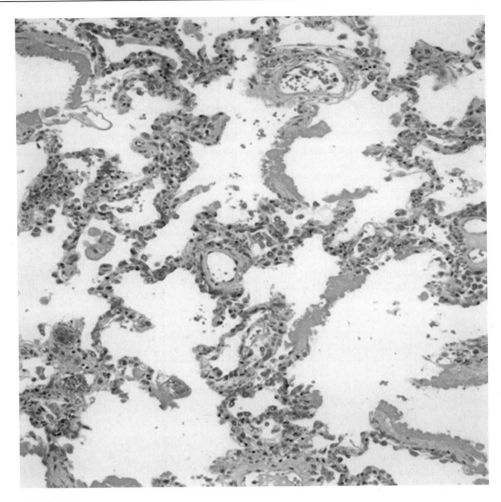

FIGURE 15-10

Fatal human monocytotropic ehrlichiosis
Lung demonstrates diffuse alveolar damage with hyaline membranes. (Generously provided by Christopher Paddock, MD, Centers for Disease Control and Prevention.)

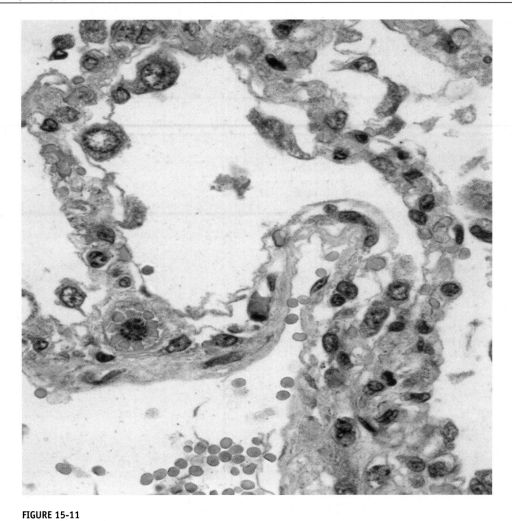

FIGURE 15-11

Ehrlichia chaffeensis **immunohistochemistry**
Immunohistochemical demonstration of antigen of *Ehrlichia chaffeensis* in circulating monocytes and interstitial macrophages of alveolar septa in human monocytotropic ehrlichiosis. (Generously provided by Christopher Paddock, MD, Centers for Disease Control and Prevention.)

EHRLICHIAL PNEUMONITIS—FACT SHEET

Definition

➠ Interstitial pneumonia associated with infection with *Ehrlichia chaffeensis*

Incidence

➠ In the southeastern and south-central U.S., the incidence of human monocytotropic ehrlichiosis (HME) varies from less than 1 to approximately 1000 cases per million population according to variations in diagnosis and reporting and whether surveillance is passive or active

Mortality

➠ The case fatality rate is 2.7%

Gender and Age Distribution

➠ HME is diagnosed in patients of all ages with substantially higher incidence in persons greater than 30 years of age and in males

Clinical Features

➠ HME patients typically have fever, headache, and myalgias
➠ Gastrointestinal, respiratory, and neurologic manifestations or rash are present in fewer than 40% of cases
➠ Leukopenia, thrombocytopenia, and elevated hepatic transaminases occur frequently

Radiologic Features

➠ Among the patients who had chest radiographs in one series, 44% had pulmonary infiltrates that have been characterized as interstitial or alveolar opacities and may be associated with pleural effusions

Prognosis and Therapy

➠ The only treatment that is established as effective is doxycycline or tetracycline, which usually results in defervescence within 24 to 48 hours

ANAPLASMA PNEUMONIA

Human granulocytic anaplasmosis (HGA) has a lower incidence of respiratory involvement than HME (Figure 15-12). The main pulmonary lesions that have been reported are those of opportunistic pneumonias.

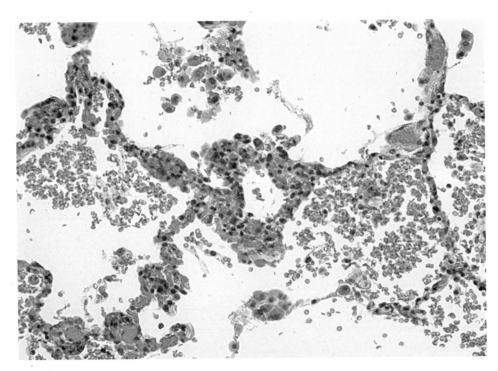

FIGURE 15-12

Human granulocytotropic anaplasmosis

Interstitial pneumonia and alveolar hemorrhages. (Generously provided by J. Stephen Dumler, MD, Johns Hopkins Medical Institutions.)

ANAPLASMA PHAGOCYTOPHILUM PNEUMONIA—FACT SHEET

Definition

➤ Interstitial pneumonitis associated with *A. phagocytophilum* infection

Incidence

➤ In endemic areas an incidence greater than 50 cases per 100,000 population has been reported

Morbidity and Mortality

➤ The case fatality rate is probably less than 0.5%, but half or more of patients are hospitalized

Gender and Age Distribution

➤ Human granulocytic araplasmosis (HGA) occurs in all age groups, but the incidence is substantially higher in persons older than 30 years and in males

Clinical Features

➤ Fever, headache, myalgias, leukopenia, thrombocytopenia, and elevated hepatic transaminases are usually present
➤ Interstitial pneumonitis has been reported in a higher proportion of European than North American HGA patients

Radiologic Features

➤ Bilateral interstitial infiltrates have been reported

Prognosis and Therapy

➤ Doxycycline is the drug of choice
➤ Rifampin has been used to treat HGA during pregnancy

SUGGESTED READING

Mycoplasma Pneumoniae

1. Clyde WA Jr. Infections of the respiratory tract due to *Mycoplasma pneumoniae*. In: Chernick V, Kendig EL Jr, eds. *Kendig's Disorders of the Respiratory Tract in Children*. 5 ed. Philadelphia, PA: WB Saunders; 1990:403-12.
2. Daxboeck F, Krause R, Wenisch C. Laboratory diagnosis of *Mycoplasma pneumoniae* infection. *Clin Microbiol Infect*. 2003;263-73.
3. Leons K, Ursi D, Goossens H, et al. Molecular diagnosis of *Mycoplasma pneumoniae* respiratory tract infections. *J Clin Microbiol*. 2003;41: 4915-23.

Chlamydia

4. Arth C, Von Schmidt B, Grossman M, Schachter J. Chlamydial pneumonitis. *J Pediatr*. 1978;93:447-9.
5. Beem MO, Saxon EM. Respiratory-tract colonization and a distinctive pneumonia syndrome in infants infected with *Chlamydia trachomatis*. *N Engl J Med*. 1977;296:306-10.
6. Grayston JT, Thom DH. The chlamydial pneumonias. *Curr Clin Top Infect Dis*. 1991;11:1-18.
7. Ito JI Jr, Comess KA, Alexander, ER, et al. Pneumonia due to *Chlamydia trachomatis* in an immunocompromised adult. *N Engl J Med*. 1982;307:95-8.

Q Fever

8. Janigan DT, Marrie TJ. Pathology of Q fever pneumonia. In: Marrie TJ, ed. *Q Fever*. Boca Raton, Fla: CRC Press; 1990:161-70.
9. Marrie TJ. Acute Q fever. In: Marrie TJ, ed. *Q Fever*. Boca Raton, Fla: CRC Press; 1990:125-60.
10. Maurin M, Raoult M. Q fever. *Clin Microbiol Rev*. 1999;12:518-53.
11. Walker DH. Pathology of Q fever. In: Walker DH, ed. *Biology of Rickettsia Diseases, Vol. II*. Boca Raton, Fla: CRC Press; 1988:17-27.

Rickettsiae

12. Raoult D, Walker DH. *Rickettsia rickettsii* (epidemic or louse-borne typhus). In: Mandell GL, Douglas RG Jr, Bennett JE, eds. *Principles and Practice of Infectious Diseases*. 6 ed. New York: Elsevier; 2004: 2303-6.
13. Walker DH. Pathology and pathogenesis of the vasculotropic rickettsioses. In: Walker DH, ed. *Biology of Rickettsial Diseases, Vol. I*. Boca Raton, Fla: CRC Press; 1985:115-38.

16 Idiopathic Interstitial Pneumonias

Andras Khoor

INTRODUCTION

Idiopathic interstitial pneumonias comprise a number of relatively rare clinicopathologic entities, which can be distinguished from one another and from other forms of diffuse interstitial lung disease by their clinical, radiologic, and histologic features. The recent American Thoracic Society/European Respiratory Society (ATS/ERS) classification, which is the result of an international consensus, encompasses the follow-ing clinicopathologic entities in order of relative frequency: idiopathic pulmonary fibrosis (IPF), non-specific interstitial pneumonia (NSIP), cryptogenic organizing pneumonia (COP), acute interstitial pneu-monia (AIP), respiratory bronchiolitis associated in-terstitial lung disease (RB-ILD), desquamative inter-stitial pneumonia (DIP), and lymphoid interstitial pneumonia (LIP) (Table 16-1). A category of unclas-sifiable interstitial pneumonia is also recognized to acknowledge that some cases of idiopathic interstitial pneumonia defy precise classification.

The ATS/ERS document also defines a set of histo-logic patterns that provide the morphologic basis for the clinicopathologic diagnoses (Table 16-1). These histo-logic patterns are distinctive, but not entirely specific. The same histology may be seen not only in the idio-pathic setting, but also in a variety of conditions of known etiology. For example, UIP (usual interstitial pneumonia) can be seen not only in patients with IPF, but also in patients with connective tissue diseases. It is recommended that the word "pattern" be added to the histologic diagnosis, when the histologic and clinico-pathologic terms would be otherwise the same. For ex-ample, "NSIP pattern," "DIP pattern," and "LIP pat-tern" are used to describe the histology, and "NSIP," "DIP," and "LIP" are used for the final clinicopathologic diagnosis.

Surgical lung biopsy is the gold standard for the diag-nosis of idiopathic interstitial pneumonias, but high-resolution computed tomography (HRCT) also plays an important role in the evaluation of these patients. Dis-tinctive HRCT findings consistent with UIP are present in approximately half of the patients with IPF. If these findings are present, a diagnosis of IPF can be made without a surgical lung biopsy. In the absence of the characteristic HRCT findings of UIP, patients with sus-pected idiopathic interstitial pneumonia are advised to undergo surgical lung biopsy. The surgical lung biopsy should include samples from at least two lobes. Trans-bronchial lung biopsy does not yield sufficient material for the diagnosis of an idiopathic interstitial pneumo-nia, with the exception of some cases of diffuse alveolar damage (DAD)/AIP and organizing pneumonia (OP)/ cryptogenic organizing pneumonia (COP). On the other hand, transbronchial lung biopsy may be used to ex-clude some other diseases, including sarcoidosis and certain infections.

IDIOPATHIC PULMONARY FIBROSIS/USUAL INTERSTITIAL PNEUMONIA (IPF/UIP)

IPF, which is known as cryptogenic fibrosing alveolitis in the British literature, is the most common idiopathic interstitial pneumonia. Lung biopsies from patients with IPF show the histologic pattern of UIP. UIP is patchy, temporally heterogeneous fibrosis, which is characterized by a spectrum of findings that ranges from normal lung to fibroblastic foci, and to scarring and honeycombing. The histologic pattern of UIP is not

TABLE 16-1

Idiopathic Interstitial Pneumonias and the Underlying Histologic Patterns

Idiopathic Interstitial Pneumonia	Histologic Pattern
Idiopathic pulmonary fibrosis	Usual interstitial pneumonia
Nonspecific interstitial pneumonia	Nonspecific interstitial pneumonia pattern
Cryptogenic organizing pneumonia	Organizing pneumonia
Acute interstitial pneumonia	Diffuse alveolar damage
Respiratory bronchiolitis-associated interstitial lung disease	Respiratory bronchiolitis
Desquamative interstitial pneumonia	Desquamative interstitial pneumonia pattern
Lymphoid interstitial pneumonia	Lymphoid interstitial pneumonia pattern

Adapted from Table 2, Travis WD, King TE, Bateman ED, et al. American Thoracic Society/European Respiratory Society international multidisciplinary consensus classification of the idiopathic interstitial pneumonias. *Am J Respir Crit Care Med.* 2002;165:277-304.

entirely specific for IPF; a similar pattern can be seen in some patients who suffer from connective tissue diseases and a few other conditions. The clinicopathologic term of IPF is appropriate only if other causes of UIP are excluded. If a lung biopsy reveals UIP in the setting of an underlying disease (e.g., rheumatoid arthritis), the final diagnosis should be UIP, and the underlying condition should be mentioned (e.g., UIP associated with rheumatoid arthritis).

A surgical lung biopsy that shows UIP in the proper clinical background is the most definitive method of establishing a diagnosis of IPF. However, approximately half of the patients with IPF have characteristic HRCT findings that are compatible with UIP. In these cases, a diagnosis of IPF can be made without a surgical lung biopsy.

CLINICAL FEATURES

The estimated incidence of IPF is 10.7 cases per 100,000 males per year and 7.4 cases per 100,000 females per year. The patients are usually over 50 years of age and present with a history of dyspnea on exertion and nonproductive cough. Bibasilar, late inspiratory, fine crackles ("velcro" rales) are found on chest auscultation. Pulmonary function tests (PFTs) reveal restriction and impairment of gas exchange. Lung volumes are typically reduced, but may be normal in patients with superimposed chronic obstructive pulmonary disease.

RADIOLOGIC FEATURES

CHEST RADIOGRAPHY

Chest radiographs in patients with IPF typically show a bilateral reticular pattern, involving mainly the lower lung zones. Less than 10 percent of the patients have a normal chest x-ray at presentation.

HIGH-RESOLUTION COMPUTERIZED TOMOGRAPHY

The most characteristic HRCT finding of UIP is the presence of reticular opacities. Honeycombing and ground-glass attenuation are also common. The findings are typically basal and peripheral in distribution. HRCT may show characteristic findings for UIP even in patients with normal radiographs.

PATHOLOGIC FEATURES

GROSS FINDINGS

The lungs tend to be small, and the visceral pleura shows retractions along the interlobular septa. The cut surfaces reveal patchy, predominantly subpleural and paraseptal fibrosis with honeycombing, and areas of intervening normal lung (Figure 16-1). The fibrosis is more severe in the lower lobes.

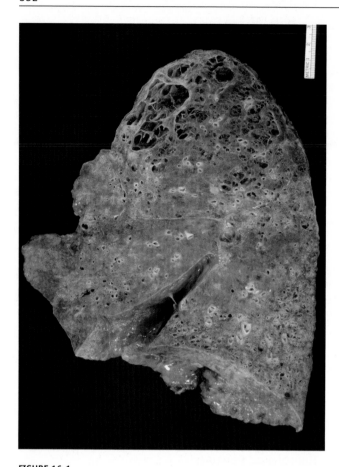

FIGURE 16-1
Usual interstitial pneumonia
The cut surface of the lung shows subpleural and paraseptal fibrosis with focal honeycombing and areas of intervening normal lung.

MICROSCOPIC FINDINGS

Microscopically, UIP is characterized by its variegated appearance; areas of fibrosis alternate with areas of normal lung (Figure 16-2). The fibrosis is subpleural and paraseptal in distribution and is temporally heterogeneous. The appearance of temporal heterogeneity is due to the presence of mature scars and immature fibroblastic foci. Scarring results in remodeling of the pulmonary architecture with formation of cystic spaces (honeycombing). The cysts may contain mucus or inflammatory cells. Fibroblastic foci, which are composed of myofibroblasts and loose connective tissue, are usually present at the interface of scars and normal lung tissue. Smooth muscle proliferation may accompany scarring. Mild interstitial chronic inflammation and scattered lymphoid aggregates may also be found. Secondary vascular changes are common and consist of medial thickening and intimal fibrosis. Biopsies from patients with the so-called "accelerated decline" or "acute exacerbation" of IPF show a combination of UIP and DAD (Figure 16-3).

DIFFERENTIAL DIAGNOSIS

Differentiating UIP/IPF from other entities involves histologic and etiologic considerations. The histologic differential diagnoses, which can often be addressed on histologic grounds alone, include the fibrosing pattern of NSIP and organizing DAD. The etiologic differential diagnoses, which must be addressed in a clinicopathologic context, include connective tissue diseases, asbestosis, hypersensitivity pneumonia, and Hermansky-Pudlak syndrome.

In the process of separating UIP from other idiopathic interstitial pneumonias (i.e., NSIP and DAD), the presence or absence of temporal heterogeneity is the single most helpful histologic finding. The fibrosing pattern of NSIP is characterized by uniform interstitial fibrosis, which may be accompanied by mild to moderate chronic inflammation. The hallmark of organizing DAD is diffuse interstitial fibroblast proliferation, which incorporates remnants of hyaline membranes into the alveolar septa. In contrast to NSIP and DAD, UIP has a variegated appearance with dense scars, scattered fibroblast foci, and areas of normal lung. Knowledge of the clinical history may also help differentiate organizing DAD from UIP. Whereas patients with UIP typically have a long history of shortness of breath and unproductive cough, patients with DAD usually present with acute respiratory failure.

Sometimes, in a patient with multiple biopsies, UIP is seen in one lobe and an NSIP pattern is seen in another lobe. In such cases, the overall histologic diagnosis should be UIP. It also occurs that a lung biopsy shows features that are indeterminate between UIP and fibrosing NSIP. In these cases, a review of the HRCT findings may prove to be useful. If the distinction between the two patterns cannot be made with certainty after the pathologic-radiologic correlation, the term "fibrosing interstitial pneumonia, not further classified" can be used. It is not appropriate to use the term "unclassifiable interstitial pneumonia" in this situation.

Connective tissue diseases, asbestosis, hypersensitivity pneumonia, and Hermansky-Pudlak syndrome usually cannot be separated from UIP/IPF without clinicopathologic correlation. However, some unusual istologic findings in a biopsy otherwise similar to UIP may prompt a clinical inquiry. The presence of prominent lymphoid aggregates, lymphoid follicles, or chronic pleuritis should raise the possibility of a connective tissue disease. Pleural plaques may be associated with asbestosis, and their presence should prompt a search for asbestos bodies and an inquiry into asbestos exposure. Vaguely formed granulomas may suggest hypersensitivity pneumonia. Hermansky-Pudlak syndrome is an autosomal recessive condition that is characterized by defects in platelet aggregation, oculocutaneous albinism, and accumulation of ceroid-filled histiocytes in many organs. Pulmonary involvement manifests as interstitial lung

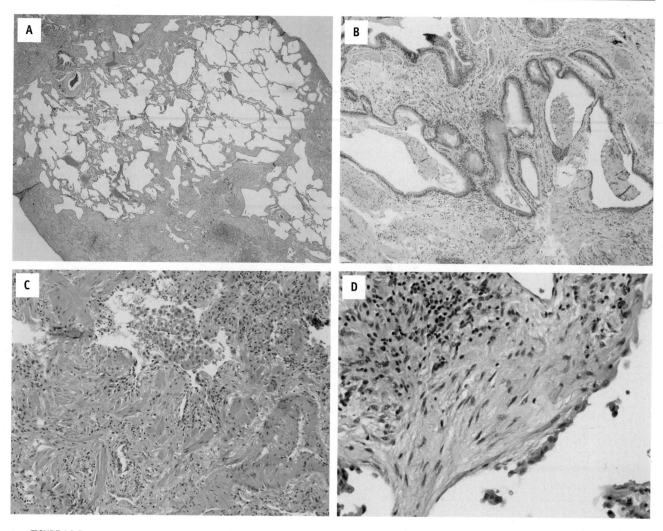

FIGURE 16-2

Usual interstitial pneumonia

(A) At low power, UIP is characterized by its variegated appearance; areas of fibrosis alternate with areas of uninvolved lung. **(B)** Focally, microscopic honeycombing can be seen. **(C)** Medium power often reveals foci of smooth muscle proliferation. **(D)** Fibroblastic foci are usually found at the interface of dense fibrosis and normal lung.

disease, which is histologically similar to UIP. However, in Hermansky-Pudlak syndrome, the fibrosis is accompanied by ceroid-filled histiocytes, which are present both in the air spaces and in the interstitium.

PROGNOSIS AND THERAPY

For patients with IPF, the mean length of survival from the time of diagnosis is between 2.5 and 3.5 years. Respiratory failure is the most frequent cause of death. Aggressive immunosuppressive and cytotoxic therapy has failed to reduce the death rate, but lung transplantation is beneficial in selected cases. Novel therapies such as γ-interferon and imatinib mesylate show some promise.

Some patients with IPF develop acute, fulminant respiratory failure. This "accelerated decline" or "acute exacerbation" of IPF has a very poor prognosis, and patients usually die within 1 week.

NONSPECIFIC INTERSTITIAL PNEUMONIA

Nonspecific interstitial pneumonia (NSIP) is both a histologic pattern and a clinicopathologic entity. NSIP pattern is characterized by mild to moderate interstitial chronic inflammation and/or temporally uniform interstitial fibrosis. Additionally, NSIP pattern lacks specific histologic features of other interstitial lung diseases (e.g., hyaline membranes of DAD). NSIP can be the

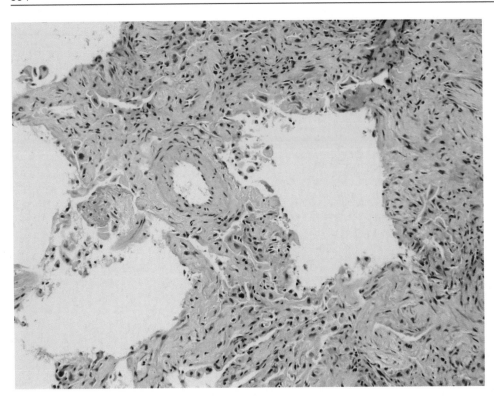

FIGURE 16-3

Usual interstitial pneumonia with "acute exacerbation"
At medium power, the pulmonary parenchyma is remodeled by dense scars of UIP. The superimposed diffuse alveolar damage is represented by remnants of hyaline membranes and loose connective tissue, which incorporates the hyaline membranes into the alveolar septa.

IDIOPATHIC PULMONARY FIBROSIS—FACT SHEET

Definition
- A chronic interstitial pneumonia of unknown etiology showing the histologic pattern of usual interstitial pneumonia in a surgical lung biopsy

Incidence
- The incidence is estimated as 10.7 cases per 100,000 males per year and 7.4 cases per 100,000 females per year

Gender and Age Distribution
- Slightly more common in males
- Patients are usually older than 50 years at onset

Clinical Features
- Insidious onset of otherwise unexplained dyspnea on exertion, and cough
- Bibasilar, inspiratory crackles (dry or "velcro" type in quality)
- Abnormal pulmonary function studies that include evidence of restriction and impaired gas exchange

Radiologic Features
- On HRCT, bibasilar reticular abnormalities with honeycombing and ground-glass attenuation

Prognosis
- The clinical course is invariably one of gradual deterioration
- The median length of survival from the time of diagnosis is between 2.5 and 3.5 years

---

USUAL INTERSTITIAL PNEUMONIA—PATHOLOGIC FEATURES

Microscopic Findings
- Temporal heterogeneity
- Dense fibrosis with "honeycomb" change
- Fibroblast foci
- Areas of normal lung
- Frequent subpleural and paraseptal distribution

Pathologic Differential Diagnosis
- Nonspecific interstitial pneumonia, fibrosing pattern
- Diffuse alveolar damage, organizing phase

Etiologic Differential Diagnosis (Clinical Conditions Associated with UIP)
- Idiopathic pulmonary fibrosis
- Connective tissue diseases
- Asbestosis
- Hypersensitivity pneumonia
- Hermansky-Pudlak syndrome

manifestation of connective tissue diseases, drug toxicity, and hypersensitivity pneumonia. The etiology of NSIP, however, is often unknown.

CLINICAL FEATURES

NSIP is less common than UIP, but occurs more frequently than the remaining idiopathic interstitial pneumonias. The average age at presentation is between 40 and 50 years, but NSIP may also occur in children. It has a slight predilection for females. Clinical symptoms of NSIP are similar to those of IPF; patients often present with dyspnea on exertion, and cough. Crackles are common findings on auscultation. PFTs usually reveal a restrictive defect with lowered diffusing capacity of the lung for carbon monoxide (DLCO). Exercise-associated gas exchange abnormalities are commonly present.

RADIOLOGIC FEATURES

CHEST RADIOGRAPHY

NSIP has no specific radiographic findings, but ground-glass opacities and areas of consolidation are common.

HIGH-RESOLUTION COMPUTED TOMOGROPHY

On HRCT, areas of ground-glass attenuation are seen in virtually all cases. Although a reticular pattern is common, it is rarely the predominant finding.

PATHOLOGIC FEATURES

Histologically, NSIP is divided into cellular and fibrosing patterns. The cellular NSIP pattern is characterized by mild to moderate interstitial chronic inflammation with a mixture of lymphocytes and plasma cells (Figure 16-4). Lymphoid aggregates are a common finding.

The hallmark of the fibrosing NSIP pattern is the presence of diffuse, temporally uniform interstitial fibrosis (Figure 16-5). This may or may not be accompanied by mild to moderate chronic inflammation. The fibrous connective tissue may be dense or loose in character, but has the same appearance throughout the lung. Honeycomb change and fibroblastic foci are either absent or inconspicuous. Superimposed organizing pneumonia may be seen focally in both the cellular and the fibrosing pattern of NSIP (Figure 16-6)

DIFFERENTIAL DIAGNOSIS

Histologic differential diagnoses for the cellular NSIP pattern include the LIP pattern and organizing pneumonia. Both cellular NSIP and LIP are characterized by the presence of chronic inflammatory cells in the alveolar septa, and separation of the two patterns is not well defined. However, in most cases of LIP, there is a marked lymphoid infiltrate, which is noticeably different from the mild to moderate chronic inflammation typically seen in NSIP. OP can be a minor component of cellular NSIP. However, cases of NSIP with an

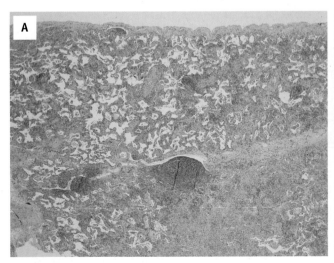
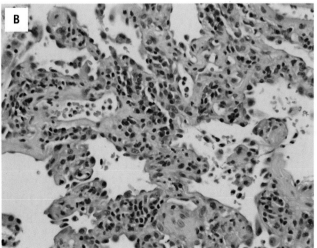

FIGURE 16-4

Cellular nonspecific interstitial pneumonia pattern

(A) At low power, the cellular NSIP pattern is characterized by a diffuse interstitial infiltrate. Scattered lymphoid aggregates may be present. **(B)** At high power, the inters the infiltrate is composed of lymphocytes and a variable number of plasma cells.

FOUNDATIONS IN DIAGNOSTIC PATHOLOGY SERIES

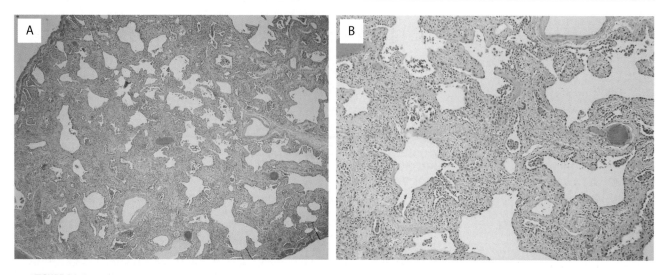

FIGURE 16-5

Fibrosing nonspecific interstitial pneumonia pattern
Fibrosing NSIP pattern is characterized by temporally uniform interstitial fibrosis. The thickened alveolar septa may also contain chronic inflammatory cells.

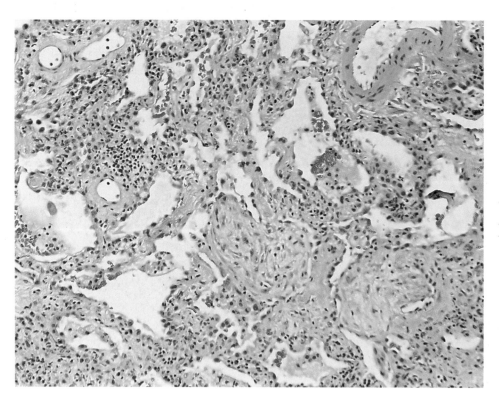

Figure 16-6

Nonspecific interstitial pneumonia pattern with a minor component of organizing pneumonia
Organizing pneumonia with fibroblastic plugs may be a minor component of the NSIP pattern.

OP component can usually be separated from cases where OP is the main cause of the respiratory illness (e.g., COP). In NSIP, the interstitial chronic inflammation is diffuse, whereas it is limited to areas of fibroblast proliferation in COP.

Histologic differential diagnoses of the fibrosing NSIP pattern include UIP and organizing DAD. Separation of fibrosing NSIP and UIP has been discussed earlier. Fibrosing NSIP and organizing DAD are similar in that they are both characterized by uniform interstitial fibrosis. Organizing DAD can be distinguished by the presence of hyaline membranes and the clinical history.

Etiologic differential diagnoses that must be considered in patients with NSIP include hypersensitivity pneumonia, connective tissue diseases, drug toxicity, infection, and immunodeficiency. Poorly formed granulomas associated with the NSIP pattern should raise the level of concern to exclude these possibilities.

NONSPECIFIC INTERSTITIAL PNEUMONIA—FACT SHEET

Definition

▸ NSIP is an idiopathic interstitial pneumonia characterized by temporally uniform interstitial chronic inflammation and/or fibrosis

Incidence

▸ Less frequent than idiopathic pulmonary fibrosis, but more common than other idiopathic interstitial pneumonias

Gender and Age Distribution

▸ No gender predominance
▸ Median age of patients is between 40 and 50 years at onset

Clinical Features

▸ Breathlessness, cough, fatigue, and weight loss are common
▸ Abnormal pulmonary function studies that include evidence of restriction and impaired gas exchange

Radiologic Features

▸ On HRCT, ground-glass attenuation is the predominant finding in the majority of cases

Prognosis and Therapy

▸ The prognosis of NSIP is more variable than that of idiopathic pulmonary fibrosis
▸ Corticosteroids produce improvement or recovery in up to 75% of patients
▸ 5 year survival with cellular NSIP is 100%
▸ With fibrosing NSIP, 5- and 10-year survival rates are 90% and 35%, respectively

NONSPECIFIC INTERSTITIAL PNEUMONIA PATTERN—PATHOLOGIC FEATURES

Microscopic Findings
Cellular Pattern

▸ Mild to moderate interstitial chronic inflammation

Fibrosing Pattern

▸ Temporally homogeneous interstitial fibrosis
▸ Chronic inflammation may or may not be present

Pathologic Differential Diagnosis
Cellular Pattern

▸ Lymphoid interstitial pneumonia pattern
▸ Organizing pneumonia

Fibrosing Pattern

▸ Usual interstitial pneumonia
▸ Diffuse alveolar damage, organizing phase

Etiologic Differential Diagnosis (Clinical Conditions Associated with NSIP Pattern)

▸ Idiopathic NSIP
▸ Hypersensitivity pneumonia
▸ Connective tissue diseases
▸ Drug toxicity
▸ Infection
▸ Immunodeficiency

PROGNOSIS AND THERAPY

NSIP is treated with corticosteroids, which results in improvement or recovery in up to 75 percent of the patients. The prognosis of cellular NSIP is better than that of fibrosing NSIP. On the other hand, fibrosing NSIP has better prognosis than UIP. Several authors have reported that the 5-year survival rate for patients with cellular NSIP approaches 100%. The 5- and 10-year survival rates for patients with fibrosing NSIP are 90% and 35%, respectively.

CRYPTOGENIC ORGANIZING PNEUMONIA

As a histopathologic pattern, OP (formerly known as bronchiolitis obliterans organizing pneumonia or BOOP) is characterized by the presence of air-space-filling fibroblastic plugs. OP can be the main lesion in the lung and the cause of the patient's respiratory illness. However, it can also be seen as a minor component of other diseases (e.g., NSIP, hypersensitivity pneumonia, eosinophilic pneumo-

nia, Wegener's granulomatosis), and as a nonspecific reaction around other lesions (e.g., abscess, neoplasm). If OP is the main lesion, the pathologist and the clinician must search to exclude a specific cause such as infection, drug reaction, connective tissue disease, or bronchial obstruction. If a specific etiology is not found, the patient is diagnosed with cryptogenic organizing pneumonia (COP) (formerly known as idiopathic BOOP).

The histologic pattern of OP can be recognized not only in a surgical lung biopsy but also in a transbronchial biopsy. However, one must be especially careful to exclude other possibilities before making a diagnosis of COP in such a small specimen. If the clinical follow-up does not show the typical prompt response to corticosteroid therapy, a surgical lung biopsy may be indicated.

CLINICAL FEATURES

COP usually presents in the fifth or sixth decade of life. The clinical presentation is acute or subacute and mimics that of a community-acquired pneumonia. Shortness of breath and nonproductive cough are the most common symptoms, but fever, malaise, and fatigue may also be present. Examination of the chest often reveals inspiratory crackles. PFTs confirm a restrictive defect. Hypoxemia is almost always found.

RADIOLOGIC FEATURES

CHEST RADIOGRAPHY

The most common chest radiographic manifestation of COP is patchy air space consolidation.

HIGH-RESOLUTION COMPUTED TOMOGRAPHY

The characteristic HRCT finding is bilateral areas of consolidation, which often show peribronchial or subpleural distribution.

PATHOLOGIC FEATURES

GROSS FINDINGS

Grossly, the lungs show scattered, ill-defined nodules.

MICROSCOPIC FINDINGS

At low-power microscopy, bronchiolocentric and peripheral areas of organization are seen with surrounding, relatively normal lung (Figure 16-7). The organizing fibrosis is composed of anastomosing intraluminal plugs

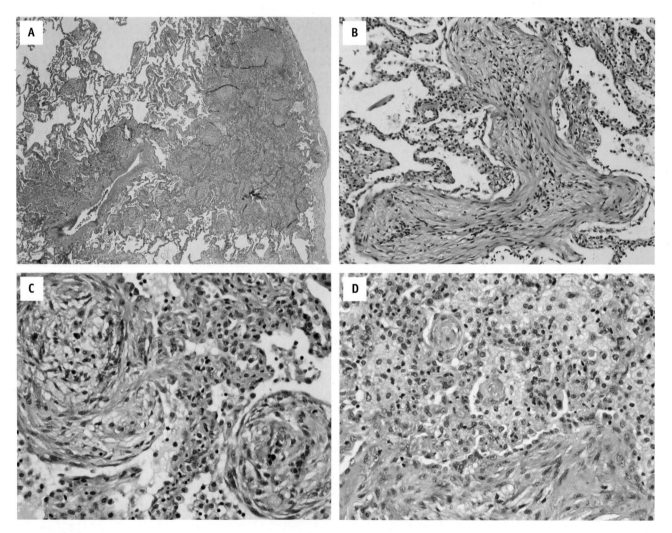

FIGURE 16-7

Organizing pneumonia
(A) At low power, the lung shows bronchiolocentric and peripheral areas of involvement. **(B)** Medium power reveals anastomosing, intraluminal plugs of loose connective tissue (fibroblastic plugs), and associated mild alveolar septal thickening. **(C)** At high power, the fibroblastic plugs may contain small collections of chronic inflammatory cells. **(D)** Lipid-laden macrophages may accumulate distal to obstructed small airways (endogenous lipid pneumonia).

of loose connective tissue (fibroblastic plugs) and involves bronchioles and peribronchiolar air spaces. The bronchiolar involvement may be absent. Within the fibroblastic plugs, there may be small collections of lymphocytes, plasma cells, and histiocytes. The architecture of the lung is well preserved, but mild interstitial chronic inflammation is present in areas of organization. Endogenous lipid pneumonia (postobstructive pneumonia) characterized by foamy, lipid-laden macrophage accumulation may develop distal to obstructed bronchioles.

DIFFERENTIAL DIAGNOSIS

OP should be differentiated from organizing DAD and constrictive bronchiolitis obliterans. Organizing DAD may show focal intraluminal fibrosis and resemble OP. The distinguishing features of organizing DAD include diffuse rather than patchy distribution, predominantly interstitial rather than purely intraluminal fibrosis, and, most importantly, hyaline membranes. OP differs from constrictive bronchiolitis obliterans. Constrictive bronchiolitis obliterans or obliterative bronchiolitis involves bronchioles and is characterized by subepithelial dense fibrosis. On the other hand, OP involves not only the bronchioles but also the surrounding alveoli and is composed of intraluminal loose connective tissue.

It is important that the pathologist searches for histologic clues to exclude the possibility that the OP is related to another lung disease, such as NSIP, hypersensitivity pneumonia, eosinophilic pneumonia, Wegener's granulomatosis, an abscess, or a neoplasm.

PROGNOSIS AND THERAPY

Approximately two-thirds of patients respond to corticosteroid therapy. Although relapses may occur, they usually respond to further corticosteroid treatment. Approximately one-third of the patients have persistent disease. For these cases, cytotoxic drugs (cyclophosphamide or azathioprine) have been used with limited success. The overall prognosis of COP is much better than that of other idiopathic interstitial pneumonias.

ACUTE INTERSTITIAL PNEUMONIA

AIP is a clinicopathologic term describing the idiopathic form of acute respiratory distress syndrome (ARDS). Historically, AIP has also been called Hamman-Rich syndrome. Lung biopsies from patients with AIP show the histologic pattern of DAD. Most diagnostic lung biopsies are performed during the organizing rather than the acute phase.

CRYPTOGENIC ORGANIZING PNEUMONIA—FACT SHEET

Definitions
→ Organizing pneumonia is a histologic pattern characterized by air-space-filling fibroblast plugs
→ COP is a clinicopathologic entity of unknown etiology with the underlying histopathological pattern of organizing pneumonia

Gender and Age Distribution
→ Equal gender distribution
→ Mean age of patients at onset is 55 years

Clinical Features
→ Patients typically present with variable degrees of cough, dyspnea, and fever of relatively short duration (usually less than 3 months)
→ Some patients give a history of an antecedent respiratory tract infection
→ Localized or widespread crackles are frequent
→ Pulmonary function tests confirm a restrictive ventilatory pattern

Radiologic Features
→ On HRCT, patchy consolidation is present in 90% of patients

Prognosis and Therapy
→ The majority of patients recover completely with administration of oral corticosteroids

---

ORGANIZING PNEUMONIA—PATHOLOGIC FEATURES

Microscopic Findings
→ Intraluminal fibroblast plugs in distal air spaces (bronchioles, alveolar ducts, and alveoli)
→ Patchy distribution
→ Uniform temporal appearance
→ Preservation of lung architecture
→ Mild interstitial chronic inflammation (confined to the area of air space fibrosis)

Pathologic Differential Diagnosis
→ Diffuse alveolar damage, organizing phase
→ Constrictive bronchiolitis obliterans

Etiologic Differential Diagnosis (Clinical Conditions Associated with Organizing Pneumonia)
→ Cryptogenic organizing pneumonia
→ Organizing infection
→ Drug reaction
→ Connective tissue diseases
→ Organization distal to bronchial obstruction
→ Minor component of other diseases (nonspecific interstitial pneumonia, hypersensitivity pneumonia, eosinophilic pneumonia, Wegener's granulomatosis)
→ Nonspecific reaction around other lesions (abscess, neoplasm)

AIP is a diagnosis of exclusion; clinical information and laboratory results are necessary to rule out known causes of DAD/ARDS. If these data are not available at the time of the biopsy, a diagnosis of "DAD, etiology undetermined" can be rendered.

CLINICAL FEATURES

Clinical features of AIP are those of ARDS. Patients typically present with a prodromal illness reminiscent of an upper respiratory tract viral infection, which is followed by acute respiratory tract failure. Cough, dyspnea, and fever are often present. Tachypnea is common, and crackles are heard on chest examination in half of the patients. PFTs reveal a restrictive pattern with reduced DLCO. Hypoxemia develops early.

RADIOLOGIC FEATURES

CHEST RADIOGRAPHY

The main radiographic finding is rapidly progressive, bilateral air space consolidation.

HIGH-RESOLUTION COMPUTED TOMOGRAPHY

HRCT shows bilateral ground-glass attenuation and areas of consolidation with air bronchograms.

PATHOLOGIC FEATURES

Lung biopsies from patients with AIP show histologic features of DAD (Figure 16-8). In the acute phase, hyaline membranes, edema, and mild interstitial acute inflammation are seen. The organizing phase is characterized by loose organizing fibrosis, which is present primarily in the alveolar septa. Remnants of hyaline membranes are usually present.

DIFFERENTIAL DIAGNOSIS

Histologically, organizing DAD is most likely to be confused with UIP, fibrosing NSIP, or OP. However, DAD is usually readily apparent in the biopsy due to the presence of hyaline membranes. Separating AIP from known causes of DAD requires clinical correlation.

PROGNOSIS AND THERAPY

There is no effective treatment for patients with AIP. Corticosteroids are commonly used, but have little impact on patient survival. Virtually all patients require mechanical ventilation, and mortality rates are high. Patients who survive the initial illness generally have a favorable outcome.

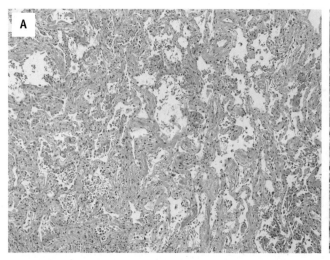 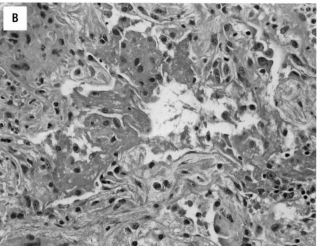

FIGURE 16-8

Acute interstitial pneumonia
Biopsies of AIP show diffuse alveolar damage (DAD), typically in the organizing phase. **(A)** At low power, organizing DAD is characterized by uniform alveolar septal thickening. **(B)** At high power, the alveolar septal thickening is due to organizing fibrosis and remnants of hyaline membranes.

ACUTE INTERSTITIAL PNEUMONIA—FACT SHEET

Definition

▸ AIP is a distinct, rapidly progressive form of idiopathic interstitial pneumonia, showing histologic characteristics of diffuse alveolar damage

▸ The term AIP is synonymous with idiopathic diffuse alveolar damage

▸ Some of the cases described by Hamman and Rich probably represented AIP

Gender and Age Distribution

▸ No gender predominance

▸ Wide age range, with a mean age of approximately 50 years

Clinical Features

▸ Patients often present with signs and symptoms suggestive of an upper respiratory tract viral infection, followed by acute respiratory failure

▸ Pulmonary function tests show a restrictive pattern

Radiologic Features

▸ The most common findings on HRCT include areas of ground-glass attenuation, bronchial dilatation, and architectural distortion

Prognosis and Therapy

▸ No proven treatment

▸ Median length of survival from the onset of illness is between 1 and 2 months

▸ Mortality rates are high (50% or more)

ACUTE INTERSTITIAL PNEUMONIA—PATHOLOGIC FEATURES

Microscopic Findings

▸ Diffuse alveolar damage (typically organizing)

Pathologic Differential Diagnosis

▸ Usual interstitial pneumonia

▸ Nonspecific interstitial pneumonia

▸ Organizing pneumonia

Etiologic Differential Diagnosis (Clinical Conditions Associated with DAD)

▸ See Chapter 9

RESPIRATORY BRONCHIOLITIS-ASSOCIATED INTERSTITIAL LUNG DISEASE (RB-ILD)

RB is a histologic pattern characterized by accumulation of pigmented macrophages within respiratory bronchioles and adjacent air spaces. It is a common, incidental lung biopsy finding in cigarette smokers. Rarely, RB is the sole histologic finding in patients who have clinical evidence of interstitial lung disease. In this situation, the clinicopathologic diagnosis of RB-ILD is applied.

CLINICAL FEATURES

RB-ILD usually affects smokers in the fourth and fifth decades of life. Rare cases are related to environmental dust rather than smoke exposure. There is no gender predilection. Presenting symptoms include cough and dyspnea. Fine, bibasilar end-inspiratory crepitations are commonly observed on chest examination. PFTs may be normal or reveal a mixed obstructive-restrictive pattern with slightly reduced DLCO. Mild hypoxemia is often present.

RADIOLOGIC FEATURES

CHEST RADIOGRAPHY

Radiographic abnormalities usually consist of ground-glass opacities and bronchial wall thickening.

HIGH-RESOLUTION COMPUTED TOMOGRAPHY

HRCT findings include bilateral ground-glass attenuation and centrilobular nodular opacities.

PATHOLOGIC FEATURES

Histologically, RB is characterized by bronchiolocentric alveolar macrophage accumulation (Figure 16-9). The macrophages are found mainly within respiratory bronchioles and alveolar ducts, although they may also extend into peribronchiolar alveoli. Large areas of intervening lung parenchyma are normal. The macrophages possess abundant cytoplasm and contain finely granular, golden-brown pigment (smoker's pigment), which stains weakly with Prussian blue. The bronchiolar walls

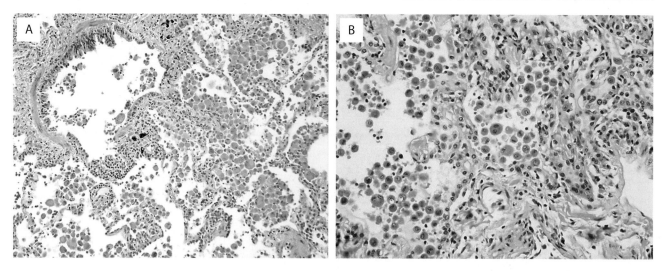

FIGURE 16-9

Respiratory bronchiolitis

(A) At low power, bronchiolocentric alveolar macrophage accumulation is observed. **(B)** At high power, the macrophages contain finely granular, golden-brown pigment (smoker's pigment).

may show mild chronic inflammation and fibrosis. Mild interstitial thickening often accompanies the macrophage accumulation, but is localized to the peribronchiolar parenchyma.

DIFFERENTIAL DIAGNOSIS

The main differential diagnosis for RB is DIP. Both DIP and RB are characterized by accumulation of finely pigmented alveolar macrophages. However, the alveolar macrophage accumulation is diffuse in DIP, whereas it is limited to the peribronchiolar parenchyma in RB.

PROGNOSIS AND THERAPY

The prognosis of RB-ILD is generally favorable. The process may be clinically stable or may improve gradually, especially with cessation of smoking. Corticosteroid therapy appears to be unnecessary in most cases. On the other hand, some patients deteriorate despite therapy.

DESQUAMATIVE INTERSTITIAL PNEUMONIA

Desquamative interstitial pneumonia (DIP) is a histologic pattern as well as a clinicopathologic entity. DIP as a histologic pattern shows considerable similarities to RB. However, the DIP pattern is a diffuse form of pigmented alveolar macrophage accumulation, whereas the

macrophages are limited to the peribronchiolar parenchyma in RB. The similarities in their histologic background and their common epidemiologic link to cigarette smoking suggest that DIP and RB-ILD represent different points along the spectrum of smoking-related interstitial lung disease.

CLINICAL FEATURES

Most patients with DIP present in the fourth and fifth decades of life; nearly 90% of them are cigarette smokers. Rare cases have been reported in children. DIP is more common in men, with a male-to-female ratio of 2:1. The most common symptoms include dyspnea and cough. Auscultation of the chest reveals crackles. PFTs confirm a restrictive pattern with reduced DLCO. Hypoxemia is common.

RADIOLOGIC FEATURES

CHEST RADIOGRAPHY

The most common chest radiographic finding is widespread ground-glass opacification.

HIGH-RESOLUTION COMPUTED TOMOGRAPHY

Ground-glass opacities can be found on HRCT in all cases of DIP. In a minority of cases, the ground-glass opacities progress to a reticular pattern, which represents fibrosis.

RESPIRATORY BRONCHIOLITIS-ASSOCIATED INTERSTITIAL LUNG DISEASE—FACT SHEET

Definition

» Respiratory bronchiolitis (RB) is a histologic term, describing pigmented macrophage accumulation in respiratory bronchioles and adjacent airspaces
» RB is a common incidental finding in lung biopsies from smokers
» Rarely, RB is the single histologic abnormality in a lung biopsy from a patient with the clinical presentation of an interstitial lung disease; in such cases, the clinicopathologic term of RB-ILD is applied

Gender and Age Distribution

» No gender predilection
» Usually affects current smokers in the fourth and fifth decades of life

Clinical Features

» There is an invariable relationship to smoking
» Nearly all patients present with mild, nonspecific respiratory complaints including cough and gradual onset of dyspnea
» The most common pulmonary function abnormality is a reduced diffusing capacity of the lung for carbon monoxide

Radiologic Features

» HRCT reveals bilateral ground-glass opacities

Prognosis

» The clinical course is characterized by relative stability in the majority of patients, especially with cessation of smoking

RESPIRATORY BRONCHIOLITIS—PATHOLOGIC FEATURES

Microscopic Findings

» Bronchiolar and peribronchiolar accumulation of pigmented alveolar macrophages
» The macrophages contain finely granular, golden-brown pigment (smoker's pigment)
» Bronchiolar walls may show mild chronic inflammation and fibrosis

Pathologic Differential Diagnosis

» Desquamative interstitial pneumonia

PATHOLOGIC FEATURES

The histologic hallmark of DIP is marked diffuse alveolar macrophage accumulation (Figure 16-10). This is accompanied by mild interstitial chronic inflammation, and typically little fibrosis. The alveolar macrophages contain smoker's pigment. As in any type of alveolar macrophage accumulation, a small number of multinucleated macrophages can be seen, but these are not a prominent finding. Intra-alveolar laminated concretions (blue bodies) may also be present.

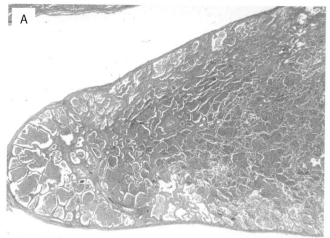

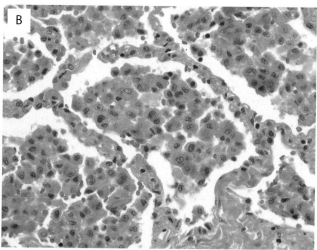

FIGURE 16-10

Desquamative interstitial pneumonia pattern
(A) At low power, the hallmark of DIP pattern is diffuse alveolar macrophage accumulation. **(B)** At high power, the macrophages contain smoker's pigment. Note the mild alveolar septal thickening.

DESQUAMATIVE INTERSTITIAL PNEUMONIA—FACT SHEET

Definition

▸ DIP is a clinicopathologic entity characterized by diffuse intra-alveolar macrophage accumulation

▸ RB-ILD and DIP represent different points along a spectrum of smoking-related interstitial lung disease

Gender and Age Distribution

▸ DIP is more common in men than in women by a ratio of 2:1

▸ It affects cigarette smokers primarily in their fourth or fifth decades of life

Clinical Features

▸ The most common pulmonary function abnormality is a reduced diffusing capacity of the lung for carbon monoxide

Radiologic Features

▸ HRCT reveals ground-glass opacities bilaterally in most patients

Prognosis and Therapy

▸ The clinical course is characterized by relative stability in the majority of patients and a partial response to corticosteroid therapy

▸ The overall survival is about 70% after 10 years

DESQUAMATIVE INTERSTITIAL PNEUMONIA PATTERN—PATHOLOGIC FEATURES

Microscopic Findings

▸ Diffuse accumulation of pigmented alveolar macrophages

▸ The macrophages contain smoker's pigment

▸ The alveolar septa may show mild chronic inflammation and mild to moderate fibrous thickening

Pathologic Differential Diagnosis

▸ Respiratory bronchiolitis

▸ DIP-like reaction

▸ Giant cell interstitial pneumonia

▸ Eosinophilic pneumonia

▸ Hemosiderosis

DIFFERENTIAL DIAGNOSIS

The histologic differential diagnoses for the DIP pattern include RB, DIP-like reaction, giant cell interstitial pneumonia, eosinophilic pneumonia, and hemosiderosis. As has been mentioned earlier, DIP pattern differs from RB by the extent of alveolar macrophage accumulation. It is diffuse in DIP, whereas it is limited to the peribronchiolar parenchyma in RB. Focal pigmented alveolar macrophage accumulation, also known as DIP-like reaction, has been described adjacent to a wide variety of lung lesions, the best known example of which is Langerhans cell histiocytosis. However, it is now believed that DIP-like reaction is related to smoking and actually represents RB. Giant cell interstitial pneumonia, which is the histologic manifestation of hard metal pneumoconiosis, may also be reminiscent of DIP. However, in giant cell interstitial pneumonia, there are numerous multinucleated giant cells, which are both histiocytic and epithelial in origin. In DIP, a few multinucleated alveolar macrophages are present, but they are usually inconspicuous. The predominant histologic feature in eosinophilic pneumonia is the filling of alveolar spaces by eosinophils admixed with variable numbers of macrophages. When macrophages are abundant and eosinophils are depleted due to previous corticosteroid therapy, eosinophilic pneumonia may resemble DIP. In such cases, the presence of focal residual eosino-

philia may be a histologic clue. Hemosiderosis, similar to DIP pattern, is characterized by pigmented alveolar macrophage accumulation. However, hemosiderin is a coarsely granular pigment, whereas smoker's pigment in DIP is finely dispersed, or "dusty."

PROGNOSIS AND THERAPY

The prognosis of DIP is generally good. Most patients improve with smoking cessation and corticosteroid therapy. The overall survival is about 70% after 10 years.

LYMPHOID INTERSTITIAL PNEUMONIA (LIP)

LIP is both a histologic pattern and a clinicopathologic syndrome. As a histologic pattern, LIP is characterized by diffuse infiltration of the alveolar septa by a dense lymphoplasmacytic infiltrate. The majority of patients with the corresponding clinicopathologic syndrome have an underlying condition. LIP is common in human immunodeficiency virus (HIV)-infected children; it is one of the two most common acquired immune deficiency syndrome (AIDS)-defining conditions in the pediatric population. It has also been reported in association with rheumatoid arthritis, Sjögren's syndrome, Hashimoto thyroiditis, pernicious anemia, chronic active hepatitis, systemic lupus erythematosus, autoimmune hemolytic anemia, primary biliary cirrhosis, myasthenia gravis, and hypogammaglobulinemia. LIP rarely presents as an idiopathic process.

CLINICAL FEATURES

The clinical presentation of LIP is typically that of the underlying disease. The rare idiopathic form has a female predilection and is usually diagnosed in the fifth decade. Patients often present with cough and dyspnea; physical examination reveals bibasilar crackles. Dysproteinemia (hyper- or hypogammaglobulinemia) is found in more than half of the cases. PFTs reveal reduced lung volumes and lowered DLCO. Hypoxemia is common.

RADIOLOGIC FEATURES

CHEST RADIOGRAPHY

Two chest radiographic patterns have been described: basilar with an alveolar component, and diffuse with associated honeycombing.

HIGH-RESOLUTION COMPUTED TOMOGRAPHY

The dominant HRCT finding is ground-glass opacity. A reticular pattern is seen in more than a third of patients.

PATHOLOGIC FEATURES

GROSS FINDINGS

Grossly, the lung is pink-tan or tan-gray and diffusely firm to palpation.

MICROSCOPIC FINDINGS

Histologically, LIP is characterized by a marked diffuse interstitial infiltrate of small lymphocytes and plasma cells (Figure 16-11). The infiltrate may be more prominent along the pleura, interlobular septa, and bronchovascular bundles. Lymphoid follicles and vaguely formed granulomas may be observed. In late stages, fibrosis may accompany the interstitial infiltrate.

ANCILLARY STUDIES

Immunohistochemical studies uncover a mixture of B and T cells, with B cells found in primary follicles and germinal centers and T cells present in the intervening areas. The plasma cells show polyclonal staining for immunoglobulin light chains. Molecular studies reveal a

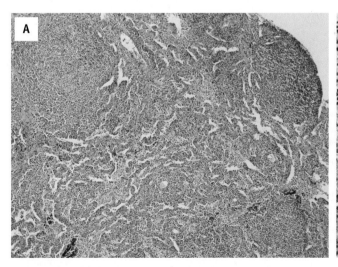
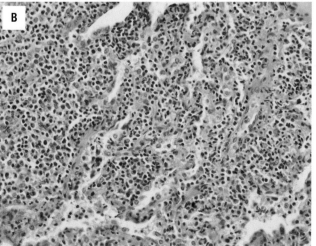

FIGURE 16-11

Lymphoid interstitial pneumonia pattern
(A) At low power, LIP pattern is characterized by a marked interstitial lymphoid infiltrate. Note the presence of lymphoid nodules. **(B)** At high power, reactive lymphocytes and a variable number of plasma cells are seen.

germ line configuration of the immunoglobulin heavy and light chain genes, and there are no clonal cytogenetic abnormalities.

DIFFERENTIAL DIAGNOSIS

LIP is considered to be part of a spectrum of pulmonary lymphoid proliferations that include follicular bronchitis/bronchiolitis, nodular lymphoid hyperplasia (pseudolymphoma), and extranodal marginal zone B-cell lymphoma of mucosa-associated lymphoid tissue (Chapter 22). When lymphoid nodules are centered on bronchovascular bundles, the disease is termed "follicular bronchitis/bronchiolitis" (or "pulmonary lymphoid hyperplasia" in the pediatric AIDS literature). In LIP, the lymphoid infiltrate extensively involves the pulmonary interstitium. Nodular lymphoid hyperplasia is a mass-like lesion, consisting of a population of reactive lymphoid cells with a variable number of plasma cells. Extranodal marginal zone B-cell lymphoma of mucosa-associated lymphoid tissue shows a central mass comprised predominantly of small lymphocytes, with peripheral tracking along lymphatic pathways. Bronchial infiltration is often associated with lymphoepithelial lesions. The neoplastic cells have the immunophenotypic features of marginal zone B-cells. Light chain restriction may be demonstrated when there is a significant plasmacytic component. Appropriate molecular studies show clonality of the immunoglobulin heavy and/or light chain genes.

PROGNOSIS AND THERAPY

Corticosteroids are the most widely used treatment and are thought to arrest or improve symptoms in a large proportion of patients. Unfortunately, more than a third of patients progress to diffuse fibrosis.

LYMPHOID INTERSTITIAL PNEUMONIA—FACT SHEET

Definition
- ‣ LIP is a clinicopathologic term used to describe benign disorders that are characterized by a prominent interstitial lymphoid infiltrate

Gender and Age Distribution
- ‣ LIP can occur in both children and adults
- ‣ Most adult patients are women in the fourth through seventh decades of life

Clinical Features
- ‣ Patients often present with cough, dyspnea, and bibasilar crackles
- ‣ Pulmonary function tests reveal reduced lung volumes, and reduced diffusing capacity of the lung for carbon monoxide

Radiologic Features
- ‣ The dominant finding is usually ground-glass opacities

Prognosis and Therapy
- ‣ Corticosteroids are the most widely used treatment
- ‣ More than a third of patients develop fibrosis

LYMPHOID INTERSTITIAL PNEUMONIA PATTERN—PATHOLOGIC FEATURES

Microscopic Findings
- ‣ Prominent diffuse interstitial infiltrate composed of polymorphic lymphocytes and plasma cells
- ‣ Lymphoid follicles are present focally

Pathologic Differential Diagnosis
- ‣ Follicular bronchiolitis
- ‣ Nodular lymphoid hyperplasia
- ‣ Extranodal marginal zone B-cell lymphoma of mucosa-associated lymphoid tissue
- ‣ Nonspecific interstitial pneumonia

Etiologic Differential Diagnosis (Clinical Conditions Associated with LIP Pattern)
- ‣ Idiopathic LIP
- ‣ Infection
- ‣ Connective tissue diseases, especially Sjögren's syndrome
- ‣ Immunodeficiency (HIV)

SUGGESTED READINGS

General

1. Travis WD, King TE, Bateman ED, et al. American Thoracic Society/ European Respiratory Society international multidisciplinary consensus classification of the idiopathic interstitial pneumonias. *Am J Respir Crit Care Med.* 2002;165:277-304.
2. Fukuoka J, Leslie KO. Chronic diffuse lung diseases. In: Leslie KO, Wick MR, eds. *Practical Pulmonary Pathology: A Diagnostic Approach.* Philadelphia, Pa: Churchill Livingstone; 2005:181-258.
3. Nicholson AG. Classification of idiopathic interstitial pneumonias: making sense of the alphabet soup. *Histopathology.* 2002;41:381-91.
4. Travis WD, Colby TC, Koss MN, Rosado-de-Christenson ML, Müller NL, King TEJ. *Non-Neoplastic Disorders of the Lower Respiratory Tract.* Washington, DC: The American Registry of Pathology; 2002, 1st ed.

Idiopathic Pulmonary Fibrosis/Usual Interstitial Pneumonia

5. Flaherty KR, Toews GB, Travis WD, et al. Clinical significance of histological classification of idiopathic interstitial pneumonia. *Eur Respir J.* 2002;19:275-83.
6. Katzenstein AL, Zisman DA, Litzky LA, Nguyen BT, Kotloff RM: Usual interstitial pneumonia: histologic study of biopsy and explant specimens. *Am J Surg Pathol.* 2002;26:1567-77.
7. Monaghan H, Wells AU, Colby TV, du Bois RM, Hansell DM, Nicholson AG. Prognostic implications of histologic patterns in multiple surgical lung biopsies from patients with idiopathic interstitial pneumonias. *Chest.* 2004;125:522-6.
8. Myers JL, Selman M. Respiratory epithelium in usual interstitial pneumonia/idiopathic pulmonary fibrosis: spark or destructive flame? *Am J Respir Crit Care Med.* 2004;169:3-5.
9. Nicholson AG, Fulford LG, Colby TV, du Bois RM, Hansell DM, Wells AU. The relationship between individual histologic features and disease progression in idiopathic pulmonary fibrosis. *Am J Respir Crit Care Med.* 2002;166:173-7.
10. Rice AJ, Wells AU, Bouros D, et al. Terminal diffuse alveolar damage in relation to interstitial pneumonias: an autopsy study. *Am J Clin Pathol.* 2003;119:709-14.
11. Wittram C. The idiopathic interstitial pneumonias. *Curr Probl Diagn Radiol.* 2004;33:189-99.

Nonspecific Interstitial Pneumonia

12. Jegal Y, Kim DS, Shim TS, et al. Physiology is a stronger predictor of survival than pathology in fibrotic interstitial pneumonia. *Am J Respir Crit Care Med.* 2005;171:639-44.
13. Katzenstein AL, Fiorelli RF. Nonspecific interstitial pneumonia/fibrosis: histologic features and clinical significance. *Am J Surg Pathol.* 1994;18:136-47.
14. Nicholson AG, Wells AU. Nonspecific interstitial pneumonia: nobody said it's perfect. *Am J Respir Crit Care Med.* 2001;164:1553-4.
15. Travis WD, Matsui K, Moss J, Ferrans VJ. Idiopathic nonspecific interstitial pneumonia: prognostic significance of cellular and fibrosing patterns: survival comparison with usual interstitial pneumonia and desquamative interstitial pneumonia. *Am J Surg Pathol.* 2000;24:19-33.

Cryptogenic Organizing Pneumonia

16. Cordier JF. Cryptogenic organizing pneumonia. *Clin Chest Med.* 2004;25:727-38.
17. Myers JL, Colby TV. Pathologic manifestations of bronchiolitis, constrictive bronchiolitis, cryptogenic organizing pneumonia, and diffuse panbronchiolitis. *Clin Chest Med.* 1993;14:611-22.
18. Nagai S, Izumi T. Bronchiolitis obliterans with organizing pneumonia. *Curr Opin Pulm Med* 1996;2:419-23.
19. Yousem SA, Lohr RH, Colby TV. Idiopathic bronchiolitis obliterans organizing pneumonia/cryptogenic organizing pneumonia with unfavorable outcome: pathologic predictors. *Mod Pathol.* 1997;10:864-71.

Acute Interstitial Pneumonia

20. Bouros D, Nicholson AC, Polychronopoulos V, du Bois RM. Acute interstitial pneumonia. *Eur Respir J.* 2000;15:412-8.
21. Vourlekis JS: Acute interstitial pneumonia. *Clin Chest Med.* 2004;25:739-47.

Respiratory Bronchiolitis Associated Interstitial Lung Disease and Desquamative Interstitial Pneumonia

22. Aubry MC, Wright JL, Myers JL. The pathology of smoking-related lung diseases. *Clin Chest Med.* 2000;21:11-35.
23. Craig PJ, Wells AU, Doffman S, et al. Desquamative interstitial pneumonia, respiratory bronchiolitis, and their relationship to smoking. *Histopathology.* 2004;45:275-82.
24. Desai SR, Ryan SM, Colby TV. Smoking-related interstitial lung diseases: histopathological and imaging perspectives. *Clin Radiol.* 2003;58:259-68.
25. Myers JL, Veal CF Jr, Shin MS, Katzenstein AL. Respiratory bronchiolitis causing interstitial lung disease: a clinicopathologic study of six cases. *Am Rev Respir Dis.* 1987;135:880-4.
26. Ryu JH, Colby TV, Hartman TE, Vassallo R. Smoking-related interstitial lung diseases: a concise review. *Eur Respir J.* 2001;17:122-32.
27. Ryu JH, Myers JL, Capizzi SA, Douglas WW, Vassallo R, Decker PA. Desquamative interstitial pneumonia and respiratory bronchiolitis-associated interstitial lung disease. *Chest.* 2005;127:178-84.
28. Vassallo R, Jensen EA, Colby TV, et al. The overlap between respiratory bronchiolitis and desquamative interstitial pneumonia in pulmonary Langerhans cell histiocytosis: high-resolution CT, histologic, and functional correlations. *Chest.* 2003;124:1199-205.

Lymphoid Interstitial Pneumonia

29. Fishback N, Koss M. Update on lymphoid interstitial pneumonitis. *Curr Opin Pulm Med.* 1996;2:429-33.
30. Kurtin PJ, Myers JL, Adlakha H, et al. Pathologic and clinical features of primary pulmonary extranodal marginal zone B-cell lymphoma of MALT type. *Am J Surg Pathol.* 2001;25:997-1008.
31. Swigris JJ, Berry GJ, Raffin TA, Kuschner WG. Lymphoid interstitial pneumonia: a narrative review. *Chest.* 2002;122:2150-64.
32. Travis WD, Galvin JR. Non-neoplastic pulmonary lymphoid lesions. *Thorax.* 2001;56:964-71.

17 Other Interstitial Lung Diseases

Roberto J. Barrios

- Hypersensitivity Pneumonitis
- Sarcoidosis
- Lymphangioleiomyomatosis
- Pulmonary Alveolar Proteinosis
- Acute Eosinophilic Pneumonia
- Chronic Eosinophilic Pneumonia

HYPERSENSITIVITY PNEUMONITIS

Hypersensitivity pneumonitis (HP) is also known as extrinsic allergic alveolitis. It can be defined as a diffuse interstitial granulomatous pneumonitis triggered by exposure to inhaled antigens (mold, bacteria, animal proteins, insect proteins) or other sometimes unknown allergen particles of small size (5 µm or smaller) in susceptible individuals. Although the list of antigens that could potentially serve as stimuli for this reaction is limitless, the individual must be immunologically reactive to the agent for the disease to develop, and exposure to the agent is necessary. The disease may be known by a great variety of names depending on the causal agent (farmer's lung, pigeon breeder's disease, ventilation pneumonitis, etc.), but the clinical presentations and pathologic findings are similar, regardless of the identity of the responsible antigen. A combination of types III and IV hypersensitivity reactions is believed to account for the pathogenesis of this condition.

CLINICAL FEATURES

Patients with HP can present with an acute, subacute, or chronic clinical picture. A patient with acute HP may report a history of abrupt onset (4 to 6 hours after exposure) of a flu-like syndrome with fever, malaise, chills, diaphoresis, headache, nonproductive cough, and dys-

pnea. There is peripheral blood leukocytosis with neutrophilia, but eosinophilia is usually not seen. These symptoms resolve without specific treatment in 1 to 3 days, but can recur with repeated exposures to the triggering agent. The subacute form of the disease is more difficult to define: usually these patients have had a history consistent with HP for several months, with multiple acute exacerbations of the disease. Patients with chronic HP present with progressive dyspnea, cough, weight loss, and anorexia, developing over a period of months or years. Some patients will recognize acute symptoms after exposures to the antigen, while others may notice a more insidious onset of dyspnea.

RADIOLOGIC FEATURES

Plain films of the chest may show parenchymal changes that become better defined on high-resolution computed tomography (HRCT) scan. HRCT during the acute and subacute phases shows bilateral ground-glass opacities and centriacinar nodules. The ground-glass infiltrates can be preferentially located in the centers of the secondary pulmonary lobules with relative sparing of the periphery. If small airway obstruction is present, air trapping can be seen on expiratory HRCT as a mosaic pattern. Patients with chronic disease show a radiological appearance that will depend on the degree of interstitial fibrosis, with a reticular pattern.

PATHOLOGIC FEATURES

GROSS FINDINGS

Only a few cases of acute HP have been described because the disease is usually not fatal during early stages, and the appearance is one of acute diffuse alveolar damage. In the subacute stage, there may be irregular areas of consolidation that tend to be centriacinar in distribution. The chronic stage has been well described and consists of interstitial fibrosis with honeycomb change in areas.

MICROSCOPIC FINDINGS

Lung biopsies are usually obtained from patients with subacute or chronic disease, while acute HP is less often seen in surgical pathology material since the patient may not seek medical attention during this stage, or the diagnosis may be made clinically. The histopathology of acute farmer's lung has been described as that of acute diffuse alveolar damage. The histopathology of the subacute and chronic manifestations of HP is well known: there is a typically bronchiolocentric interstitial pneumonitis (Figure 17-1), with interstitial lymphoplasmacytic infiltrates (Figure 17-2), cellular bronchiolitis, and poorly formed (loose), non-necrotizing granulomas. Isolated giant cells (Figure 17-2) with occasional cholesterol clefts and Schaumann's bodies may be found. As a rule, these granulomas are small and poorly defined. Stains for microorganisms (fungi, acid fast organisms) will usually not reveal these agents. Obliterative bronchiolitis can also be present in occasional examples.

While the triad of interstitial pneumonitis, cellular bronchiolitis, and ill-defined granulomas is seen in 80% of the well documented cases of HP, some cases will demonstrate only one or two of these features, and in these cases, it is particularly important to demonstrate a linkage between exacerbations and exposures to the triggering agent. Occasional areas of organizing pneumonia are commonly seen (Figure 17-3), in combination with the other findings. In some cases, there are collections of foamy macrophages (Figure 17-4)

which may represent small foci of endogenous lipid pneumonia, although it has been suggested that some antigens (such as those seen in pigeon breeder's disease) may be present in some of these foamy cells. If exposure to the inciting antigen is avoided, the granulomatous lesions resolve in 4 to 6 months, but persistent exposure results in progression of the disease to interstitial fibrosis that may resemble a nonspecific interstitial pneumonia (NSIP) or usual interstitial pneumonia (UIP) pattern.

CYTOLOGIC FINDINGS

Bronchoalveolar lavage characteristically shows increased CD8+ T-cells.

ANCILLARY STUDIES

IMMUNOHISTOCHEMISTRY

There is a predominance of CD3+ CD8+ T-cells over CD4+ T-cells and B-cells.

ULTRASTRUCTURAL STUDIES

Although electron microscopy is not necessary to make the diagnosis of hypersensitivity pneumonitis, by electron microscopy it is possible to find intra-alveolar

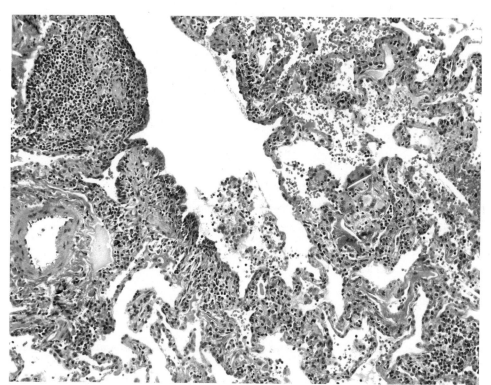

FIGURE 17-1

Hypersensitivity pneumonitis
A respiratory bronchiole shows mild lymphoplasmacytic infiltrates in its wall, with a lymphoid aggregate. Similar chronic inflammatory infiltrates extend into adjacent alveolar septa. A cluster of multinucleated giant cells is present, with a cholesterol cleft in the cytoplasm of one giant cell.

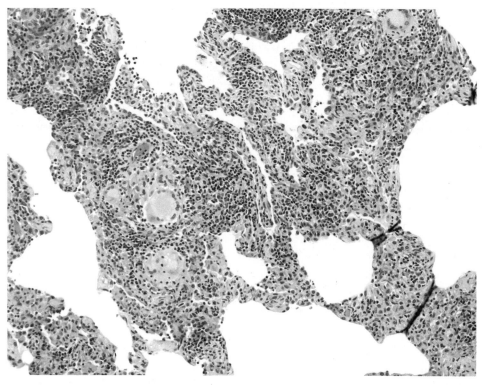

FIGURE 17-2

Hypersensitivity pneumonitis
Dense interstitial lymphoplasmacytic infiltrates with scattered multinucleated giant cells are present.

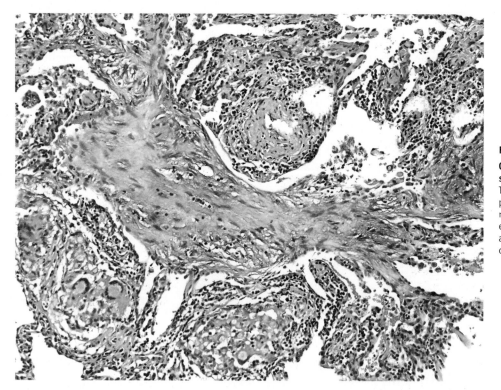

FIGURE 17-3

Organizing pneumonia in hypersensitivity pneumonitis
This alveolar duct is largely filled by a plug of connective tissue. Interstitial regions of adjacent alveolar septa are expanded by lymphocytic infiltrates, and occasional multinucleated giant cells are seen.

clusters of loose connective tissue attached to alveolar walls, which have been called buds. These foci contain a small number of macrophages, fibroblasts, and myofibroblasts, and represent the reparative stage of an exudative process. No immune complexes have been seen in most patients.

DIFFERENTIAL DIAGNOSIS

The differential diagnosis for hypersensitivity pneumonitis includes many diffuse interstitial lung diseases including infections, sarcoidosis, bronchiolitis obliterans,

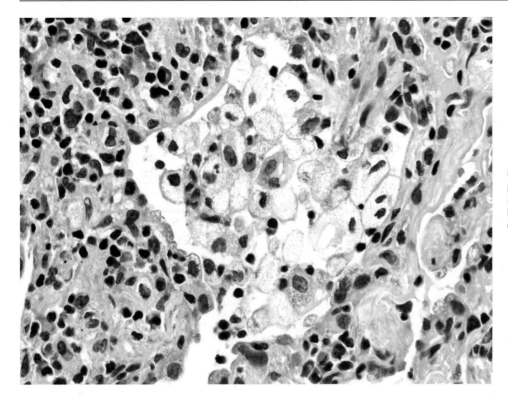

FIGURE 17-4
Hypersensitivity pneumonitis
Foamy macrophages occupy an alveolar space, perhaps representing endogenous lipid pneumonia.

UIP, and NSIP. Infections, particularly due to mycobacterial, fungal, and respiratory viruses, should always be ruled out by cultures, special stains, and clinical correlation. Hot tub lung is caused by a mycobacterial infection (*M. avium* complex) and histologically resembles HP, but cultures demonstrate the organism. Sarcoidosis is usually associated with well formed granulomas that follow the lymphatic routes and the interlobular septa. Bronchiolitis obliterans can be caused by other types of lung injury, as well as HP, and manifests dense subepithelial fibrosis in bronchioles, causing luminal obstruction. Variable degrees of inflammation can accompany the fibrosis, but there is usually little or no interstitial pneumonia, and granulomas are absent in non-HP-associated cases. The cellular pattern of NSIP can be seen in patients with a history of exposure to organic antigens. The pathologist should keep in mind that NSIP is a histologic pattern, and although it can be idiopathic, some well documented cases of HP have been associated with a biopsy diagnosis of NSIP. Drugs such as mesalamine, methotrexate, and others, can also serve as stimuli for reactions that have features of HP, usually NSIP and granulomas. The differential diagnosis should also include lymphoid interstitial pneumonia in cases in which the lymphocytic infiltrate is very prominent. In rare cases, lymphocytic interstitial pneumonia can be a manifestation of HP.

PROGNOSIS AND THERAPY

The long-term prognosis of patients with HP depends on several factors including the type and duration of antigen exposure and the response of the individual to immunologic injury. Acute and subacute cases, in which the offending antigen is identified and avoided and the patient receives adequate treatment, generally show a good prognosis. Corticosteroids are a mainstay of therapy and will produce improvement in most subacute and chronic cases. A subset of patients with chronic HP, however, will have developed significant interstitial fibrosis by the time the diagnosis is made, and these individuals may not respond to corticosteroids and avoidance of the responsible agent.

SARCOIDOSIS

Sarcoidosis is a multisystem granulomatous disease of unknown etiology that is characterized pathologically by the presence of non-necrotizing granulomas. The minimal criteria for a diagnosis of sarcoidosis include consistent clinical features, the histologic finding of non-necrotizing

HYPERSENSITIVITY PNEUMONITIS—FACT SHEET

Definition

▸ Diffuse interstitial granulomatous pneumonitis, caused by exposure to inhaled organic antigens or other particles of small size in susceptible individuals

▸ Large number of syndromes associated with specific triggering agents; major categories of agents include fungi, bacteria, and animal proteins

Incidence and Location

▸ Worldwide distribution

▸ Prevalence varies depending on geographic location and shows a seasonal variation for some syndromes

▸ Exposures are occupational in some cases (e.g., farmer's lung, bagassosis, bird handler's lung)

Morbidity and Mortality

▸ Low mortality

▸ Morbidity depends on chronicity of exposure: prompt antigen withdrawal will produce improvement in most acute and subacute cases, while the prognosis is more variable in chronic cases

Gender, Race, and Age Distribution

▸ There is no predilection for specific gender, racial, or age groups, although HP is infrequent in children

Clinical Features

▸ Acute form presents as a flu-like syndrome 4 to 5 hours after antigen exposure, and is usually self-limited

▸ Subacute and chronic forms present with chronic cough, dyspnea, and malaise for weeks or months (subacute), or months to years (chronic); exacerbations of cough and fever may be noted during exposures to antigens

▸ Diagnosis is made on the basis of clinical history, biopsy, and exclusion of other entities in the differential diagnosis

Radiologic Features

▸ Acute and subacute phases: bilateral ground-glass opacities and centriacinar nodules; the ground-glass infiltrates can be preferentially located in the centers of the secondary pulmonary lobules with relative sparing of the periphery

▸ Chronic disease: variable degrees of interstitial fibrosis with a reticular pattern and/or honeycomb change

Prognosis and Therapy

▸ Acute and subacute forms usually resolve with antigen avoidance, and corticosteroid therapy is also administered to many patients to promote resolution

▸ Chronic cases vary in the degree of interstitial fibrosis, so therapeutic responsiveness to antigen avoidance and corticosteroid therapy is more variable. Many patients, however, will experience improvement with these approaches

HYPERSENSITIVITY PNEUMONITIS—PATHOLOGIC FEATURES

Gross Findings

▸ Acute phase: pattern of diffuse acute alveolar damage

▸ Subacute phase: patchy consolidation with a predominantly centriacinar distribution

▸ Chronic stage: patchy or more diffuse interstitial fibrosis with areas of honeycombing

Microscopic Findings

▸ Triad of interstitial pneumonitis (typically bronchiolocentric), cellular bronchiolitis, and poorly formed granulomas is seen in approximately 80% of patients; other patients may show only one or two of these features

▸ Organizing pneumonia may be present

▸ Alveolar collections of lipid-laden macrophages may be present

▸ Obliterative bronchiolitis may be present

Cytologic Findings

▸ Increased CD8+ T-cells in bronchoalveolar lavage

Immunohistochemical Features

▸ Predominance of CD3+ CD8+ T-cells over CD4+ T-cells and B-cells

Pathologic Differential Diagnosis

▸ Infections

▸ Sarcoidosis

▸ Drug reactions with HP-like features

▸ Nonspecific interstitial pneumonia due to causes other than HP

▸ Usual interstitial pneumonia

▸ Bronchiolitis obliterans

▸ Lymphoid interstitial pneumonia

been conclusively proven to be responsible for the disease. The disease is most likely multifactorial, with a genetic predisposition determined by the varying effects of several genes and the interaction of the susceptible host with environmental agents. There is significant heterogeneity in disease presentation and severity among different ethnic and racial groups and a linkage to specific HLA types. There are several alleles that seem to confer susceptibility to disease (HLA DR 11, 12, 14, 15, 17) and some that seem to be protective (HLA DR1, DR4, and possibly HLA-DQB1*0201).

CLINICAL FEATURES

The lung and hilar lymph nodes represent the most common sites of involvement by sarcoidosis. Symptoms resulting from parenchymal lung involvement include dyspnea and cough. Pulmonary function abnormalities are found in nearly all symptomatic patients and in some patients who are asymptomatic. Physiologic abnormalities in patients with symptomatic sarcoidosis typically consist of a reduction in DL_{co} and vital capacity without

granulomas, and exclusion of other potential etiologies that may explain the granulomatous inflammation. Sarcoidosis represents an exaggerated Th1-type immune response that is probably triggered by an unidentified antigen or antigens at sites of disease activity. Although many potential antigenic causes have been studied, none has yet

airflow obstruction. The DL_{co} typically becomes abnormal before the vital capacity becomes abnormal, but both are usually affected in persons with moderate or severe symptoms. Airflow obstruction is relatively uncommon except in patients with advanced disease or with endobronchial involvement of larger airways. In rare instances, diffuse endobronchial granulomas in small airways lead to a predominantly obstructive pattern.

Intrathoracic sarcoidosis is diagnosed most easily by bronchoscopy with lung biopsy. The yield of bronchoscopic biopsy depends on the radiographic stage. In patients with pulmonary infiltrates (stages II and III), bronchoscopic lung biopsy demonstrates non-necrotizing granulomas in approximately 90% of cases. In stage I disease, the yield is 60% to 70%. If a diagnosis is not established by bronchoscopy and lung biopsy, mediastinoscopy is indicated and will provide a diagnosis in over 95% of cases in which mediastinal adenopathy is present. Needle aspiration procedures can also be useful for retrieving granulomas. Biopsy of extrapulmonary tissues can also be performed for diagnosis when clinically indicated (e.g., in patients with peripheral lymph node enlargement or skin lesions).

RADIOLOGIC FEATURES

Sarcoidosis is characterized by bilateral hilar lymphadenopathy and diffuse infiltrative lung disease. The changes have been classified according to a five-stage system as follows: stage 0, normal chest radiograph (8% of cases at presentation); stage I, bilateral hilar lymphadenopathy alone (40% of cases); stage II, bilateral hilar lymphadenopathy and diffuse infiltrative lung disease (37% of cases); stage III, diffuse infiltrative lung disease alone (10% of cases); and stage IV, lung fibrosis, often with upper lobe cystic disease (5% of cases).

PATHOLOGIC FEATURES

GROSS FINDINGS

The gross findings depend on the stage of the disease. Yellowish nodules corresponding to granulomas can be seen along the interlobular septa and bronchovascular areas of the lung, as well as on a cut section of involved lymph nodes. In advanced stages, interstitial fibrosis and honeycomb changes can develop.

MICROSCOPIC FINDINGS

The classical histopathological lesion in sarcoidosis is the non-necrotizing granuloma. Granulomas are usually small, compact, well circumscribed (Figure 17-5), generally unassociated with diffuse interstitial pneumonitis (unlike hypersensitivity pneumonitis), and often follow lymphatic and bronchovascular routes (Figures 17-6, 17-7). Granulomas can often be found in the bronchial mucosa, accounting for the high percentage of cases that can be diagnosed by bronchoscopic lung biopsy

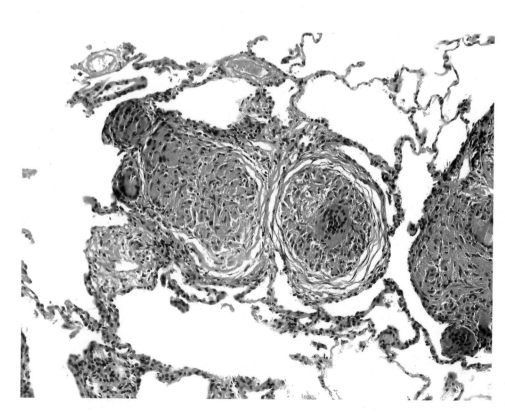

FIGURE 17-5
Sarcoidosis
Granulomas are classically compact and non-necrotizing.

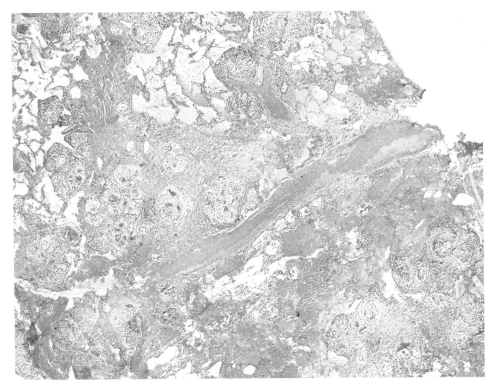

FIGURE 17-6

Sarcoidosis

Granulomas are often distributed along lymphatic routes, as is illustrated here.

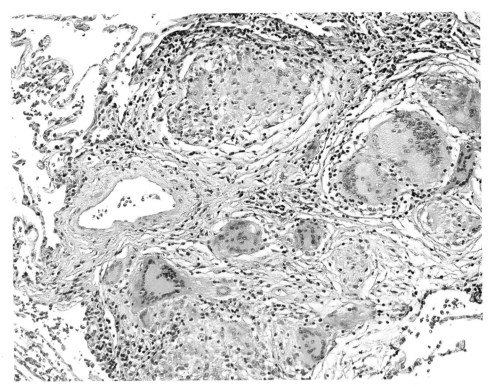

FIGURE 17-7

Sarcoidosis

Multinucleated giant cells and a small granuloma lie adjacent to a lymphatic.

(Figure 17-8). Granulomatous pulmonary angiitis is a frequent manifestation of sarcoidosis (Figure 17-9). Although the granulomas in sarcoidosis are usually described as non-necrotizing, small foci of necrosis have been reported in 6-39% of cases. Schaumann's bodies, also known as conchoidal bodies, are lamellated calcifica-tions that are often seen in giant cells in the sarcoidal granulomas as well as other types of granulomatous le-sions. Asteroid bodies are seen in 2-9% of granu-lomas from patients with sarcoidosis; these structures are seen within giant cells and consist of 5-30 μm stellate inclusions with numerous rays radiating from a central

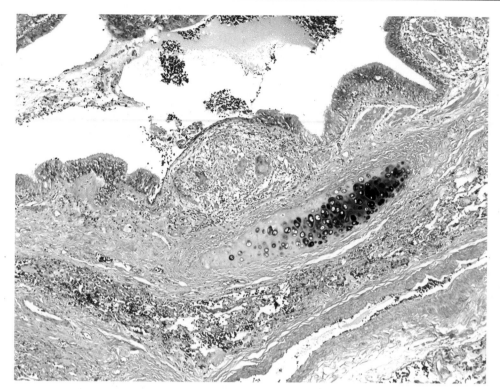

FIGURE 17-8
Sarcoidosis
Bronchial granulomas are commonly found in sarcoidosis, as is shown here, accounting for the high utility of bronchoscopy in establishing the diagnosis.

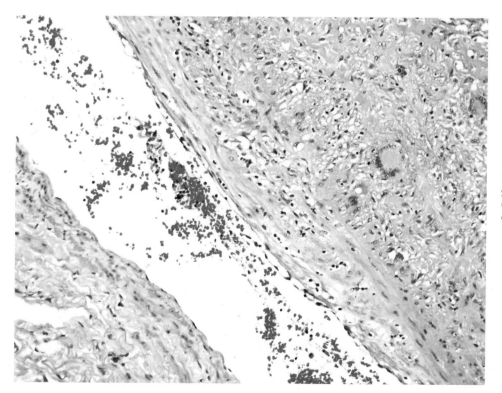

FIGURE 17-9
Sarcoidosis
Granulomatous angiitis is another common finding in sarcoidosis.

core. Oxalate crystals, which are birefringent under polarized light, may also be found. Over time, the granulomas become hyalinized (Figure 17-10), and dense interstitial fibrosis can develop. Stains for acid-fast organisms and fungi should be performed, and will be negative.

Cytologic Findings

Cytology samples, especially needle aspirates, may yield non-necrotizing granulomas (Figure 11).

Differential Diagnosis

The differential diagnosis includes other granulomatous pulmonary disorders. Demonstration of an infectious agent in a granuloma by a special stain precludes a diagnosis of sarcoidosis. Similarly, isolation of a compatible agent by culture should deter one from a diagnosis of sarcoidosis. In hypersensitivity pneumonitis, granulomas are usually more poorly formed than in sarcoidosis, and are usually accompanied by interstitial pneumonia and cellular bronchiolitis. Small, well circumscribed non-necrotizing sarcoidal granulomas are exceedingly uncommon in Wegener's granulomatosis, which is characterized by vasculitis and zones of geographic necrosis with granulomatous rims. Recently, interferon therapy has been associated with development of a granulomatous reaction that is histologically similar to sarcoidosis. Other drugs can also potentially produce a granulomatous pneumonitis, but the pattern is usually more like HP than sarcoidosis. Finally, berylliosis, an uncommon occupational lung disease associated with exposure to beryllium, manifests a granulomatous reaction pattern similar to sarcoidosis, but patients will have a history of exposure to the substance.

Prognosis and Therapy

The natural history of sarcoidosis is highly variable. In 60-70% of all cases, spontaneous remission will occur, and in 10-30%, the disease will follow a progressive course. The mortality rate is up to 10%, and death usually results from progressive lung disease, neurosarcoidosis, or cardiac disease. Other adverse prognostic features include chronic uveitis, onset after 40 years of age, hypercalcemia or nephrocalcinosis, nasal mucosal involvement, and cystic bone disease.

The treatment of patients with sarcoidosis has been a controversial issue. Many patients have mild disease that does not require systemic treatment. Although some authors believe that corticosteroid treatment induces the chronic fibrotic form of the disease, they are still used in many centers, but clinical trials have not shown a significant difference between treated and untreated groups. The use of methotrexate, azathioprine, and hydroxychloroquine as second-line agents has become the standard for most patients with symptomatic

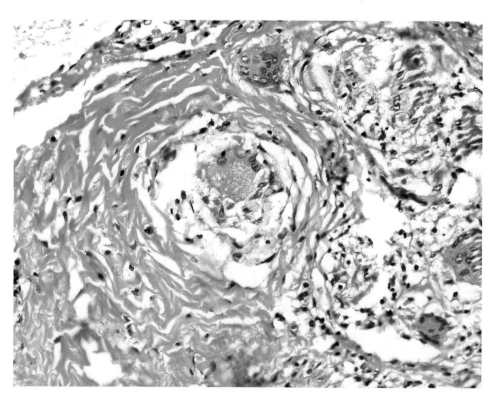

FIGURE 17-10
Sarcoidosis
Perigranulomatous hyalinization develops over time in sarcoidosis.

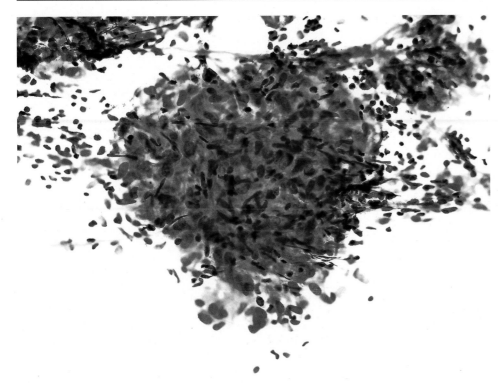

FIGURE 17-11
Sarcoidosis
This transbronchial needle aspirate yielded a small non-necrotizing granuloma.

sarcoidosis. Tumor necrosis factor-modifiers, including pentoxifylline, thalidomide, etanercept, and infliximab, are under investigation.

LYMPHANGIOLEIOMYOMATOSIS

Lymphangioleiomyomatosis (LAM), also known as lymphangiomyomatosis, is a diffuse infiltrative lung disease characterized by proliferation of modified smooth muscle cells that characteristically co-express muscle and melanocytic markers. It may occur as a sporadic disease or as a component of tuberous sclerosis complex (TSC), and may be associated with other lesions in the family of perivascular epithelioid cell neoplasms (PEComas) including angiomyolipoma and clear cell "sugar" tumor of the lung (CCST).

CLINICAL FEATURES

LAM is a disease that, as a rule, affects women in the reproductive years (average 32-34 years). Patients usually complain of progressive dyspnea. Classical complications of this disease are repeated pneumothorax, chylous effusions, and hemorrhage that leads to hemoptysis. Pulmonary function studies show an obstructive or mixed pattern with decreased diffusing capacity. The total lung capacity is usually increased. These features differ from what one would expect in most interstitial diseases (small lungs and restrictive pattern). Lesions identical to LAM are seen in 1-3% of patients with TSC. TSC has been linked to a germline mutation affecting 1 of 2 tumor suppressor genes: TSC1 on chromosome 9q34 (which encodes hamartin) and TSC2 on chromosome 16p13 (which encodes tuberin).

RADIOLOGIC FEATURES

The lungs are usually large and display diffuse cystic changes.

PATHOLOGIC FEATURES

GROSS FINDINGS

The classical gross findings consist of bilateral, diffuse cystic changes in which the cysts vary from a few millimeters to several centimeters in diameter. The cysts are separated by normal lung tissue in early lesions, but in advanced cases the cut surface may be diffusely cystic and resemble bullous emphysema or honeycomb lung.

SARCOIDOSIS—FACT SHEET

Definition

▸ Sarcoidosis is a multisystem granulomatous disease of unknown etiology that is characterized pathologically by the presence of non-necrotizing granulomas

Incidence and Location

▸ Worldwide distribution
▸ Prevalence of 10-40 per 100,000 is reported in the United States and Europe

Morbidity and Mortality

▸ Death attributable directly to the disease is seen in up to 10% of those affected
▸ In most individuals, the disease remains relatively stable, but 10-30% of patients have a progressive course

Gender, Race, and Age Distribution

▸ Females are slightly more often affected than males
▸ In the United States, the prevalence is higher in African-Americans, but in Europe the disease primarily affects Caucasians
▸ Rare among Inuit, Canadian Indians, New Zealand Maoris, and Southeast Asians and in several countries of Latin America
▸ Most common in middle age

Clinical Features

▸ Dyspnea and cough are associated with lung parenchymal involvement
▸ Other symptoms depend upon the organ systems involved and the severity of involvement

Radiologic Features

▸ Presentation depends upon the stage of the disease
▸ Hilar lymphadenopathy and interstitial reticular, reticulonodular, or nodular infiltrates, often following lymphatic routes, are typical
▸ Pleural effusion in 10% of cases
▸ Nodular sarcoidosis is an uncommon variant that presents with nodules up to 5 cm in diameter, which may be cavitary

Prognosis and Therapy

▸ Spontaneous remissions in a large number of patients
▸ Chronic progressive disease in 10-30%
▸ Mortality rates up to 10% have been reported
▸ Corticosteroids are commonly used for treatment, and a variety of second-line agents are also available

SARCOIDOSIS—PATHOLOGIC FEATURES

Gross Findings

▸ Changes may be minimal in early disease, but with progression, yellowish nodules may be visible along the interlobular septa and bronchovascular areas
▸ In advanced disease, there is diffuse interstitial fibrosis and honeycomb change
▸ Involved lymph nodes may demonstrate replacement by yellowish nodules or fibrosis

Microscopic Findings

▸ Multiple well circumscribed non-necrotizing granulomas in multiple organs
▸ Granulomas tend to show a lymphangitic and perivascular distribution in the lung
▸ Granulomatous vasculitis may be present
▸ Although granulomas are usually non-necrotizing, foci of necrosis in granulomas are not uncommon
▸ No microorganisms identified on acid-fast and fungal stains

Pathologic Differential Diagnosis

▸ Granulomatous infections, particularly mycobacterial and fungal infections
▸ Hypersensitivity pneumonitis
▸ Drug reactions
▸ Wegener's granulomatosis

MICROSCOPIC FINDINGS

The histopathologic diagnostic feature is the presence of proliferations of modified smooth muscle cells. At low magnification, the pulmonary parenchyma demonstrates cystically enlarged air spaces (Figure 17-12). Rupture of these cysts gives rise to the characteristic presentation of pneumothorax. The smooth muscle cells are usually observable in the walls of the cysts, where they appear as bundles of plump and spindle-shaped cells with pale eosinophilic cytoplasm and elongate nuclei (Figure 17-13), and in some areas, may take on an "epithelioid" appearance (Figure 17-14). Alveolar and bronchiolar walls are infiltrated by these cells. Proliferation of these peculiar smooth muscle cells is also seen in lymphatics (this explains why some patients present with chylothorax) and small veins, the latter associated with foci of hemosiderin deposition. Hyperplasia of alveolar type II cells may accompany these findings (Figure 17-15).

ANCILLARY STUDIES

IMMUNOHISTOCHEMISTRY

As expected, smooth muscle cell antibodies such as smooth muscle actin label the proliferating cells. Estrogen and progesterone receptors may also be detectable in some of the proliferating smooth muscle cells (Figure 17-16). Approximately 17-67% of the cells show positivity for HMB-45 (human melanin black-45) (Figure 17-17).

ULTRASTRUCTURAL STUDIES

By electron microscopy, the proliferating cells show characteristics of smooth muscle cells, with dense bodies and with abundant intracytoplasmic glycogen.

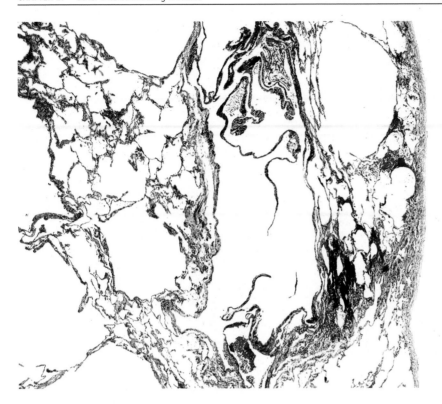

FIGURE 17-12
Lymphangioleiomyomatosis
Subpleural air spaces are cystically enlarged (Masson trichrome).

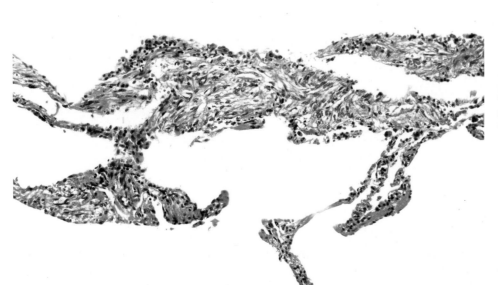

FIGURE 17-13
Lymphangioleiomyomatosis
These cytologically bland, spindle-shaped, modified smooth muscle cells are characteristic of lymphangioleio-myomatosis.

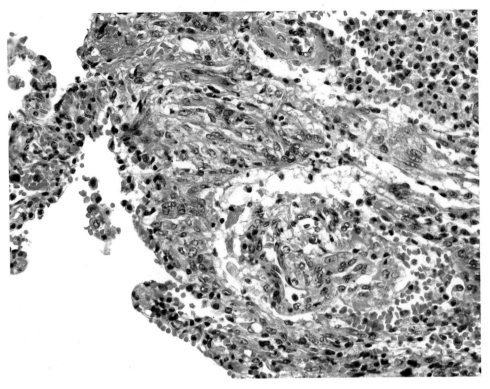

FIGURE 17-14

Lymphangioleiomyomatosis
The modified smooth muscle cells can have an epithelioid appearance, as is shown in this view.

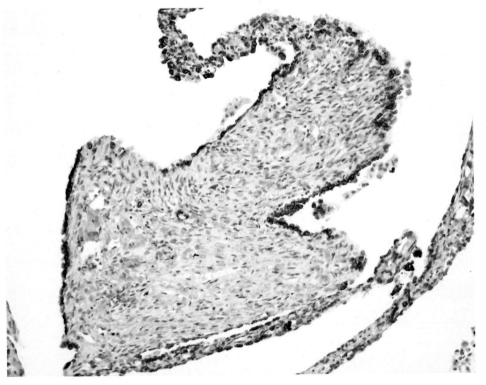

FIGURE 17-15

Lymphangioleiomyomatosis
Hyperplastic type II cells, immunopositive for cytokeratin, line the expanded alveolar septum.

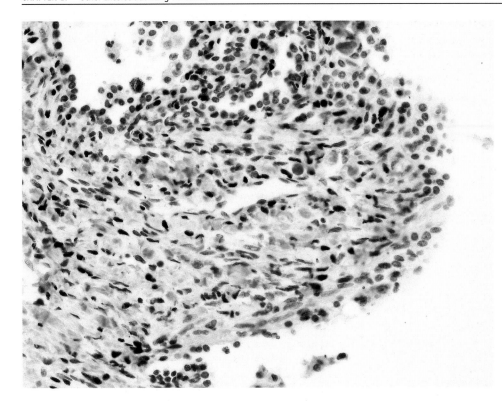

FIGURE 17-16

Lymphangioleiomyomatosis
Nuclear staining for estrogen receptor is often observed in the smooth muscle cells.

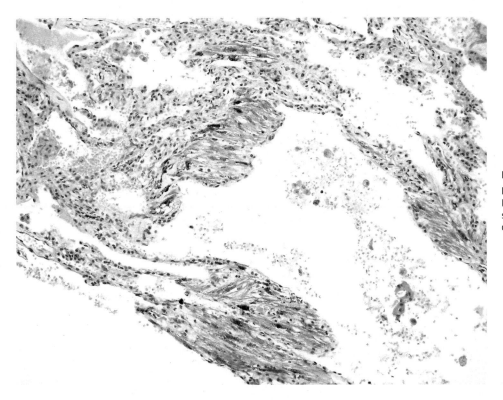

FIGURE 17-17

Lymphangioleiomyomatosis
Expression of HMB-45 by the modified smooth muscle cells is an important diagnostic feature.

DIFFERENTIAL DIAGNOSIS

In a woman of reproductive age who presents with diffuse cystic lung disease, this diagnosis must be seriously considered. Performance of an HMB45 stain can be very helpful for highlighting the modified smooth muscle cells in subtle cases or in cases with limited tissue. Histologically, LAM must be distinguished from advanced interstitial fibrosis, which is frequently associated with proliferation of histologically normal smooth muscle cells ("muscular cirrhosis" of the lung) that do not show the more cellular and glycogenated appearance of the modified smooth muscle cells in LAM. Furthermore, HMB45 staining will be negative in the smooth muscle cells that one encounters in interstitial fibrosing conditions, while in LAM it will often be expressed by the smooth muscle cells. Grossly, the cystic changes may prompt consideration of honeycomb lung or bullous emphysema, but again, microscopic recognition of the characteristic HMB45-positive modified smooth muscle cells will allow for differentiation between LAM and these entities.

PROGNOSIS AND THERAPY

LAM is usually progressive and leads to increasing respiratory disability over time. Although earlier series showed a high mortality rate within several years of diagnosis, a more recent national study reported a 10-year survival of 91% from onset of symptoms. Hormonal manipulation has been tried on the basis of expression of estrogen and progesterone receptors in the proliferating cells, with oophorectomy and Tamoxifen, but the success rate has not been promising. Progesterone therapy also does not appear to slow the decline in lung function in LAM. Although lung transplantation has been performed in some patients, recurrence of LAM in the transplanted lung has been reported, and the recurrent LAM cells appear to be derived from the recipient.

PULMONARY ALVEOLAR PROTEINOSIS

Pulmonary alveolar proteinosis (PAP), also known as alveolar lipoproteinosis or alveolar phospholipoproteinosis, is a rare congenital or acquired condition characterized by alveolar accumulation of surfactant components with minimal interstitial inflammation or fibrosis. The intra-alveolar material is seen as finely granular eosinophilic deposits that stain with periodic acid-Schiff (PAS) stain. The granulocyte-macrophage colony-stimulating factor (GM-CSF) pathway is important in the disease pathogenesis of both the acquired and congenital forms of PAP. Many patients with the acquired idiopathic form have antibodies against GM-CSF that seem to interfere with surfactant clearance by alveolar macrophages. Several mutations of the genes encoding GM-CSF receptor subunits or surfactant proteins have been discovered in patients with the congenital form of PAP.

CLINICAL FEATURES

PAP is primarily a disease of the fourth and fifth decades of life. There is a male predominance. There is a congenital form of PAP and an acquired form that can be idiopathic or secondary. The congenital form is discussed in another chapter. The secondary form of PAP can be associated with acute silicosis and other inhalational syndromes, immunodeficiency disorders, hematopoietic neoplasia, myelodysplastic and myeloproliferative syndromes, respiratory infections, lysinuric protein intolerance, and lung transplantation. Clinical features include progressive breathlessness, cough, fatigue, and malaise. Alveolar proteinosis has a variable clinical course ranging from spontaneous resolution to death with pneumonia or respiratory failure.

RADIOLOGIC FEATURES

The chest radiograph typically shows bilateral, symmetrical, alveolar-filling opacities with a nodular pattern that tend to involve perihilar regions and lower lobes and spare the costophrenic angles and the apices. High-resolution computed tomography (HRCT) reveals a bilateral ground-glass appearance with interlobular septal thickening that has been described as "crazy paving."

PATHOLOGIC FEATURES

GROSS FINDINGS

The lungs in PAP are very heavy and viscid, and a yellowish milky material is seen exuding from the air spaces. Occasional small yellow nodules are also seen on cut surface.

MICROSCOPIC FINDINGS

Characteristically, there is diffuse filling of the alveolar spaces and terminal bronchioles with an eosinophilic, finely granular, acellular material with occasional aggregates of foamy macrophages (Figures 17-18, 17-19). The intra-alveolar material is PAS-positive (Figure 17-20). Although there may be a mild

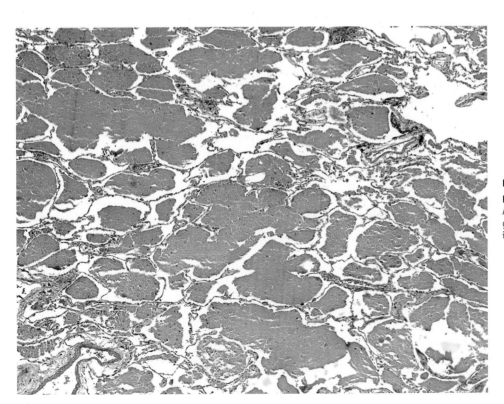

FIGURE 17-18
Pulmonary alveolar proteinosis
Alveolar spaces are filled with finely granular eosinophilic material, and interstitial changes are minimal.

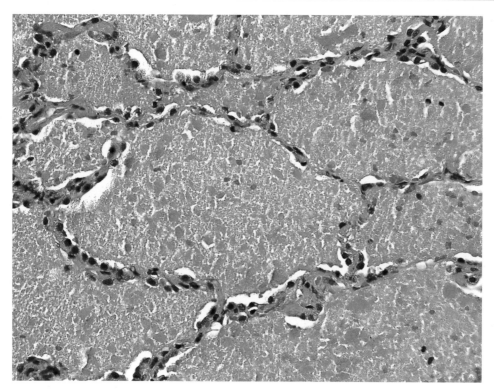

FIGURE 17-19
Pulmonary alveolar proteinosis
Granular eosinophilic exudate fills the alveoli.

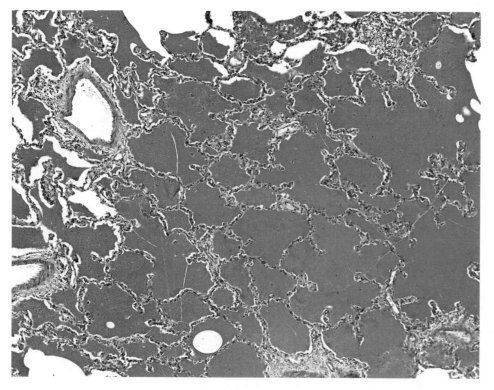

FIGURE 17-20
Pulmonary alveolar proteinosis
The exudate stains with a periodic acid-Schiff stain.

interstitial lymphocytic infiltrate, this is not a prominent feature. The alveolar architecture is usually well preserved, except in advanced cases in which pulmonary fibrosis has developed.

CYTOLOGIC FINDINGS

In approximately 75% of clinically suspected cases, a characteristic "milky" material can be obtained from bronchoalveolar lavage (BAL). Cytologic examination of this fluid reveals large amounts of granular, acellular, eosinophilic proteinaceous material (Figure 17-21).

ANCILLARY STUDIES

IMMUNOHISTOCHEMISTRY

The material that fills the air spaces is immunoreactive for surfactant components.

ULTRASTRUCTURAL STUDIES

Electron microscopic examination of tissues or bronchoalveolar lavage fluid reveals the presence of concentrically laminated phospholipid structures (lamellar

bodies), representing surfactant, identical to those seen in type II pneumocytes.

DIFFERENTIAL DIAGNOSIS

The microscopic differential diagnosis includes other conditions in which the alveoli are filled with an eosinophilic material: pulmonary edema, *Pneumocystis* pneumonia, and conditions associated with abundant mucin in alveoli. Pulmonary edema is usually seen as a thinner, homogeneous eosinophilic material that lacks the coarse granules, cholesterol clefts, and foamy macrophages of PAP. The eosinophilic material seen in *Pneumocystis* pneumonia shows a honeycomb pattern in which the small spaces in the aggregates of exudate are filled with cysts that can be highlighted with a methenamine silver stain. It should be noted, however, that alveolar proteinosis can occur in association with *Pneumocystis* pneumonia (Figure 17-22), both predisposed to by a third immunocompromising condition. Intra-alveolar accumulation of mucin may occur in cases of mucinous adenocarcinomas or in a setting of mucostasis due to bronchiectasis or asthma. In these conditions, the eosinophilic material is paler, not granular and dense, lacks cholesterol clefts, and stains with mucicarmine.

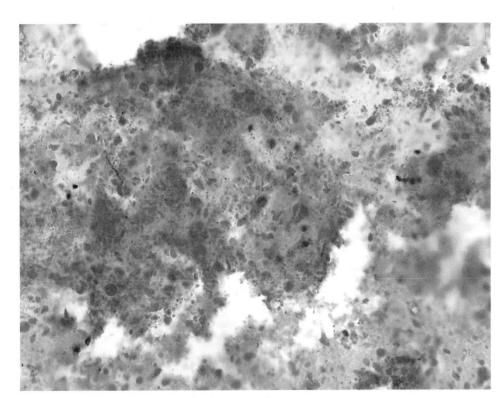

FIGURE 17-21

Pulmonary alveolar proteinosis
Bronchoalveolar lavage characteristically yields large amounts of the granular exudate.

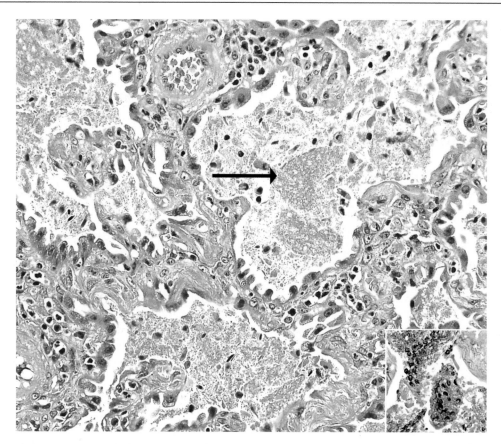

FIGURE 17-22

Pneumocystis jiroveci **pneumonia and pulmonary alveolar proteinosis**

Aggregates (arrow) of honeycomb exudate reflect the existence of *Pneumocystis jiroveci* pneumonia associated with a background of alveolar proteinosis. The inset, taken from the same case, shows the organisms stained with methenamine silver.

PROGNOSIS AND THERAPY

The clinical course of PAP is highly variable and falls into one of three categories: stable but with persistent symptoms, progressive deterioration, or spontaneous improvement. In a retrospective analysis of 343 cases, the 5-year survival rate was about 75%. Of the deaths in that study, 72% were directly due to respiratory failure from PAP, and 20% were due to PAP complicated by uncontrolled infection. Although patients with PAP are vulnerable to the common respiratory pathogens, they are also predisposed to opportunistic infections, particularly with *Nocardia*. Performance of organism stains and cultures is helpful for evaluating for superimposed infections.

Approaches to therapy of PAP have included bilateral whole-lung lavage and, recently, the use of GM-CSF for patients with acquired PAP. Recent studies evaluating GM-CSF as a therapy for PAP have shown improvement in at least half of the acquired cases, but the congenital form of the disease does not respond to therapy with GM-CSF. Corticosteroids have no value and may increase the risk of infections. Spontaneous remissions

have been reported, but progression to advanced fibrotic disease has also been observed.

ACUTE EOSINOPHILIC PNEUMONIA

Acute eosinophilic pneumonia (AEP) is characterized by the rapid onset of an acute pulmonary syndrome resembling the acute respiratory distress syndrome (ARDS) or an infectious pneumonia, with significant pulmonary eosinophilia.

CLINICAL FEATURES

This disorder can arise at any age, usually in a previously healthy person. Associations with cigarette smoking and allergic rhinitis have been described, and in a few cases, AEP appears to represent a drug reaction, but in most cases an etiologic factor cannot be defined. Symptoms include a rapid onset of pleuritic pain, shortness of

PULMONARY ALVEOLAR PROTEINOSIS—FACT SHEET

Definition

➤ Pulmonary alveolar proteinosis (PAP) is an acquired or congenital condition characterized by alveolar accumulation of surfactant; in some patients, it is associated with abnormalities in the granulocyte-macrophage colony-stimulating factor (GM-CSF) pathway or surfactant gene mutations

Incidence and Location

➤ Rare
➤ Worldwide distribution

Mortality

➤ 5-year survival rate of approximately 75%
➤ Deaths are due to PAP-induced pulmonary failure, superimposed infection, or underlying disease

Gender and Age Distribution

➤ More common in men (4:1 male-to-female ratio)
➤ Patients of all ages can be affected, but the prevalence is highest between 30 and 50 years of age
➤ Rare familial cases

Clinical Features

➤ Progressive dyspnea, cough, fatigue, and malaise

Radiologic Features

➤ Chest radiograph typically shows bilateral, symmetric, alveolar-filling opacities with a nodular pattern that tend to involve perihilar regions and lower lobes and spare the costophrenic angles and the apices
➤ HRCT reveals a bilateral ground-glass appearance with interlobular septal thickening that has been described as "crazy paving"

Prognosis and Therapy

➤ Highly variable course
➤ Spontaneous remission can occur
➤ Treatment approaches include bilateral whole-lung lavage and GM-CSF therapy

PULMONARY ALVEOLAR PROTEINOSIS—PATHOLOGIC FEATURES

Gross Findings

➤ Heavy and viscid lungs, with yellowish milky material in air spaces on cut surface and occasional yellow nodules
➤ If superimposed infection is present, additional abnormalities (usually consolidation) corresponding to the infection may also be present

Microscopic Findings

➤ Filling of the alveolar spaces and bronchioles with an eosinophilic, finely granular acellular material that is PAS-positive
➤ Absence of significant interstitial inflammation in uncomplicated cases
➤ Scattered aggregates of foamy macrophages in air spaces
➤ Variable degrees of interstitial fibrosis
➤ Features of superimposed infection may be present (acute inflammatory infiltrates, granulomas, necrosis, etc.)

Immunohistochemical Findings

➤ Alveolar material stains for surfactant components

Ultrastructural Features

➤ Concentrically laminated phospholipid structures (lamellar bodies)

Pathologic Differential Diagnosis

➤ Pulmonary edema
➤ *Pneumocystis* pneumonia
➤ Alveolar mucin accumulations

---

breath, myalgias, and fever, with severe hypoxemia. Bronchoalveolar lavage (BAL) and pleural fluids demonstrate substantial eosinophilia (usually more than 25% of cells), and peripheral blood eosinophilia may or may not be observed.

RADIOLOGIC FEATURES

Chest radiographs show extensive bilateral alveolar and interstitial opacities. Pleural effusions are commonly present. With treatment, the radiographic changes resolve rapidly, often within 3 weeks.

PATHOLOGIC FEATURES

MICROSCOPIC FINDINGS

Findings of diffuse alveolar damage are accompanied by interstitial and alveolar infiltrates of eosinophils (Figure 17-23), which may vary in density from area to area, and in some areas be relatively inconspicuous. In the acute phase, edema and hyaline membranes are noted. In the organizing phase, hyaline membranes are replaced by proliferating fibroblasts in the interstitium and alveoli, with restoration of the alveolar lining by hyperplastic pneumocytes, and variable degrees of collagen deposition.

CYTOLOGIC FINDINGS

BAL and pleural fluids contain large numbers of eosinophils, accounting for more than 25% of cells. In the BAL fluid, other findings of diffuse alveolar damage (fragments of hyaline membranes, reactive pneumocytes) may also be seen.

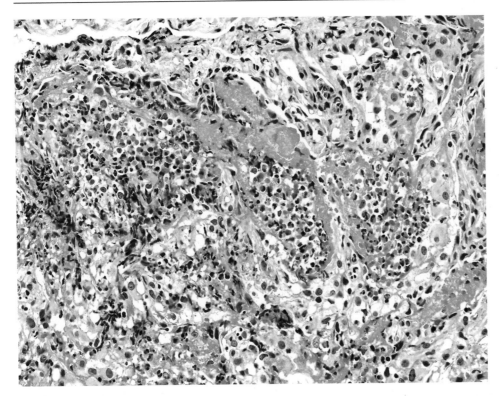

FIGURE 17-23
Acute eosinophilic pneumonia
Hyaline membranes lie along alveolar septa, and air spaces are filled by eosinophils and macrophages.

ACUTE EOSINOPHILIC PNEUMONIA—FACT SHEET

Definition

▸▸ A disorder characterized by the rapid onset of an acute pulmonary syndrome resembling the acute respiratory distress syndrome (ARDS) or an infectious pneumonia, with significant pulmonary eosinophilia

Incidence

▸▸ Rare
▸▸ A recent report describes 18 cases of AEP among 183,000 military personnel deployed in or near Iraq, with an incidence of 9.1 per 100,000 person-years

Mortality

▸▸ Death is uncommon if AEP is diagnosed and treated

Gender and Age Distribution

▸▸ Male predominance
▸▸ Can occur at any age, but the average age at presentation is 30 years

Clinical Features

▸▸ Rapid onset of respiratory failure requiring mechanical ventilation
▸▸ Symptoms include pleuritic pain, shortness of breath, myalgia, and fever
▸▸ Most cases are idiopathic, but subsets are associated with smoking, allergic rhinitis, or drug administration

Radiologic Features

▸▸ Extensive bilateral opacification and pleural effusions

Prognosis and Therapy

▸▸ Corticosteroids remain the mainstay of therapy and produce rapid recovery
▸▸ Relapses have not been reported

ACUTE EOSINOPHILIC PNEUMONIA—PATHOLOGIC FEATURES

Microscopic Findings

▸▸ Acute or organizing diffuse alveolar damage accompanied by interstitial and alveolar infiltrates of eosinophils

Cytologic Findings

▸▸ Increased numbers of eosinophils (more than 25% of cells) in bronchoalveolar lavage and pleural fluids

Pathologic Differential Diagnosis

▸▸ Other causes of diffuse alveolar damage
▸▸ Chronic eosinophilic pneumonia
▸▸ Churg-Strauss syndrome

DIFFERENTIAL DIAGNOSIS

Other causes of diffuse alveolar damage (DAD) should be considered in the differential diagnosis, but usually do not manifest the degree of eosinophilia characteristic of AEP. It is most important to evaluate for infections, since the current treatment of AEP utilizes corticosteroids. An exacerbation of chronic eosinophilic pneumonia (CEP) may also be considered in the differential diagnosis, but patients with CEP will usually have a history of multiple similar episodes in the past, and a background of subacute and/or chronic parenchymal changes (organizing pneumonia, interstitial fibrosis) is frequently seen in CEP. Churg-Strauss syndrome represents another potential consideration, since eosinophilic pneumonia is often seen in the context of this syndrome. The finding of vasculitis is helpful for diagnosis of Churg-Strauss syndrome, as is the fulfillment of other clinical criteria for this diagnosis (discussed in another chapter).

PROGNOSIS AND THERAPY

Corticosteroid therapy typically produces rapid and complete recovery.

CHRONIC EOSINOPHILIC PNEUMONIA

Chronic eosinophilic pneumonia (CEP) is a distinctive, chronic, relapsing pulmonary disorder associated with peripheral blood and pulmonary eosinophilia, which responds rapidly to corticosteroid therapy, and which may be idiopathic or triggered by exposure to one of numerous potential triggers.

CLINICAL FEATURES

CEP is characterized by progressive respiratory and systemic symptoms developing over weeks or months, with a mean interval of 4 months between the onset of symptoms and the diagnosis. The most common manifestations are dyspnea, cough, and chest pain, often accompanied with fatigue, malaise, fever, and weight loss. Hemoptysis and pleural effusions are uncommon. Physical examination may reveal wheezes or crackles. Peripheral blood eosinophilia is usually present. Patients may experience exacerbations of these abnormalities superimposed upon the chronic course of the disease.

The disorder is more common in females than males. Although it can develop at any age, middle age is most common. Asthma, chronic rhinitis, or sinusitis is present in many patients. A broad range of etiologic agents have been identified, including a wide variety of drugs, parasites, bacteria, fungi, metal salts, and other materials. In many patients, however, a triggering agent cannot be pinpointed.

RADIOLOGIC FEATURES

Typical findings include peripheral alveolar opacities with ill-defined margins and a density varying from ground-glass to air-space consolidation. Migration of the infiltrates over time is highly suggestive of the diagnosis. A pattern of "photographic negative of pulmonary edema" is considered characteristic but is not always found. The infiltrates usually disappear rapidly after corticosteroid treatment, but may recur, sometimes in the same areas, after therapy is discontinued.

PATHOLOGIC FEATURES

GROSS FINDINGS

There are irregular, patchy areas of consolidation, often subpleural.

MICROSCOPIC FINDINGS

CEP is characterized by dense infiltrates of eosinophils, often accompanied by variable numbers of macrophages, in alveoli (Figures 17-24 and 17-25). Occasional multinucleated giant cells are seen. Eosinophil abscesses are common, and consist of a central area of necrosis surrounded by histiocytes with a palisaded arrangement, mixed with eosinophils (Figure 17-26). In addition, there is an interstitial inflammatory infiltrate composed of eosinophils, lymphocytes, and plasma cells. Organizing pneumonia is commonly found in association with these findings (Figure 17-27), and sarcoid-like granulomas may be seen in up to 10% of the cases. Vascular infiltration by eosinophils has been described, but a necrotizing vasculitis should not be present. In some patients, significant interstitial fibrosis and honeycomb changes can develop, resembling UIP. Histochemical stains for fungi should be performed to evaluate for these agents as potential causes of the CEP.

Corticosteroid therapy reduces the number of intact eosinophils, potentially obscuring the diagnosis. Knowledge of the patient's treatment history, clinical and radiographic findings, and peripheral blood white blood

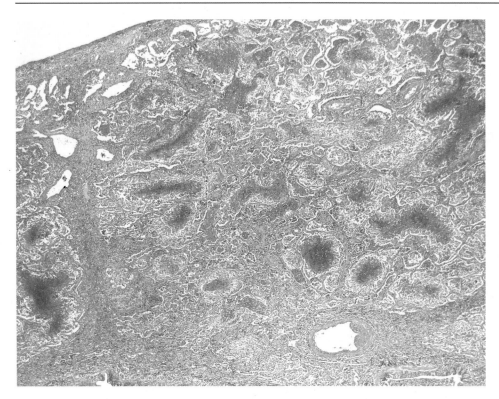

FIGURE 17-24
Chronic eosinophilic pneumonia
The peripheral lung tissue shows dense parenchymal consolidation.

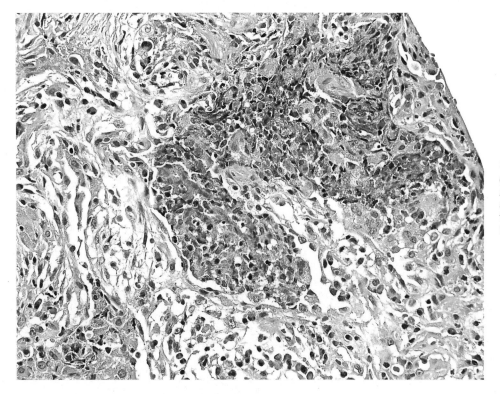

FIGURE 17-25
Chronic eosinophilic pneumonia
Alveoli contain numerous eosinophils and macrophages, and the interstitium is edematous and infiltrated by eosinophils as well.

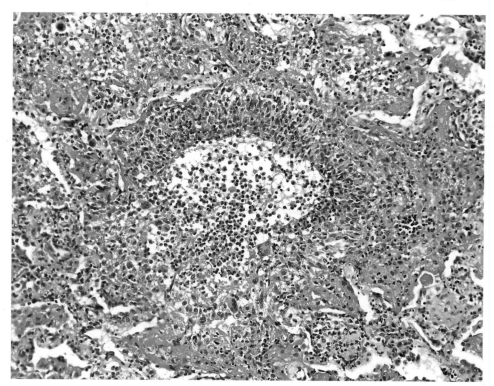

FIGURE 17-26

Chronic eosinophilic pneumonia
This eosinophil microabscess consists of a centrally necrotic collection of eosinophils and histiocytes, with palisading of the histiocytes, and occasional multinucleated giant cells. Adjacent alveoli contain eosinophils and fibrinous exudate.

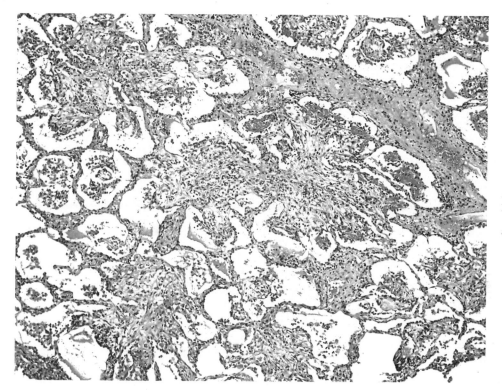

FIGURE 17-27

Organizing pneumonia in chronic eosinophilic pneumonia
In this case of chronic eosinophilic pneumonia, the fibrinous exudate in alveoli is undergoing organization.

cell differential count can be helpful for supporting an interpretation of "treated CEP."

CYTOLOGIC FINDINGS

Sputum and BAL fluid contain markedly increased numbers of eosinophils.

DIFFERENTIAL DIAGNOSIS

Corticosteroid therapy may interfere with diagnosis of CEP since it will produce a reduction in intact eosinophils and can cause significant eosinophil degeneration with karyorrhexis. The degenerated, fragmented cells can be misinterpreted as neutrophils, yielding a diagnosis of abscess with an implication of bacterial infection, which prompts a different therapeutic response than CEP. Acute eosinophilic pneumonia has a more abbreviated clinical course and does not show the subacute and chronic histologic changes of CEP. Desquamative interstitial pneumonia (DIP) is another important differential diagnostic consideration, particular in macrophage-rich cases or corticosteroid-treated eosinophil-depleted cases, but the chest radiographic findings differ from CEP, and DIP will not be associated with peripheral blood eosinophilia, unlike CEP. Churg-Strauss syndrome often includes a component of eosinophilic pneumonia as one of its manifestations. The finding of necrotizing vasculitis in the context of an eosinophilic pneumonia should prompt consideration of this syndrome and stimulate evaluation for the other clinical and laboratory findings associated with this disorder. Langerhans cell histiocytosis may also be considered in the differential diagnosis, but demonstration of clusters of S100- and CD1a-positive Langerhans cells can separate the two disorders. Also, significant degrees of peripheral blood and BAL fluid eosinophilia are not found in association with Langerhans cell histiocytosis. Lastly, pneumothorax causes eosinophilic pleuritis, and the eosinophils may extend into the subpleural lung parenchyma. In these cases, knowledge of the clinical picture and lack of peripheral blood eosinophilia will be helpful for determining the nature of the process.

CHRONIC EOSINOPHILIC PNEUMONIA—FACT SHEET

Definition

▸ A distinctive, chronic, relapsing pulmonary disorder associated with peripheral blood and pulmonary eosinophilia, which responds rapidly to corticosteroid therapy, and which may be idiopathic or triggered by a wide variety of drugs, parasites, bacteria, fungi, metal salts, and other materials

Incidence and Location

▸ Uncommon
▸ Worldwide distribution

Mortality

▸ Deaths are extremely rare

Gender and Age Distribution

▸ Occurs predominantly in women (2:1 female-to-male ratio)
▸ Mean age of 45 years at diagnosis

Clinical Features

▸ Symptoms include dyspnea, cough, and chest pain, often accompanied with fatigue, malaise, fever, and weight loss, developing over a period of months
▸ Peripheral blood eosinophilia is usually present
▸ Coexisting asthma, chronic rhinitis, or sinusitis is common
▸ Etiologic agents include a wide variety of drugs, parasites, bacteria, fungi, viruses, metal salts, fumes, and other allergens; other cases are idiopathic

Radiologic Features

▸ Peripheral alveolar opacities, with a distribution described as a "negative image of pulmonary edema," that may change location over time

Prognosis and Therapy

▸ Responds rapidly to corticosteroids, but may require prolonged treatment to reduce recurrences

---

CHRONIC EOSINOPHILIC PNEUMONIA—PATHOLOGIC FEATURES

Gross Findings

▸ Irregular areas of consolidation, usually peripheral and bilateral

Microscopic Features

▸ Predominantly intra-alveolar collections of eosinophils, variable numbers of macrophages, and occasional multinucleated giant cells
▸ Eosinophil abscesses with central necrosis surrounded by palisaded histiocytes and eosinophils
▸ Organizing pneumonia is common
▸ Sarcoid-like granulomas may be seen in up to 10% of cases
▸ Vascular infiltration by eosinophils, but not necrotizing vasculitis, can be present
▸ Variable degrees of interstitial fibrosis and honeycomb change

Pathologic Differential Diagnosis

▸ Acute eosinophilic pneumonia
▸ Desquamative interstitial pneumonia (especially after corticosteroid administration)
▸ Churg-Strauss syndrome
▸ Langerhans cell histiocytosis
▸ Eosinophil infiltrates secondary to pneumothorax

PROGNOSIS AND THERAPY

Deaths due to CEP are extremely rare. Typically, the infiltrates and symptoms disappear soon after corticosteroid administration. It is common, however, for patients with CEP to require prolonged treatment with corticosteroids in order to avoid relapses. Patients with asthma appear to have a lower incidence of recurrence, perhaps due to use of inhaled corticosteroids as part of their asthma treatment.

SUGGESTED READINGS

Hypersensitivity Pneumonitis

1. Agostini C, Trentin L, Facco M, Semenzato G. New aspects of hypersensitivity pneumonitis. *Curr Opin Pulm Med.* 2004;10:378-82.
2. Barrios R, Selman M, Franco R, Chapela R, Lopez JS, Fortoul TI. Subpopulations of T-cells in lung biopsies from patients with pigeon breeder's disease. *Lung.* 1987;165:181-7.
3. Katzenstein AL, Fiorelli RF. Nonspecific interstitial pneumonia/fibrosis: histologic features and clinical significance. *Am J Surg Pathol.* 1994;18:136-47.
4. Khoor A, Leslie KO, Tazelaar HD, Helmers RA, Colby TV. Diffuse pulmonary disease caused by nontuberculous mycobacteria in immunocompetent people (hot tub lung). *Am J Clin Pathol.* 2001;115:755-62.
5. Kokkarinen JI, Tukiainen HO, Terho EO. Effect of corticosteroid treatment on the recovery of pulmonary function in farmer's lung. *Am Rev Respir Dis.* 1992;145:3-5.
6. Pipavath S, Godwin JD. Imaging of interstitial lung disease. *Clin Chest Med.* 2004;25:455-65.
7. Richerson HB. Hypersensitivity pneumonitis—pathology and pathogenesis. *Clin Rev Allergy.* 1983;1:469-86.
8. Richerson HB. Immune complexes and the lung: a skeptical review. *Surv Synth Pathol Res.* 1984;3:281-91.
9. Schuyler M. Hypersensitivity pneumonitis. In: Crapo JD, Glassroth J, Karlinsky J, King T, eds. *Baum's Textbook of Pulmonary Disease.* 7 ed. Lippincott Williams & Wilkins; 2004.
10. Yi ES. Hypersensitivity pneumonitis. *Crit Rev Clin Lab Sci.* 2002;39: 581-629.

Sarcoidosis

11. Baughman RP. Pulmonary sarcoidosis. *Clin Chest Med.* 2004;25: 521-30.
12. Gal AA, Koss MN. The pathology of sarcoidosis. *Curr Opin Pulm Med.* 2002;8:445-551.
13. Gurrieri C, Bortoli M, Brunetta E, Piazza F, Agostini C. Cytokines, chemokines and other biomolecular markers in sarcoidosis. *Sarcoidosis Vasc Diffuse Lung Dis.* 2005;22:S9-14.
14. King Jr TE. Clinical advances in the diagnosis and therapy of the interstitial lung diseases. *Am J Respir Crit Care Med.* 2005;172:268-79.
15. Moller DR, Chen ES. What causes sarcoidosis? *Curr Opin Pulm Med.* 2002;8:429-34.

Lymphangioleiomyomatosis

16. Flieder DB, Travis WD. Clear cell "sugar" tumor of the lung: association with lymphangioleiomyomatosis and multifocal micronodular pneumocyte hyperplasia in a patient with tuberous sclerosis. *Am J Surg Pathol.* 1997;21:1242-7.
17. Folpe AL, Mentzel T, Lehr HA, Fisher C, Balzer BL, Weiss SW. Perivascular epithelioid cell neoplasms of soft tissue and gynecologic origin: a clinicopathologic study of 26 cases and review of the literature. *Am J Surg Pathol.* 2005;29:1558-75.
18. Johnson SR, Whale CI, Hubbard RB, Lewis SA, Tattersfield AE. Survival and disease progression in UK patients with lymphangioleiomyomatosis. *Thorax.* 2004;59:800-3.

19. Karbowniczek M, Astrinidis A, Balsara BR, et al. Recurrent lymphangiomyomatosis after transplantation: genetic analyses reveal a metastatic mechanism. *Am J Respir Crit Care Med.* 2003;167:976-82.
20. Moss J, editor. *LAM and Other Diseases Characterized By Smooth Muscle Proliferation, Lung Biology in Health and Disease.* New York: Marcel Dekker; 1999.
21. Smolarek TA, Wessner LL, McCormack FX, Mylet JC, Menon AG, Henske EP. Evidence that lymphangiomyomatosis is caused by TSC2 mutations: chromosome 16p13 loss of heterozygosity in angiomyolipomas and lymph nodes from women with lymphangiomyomatosis. *Am J Hum Genet.* 1998;62:810-5.
22. Taveira-DaSilva AM, Stylianou MP, Hedin CJ, Hathaway O, Moss J. Decline in lung function in patients with lymphangioleiomyomatosis treated with or without progesterone. *Chest.* 2004;126:1867-74.

Pulmonary Alveolar Proteinosis

23. Ioachimescu OC, Kavuru MS. Pulmonary alveolar proteinosis. *Chron Respir Dis.* 2006;3:149-59.
24. Pascual J, Gomez Aguinaga MA, Vidal R, et al. Alveolar proteinosis and nocardiosis: a patient treated by bronchopulmonary lavage. *Postgrad Med J.* 1989;65:674-7.
25. Presneill JJ, Nakata K, Inoue Y, Seymour JF. Pulmonary alveolar proteinosis. *Clin Chest Med.* 2004;25:593-613.
26. Seymour JF, Presneill JJ. Pulmonary alveolar proteinosis: progress in the first 44 years. *Am J Respir Crit Care Med.* 2002;166:215-35.
27. Singh G, Katyal SL, Bedrossian CW, Rogers RM. Pulmonary alveolar proteinosis: Staining for surfactant apoprotein in alveolar proteinosis and in conditions simulating it. *Chest.* 1983;83:82-6.
28. Venkateshiah SB, Yan TD, Bonfield TL, et al. An open-label trial of granulocyte macrophage colony stimulating factor therapy for moderate symptomatic pulmonary alveolar proteinosis. *Chest.* 2006;130:227-37.
29. Wang BM, Stern EJ, Schmidt RA, Pierson DJ. Diagnosing pulmonary proteinosis: a review and an update. *Chest.* 1997;111:460-6.
30. Yousem SA. Alveolar lipoproteinosis in lung allograft recipient. *Hum Pathol.* 1997;28:1383-6.

Acute Eosinophilic Pneumonia

31. Allen J. Acute eosinophilic pneumonia. *Semin Respir Crit Care Med.* 2006;27:142-7.
32. Allen JN, Magro CM, King MA. The eosinophilic pneumonias. *Semin Respir Crit Care Med.* 2002;23:127-34.
33. Cottin V, Cordier JF. Eosinophilic pneumonias. *Allergy.* 2005;60: 841-57.
34. Pope-Harman AL, Davis WB, Allen ED, Christoforidis AJ, Allen JN. Acute eosinophilic pneumonia: a summary of 15 cases and review of the literature. *Medicine (Baltimore).* 1996;75:334-42.
35. Shorr AF, Scoville SL, Cersovsky SB, et al. *JAMA.* 2004;292:2997-3005.
36. Tazelaar HD, Linz LJ, Colby TV, Myers JL, Limper AH. Acute eosinophilic pneumonia: histopathologic findings in nine patients. *Am J Respir Crit Care Med.* 1997;155:296-302.

Chronic Eosinophilic Pneumonia

37. Alberts WM. Eosinophilic interstitial lung disease. *Curr Opin Pulm Med.* 2004;10:419-24.
38. Carrington CB, Addington WW, Goff AM, et al. Chronic eosinophilic pneumonia. *N Engl J Med.* 1969;280:787-98.
39. Liebow AA, Carrington CB. The eosinophilic pneumonias. *Medicine (Baltimore).* 1969;48:251-85.
40. Jederlinic PJ, Sicilian L, Gaensler EA. Chronic eosinophilic pneumonia: a report of 19 cases and a review of the literature. *Medicine (Baltimore).* 1988;67:154-62.
41. Olopade CO, Crotty TB, Douglas WW, Colby TV, Sur S. Chronic eosinophilic pneumonia and idiopathic bronchiolitis obliterans organizing pneumonia: comparison of eosinophil number and degranulation by immunofluorescence staining for eosinophil-derived major basic protein. *Mayo Clin Proc.* 1995;70:137-42.
42. Saitoh K, Shindo N. Electron microscopic study of chronic eosinophilic pneumonia. *Pathol Int.* 1996;46:855-61.

18

Environmental- and Toxin-Induced Lung Diseases

Allen R. Gibbs • R.L. Attanoos

- **Introduction**
- **Asbestosis and Other Asbestos-Related Lung Pathology**
- **Silicosis**
- **Coal Workers' Pneumoconiosis**
- **Hard Metal Pneumoconiosis**
- **Berylliosis**
- **Siderosis**
- **Silicatosis**
- **Toxic Gases and Fumes**
- **Intravenous Talcosis and Other Consequences of Intravenous Drug Abuse**

INTRODUCTION

Exposures to environmental agents can result in a wide spectrum of pulmonary pathologic patterns (Table 18-1). The majorities of reactions seen nowadays are chronic due to exposure to the mineral(s) over a period of many years and have latencies often exceeding several decades. Acute reactions are usually now the result of industrial accidents where exposures are relatively brief but extremely high. Occupational histories in these types of cases need to be detailed and complete, since the offending exposure may be quite early in an individual's career.

Some definitions are useful. Fumes are generated by vaporization of a metal, subsequent oxidation, and condensation to form very small particles ranging from 0.1 to 0.4 microns. Dusts are solid aerosols derived from mechanical manipulation of rocks such as grinding, drilling, blasting, and milling, and the particles are generally larger than those in fumes. Pneumoconiosis is a non-neoplastic lung disease caused by exposure to dust. In the macular and nodular pneumoconioses, there is a conventional and arbitrary subdivision into simple and complicated. If lesions greater than 1 cm in diameter are present (so-called progressive massive fibrosis), then the process is referred to as "complicated," whereas if lesions measure 1 cm or less, at most, the process is designated "simple."

The type of pathologic reaction to a material depends on the properties of the mineral, including size, shape, and durability (biopersistence), and on cumulative exposure. Exposures can result from direct handling of the material, but also indirect exposure, such as through washing the contaminated work clothes of a directly exposed member of the household (para-occupational).

ASBESTOSIS AND OTHER ASBESTOS-RELATED LUNG PATHOLOGY

Asbestos minerals are naturally occurring fibrous silicates, that have been used extensively in several thousand products including textiles, insulation products, cement, friction materials, and construction. Asbestos minerals comprise two separate mineralogical groups: serpentine and amphibole. The only member of the serpentine group is chrysotile (white) asbestos, whichcomprises 90-95% of the asbestos used in the United States. The amphibole group includes amosite (brown) and crocidolite (blue), which are the major commercial forms, and actinolite, and tremolite. The amphiboles have a much greater tendency to cause asbestos-related diseases than chrysotile, because they possess much greater biopersistence in the lungs than chrysotile, which appears to be cleared within weeks to months after exposure.

Exposure(s) to asbestos may result in pulmonary fibrosis (asbestosis), lung cancer, pleural effusions, parietal pleural plaques, rounded atelectasis, diffuse pleural fibrosis, and mesothelioma. It should be noted that the pleural sequelae can occur at much lower exposures than those required to produce asbestosis and asbestos-related lung cancers.

CLINICAL FEATURES

Theoretically, the definition of asbestosis is simple: diffuse interstitial pulmonary (not pleural) fibrosis caused by asbestos exposure. However, there are problems in applying the definition and assessing exposure in many

TABLE 18-1

Pleuropulmonary Reactions to Environmental Agents

Reactions	Agents
Asthma	Isocyanates, metals
Bronchiolitis	Nitrogen dioxide
Macular/nodular pneumoconiosis	Coal, silica, silicates
Diffuse interstitial fibrosis	Asbestos, hard metal
Granulomatous	Beryllium
Diffuse alveolar damage	Toxic fumes
Desquamative interstitial pneumonia	Silica, silicates, hard metal
Giant cell interstitial pneumonia	Hard metal
Alveolar proteinosis	Silica
Emphysema	Coal, cadmium
Pleural plaque	Asbestos, talc
Lung cancer	Asbestos, nickel, arsenic, chromium compounds
Mesothelioma	Asbestos

PATHOLOGIC FEATURES

GROSS FINDINGS

In symptomatic cases, the lungs are usually reduced in size, with bosselation of the pleural surfaces. Cut sections of the lung will reveal fine honeycomb changes that are most marked in the lower zones and subpleural regions (Figure 18-1). In lesser degrees of asbestosis, the lungs can feel indurated without obvious honeycombing, or may appear normal on gross examination. Concomitantly, there is often thickening of the visceral and parietal pleura and/or plaques but these do not correlate with the extent of the lung parenchymal abnormalities.

MICROSCOPIC FINDINGS

The diagnosis of asbestosis is usually made from evaluation of a surgical tissue sample or autopsy sample, rather than a transbronchial biopsy. Transbronchial biopsies are generally not satisfactory for diagnosis of

cases, and therefore there are no accurate data for the incidence and prevalence of asbestosis by country. However, in industrialized nations where control of dust emissions has been exercised, the incidence of symptomatic asbestosis has declined considerably. Clinical cases of asbestosis are usually seen in the context of prolonged substantial direct exposures several decades ago, and the latency from first exposure to presentation is typically over 20 years. The onset of symptoms is insidious, with breathlessness on effort, and any progression, if it occurs, takes place over many years. Cough may occur in the later stages, and finger clubbing develops in about half of those with advanced fibrosis. Fine inspiratory crackles are present bilaterally at the lung bases and extend to the middle and upper zones with disease progression. Finally, cor pulmonale and death may result. Lung function tests usually show a restrictive pattern.

RADIOLOGIC FEATURES

On chest radiographs, asbestosis typically results in irregular small opacities, first at the lung bases and later in the middle and upper zones. In the later stages, honeycombing may occur. In about one-third there is also pleural thickening, with or without calcification. High-resolution computed tomography (HRCT) is more sensitive than standard chest radiographs for detecting the changes of asbestosis, but the findings are not specific.

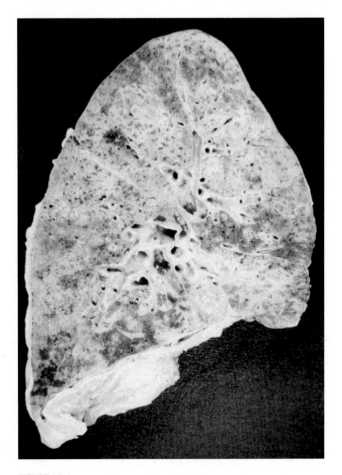

FIGURE 18-1

Asbestosis

Cut section of a contracted lung showing fine honeycombing that is most marked in the lower zones.

asbestosis. The histologic features are similar to those of idiopathic interstitial fibrosis with the additional finding of asbestos bodies. There is a commonly used light microscopic grading system (Table 18-2), and clinical symptoms and radiologic changes are usually found only in the higher grades. The earliest changes are seen around the respiratory bronchioles, but as the disease progresses, the fibrosis extends along alveolar walls and alveolar ducts to link up with other lesions (Figure 18-2). Eventually, severe disorganization of lung architecture occurs, with honeycomb changes (Figure 18-3). Other features less commonly encountered are foreign body giant cells around the asbestos bodies, osseous metaplasia, and pulmonary blue bodies (Figure 18-4).

An asbestos body is characterized by a clear fibrous core coated by iron-protein-mucopolysaccharide material which forms a golden-brown, beaded, dumbbell or drumstick-shaped structure (Figure 18-5). When these cores have been examined by analytical techniques, they are almost always amphibole fibers. The Prussian blue stain can be used to highlight the asbestos bodies because of the iron content. Care has to be taken in identifying them because other materials can be coated to form ferruginous bodies, but usually their cores are different and are not clear (Figure18-6). Although there is no universally agreed upon number of asbestos bodies needed to make a diagnosis of asbestosis, a general guideline is that 2 or more per cm^2 should be present to make a confident diagnosis.

TABLE 18-2
Light Microscopic Grading Scheme for Asbestosis

Grade 0	No peribronchiolar fibrosis or less than half of bronchioles involved
Grade 1	Fibrosis confined to the walls of respiratory bronchioles and first adjacent tier of alveoli
Grade 2	Fibrosis around respiratory bronchioles which extends into adjacent alveolar ducts and alveoli but does not join up with fibrosis extending from other respiratory bronchioles
Grade 3	Fibrosis that links up adjacent respiratory bronchioles but with little architectural distortion
Grade 4	Honeycomb changes

Modified from CAP-NIOSH and Sporn-Roggli schema: Craighead JE et al. *Arch Pathol Lab Med*. 1982;106:544-596; Roggli VL et al. *Pathology of Asbestos-Associated Diseases*. 2nd ed. Springer, 2004.

ANCILLARY STUDIES

Mineral analysis of bronchoalveolar lavage (BAL) or lung tissue shows high asbestos fiber/body burdens in cases of asbestosis. A normal count would provide strong evidence against a diagnosis of asbestosis. In a

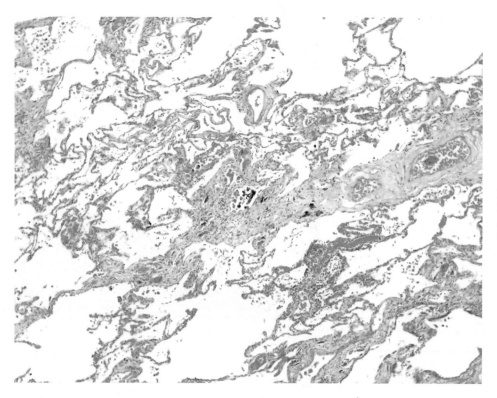

FIGURE 18-2

Asbestosis

Slight interstitial fibrosis (grade 2) extending out from respiratory bronchioles, but with good preservation of lung architecture.

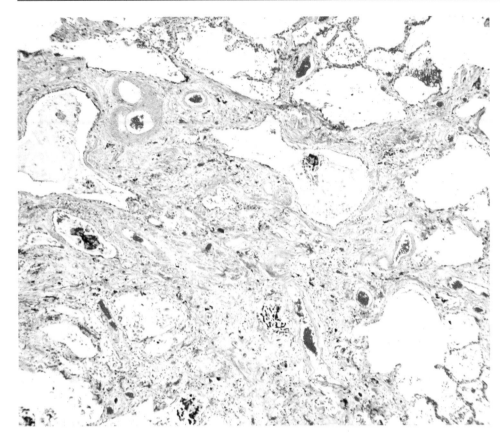

FIGURE 18-3

Asbestosis

Severe interstitial fibrosis with disorganization of lung architecture.

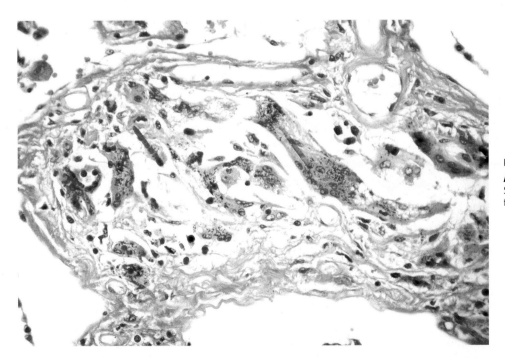

FIGURE 18-4

Asbestosis

Several asbestos bodies and associated foreign body giant cell reaction.

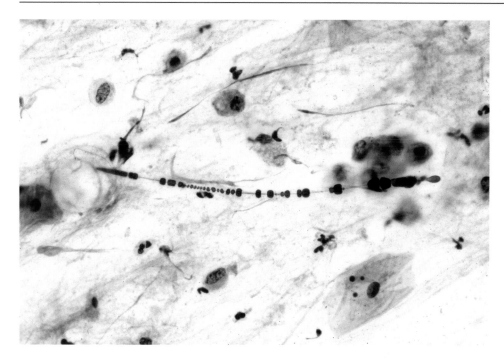

FIGURE 18-5
Asbestosis
An asbestos body showing a clear fibrous core coated by iron-containing material.

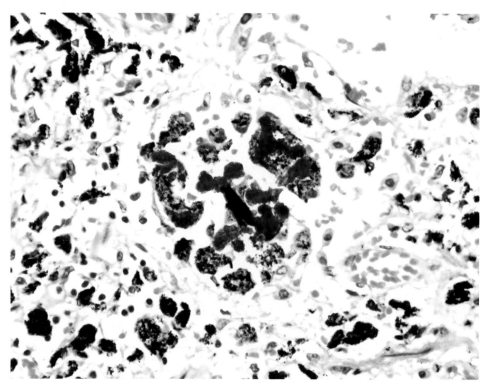

FIGURE 18-6
Coal workers' pneumoconiosis
"Coal bodies" formed on black and brown irregularly shaped material.

setting of asbestosis, the BAL usually shows a concentration greatly above 1 fiber per ml. It is distinctly unusual for a case of diffuse interstitial fibrosis without asbestos bodies on light microscopy to show lung tissue concentrations of asbestos fibers in the range usually associated with asbestosis.

DIFFERENTIAL DIAGNOSIS

In advanced cases, the major differential diagnoses include idiopathic pulmonary fibrosis, chronic extrinsic allergic alveolitis, sarcoidosis, Langerhans cell histiocytosis, and other mineral-dust-induced pneumoconioses such as silicosis and siderosis. Asbestosis is usually associated with the presence of numerous asbestos bodies and this separates it from idiopathic pulmonary fibrosis and the other conditions listed above. Also, the presence of fibroblast foci is uncommon in asbestosis. Granulomas or Langerhans cell aggregates with mixed inflammation would be compatible with diagnoses of sarcoidosis and Langerhans cell histiocytosis, respectively. For diagnosis

of the other mineral-induced pneumoconioses such as silicosis and siderosis, characteristic features should be present, such as silicotic nodules in silicosis and pseudo-asbestos bodies with yellow or black cores in welders' siderosis.

There are considerable problems in separating grade 1 and 2 lesions of asbestosis from peribronchiolar fibrosis due to cigarette smoking, urban pollution, and mineral-dust-induced lesions. These grades of fibrosis are frequent in non-asbestos exposed individuals, on the order of 40% of the general population.

PROGNOSIS AND THERAPY

There is no specific therapy, and treatment is symptomatic. Progression is slow, but not invariable, and is dependent on cumulative exposure and fiber type. Today, it is uncommon to see fatal cases of asbestosis. However, there is an increased risk of mesothelioma in these patients as well as lung cancer, the latter due to the synergy between asbestos exposure and smoking.

SILICOSIS

Silicosis is a chronic, diffuse, interstitial, nodular lung disease resulting from relatively high-dose crystalline silica exposures taking place over many years. Silica generally comprises more than 10% of the dust, and the remainder consists of other silicates, coal, or iron oxide,

---

ASBESTOSIS—FACT SHEET

Definition
▸ Diffuse pulmonary interstitial fibrosis caused by asbestos exposure

Incidence
▸ There are no reliable data for the incidence of asbestosis in the various countries

Morbidity and Mortality
▸ Morbidity and mortality depends on the severity of fibrosis
▸ In industrialized countries, death due to asbestosis is very uncommon

Gender and Age Distribution
▸ More common in males because of occupation
▸ Onset is usually in the middle-aged or elderly

Clinical Features
▸ Insidious presentation with shortness of breath and later cough
▸ Fine crackles over the bases of the lungs and sometimes finger clubbing
▸ Restrictive pattern on pulmonary function testing

Radiologic Features
▸ Small, irregular opacities more prevalent in the lower zones
▸ Honeycombing in advanced cases
▸ Frequent coexisting pleural changes include thickening, plaques, and rounded atelectasis

Prognosis and Therapy
▸ Usually slowly progressive, if at all, nowadays
▸ No specific treatment
▸ Increased risk of associated lung cancer

ASBESTOSIS—PATHOLOGIC FEATURES

Gross Findings
▸ Contracted lungs with bosselated surfaces in advanced cases
▸ Cut sections reveal fine honeycombing that is most marked in the lower zones and subpleural regions

Microscopic Findings
▸ Various grades of interstitial fibrosis ranging from peribronchiolar to diffuse with linking up of adjacent foci and disorganization of lung architecture
▸ Asbestos bodies
▸ Foreign-body giant cells
▸ Foci of ossification

Pathologic Differential Diagnosis
▸ Usual interstitial pneumonia
▸ Nonspecific interstitial pneumonia, fibrotic
▸ Langerhans cell histiocytosis
▸ Chronic hypersensitivity pneumonitis

depending on the source. Exposure can occur during extraction of stone (tunneling, mining, and quarrying), processing of stone or sand, abrasive use of silica or sand (for example, sand blasting and foundry casting), production of fine silica powder, and use of sand or silica in glass and ceramic manufacture. The chronic form of the disease is the most frequently observed, but severe disabling forms are infrequent now in developed countries because of improved industrial hygiene. Complications include tuberculosis, scleroderma, and, more debatably, lung cancer. Where the silica content of the dust is below 10%, mixed-dust pneumoconiosis rather than silicosis may result. The acute form (silicoproteinosis) is rarely seen because it is associated with very high exposures to very fine particulates, as can result from silica sandblasting, and it can develop within a few weeks or months of first exposure to the dust.

CLINICAL FEATURES

Symptoms and signs are nonspecific and include productive cough and slowly progressive shortness of breath on exertion. Presentation is usually in adults more than 40 years of age and frequently occurs several years after exposure has ceased. Clinical diagnosis relies on the occupational history, appropriate radiologic changes, and exclusion of other possible causes. Respiratory function is often normal in the early stages, but a mixed pattern of obstruction and restriction is seen with advanced disease.

RADIOLOGIC FEATURES

Typical radiographic changes of silicosis are diffuse nodular opacities, with predominance in the upper zones, and enlargement of mediastinal and hilar lymph nodes with peripheral calcification ("egg-shell"). Parenchymal lung lesions over 1 cm are designated "progressive massive fibrosis." Pleural fibrosis frequently accompanies progressive massive fibrosis in silicosis.

PATHOLOGIC FEATURES

GROSS FINDINGS

The typical appearance is that of well demarcated, round, hard, grey-to-black nodules measuring a few millimeters in size or more, most prevalent in the upper zones of the lobes (Figure 18-7). Larger nodules measuring up to several centimeters may be present, but these are less numerous than the smaller nodules and occur at later stages of the disease. When the nodules exceed

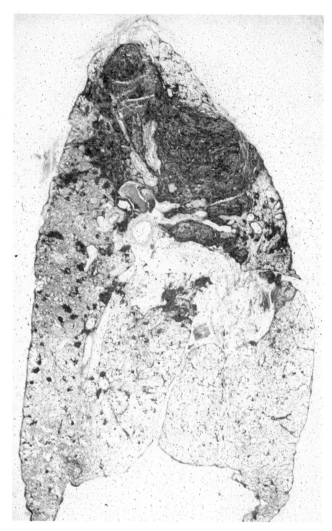

FIGURE 18-7
Silicosis
Typical well demarcated, round, whorled nodules.

1 cm in diameter, the term "progressive massive fibrosis" (PMF) may be used, and indicates more severe disease. Cavitation can occur, usually as a result of ischemia, but mycobacterial infection should be looked for because silica exposure does predispose to mycobacterial infection. Macular lesions may also be seen.

MICROSCOPIC FINDINGS

In individuals exposed to dusts containing mixtures of silica and silicates, there is usually a combination of 3 types of lesions: dust macules, mixed-dust fibrotic nodules, and classical silicotic nodules, the latter predominating in classical silicosis, whereas the mixed-dust fibrotic nodules predominate in mixed-dust fibrosis (Figures 18-8, 18-9, 18-10). Macules are interstitial collections of dust-containing macrophages with little or no associated fibrosis and as such are similar to those seen in coal workers' pneumoconiosis and silicatosis. The

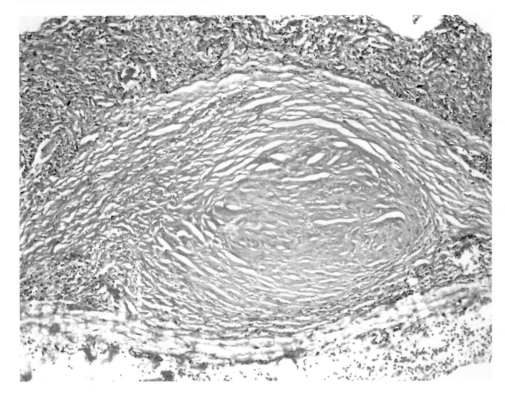

FIGURE 18-8

Silicosis

Typical whorled silicotic nodule with central collagenous area surrounded by cellular area containing numerous particles.

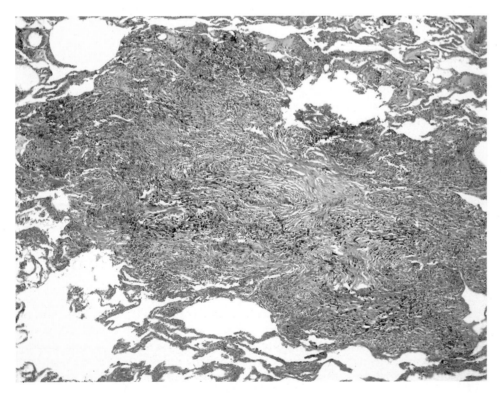

FIGURE 18-9

Silicosis

Mixed-dust fibrotic nodule which is stellate and shows haphazardly arranged collagen at the center.

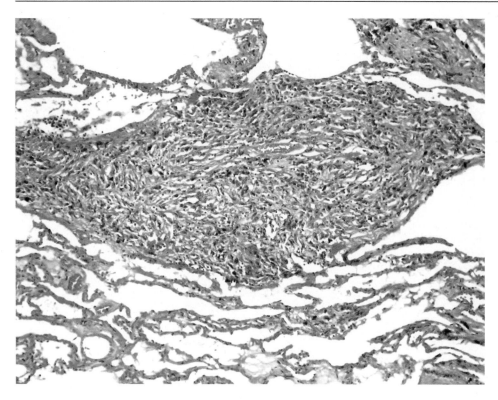

FIGURE 18-10
Silicosis
Macule containing numerous particle-laden macrophages with little collagen.

classical silicotic nodule is circumscribed with hyalin-ized whorled collagen centrally and a cellular periphery consisting of lymphocytes and macrophages containing dust particles. The center may show necrosis with vari-able amounts of calcification. When examined under polarized light, the weakly birefringent silica particles can be seen throughout the nodule, whereas the more strongly birefringent silicate particles are more prevalent at the periphery of the nodule. PMF lesions of silicosis are typically formed by coalescence of individual nod-ules that can still be identified (Figure 18-11). Hilar lymph nodes often contain silicotic nodules, but if lung lesions are absent, the patient should not be diagnosed with silicosis. Mixed-dust fibrotic nodules are palpable, stellate lesions with central variably collagenized areas. Macules and mixed-dust fibrotic nodules tend to spread diffusely into the adjacent interstitium. Caplan's-type lesions (see below) are occasionally seen in silicosis.

Acute silicosis shows a lipoproteinosis picture, the alveolar spaces being filled with acellular, finely granu-lar, eosinophilic PAS-positive material. Sometimes, but not always, immature silicotic nodules may be seen within the interstitium.

DIFFERENTIAL DIAGNOSIS

The typical whorled fibrotic nodules, when numerous, are virtually pathognomonic of silicosis. In these cases, it should not be difficult to establish an occupational source for the exposure(s). Occasional isolated nodules may be mimicked by healed tuberculous lesions, sar-coidosis lesions, Caplan's lesions, and rheumatoid nod-ules. The presence of polarizable particles, particularly at the periphery of the nodule, helps to establish a diag-nosis of silicotic or mixed-dust fibrotic nodule. In diffi-cult cases, mineralogical analysis of the lung tissues may be necessary to establish the diagnosis.

PROGNOSIS AND THERAPY

Management has largely concentrated on prevention with dust control measures. Treatment is symptomatic, since there is no specific therapy. Progression is typi-cally slow and may not cause too severe a degree of im-pairment in elderly patients, but transplantation may be necessary in younger individuals with severe progres-sive disease.

COAL WORKERS' PNEUMOCONIOSIS

Coal workers' pneumoconiosis (CWP) results from ex-posure to coal dust, which usually occurs during the mining process. Cases have also been described, how-ever, in coal trimmers employed in loading coal onto ships. Coals are complex materials rich in carbon but

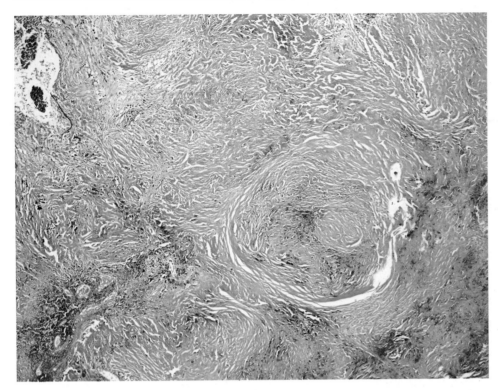

FIGURE 18-11
Silicosis
Progressive massive fibrosis lesion composed of fused individual silicotic nodules.

SILICOSIS—FACT SHEET

Definition
▸ Silicosis is a predominantly nodular pneumoconiosis caused by exposure to dusts containing a substantial proportion of crystalline silica

Incidence
▸ It is estimated that in the U.S. the rate is about 500 cases per 100,000, and there is a population of 200,000 at risk
▸ The acute form (silicoproteinosis) is rarely seen nowadays

Mortality
▸ About 200 cases per annum are recorded on death certificates in the U.S.

Gender and Age Distribution
▸ Primarily seen in middle-aged or elderly males because of long latency and occupation

Clinical Features
▸ Insidious onset of shortness of breath and productive cough

Radiologic Features
▸ Diffuse nodular opacities with a predominance in the upper zones and enlargement of mediastinal and hilar lymph nodes with peripheral calcification ("egg-shell")

Prognosis and Therapy
▸ Progression is typically slow
▸ Treatment is symptomatic since there is no specific therapy

SILICOSIS—PATHOLOGIC FEATURES

Gross Findings
▸ Combinations of macules and nodules, most marked in the upper zones
▸ Progressive massive fibrosis lesions can occur and may cavitate

Microscopic Findings
▸ Dust macules, mixed-dust fibrotic nodules and classical silicotic nodules, the latter predominating in classical silicosis, whereas the mixed-dust fibrotic nodules predominate in mixed-dust fibrosis
  ▸ Macule: interstitial collection of dust-containing macrophaes with little or no associated fibrosis
  ▸ Silicotic nodule: circumscribed nodule with central hyalinized whorled collagen and a cellular periphery of lymphocytes and macrophages containing dust particles
  ▸ Mixed dust fibrotic nodule: variably pigmented nodule with whorled collagen at its center and a peripheral cuff of macrophages that extend out into the adjacent interstitial areas (not as well circumscribed as the silicotic nodule)
▸ On polarized light, the weakly birefringent silica particles can be seen throughout the nodules, whereas the more strongly birefringent silicate particles are more prevalent at the periphery of the nodules
▸ Progressive massive fibrosis lesions of silicosis are typically formed by coalescence of individual nodules which can still be identified
▸ Hilar lymph nodes commonly contain silicotic nodules, but if lung lesions are absent they should not be considered diagnostic of silicosis

Pathologic Differential Diagnosis
▸ When numerous, the typical whorled fibrotic nodules are virtually pathognomonic of silicosis
▸ Occasional isolated nodules may be mimicked by healed tuberculous lesions, sarcoid lesions, Caplan lesions, and rheumatoid nodules

also containing some silica, a range of silicates, and some trace elements including titanium and beryllium. Based on calorific value, coals are ranked into low, medium, and high groups. The incidence of CWP varies from mine to mine and even within mines according to cumulative exposure, particle-size distribution, coal rank, and the concentration of silica and other clay minerals such has mica and illite. In addition to the dust-derived lesions, exposure to coal dust results in chronic bronchitis and emphysema.

CLINICAL FEATURES

Despite the presence of abnormal radiologic changes, affected individuals may be asymptomatic. With more severe disease, however, individuals may complain of cough, often with black sputum, and shortness of breath. Symptoms are usually associated with more advanced stages of PMF rather than simple pneumoconiosis. Pulmonary function tests typically show an obstructive pattern in the advanced stages of PMF, due to concomitant emphysema. Symptomatic CWP is not usually seen with coal dust exposures spanning less than 20 years, and is associated with underground working. Caplan's lesions can arise in coal workers with rheumatoid arthritis and develop more quickly than conventional PMF lesions.

RADIOLOGIC FEATURES

The typical pattern is one of small, rounded opacities that are most prevalent in the upper zones. PMF lesions may occur, are predominant in the upper lobes, and may cavitate. Irregular opacities tend to occur at the bases and appear to largely be the result of emphysema. Caplan's lesions are multiple large, round opacities frequently set in a background of few small opacities or a clear lung field.

PATHOLOGIC FEATURES

GROSS FINDINGS

The earliest lesions are the nonpalpable, stellate, black macules, which measure a few millimeters in size and are scattered through the lungs with upper-zone predominance (Figure 18-12). At their smallest—about 1 mm—they merge with the black lesions seen in urban dwellers. In severe cases, macules may occur in most of the lung lobules and are often accompanied by variable degrees of emphysema. Superimposed upon these

macular lesions may be a lesser number of palpable stellate or rounded fibrotic nodules which are larger than the macules. Lesions above 1 cm are designated as PMF lesions and may cavitate (Figure 18-13). In contrast to silicosis, the lesions in CWP are usually soft and not made up of confluent separate nodules. Other features are blackening of the interlobular septa and pleura as a result of coal dust deposition, and enlargement and blackening of bronchial, hilar, and mediastinal lymph nodes. Emphysema, mainly of the centrilobular type, will frequently be present since coal dust accumulation has an additive effect with cigarette smoking. Caplan's nodules are concentric, usually over 0.5 cm in diameter, scattered irregularly throughout the lungs, and may show necrosis (Figure 18-14); the background lung tissue often shows relatively little evidence of pneumoconiosis.

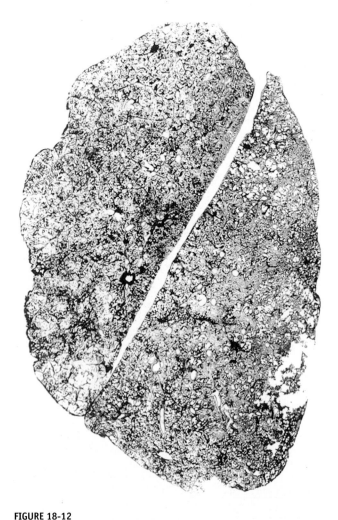

FIGURE 18-12

Coal workers' pneumoconiosis

Simple CWP showing numerous macules with associated emphysema.

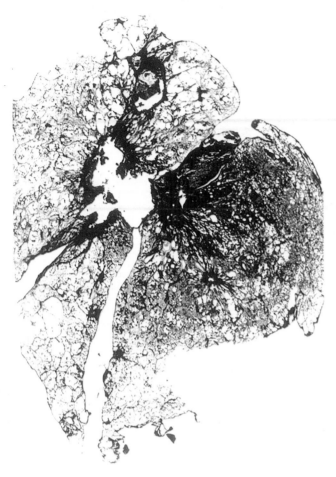

FIGURE 18-13

Coal workers' pneumoconiosis
Complicated CWP demonstrating extensive particle deposition, parenchymal contraction due to associated scarring, and emphysematous changes.

MICROSCOPIC FINDINGS

Macules consist of collections of free and intracellular coal dust particles around respiratory bronchioles with little or no fibrosis (Figures 18-15, 18-16). They are often associated with centrilobular emphysema, often referred to as focal in this context. Dust-containing macrophages may be present in alveolar spaces, and there may be dust deposition along the interlobular septa and pleura. Nodules consist of large quantities of coal dust mixed with irregularly distributed collagen (Figure 18-16). PMF lesions, by definition, exceed 1 cm in diameter and show variable amounts of collagen and necrosis. Vascular obliteration due to infiltration of dust-laden cells may be present in PMF. Caplan's lesions are basically necrobiotic nodules with concentric alternating zones of dust, cells (macrophages, neutrophils, fibroblasts, and occasional giant cells), and circumferentially arranged collagen fibers, fibroblasts, and plasma cells. The fibroblasts adjacent to the necrosis are often palisaded. Ferruginous bodies with black cores are not unusual in CWP, and can potentially be mistaken for asbestos bodies.

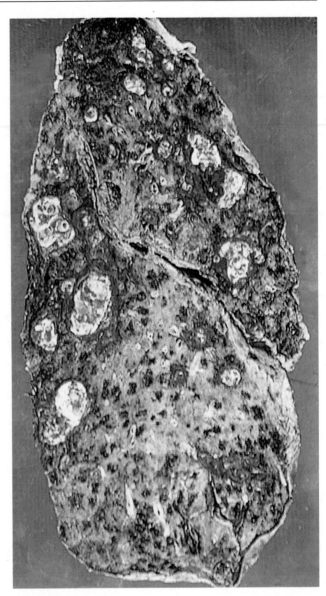

FIGURE 18-14

Coal workers' pneumoconiosis
Typical nodular Caplan lesions, including some with central necrosis, with a background of CWP.

DIFFERENTIAL DIAGNOSIS

Dust-induced lesions similar to the macules of CWP may occur in urban dwellers and those cooking with biogenic fuels in closed spaces. However, the presence of lesions measuring 2 mm or more, and a history of working more than 10 years in coal mines, will establish the diagnosis of CWP. In cases with numerous ferruginous bodies, the changes may be mistaken for asbestosis, but the appearance of the cores (black with coal and clear with asbestos) will clarify the diagnosis.

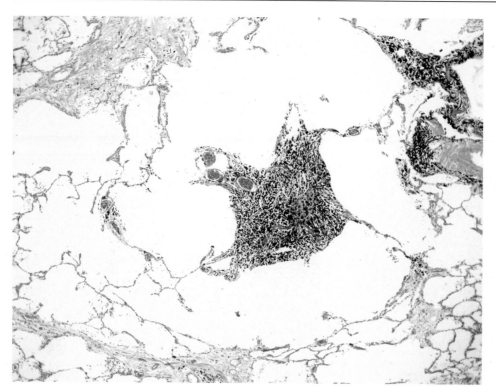

FIGURE 18-15

Coal workers' pneumoconiosis
Macule consisting of a collection of coal dust particles adjacent to a respiratory bronchiole (not seen in this view).

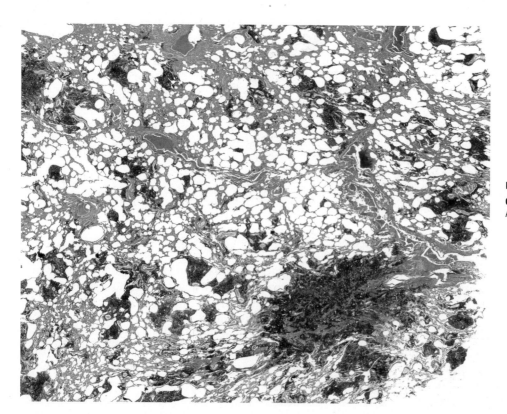

FIGURE 18-16

Coal workers' pneumoconiosis
A nodule and numerous macules.

PROGNOSIS AND THERAPY

Management has largely concentrated on prevention with dust control measures. Treatment is symptomatic since there is no specific therapy. If CWP is detected at an early stage, progression is unlikely to occur if there is no further exposure. On the other hand, PMF frequently progresses after cessation of exposure, and death may result from respiratory failure. There is no reduction in life expectancy with simple pneumoconiosis, but about 4% of deaths in coal miners are directly due to complicated CWP.

HARD METAL PNEUMOCONIOSIS

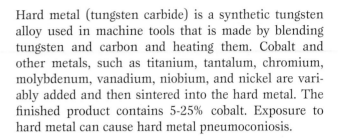

Hard metal (tungsten carbide) is a synthetic tungsten alloy used in machine tools that is made by blending tungsten and carbon and heating them. Cobalt and other metals, such as titanium, tantalum, chromium, molybdenum, vanadium, niobium, and nickel are variably added and then sintered into the hard metal. The finished product contains 5-25% cobalt. Exposure to hard metal can cause hard metal pneumoconiosis.

CLINICAL FEATURES

Exposures ranging from a few months to several years, but usually exceeding 10 years, have induced pneumoconiosis. The clinical features of hard metal pneumoconiosis are variable and may be complicated by asthma or hypersensitivity pneumonitis because inhalation of cobalt can also induce these other conditions.

COAL WORKERS' PNEUMOCONIOSIS—FACT SHEET

Definition

▸▸ Coal workers' pneumoconiosis is a macular and nodular pneumoconiosis that results from exposure to coal dust, which usually occurs during the mining process

Incidence

▸▸ The incidence of this disorder has declined in recent decades due to better dust control
▸▸ Annually, about 1-2% of active and retired coal miners receive compensation for pneumoconiosis

Mortality

▸▸ There is no reduction in life expectancy with simple CWP, but about 4% of those with complicated CWP die directly as a result of it

Gender and Age Distribution

▸▸ Typically seen in middle-aged and elderly men because of long latency and occupation

Clinical Features

▸▸ The individual may be asymptomatic even with radiologic changes, but as the severity of disease worsens, the individual may complain of cough, often with black sputum, and shortness of breath
▸▸ Symptoms are usually associated with more advanced stages of progressive massive fibrosis rather than simple pneumoconiosis
▸▸ Pulmonary function tests will typically show an obstructive pattern in the advanced stages of progressive massive fibrosis due to concomitant emphysema

Radiologic Features

▸▸ The typical pattern is one of small, rounded opacities that are most prevalent in the upper zones
▸▸ Progressive massive fibrosis lesions may occur, are predominant in the upper lobes, and may cavitate

Prognosis and Therapy

▸▸ If CWP is detected at an early stage, progression is unlikely to occur if there is no further exposure
▸▸ Progressive massive fibrosis frequently progresses after removal from exposure, and death may result from respiratory failure
▸▸ Treatment is symptomatic since there is no specific therapy

---

COAL WORKERS' PNEUMOCONIOSIS—PATHOLOGIC FEATURES

Gross Findings

▸▸ Stellate, black macules, which measure a few millimeters in size and are scattered through the lungs with upper-zone predominance; they are often associated with variable degrees of emphysema
▸▸ Superimposed upon these macular lesions may be a lesser number of palpable stellate and/or rounded fibrotic nodules
▸▸ Lesions measuring more than 1 cm are designated as progressive massive fibrosis lesions and may cavitate

Microscopic Findings

▸▸ Macules consist of collections of free and intracellular coal dust particles around respiratory bronchioles, with little or no fibrosis; centrilobular emphysema is often associated with macules and is often referred to as focal, in this context
▸▸ Dust-containing macrophages may be present in alveolar spaces and there may be dust deposition along the interlobular septa and pleura
▸▸ Nodules consist of large quantities of coal dust mixed with irregularly distributed collagen
▸▸ Progressive massive fibrosis lesions show large quantities of coal dust, variable amounts of irregularly distributed collagen, and sometimes necrosis

Pathologic Differential Diagnosis

▸▸ Dust lesions similar to the macules of CWP may occur in urban dwellers and individuals cooking with biogenic fuels in closed spaces
▸▸ The presence of numerous ferruginous ("coal") bodies may cause confusion with asbestosis, but close attention to the appearance of the cores will establish the diagnosis

RADIOLOGIC FEATURES

Radiologic changes are similar to those seen in the various types of idiopathic diffuse interstitial pneumonias, and are predominantly lower- or mid-zonal.

PATHOLOGIC FEATURES

A number of histopathologic responses have resulted from exposure to hard metal, including diffuse interstitial fibrosis, desquamative interstitial pneumonia, hypersensitivity pneumonitis, and asthma, but giant cell interstitial pneumonia (GIP) is considered almost pathognomonic. GIP is characterized by patchy interstitial chronic inflammation with a centrilobular accentuation, numerous intra-alveolar collections of macrophages (as in desquamative interstitial pneumonia), bizarre syncytial giant cells derived from the alveolar epithelium, and foreign body giant cells that often contain macrophages and neutrophils in their cytoplasm (Figures 18-17, 18-18). There is often black particulate material in macrophages and giant cells. Variable degrees of fibrosis may be seen.

DIFFERENTIAL DIAGNOSIS

GIP is virtually pathognomonic of hard metal pneumoconiosis, although there are rare cases which appear to be idiopathic. Cases lacking the typical giant cells, with patterns of diffuse interstitial fibrosis or desquamative interstitial pneumonia, may require mineralogical analysis. Since it is not present in the normal population, demonstration of tungsten (rarely cobalt) in the lung is strong supportive evidence for the diagnosis of hard metal pneumoconiosis.

PROGNOSIS AND THERAPY

There is no specific treatment for hard metal pneumoconiosis. If the patient is removed from exposure relatively early in the disease, recovery may occur, but if the disease

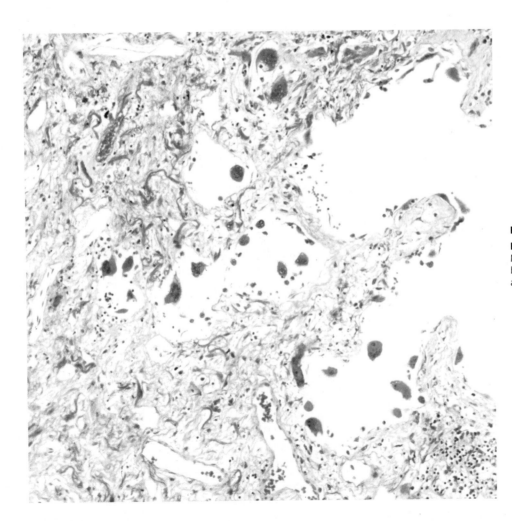

FIGURE 18-17

Hard metal pneumoconiosis
Multiple multinucleated giant cells in a background of interstitial fibrosis and architectural changes.

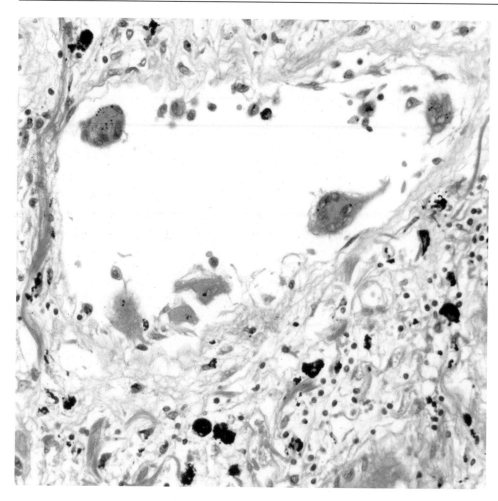

FIGURE 18-18
Hard metal pneumoconiosis
Multinucleated giant cells containing particulate material, in an alveolar space adjacent to a fibrotic alveolar septum.

presents relatively late, permanent fibrosis may result and can cause death. Once diagnosed, the affected individual should not be further exposed to hard metal dust. Corticosteroid treatment is often beneficial in patients with the GIP and desquamative interstitial pneumonia forms of disease, but is often ineffective in those with established fibrosis.

BERYLLIOSIS

Beryllium is used in many industries because of its excellent thermal and electrical conductivity properties and its lightness. Berylliosis, the pneumoconiosis stemming from exposure to beryllium, has been described in a number of settings including fluorescent lamp manufacture, metal and ceramic work, and the aerospace and nuclear industries. Exposure to beryllium compounds can result in acute and chronic lung

diseases. The acute form is very rare nowadays since it results from high exposures to dusts, fumes, or mists. The chronic form follows limited or prolonged exposure to relatively low doses (sometimes as a bystander), involves hypersensitivity reactions, and is a multisystem disease similar to sarcoidosis.

CLINICAL FEATURES

The latent period for chronic berylliosis has been variously described as ranging from 1 month to more than 40 years, but is usually many years. The disorder has an insidious onset closely mimicking sarcoidosis. Approximately one-half of cases develop during the period of exposure, and another third within 5 years after cessation of exposure. Some cases are discovered incidentally during routine surveillance of at-risk workers, whereas others present with progressive dyspnea and cough. Skin lesions may occur.

RADIOLOGIC FEATURES

Radiologic abnormalities are nonspecific and similar to sarcoidosis, with small opacities or larger nodules, with or without reticular shadows that predominate in the upper zones of the lungs.

PATHOLOGIC FEATURES

GROSS FINDINGS

In severe chronic cases coming to autopsy, the lungs appear contracted with bosselated pleural surfaces. The cut surfaces show honeycombing, which is most marked in the upper zones.

MICROSCOPIC FINDINGS

The acute form results in diffuse alveolar damage and the chronic form usually displays noncaseating granulomas resembling those of sarcoidosis and interstitial infiltrates of lymphocytes and plasma cells that tend to be more conspicuous than in sarcoidosis (Figure 18-19). Cells may contain Schaumann's and asteroid bodies, and confluent masses of granulomas may develop. Variable degrees of diffuse interstitial fibrosis occur and large,

hyalinized fibrotic nodules may be present. Sometimes, after many years, only diffuse interstitial fibrosis is seen, without granulomas, but Schaumann's bodies are often present to hint at the previous presence of granulomas (Figure 18-20). Granulomas and fibrotic nodules may be seen in the hilar lymph nodes and other organs.

DIFFERENTIAL DIAGNOSIS

Due to its histologic and radiologic similarities, sarcoidosis is the most important differential diagnostic consideration. Diagnosis of chronic berylliosis is supported by a significant history of exposure to beryllium, detection of beryllium in tissues, and evidence of sensitivity to beryllium as measured by lymphocyte transformation tests of blood or cells obtained by bronchoalveolar lavage.

PROGNOSIS AND THERAPY

There is no specific treatment for berylliosis, and the disease course cannot be predicted. Systemic corticosteroids may be beneficial in the short-term treatment of respiratory symptoms, but their effect on long-term prognosis is unknown. Cor pulmonale due to extensive pulmonary fibrosis can occur in some patients.

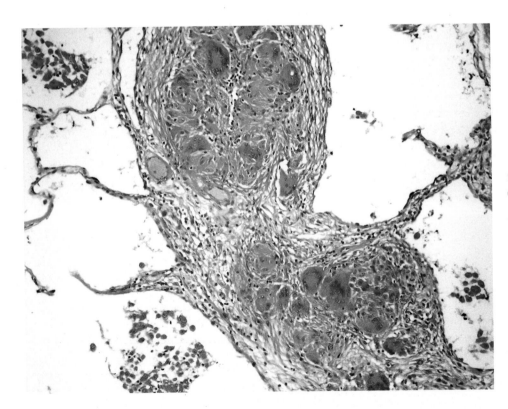

FIGURE 18-19
Chronic berylliosis
Numerous well demarcated, non-caseating, sarcoid-like granulomas.

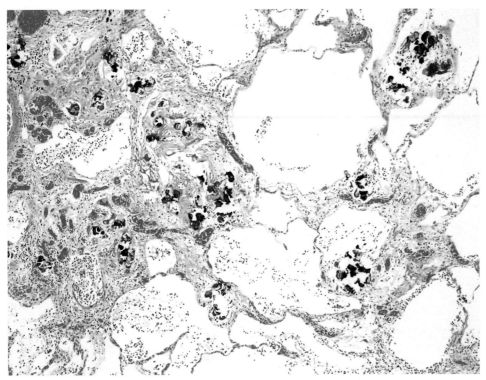

FIGURE 18-20
Chronic berylliosis
Extensive interstitial fibrosis with focal collections of Schaumann's bodies.

SIDEROSIS

Chronic exposure to dusts predominantly containing iron dust, iron oxide dust, or iron fumes with little or no silica, can lead to a condition called siderosis. Arc welders' pneumoconiosis is an example of a disorder that falls under this heading, but siderosis can also be seen in silver polishers, ochre workers, and others exposed to high concentrations of iron oxide. The particles are weakly fibrogenic and therefore usually cause little functional impairment despite the presence of opacities on chest radiographs. On light microscopy, siderosis is characterized by the accumulation of dark-brown, dust-laden macrophages with little associated fibrosis (Figures 18-21, 18-22). There are also ferruginous bodies containing black cores.

SILICATOSIS

The nonfibrous silicates are a large group of minerals which are extensively used in industry and include kaolin, talc, mica, and fuller's earth. They are less fibrogenic than asbestos and silica. However, they can cause pneumoconiosis (silicatosis) when exposures are prolonged and heavy, and where the silica content is usually less than 1%. Specific examples include kaolinosis,

talcosis, mica pneumoconiosis, and fuller's earth pneumoconiosis. Chest radiographs usually show small, rounded opacities and occasionally PMF.

These disorders show common histopathologic features. Grossly there are usually soft, stellate, grey lesions which can cavitate. Sometimes honeycombing is present. Microscopically, there are interstitial collections of macrophages containing strongly birefringent particles when viewed under polarized light. These macrophages and particles are seen at first around respiratory bronchioles, but later extend along alveolar ducts and alveolar walls to link up, and may result in diffuse interstitial collections with fine fibrosis. Foreign-body giant cells and ferruginous bodies formed on strongly birefringent particles are frequently present (Figures 18-23, 18-24). The changes must be distinguished from asbestosis, but there is usually a strong occupational history of nonfibrous silicate exposure (for example, kaolin mining, mica grinding, etc.) to assist in making the correct diagnosis, and polarization of the sections will reveal the strongly birefringent particles. In difficult cases, mineralogical analysis will provide the answer.

TOXIC GASES AND FUMES

Many different agents, either alone or in combination, can cause lung injury with a variety of manifestations.

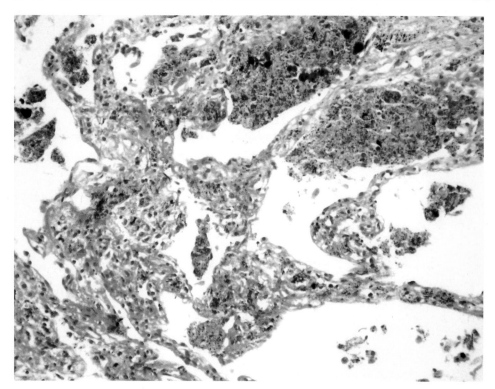

FIGURE 18-21

Siderosis
An arc welder's lung showing abundant brown and black particulate material with little associated fibrosis.

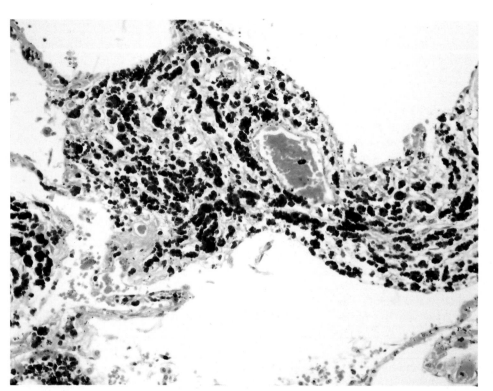

FIGURE 18-22

Siderosis
An arc welder's lung showing numerous brown and black particulate deposits and ferruginous bodies with black cores, with little associated fibrosis.

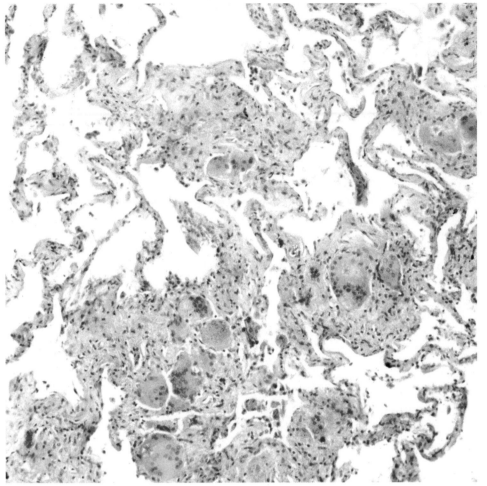

FIGURE 18-23
Talcosis
Interstitial multinucleated giant cells with interstitial fibrosis and a ferruginous body.

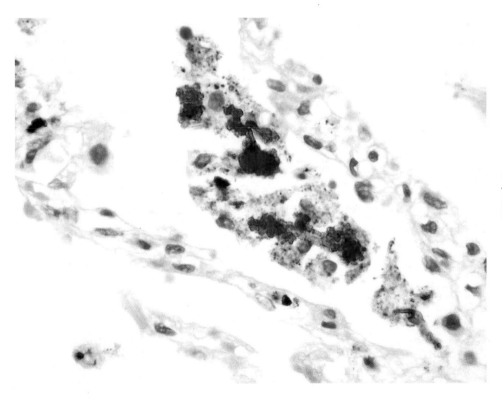

FIGURE 18-24
Talcosis
Several ferruginous bodies in an alveolar space.

CLINICAL FEATURES

There are three main presentations:
1. "Metal fume fever" resembles a mild, self-limiting, flu-like illness with onset about 4 to 8 hours after exposure to metal fumes. Zinc can trigger this type of reaction.
2. Many agents cause irritation of the upper respiratory tract and/or diffuse alveolar damage. The solubility, concentration, duration of exposure, and depth of inhalation influence whether injury occurs predominantly in the upper respiratory tract and larger airways or in the small airways and lung parenchyma. Highly water-soluble agents such as NH_3, SO_2, and HCl affect mainly the upper respiratory tract, whereas less water-soluble agents, such as oxides of nitrogen, affect the lung parenchyma and small airways. Table 18-3 shows some of the fumes and gases that have resulted in diffuse alveolar damage (toxic pneumonitis, chemical pneumonitis).
3. Subacute inflammation occurs after weeks or months of exposure to the offending agent. Examples include the Ardystil syndrome, caused by spraying of textiles with dyes containing Acramin FWR and Acramin FWN, and nylon flock workers' lung, caused by synthetic organic microfibers.

RADIOLOGIC FEATURES

Chest radiographs are usually normal or, as in metal fume fever, demonstrate transient infiltrates. With diffuse alveolar damage, there is interstitial and alveolar edema with patchy infiltrates. In the Ardystil syndrome, patchy infiltrates or micronodules are seen, and interstitial changes of variable severity occur with nylon flock workers' lung.

TABLE 18-3

Fumes and Gases Associated with Diffuse Alveolar Damage

Irritant gases:	NH_3, SO_2, HCl, Cl_2, H_2S, oxides of nitrogen, phosgene
Organic chemicals:	Aldehydes, isocyanates, amines, paraquat
Metallic compounds:	Cadmium, beryllium, mercury, nickel
Complex mixtures:	Fire smoke, pyrolysis products from plastics

PATHOLOGIC FEATURES

There are no documented changes in metal fume fever. Features of diffuse alveolar damage are described in Chapter 9 (Figure 18-25). In the Ardystil syndrome, organizing pneumonia is characteristic. In nylon flock workers' pneumoconiosis, there is lymphocytic bronchiolitis and lymphoid hyperplasia. Small airway injury by a variety of agents can lead to obliterative bronchiolitis.

PROGNOSIS AND THERAPY

The prognosis varies with the type and severity of the lung injury. For most agents, therapy is supportive.

INTRAVENOUS TALCOSIS AND OTHER CONSEQUENCES OF INTRAVENOUS DRUG ABUSE

Intravenous drug usage can lead to multiple types of infectious and noninfectious pulmonary complications. Among these are lesions resulting from the delivery of insoluble minerals to the lung, which are contained in drugs intended for oral use. These materials include talc, microcrystalline cellulose, and cornstarch. When relatively small quantities are present, histologic responses may be subtle, but become more conspicuous with greater quantities. Foreign-body granulomas, interstitial fibrosis, massive fibrosis, thrombotic pulmonary hypertensive lesions, and emphysema may result. Refractile particles situated around small pulmonary blood vessels are suggestive of intravenous drug abuse. Viewing the lesions with polarized light will demonstrate the inciting particles, which are large, pale-yellow, and platy in the case of talc, elongated and crystalline with cellulose (positive with PAS with diastase, methenamine silver, and Congo Red), and round with a Maltese-cross arrangement with cornstarch (Figure 18-26). Particles larger than 5 microns are frequently present, providing a clue that the particles were delivered via the bloodstream rather than through the airways. Individuals with massive fibrotic lesions and diffuse interstitial fibrosis usually have marked decrements in lung function which may be life-threatening. When emphysema is present, it is usually of the panacinar type, and shows greater severity in the lower zones. It has most frequently been associated with methylphenidate (Ritalin) abuse.

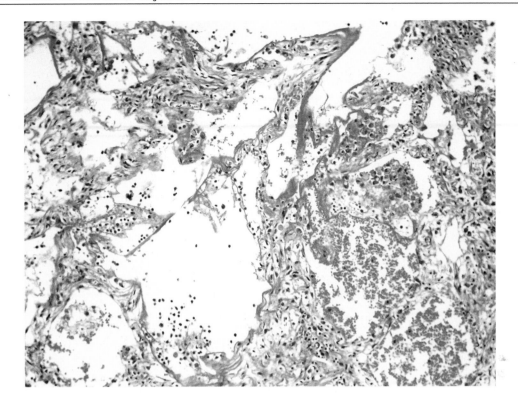

FIGURE 18-25

Acute cadmium toxicity
Diffuse alveolar damage with well developed hyaline membranes, in a patient who had welded cadmium-coated bolts a few days earlier, a few hours after which he developed respiratory failure. Large quantities of cadmium were present in the lungs.

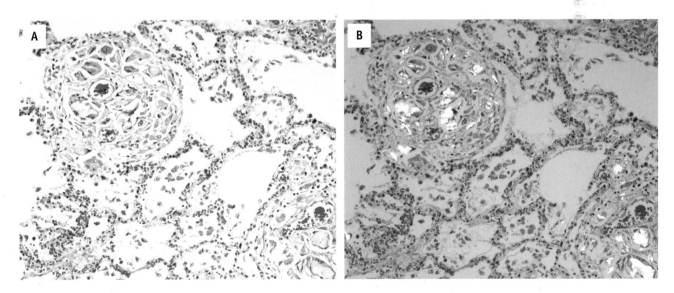

FIGURE 18-26

Intravenous talcosis
(A) Pale-yellow plate-like talc particles adjacent to blood vessels, many in giant cells. (B) A view under polarized light.

SUGGESTED READINGS

1. Churg A, Green FHY. *Pathology of Occupational Lung Disease*. 2nd ed. Baltimore: Williams and Wilkins; 1998.
2. Gibbs AR. Occupational lung disease. In: Hasleton PS, ed. *Spencer's Pathology of the Lung*. 5 ed. New York: McGraw Hill; 1996:461-506.
3. Gibbs AR, Pooley FD, Griffiths DM, et al. Talc pneumoconiosis: a pathologic and mineralogic study. *Hum Pathol*. 1992;23:1344-54.
4. Hendrick DJ, Sherwood Burge P, Beckett WS, Churg A. *Occupational Disorders of the Lung*. London: W B Saunders; 2002.
5. Hendrick DJ. Toxic lung injury: inhaled agents. In : Gibson GJ, Geddes DM, Costabel U, Sterk PJ, Corrin B, eds. *Respiratory Medicine*. 3rd ed. Edinburgh: Saunders; 2003:807-24.
6. Honma K, Abraham JL, Chiyotani K, et al. Proposed criteria for mixed-dust pneumoconiosis: definition, descriptions, and guidelines for pathologic diagnosis and clinical correlation. *Hum Pathol*. 2004;35:1515-23.
7. Kern DG, Crausman RS, Durand KTH, et al. Flock worker's lung: chronic interstitial lung disease in nylon flocking industry. *Ann Intern Med*. 1998;129:261-72.
8. Kolanz ME. Introduction to beryllium: uses, regulatory history, and disease. *Appl Occup Environ Hyg*. 2001;16:559-67.
9. Moya C, Anto JM, Newman Taylor AJ, The Collaborative Group for the Study of Toxicity in Textile Aerographic Factories: outbreak of organizing pneumonia in textile printing sprayers. *Lancet*. 1994;344:962-3.
10. Nemery B, Verbaken EK, Demedts M. Giant cell interstitial pneumonia (hard metal lung disease, cobalt lung). *Semin Respir Crit Care Med*. 2001;22:435-48.
11. Roggli VL, Oury TD, Sporn TA. *Pathology of Asbestos-Associated Diseases*, 2nd ed. New York: Springer; 2004.
12. Rossman MD. Chronic beryllium disease: a hypersensitivity disorder. *Appl Occup Environ Hyg*. 2001;1:615-8.

19 Drug Reactions and Other Iatrogenic Pulmonary Diseases

Ashley Allison • Dani S. Zander

INTRODUCTION

Iatrogenic lung injury can be induced by a wide variety of agents. A large number of therapeutic drugs, imaging contrast agents, blood products, and radiation have been implicated in the causation of a spectrum of patterns of pulmonary injury, and it is a certainty that more will be identified as time goes on. Adverse drug reactions have been estimated to occur in approximately 5% of all patients receiving any drug and are responsible for up to 0.03% of all hospital deaths. One large study estimated that up to 7% of Americans experienced serious or fatal drug reactions in the year 1994. Although less frequent than liver or cutaneous manifestations, pulmonary involvement deserves special attention due to the potential for severe disease presentations. Fortunately, most outcomes are favorable with withdrawal of the offending agent and, in some cases, immunosuppressive therapy.

In recent years, much attention has been directed to identifying potentially harmful drugs and understanding the complex and varied mechanisms of injury. Some reports published in the 1960s included fewer than 20 drugs which were believed to cause lung injury. Currently, more than 300 drugs have been implicated, spanning virtually all areas of medicine from family practice to oncology. The drugs associated with the highest rate of occurrence of adverse pulmonary reactions include the chemotherapeutic agents, nitrofurantoin, and amiodarone, but essentially any drug can be a potential cause of an idiosyncratic reaction.

Establishing a definite linkage between a potential etiologic agent and the lung injury is not always achievable, so in some cases a particular agent may be considered as a "probable" or "possible" cause of the lung injury encountered. Evaluation of patients for these complications should include a comprehensive review of all therapeutic agents being administered, their dosages, and the temporal relationships between initiation and cessation of the agents and the evolution of the patient's symptomatology. In general, evidence of a temporal association between drug usage and development of symptoms, and conversely, drug cessation and improvement in symptoms, supports linking a specific agent to a patient's respiratory disease.

For many agents, considerable data exist regarding the manifestations of drug-related lung injury. Correlation of an individual's clinical and radiologic picture with this literature, for potentially causative agents, is important. Co-existing medical conditions can affect patient presentation, as can simultaneous treatment with multiple agents. For immunocompromised patients, opportunistic infections are usually considered in the differential diagnosis and should be carefully evaluated for before the lung injury is attributed solely to an adverse drug effect. Although the diagnosis of drug-related pulmonary injury is often made clinically, lung biopsy can be helpful for establishing that compatible (although usually not specific) histologic findings are evident and excluding the presence of infection, recurrent disease, or another type of lung disease altogether.

Risk factors for pulmonary toxicity are not well understood, for many agents. Drug dosage may be important for some drugs (amiodarone, nitrosoureas), but is not always predictive even for these agents; amiodarone has been reported to induce drug reactions in what is considered to be a safe, low dosage of less then 200 mg. Other risk factors that apply to individual agents may include advanced age, renal dysfunction causing decreased drug elimination and elevated drug levels, rapid infusion with resultant elevated blood levels, and concurrent administration of an agent (for example, a chemotherapeutic drug) with potential pulmonary toxicity to a patient receiving high concentrations of oxygen or radiation therapy. Mechanisms of injury also vary for different agents. Cellular toxicity is caused by some agents or their metabolites, such as the chemotherapeutic agents, but host immune and allergic reactions play important roles in the genesis of the lung injury caused by many agents.

If the probable offending agent can be discontinued without significant adverse effects, treatment of the putative drug reaction will usually begin with withdrawal of the agent. For patients with mild reactions of a relatively short duration, this may be sufficient treatment. However, for some reactions that do not resolve with drug cessation, corticosteroids may also be administered.

Although the list of agents linked to pulmonary reactions is extensive, this chapter will focus upon several of the more common agents. Table 19-1 provides a list of the more common therapeutic drugs causing lung injury, and an overview of the more common histopathologic patterns of lung injury associated with drug reactions is shown in Table 19-2. Figures 19-1 through 19-8 show examples of some of these histopathologic patterns. A more complete list of drugs, the types of pulmonary reactions they induce, and an extensive catalog of reference material is available online at *http://www.pneumotox.com*.

AMIODARONE

Amiodarone, an amphophilic benzofuran derivative, is used in the treatment of refractory cardiac arrhythmias. Unfortunately, however, toxic effects on multiple organs including lung, skin, thyroid, eye, and liver have been associated with administration of this drug. Amiodarone pulmonary toxicity (APT) produces a number of characteristic pathologic changes in the lung that can result in respiratory insufficiency of variable severity, or even, uncommonly, in death. Amiodarone and its metabolite, desethylamiodarone, accumulate in tissues, including the lung, and are retained intracellularly in lysosomes, where they interfere with turnover of endogenous phospholipids. The accumulation of lipid imparts a foamy appearance to the cytoplasm of these cells, which is particularly conspicuous in alveolar macrophages of treated patients.

The cumulative prevalence of APT has been estimated between 1-15% of the treated population, and there appears to be some degree of linkage between higher dosages, longer durations of treatment, and an increased risk of developing APT. Nonetheless, patients receiving low dosages (up to 200 mg/day) can still

TABLE 19-1
Medicinal Drugs Associated with Adverse Pulmonary Effects*

Anticonvulsants	Carbamazepine
	Phenytoin
Antidepressants	Fluoxetine
	Tricyclic antidepressants
Anti-inflammatory agents	Aspirin
	Gold
	Methotrexate
	Penicillamine
Antimicrobial agents	Amphotericin B
	Isoniazid
	Minocycline
	Nitrofurantoin
	Sulfonamides
Appetite suppressants	Fenfluramine-phentermine
Cardiovascular agents	Amiodarone
	Angiotensin-converting enzyme Inhibitors
	Anticoagulants
	Beta-blockers
	Hydralazine
	Hydrochlorothiazide
Chemotherapeutic agents	Azathioprine
	Bleomycin
	Busulfan
	Chlorambucil
	Cyclophosphamide
	Cytosine arabinoside
	Docetaxel
	Etoposide
	Fludarabine
	Gemcitabine
	Imatinib mesylate
	Irinotecan
	Melphalan
	Methotrexate
	Mitomycin C
	Nitrosoureas
	Paclitaxel
Endocrine agents	Bromocriptine
	Propylthiouracil
Immunomodulatory agents	Azathioprine
	Interferons
	Interleukin-2
	Sirolimus

*A more comprehensive list can be found at *http://www.pneumotox.com*.

TABLE 19-2

Histopathologic Patterns Associated with Pulmonary Drug Reactions*

Primarily conducting airway-centered injury patterns	Asthma
	Bronchiectasis
Primarily distal parenchymal injury patterns	Pulmonary edema
	Diffuse alveolar damage
	Hypersensitivity pneumonia
	Interstitial pneumonia patterns—nonspecific, usual, lymphoid
	Organizing pneumonia
	Bronchiolitis obliterans
	Alveolar collections of foamy histiocytes
	Eosinophilic pneumonia
	Alveolar hemorrhage
	Panacinar emphysema and bullous lung disease
	Alveolar proteinosis-like exudates
	Obliterative fibrosis
Primarily vascular injury patterns	Pulmonary arterial hypertension
	Pulmonary veno-occlusive disease
	Small vessel vasculitis with alveolar hemorrhage
	Thrombotic and embolic phenomena
	Foreign-body giant cell reaction to intravenously administered drug preparations

*Detailed histopathologic descriptions of these injury patterns are found in the sections of the book devoted to these patterns. Combinations of the above patterns can also occur.

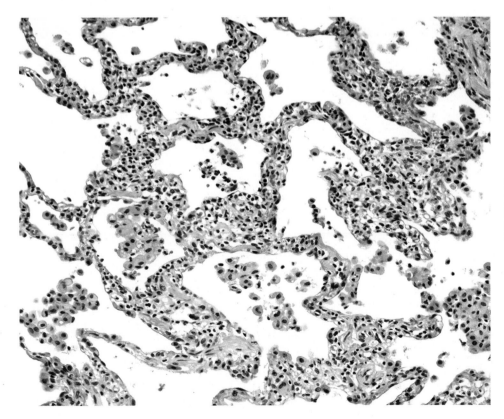

FIGURE 19-1

Nonspecific interstitial pneumonia
Many drugs produce this type of reaction pattern, which is characterized by diffuse interstitial lymphocytic infiltrates.

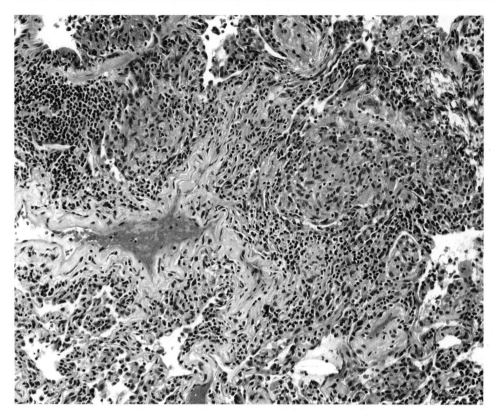

FIGURE 19-2

Hypersensitivity pneumonia
This example demonstrates granuloma formation as well as interstitial mononuclear cell infiltrates.

develop APT, albeit at a lower rate than those treated with higher dosages. Other potential risk factors for APT that have been suggested include a preexisting abnormal chest radiograph or poor pulmonary reserve, exposure to elevated oxygen concentrations, mechanical ventilation, and parenteral injection of iodinated contrast media. Men are affected more frequently than women, and the likelihood of APT appears to increase with age.

A typical presentation of APT includes an insidious onset of dyspnea, dry cough, chest pain, and malaise. Onset can occur at any point between a few days after administration of the loading dose of amiodarone to more than a decade after treatment was started. Development after cessation of therapy can also occur, but is rare. Most reactions develop, however, during the first 2.5 years after initiation of drug therapy. Radiologic features include alveolar, interstitial, or mixed alveolar-interstitial opacities, and an asymmetrical distribution of lung involvement is common. Subpleural masses are seen in a minority of patients, and pleural thickening or effusion may also be evident. Pulmonary function testing reveals a decrease in the carbon monoxide diffusing capacity. The clinical differential diagnosis may include a worsening of heart failure with cardiogenic pulmonary edema, infection, pulmonary infarcts, eosinophilic pneumonia, other drug reactions, aspiration, lymphoma, and bronchioloalveolar carcinoma. If other etiologies for the

lung disease can be eliminated, and APT is judged to be the most likely diagnosis, treatment usually involves withdrawal of the drug, provided that the drug can be discontinued. Clearance from tissues, however, is slow, and visible clinical improvement may take weeks or months. Corticosteroid therapy is also commonly administered, often for long periods of time; premature discontinuation of the corticosteroids may lead to a recurrence of symptoms. Together, this approach will produce radiographic resolution in approximately 85% of patients. In a small number of patients, pulmonary fibrosis develops. The mortality rate for APT has been reported to lie between 21% and 33% in hospitalized patients with APT.

Lung biopsy is usually obtained in patients for whom the diagnosis of APT is uncertain, in whom the amiodarone cannot be discontinued without risks, or who do not show improvement by 1 to 2 months after discontinuation of amiodarone and institution of corticosteroid therapy. Histologic evaluation can determine whether compatible features are present and also whether another process (especially an infection or heart failure) exists or coexists with APT. Biopsy characteristically shows features of a chronic interstitial pneumonia accompanied by lipid-laden macrophages and lipid inclusions in other cell types (Figure 19-9). The lipid-laden macrophages are usually conspicuous in alveolar spaces, and cytoplasmic lipid vacuoles can also be seen in pneumocytes, interstitial cells, and

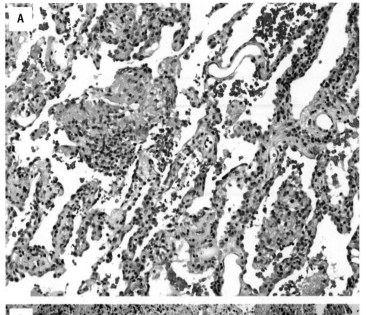

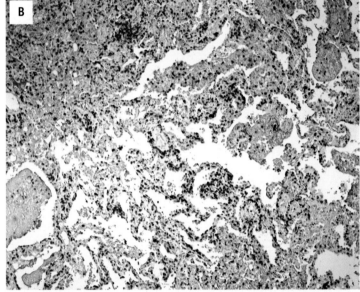

FIGURE 19-3

Gleevec-associated lung injury

(A) Mild interstitial mononuclear cell infiltrates, intra-alveolar fibrin, and an early granuloma are observed in this case of Gleevec-associated lung injury, compatible with a hypersensitivity pneumonia pattern. (B) CD3+ lymphocytes (T-cells) predominate, and few CD20+ B-cells are present (C).

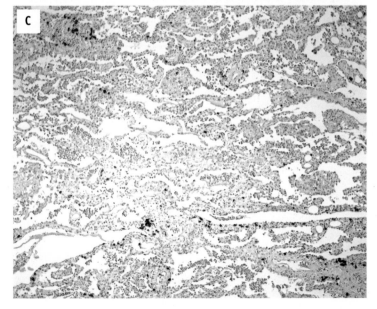

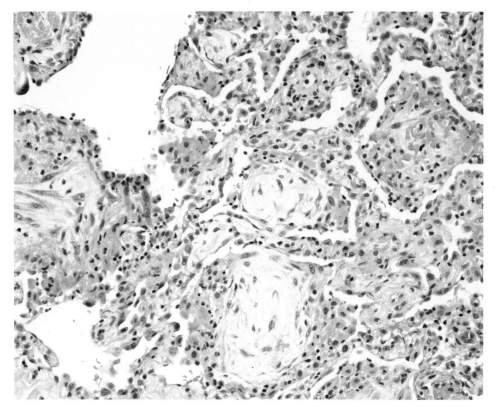

FIGURE 19-4

Organizing pneumonia
Alveolar filling by granulation tissue is characteristic of organizing pneumonia. Organizing pneumonia can be seen as an isolated finding in association with a drug reaction, or can be found in combination with other histologic changes such as hypersensitivity pneumonia or eosinophilic pneumonia.

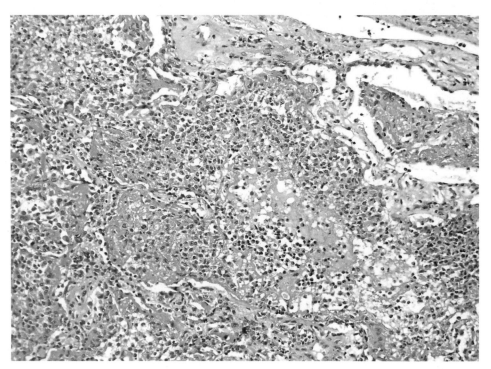

FIGURE 19-5

Eosinophilic pneumonia
Alveoli contain large numbers of eosinophils and macrophages, with admixed fibrinous material and an occasional giant cell. Focal interstitial fibrosis is present. Clinically, this represented an acute exacerbation of a chronic eosinophilic pneumonia.

endothelial cells. Variable numbers of interstitial mononuclear inflammatory cells, primarily lymphocytes, are present, and interstitial edema or fibrosis with type 2 pneumocyte proliferation may be evident. Organizing pneumonia, characterized by myxoid fibroblastic tissue in distal airways and alveoli, is another frequent

finding, and the severity and extensiveness of interstitial and alveolar fibrosis is variable.

In some patients presenting with features of the acute respiratory distress syndrome, a complication occurring almost entirely in patients receiving amiodarone after thoracic surgery, a histologic picture of diffuse alveolar

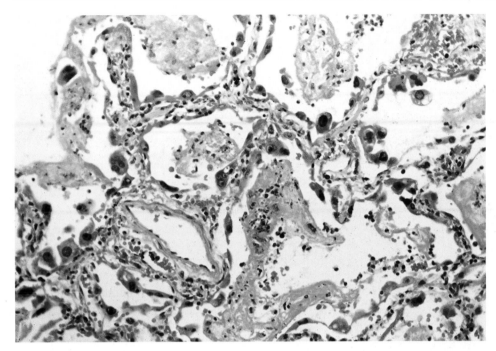

FIGURE 19-6
Busulfan-associated lung injury
The alveolar septa are slightly thickened and mildly inflamed, and fibrinous material with inflammatory cells occupies alveolar spaces. Type 2 pneumocyte proliferation with prominent cytoatypia (nuclear hyperchromasia and enlargement) is present.

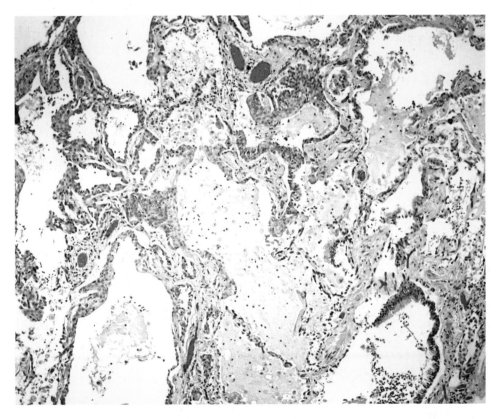

FIGURE 19-7
Chemotherapy-associated lung injury
This patient received multiagent chemotherapy and developed bilateral honeycomb changes. Note the interstitial fibrosis, remodeling, and bronchiolar metaplasia of the alveolar lining.

damage can be seen (Chapter 9). Alveolar hemorrhage is another less common feature.

Bronchoalveolar lavage fluid typically shows foamy macrophages. These cells reflect drug use, but are not specific for drug toxicity, since they are seen in settings with and without clinical and radiologic evidence of

APT. Lymphocytosis, with increased CD8+ lymphocytes, has been reported, as have increased neutrophils.

Ultrastructural analysis can be performed on tissue or cells from the bronchoalveolar lavage fluid, and reveals membrane-bound cytoplasmic inclusions composed of densely packed whorls of thin lamellae, similar

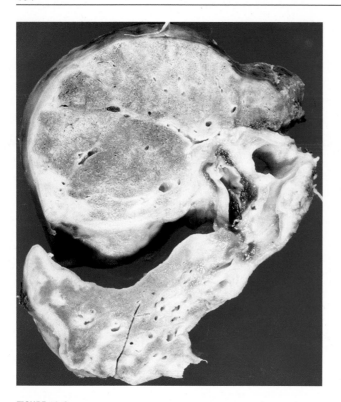

FIGURE 19-8

Bischloronitrosourea (BCNU)-associated pulmonary fibrosis
Marked interstitial fibrosis, most prominent subpleurally, distorts the upper and lower lobes.

to surfactant lamellar bodies. However, these inclusions can be seen in macrophages, endothelial cells, interstitial cells, and pneumocytes.

CHEMOTHERAPEUTIC AGENTS

Many chemotherapeutic agents have been associated with lung injury. Bleomycin, methotrexate, cyclophosphamide, busulfan, and a variety of other agents are recognized for their roles in triggering lung injury, which can range from mild to severe and potentially fatal. Pulmonary toxicity is estimated to develop in less than 10% of patients receiving chemotherapeutic agents, however. Usual symptoms include dyspnea, cough, and often fever. Although acute presentations can occur, symptoms more frequently begin weeks to as long as years after initiation of the agent(s). Radiologic changes commonly include diffuse interstitial infiltrates or a mixed interstitial-alveolar pattern, and lung function studies typically show reduction in diffusing capacity. Naturally, these changes depend upon the specific pattern of lung injury displayed and its severity.

The differential diagnosis includes the various entities that can be associated with each of these specific histologic patterns. Evaluation for infections is a high priority in these patients, and appropriate organism stains and cultures should be performed. Respiratory viral infections can produce diffuse alveolar damage with pneumocyte atypia, so these agents may be considered in the differential diagnosis for biopsies with those findings, but can be diagnosed by culture or other methodologies (Chapters 13 and 38).

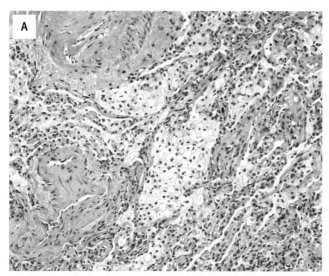
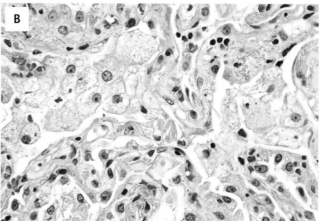

FIGURE 19-9

Amiodarone pulmonary toxicity
(A) and **(B)** Foamy macrophages fill alveolar spaces, and minimal interstitial inflammation is present.

AMIODARONE-ASSOCIATED PULMONARY TOXICITY—FACT SHEET

Incidence and Risk Factors

» Cumulative prevalence estimated at 1-15% of the treated population

» Toxicity appears to be more common with higher dosages, but can also develop in patients treated with low dosages (up to 200 mg/day)

» Other suggested risk factors include increased age, a preexisting abnormal chest radiograph or poor pulmonary reserve, exposure to elevated oxygen concentrations and mechanical ventilation, and parenteral injection of iodinated contrast media

Clinical Features

» Men are more frequently affected than women

» Insidious onset of dyspnea, dry cough, chest pain, and malaise is usual

» Onset is typically weeks to years after beginning the medication, but can occur at any point from a few days after initiation of therapy to more than a decade after treatment was begun, and rare cases develop after the drug has been discontinued

Radiologic Features

» Radiologic findings include variably severe interstitial and/or alveolar infiltrates, patchy or diffuse, involving one or both lungs

» Pleural effusions are common

Prognosis and Therapy

» Treatment usually involves discontinuation of the drug, and corticosteroids are also commonly administered, often for prolonged periods

» Premature discontinuation of corticosteroid therapy may precipitate a relapse

» Clinical and radiologic improvement can take weeks or months, due to the slow clearance of the drug from tissues

» Radiologic resolution occurs in approximately 85% of patients

» Degree of persistent respiratory compromise depends upon the extent of pulmonary fibrosis

» Mortality rate reportedly lies between 21% and 33% for patients hospitalized for drug toxicity

AMIODARONE-ASSOCIATED PULMONARY TOXICITY—PATHOLOGIC FEATURES

Histologic Findings

» Numerous lipid-laden macrophages in alveolar spaces

» Pneumocytes, interstitial cells, and endothelial cells may demonstrate cytoplasmic lipid vacuoles

» Variably intense lymphocytic interstitial infiltrate

» Variable degrees of interstitial edema or fibrosis with type 2 pneumocyte proliferation

» Other patterns may include organizing pneumonia and diffuse alveolar damage

Cytologic Findings (Bronchoalveolar Lavage)

» Foamy macrophages

» Lymphocytosis with increased CD8+ lymphocytes and/or neutrophilia

Ultrastructural Findings

» Membrane-bound cytoplasmic inclusions composed of densely packed whorls of thin lamellae, similar to surfactant lamellar bodies, in macrophages, endothelial cells, interstitial cells, and pneumocytes

Differential Diagnosis

» Infections, especially those that can cause an interstitial pneumonia (viruses, *Mycoplasma, Chlamydia,* fungi) or macrophage infiltrates (mycobacteria, fungi, Whipple's disease, malakoplakia)

» Lipoid pneumonia due to aspiration (exogenous) or airway obstruction (endogenous)

» Storage diseases

» Other causes of diffuse alveolar damage (Chapter 9)

BLEOMYCIN

Among the chemotherapeutic agents, bleomycin is the most prevalent cause of pulmonary disease. It is an antibiotic agent that produces cytotoxicity by induction of free radicals, which causes breaks in DNA, leading to cell death. Its inactivating enzyme, bleomycin hydrolase, is relatively deficient in the lungs and skin, which predisposes to toxic manifestations predominantly in these sites. Reported risk factors for pulmonary toxicity include advanced age, uremia, drug dosage over 450 U, high inspired oxygen concentrations, concomitant thoracic radiation therapy, and concurrent use of cyclophosphamide. Up to 20% of patients treated with bleomycin have been reported to develop clinical lung disease, and the mortality rate may be as high as 3% of all patients treated with bleomycin. Treatment usually

includes discontinuation of bleomycin and administration of corticosteroids.

Interstitial pneumonia is the most common manifestation of pulmonary toxicity. The pathologic features reflect a progression of cellular injury, with features of diffuse alveolar damage (Chapter 9). Early changes include vascular endothelial injury, interstitial edema, and pneumocyte necrosis. This is followed by proliferation of type 2 pneumocytes, which may show marked atypia, and often prominent metaplastic epithelial changes (Figure 19-10). Abundant macrophages may be seen in alveolar spaces, and there is usually a mild mixed inflammatory interstitial infiltrate. Fibroblast proliferation occurs, with resultant interstitial and alveolar fibrosis. The advanced process can resemble usual interstitial pneumonia (Chapter 16).

Other histologic presentations can include eosinophilic pneumonia (Chapter 17) and organizing pneumonia. In some patients, lesions can have a more nodular

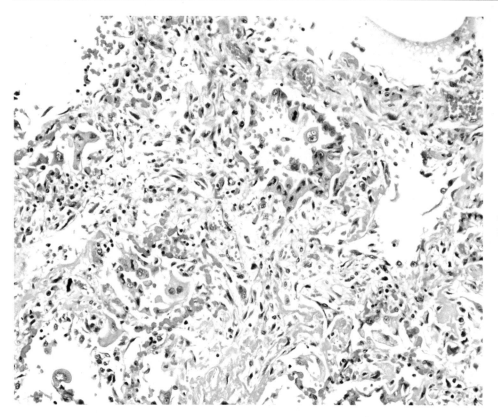

FIGURE 19-10
Bleomycin pulmonary toxicity
Organizing diffuse alveolar damage with pneumocyte cytoatypia is observed.

radiographic appearance, which may raise the question of tumor metastasis.

CYCLOPHOSPHAMIDE

Cyclophosphamide, an alkylating agent, is a cornerstone of many chemotherapeutic regimens for treatment of a wide variety of malignancies and inflammatory conditions such as glomerulonephritis and Wegener's granulomatosis. The frequency of clinically significant lung injury is difficult to estimate, since other potential causes of lung injury frequently exist in patients with potential cyclophosphamide toxicity, but appears to be less than 1%. Both early- and late-onset pneumonitis have been described in association with this agent. With early onset pneumonitis, symptoms of cough, dyspnea, and fever develop within 1 to 6 months after drug exposure. Patients frequently improve with discontinuation of the drug and use of corticosteroids. In contrast, late-onset pneumonitis and fibrosis develop after prolonged treatment with cyclophosphamide over months to years, and can occur even after discontinuation of the drug. Insidious onset of cough and dyspnea

with radiographic evidence of pleural thickening and restrictive changes on pulmonary function testing are characteristic. Progressive respiratory failure may lead to death in patients with this form of drug toxicity. Although clear-cut risk factors have not been identified, men may be at higher risk than women for this complication. Histologic manifestations that have been linked to cyclophosphamide include diffuse alveolar damage (Chapter 9) (Figure 19-11), organizing pneumonia, and alveolar hemorrhage. Pneumocyte atypia may be present.

METHOTREXATE

Methotrexate is used in the therapy of multiple inflammatory and neoplastic disorders and acts via inhibition of dihydrofolate reductase, leading to interference with DNA synthesis, repair, and cellular replication. It is generally given in low doses as an anti-inflammatory agent to treat disorders such as rheumatoid arthritis, psoriasis, and other autoimmune disorders, and in higher doses as a chemotherapeutic agent. In patients who are receiving methotrexate for treatment of rheumatoid arthritis, the

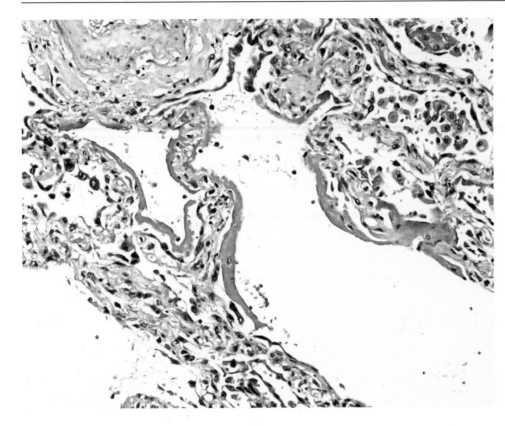

FIGURE 19-11
Cyclophosphamide-associated lung injury
Conspicuous hyaline membranes indicate the presence of diffuse alveolar damage. Pneumocyte atypia is focal.

likelihood of developing pulmonary complications appears to lie between 0.3% and 11.6%. Most complications develop within 2 years of starting therapy, but onset as early as 1 month after initiation of therapy has been reported, and in rare patients the pneumonitis has appeared after discontinuation of the drug. In patients with rheumatoid arthritis, symptoms of shortness of breath, cough, and fever are usually present for several weeks before diagnosis, but more acute presentations also occasionally occur. Radiologic findings usually include bilateral interstitial infiltrates, and, in some cases, alveolar infiltrates are also observed. Most patients will improve with discontinuation of the methotrexate, and corticosteroid therapy has also been suggested to accelerate recovery. The reported mortality rate is approximately 17%. In patients who are rechallenged with methotrexate after an initial pulmonary event, recurrent lung disease can also develop.

The histologic patterns observed have features of hypersensitivity pneumonia (Chapter 17), nonspecific interstitial pneumonia (Chapter 16), or diffuse alveolar damage (Chapter 9). Mononuclear cell interstitial infiltrates and fibrosis are commonly seen, often in combination with poorly formed granulomas or multinucleated giant cells. Hyaline membranes are present with a diffuse alveolar damage pattern. Tissue eosinophil infiltrates can also be seen in occasional patients. Bronchoalveolar lavage typically demonstrates a lymphocytosis and, in some cases, neutrophilia.

Histopathologic evaluation is important for its demonstration of appropriate histopathology, as well as for evaluation for other processes considered in the differential diagnosis. In patients whose biopsies show characteristics of hypersensitivity pneumonia, information about exposures to other triggers of hypersensitivity pneumonia should be sought. Documentation of a temporal relationship between drug initiation and onset of symptoms, and between drug withdrawal and improvement in symptoms, can be helpful for establishing a linkage between the lung disease and the drug. If granulomas are the primary finding, sarcoidosis and granulomatous infections may be considered. Since many patients receiving this drug have some degree of iatrogenic immunocompromise, infection is usually a significant clinical consideration, and evaluation of histopathology and culture results for evidence of infection will be important. In biopsies showing only a nonspecific interstitial pneumonia, the differential diagnosis will include the spectrum of disorders associated with this histologic pattern (Chapter 16). Pulmonary involvement by the underlying disease can also be considered in the differential diagnosis. Collagen vascular diseases can be associated with

---

pulmonary pathology that overlaps with some features of methotrexate-related drug injury (Chapter 36).

MESALAMINE

Mesalamine (5-aminosalicylic acid), is an anti-inflammatory medication widely used for the treatment of inflammatory bowel diseases (IBD). It represents the effective moiety of its predecessor, sulfasalazine, which consists of mesalamine bound to sulfapyridine, a transport molecule. Relatively few cases of mesalamine-associated lung injury have been reported, and the prevalence of this complication appears to be quite low. Nonetheless, mesalamine-associated lung injury often enters into the differential diagnosis for pulmonary disease in patients with IBD who are treated with mesalamine. Since the therapeutic approach differs from other entities that may be considered (infections, IBD-associated lung disease), awareness of this entity can be important.

The pathogenesis of mesalamine-associated lung injury is not well understood, but immunologic mechanisms appear to play a role based on the histologic response pattern and evidence obtained from lymphocyte stimulation testing. Concomitant immunomodulatory therapy, however, does not appear to prevent development of lung disease. A relationship between dosage and pulmonary toxicity has not been shown, and there are no recognized risk factors for development of lung injury. Women are affected more often than men.

A typical clinical presentation involves the insidious onset of low-grade fever, dry cough, fatigue, and dyspnea. Onset can range from days to years after initiation of mesalamine therapy, and the mean time of onset is approximately 11 months after the initiation of therapy. Variable degrees of hypoxemia, sometimes requiring supplemental oxygen therapy, are observed. Peripheral blood and bronchoalveolar lavage fluid eosinophilia have been described in some patients. The radiologic findings are nonspecific and include unilateral or bilateral interstitial infiltrates, consolidation, and, less commonly, pleural effusions.

Pathologic features resemble those of hypersensitivity pneumonitis and include interstitial lymphocytic or lymphoplasmacytic infiltrates; alveolar fibrinous exudates, granulation tissue, and fibrosis; and poorly formed nonnecrotizing granulomas and multinucleated giant cells (Figure 19-12). Individual biopsies may demonstrate one or more of these features. Other variably present abnormalities include hyaline membranes, alveolar eosinophil infiltrates, and lymphocytic airway inflammation and granulation tissue. Although there is some overlap between pulmonary involvement by IBD (Chapter 36) and mesalamine-induced pulmonary reactions, predominant involvement of the alveolar parenchyma favors a reaction to mesalamine, while predominance of larger airway abnormalities favors pulmonary involvement by IBD, and acute inflammatory infiltrates are more common in association with IBD. Other potential causes of hypersensitivity pneumonia should also be considered in the differential diagnosis, and if the pattern is one of isolated nonspecific interstitial pneumonia or organizing pneumonia (Chapter 16), then the histologic differential diagnosis for these conditions applies.

Treatment consists of drug withdrawal, and in some patients, corticosteroids have been used concurrently. Most patients experience symptomatic and radiographic improvement within weeks or months.

NITROFURANTOIN

Nitrofurantoin, a synthetic, broad-spectrum antibacterial agent, is used in the treatment of urinary tract infections. Although it is a commonly cited medicinal

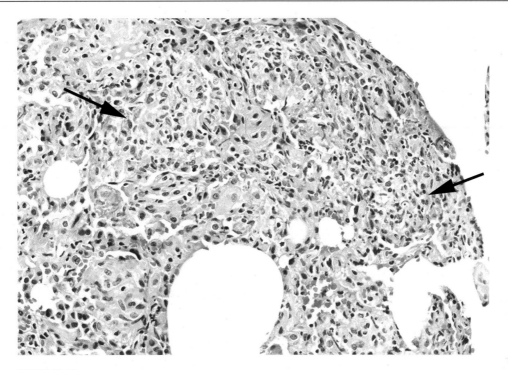

FIGURE 19-12

Mesalamine-associated lung injury

Poorly formed granulomas (arrows) lie in alveolar spaces, and other areas of the biopsy demonstrate mild interstitial mononuclear cell infiltrates, features compatible with a hypersensitivity pneumonia reaction pattern. This patient's lung disease resolved completely with discontinuation of mesalamine and corticosteroid therapy.

cause of adverse pulmonary reactions, associated lung injury appears to be rare, estimated at 0.001% of courses of therapy. Immunologic mechanisms and oxidant-related injury have been postulated to play a role in the pathogenesis of nitrofurantoin-associated lung disease.

Acute, subacute, and chronic presentations have been described. The acute form is more common than the chronic form, usually develops within 2 weeks of initiating treatment, and can present with bronchospasm or with symptoms including fever, dyspnea, cough, rash, arthralgia, fatigue, and peripheral eosinophilia.

MESALAMINE-ASSOCIATED PULMONARY TOXICITY—FACT SHEET

Incidence and Risk Factors

‣ Rare, incidence may be under-reported
‣ No known risk factors

Clinical and Radiologic Findings

‣ Insidious onset of low-grade fever, dyspnea, dry cough, and fatigue
‣ Onset typically months after beginning therapy, however, may range from days to years
‣ Radiologic features vary and can include unilateral or bilateral interstitial infiltrates, consolidation, and pleural effusions

Prognosis and Therapy

‣ Treatment involves discontinuation of the drug, and corticosteroids have been administered in some cases
‣ Resolution of clinical and radiologic abnormalities typically occurs within weeks or months of drug cessation

---

MESALAMINE-ASSOCIATED PULMONARY TOXICITY—PATHOLOGIC FEATURES

Histologic Findings (one or more may be represented in individual cases)

‣ Interstitial lymphocytic or lymphoplasmacytic infiltrates
‣ Alveolar fibrinous exudates, granulation tissue, and fibrosis
‣ Poorly formed non-necrotizing granulomas and multinucleated giant cells
‣ Less-commonly observed features can include hyaline membranes, alveolar eosinophil infiltrates, and lymphocytic airway inflammation and granulation tissue

Differential Diagnosis

‣ Pulmonary involvement by inflammatory bowel disease (Chapter 36)
‣ Infections, especially those that can cause interstitial pneumonia or granulomas (viruses, *Mycoplasma, Chlamydia,* mycobacteria, fungi)
‣ Other causes of hypersensitivity pneumonia (Chapter 17)
‣ Other causes of organizing pneumonia (Chapter 16)
‣ Other causes of nonspecific or usual interstitial pneumonia (Chapter 16)

Discontinuation of the drug usually produces improvement. Subacute or chronic lung injury occurs less often, usually after months or years of drug use, and the prognosis with cessation of drug usage and corticosteroid therapy is variable. Symptoms include insidious onset of dyspnea and cough. Ground-glass opacities are frequently seen, and other radiographic findings may include subpleural irregular linear opacities and patchy consolidation. Histologic findings described in association with nitrofurantoin include acute lung injury (Chapter 9), nonspecific interstitial pneumonia (Chapter 16) (Figure 19-13), desquamative interstitial pneumonia (Chapter 16), organizing pneumonia, vasculitis, and mixed inflammatory cell infiltrates including eosinophils.

SIROLIMUS

Sirolimus has become an important immunosuppressive drug for treatment of transplant patients with renal dysfunction. Associated pulmonary abnormalities have been increasingly recognized since 2000, developing most commonly in renal transplant recipients, with

---

NITROFURANTOIN-ASSOCIATED PULMONARY EFFECTS—FACT SHEET

Incidence
- Develops in approximately 0.001% of courses of therapy

Clinical Features
- Acute, subacute, and chronic presentations
- Acute form is most common, with onset of bronchospasm or fever, dyspnea, cough, rash, arthralgia, fatigue, and peripheral eosinophilia, typically beginning 7 to 14 days after starting therapy
- Insidious onset of dyspnea and cough with subacute and chronic injury

Radiologic Features
- Ground-glass opacities are frequently seen, and other radiographic findings may include subpleural irregular linear opacities and patchy consolidation

Histopathologic Reaction Patterns
- Acute lung injury (Chapter 9)
- Nonspecific interstitial pneumonia (Chapter 16)
- Desquamative interstitial pneumonia (Chapter 16)
- Organizing pneumonia (Chapter 16)
- Vasculitis (Chapter 8)
- Mixed inflammatory cell infiltrates including eosinophils

Prognosis and Therapy
- Discontinuation of the drug usually leads to improvement with acute presentations
- With chronic cases, prognosis with drug cessation and corticosteroids is variable

---

fewer cases observed among other solid organ transplant recipients. Reports suggest that toxicity is linked to higher dosages, and an immunologic basis for drug toxicity has also been suggested. Dyspnea on exertion, dry cough, fatigue, and fever are common symptoms, and hemoptysis and weight loss occur less frequently. Time of onset varies, with some cases appearing more than a year after starting therapy. Radiologic studies usually show bilateral patchy air space disease, and biopsies reveal organizing pneumonia, interstitial lymphocytic infiltrates, non-necrotizing granulomas, and/or diffuse alveolar hemorrhage (Figure 19-14). The prognosis is usually favorable with resolution of symptoms following cessation of drug administration.

RADIATION

External beam radiation therapy is frequently and successfully used in the treatment of thoracic malignancies such as lung and breast carcinoma, thymoma, and lymphoma. However, the lungs are highly susceptible to the damaging effects of radiation, and the concomitant or sequential use of certain chemotherapeutic agents may potentiate these effects. Radiation-induced lung toxicity is the result of direct cytotoxic effects of ionizing radiation and indirect damage secondary to inflammation and oxidant injury, and is a dose-limiting factor for radiation therapy. Clinically recognizable radiation-induced lung damage occurs in 5-15% of patients treated, and reports suggest that the risk of development of radiation fibrosis is related to the volume of lung irradiated above a threshold of 20-30 Gy.

The clinical picture can vary considerably, depending on severity. A typical presentation includes an insidious onset of dyspnea, cough, and fever within 2 to 3 months after completion of radiation therapy. Rarely, reactions may occur within 2 weeks of therapy or many months after completion. Although mild cases may spontaneously resolve, many patients are treated with corticosteroids, with resolution of symptoms within weeks for the majority. In severe cases, patients can progress to chronic pulmonary fibrosis with respiratory compromise; however, death due to radiation-induced pulmonary disease is very rare.

Radiologic findings in the acute phase are highly variable, ranging from subtle interstitial or alveolar opacities to patchy or homogeneous areas of consolidation. Both acute and chronic changes are usually limited to the area of radiation field. High resolution computed tomography scan typically shows more extensive involvement than is apparent on chest radiograph.

Although the diagnosis is often made clinically, pathologic confirmation may be necessary to rule out other

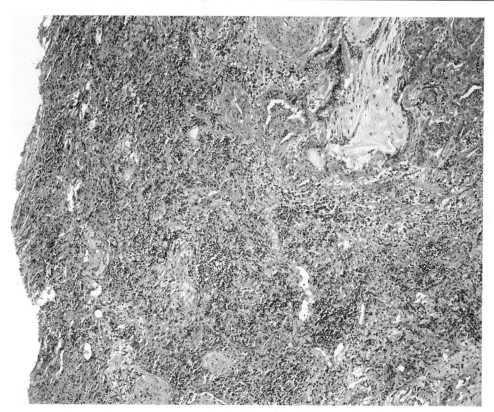

FIGURE 19-13

Nitrofurantoin lung toxicity
There is diffuse, marked interstitial infiltration by mononuclear inflammatory cells, primarily lymphocytes, and a background of interstitial fibrosis.

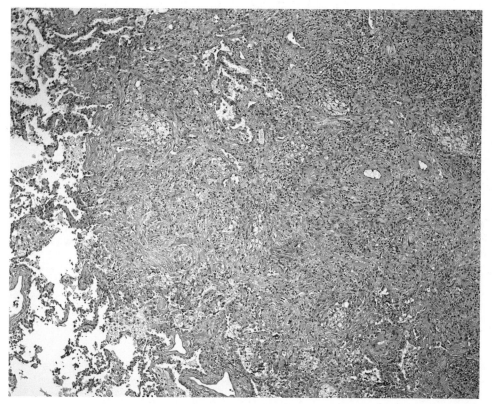

FIGURE 19-14

Sirolimus pneumonia
Nodules of organizing pneumonia with hemosiderin-laden macrophages were noted in this wedge biopsy from a renal transplant patient. Infection was suspected clinically, but all cultures and serologic studies were negative.

potential causes of pulmonary disease in this patient population, particularly infections and recurrent or metastatic malignancy. Biopsy of acute radiation pneumonitis shows changes of diffuse alveolar damage (Chapter 9). Subsequently, organization occurs with fibroblast proliferation, variable degrees of interstitial and alveolar fibrosis, and vascular intimal fibrosis with foamy macrophages. Interstitial lymphocytic infiltrates and organizing pneumonia have also been described (Figure 19-15A). Contiguous scarring can replace much of the normal parenchymal architecture (Figure 19-15B), and areas of scarring may also show elastotic changes similar to those frequently seen in the lung apices. Cells with nuclear enlargement, hyperchromasia, and nuclear irregularity are also commonly observed in the areas of injury (Figure 19-15A).

ILLICIT DRUG USE

Illicit drug use remains a major societal problem. A survey conducted in 2000 indicated that 39% of the United States population aged 12 or older had used illicit drugs at least once in their lifetime, 11% during the preceding year, and 6% within the preceding month. Both inhaled and intravenously injected drugs have the potential to cause significant lung injury, and the patterns of injury and severity depend upon the individual agents, the concentrations and routes of administration, effects of other substances used concurrently (tobacco, other illicit preparations), and idiosyncratic factors.

RADIATION PNEUMONITIS—FACT SHEET

Incidence and Risk Factors

▸ Occurs in 5-15% of patients receiving radiation therapy
▸ Risk appears to be related to the volume of lung irradiated above a threshold of 20-30 Gy
▸ Increased risk with concomitant or sequential use of some chemotherapeutic agents

Clinical Features

▸ Insidious onset of dyspnea, cough, and fever
▸ Onset typically 2 to 3 months after completion of therapy (ranges from 2 weeks to many months)

Radiologic Features

▸ Radiographic changes are usually limited to the radiation field, and range from vague interstitial or alveolar infiltrates to discrete patchy or diffuse pulmonary consolidation

Microscopic Findings

▸ Diffuse alveolar damage (Chapter 9)
▸ Variable degrees of organizing pneumonia (Chapter 16) and interstitial lymphocytic infiltrates
▸ Variable degrees of interstitial, alveolar, and replacement fibrosis
▸ Vascular intimal fibrosis with foamy macrophages
▸ Cells with nuclear enlargement, hyperchromasia, and nuclear irregularity

Prognosis and Therapy

▸ Mild disease may resolve spontaneously, but symptomatic or severe disease is generally treated with corticosteroids to produce resolution of symptoms within weeks for the majority of patients
▸ Some patients develop variable degrees of pulmonary fibrosis, which is the main determinant of the degree of persistent respiratory compromise
▸ Death due to radiation-induced pulmonary disease is rare

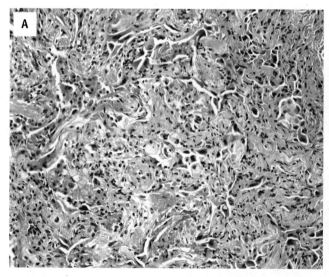 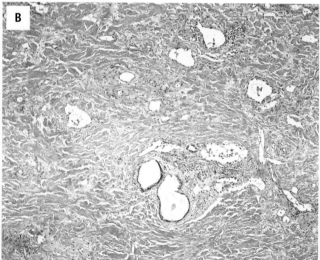

FIGURE 19-15

Radiation pneumonitis
(A) Organizing pneumonia with fibrosis and pneumocyte atypia is seen. **(B)** Dense fibrous tissue replaces most of the normal architectural elements in this area of the radiation field.

Although heroin and cocaine are the most commonly used intravenous drugs, other drugs normally consumed orally can also be crushed and injected. Pulmonary edema is a well recognized sequel to heroin overdose. The frequency of this complication appears to have declined over the last several decades, to approximately 2% of patients with heroin overdose. Mechanical ventilation is often needed, but in most patients the process resolves within days. Foreign body granulomas commonly result from injection of drugs, triggered by the relatively poorly digestible materials used to dilute the drugs or present in the crushed pills (Chapter 18). The granulomas usually lie in and adjacent to blood vessels, and examination under polarized light can be helpful to highlight the foreign materials, usually in the cytoplasm of multinucleated giant cells and macrophages. Pulmonary hypertensive changes may accompany the granulomas or occur independently. Septic pulmonary emboli originating from tricuspid valve endocarditis represent another potential consequence of intravenous drug abuse. Cases of alveolar hemorrhage associated with intravenous cocaine use have been described. Aspiration pneumonia is predisposed to by mental status compromise occurring with intoxication. Early development of emphysema has been observed in some young users of intravenous drugs, particularly associated with methylphenidate.

Pneumothoraces and empyemas, whose development is usually linked to attempted injection into the internal jugular vein, have also been reported.

Inhalational drugs are introduced via smoking (most often marijuana and cocaine) or nasal routes (usually cocaine and, less often, heroin). Marijuana's effects upon the airways appear similar to those of tobacco smoking, and can include physiologic evidence of increased airway resistance and histopathologic findings of airway inflammation, edema, goblet cell hyperplasia, and in some cases, bullae. "Crack" is cocaine alkaloid mixed with a solvent, which is then evaporated, and the drug is then usually smoked in a pipe or can be mixed with tobacco or marijuana in the form of a cigarette. Associated pulmonary pathology can include abundant carbonaceous deposits, thermal airway injury, organizing pneumonia, aspirated materials (parts of pipes, nasal septa), pulmonary hemorrhage, edema, interstitial pneumonia, eosinophil infiltrates, foreign body granulomas, pulmonary infarction, airway epithelial changes (basal cell hyperplasia, squamous metaplasia, epithelial flattening with ciliary loss), and consequences of barotrauma (Figure 19-16A,B). Inhalation of smoke from heroin heated over a flame can cause severe asthma exacerbations and obstructive changes on pulmonary function testing. Panacinar emphysema has been associated with chronic glue sniffing.

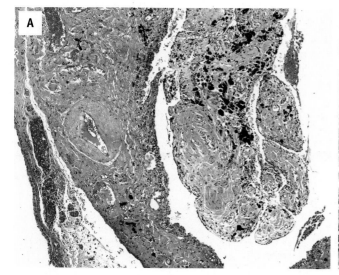
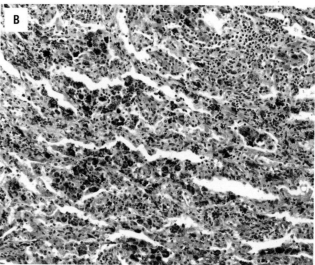

FIGURE 19-16

Crack cocaine abuse

(A) This lung has thick-walled apical bullae with abundant pigment-laden macrophages in their walls. **(B)** Elsewhere in the same lung, more pigment-laden macrophages are accompanied by interstitial lymphocytic infiltrates.

SUGGESTED READINGS

General Information

1. Camus P, Bonniaud P, Fanton A, Camus C, Baudaun N, Foucher P. Drug-induced and iatrogenic infiltrative lung disease. *Clin Chest Med.* 2004;25:479-519.
2. Camus P, Fanton A, Bonniaud P, Camus C, Foucher P. Interstitial lung disease induced by drugs and radiation. *Respiration.* 2004;71:301-326.
3. Davies PDB. Drug-induced lung disease. *Br J Dis Chest.* 1969;LXIII 2:57-70.
4. Delaunois LM. Mechanisms in pulmonary toxicology. *Clin Chest Med.* 2004;25:1-14.
5. Dementer SL, Ahmad M, Tomashefski JF. Drug-induced pulmonary disease. *Cleve Clin Q.* 1979;46:89-124.
6. Flieder DB, Travis WD. Pathologic characteristics of drug-induced lung disease. *Clin Chest Med.* 2004;25:37-45.
7. Foucher P, Camus P, Groupe d'Etudes de la Pathologie Pulmonaire Iatrogène. Pneumotox on line [homepage]. Available at: *http://www.pneumotox.com.*
8. Lazarou J, Pomeranz BM, Corey PN. Incidence of adverse drug reactions in hospitalized patients: a meta-analysis of prospective studies. *JAMA.* 1998;279:1200-5.
9. Myers JL. Pathology of drug-induced lung disease. In: Katzenstein AL, ed. *Katzenstein and Askin's Surgical Pathology of Non-neoplastic Lung Disease,* 3rd ed. Philadelphia: WB Saunders; 1997:81-111.
10. Ozkan M, Dweik R, Ahmad M. Drug-induced lung disease. *Clev Clin J Med.* 2001;68:782-95.
11. Rosenow EC. The spectrum of drug-induced pulmonary disease. *Ann Intern Med.* 1972;77:977-91.
12. Sostman HD, Matthay RA, Putman CE. Cytotoxic drug-induced lung disease. *Am J Med.* 1977;62:608-15.
13. Travis WD, Colby TV, Koss MN, Rosado-de-Christenson ML, Muller NL, King TE. Drug and radiation reactions. In: *Non-Neoplastic Disorders of the Lower Respiratory Tract.* First Series, Fascicle 2. Washington, DC: American Registry of Pathology and the Armed Forces Institute of Pathology; 2002:321-50.

Amiodarone

14. Camus P, Martin WJ II, Rosenow EC. Amiodarone pulmonary toxicity. *Clin Chest Med.* 2004;25:65-75.
15. Kennedy JI, Myers JL, Plumb VJ, Fulmer JD. Amiodarone pulmonary toxicity: clinical, radiologic, and pathologic correlations. *Arch Intern Med.* 1987;147:50-5.
16. Myers JL, Kennedy JI, Plumb VJ. Amiodarone lung: pathologic findings in clinically toxic patients. *Hum Pathol.* 1987;18:349-54.
17. Ott MC, Khoor A, Leventhal JP, Paterick TE, Burger CD. Pulmonary toxicity in patients receiving low-dose amiodarone. *Chest.* 2003;123:646-51.
18. Stein B, Zaatari GS, Pine JR. Amiodarone pulmonary toxicity: clinical, cytologic and ultrastructural findings. *Acta Cytol.* 1987;31:357-61.

Chemotherapeutic Agents

19. Ben Arush MW, Roguin A, Zamir E, et al. Bleomycin and cyclophosphamide toxicity simulating metastatic nodules to the lungs in childhood cancer. *Pediatr Hematol Oncol.* 1997;14:381-6.
20. Cannon GW. Methotrexate pulmonary toxicity. *Rheum Dis Clin North Am.* 1997;23:917-37.
21. Cohen MB, Austin JH, Smith-Vaniz A, Lutzky J, Grimes MM. Nodular bleomycin toxicity. *Am J Clin Pathol.* 1989;92:101-4.
22. Imokawa S, Colby TV, Leslie KO, Helmers RA. Methotrexate pneumonitis: review of the literature and histopathological findings in nine patients. *Eur Respir J.* 2000;15:373-81.
23. Kremer JM, Alarcon GS, Weinblatt ME, et al. Clinical, laboratory, radiographic, and histopathologic features of methotrexate-associated lung injury in patients with rheumatoid arthritis: a multicenter study with literature review. *Arthritis Rheum.* 1997;40:1829-37.
24. Limper AH. Chemotherapy-induced lung disease. *Clin Chest Med.* 2004;25:53-64.
25. Lock BJ, Eggert M, Cooper JA Jr. Infiltrative lung disease due to noncytotoxic agents. *Clin Chest Med.* 2004;25:47-52.
26. Luna MA, Bedrossian CWM, Lichtiger B, Salem PA. Interstitial pneumonitis associated with bleomycin therapy. *Am J Clin Pathol.* 1972;58:501-10.
27. Malik SW, Myers JL, DeRemee RA, Specks U. Lung toxicity associated with cyclophosphamide use: two distinct patterns. *Am J Respir Crit Care Med.* 1996;154:1851-6.
28. Santrach PJ, Askin FB, Wells RJ, Azizkhan RG, Merten DF. Nodular form of bleomycin-related pulmonary injury in patients with osteogenic sarcoma. *Cancer.* 1989;64:806-11.
29. Sleijfer S. Bleomycin-induced pneumonitis. *Chest.* 2001;120:617-624.
30. Smith JG. The histopathology of pulmonary reactions to drugs. *Clin Chest Med.* 1990;11:95-117.
31. Yousem SA, Lifson JD, Colby TV. Chemotherapy-induced eosinophilic pneumonia: relation to bleomycin. *Chest.* 1985;88:103-6.

Illicit Drugs

32. Gotway MB, Marder SR, Hanks DK, et al. Thoracic complications of illicit drug use: an organ system approach. *Radiographics.* 2002;22 (Spec No): S119-35.
33. Laposata EA, Mayo GL. A review of pulmonary pathology and mechanisms associated with inhalation of freebase cocaine ("crack"). *Am J Forensic Med Pathol.* 1993;14:1-9.
34. Substance Abuse and Mental Health Services Administration. Summary of findings from the 2000 national household survey on drug abuse. Rockville: Office of Applied Studies; 2001 [NHSDA Series H-13, DHHS Publication #(SMA) 01-3549].
35. Wolff AJ, O'Donnell AE. Pulmonary effects of illicit drug use. *Clin Chest Med.* 2004;25:203-16.

Mesalamine

36. Casey MB, Tazelaar JD, Myers JL, et al. Noninfectious lung pathology in patients with Crohn's disease. *Am J Surg Pathol.* 2003;27:213-9.
37. Foster RA, Zander DS, Mergo PJ, Valentine JF. Mesalamine-related lung disease: clinical, radiographic, and pathologic manifestations. *Inflamm Bowel Dis.* 2003;9:308-15.

Nitrofurantoin

38. Cameron RJ, Kolbe J, Wilsher ML, Lambie N. Bronchiolitis obliterans organizing pneumonia associated with the use of nitrofurantoin. *Thorax.* 2000;55:249-51.
39. Castleman B, Scully RE, McNeely BU. Case records of the Massachusetts General Hospital. *N Engl J Med.* 1974;290:1309-14.
40. D'Arcy PF. Nitrofurantoin. *Drug Intell Clin Pharm.* 1985;19:540-7.
41. Holmberg L, Boman G, Bottiger LE, Eriksson B, Spross R, Wessling A. Adverse reactions to nitrofurantoin: analysis of 921 reports. *Am J Med.* 1980;69:733-8.
42. Mendez JL, Nadrous HF, Hartman TE, Ryu JH. Chronic nitrofurantoin-induced lung disease. *Mayo Clin Proc.* 2005;80:1298-302.
43. Rossi SE, Erasmus JJ, McAdams HP, Sporn TA, Goodman PC. Pulmonary drug toxicity: radiologic and pathologic manifestations. *Radiographics.* 2000;20:1245-59.
44. Schattner A, Von der Walde J, Kozak N, Sokolovskaya N, Knobler H. Nitrofurantoin-induced immune-mediated lung and liver disease. *Am J Med Sci.* 1999;317:336-40.
45. Smith JG. The histopathology of pulmonary reactions to drugs. *Clin Chest Med.* 1990;11: 95-117.

Radiation

46. Abratt RP, Morgan GW. Lung toxicity following chest irradiation in patients with lung cancer. *Lung Cancer.* 2002;35:103-9.
47. Abratt RP, Morgan GW, Silvestri G, Willcox P. Pulmonary complications of radiation therapy. *Clin Chest Med.* 2004;25:167-77.

48. Travis WD, Colby TV, Koss MN, Rosado-de-Christenson ML, Muller NL, King TE. Drug and radiation reactions. In: *Non-Neoplastic Disorders of the Lower Respiratory Tract*. First Series, Fascicle 2. Washington, DC: American Registry of Pathology and the Armed Forces Institute of Pathology; 2002:340-7.

Sirolimus

49. McWilliams TJ, Levvey BJ, Russell PA, et al. Interstitial pneumonitis associated with sirolimus: a dilemma for lung transplantation. *J Heart Lung Transplant*. 2003;22:210-3.

50. Morelon E, Stern M, Israel-Biet D, et al. Characteristics of sirolimus-associated interstitial pneumonitis in renal transplant patients. *Transplantation*. 2001;72:787-90.

51. Pham PT, Pham PC, Danovitch GM, et al. Sirolimus-associated pulmonary toxicity. *Transplantation*. 2004;77:1215-20.

52. Vlahakis NE, Rickman OB, Morgenthaler T. Sirolimus-associated diffuse alveolar hemorrhage. *Mayo Clin Proc*. 2004;79:541-5.

20 Emphysema and Diseases of Large Airways

Linda K. Green

INTRODUCTION

The disorders included in this chapter are grouped under the heading "obstructive lung diseases." These diseases share the characteristic of increased resistance to airflow, which can be caused by either an increase in the resistance of the conducting airways or an increase in lung compliance due to emphysematous lung destruction, or both. Obstructive lung diseases include emphysema, chronic bronchitis, asthma, and bronchiectasis. Although these diseases have distinctive clinical and pathologic features, patients can show features of more than one of these disorders. The combination of emphysema and chronic bronchitis is particularly frequent, due to the strong linkages of these diseases to a common etiologic factor, tobacco smoking. The term "chronic obstructive pulmonary disease" (COPD) is commonly used to refer to both processes, and is defined physiologically by airflow limitation measured during forced expiration. A component of asthma may also contribute to COPD in some patients. Small airway abnormalities also form part of the constellation of changes contributing to airflow limitation in smokers, and are discussed in more depth in chapter 21.

EMPHYSEMA

Emphysema is a disorder characterized by abnormal permanent enlargement of air spaces distal to the terminal bronchiole, with destruction of their walls and with-

out obvious fibrosis. It is often associated with chronic bronchitis and produces physiologic airflow obstruction. There are four described variants that affect different regions of the pulmonary lobule: (1) centriacinar or centrilobular, (2) panacinar or panlobular, (3) paraseptal, and (4) irregular. Centriacinar emphysema is the most common form of emphysema and is most closely associated with long-standing tobacco use. Panacinar emphysema is characteristic of α-1-antitrypsin (A1AT) deficiency. Irregular emphysema occurs at the periphery of large scars or other focal lesions. Patients may have more than one type; mixtures of centriacinar and paraseptal emphysema are common in smokers, and centriacinar emphysema can progress in smokers to involve whole acini. Large bullae can also develop, compress adjacent lung tissue, and further compromise ventilation, or these structures may spontaneously rupture, leading to a pneumothorax.

The pathogenesis of emphysema has received extensive study and remains a subject of continued investigation. The protease-antiprotease theory suggests that emphysema results from an imbalance between activities of proteases (especially elastase) and antiproteases. Supporting this theory is the association between human A1AT deficiency and emphysema, and the observation that exposure of the lungs of experimental animals to certain proteolytic enzymes can reproduce lesions of emphysema. The inflammatory response triggered by smoking may play an important role in pathogenesis; smokers with severe emphysema appear to accumulate substantially increased numbers of neutrophils, macrophages, T lymphocytes, and eosinophils compared to smokers with normal lung function. Neutrophil and macrophage activation is believed to occur, with release of proteases, especially elastase. Inactivation of antiproteases by reactive oxygen species introduced via tobacco smoke and activated neutrophils has also been described, further promoting tissue injury.

A1AT is a serine protease inhibitor synthesized by the liver and secreted into the blood. Its major function is the inhibition of neutrophil proteases, and it represents the most important inhibitor of protease activity in the lung. The A1AT gene is located on the long arm of chromosome 14 (SERPINA 1 gene with at least 70 alleles), and manifests an autosomal codominant pattern of allelic expression. The PiMM phenotype is the most common phenotype, occurring in 90% of the general population. Individuals homozygous for PiZ (PiZZ) have markedly reduced A1AT activity and are the most commonly affected by symptomatic emphysema, with 80-90% eventually developing emphysema. Heterozygous PiSZ individuals have 30-35% of normal activity and are at a higher risk as well. Tobacco smoking accelerates the progression of emphysema in patients with A1AT deficiency.

CLINICAL AND LABORATORY FEATURES

In the United States, 4-5% of males and 1-3% of females are estimated to have emphysema. The most important environmental cause is tobacco smoking, and A1AT deficiency accounts for another significant subset of patients with emphysema. Patients typically develop symptoms after age 50. Dyspnea is characteristic, while cough is not usually conspicuous unless there is coexisting chronic bronchitis. Respiratory rate increases, with use of accessory respiratory muscles. Thoracic examination may reveal a "barrel chest" due to hyperinflation, diffusely decreased breath sounds, hyperresonance on percussion, and prolonged inspiration. Clinical laboratory testing may include measurement of A1AT level, genotyping of A1AT in patients with A1AT levels greater than 7 mmol/L, hemoglobin/hematocrit measurement to detect polycythemia, and arterial blood gas testing. Pulmonary function testing shows reduction in forced expiratory volume in 1 second (FEV_1), as a reflection of airflow obstruction.

RADIOLOGIC FEATURES

Chest radiographs reveal hyperinflation with hyperlucency, rapidly tapering vascular shadows, "pushed down" diaphragms, and a long, narrow heart shadow. High resolution computed tomography (HRCT) is a more sensitive and specific test for emphysema (Figure 20-1) and will reveal bullae that may be less apparent on routine x-rays. However, HRCT is not part of routine evaluation, and is usually done in instances when lung volume reduction surgery is planned or if another abnormality (e.g., a lung cancer) is suspected.

PATHOLOGIC FEATURES

GROSS FINDINGS

The lungs usually appear enlarged and hyperinflated and have less than normal weight. Blebs or large, air-filled bullae (Figure 20-2) may be present, particularly in the

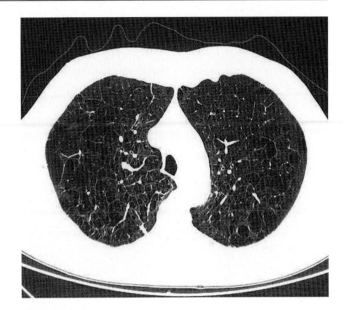

FIGURE 20-1
Emphysema
High-resolution computed tomography shows hyperinflated lungs with extensive emphysematous changes.

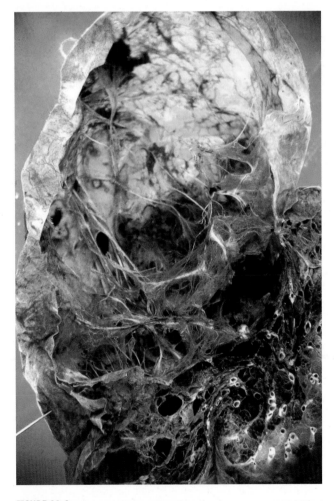

FIGURE 20-2
Emphysema
This inflated formalin-fixed lung demonstrates severe emphysema with bullae.

apices. In centriacinar emphysema, enlarged air spaces are visible in the centers of the lobules, and are surrounded by normal-appearing parenchyma (Figure 20-3). This type of emphysema is usually most pronounced in the central regions of the upper lobes. The walls of the enlarged air spaces often have a blackened appearance. In AIAT deficiency, panacinar emphysema is usually most severe in the lung bases and involves the entire lobule. Paraseptal emphysema appears as enlarged air spaces along interlobular septa and pleura. In irregular emphysema, the abnormal air spaces lie adjacent to focal lesions such as scars. Combinations of more than one type of emphysema are common, and bullae (emphysematous air spaces measuring more than 1.0 cm in diameter) may develop in any type.

MICROSCOPIC FINDINGS

Histologically, there is alveolar wall destruction with isolated or "free-floating" portions of septae that appear to be disconnected from other parenchymal structures (Figure 20-4). Enlargement of alveolar sacs without airway destruction can occur secondary to subtotal airway obstruction or as an artifact caused by overinflation with formalin, and should not be overdiagnosed as emphysema. In centriacinar emphysema, air space enlargement occurs in the proximal portion of the acinus/lobule (primarily at the level of the respiratory bronchiole), and distal alveoli are relatively spared. A small artery is

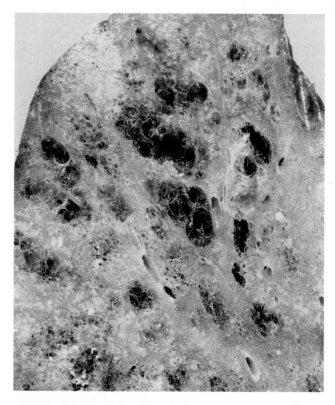

FIGURE 20-3
Emphysema
This upper lobe demonstrates emphysema that is predominantly centriacinar in distribution. Enlarged air spaces have darkened walls. (Courtesy of Dr. Dani Zander, Penn State M.S. Hershey Medical Center, Hershey, Pennsylvania.)

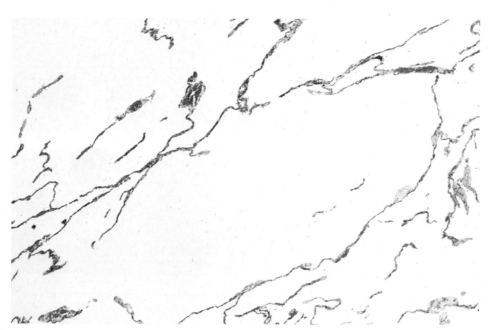

FIGURE 20-4
Emphysema
Air spaces are enlarged, with loss of alveolar septae and "free-floating" fragments of alveolar walls that appear unattached to adjacent structures.

often seen adjacent to the enlarged air space, and represents a clue to the centriacinar location of the emphysema. Groups of pigment-containing macrophages are also frequently seen in peribronchiolar regions. Panacinar emphysema results in diffuse acinar destruction and air space enlargement, involving all portions of the acinus/lobule. In paraseptal emphysema, the centriacinar structures are preserved, and the site of emphysematous air space enlargement lies adjacent to an interlobular septum or the pleura. In irregular emphysema, the emphysematous air spaces lie adjacent to a focal lesion, usually a scar.

PROGNOSIS AND THERAPY

Emphysematous destruction of air space structures is irreversible and can lead to death, directly or as a consequence of a complication such as bullous rupture with tension pneumothorax or hemorrhage. Goals of therapy include improving quality of life and preventing further damage. For smokers, smoking cessation is the most essential part of a comprehensive treatment plan.

CHRONIC BRONCHITIS

CLINICAL FEATURES

Chronic bronchitis is defined by clinical manifestations of a chronic productive or mucus-producing cough on most days of the month for at least 3 months in at least 2 consecutive years, with no other identifiable cause. In the United States, this disorder affects 4-5% of the population, most over the age of 45. Chronic bronchitis is associated with airflow obstruction, which is demonstrable by pulmonary function testing. It can occur as an isolated condition, but is often associated with emphysema

---

EMPHYSEMA—FACT SHEET

Definition
- Disorder characterized by abnormal permanent enlargement of air spaces distal to the terminal bronchiole, with destruction of their walls and without obvious fibrosis

Incidence
- Estimated to affect 5-8% of the U.S. population
- Primarily affects smokers and individuals with A1AT deficiency

Morbidity and Mortality
- A component of chronic obstructive pulmonary disease, which is the 4th leading cause of death in the United States
- Can lead to pulmonary hypertension and cor pulmonale especially if concurrent chronic bronchitis exists
- Can cause death from respiratory failure or rupture of bullae with tension pneumothorax or hemorrhage

Gender and Age Distribution
- Male predominance (male-to-female ratio = 2:1)
- Symptoms in smokers usually develop after age 50, but can occur earlier in A1AT deficiency, especially with concurrent smoking

Clinical Features
- Dyspnea is characteristic
- If coexisting chronic bronchitis is present, individuals will have a productive cough
- Physical examination: "barrel" chest, decreased breath sounds, prolonged inspiration
- Spirometry: decreased forced expiratory volume in 1 second (FEV_1)
- With advancing disease, hypoxemia develops

Radiologic Features
- Hyperinflated lungs, tapering vascular shadows with hyperlucency, "pushed down" diaphragms, bullae

Prognosis and Therapy
- Damage is irreversible
- Smoking cessation is central to treatment plan, to avoid progression
- A1AT deficiency is treated with A1AT replacement therapy
- Surgical therapies include bullectomy, lung volume reduction therapy, and lung transplantation

---

EMPHYSEMA—PATHOLOGIC FEATURES

Gross Findings
- Enlarged and hyperinflated lungs
- Bullae may be present, especially in the apical regions in smokers
- Several types of emphysema, which can occur in combinations and with varying severities:
  - Centriacinar (centrilobular): enlarged air spaces in centers of lobules (primarily at the level of the respiratory bronchiole), often with blackened walls, surrounded by unaffected parenchyma; upper lobes affected more than lower lobes
  - Panacinar (panlobular): air space enlargement throughout the lobule; in A1AT deficiency, lower lobes are affected more than upper lobes
  - Paraseptal: enlarged air spaces along interlobular septae and pleura
  - Irregular: Localized air space enlargement adjacent to a focal lesion, usually a scar

Microscopic Findings
- Alveolar wall destruction with "free-floating" portions of septae that appear disconnected from other parenchymal structures, leading to air space enlargement

Pathologic Differential Diagnosis
- Overinflation secondary to partial airway obstruction, or due to artifactual overinflation with formalin

or asthma. Direct bronchial damage related to tobacco use, bacterial and viral infections, allergic injury, and environmental pollution have been implicated in its pathogenesis. Periodic symptomatic exacerbations are common and are usually precipitated by infections.

RADIOLOGIC FEATURES

Radiologic studies often show bronchial wall thickening, but this finding is nonspecific.

PATHOLOGIC FEATURES

Gross findings include abundant mucus or mucopurulent secretions in airways, thickening of bronchial walls, and sometimes hyperemic mucosa, especially if superimposed airway infection is present (Figure 20-5).

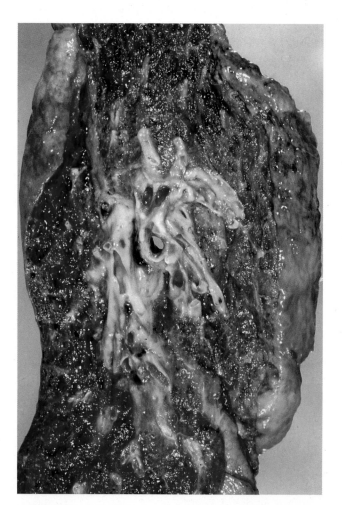

FIGURE 20-5
Chronic bronchitis
This lung shows thickened bronchi with hyperemic mucosae and peribronchial fibrosis.

Microscopically, increased intraluminal mucus is characteristic, primarily due to enlargement of the mucous glands in the bronchial wall, and also contributed to by the increased numbers of goblet cells in the surface epithelium (Figures 20-6, 20-7). The ratio of the thickness of the submucosal gland layer to the distance between the basal lamina of the mucosa and inner perichondrium is known as the "Reid Index." This ratio is increased in chronic bronchitis (normal is approximately 0.4). Chronic inflammatory cell infiltrates are typically observed in the mucosa and submucosa of bronchi and bronchioles, and lymphoid aggregates of bronchial-associated lymphoid tissue (BALT) may be seen in the walls of small airways and contribute to luminal narrowing. Other findings may include submucosal and adventitial fibrosis in bronchi and bronchioles, squamous metaplasia, reserve cell hyperplasia, and thickening of the bronchial basement membrane. Bronchioles often contain goblet cells, which do not exist in this location in normal lungs. Bronchiolar abnormalities (small airway diseases) are discussed more thoroughly in chapter 21.

PROGNOSIS AND THERAPY

Treatment is aimed at reducing bronchial irritation and treating infections. For smokers, smoking cessation is strongly advised. With advanced disease, patients develop hypoxemia, which can lead to pulmonary hypertension and cor pulmonale. Death is also commonly caused by respiratory failure associated with a bacterial pneumonia.

ASTHMA

Asthma is an increasingly common clinical syndrome that has significant worldwide medical and economic impact. In 1997, it was defined by the National Asthma Education and Prevention Program Expert Panel in the following manner:

"Asthma is a chronic inflammatory disorder of the airways in which many cells and cellular elements play a role, in particular, mast cells, eosinophils, T lymphocytes, neutrophils, and epithelial cells. In susceptible individuals, this inflammation causes recurrent episodes of wheezing, breathlessness, chest tightness, and cough, particularly at night and in the early morning. These episodes are usually associated with widespread but variable airflow obstruction that is often reversible either spontaneously or with treatment. The inflammation also causes an associated increase in the existing bronchial hyperresponsiveness to a variety of stimuli."

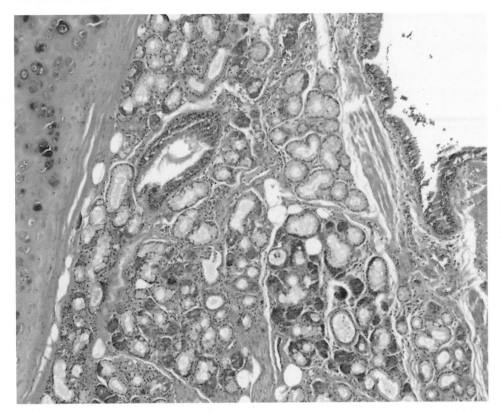

FIGURE 20-6

Chronic bronchitis
This bronchus has a markedly thickened submucosal gland layer. (Courtesy of Dr. Dani Zander, Penn State M.S. Hershey Medical Center, Hershey, Pennsylvania.)

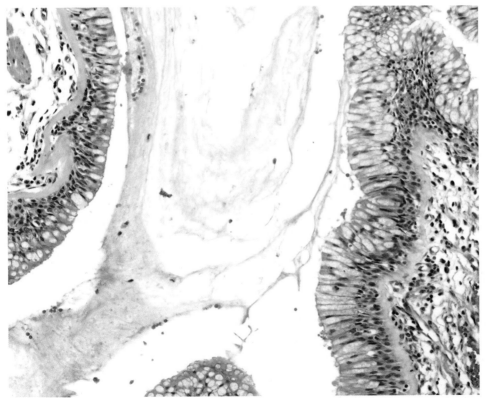

FIGURE 20-7

Chronic bronchitis
Goblet cell hyperplasia is conspicuous, and the basement membrane of the airway is thickened. The airway lumen contains abundant mucus.

CHRONIC BRONCHITIS—FACT SHEET

Definition

▸ Clinically defined by a chronic productive or mucus-producing cough on most days of the month for at least 3 months in at least 2 consecutive years, with no other identifiable cause

Incidence

▸ Affects 4-5% of the U.S. population

Morbidity and Mortality

▸ A component of chronic obstructive pulmonary disease, which is the 4th leading cause of death in the United States and has a mortality rate of 50% at 10 years after diagnosis
▸ Can lead to pulmonary hypertension and cor pulmonale
▸ Can also cause death from respiratory failure due to severe disease, often with superimposed respiratory tract infection

Gender and Age Distribution

▸ Female-dominant (male-to-female ratio = 1:2)
▸ Most affected individuals are more than 45 years of age

Clinical Features

▸ Associated with smoking (more than 90%); exposure to dusts, fumes, or toxins; airway infections; allergic airway injury
▸ Symptoms include cough with excessive sputum production, dyspnea
▸ Superimposed respiratory tract infections are common, and can be associated with worsening respiratory symptoms, fever, chills
▸ Spirometry: decreased forced expiratory volume in 1 second (FEV_1)
▸ With advancing disease, hypoxemia develops

Radiologic Features

▸ Nonspecific but may show bronchial wall thickening

Prognosis and Therapy

▸ High long-term mortality with death related to respiratory failure from exacerbations and infections
▸ Treatment strategies are geared toward reducing bronchial irritation and treating infections: smoking cessation, antibiotics for infections, bronchodilators, supplemental oxygen

---

CHRONIC BRONCHITIS—PATHOLOGIC FEATURES

Gross Findings

▸ Airways are filled with abundant mucus or mucopurulent secretions
▸ Bronchial walls often appear thickened, and the mucosal surfaces hyperemic

Microscopic Findings

▸ Abundant mucus in bronchial and bronchiolar lumens, with variable acute inflammation depending upon the presence or absence of infection
▸ Enlargement of the mucous glands in the bronchial wall
▸ Increased bronchial goblet cells, goblet cell metaplasia of bronchioles
▸ Chronic inflammatory infiltrates in the mucosa and submucosa of bronchi and bronchioles
▸ Increased bronchial-associated lymphoid tissue (BALT) in small airways
▸ Submucosal and adventitial fibrosis in bronchi and bronchioles
▸ Squamous metaplasia and reserve cell hyperplasia
▸ Thickening of the bronchial basement membrane

CLINICAL FEATURES

In the United States, asthma affects 5-10% of the population. Recent trends suggest an increase in the prevalence of asthma, especially in children less than 6 years of age. Although a variety of explanations have been put forth to account for the increasing frequency of this condition, there is currently no clear answer. The disease is most prevalent in the very young, with two-thirds of patients diagnosed prior to the age of 18 years. In many of these children, the condition becomes inapparent by early adulthood. Symptoms include wheezing, cough, shortness of breath, chest tightness, and sputum production. These symptoms vary in severity and frequency between individuals. In the usual case, an acute episode lasts up to several hours and responds to bronchodilators. Some patients have persistence of mild wheezing and cough chronically. The most severe form of asthma is status asthmaticus, in which the episode can persist for days. Triggering agents include a broad spectrum of allergens, respiratory tract infections, medications, gastroesophageal reflux, exercise, cold, and stress. Physical examination reveals end-expiratory wheezing or a prolonged expiratory phase. Peripheral blood eosinophilia greater than 4% is common. Spirometry shows reduction in the FEV_1/FVC ratio that improves with bronchodilators.

RADIOLOGIC FEATURES

In most patients, chest x-ray reveals normal lungs or hyperinflation.

Multiple classification systems for asthma have been published, based on symptomatic severity, therapeutic responsiveness, triggering agent(s) and pathogenesis. Atopic asthma is the most common type of asthma and involves stimulation of Th2 responses by inhaled antigens, leading to type I immunoglobulin-E-mediated hypersensitivity reactions. Other major types of asthma include nonatopic asthma (most often prompted by a respiratory tract infection), drug-induced asthma, and occupational asthma. Airflow obstruction results from bronchoconstriction via IgE-dependent reactions to aeroallergens or other stimulatory mechanisms; airway edema; luminal filling of airways by mucus, exudates, and cell debris; and chronic changes due to airway remodeling.

PATHOLOGIC FEATURES

In patients who have died of status asthmaticus, gross examination of the lungs shows areas of overinflation alternating with areas of atelectasis and mucus plugging. Microscopically, bronchial and bronchiolar walls are infiltrated by a mixture of inflammatory cells, typically including a prominent component of eosinophils (Figure 20-8). Mucus plugging is often present with inflammatory cells in the mucus, especially eosinophils. In the mucus, Charcot-Leyden crystals are commonly seen, as are detached tufts of ciliated columnar cells (Creola bodies) (Figure 20-9). Other histologic findings include muscular hyperplasia in airways, epithelial cell injury and loss, goblet cell hyperplasia in bronchi, thickening of the submucosal mucous glands, thickening of airway basement membranes, reserve cell hyperplasia, squamous metaplasia, and goblet cell metaplasia in bronchioles.

DIFFERENTIAL DIAGNOSIS

Many of the histologic changes in asthma overlap with those of chronic bronchitis, but the presence of conspicuous eosinophilia and smooth muscle hypertrophy favor asthma. That said, some patients with chronic bronchitis also have an allergic component to their airway disease and demonstrate airway eosinophilia. Asthma can also be associated with other diseases including allergic bronchopulmonary fungal diseases, eosinophilic pneumonia (Chapter 17), and Churg-Strauss syndrome (Chapter 8). Performance of a fungal stain is helpful for evaluating for bronchial colonization by fungi as occurs in allergic bronchopulmonary aspergillosis and other fungal diseases. Eosinophilic pneumonia demonstrates alveolar infiltrates of eosinophils, and may coexist with asthma. Asthma is one of multiple criteria used for diagnosis of Churg-Strauss syndrome. Histologically, in this disorder, asthmatic changes are accompanied by vasculitis.

PROGNOSIS AND THERAPY

Complications associated with asthma include pneumonia, pneumothorax, pneumomediastinum, and respiratory failure requiring intubation and mechanical ventilation. Management of asthma usually entails: (1) sequential objective measurement of lung function, (2) environmental control measures, (3) comprehensive pharmacologic therapy, and (4) patient education. Therapeutic goals include control of symptoms, prevention of exacerbations, optimization of pulmonary function, maintenance of activity, avoidance of adverse effects of medications, and prevention of irreversible airflow limitation and asthma-related mortality.

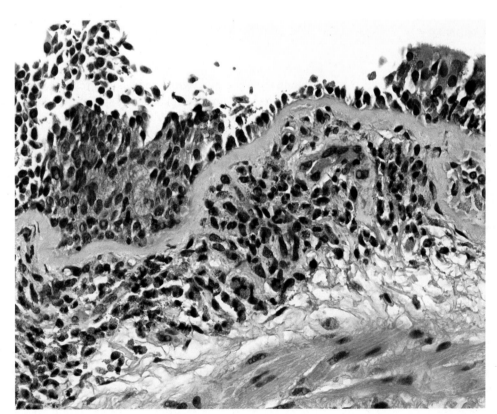

FIGURE 20-8

Asthma

The bronchial wall is infiltrated by inflammatory cells, including numerous eosinophils. Airway epithelial injury and cell loss are evident.

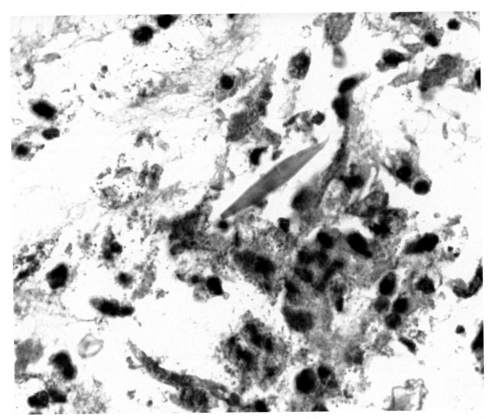

FIGURE 20-9

Asthma

A rhomboid Charcot-Leyden crystal lies in a background of degenerating eosinophils.

ALLERGIC BRONCHOPULMONARY ASPERGILLOSIS

Allergic bronchopulmonary aspergillosis (ABPA) is an allergic lung disorder most often triggered by the common fungus *Aspergillus fumigatus,* and occasionally by other aspergillus species. It primarily occurs in patients with asthma or cystic fibrosis, and rarely in patients with chronic granulomatous disease or the hyper-immunoglobulin E syndrome, or without clinical features of any of these disorders. In ABPA, airway injury is caused by a combination of direct fungal injury via fungal proteases and an antigen-induced Th2-type response with cytokine and chemokine release, eosinophil infiltration, and growth factor secretion promoting airway remodeling. Enhanced susceptibility is associated with HLA-DR2 and/or DR5. Occasionally, similar clinicopathologic syndromes can be caused by other fungi ("allergic bronchopulmonary fungal disease") including species of *Candida, Curvularia, Helminthosporium, Torulopsis, Bipolaris, Cladosporium, Saccharomyces, Schizophyllum,* and *Trichosporon.*

CLINICAL AND LABORATORY FEATURES

Patients with ABPA often experience a worsening of asthmatic symptoms, with shortness of breath, wheezing, and production of thick, brown sputum or mucus plugs. The incidence of ABPA is approximately 1-2% in patients with persistent asthma, and 1-15% in patients with cystic fibrosis. Features of ABPA include the following: asthma, lung infiltrates, central bronchiectasis, immediate reactivity to cutaneous injections of small doses of *A. fumigatus,* elevated total serum IgE, precipitating antibodies to *A. fumigatus,* and peripheral blood eosinophilia. If central bronchiectasis is present, essential criteria include the presence of asthma, immediate cutaneous reactivity to *Aspergillus* antigens, and serum IgE greater than 417 IU per mL.

RADIOLOGIC FEATURES

In ABPA, chest radiographic abnormalities include fleeting alveolar and subsegmental or lobar infiltrates that are often bilateral and predominantly in the

ASTHMA—FACT SHEET

Definition

▸ National Asthma Education and Prevention Program Expert Panel (1997): "Asthma is a chronic inflammatory disorder of the airways in which many cells and cellular elements play a role, in particular, mast cells, eosinophils, T lymphocytes, neutrophils, and epithelial cells. In susceptible individuals, this inflammation causes recurrent episodes of wheezing, breathlessness, chest tightness, and cough, particularly at night and in the early morning. These episodes are usually associated with widespread but variable airflow obstruction that is often reversible either spontaneously or with treatment. The inflammation also causes an associated increase in the existing bronchial hyperresponsiveness to a variety of stimuli."

Incidence

▸ Affects 5-10% of the U.S. population, and is increasing

Morbidity and Mortality

▸ Responsible for more than 11 million hospital visits per year
▸ Accounts for more than 5,000 deaths annually, and may contribute to more

Gender, Race, and Age Distribution

▸ Male predominance (male-to-female ratio = 2:1) until puberty (male-to-female ratio = 1:1)
▸ Higher frequency in children, with two-thirds of individuals diagnosed before age 18
▸ May have a higher prevalence in African-American children

Clinical Features

▸ Symptoms include wheezing, breathlessness, cough, chest tightness, and sputum production
▸ Typical acute episode lasts up to several hours and responds to bronchodilators
▸ Some patients have persistence of mild symptoms between acute exacerbations
▸ Symptoms may be triggered by exposure to allergens, respiratory tract infections, exercise, medications, air pollution, cold, stress
▸ Physical examination reveals an increased respiratory rate and end-expiratory wheezing
▸ Spirometry shows a reduced FEV_1/FVC ratio that improves with bronchodilators

Radiologic Features

▸ Chest x-ray can appear normal or show hyperinflation or occasionally atelectasis

Prognosis and Therapy

▸ Symptoms often disappear as children become adults
▸ Most patients with asthma can achieve symptomatic control and improvement of lifestyle through patient education, avoidance of potential triggers, and pharmacologic therapy with anti-inflammatory agents and bronchodilators

ASTHMA—PATHOLOGIC FEATURES

Gross Findings

▸ In fatal status asthmaticus, there are areas of overinflation and atelectasis, and filling of bronchi and bronchioles with mucus

Microscopic Findings

▸ Mixed inflammatory cell infiltrates (with eosinophils) in bronchi and bronchioles
▸ Smooth muscle hypertrophy in airways
▸ Goblet cell hyperplasia in bronchi, goblet cell metaplasia of bronchioles
▸ Enlarged bronchial submucosal glands
▸ Mucus plugging of airways with mixed inflammation including eosinophils and Charcot-Leyden crystals
▸ Epithelial cell injury and loss, reserve cell hyperplasia, squamous
▸ Thickened bronchial basement membranes

Cytologic Findings (Bronchial Brushings and Washings)

▸ Inflammation with prominent eosinophils
▸ Charcot-Leyden crystals
▸ Creola bodies
▸ Goblet cell hyperplasia

Pathologic Differential Diagnosis

▸ Chronic bronchitis
▸ Eosinophilic pneumonia
▸ Churg-Strauss syndrome

upper lobes; cystic bronchiectasis and mucus plugs; and thickened bronchial walls (Figure 20-10). There may also be pleural thickening, atelectasis, scarring, and air trapping.

PATHOLOGIC FEATURES

Classic pathologic findings include bronchiectasis, mucoid impaction of bronchi, bronchocentric granulomas, eosinophilic pneumonia, and chronic or exudative bronchitis. Mucoid impaction is manifested by filling of the ectatic bronchial lumen by mucus intermixed with inflammatory cells, including numerous eosinophils (Figure 20-11). It may be organized as "allergic mucin," with a layered pattern of cells, cellular debris, Charcot-Leyden crystals, and mucus. *Aspergillus* hyphae are found in the luminal mucoid material (colonizers), but may be difficult to locate due to small numbers and fragmentation (Figure 20-12). The histologic changes in the adjacent bronchial wall are usually those of asthma, and direct invasion by the fungus is usually absent. In bronchocentric granulomatosis, necrotizing granulomas with or without fungi are centered upon

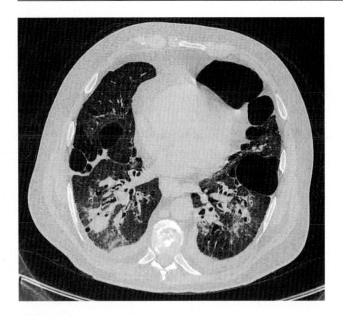

FIGURE 20-10

Allergic bronchopulmonary aspergillosis
The CT scan demonstrates bronchiectasis and bilateral lung parenchymal infiltrates.

DIFFERENTIAL DIAGNOSIS

None of the major pathologic manifestations of ABPA is restricted to this disorder. Mucoid impaction can also occur in settings of airway obstruction due to neoplasms and other infections. Bronchocentric granulomatosis can represent a response to infections with mycobacteria, other genera of fungi, or *Echinococcus.* Eosinophilic pneumonia has many different associations (Chapter 17).

PROGNOSIS AND THERAPY

The treatment of ABPA includes corticosteroids and antifungal agents. This approach will usually reduce airway inflammation and fungal colonization of airways.

small airway lumens; an elastic stain can be helpful to outline the residuum of the airway wall (Figures 20-13, 20-14). Eosinophilic pneumonia is characterized by alveolar infiltrates of eosinophils and macrophages (Chapter 17).

BRONCHIECTASIS

Bronchiectasis refers to permanent dilatation of bronchi and bronchioles usually caused by inflammatory damage to the structural elements of the airway walls. These airways are typically easily collapsible and partially or completely filled with mucopurulent

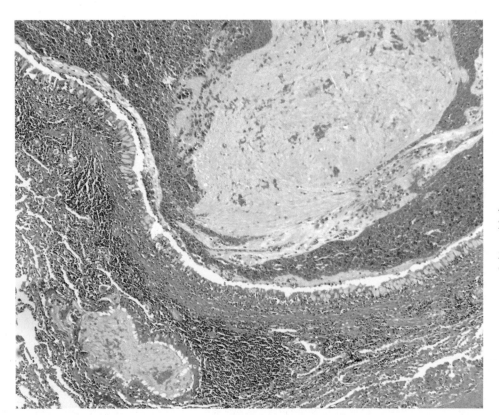

FIGURE 20-11

Allergic bronchopulmonary aspergillosis—mucoid impaction
The bronchial lumen is filled with allergic mucin. (Courtesy of Dr. Dani Zander, Penn State M.S. Hershey Medical Center, Hershey, Pennsylvania.)

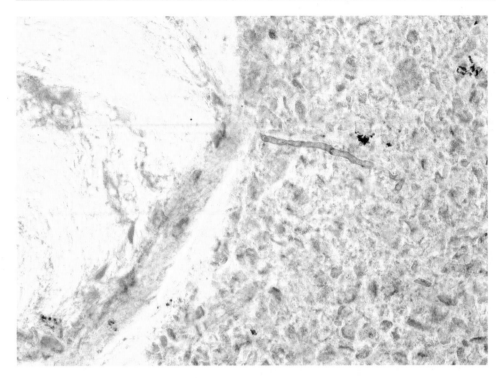

FIGURE 20-12

Allergic bronchopulmonary aspergillosis—mucoid impaction
A fragmented *Aspergillus* hyphus is highlighted by this methenamine silver stain.

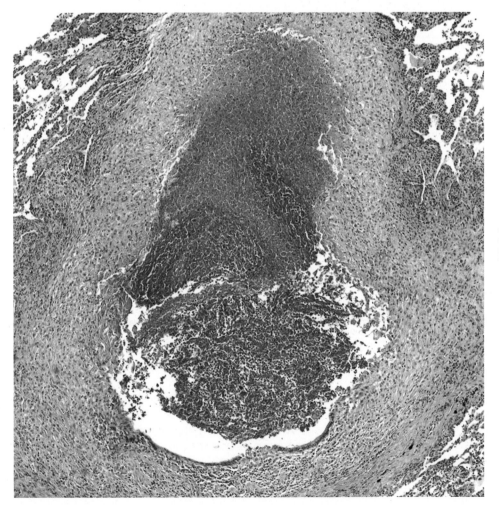

FIGURE 20-13

Allergic bronchopulmonary aspergillosis—bronchocentric granulomatosis
This small airway is markedly distorted by necrotizing granulomatous inflammation.

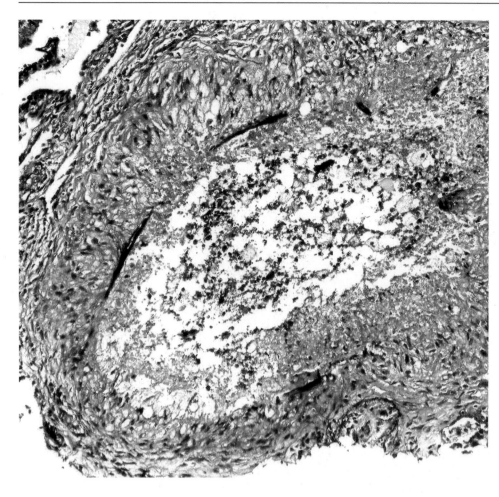

FIGURE 20-14

Allergic bronchopulmonary aspergillosis—bronchocentric granulomatosis
An elastic stain helps to delineate the existence of a small airway that has been obscured by the necrotizing granulomatous inflammation.

exudates, resulting in impairment of clearance and airflow obstruction. Airway obstruction is also a common antecedent of bronchiectasis. A foreign body, inspissated mucus plug (in cystic fibrosis, for example), neoplasm, intraluminal inflammatory process, or source of extrinsic compression (neoplasm or enlarged lymph node) can produce obstruction, interfere with airway clearance, and predispose to the chronic destructive inflammation that leads to bronchiectasis. Airway injury results from products of inflammatory cells as well as direct damage inflicted by the infectious agents and their secreted products. If the obstruction and associated inflammation are relieved early in the process, the damage may be reversible. With persistence over time, however, there will be loss of smooth muscle, elastic fibers, and cartilage, with replacement fibrosis and changes that are not reversible.

With localized obstruction, the resulting bronchiectasis will generally be limited to the obstructed airway(s). Other etiologies of bronchiectasis can affect multiple airways. Severe and chronic airway infections (especially *Staphylococcus* sp., *Klebsiella* sp., pertussis,

measles) can damage single or multiple airways and cause bronchiectasis. Hereditary disorders including cystic fibrosis, ciliary disorders, and immune deficiencies predispose to chronic airway infections that can lead to more diffuse examples of bronchiectasis. Bronchiectasis can also occasionally be associated with aspiration, right middle lobe syndrome, Young's syndrome, congenital anatomic defects such as bronchopulmonary sequestration, rheumatoid arthritis, Sjögren's syndrome, panbronchiolitis, lung and bone marrow transplantation, and ABPA.

CLINICAL FEATURES

Although bronchiectasis can declare itself at any age, it usually has its origins during the first two decades of life. A productive cough is characteristic, and daily sputum measurement can be used as a measure of the severity of disease (less than 10 mL/d is mild, 10-150 mL/d is moderate, greater than 150 mL/d is severe). Other symptoms include hemoptysis, shortness of breath, and fevers.

ALLERGIC BRONCHOPULMONARY ASPERGILLOSIS—FACT SHEET

Definition

» An allergic inflammatory disorder of the airways triggered by inhaled *Aspergillus*, which can lead to bronchiectasis and lung parenchymal injury
» If central bronchiectasis is present, essential criteria include the following:
  » Presence of asthma
  » Immediate cutaneous reactivity to *Aspergillus* antigens
  » Serum IgE greater than 417 IU/mL

Incidence

» Occurs in 1-2% of individuals with persistent asthma
» Occurs in 1-15% of people with cystic fibrosis
» Rarely develops in patients with chronic granulomatous disease or hyper-IgE syndrome
» Rare in people without clinical features of any of these processes

Morbidity

» Usually treatable when recognized, but patients develop bronchiectasis and parenchymal fibrosis of variable severity

Gender and Age Distribution

» Male predominant (male-to-female ratio = 3:1)
» Onset is often in childhood, but the disorder can remain occult for years or decades

Clinical and Laboratory Features

» Asthmatic symptoms of wheezing and cough usually worsen, and individuals may produce thick brown sputum or mucus plugs containing *A. fumigatus*, which is detectable by histochemical stains and cultures
» Immediate cutaneous reactivity to small doses of *Aspergillus*
» Peripheral blood eosinophilia
» Elevated total serum IgE
» Precipitating antibodies to *Aspergillus*

Radiologic Features

» Pulmonary infiltrates, cystic bronchiectasis with mucus plugs, and thickened bronchial walls

Prognosis and Therapy

» Treatment with corticosteroids and antifungal agents usually produces clinical improvement

ALLERGIC BRONCHOPULMONARY ASPERGILLOSIS—PATHOLOGIC FEATURES

Gross Findings

» Central bronchiectasis with mucoid impaction
» Parenchymal consolidation and fibrosis

Microscopic Findings

» Mucoid impaction of bronchi: airway filling by "allergic mucin" with a layered pattern of cells (especially eosinophils), cellular debris, Charcot-Leyden crystals, *Aspergillus* hyphae (more extensive description of fungal morphology in Chapter 12)
» Asthmatic changes in airways, often with accompanying features of bronchiectasis
» Bronchocentric granulomas: necrotizing granulomas centered upon small airway lumens; distorted airways can be located with an elastic stain, and a fungal stain may highlight *Aspergillus* hyphae
» Eosinophilic pneumonia: eosinophil and macrophage infiltrates in alveoli with variable organization

Cytologic Findings (Bronchial Brushings and Washings, Bronchoalveolar Lavage)

» Numerous eosinophils (can be distinguished more easily from neutrophils on a Diff-Quik stain than on a Papanicolaou stain), abundant mucus, cellular debris, Charcot-Leyden crystals
» *Aspergillus* hyphae with degenerative changes and fragmentation

Pathologic Differential Diagnosis

» Mucoid impaction also occurs in settings of airway obstruction by neoplasms or other infectious processes
» Bronchocentric granulomas can also be associated with infections with mycobacteria, other genera of fungi, and *Echinococcus*
» Eosinophilic pneumonia can be associated with a wide variety of infectious and noninfectious agents (Chapter 17)
» Clinicopathologic syndromes ("allergic bronchopulmonary fungal diseases" or "allergic bronchopulmonary mycoses") similar to ABPA can be triggered by fungi other than *Aspergillus* (species of *Candida*, *Curvularia*, *Helminthosporium*, *Torulopsis*, *Bipolaris*, *Cladosporiosis*, *Saccharomyces*, *Schizophyllum*, *Trichosporon*)

RADIOLOGIC FEATURES

High resolution computed tomography (HRCT) will demonstrate this condition, with a sensitivity of 96% and a specificity of 93%. Chest x-ray is less sensitive. Atelectasis or infiltrates in the affected lung segment or lobe are also commonly present.

PATHOLOGIC FEATURES

GROSS FINDINGS

In some cases, the distribution of the bronchiectasis is related to its etiology (predilection for upper lobes in tuberculosis and ABPA, lower lobes in bacterial and viral

While the incidence of bronchiectasis is not known because the symptoms are not specific and minor forms of the condition go unrecognized, it appears to have declined with widespread immunization (pertussis) and effective antibiotic treatment of airway infections. Potential complications include recurrent pneumonia, empyema, pneumothorax, and lung abscesses.

infections, all lobes in cystic fibrosis and immune deficiencies) (Figures 20-15, 20-16). The shapes of the dilated sections of bronchi can be described as saccular, cystic, or cylindrical. The airway wall may appear thickened, and mucoid or mucopurulent secretions are frequently seen in the airway lumens. The mucosal surfaces can show ulcerations, irregularities, and hyperemia. Consolidation of the lung parenchyma can accompany the bronchiectasis, and the pleura may appear thickened.

MICROSCOPIC FINDINGS

The bronchial wall typically demonstrates prominent chronic inflammation with lymphoid follicles and germinal centers (Figure 20-17), and varying degrees of neutrophil infiltration. Epithelial ulceration is common (Figure 20-18). As the process advances, there is loss of smooth muscle and cartilage, formation of granulation tissue, and, eventually, dense fibrosis of the bronchial wall (Figure 20-17). Coexisting findings may include adjacent organizing pneumonia and pulmonary hypertensive changes. If tuberculosis is responsible for the bronchiectasis, granulomatous inflammation can also be seen. Ectatic bronchi may also contain fungi, usually *Aspergillus* (Figure 20-18), which may be a component of mucoid impaction in ABPA or organized as an aspergilloma (Chapter 12).

PROGNOSIS AND THERAPY

More effective approaches to prevention and treatment of airway infections have decreased the incidence of bronchiectasis in the United States. Antibiotics and chest physiotherapy are the mainstays of therapy. In patients whose symptoms are poorly controlled by antibiotics, surgery can be performed to remove the affected area, and selected vessel embolization can be done for significant hemoptysis. Lung transplantation can also be considered as a therapy for advanced cases. In fatal cases, mortality is usually related to progressive respiratory failure and cor pulmonale, infection, or occasionally massive hemorrhage from an eroded blood vessel.

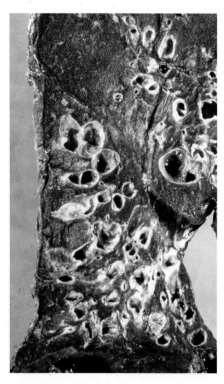

FIGURE 20-15
Bronchiectasis
Bronchi are markedly dilated.

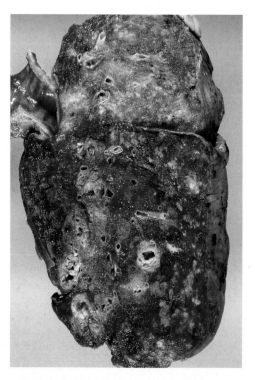

FIGURE 20-16
Bronchiectasis
This lung shows thickening and dilatation of some bronchi as well as pneumonia.

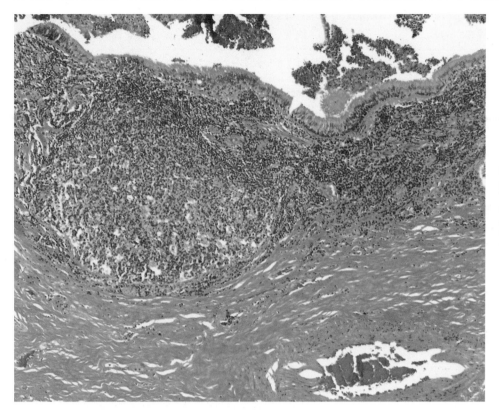

FIGURE 20-17

Bronchiectasis
The bronchial wall is distorted by chronic inflammation with germinal center formation, and dense fibrosis. Note the absence of cartilage, smooth muscle, and submucosal glands.

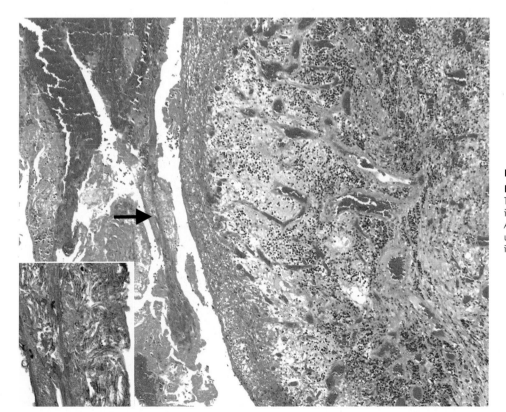

FIGURE 20-18

Bronchiectasis
This bronchus demonstrates ulceration, inflammation, and granulation tissue. *Aspergillus* hyphae focally overlie the ulcerated mucosal surface (arrow and inset).

BRONCHIECTASIS—FACT SHEET

Definition

» Permanent dilatation of bronchi and bronchioles usually caused by inflammatory damage to the structural elements of the airway walls

Incidence

» Not known, but has declined since the introduction of immunizations and antibiotics in the United States
» A major cause of morbidity in less developed countries
» Etiologies and associations include airway obstruction (foreign body, inspissated mucus plug, neoplasm, intraluminal inflammatory process, extrinsic compression), severe and chronic airway infections, hereditary disorders (cystic fibrosis, ciliary disorders, immune deficiencies), aspiration, right middle lobe syndrome, Young's syndrome, congenital anatomic defects such as bronchopulmonary sequestration, rheumatoid arthritis, Sjögren's syndrome, panbronchiolitis, lung and bone marrow transplantation, ABPA

Mortality

» Death rate of 1,000 patients per year in the United States
» Mortality is related to progressive respiratory failure and cor pulmonale, infection, or occasionally massive hemorrhage from an eroded blood vessel

Gender, Race, and Age Distribution

» No significant gender or racial predilection
» Process often begins in childhood
» Diagnosis can be made during childhood or adulthood

Clinical Features

» Symptoms include daily viscid sputum production, hemoptysis, shortness of breath, fevers
» Hypoxemia can develop with advancing disease

Radiologic Features

» High resolution computed tomography is very effective for showing the airway dilatation and wall thickening
» Atelectasis and lung infiltrates are common accompaniments

Prognosis and Therapy

» Prognosis is related to potential complications including pneumonia, abscesses, empyema, pneumothorax, and hemoptysis
» Standard therapy includes antibiotics and chest physiotherapy
» Surgical excision of the affected area or selected vessel embolization can be done for significant hemoptysis
» Lung transplantation can be performed for advanced disease

BRONCHIECTASIS—PATHOLOGIC FEATURES

Gross Findings

» Dilated airways filled with mucoid or mucopurulent secretions
» Airway wall may appear thickened
» Mucosal surfaces can show ulcerations, irregularities, and hyperemia
» Consolidation of the lung parenchyma may accompany the bronchiectasis, and the pleura may appear thickened

Microscopic Findings

» Prominent chronic inflammatory infiltrates with variable degrees of neutrophil infiltration and often lymphoid aggregates with germinal centers
» Reactive changes in the respiratory epithelium, reserve cell hyperplasia, squamous metaplasia
» Epithelial ulceration is common
» Loss of airway smooth muscle, elastic fibers, and cartilage, with formation of granulation tissue and eventually dense fibrosis of the airway wall
» Other accompanying findings may include organizing pneumonia and pulmonary hypertensive changes
» If secondary to tuberculosis, granulomatous inflammation can be seen (acid-fast stains may be helpful for identification)
» Fungi, usually *Aspergillus*, may colonize ectatic bronchi either as an aspergilloma or as a component of mucoid impaction in ABPA (fungal stains may be helpful for identification)

Cytologic Findings (Bronchial Brushings and Washings)

» Mixed inflammation, cellular debris, mucus, reactive respiratory epithelial cells, squamous metaplasia

Pathologic Differential Diagnosis

» Depending upon the clinical information, a variety of testing may be done to determine the etiology of the bronchiectasis:
  » Bronchoscopy—to evaluate for airway obstruction and remove a foreign body, if one is present
  » Cultures—to evaluate for severe and chronic airway infections caused by bacteria, mycobacteria, and fungi
  » Sweat chloride test and genetic testing—to evaluate for cystic fibrosis
  » Ciliary motility and ultrastructural studies—to evaluate for ciliary disorders
  » Complete blood count, peripheral blood differential count, immunoglobulin assays, cellular immune deficiency assays—to evaluate for immune deficiencies and ABPA
  » Testing for immediate cutaneous reactivity to *Aspergillus* antigens—to evaluate for ABPA
  » Autoimmune serologic studies—to evaluate for rheumatoid arthritis and Sjögren's syndrome
  » Radiographic and angiographic studies—to evaluate for right middle lobe syndrome and congenital anatomic defects such as bronchopulmonary sequestration

SUGGESTED READINGS

Emphysema

1. Bohadana A, Teculescu D, Martinet Y. Mechanisms of chronic airway obstruction in smokers. *Respir Med*. 2004;98:139-51.
2. Churg A, Wright JL. Proteases and emphysema. *Curr Opin Pulm Med*. 2005;11:153-9.
3. Grumelli S, Corry DB, Song LZ, et al. An immune basis for lung parenchymal destruction in chronic obstructive pulmonary disease and emphysema. *PLoS Med*. 2004;1:e8.
4. Hogg JC. Pathophysiology of airflow limitation in chronic obstructive pulmonary disease. *Lancet*. 2004;364:709-21.
5. Pinkard NB. Enlarged airspaces. In Cagle PT, ed. *Diagnostic Pulmonary Pathology*. New York: Marcel Dekker, Inc; 2000:349-52.
6. Retamales I, Elliott WM, Meshi B, et al. Amplification of inflammation in emphysema and its association with latent adenoviral infection. *Am J Respir Crit Care Med*. 2001;164:469-73.
7. Snider G, et al. The definition of emphysema: report of a National Heart, Lung, and Blood Institute, Division of Lung Diseases workshop. *Am Rev Respir Dis*. 1985;132:182-85.
8. Stavngaard T, Shaker SB, Dirksen A. Quantitative assessment of emphysema distribution in smokers and patients with alpha(1)-antitrypsin deficiency. *Respir Med*. 2005;100:94-100.
9. Tomashefski JF Jr, Crystal RG, Weidemann HP, et al. The bronchopulmonary pathology of alpha-1 antitrypsin (AAT) deficiency: findings of the Death Review Committee of the national registry for individuals with severe deficiency of alpha-1 antitrypsin. *Hum Pathol*. 2004;35:1452-61.

Chronic Bronchitis

10. American Thoracic Society. Standards for the diagnosis and care of patients with chronic obstructive pulmonary disease. *Am J Respir Crit Care Med*. 1995;152: S77-S121.
11. Hogg JC. Pathophysiology of airflow limitation in chronic obstructive pulmonary disease. *Lancet*. 2004;364:709-21.
12. Liu X, Driskell RR, Engelhardt JF. Airway glandular development and stem cells. *Curr Top Dev Biol*. 2004;64:33-56.
13. Llor C, Naberan K, Cots JM, et al. Economic evaluation of the antibiotic treatment of exacerbations of chronic bronchitis and COPD in primary care. *Int J Clin Pract*. 2004;58:937-44.
14. Miravitlles M, Llor C, Naberan K, et al, for the EFEMAP study group. Variables associated with recovery from acute exacerbations of chronic bronchitis and chronic obstructive pulmonary disease. *Respir Med*. 2005;99:955-65.
15. Orlandi I, Moroni C, Camiciottoli G, et al. Chronic obstructive pulmonary disease: thin-section CT measurement of airway wall thickness and lung attenuation. *Radiology*. 2005;234:604-10.
16. Schmier JK, Halpern MT, Higashi MK, et al. The quality of life impact of acute exacerbations of chronic bronchitis (AECB): a literature review. *Qual Life Res*. 2005;14:329-47.
17. Sethi S, Murphy TF. Acute exacerbations of chronic bronchitis: new developments concerning microbiology and pathophysiology: impact on approaches to risk stratification and therapy. *Infect Dis Clin North Am*. 2004;18:861-2.
18. Sunyer J, Zock JP, Kromhout H, et al. Lung function decline, chronic bronchitis and occupational exposures in young adults. *Am J Respir Crit Care Med*. 2005;172:1139-45.

Asthma

19. Bai TR, Knight DA. Structural changes in the airways in asthma: observations and consequences. *Clin Sci*. 2005;108:463-77.
20. Bochner B, Busse W. Allergy and asthma. *J Allergy Clin Immunol*. 2005;115:953-9.
21. Chan-Yeung M. Occupational asthma: the past 50 years. *Can Respir J*. 2004;11:21-6.
22. Guinee DG. Pulmonary eosinophilia. In: Cagle PT, ed. *Diagnostic Pulmonary Pathology*. New York: Marcel Dekker, Inc; 2000:208-11.
23. Kenyon NJ, Jarjour NN. Severe asthma. *Clin Rev Allergy Immunol*. 2003;25:131-49.
24. Kheradmand F, Rishi K, Corry DB. Environmental contributions to the allergic asthma epidemic. *Environ Health Perspect*. 2002;110:553-6.
25. McFadden ER. Exercise-induced airway obstruction. *Clin Chest Med*. 1995;16:671-82.
26. McFadden ER, Warren EL: Observations in asthma mortality. *Ann Intern Med*. 1997;127:142-7.
27. National Asthma Education and Prevention Program. Expert Panel Report 2: Guidelines for the Diagnosis and Management of Asthma. Bethesda, MD: National Institutes of Health. Publication No. 97-4051. 1997.
28. National Asthma Education and Prevention Program. Expert Panel Report: Guidelines for the Diagnosis and Management of Asthma. Update of Selected Topics—2002. Bethesda, MD: National Institutes of Health. Publication No. 02-5074. 2003.

Allergic Bronchopulmonary Aspergillosis

29. Greenberger PA. Allergic bronchopulmonary aspergillosis. *J Allergy Clin Immunol*. 2002;110:685-92.
30. Hamill RJ. Infectious diseases: mycotic. In: Tierney LM, McPhee SJ, Papadakis, MA, eds. *Current Medical Diagnosis and Treatment*. 37 ed. Stamford: Appleton & Lange, 1997.
31. Knutsen AP. Lymphocytes in allergic bronchopulmonary aspergillosis. *Front Biosci*. 2003;8:d589-d602.
32. Marr KA, Patterson T, Denning D. Aspergillosis: pathogenesis, clinical manifestations, and therapy. *Infect Dis Clin North Am*. 2002;16:875-94.
33. Soubani AO, Chandrasekar PH. The clinical spectrum of pulmonary aspergillosis. *Chest*. 2002;121:1988-99.
34. Wark PA, Gibson PG. Allergic bronchopulmonary aspergillosis: new concepts of pathogenesis and treatment. *Respirology*. 2001;6:1-7.
35. Zander DS. Allergic bronchopulmonary aspergillosis: an overview. *Arch Pathol Lab Med*. 2005;129:924-8.

Bronchiectasis

36. Cowan MJ, Gladwin MT, Shelhamer JH. Disorders of ciliary motility. *Am J Med Sci*. 2001;321:3-10.
37. Dogru D, Nik-Ain A, Kiper N, et al. Bronchiectasis: the consequence of late diagnosis in chronic respiratory symptoms. *J Trop Pediatr*. 2005; 51:362-5.
38. Fujita J, Ohtsuki Y, Shigeto E, et al. Pathological findings of bronchiectasis caused by Mycobacterium avium intracellulare complex. *Respir Med*. 2003;97:933-8.
39. Pasteur MC, Helliwell SM, Houghton SJ, et al. An investigation into causative factors in patients with bronchiectasis. *Am J Respir Crit Care Med*. 2000;162:1277-84.
40. Pifferi M, Caramella D, Bulleri A, et al. Pediatric bronchiectasis: correlation of HRCT, ventilation and perfusion scintigraphy, and pulmonary function testing. *Pediatr Pulmonol*. 2004;38:298-303.
41. Redding G, Singleton R, Lewis T, et al. Early radiographic and clinical features associated with bronchiectasis in children. *Pediatr Pulmonol*. 2004;37:297-304.
42. Remy-Jardin A, Amara A, Campistron P, et al. Diagnosis of bronchiectasis with multislice spiral CT: accuracy of 3 mm thick structured sections. *Eur Radiol*. 2003;13:1165-71.
43. Valery PC, Torzillo PJ, Mulholland K, et al. Hospital-based case-control study of bronchiectasis in indigenous children in Central Australia. *Pediatr Infect Dis J*. 2004;23:902-8.

21 Diseases of Small Airways

Armando E. Fraire • Roberto J. Barrios

INTRODUCTION

Bronchiolitis is a general term used to describe inflammatory lung diseases primarily affecting the small conducting airways and often (but not always) sparing the more distal lung parenchyma. Bronchiolitis occurs in a wide variety of clinical settings (Table 21-1) and manifests varied histopathologic changes, resulting in an equally varied and sometimes confusing terminology. Diseases of small airways involve airways of 2 mms in diameter or less, roughly corresponding to ninth-generation airways. Their fundamental histopathologic feature is complete or partial luminal obstruction brought about by bronchiolar wall thickening and inflammation, intraluminal growth or peribronchiolar fibrosis. This can translate into physiologic changes of obstruction, but, not uncommonly, restrictive defects may accompany these changes or occur alone. Radiographic characteristics of bronchiolitis include bronchiolar wall thickening, bronchiolar dilatation and luminal impaction due to either secretions or cellular or fibrotic intraluminal tissue. Impaction is manifested radiographically as 2-4 mm nodular or linear branching centrilobular opacities on computed tomography of the chest. It can produce a tree-in-bud radiographic pattern, which is regarded as typical of bronchiolitis, in which branching linear structures have more than one contiguous branching site, somewhat resembling the childhood toy "jacks."

By definition, bronchioles are airways that do not have cartilage in their walls. The membranous (or terminal) bronchioles serve purely an air conducting function (Figure 21-1), while the respiratory bronchioles, which bear alveoli, also participate in gas exchange. Diseases affecting small airways may originate intrinsically within the bronchioles or may result from extension of diseases that involve primarily the bronchi (bronchitis, bronchiectasis) or the lung parenchyma (bronchopneumonia). As noted, this group of diseases has a broad spectrum of etiologies that includes infectious and non-infectious agents such as bacteria, viruses, toxic fumes, and inhaled dusts. Some diseases of small airways are associated with connective tissue disorders, others result from drug usage, and others occur in the clinical setting of organ transplantation. Given the histologic overlap between the manifestations of this spectrum of conditions, it is sometimes difficult to determine a specific cause of the bronchiolitis in an individual case. Bronchiolitis may also represent one of several features of another pulmonary disorder, such as hypersensitivity pneumonia or respiratory bronchiolitis-interstitial lung disease.

Diseases of small airways have been classified according to etiology or clinical setting, and also by histopathology (Tables 21-1, 21-2). This chapter will discuss the major clinicopathologic entities classified as small airway diseases.

ACUTE BRONCHIOLITIS

The term "acute bronchiolitis" is commonly used, clinically, to describe an illness in infants and children characterized by acute wheezing and signs of respiratory infection. It can also be used, histologically, to refer to acute inflammatory and sometimes necrotizing injury to the bronchiolar epithelium. The bronchiolar epithelium is vulnerable to acute injury by infectious agents (especially respiratory viruses, but also bacteria, *Mycoplasma,* *Chlamydia,* fungi, and mycobacteria) and inhaled toxic fumes and vapors. Acute injury to the bronchioles can also be seen in settings of asthma, aspiration, bronchiectasis, inflammatory bowel disease, and connective tissue

TABLE 21-1

Clinical Syndromes Associated with Bronchiolitis

Inhalational Injury	Postinfectious	Drug or Chemical Induced Reactions	Idiopathic
Toxic fume inhalation	Viral:	Hexamethonium	No associated diseases:
Grain dusts	Respiratory syncytial virus	L-Tryptophan	Cryptogenic bronchiolitis
Irritant gases	Adenovirus types 1,2,3,5,6,7,21	Busulfan	Respiratory bronchiolitis-associated interstitial
Mineral dusts	Rhinovirus	Free-base cocaine	lung disease
Fumes (e.g., welding)	Parainfluenza	Gold	Cryptogenic organizing pneumonia (also called
Cigarette smoke	Influenza	Cephalosporin	bronchiolitis obliterans organizing pneumonia)
	Paramyxovirus (measles or mumps)	Sulfasalazine	Diffuse panbronchiolitis
	Varicella zoster	Amiodarone	Associated with other diseases
	Cytomegalovirus	Acebutolol	Associated with organ transplantation:
	Human immunodeficiency virus	Sulindac	Bone marrow
	Other infectious agents:	Paraquat poisoning	Heart-lung
	Mycoplasma pneumoniae		Lung
	Legionella pneumophila		Associated with connective tissue disease:
	Serratia marcescens		De novo process
	Bordetella pertussis		Drug reaction
	Streptococcus group B, beta-		Idiopathic pulmonary fibrosis
	hemolytic		Hypersensitivity pneumonitis
	Nocardia asteroides		Malignant histiocytosis
			Chronic eosinophilic pneumonia
			Acute respiratory distress syndrome
			Vasculitis, especially Wegener's
			granulomatosis
			Chronic thyroiditis
			Irradiation pneumonitis
			Aspiration pneumonitis
			Distal to bronchial obstruction, "obstructive
			pneumonitis"
			Ulcerative colitis

From King TE Jr. Overview of bronchiolitis. *Clin Chest Med.* 1993;14:607-610, with permission.

disorders. The clinical, radiographic, and pathologic features described below apply primarily to acute viral bronchiolitis, but overlap to some extent with acute bronchiolar injury due to bacterial infections or inhaled toxic substances.

CLINICAL FEATURES

Most patients present with an acute onset of fever, tachypnea, dyspnea, prolonged expiration, and wheezing. In infants, nasal flaring and chest retractions may be seen. Crackles are usually heard on auscultation. Adults and children can be affected, and age predilections depend upon the specific etiologic agent. Infectious agents that cause acute bronchiolitis and its potential sequel, obliterative bronchiolitis, are discussed in more detail in other chapters. In brief, respiratory syncytial viruses (RSV) are responsible for annual outbreaks of bronchiolitis and pneumonia, primarily in infants and young children. Adenovirus and parainfluenza viruses can also produce acute bronchiolitis in children and adults, but more commonly cause upper respiratory tract infections. Cases of acute bronchiolitis caused by *M. pneumoniae, C. trachomatis,* and *C. pneumoniae* have been described in adults and children. Toxic inhalational exposures occur primarily in the adult population.

PULMONARY FUNCTION TESTING

Obstructive ventilatory defects can be observed.

RADIOLOGIC FEATURES

Radiographic studies show variable changes including centrilobular nodules, diffuse bilateral reticulonodular opacities, linear or ground-glass opacities, or patchy

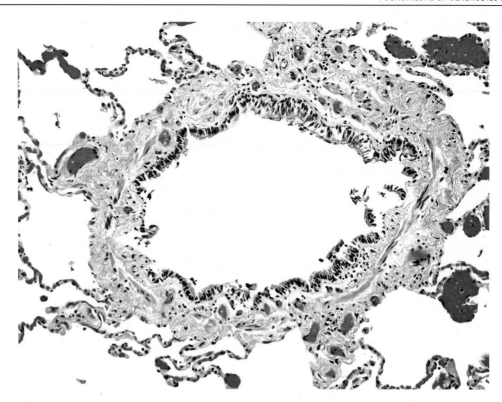

FIGURE 21-1

Normal membranous (terminal) bronchiole with ciliated columnar epithelium
The basement membrane is thin, and there is a circumferential layer of smooth muscle that can be distinguished from the connective tissue that surrounds the airway and is contiguous with the alveolar septa. The focal detachment of the epithelium is artifactual.

pneumonic consolidation. Hyperinflation is particularly common in children. Atelectasis can also be observed.

PATHOLOGIC FEATURES

Pathologic features of acute infectious bronchiolitis are primarily those of an acute bronchiolitis, with neutrophilic infiltration of the bronchiolar epithelium and the surrounding peribronchiolar tissues (Figure 21-2). Epithelial or mucosal necrosis may be present (Figure 21-3), and neutrophils and fibrinous material can accumulate in the lumens of bronchioles and alveolar ducts. Similar changes can occur in bronchiolar injuries associated with toxic inhalations, although some examples may show lesser degrees of inflammatory cell infiltration and more hypocellular necrosis. In cases of RSV infection, this phase is often followed by a pronounced regenerative hyperplasia of the bronchiolar epithelium, in which the epithelium develops small papillary projections extending into the bronchiolar lumens (Figure 21-4). Over time, the mural or luminal exudates can resolve or become organized and fibrotic, producing luminal obstruction. In the latter case, the process is then referred to as bronchiolitis obliterans, or obliterative

bronchiolitis. At these later points, lymphocytes and plasma cells can be seen in the fibrous tissue, and complete or partial loss of the bronchiolar epithelium is common. Other secondary changes include inflammation of alveolar walls and the presence of foamy macrophages in the peribronchiolar alveoli (endogenous lipoid pneumonia).

DIFFERENTIAL DIAGNOSIS

Acute bronchiolitis is often recognized from its clinical and radiographic features, and biopsy is usually not necessary. Biopsy is more commonly performed in severe or atypical cases, or in immunocompromised patients who may have multiple potential etiologies (with differing treatments) for their respiratory illnesses. For the most part, the histologic appearance does not point to a specific etiology, although there are exceptions. RSV and parainfluenza can produce multinucleated giant cells and intracytoplasmic inclusions (Figure 21-4, also discussed in Chapter 13). "Smudge cells" and intranuclear inclusions may indicate adenovirus. Immunohistochemical staining for respiratory viruses can be helpful, as can cultures, immunofluorescence staining, or molecular, serologic, or antigenic testing. Patient age

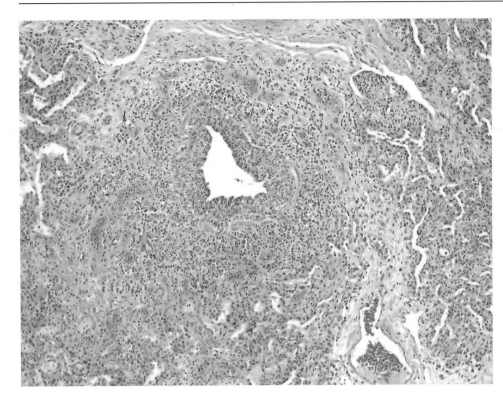

FIGURE 21-2

Acute bronchiolitis

Note dense acute inflammatory infiltrate within the bronchiolar epithelium. The peribronchiolar tissues are also inflamed.

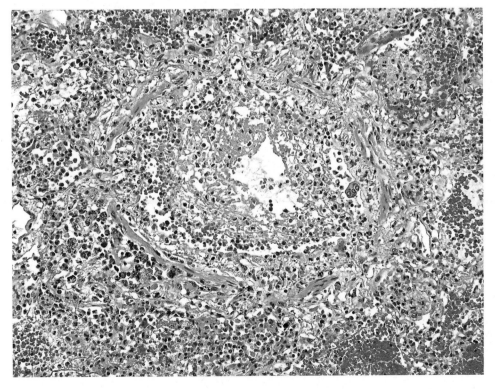

FIGURE 21-3

Acute bronchiolitis secondary to adenovirus

This severe case of acute necrotizing bronchiolitis developed in a solid organ transplant recipient. The bronchiolar mucosa shows extensive necrosis and inflammation with loss of the epithelium; only a small group of epithelial cells is visible. The smooth muscle is important for identifying this structure as a bronchiole. This type of injury may evolve into constrictive bronchiolitis.

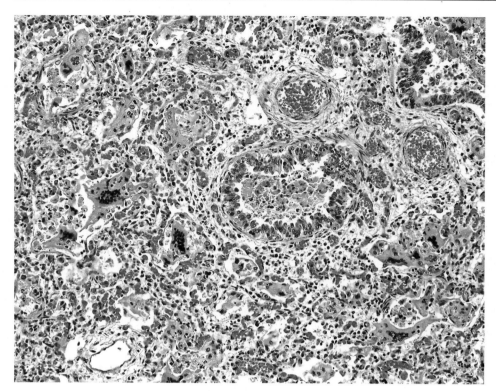

FIGURE 21-4

Bronchiolitis due to respiratory syncytial virus
Two bronchioles (central, top right) display epithelial hyperplasia, with formation of small papillary projections. Their lumens are partially obstructed by fibrinous and cellular exudate. In the adjacent lung parenchyma, the characteristic multinucleated cells are present.

ACUTE BRONCHIOLITIS—FACT SHEET

Definition

▸ Acute bronchiolar injury secondary to acute exposure to a variety of infectious and noninfectious agents

Incidence and Location

▸ Common clinical syndrome, often treated symptomatically without need for biopsy
▸ Worldwide distribution

Morbidity and Mortality

▸ Mortality is less than 1% overall
▸ Immunocompromised patients with respiratory viral infections have a higher mortality, especially with adenovirus
▸ Obliterative bronchiolitis is a potential consequence, and is a cause of chronic respiratory dysfunction

Gender, Race, and Age Distribution

▸ Affects both genders
▸ No specific racial predilection
▸ Age distribution depends upon particular cause

Clinical Features

▸ Symptoms include fever, tachypnea, dyspnea, prolonged expiration, wheezing
▸ Etiologies include infectious agents (especially respiratory viruses, but also bacteria, *Mycoplasma, Chlamydia,* fungi, and mycobacteria) and inhaled toxic fumes and vapors
▸ This injury pattern can also be seen in settings of asthma, aspiration, bronchiectasis, inflammatory bowel disease, and connective tissue disorders

---

ACUTE BRONCHIOLITIS—PATHOLOGIC FEATURES

Microscopic Findings

▸ Neutrophilic infiltration of the bronchiolar epithelium, with or without epithelial or mucosal necrosis, and fibrinous material in airway lumens
▸ With time, luminal exudates resolve or organize
▸ With respiratory syncytial virus infection, bronchiolar epithelial hyperplasia may be conspicuous
▸ Viral changes may be present (Chapter 13)

Immunohistochemistry

▸ Can be helpful for identification of specific respiratory viruses (respiratory syncytial virus, adenovirus, parainfluenza, influenza)

Pathologic Differential Diagnosis

▸ Spectrum of etiologies including infectious agents and noninfectious etiologies
▸ Diffuse panbronchiolitis
▸ Obliterative bronchiolitis

---

and history are also important for defining more likely etiologic agents.

The differential diagnosis may also include diffuse panbronchiolitis, which can include a component of acute inflammation but also shows characteristic centrilobular accumulations of foamy macrophages in interstitial regions and airspaces. Constrictive bronchiolitis may also show acute inflammatory infiltrates in bronchiolar mucosae, but will feature dense, mature collagenous

Pulmonary Function Tests
➤ Obstructive ventilatory defects can be observed

Radiologic Features
➤ Variable changes including centrilobular nodules, diffuse bilateral reticulonodular opacities, linear or ground-glass opacities, or patchy pneumonic consolidation
➤ Hyperinflation is particularly common in children
➤ Atelectasis can also be observed

Prognosis and Therapy
➤ The prognosis is variable, depending upon the diffuseness and severity of the injury
➤ Most patients have relatively mild symptoms and can be given supportive care, leading to full recovery
➤ With more severe disease, supplemental oxygen, antimicrobial therapy, corticosteroids, or bronchodilators may be administered

thickening of the bronchiolar wall, which will not be observed in acute bronchiolitis.

PROGNOSIS AND THERAPY

The prognosis is variable, depending upon the diffuseness and severity of the injury. Most patients have relatively mild symptoms and can be given supportive care. With more severe disease, supplemental oxygen, antimicrobial therapy, corticosteroids, or bronchodilators may

be administered. Overall, the mortality rate is less than 1%, but mortality associated with the respiratory viral infections appears to be higher with immunocompromise. Evolution of acute bronchiolitis into obliterative bronchiolitis occurs in some patients, particularly after adenovirus infection and after some toxic inhalations.

CONSTRICTIVE BRONCHIOLITIS

Constrictive bronchiolitis (CB), also known as bronchiolitis obliterans or obliterative bronchiolitis, is characterized clinically by chronic cough, dyspnea, limitation of airflow, and lack of response to bronchodilators and prednisone. Its main histopathologic features are irreversible mural and luminal fibrotic scarring of bronchioles with narrowing or obliteration of the airway lumens. CB occurs in a variety of clinical settings, often as a complication of lung or bone marrow transplantation; after exposure to inhaled toxic agents such as nitrogen dioxide, sulfur dioxide, ammonia, chlorine, and phosgene; with usage of some drugs such as gold, penicillamine and lomustine; as a sequel to infections with adenovirus and other respiratory viruses; and in the setting of systemic disorders such as rheumatoid arthritis, systemic sclerosis, ulcerative colitis, and ankylosing spondylitis. In the Far East, an outbreak of CB occurring in association with consumption of tea leaves of *Sauropus androgynous* (as an appetite suppressant) has been reported. Another rare syndrome, the Swyer-James syndrome (also known as MacLeod's syndrome)

TABLE 21-2

Comparison of Key Pathologic, Radiographic, and Physiologic Features in Proliferative and Constrictive Bronchiolitis Obliterans

Key Features	Proliferative Bronchiolitis	Constrictive Bronchiolitis
Histopathologic manifestations	Common finding Nonspecific reparative reaction to bronchiolar injury Organizing intraluminal exudate Most prominent in alveolar ducts Inflammatory changes in surrounding alveolar walls Foamy macrophages in alveoli	Very uncommon finding Obliterans not a constant feature Variety of histologic changes: bronchiolar inflammation to progressive concentric fibrosis; smooth muscle hyperplasia; bronchiolectasis with mucous stasis; distortion and fibrosis of small airway walls with bronchiolar metaplasia extending onto peribronchiolar alveolar septa Follicular bronchitis Cellular bronchiolitis
Radiographic abnormalities	Bilateral patchy air space opacities Interstitial opacities Small, rounded opacities Opacities may be migratory	May be normal Progressive increase in lung volume on serial radiographs High-resolution CT scan may show marked heterogeneity of lung density
Pulmonary function	Restrictive defect	Obstructive defect with hyperinflation

From King TE Jr. Overview of bronchiolitis. *Clin Chest Med.* 1993;14:607-610, with permission.

is characterized by CB in association with recurrent pulmonary infections, decreased exercise tolerance, and unilateral hyperlucency on chest radiographs. Some cases of CB are idiopathic.

The pathogenesis of this process is not well understood. Streichenberger, et al., studied the complex interaction between lysyl oxidase (LOX), the main collagen-cross-linking enzyme, and protein matrix components (tenascin, fibronectin) of the extracellular matrix, and identified three stages of the disease (inflammatory, fibroinflammatory, and fibrotic), suggesting that persistence of LOX might account for the irreversibility of the fibrotic process in the later stages of the disease. In the transplant literature, there is information about the roles of lymphocytes and fibroblasts, as well as a variety of mediators (growth factors, adhesion molecules, oxidants, and others) in the genesis of this process.

PULMONARY FUNCTION TESTING

Obstructive ventilatory defects are observed, without significant response to bronchodilators. In the setting of lung transplantation, progressive airway obstruction is characterized by decreasing FEV_1 (bronchiolitis obliterans syndrome).

RADIOLOGIC FEATURES

Chest radiographs may be normal or show nonspecific changes such as hyperinflation, peripheral attenuation of vascular margins, and sometimes nodular or reticulonodular opacities. Bronchial wall thickening and bronchiectasis can occasionally be seen.

PATHOLOGIC FEATURES

Typically, bronchioles in CB have thickened fibrotic hypocellular walls with concurrent luminal narrowing (Figure 21-5). The mature collagen is often circumferential in distribution, but not always so. In the fibrotic walls, a variably dense mononuclear inflammatory infiltrate including lymphocytes (usually predominantly T-cells, with fewer B-cells) and plasma cells may be seen. The dense collagen may replace some or all of the bronchiolar smooth muscle and extend out into peribronchiolar tissues. As the fibrosis progresses, the lumen can eventually become obliterated (Figure 21-6). The bronchiolar respiratory epithelium may have a reactive or attenuated appearance, with squamous metaplasia, or resemble type II pneumocytes.

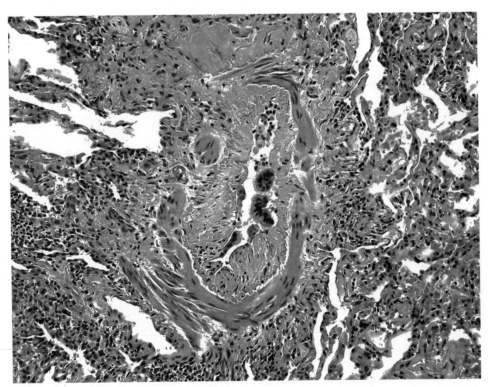

FIGURE 21-5
Constrictive bronchiolitis
There is circumferential collagen deposition, causing thickening of the bronchiolar wall and narrowing of the lumen.

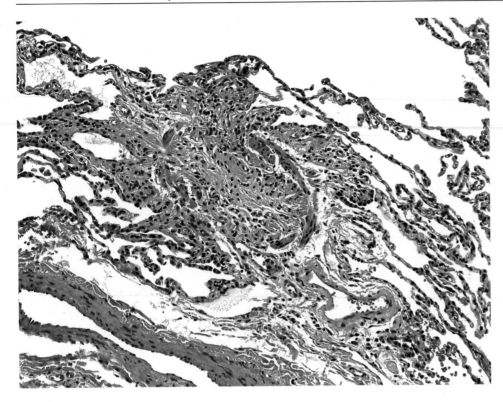

FIGURE 21-6
Constrictive bronchiolitis
The lumen of this bronchiole is completely filled by mature collagen.

Trichrome stains are helpful for assisting in the identification of obliterated bronchioles by highlighting their muscle coats, when their lumens have been replaced by fibrotic scars, and by clarifying the presence and degree of fibrosis. A Verhoeff-van Gieson elastic stain is also helpful for identifying the obstructed airways, by highlighting the elastic layer of the obliterated bronchioles. Another clue to the diagnosis lies in finding a small pulmonary artery branch that is unpaired with a bronchiole. Since the pulmonary arteries and the airways travel together, the absence of a bronchiole adjacent to a small artery should prompt consideration of obliterative bronchiolitis as a diagnostic possibility.

DIFFERENTIAL DIAGNOSIS

CB can overlap clinically and radiographically with organizing pneumonia, which can include a component of bronchiolar connective tissue. In organizing pneumonia, the connective tissue is usually young and fibroblastic, with little if any dense collagen, and occupies the lumen of the bronchiole rather than developing in the airway wall, as it does in CB. A subset of cases of organizing pneumonia, however, will develop substantial fibrosis with a component of obliterative bronchiolitis. In these cases, the luminal fibrosis often retains the appearance of a polypoid structure (Figure 21-7). In organizing pneumonia, the young connective tissue typically extends into adjacent alveoli, and may be accompanied by a chronic inflammatory infiltrate in the connective tissue, bronchiolar walls, and alveolar septa. In contrast, CB is characterized by a distinctive pattern of dense, highly collagenized fibrosis that is located in the bronchiolar wall, often with a circumferential distribution. Alternatively, CB can manifest with complete cicatrization of the bronchiolar lumen, again with a densely collagenized appearance.

Determination of the etiology of the CB is usually approached by evaluation of the clinical history, with a search for risk factors. By definition, the histologic lesion is usually advanced and does not usually offer information about the insult that was responsible for creating it.

PROGNOSIS AND THERAPY

The course of CB is usually progressive, often ending in respiratory failure. A variety of medications including corticosteroids, azathioprine, cyclosporine, methotrexate, ganciclovir, and OKT-3 have been used with variable, but generally unsuccessful, results. Corticosteroids and immunosuppressive drugs usually do not stop the evolution of the disease towards chronic respiratory insufficiency, and for many patients, lung transplantation

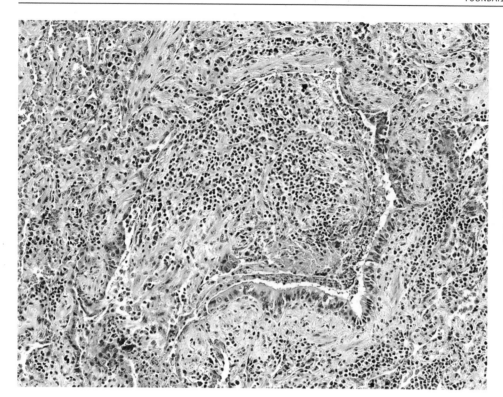

FIGURE 21-7
Obliterative bronchiolitis, probably arising from organizing pneumonia
The lumen of this bronchiole is totally obstructed by connective tissue with a dense chronic inflammatory infiltrate.

CONSTRICTIVE BRONCHIOLITIS—FACT SHEET

Definition
▸ A bronchiolar disease characterized clinically by chronic cough and dyspnea, functionally by limitation of air flow, and histopathologically by mural and peribronchiolar fibrosis

Incidence and Location
▸ The actual incidence is not known, but CB is more prevalent in the setting of organ transplantation, exposure to toxic agents, connective tissue disorders, and after viral infections
▸ Worldwide distribution

Morbidity and Mortality
▸ High mortality rate
▸ Most important cause of mortality in long-term survivors of lung transplantation
▸ Frequently complicated by superimposed infections

Gender, Race, and Age Distribution
▸ Affects adults and children of both genders
▸ No evident racial predilection

CONSTRICTIVE BRONCHIOLITIS—PATHOLOGIC FEATURES

Microscopic Findings
▸ Bronchioles have thickened fibrotic hypocellular walls with concurrent luminal narrowing; complete replacement of the lumen by mature collagen may occur
▸ The mature collagen is often circumferential in distribution, but not always so; it may replace some or all of the bronchiolar smooth muscle and extend out into peribronchiolar tissues
▸ The bronchiolar epithelium may have a reactive or attenuated appearance, with squamous metaplasia, or resemble type II pneumocytes
▸ Trichrome and elastic van Gieson stains are helpful for assisting in the identification of obliterated bronchioles by highlighting their muscle coats (trichrome stain) or the bronchiolar elastica (elastic van Gieson), as well as for enhancing the visibility of the fibrous tissue

Immunohistochemistry
▸ Most cases show a predominance of T-cells, with fewer B-cells

Pathologic Differential Diagnosis
▸ Although there are numerous antecedents to CB, the specific cause of an individual case cannot usually be determined histologically
▸ Organizing pneumonia with fibrosis

remains the only option. However, new immunomodulatory agents are under investigation for treatment of this condition, and preliminary results with etanercept, a tumor necrosis factor (TNF)-α inhibitor, combined with methotrexate, have shown benefit for CB associated with rheumatoid arthritis. Surgery has a very limited role in the management of CB, but new surgical therapeutic modalities such as lung volume reduction surgery (LVRS) may offer relief of symptoms in some cases.

FOLLICULAR BRONCHIOLITIS

Follicular bronchiolitis (FB) is primarily characterized by the accumulation of nodular lymphoid aggregates (with or without germinal centers) in the walls of the bronchioles, peribronchial tissues and immediate adjacent alveolar septa. FB can be idiopathic or occur in association with a number of conditions such as congenital and acquired immunodeficiency states; connective tissue diseases, particularly rheumatoid arthritis and Sjögren's syndrome; pulmonary infections; bronchiectasis; some hypersensitivity conditions; and a list of other disorders.

CLINICAL FEATURES

FB occurs in adults and children. Symptoms are nonspecific and include progressive dyspnea, fever, cough, and recurrent upper respiratory infections. In some patients, the dominant clinical features may be those of an underlying disorder: joint pain in rheumatoid arthritis, the sicca syndrome in Sjögren's syndrome, and polymicrobial infections in patients with the acquired immune deficiency syndrome. Peripheral blood eosinophilia, as reported by Yousem in a subset of patients with FB, suggested an underlying hypersensitivity state. In cases showing overlap with lymphocytic interstitial pneumonia (LIP), dysproteinemia may be observed.

PULMONARY FUNCTION TESTING

Pulmonary function testing yields variable results (obstructive, restrictive, or mixed ventilatory defects).

RADIOLOGIC FEATURES

FB is characterized radiographically by bilateral nodular or reticulonodular opacities, without formation of dominant masses. High-resolution computed tomography shows a centrilobular location of the nodular opacities with branching lines, as well as patchy ground-glass opacities.

PATHOLOGIC FEATURES

Knowledge of the gross appearance of FB is limited. However, some authors report numerous minute nodules, about 1-2 mm in diameter, located adjacent to small airways. Microscopically, dense lymphoid or lymphoplasmacytic infiltrates are seen encircling small airways (Figure 21-8). In addition, lymphoid follicles with well defined germinal centers may partially or completely surround bronchioles. In cases with exuberant lymphoid proliferation, compression of bronchioles may occur, with resultant endogenous lipoid pneumonia. In these instances, numerous lipid-laden macrophages will be found filling the neighboring air spaces.

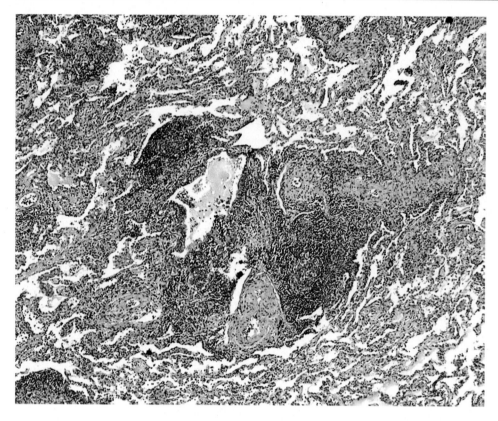

FIGURE 21-8
Follicular bronchiolitis
The bronchiole is surrounded by a dense lymphoid infiltrate with germinal centers.

Few studies have investigated the nature of the lymphoid cells in FB, and report a mixture of T- and B-cells. In the setting of rheumatoid arthritis, Sato, et al., have characterized the lymphoid tissue of FB as showing B-cells that express surface IgM in follicular areas, with numerous associated T-cells, particularly CD4+ cells. In another study of lymphocytic bronchiolitis in children by Maurd et al., the cellular infiltrate was mainly composed of T-cells with a predominance of CD8+ cells.

DIFFERENTIAL DIAGNOSIS

FB overlaps with lymphocytic interstitial pneumonia (LIP) and nodular lymphoid hyperplasia of the lung (NLH). These three conditions are believed by some to represent variations on a single theme (lymphoid hyperplasia), and also show overlapping clinical associations. The differential diagnosis is discussed more extensively in Chapter 22. In brief, radiographically, NLH forms a mass lesion, while both FB and LIP present with a more diffuse pattern of abnormalities. Histologically, FB demonstrates a predominantly bronchiolar localization of the lymphoid infiltrates, while predominant interstitial involvement is characteristic

of LIP. FB differs from another closely related condition, follicular bronchitis, only in regard to the caliber of the involved airways. Follicular bronchiectasis, as seen in conditions such as cystic fibrosis, demonstrates lymphoid follicle formation in the damaged, ectatic bronchi. Hypersensitivity pneumonitis may show prominent peribronchiolar lymphoid follicles, but also usually shows incomplete or poorly formed granulomas and an interstitial inflammatory component that is more intense than that seen in FB. Rare cases of diffuse panbronchiolitis may show prominent lymphoid hyperplasia with germinal centers, similar to FB, but can be distinguished by the concomitant presence of centrilobular interstitial and air space collections of foamy macrophages.

PROGNOSIS AND THERAPY

Although this condition can be a source of morbidity, primarily due to chronic cough, it does not appear to be a direct cause of death in affected patients. Corticosteroids are the principal treatment modality, but response to therapy is quite variable. Erythromycin has also been used with benefit to treat patients with chronic cough due to rheumatoid arthritis-associated FB.

FOLLICULAR BRONCHIOLITIS—FACT SHEET

Definition

>> A form of bronchiolitis characterized by accumulation of nodular aggregates of lymphoid tissue with or without germinal centers

Incidence and Location

>> Uncommon disorder
>> No specific geographic distribution is recognized

Morbidity and Mortality

>> FB does not appear to be a direct cause of death in affected patients, and the primary morbidity is due to chronic cough
>> Pediatric patients with the idiopathic disorder tend to improve with age, but residual mild obstructive lung disease has been reported

Gender, Race, and Age Distribution

>> Occurs in adults and children of both genders
>> No racial predilection is recognized

Clinical Features

>> Symptoms include fever, cough, and dyspnea, as well as symptoms related to an associated underlying condition
>> Associated conditions include congenital and acquired immunodeficiency states; connective tissue diseases, particularly rheumatoid arthritis and Sjögren's syndrome; pulmonary infections; bronchiectasis; some hypersensitivity conditions; and other disorders
>> Some cases are idiopathic

Pulmonary Function Tests

>> Most patients show evidence of obstructive, restrictive, or mixed ventilatory defects

Radiologic Features

>> Chest radiograph reveals bilateral nodular or reticulonodular opacities
>> High-resolution computed tomography shows centrilobular nodular opacities with branching lines, as well as patchy ground-glass opacities

Prognosis and Therapy

>> Corticosteroids are the principal treatment modality, but response to therapy is variable
>> Erythromycin has also been used with benefit to treat patients with chronic cough due to rheumatoid arthritis-associated FB

FOLLICULAR BRONCHIOLITIS—PATHOLOGIC FEATURES

Gross Findings

>> Numerous minute nodules, about 1-2 mm in diameter, located adjacent to small airways

Microscopic Findings

>> Lymphoid tissue, with or without germinal centers, partially or completely surrounding bronchioles, and sometimes causing compression of the bronchiolar lumens
>> Secondary endogenous lipoid pneumonia may be present (lipid-laden macrophages in adjacent air spaces)

Immunohistochemistry

>> Mixture of T- and B-cells

Pathologic Differential Diagnosis

>> Lymphocytic interstitial pneumonia
>> Nodular lymphoid hyperplasia
>> Follicular bronchitis
>> Bronchiectasis
>> Hypersensitivity pneumonitis
>> Diffuse panbronchiolitis

interstitial pneumonia (DIP). All of these disorders are highly linked to cigarette smoking and share the feature of pigmented macrophages in air spaces, but the anatomic distributions of the macrophage infiltrates differ: bronchiolar in RB, bronchiolar and peribronchiolar in RB-ILD, and primarily alveolar in DIP. Interstitial fibrosis can accompany the macrophage infiltrates in these conditions, and its distribution usually parallels the distribution of the macrophages.

CLINICAL FEATURES

Patient ages range from the late 20s to the 60s, but most often patients with RB are middle-aged. Both genders can be affected. Most patients with RB are either current cigarette smokers or former smokers. Interestingly, in some patients, the bronchiolitis was noted to persist for years after cessation of smoking. Symptoms can include dyspnea and cough, or patients can be asymptomatic. Physical exam may show rales and/or digital clubbing.

PULMONARY FUNCTION TESTING

Functional abnormalities in RB may be minimal, but a combined pattern of restrictive and obstructive changes is likely to be present. Decreased diffusing capacity may

RESPIRATORY BRONCHIOLITIS

A distinct small airway disease occurring almost exclusively in cigarette smokers, respiratory bronchiolitis (RB) is characterized histopathologically by accumulations of pigment-laden macrophages within membranous and respiratory bronchioles. There are also rare case reports of RB developing in nonsmokers exposed to asbestos and nonasbestos dusts, or fumes. RB bears a close relationship to respiratory bronchiolitis-associated interstitial lung disease (RB-ILD) and to desquamative

also be present, particularly in cases with more interstitial involvement (RB-ILD).

RADIOLOGIC FEATURES

The chest radiograph can be normal or show diffuse bilateral lesions, including poorly defined centrilobular nodules or ground-glass opacities, which can be better visualized on high-resolution computed tomography.

PATHOLOGIC FEATURES

Histopathologic changes are seen primarily in respiratory bronchioles, but may extend into alveolar ducts. The main histopathologic changes are accumulations of tan-colored macrophages, with or without black cytoplasmic dust particles, located within the airway lumina (Figure 21-9). Frequently, the pigmented macrophages will extend into surrounding alveoli, giving rise to a picture of RB-ILD (Figure 21-10). On iron stain, the cytoplasm of the tan-colored macrophages is faintly positive with a dusty appearance, distinct from the much coarser and brightly staining granules of hemosiderin pigment (Figure 21-11). The bronchiolar walls may

show mild lymphocytic inflammation and fibrosis. Goblet cell metaplasia may be seen in some cases.

Immunohistochemistry plays no role in the diagnosis of RB, which is a morphologic diagnosis, but immunostains for histiocytic markers such as CD68 may be used to semiquantitate the number of macrophages and to outline their distribution. Trichrome stains help to estimate the extent of any fibrosis that may present. Ultrastructurally, the macrophages in RB contain lysosomes and phagolysosomes with many elongated intracytoplasmic needle-shaped inclusions. These inclusions are thought to originate in cigarette smoke.

DIFFERENTIAL DIAGNOSIS

RB is related to desquamative interstitial pneumonia (DIP) and has in fact been suggested by some to represent an early phase of DIP, in which the bronchioles, rather than the alveoli, are preferentially filled with pigment-laden macrophages. Nonetheless, these disorders are currently classified separately. Useful points to keep in mind when considering this differential diagnosis include the fact that in DIP, there is uniform involvement of lung parenchyma, mild or moderate fibrotic thickening of alveolar walls, mild interstitial chronic inflammation, and a more extensive and intense alveolar macrophage

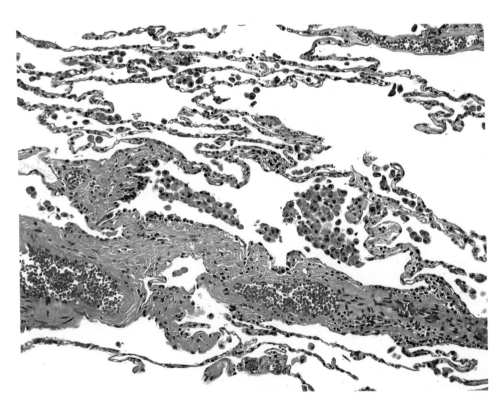

FIGURE 21-9

Respiratory bronchiolitis
Numerous pigmented macrophages occupy the lumen of this respiratory bronchiole.

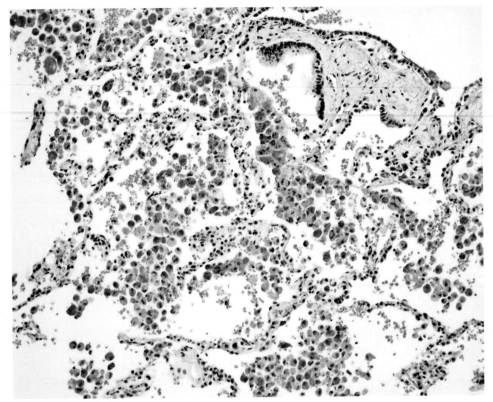

FIGURE 21-10
Respiratory bronchiolitis
Large numbers of pigment-laden macrophages extend from the respiratory bronchiole into peribronchiolar alveolar spaces.

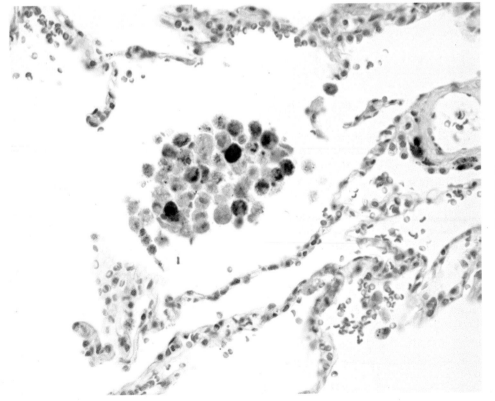

FIGURE 21-11
Respiratory bronchiolitis
Note the fine iron-positive pigment in the cytoplasm of these macrophages (Perl's iron stain).

RESPIRATORY BRONCHIOLITIS—FACT SHEET

Definition

» A distinctive small airway disease occurring almost exclusively in cigarette smokers, characterized histopathologically by accumulations of pigment-laden macrophages within membranous and respiratory bronchioles

Incidence and Location

» Common finding in cigarette smokers
» Worldwide distribution

Morbidity and Mortality

» Morbidity is symptomatic (dyspnea and cough)
» No associated mortality

Gender, Race, and Age Distribution

» No evident gender or racial predilection
» Usually affects middle-aged people, but the age range is broad

Clinical Features

» Some patients are asymptomatic, but most have dyspnea and cough
» Physical examination may show rales or digital clubbing

Pulmonary Function Tests

» Typically show combined restrictive and obstructive abnormalities

Radiologic Features

» Chest radiograph can be normal or show diffuse bilateral lesions including poorly defined centrilobular nodules or ground-glass opacities, which can be better visualized on high-resolution computed tomography

Prognosis and Therapy

» The prognosis is favorable
» Smoking cessation is the mainstay of treatment, and corticosteroids have also been used in some cases

---

RESPIRATORY BRONCHIOLITIS—PATHOLOGIC FEATURES

Microscopic Findings

» Aggregates of tan, dust-laden macrophages located within bronchiolar lumina and extending into adjacent alveolar spaces
» May show mild bronchiolar or peribronchiolar fibrosis and chronic inflammation

Ultrastructural Findings

» Macrophages contain lysosomes and phagolysosomes with many elongated intracytoplasmic needle-shaped inclusions, which are thought to originate from cigarette smoke

Pathologic Differential Diagnosis

» Desquamative interstitial pneumonia
» Asbestos-related airway disease with bronchiolar fibrosis
» Langerhans cell histiocytosis

PROGNOSIS AND THERAPY

The prognosis of RB is favorable. Most patients symptomatically respond to smoking cessation. More severely symptomatic patients may benefit from combined cessation therapy and corticosteroid regimens. Experience with transplanted lungs, however, shows that despite smoking cessation, the macrophage collections may persist for years in the lungs.

DIFFUSE PANBRONCHIOLITIS

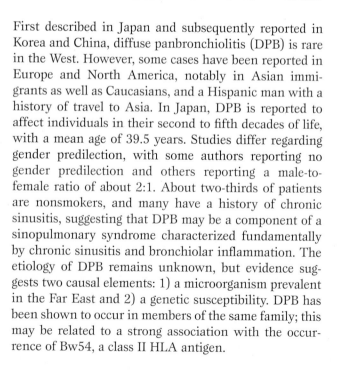

First described in Japan and subsequently reported in Korea and China, diffuse panbronchiolitis (DPB) is rare in the West. However, some cases have been reported in Europe and North America, notably in Asian immigrants as well as Caucasians, and a Hispanic man with a history of travel to Asia. In Japan, DPB is reported to affect individuals in their second to fifth decades of life, with a mean age of 39.5 years. Studies differ regarding gender predilection, with some authors reporting no gender predilection and others reporting a male-to-female ratio of about 2:1. About two-thirds of patients are nonsmokers, and many have a history of chronic sinusitis, suggesting that DPB may be a component of a sinopulmonary syndrome characterized fundamentally by chronic sinusitis and bronchiolar inflammation. The etiology of DPB remains unknown, but evidence suggests two causal elements: 1) a microorganism prevalent in the Far East and 2) a genetic susceptibility. DPB has been shown to occur in members of the same family; this may be related to a strong association with the occurrence of Bw54, a class II HLA antigen.

accumulation, whereas in RB the process is bronchiolocentric, the macrophages are found primarily within small airways, and parenchymal involvement is limited or nonexistent. There are cases, however, in which the histology seems to fall between these two disorders. Asbestos-related airway disease with bronchiolar fibrosis is another consideration in the differential diagnosis of RB. The clinical history and occupational background and a careful search for asbestos fibers aided by iron stains (to visualize ferruginous bodies) should facilitate the diagnosis. Langerhans cell histiocytosis (LCH) is also associated with cigarette smoking and is characterized by prominent macrophage accumulations in the lung. These macrophage accumulations often surround the stellate nodules of LCH. In LCH, unlike RB, clusters of S100+, CD1a+ Langerhans cells with the characteristic nuclear infoldings will usually be apparent, and are often associated with a mixture of accompanying inflammatory cells including eosinophils.

CLINICAL FEATURES

The clinical presentation is nonspecific. In its early stages, DPB can manifest as cough, sputum production, and labored breathing. Later, as the disease becomes more established, fever ensues along with increased sputum production and worsening dyspnea. Digital clubbing can be present. A history of chronic paranasal sinusitis is obtained from the majority of patients.

PULMONARY FUNCTION TESTING

Pulmonary function tests show a pattern of obstruction, but in some cases slight or moderate restrictive impairment can be seen. Increases in residual volume and the ratio of residual volume to total lung capacity are observed.

RADIOLOGIC FEATURES

On chest radiograph, bilateral diffuse nodular or reticulonodular infiltrates are seen in about 70% of patients at presentation, and more than 90% at later stages. Hyperinflation can be prominent. On computed tomography, diffuse, small, rounded and linear opacities with dilated bronchioles are usually noted, and are helpful in making or supporting a suspected diagnosis of DPB.

LABORATORY FEATURES

Important laboratory findings include hypoxemia, leukocytosis, and increased sedimentation rate, C-reactive protein, and immunoglobulins G and A. A characteristic feature is a persistent elevation of cold agglutinins. Tests for anti-mycoplasma antibodies, however, are usually negative.

PATHOLOGIC FEATURES

Grossly, multiple yellow nodules measuring 2-4 mm in diameter are seen bilaterally in centrilobular locations. Histopathologically, there is thickening of the walls of respiratory and terminal bronchioles due to infiltration by lymphocytes, histiocytes, and plasma cells, which are also found in the bronchiolar lumen. Lymphoid aggregates can be seen, and intraluminal neutrophils can be prominent. Characteristically, accumulations of foamy macrophages (xanthoma cells) are found in the interstitium and air spaces in centrilobular areas (Figures 21-12, 21-13). In advanced stages, constriction of bronchioles,

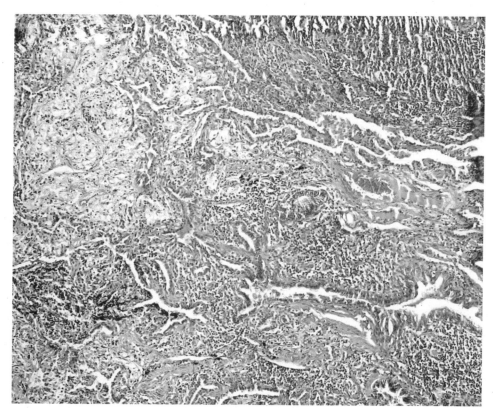

FIGURE 21-12
Diffuse panbronchiolitis
Foamy macrophage infiltrates distort the interstitial regions adjacent to a respiratory bronchiole. There is a dense accompanying lymphocytic infiltrate. (From Aslan AT, et al. Childhood diffuse panbronchiolitis: a case report. *Pediatr Pulmonol.* 2005;40:354-357, with permission.)

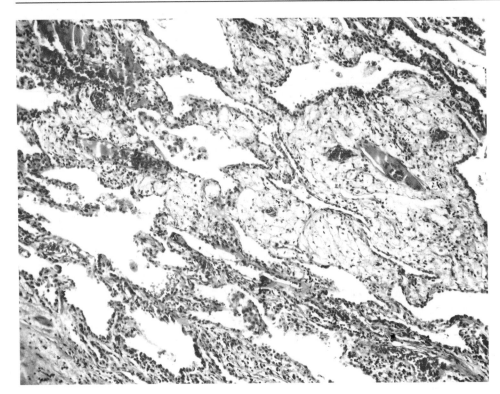

FIGURE 21-13

Diffuse panbronchiolitis
Foamy macrophages expand the interstitial regions. (From Aslan AT, et al. Childhood diffuse panbronchiolitis: a case report. *Pediatr Pulmonol*. 2005;40: 354-357, with permission.)

DIFFUSE PANBRONCHIOLITIS—FACT SHEET

Definition

▸ A clinicopathologic entity occurring primarily in the Far East and Asia, characterized by chronic inflammation of bronchioles with accumulation of foamy histiocytes in the septa of peribronchiolar alveoli, and an association with chronic sinus disease

Incidence and Location

▸ Rare disease that is largely restricted to the Far East and Asia, particularly Japan
▸ Only small numbers of cases reported in the West

Morbidity and Mortality

▸ Overall survival at 5 years is approximately 50%, and at 10 years approximately 25%
▸ Death is usually due to cor pulmonale and respiratory failure
▸ Debilitating bronchiectasis and cystic lung changes develop in advanced cases
▸ When secondary infections with *H. influenzae* or *S. pneumoniae* occur, purulent sputum production increases, and dyspnea may worsen

Gender, Race, and Age Distribution

▸ Most patients are Asian; fewer cases in Caucasians and Blacks
▸ Studies differ regarding gender predilection, with some authors reporting a male-to-female ratio of about 2:1
▸ In Japan, affected individuals are in their second to fifth decades of life, with a mean age of 39.5 years

---

DIFFUSE PANBRONCHIOLITIS—PATHOLOGIC FEATURES

Gross Findings

▸ Multiple centrilobular, yellow nodules measuring 2-4 mm in diameter, in both lungs

Microscopic Findings

▸ Infiltration of the walls of respiratory and terminal bronchioles by lymphocytes, histiocytes, and plasma cells, which are also found in the bronchiolar lumens
▸ Characteristic accumulations of foamy macrophages (xanthoma cells) in the interstitium and air spaces in centrilobular areas
▸ Lymphoid aggregates can be seen
▸ Intraluminal neutrophils can be prominent
▸ In advanced stages, constriction of bronchioles, more proximal bronchiolectasis and greater involvement of alveoli can occur

Pathologic Differential Diagnosis

▸ Aspiration of oily material (exogenous lipoid pneumonia)
▸ Endogenous lipoid pneumonia due to airway obstruction
▸ Cystic fibrosis
▸ Bronchiectasis
▸ Follicular bronchiolitis
▸ Obliterative bronchiolitis

DIFFUSE PANBRONCHIOLITIS—FACT SHEET—cont'd

Clinical Features

▸ Symptoms include cough, sputum production, dyspnea, fever, and sometimes digital clubbing

▸ A history of chronic paranasal sinusitis is obtained from the majority of patients

▸ Rare familial cases, possibly related to a strong association with the occurrence of Bw54, a class II HLA antigen

Pulmonary Function Tests

▸ Pulmonary function tests show a pattern of obstruction, but in some cases a slight or moderate restrictive impairment can be seen

▸ Increases in residual volume and the ratio of residual volume to total lung capacity are also observed

Radiologic Features

▸ Bilateral diffuse nodular or reticulonodular infiltrates on chest radiograph, sometimes with prominent hyperinflation

▸ On computed tomography, diffuse, small, rounded, and linear opacities with dilated bronchioles

Laboratory Features

▸ Hypoxemia, leukocytosis, increased sedimentation rate, C-reactive protein, and immunoglobulins G and A

▸ Persistent elevation of cold agglutinins is characteristic

▸ Tests for anti-mycoplasma antibodies are usually negative

Prognosis and Therapy

▸ DPB is a progressive illness with a poor prognosis

▸ Long-term, low-dose erythromycin therapy is useful for treatment of associated infections

▸ Lung transplantation is indicated in advanced cases, but recurrence of DPB in the allograft has been reported

more proximal bronchiolectasis and greater involvement of alveoli can occur.

DIFFERENTIAL DIAGNOSIS

As noted above, the distinctive histopathologic feature of DPB is the centriacinar accumulation of foamy macrophages occurring in association with the other bronchiolar inflammatory changes. While foamy macrophages can accumulate in alveoli in settings of airway obstruction or aspiration of oily substances (lipoid pneumonia), they are usually located preferentially in air spaces rather than in the interstitium, as they are in DPB. Histologic changes similar to DPB have been described in cystic fibrosis, bronchiectasis, and other types of bronchiolitis. In these instances, features that are particularly important in facilitating the distinction are (1) the association of DPB with sinusitis, (2) the presence of multiple small nodules in both lungs on radiographic images, and (3) presence of cold

agglutinins in serum. While peribronchiolar lymphoid hyperplasia is typically seen in follicular bronchiolitis (FB), a rare case of DPB will present with this feature, but the interstitial foamy macrophages of DPB are not seen in FB.

PROGNOSIS AND THERAPY

DPB is a chronic progressive illness with a poor prognosis. The reported overall survival at 5 years is approximately 50%, and at 10 years approximately 25%. Debilitating bronchiectasis and cystic lung changes develop in advanced cases. When secondary infections with *H. influenzae* or *S. pneumoniae* occur, purulent sputum production increases, and worsening of dyspnea may develop. Death is usually due to cor pulmonale and respiratory failure. Long-term low dose erythromycin therapy has significantly improved the prognostic outlook, however, and now constitutes a major form of treatment. Lung transplantation has been performed in some cases. One case report, however, documented recurrence of DPB in the allograft.

MINERAL DUST AIRWAY DISEASE

The development of parenchymal fibrosis following exposure to mineral dusts is well known, and is discussed in Chapter 18. Less well known, however, is the development of bronchiolar injury, usually fibrosis, secondary to deposition of mineral dusts, particularly in respiratory bronchioles and sometimes alveolar ducts. The term "dust" conveys different meanings to different people. In this section, "dust" is defined according to Greenberg, namely, particulates formed from solid organic and inorganic materials, reduced in size through a mechanical process such as crushing, drilling, grinding, blasting, or pulverization. Generally, airborne dusts range in size from 0.1 to 25 microns and are thus small enough to enter small distal airways. Dusts that can cause bronchiolar damage include asbestos, talc, mica, silica, silicates, coal, aluminum oxide, and iron oxide, among others. Exposure to dusts can also trigger hypersensitivity pneumonitis, which is discussed in Chapter 17, and the organic dust toxic syndrome (ODTS). ODTS can be defined as an acute inflammatory condition affecting airways and alveoli, which is caused by inhalation of one or more agents in organic dusts. With heavy exposure, nonspecific symptoms, such as fever and malaise, may occur. ODTS occurs in subjects without evidence of hypersensitivity, and with a high enough exposure concentration, all exposed individuals may develop the syndrome.

CLINICAL FEATURES

The usual clinical manifestations are those of a chronic bronchiolitis, and consist of gradual worsening of cough and dyspnea. In some instances, particularly following exposure to high levels of organic dust containing fungal spores and hyphae, an acute presentation (influenza-like symptoms with crackles on auscultation) is observed. These latter cases are basically cases of mycotoxicosis and are described in the literature as examples of mill or grain fever.

RADIOLOGIC FEATURES

Tiny, poorly defined, punctate, centrilobular opacities can be seen on chest radiographs and high-resolution computed tomography.

MINERAL DUST AIRWAY DISEASE—FACT SHEET

Definition
▸ Bronchiolar injury, usually fibrosis, secondary to deposition of mineral dusts including asbestos, talc, mica, silica, silicates, coal, aluminum oxide, iron oxide, and others

Incidence
▸ Not known with certainty, but probably quite common in specific cohorts of occupationally exposed individuals

Morbidity and Mortality
▸ Little information available

Gender, Race, and Age Distribution
▸ Adults with significant exposure histories
▸ No known gender or racial predilection

Clinical Features
▸ Usual manifestations include the gradual worsening of cough and dyspnea
▸ Exposure to high levels of organic dust containing fungal spores and hyphae may result in an acute presentation (influenza-like symptoms with crackles on auscultation)

Pulmonary Function Tests
▸ Obstructive ventilatory defects can be associated with this type of bronchiolar injury

Radiologic Features
▸ Tiny, poorly defined, punctate, centrilobular opacities

Prognosis and Therapy
▸ Little information is available regarding prognosis
▸ Treatment is removal from exposure and supportive measures
▸ Antimicrobial agents are used to treat superimposed infections

---

PULMONARY FUNCTION TESTING

Obstructive ventilatory defects can be associated with this type of bronchiolar injury.

PATHOLOGIC FEATURES

Only a few cases of "grain fever" have been examined microscopically, and they display neutrophil infiltrates affecting bronchioles, alveoli, and interstitium, with or without spores. The more common forms of dust-related bronchiolar injury are characterized by fibrosis of the bronchiolar walls. The degree of fibrosis appears to be closely related to dust burden, and its extent can be assessed with trichrome stains. In the setting of asbestos exposure, a distinctive lesion reported by Churg is that of marked fibrosis and pigmentation of the respiratory bronchioles. Iron staining of tissues is helpful for highlighting asbestos fibers coated with iron-rich proteinaceous compounds (ferruginous bodies). Examination of tissues under polarized light can reveal refractile silicates in smokers or others with silicate exposure.

DIFFERENTIAL DIAGNOSIS

Other causes of obliterative bronchiolitis can produce similar bronchiolar fibrosis, but identification of dust particles will help in distinguishing dust-related causes from other causes of obliterative bronchiolitis. Separation from hypersensitivity pneumonitis should present little difficulty, particularly if granulomas are present and the clinical background is appropriate.

MINERAL DUST AIRWAY DISEASE—PATHOLOGIC FEATURES

Microscopic Findings
▸ Fibrous thickening of bronchiolar walls, which can be highlighted with trichrome stains
▸ Asbestos exposure is associated with a distinctive lesion characterized by marked fibrosis and pigmentation of the respiratory bronchioles
▸ Iron staining of tissues is helpful for identifying ferruginous bodies
▸ Examination of tissues under polarized light can reveal refractile silicates in smokers and others exposed to silicates

Pathologic Differential Diagnosis
▸ Other causes of obliterative bronchiolitis
▸ Hypersensitivity pneumonitis

PROGNOSIS AND THERAPY

Treatment is limited to removal from exposure, along with supportive measures. Antimicrobial agents are used to treat superimposed infections. Little information is available regarding prognosis.

PERIBRONCHIOLAR METAPLASIA

While not strictly a form of bronchiolitis, we discuss peribronchiolar metaplasia (PBM) in this chapter due to the fact that it is an abnormality affecting the bronchioles. PBM is a fairly commonly observed proliferation of the bronchiolar epithelium that extends into adjacent peribronchiolar alveoli, hypothetically via the canals of Lambert. PBM can be seen in a spectrum of interstitial lung diseases, in association with thromboembolism or lung cancer, or as an isolated, primary abnormality in patients with a clinical presentation of interstitial lung disease. This section focuses upon the latter form of PBM, in which it represents a primary cause of interstitial lung disease. PBM has also been referred to as alveolar bronchiolization and "lambertosis," and has been believed to represent a reparative phenomenon resulting from injury to small airways. The cause of this injury is usually unknown, but an association with connective tissue diseases has been observed, and hypersensitivity pneumonitis was not ruled out in some reported cases with isolated granulomas. Cases with similar histologic features have also been reported in series under the headings of "centrilobular fibrosis," "idiopathic bronchiolocentric interstitial pneumonia" and "airway-centered interstitial fibrosis."

The incidence, prevalence, level of proliferative activity, and possible preneoplastic potential of PBM are poorly documented. We examined 240 glass tissue slides from 66 consecutive adult noncancer autopsies and 171 glass tissue slides from 79 surgical resections for lung cancer, and identified four cases of PBM. As a primary cause of interstitial lung disease, however, it appears to be uncommon.

CLINICAL FEATURES AND PULMONARY FUNCTION TESTING

In Fukuoka's series of 15 cases of PBM as a cause of interstitial lung disease, 13 patients were women and 2 were men. Ages ranging from 44 to 74 years, with a mean of 56.7 years. The chief complaints were dyspnea, cough, shortness of breath, and dyspnea on exertion, and one patient was asymptomatic. Associated conditions included rheumatoid arthritis and mixed connective tissue disease, and some patients had serologic (ANA, c-ANCA) abnor-

malities without clinical disease. Histories included welding with toxic fume and asbestos exposure in one patient, and pigeon exposure in another patient. Pulmonary function testing revealed heterogeneous results: obstructive, restrictive, mixed, and normal findings were obtained.

In the series of Yousem and Dacic, which included 10 patients with idiopathic bronchiolocentric interstitial pneumonia, there was a marked predilection for women (80%) in middle age (40-50 years). Pulmonary function testing revealed restrictive defects. The series of Churg and colleagues included 12 patients with airway-centered interstitial fibrosis who presented with chronic cough and dyspnea, showed a 2-to-1 female predominance, and a peak disease occurrence between the ages of 40 and 65 years of age. Restrictive changes were observed on pulmonary function testing.

RADIOLOGIC FEATURES

In Fukuoka's series, computed tomography (CT) showed mosaic attenuation, ground-glass opacities, and air trapping. Interstitial disease was reported in Yousem and Dacic's series, and in Churg and colleagues' series, CT scans showed peribronchovascular interstitial thickening and traction bronchiectasis with thickened airway walls and surrounding fibrosis, conglomerate fibrotic masses, bronchiolectasis, and/or honeycombing.

PATHOLOGIC FEATURES

Histologically, PBM is a nodular peribronchiolar proliferation of the bronchiolar epithelium growing along thickened peribronchiolar alveolar septa; bronchiolar walls also appear fibrotic and thickened (Figure 21-14). The bronchiolar epithelium varies from cuboidal to low columnar, with or without cilia (Figure 21-15), usually without goblet cells. The percentage of bronchioles affected ranged from 37-100% in Fukuoka's series. Other findings may include peribronchiolar fibrosis, inflammation, minor constrictive changes in bronchioles, and dilatation. Granulomas were reported in some of Fukuoka's cases, but not in Yousem's or Churg's cases. Also, the patient groups in Yousem's and Churg's studies may have included patients with significant interstitial fibrosis beyond the peribronchiolar region, unlike the series of Fukuoka and colleagues, in which patients with this finding were excluded.

Rarely, the bronchiolar epithelium may be cytologically atypical, raising the possibility of a precursor (preneoplastic) form of hyperplasia. Evaluation of p53, Ki67 and Her2neu in cases of PBM reveals a low level of proliferative activity and an uncertain, but probably low level, of preneoplastic potential (Stachurski and Fraire, unpublished data).

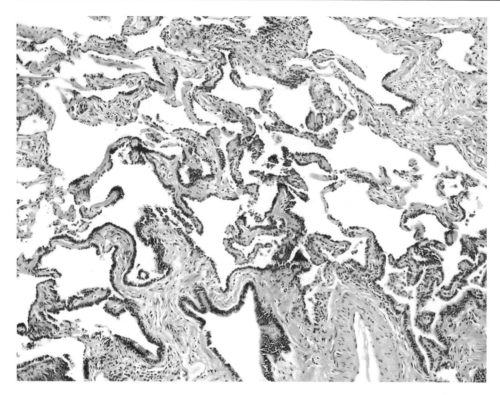

FIGURE 21-14
Peribronchiolar metaplasia
Note the extension of the bronchiolar epithelium along peribronchiolar alveolar walls, which also demonstrate some interstitial fibrosis.

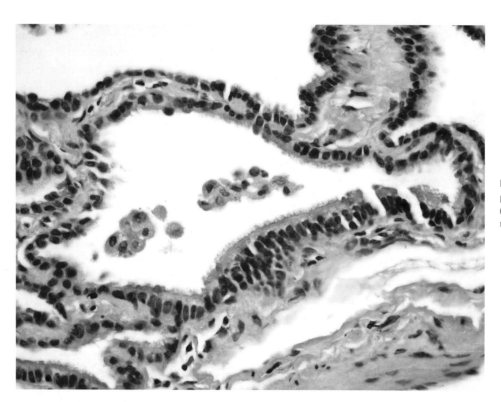

FIGURE 21-15
Peribronchiolar metaplasia
Cilia are evident in this higher-magnification view.

DIFFERENTIAL DIAGNOSIS

As noted earlier, PBM can occur in the context of other interstitial lung diseases, including usual interstitial pneumonia, nonspecific interstitial pneumonia, desquamative interstitial pneumonia, respiratory bronchiolitis, and hypersensitivity pneumonia. If one of these interstitial lung diseases is present, PBM should not be presented as the primary diagnosis. These diseases show a spectrum of interstitial fibrosis and/or inflammatory changes that are not part of

PERIBRONCHIOLAR METAPLASIA—FACT SHEET

Definition

» A proliferation of the bronchiolar epithelium that extends into adjacent peribronchiolar alveoli, and can be a cause of interstitial lung disease

Incidence

» The incidence is unknown, but PBM as a primary cause of interstitial lung disease appears to be uncommon

Mortality

» The mortality varies between reports, which likely include differing patient populations:
  » In Fukuoka's series, all patients with follow-up information were alive
  » In the series published by Yousem and Dacic, death due to disease occurred in 33% of patients, and 56% had persistent or progressive disease
  » In Churg's series, one-third of patients died due to disease progression

Gender, Race, and Age Distribution

» Female predominance
» Patients are typically between 40 and 70 years of age
» No racial predilection has been noted

Clinical Features

» Symptoms include dyspnea, cough, shortness of breath, and dyspnea on exertion
» Patients can be asymptomatic
» Co-existing conditions reported include rheumatoid arthritis and mixed connective tissue disease, as well as serologic (ANA, c-ANCA) abnormalities without clinical disease

Pulmonary Function Tests

» Obstructive, restrictive, mixed, or normal findings

Radiologic Features

» In Fukuoka's series, computerized tomography showed mosaic attenuation, ground-glass opacities, and air trapping
» Interstitial disease was reported in Yousem and Dacic's series
» In Churg and colleagues' series, CT scans showed peribronchovascular interstitial thickening and traction bronchiectasis with thickened airway walls and surrounding fibrosis, conglomerate fibrotic masses, bronchiolectasis, and/or honeycombing

Prognosis and Therapy

» The prognosis of this disorder has varied significantly between reports
» In Churg's series, all of the patients were treated with corticosteroids, with variable responses including improvement, stabilization, and worsening of disease

PERIBRONCHIOLAR METAPLASIA—PATHOLOGIC FEATURES

Microscopic Findings

» Nodular peribronchiolar proliferation of bronchiolar epithelium along thickened peribronchiolar alveolar septa
» Bronchiolar walls appear fibrotic and thickened
» The bronchiolar epithelium varies from cuboidal to low columnar, with or without cilia, usually without goblet cells
» 37-100% of bronchioles can be affected
» Other findings may include peribronchiolar fibrosis, inflammation, minor constrictive change in bronchioles, and dilatation
» Granulomas were reported in some of Fukuoka's cases, but not in Yousem's or Churg's cases

Pathologic Differential Diagnosis

» PBM can occur in the context of other interstitial lung diseases, including usual interstitial pneumonia, nonspecific interstitial pneumonia, desquamative interstitial pneumonia, respiratory bronchiolitis, and hypersensitivity pneumonia
» Atypical adenomatous hyperplasia
» Bronchioloalveolar carcinoma and other histologic subtypes of adenocarcinoma

itis and bronchiolocentric interstitial lymphocytic infiltrates. The histologic differential diagnosis also includes atypical adenomatous hyperplasia (AAH), but AAH is not invariably bronchiolocentric, tends to display a cuboidal cell composition rather than the spectrum of cell types seen in PBM, and usually shows more cytoatypia than PBM. Bronchioloalveolar carcinoma and other histologic subtypes of adenocarcinoma may also be considered in the differential diagnosis, but these entities also do not manifest the bronchiolocentricity of PBM, have more cytoatypia, and often display a variety of architectural patterns (acinar, papillary, solid) that PBM lesions do not show.

PROGNOSIS AND THERAPY

The prognosis of this disorder has varied significantly between reports, but as discussed above, these are some clinical and histologic dissimilarities in the cases included. In Fukuoka's series, all patients with follow-up information were alive, and almost half had experienced improvement in their symptoms. In the series published by Yousem and Dacic, death due to disease occurred in 33% of patients, and 56% had persistent or progressive disease. In Churg's series, all of the patients were treated with corticosteroids, with variable responses including improvement, stabilization, and worsening of disease. One-third of patients died due to disease progression.

the spectrum of PBM. Chronic hypersensitivity pneumonia may be the most difficult to separate from PBM, especially if one accepts the presence of granulomas within the spectrum of lesions defined as PBM. Other features that would favor hypersensitivity pneumonia include chronic (lymphocytic) bronchiol-

SUGGESTED READINGS

General References

1. Colby TV, Churg AC. Patterns of pulmonary fibrosis. In: Sommers SC, Rosen PIP, Fechner RE eds. *1986 Pathology Annual*. Norwalk: Appleton-Century-Crofts; 1986:277.
2. Colby TV, Myers JL. The clinical and histologic spectrum of bronchiolitis obliterans including bronchiolitis obliterans organizing pneumonia (BOOP). *Semin Respir Med*. 1992;13:119-33.
3. Epler GR, Colby TV. The spectrum of bronchiolitis obliterans. *Chest*. 1983;83:161-2.
4. King TE. Overview of bronchiolitis. *Clin Chest Med*. 1993;3:607-10.
5. Lynch DA. Imaging of small airways diseases. *Clin Chest Med*. 1993;4:623-34.
6. Ryu JH, Myers JL, Swensen SJ. Bronchiolar disorders. *Am J Respir Crit Care Med*. 2003 Dec 1;168:1277-92.
7. Visscher DW, Myers JL. Bronchiolitis: the pathologist's perspective. *Proc Am Thorac Soc*. 2006;3:41-7.

Acute Bronchiolitis

8. Akpinar-Elci M, Travis WM, Lynch DA, et al. Bronchiolitis obliterans syndrome in popcorn production plant workers. *Eur Respir J*. 2004;24:298-302.
9. Andersen P. Pathogenesis of lower respiratory tract infections due to Chlamydia, Mycoplasma, Legionella, and viruses. *Thorax*. 1998;53:302-7.
10. Boag AH, Colby TV, Fraire AE, et al. Lung disease in nylon flock workers: pathologic features of a distinctive lesion of lymphocytic bronchiolitis and peribronchiolitis with lymphoid hyperplasia. *Am J Surg Pathol*. 1999;23:1539-45.
11. Ezri T, Kunichezky S, Eliraz A, et al. Bronchiolitis obliterans: current concepts. *Q J Med*. 1994;87:1-10.
12. Fraser RS, Müller NK, Colman N, Paré PD, eds. *Fraser and Parés Diagnosis of Diseases of the Chest*. 4th ed. Philadelphia, London, Toronto: WB Saunders Co, 1999.
13. Ramirez RJ, Dowell AR. Silo-fillers disease: nitrogen dioxide induced lung injury. Long-term follow-up and review of the literature. *Ann Intern Med*. 1971;74:569-76.

Constrictive Bronchiolitis

14. Aguayo S, Miller Y, Waldron JJ, et al. Brief report: idiopathic diffuse hyperplasia of pulmonary neuroendocrine cells and airways disease. *N Engl J Med*. 1992;327:1285-8.
15. Bloch KE, Weder W, Bochler A, et al. Successful lung volume reduction surgery in a child with severe airflow obstruction and hyperinflation due to constrictive bronchiolitis. *Chest*. 2002;122:747-50.
16. Cortot AB, Cottin B, Miossec P, et al. Improvement of refractory rheumatoid arthritis: associated constrictive bronchiolitis with etanercept. *Respir Med*. 2005;99:511-14.
17. Schlesinger C, Meyer CA, Veeraraghavan S, et al. Constrictive (obliterative) bronchiolitis: diagnosis, etiology, and a critical review of the literature. *Ann Diagn Pathol*. 1998;2:321-34.
18. Streichenberger N, Peyrol S, Philit F, et al. Constrictive bronchiolitis obliterans: characterisation of fibrogenesis and lysyl oxidase expression patterns. *Virchows Arch*. 2001;439:78-84.
19. Ward H, Fischer KL, Waghray R, et al. Constrictive bronchiolitis and ulcerative colitis. *Can Respir J*. 1999;6:197-200.

Follicular Bronchiolitis

20. Chatte G, Streichenberger N, Boillot O, et al. Lymphocytic bronchitis/bronchiolitis in a patient with primary biliary cirrhosis. *Eur Respir J*. 1995;8:176-9.
21. Constantopoulos SH, Drosos AA, Maddison PJ, et al. Xerotrachea and interstitial lung disease in primary Sjögren's syndrome. *Respiration*. 1984;46:310-4.
22. Fortoul TI, Cano Valle F, et al. Follicular bronchiolitis in association with connective tissue diseases. *Lung*. 1985;63:305-14.
23. Hayakawa H, Sato A, Imokawa S, Toyoshima M, Chida K, Iwata M. Bronchiolar disease in rheumatoid arthritis. *Am J Respir Crit Care Med*. 1996;154:1531-6.
24. Kinane BT, Mansell AL, Zwerdling RG, Lapey A, Shannon DC. Follicular bronchitis in the pediatric population. *Chest*. 1993;104:1183-6.

25. Mauad T, van Schadewijk A, Schrumpf J, et al. Lymphocytic inflammation in childhood bronchiolitis obliterans. *Pediatr Pulmonol*. 2004;38:233-9.
26. Romero S, Barroso E, Gil J, Aranda I, Alonso S, Garcia-Pachon E. Follicular bronchiolitis: clinical and pathologic findings in six patients. *Lung*. 2003;181:309-19.
27. Sato A, Hayakawa H, Uchiyama H, et al. Cellular distribution of bronchus-associated lymphoid tissue in rheumatoid arthritis. *Am J Respir Crit Care Med*. 1996;154:1903-7.
28. Yousem SA, Colby TV, Carrington CB. Follicular bronchitis/bronchiolitis. *Hum Pathol*. 1985;16:700-6.
29. Yousem SA. Lymphocytic bronchitis/bronchiolitis in lung allograft recipients. *Am J Surg Pathol*. 1993;17:491-6.

Respiratory Bronchiolitis

30. Aubry MC, Wright JL, Myers JL. The pathology of smoking related lung diseases. *Clin Chest Med*. 2000;21:11-35.
31. Fraig M, Shreesha U, Savici D, et al. Respiratory bronchiolitis: a clinico-pathologic study in current smokers, ex-smokers, and never-smokers. *Am J Surg Pathol*. 2002;26:647-53.
32. Myers JL, Veal CF Jr, Shin MS, et al. Respiratory bronchiolitis causing interstitial lung disease: a clinicopathologic study of six cases. *Am Rev Respir Dis*. 1987;135:880-4.
33. Nagai S, Hoshino Y, Hayashi M, et al. Smoking-related interstitial lung diseases. *Curr Opin Pulm Med*. 2000;6:415-9.
34. Ryu JH, Colby TV, Hartman TE, et al. Smoking-related interstitial lung diseases: a concise review. *Eur Respir J*. 2001;17:122-32.
35. Travis WD, King TE, Bateman ED, et al. American Thoracic Society International multidisciplinary consensus classification of the idiopathic interstitial pneumonias. *Am J Respir Crit Care Med*. 2002;265:277-304.
36. Yousem SA, Colby TV, Gaensler EA. Respiratory bronchiolitis-associated interstitial lung disease and its relationship to desquamative interstitial pneumonia. *Mayo Clin Proc*. 1989;64:1373-80.

Diffuse Panbronchiolitis

37. Aslan AT, Ozcelik U, Talim B, et al. Childhood diffuse panbronchiolitis: a case report. *Pediatr Pulmonol*. 2005;40:354-7.
38. Chern MSHK, Yuen Y, Hsu YT, et al. Radiology of diffuse panbronchiolitis: experience in VGH-Taipei. *Chung Hua I Hsueh Tsa Chih Taipei*. 1992;50:469-74.
39. Fitzgerald JE, King TE Jr, Lynch DA, et al. Diffuse panbronchiolitis in the United States. *Am J Respir Crit Care Med*. 1996;154:497-503.
40. Fraser RS, Müller NK, Colman N, Paré PD, eds. *Fraser and Parés Diagnosis of Diseases of the Chest*. 4th ed. Philadelphia, London, Toronto: WB Saunders Co; 1999.
41. Homma H. Diffuse panbronchiolitis (diffuse respiratory bronchiolitis)—a disease of the lung. *Nippon Naika Gakkai Zasshi* 1976;65:645-59.
42. Hu H, Liu Y, Cai Z, et al. A case of diffuse panbronchiolitis. *Chinese Med*. 1996;109:949-52.
43. Iwata M, Sato A, Colby TV. Diffuse panbronchiolitis. In: Epler GR, ed. *Diseases of the Bronchioles*. New York: Raven Press; 1994:153-80.
44. Kim YW, Han SK, Shim YS, et al. The first report of diffuse panbronchiolitis in Korea: five case reports. *Intern Med*. 1992;31:695-701.

Mineral Dust Airway Disease

45. Akira M, Higashihara T, Yokoyama K. Radiographic typing of pneumoconiosis: thin-section CT. *Radiology*. 1989;171:117-23.
46. Churg A. Mineral dust induced bronchiolitis. In: Epler GR, ed. *Diseases of the Bronchioles*. New York: Raven Press; 1994:27-41.
47. Churg A, Wright JL. Small-airway lesions in patients exposed to nonasbestos mineral dusts. *Hum Pathol*. 1983;14:688-93.
48. Churg A, Wright JL, Wiggs B, et al. Small airways disease and mineral dust exposure: prevalence, structure, and function. *Am Rev Respir Dis*. 1985;131:139-43.
49. Keith I, Day R, Lemaire S, et al. Asbestos-induced fibrosis in rats: increase in lung mast cells and autocoid contents. *Lung Res*. 1987;13:311-27.
50. Kennedy SM, Wright JL, Mullen JB, Pare PD, Hogg JC. Pulmonary function and peripheral airway disease in patients with mineral dust or fume exposure. *Am Rev Respir Dis*. 1985;132:1294-9.

51. Pinkerton KE, Green FH, Saiki C, et al. Distribution of particulate matter and tissue remodeling in the human lung. *Environ Health Perspect.* 2000;108:1063-9.

Peribronchiolar Metaplasia

52. Berkheiser SW. Bronchiolar proliferations and metaplasia associated with thromboembolism: a pathological and experimental study. *Cancer.* 1963;16:205-11.
53. Churg A, Myers J, Suarez T, et al. Airway-centered interstitial fibrosis. A distinct form of aggressive diffuse lung disease. *Am J Surg Pathol.* 2004;28:62-8.

54. Fukuoka J, Franks TJ, Colby TV, et al. Peribronchiolar metaplasia: a common histologic lesion in diffuse lung disease and a rare cause of interstitial lung disease: clinicopathologic features of 15 cases. *Am J Surg Pathol.* 2005;29:948-54.
55. Jensen-Taubman SM, Steinberg SM, Linnoila RI. Bronchiolization of the alveoli in lung cancer: pathology, patterns of differentiation and onco-gene expression. *Int J Cancer.* 1998;75:489-96.
56. Lambert MW. Accessory bronchiole: alveolar communications. *J Pathol Bacteriol.* 1955;30:311-7.
57. Nettesheim P, Szakal AK. Morphogenesis of alveolar bronchiolization. *Lab Invest.* 1972;26:210-91.
58. Yousem SA, Dacic S. Idiopathic bronchiolocentric interstitial pneumonia. *Mod Pathol.* 2002;15:1148-53.

22

Lymphoid Lesions of the Lung

Donald G. Guinee, Jr.

INTRODUCTION

Pulmonary lymphoproliferative disorders encompass of a spectrum of benign and malignant lymphoid proliferations. Benign proliferations include intraparenchymal lymph nodes, follicular bronchiolitis, lymphoid interstitial pneumonia (LIP) (sometimes encompassed under the term "diffuse lymphoid hyperplasia"), and localized "nodular" lymphoid hyperplasia. Malignant lymphoproliferative disorders include pulmonary marginal zone B-cell lymphoma of mucosa-associated lymphoid tissue (MALT), pulmonary lymphomatoid granulomatosis, post-transplant lymphoproliferative disorder, diffuse large B-cell lymphoma, primary pulmonary Hodgkin lymphoma, intravascular lymphoma, and secondary involvement of

the lung by leukemia and lymphoma. Other rare types of lymphoproliferative disorders may also rarely present primarily within the lung and include extramedullary plasmacytoma and primary pulmonary Ki-1+ anaplastic large cell lymphoma. Two distinctive types of lymphoma may develop within the pleural cavity and include primary effusion lymphoma and pyothorax-associated lymphoma.

INTRAPARENCHYMAL LYMPH NODE

Pulmonary lymph nodes may be biopsied to exclude the possibility of carcinoma. This possibility has been enhanced by their increased detection on radiographic imaging procedures.

CLINICAL FEATURES

Intraparenchymal lymph nodes are often discovered as an incidental finding on radiographic studies. Patients are usually asymptomatic or have symptoms related to other types of disease. Most patients are smokers, a habit which is postulated to predispose them to development of these lymph nodes. In one study, intraparenchymal lymph nodes were found in 18% of patients undergoing autopsy.

RADIOLOGIC FEATURES

Intrapulmonary lymph nodes usually appear as single or multiple well circumscribed nodules in a subpleural or paraseptal location. They may occasionally have radiographic features which are worrisome for either primary or metastatic disease (e.g., spiculation, pleural indentation, fuzzy margins, and vascular involvement) (Figure 22-1).

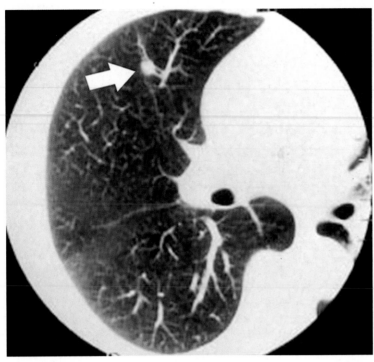 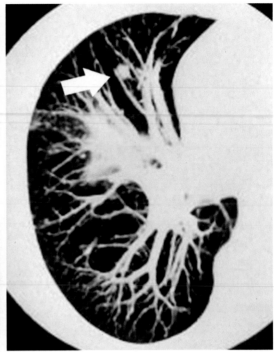

FIGURE 22-1

CT scan of intraparenchymal lymph node (arrow)

Radiographically, this nodule has a rough border and was accordingly resected to exclude carcinoma. (From Yokomise H, Ike O, et al. Importance of intrapulmonary lymph nodes in the differential diagnosis of small pulmonary nodular shadows. *Chest*. 1998;113:703-706, with permission.)

PATHOLOGIC FEATURES

GROSS FINDINGS

Intraparenchymal lymph nodes appear as solid, subpleural, round or ovoid nodules beneath the pleural surface or adjacent to interlobular septa. In one series, they ranged in size from 7 to 12 mm in maximum diameter.

MICROSCOPIC FINDINGS

Histologically, intrapulmonary lymph nodes appear similar to lymph nodes in other areas of the body. They contain both primary and secondary germinal centers (Figure 22-2). Histiocytes containing anthracotic pigment are often prominent in nodal sinuses.

DIFFERENTIAL DIAGNOSIS

Intrapulmonary lymph nodes are usually histologically distinct and not readily confused with other entities. Metastatic carcinoma should be sought in patients with known lung cancer. Intrapulmonary thymoma and nodular lymphoid hyperplasia may occasionally enter the

differential diagnosis. Intrapulmonary thymoma is histologically similar to mediastinal thymoma. Unlike intrapulmonary lymph nodes, thymomas are usually larger (0.5 to 12 cm) and contain variable mixtures of lymphocytes and epithelial cells, usually subdivided into lobules by fibrous bands. If needed, immunohistochemical staining for cytokeratin will highlight admixed epithelial cells and readily discriminate between these two entities. Although nodular lymphoid hyperplasia shares some histologic features with intrapulmonary lymph nodes, lesions of nodular lymphoid hyperplasia are usually larger lesions (2-4 cm), lack the architecture of a lymph node, contain variable amounts of fibrosis, and may efface the underlying pulmonary parenchyma.

LYMPHOID HYPERPLASIA

The term lymphoid hyperplasia encompasses follicular bronchiolitis and lymphoid interstitial pneumonia (LIP) as part of a spectrum of reactive hyperplasia of bronchus-associated lymphoid tissue (BALT). BALT is part of the spectrum of mucosa-associated lymphoid tissue (MALT), which also occurs in the thyroid, salivary glands, and gastrointestinal tract. In the lung, BALT occurs as aggregates of lymphoid tissue along

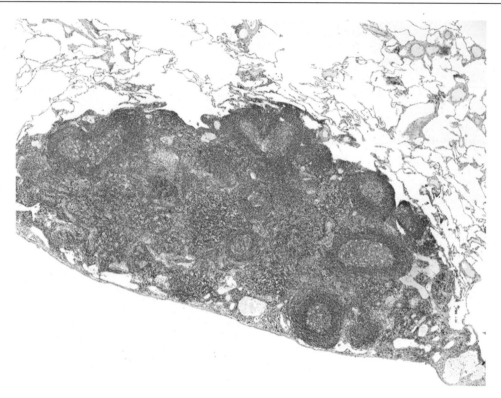

FIGURE 22-2

Intraparenchymal lymph node, low-power view
Note the subpleural location and reactive germinal centers. (Case provided courtesy of Dr. David Dail, Virginia Mason Medical Center, Seattle, Washington.)

INTRAPARENCHYMAL LYMPH NODE—FACT SHEET

Definition
- Lymph nodes occurring within the pulmonary parenchyma

Incidence
- Up to 18% of lungs at autopsy

Gender, Race and Age Distribution
- Found in males and females of any race
- Tend to be found in older individuals

Clinical and Radiologic Features
- Identified as single or multiple subpleural or paraseptal nodules on chest x-ray and CT scan
- Resected to exclude the possibility of carcinoma

Prognosis and Therapy
- Benign incidental finding with no morbidity or mortality
- No treatment is required

INTRAPARENCHYMAL LYMPH NODE—PATHOLOGIC FEATURES

Gross Findings
- Solid, round, or oval-shaped nodule(s) in a subpleural or paraseptal distribution

Microscopic Findings
- Appear similar to normal lymph nodes with primary and secondary follicles and sinus histiocytosis
- Deposits of anthracotic material are often prominent
- Metastatic carcinoma should be sought in patients with known lung cancer

Pathologic Differential Diagnosis
- Intrapulmonary thymoma
- Nodular lymphoid hyperplasia

---

bronchioles and lymphatics. Although follicular bronchiolitis and LIP have distinct histologic patterns, they frequently coexist, and their clinical associations are similar. Interaction of inhaled antigens with lymphocytes of BALT may initiate both T-cell and B-cell effector mechanisms important to normal pulmonary homeostasis. The histologic pattern of lymphoid hyperplasia, therefore, presumably reflects the different types of cellular responses. LIP is characterized by an interstitial expansion predominantly of T-lymphocytes, whereas follicular bronchiolitis consists predominantly of B-cell follicles adjacent to bronchi and bronchioles.

Cases of LIP with prominent peribronchial follicles and germinal centers reflect both a B- and T-cell response. The association of LIP with chronic infections (Epstein-Barr virus [EBV] and human immunodeficiency virus [HIV]), autoimmune diseases, drug reactions, and bone marrow transplantation presumably reflects the effects of long-standing antigenic stimulation occurring in these settings.

FOLLICULAR BRONCHIOLITIS

Follicular bronchiolitis is one pattern of hyperplasia of BALT. Follicular bronchiolitis is thought to represent hyperplasia of the BALT in response to variable antigenic stimuli. In support of this view, lesions similar to follicular bronchiolitis have been induced in experiments with animals exposed to *Mycoplasma pneumoniae*, respiratory syncytial virus, and intratracheal installation of bacille Calmette-Guérin.

CLINICAL FEATURES

Follicular bronchiolitis occurs in children and adults, although adults are affected most often (median age of 44). Symptoms associated with this pattern of pulmonary disease include progressive dyspnea and cough, sometimes accompanied by fever, weight loss, or recurrent pneumonia. Obstructive or restrictive defects may be present on spirometry. Most cases of follicular bronchiolitis are associated with an underlying connective tissue disease (e.g., rheumatoid arthritis or Sjögren's syndrome), an underlying immunodeficiency state, or hypersensitivity disorder. Occasional cases are idiopathic. Peripheral blood eosinophilia has been noted in some idiopathic cases.

Follicular bronchiolitis may also occur as a secondary finding in patients with bronchiectasis, chronic infections, chronic bronchitis, or cystic fibrosis. In these cases, the pathologic and clinical features of the disease are dominated by the primary disease process.

RADIOLOGIC FEATURES

Bilateral reticular or reticulonodular infiltrates are usually present on chest x-ray. High-resolution CT scan shows bilateral small (less than 3 mm) centrilobular and sometimes peribronchial nodules. Occasional larger (3-12 mm) nodules and focal areas of ground-glass opacity are present in some patients (Figure 22-3).

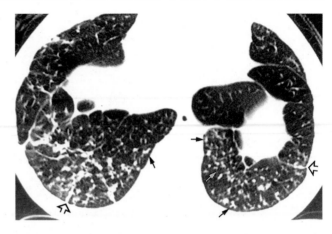

Figure 22-3

Thin section CT scan of follicular bronchiolitis in a 61-year-old male with collagen vascular disease

Several well defined clusters of nodules are present (solid arrows) and adjacent to the pleura or interlobular septa. Mild septal thickening is also present (open arrows). (From Howling SJ, Hansell DM, Wells AU, et al. Follicular bronchiolitis: thin-section CT and histologic findings *Radiology*. 1999;212: 637-642, with permission.)

PATHOLOGIC FEATURES

GROSS FINDINGS

Gross features of follicular bronchiolitis are nondescript. Cases in which follicular bronchiolitis is a secondary finding are dominated by the gross features of the primary disease (e.g., bronchiectasis, associated abscess, etc).

MICROSCOPIC FINDINGS

Follicular bronchitis/bronchiolitis consists of lymphoid follicles, often with prominent germinal centers, in a peribronchiolar or peribronchial distribution (Figure 22-4A). The hyperplastic follicles often reside between bronchioles and pulmonary arteries, and can compress the bronchiolar lumens (Figure 22-4B). Lymphocytes may be present in the adjacent bronchiolar epithelium. Lymphoid follicles may also be present in a lymphangitic distribution along the interlobular septa and beneath the pleura (Figure 22-4A). These findings can also be present in patients with LIP (see below), and there are cases where both of these patterns occur concurrently.

ANCILLARY STUDIES

IMMUNOHISTOCHEMISTRY

Like germinal centers in reactive lymph nodes, cells in the reactive germinal centers in follicular bronchiolitis express CD20 and lack BCL-2.

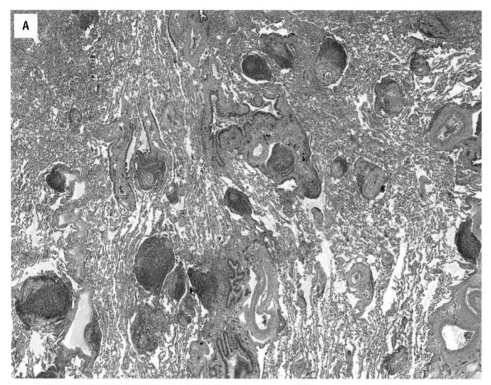

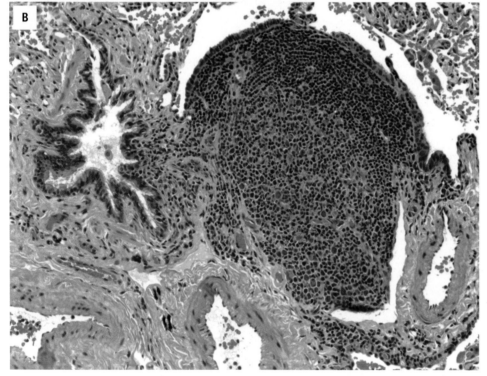

FIGURE 22-4
Follicular bronchiolitis
(A) Diffuse lymphoid hyperplasia. Low-power view shows numerous reactive germinal centers adjacent to bronchioles and along interlobular septa. Given the additional involvement along interlobular septa and pleura, some pathologists would use the term "diffuse lymphoid hyperplasia." **(B)** Intermediate-power view shows a reactive germinal center present between a terminal bronchiole and pulmonary arteriole.

DIFFERENTIAL DIAGNOSIS

The differential diagnosis of follicular bronchiolitis includes LIP, low-grade lymphoma of BALT, pulmonary involvement by chronic lymphocytic leukemia and nodular lymphoid hyperplasia. Although (LIP) may show peribronchial and peribronchiolar lymphoid follicles

(e.g., focal areas of follicular bronchiolitis), this feature is usually overshadowed by the conspicuous diffuse chronic interstitial inflammatory infiltrate that defines this pattern. While there may be focal involvement of alveolar septa by a chronic interstitial inflammatory infiltrate in follicular bronchiolitis, it is not a prominent feature. Nonetheless, there is substantial overlap between the histologic patterns and clinical conditions associated with follicular bronchiolitis and LIP, and in some cases, the distinction is somewhat arbitrary. Low-grade lymphoma of the BALT may have follicles with germinal center formation. However, these lymphomas usually contain confluent areas of monomorphous lymphocytes without germinal centers. Lymphoid cells may permeate cartilage and cause effacement of other normal structures. Similarly, pulmonary involvement by chronic lymphocytic leukemia is distinguished by a monomorphous infiltrate of small lymphocytes with a lymphatic distribution. In contrast to follicular bronchiolitis, nodular lymphoid hyperplasia usually presents as a well demarcated mass consisting of a confluent proliferation of germinal centers admixed with sheets of interfollicular plasma cells.

PROGNOSIS AND THERAPY

The prognosis of idiopathic cases of follicular bronchiolitis is generally good, but may be worse in patients under age 30. Patients are usually treated with cortico-steroids, with variable results. In patients with follicular bronchiolitis associated with a collagen vascular disease or immunodeficiency, treatment is directed at the underlying cause.

LYMPHOID INTERSTITIAL PNEUMONIA

Lymphoid interstitial pneumonia (LIP) is a histologic pattern of lung disease characterized by a diffuse, interstitial, polymorphous, predominantly mononuclear inflammatory cell infiltrate. It was first described by Liebow and others in the early 1970s, although many of the original cases would now be considered examples of low-grade lymphoma of BALT. As in the preceding discussion on follicular bronchiolitis, LIP is considered part of the spectrum of pulmonary lymphoid hyperplasia.

CLINICAL FEATURES

Females are affected more often than males. The disease usually affects older individuals with a median age of diagnosis in the fifth to sixth decade. Clinical symptoms include chronic cough and dyspnea, weight loss, and fatigue. Fever, chest pain, and hemoptysis are less common. Laboratory studies may reveal a polyclonal gammopathy or, less frequently, hypogammaglobulinemia or monoclonal gammopathy. Pulmonary function studies most often show a restrictive pattern.

LIP may be associated with or represent the pulmonary manifestation of, a number of diseases including collagen vascular diseases (e.g., Sjögren's syndrome,

---

FOLLICULAR BRONCHIOLITIS—FACT SHEET

Definition

➤ Distinct histopathologic pattern of hyperplasia of BALT, characterized by development of primary and secondary germinal centers in a peribronchiolar distribution

Incidence

➤ Rare
➤ Most cases are associated with an underlying connective tissue disease (e.g., rheumatoid arthritis and Sjögren's syndrome), immunodeficiency state, or hypersensitivity disorder

Gender and Age Distribution

➤ Females and males affected equally
➤ Affects adults most often (median age is 44), but may affect children

Clinical Features and Pulmonary Function Testing

➤ Symptoms include progressive dyspnea and cough, sometimes accompanied by fever, weight loss, or recurrent pneumonia
➤ Spirometry may show either obstructive or restrictive defects

Radiologic Features

➤ Chest x-ray: bilateral reticular or reticulonodular infiltrates
➤ High-resolution CT scan: bilateral small (less than 3 mm) centrilobular and sometimes peribronchial nodules; occasionally larger (3-12 mm) nodules and focal areas of ground-glass opacity may be present

Prognosis and Therapy

➤ Prognosis is variable but generally good, rarely a cause of death
➤ Treatment consists of corticosteroids, with variable responsiveness
➤ In patients with associated collagen vascular disease or immunodeficiency, treatment is directed at the underlying cause

---

FOLLICULAR BRONCHIOLITIS—PATHOLOGIC FEATURES

Microscopic Findings

➤ Primary and secondary lymphoid follicles in a peribronchiolar or peribronchial location
➤ Lymphoid follicles also often present along interlobular septa and pleura in a lymphatic distribution

Immunohistochemistry

➤ Lymphoid follicles stain for pan-B-cell markers (CD20) and lack staining for BCL-2

Pathologic Differential Diagnosis

➤ Lymphoid interstitial pneumonia
➤ Low-grade lymphoma of BALT
➤ Pulmonary involvement by chronic lymphocytic leukemia
➤ Nodular lymphoid hyperplasia

rheumatoid arthritis), other autoimmune disorders (e.g., autoimmune hemolytic anemia), immunodeficiency disorders (e.g. acquired immunodeficiency syndrome [AIDS], common variable immune deficiency), and infections. It can develop as a drug reaction and in a setting of allogeneic bone marrow transplantation (Table 22-1). LIP is prevalent in children (but not adults) with AIDS and since 1987 has been considered an AIDS-defining illness in those less than 13 years old. Cases of idiopathic LIP are rare.

RADIOLOGIC FEATURES

Chest radiographs show patchy bilateral reticulonodular infiltrates with a predilection for the lower lobes. On high-resolution CT scan, areas of ground-glass opacity are often accompanied by poorly defined centrilobular and subpleural nodules (Figure 22-5). Occasionally cystic spaces and lymph node enlargement may also be identified.

PATHOLOGIC FEATURES

MICROSCOPIC FINDINGS

LIP is characterized by a dense, interstitial, predominantly mononuclear cell infiltrate which diffusely expands alveolar septa (Figure 22-6A). The infiltrate consists primarily of lymphocytes, histiocytes, and plasma cells (Figure 22-6B). In some cases, there are germinal centers along bronchovascular bundles and septa. The histologic features in these cases overlap with the pattern of follicular bronchiolitis. Other findings occasionally encountered include poorly formed granulomas and multinucleated giant cells, and secondary alveolar changes can include collections of proteinaceous fluid, scattered mononuclear inflammatory cells and foamy macrophages or giant cells. In later lesions, there may be variable amounts of fibrosis and even honeycombing, ultimately resulting in end-stage lung disease.

ANCILLARY STUDIES

IMMUNOHISTOCHEMISTRY

Interstitial lymphocytes consist predominantly of CD3-expressing T-cells, while germinal centers in bronchovascular bundles are comsposed predominantly of CD20-expressing B-cells. Accompanying plasma cells are polyclonal, and express kappa or lambda in similar proportions.

TABLE 22-1
Clinical Conditions Associated with the LIP Pattern

Collagen vascular diseases	Sjögren's syndrome Rheumatoid arthritis Systemic lupus erythematosus
Other immunological disorders	Autoimmune hemolytic anemia Pernicious anemia Myasthenia gravis Hashimoto's thyroiditis Primary biliary cirrhosis Celiac sprue Dysproteinemia
Immunodeficiency	AIDS, particularly in children Common variable immunodeficiency
Infections	*Pneumocystis jiroveci* *Legionella* pneumonia Chronic active hepatitis
Drug induced/toxic exposure	Dilantin (phenytoin)
Allogeneic bone marrow transplantation	
Familial	
Idiopathic	

From Travis WD, Galvin JR, et al. Non-neoplastic pulmonary lymphoid lesions. *Thorax.* 2001;56:964-971, with permission.

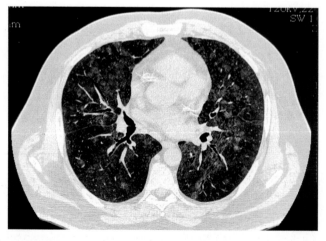

FIGURE 22-5

Thin section CT scan of LIP in a 41-year-old male with HIV
There are patchy ground-glass opacities and ill-defined centrilobular nodules affecting all lobes. (From Swigris JJ, et al. *Chest.* 2002;122;2150-2164, with permission.)

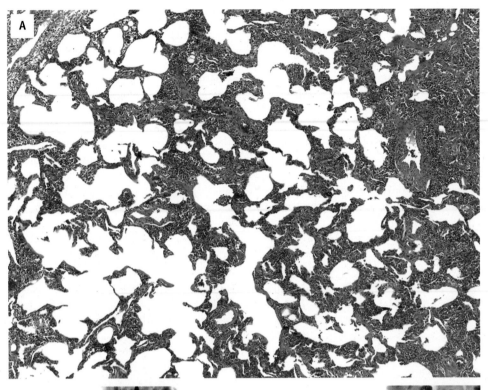

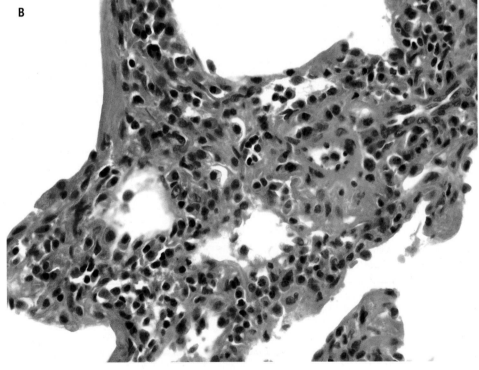

FIGURE 22-6

Lymphoid interstitial pneumonia
(A) Low-power view shows diffuse expansion of alveolar septa by a cellular inflammatory infiltrate. **(B)** High-power view shows that the interstitial infiltrate is composed of lymphocytes, histiocytes, and plasma cells.

MOLECULAR ANALYSIS

A polyclonal pattern is typically present on polymerase chain reaction for immunoglobulin heavy chain gene rearrangement. Occasional cases may show oligoclonal bands. Identification of a clonal B-cell pattern should prompt consideration of a low-grade lymphoma.

DIFFERENTIAL DIAGNOSIS

The differential diagnosis of LIP is broad. It includes all disorders in which there is a prominent lymphoid infiltrate: low-grade lymphoma of BALT, pulmonary involvement by chronic lymphocytic leukemia, angio-immunoblastic lymphadenopathy, nodular lymphoid hyperplasia, follicular bronchiolitis, hypersensitivity pneumonitis, nonspecific interstitial pneumonitis, and, in chronic forms, usual interstitial pneumonitis. Pulmonary involvement by low-grade lymphoma or chronic lymphocytic leukemia is distinguished from LIP by the monomorphism of the lymphoid infiltrate. Infiltration of bronchial cartilage and pleura may be present in low-grade lymphoma of BALT, but are absent in LIP. In cases where morphologic distinction is difficult, immunohistochemical stains and polymerase chain reaction (PCR) analysis for IgH heavy chain rearrangement can be helpful. Interstitial lymphocytes in low-grade lymphomas of the BALT and chronic

lymphocytic leukemia consist predominantly of B-cells that express CD20. Kappa or lambda light chain restriction can sometimes be demonstrated by immunohistochemical staining of associated plasma cells. PCR analysis for IgH chain gene rearrangements will frequently show a clonal rearrangement.

Angioimmunoblastic lymphadenopathy can occasionally involve the lung in a diffuse pattern. However, this disorder is usually suspected based on the clinical and radiographic features which include generalized lymphadenopathy combined with hepatosplenomegaly, autoimmune hemolytic anemia and skin rash. Nodular lymphoid hyperplasia is readily distinguished from LIP by its presentation as a well demarcated mass, as opposed to the diffuse interstitial involvement of LIP. Although follicular bronchiolitis may show focal extension of the lymphoid cells into the peribronchiolar interstitium, the diffuse interstitial involvement seen in LIP is lacking. Nonetheless, many cases of LIP have associated lymphoid follicles with germinal centers along bronchioles and, in occasional cases, the histologic features overlap, making the distinction between the two somewhat subjective. Hypersensitivity pneumonitis can be distinguished from LIP by its patchy peribronchiolar accentuation, patchy poorly formed granulomas, and

---

LYMPHOID INTERSTITIAL PNEUMONIA (LIP)—FACT SHEET

Definition
➤ Histopathologic pattern in the spectrum of pulmonary lymphoid hyperplasia, characterized by a diffuse, interstitial, polymorphous, predominantly mononuclear inflammatory cell infiltrate

Incidence
➤ Rare disorder that is often associated with other conditions, including connective tissue diseases (e.g., Sjögren's syndrome, rheumatoid arthritis), other autoimmune disorders (e.g., autoimmune hemolytic anemia), immunodeficiency (e.g., acquired immunodeficiency syndrome [AIDS], common variable immune deficiency), infections, drug usage, and allogeneic bone marrow transplantation
➤ Idiopathic LIP is extremely rare

Gender and Age Distribution
➤ Women are affected more often than men
➤ Usually develops in older patients but may occur at all ages from infants to very old; median age at diagnosis is in the fifth to sixth decade
➤ Considered an AIDS-defining illness in children less than 13 years old

Clinical Features, Pulmonary Function Testing, and Laboratory Studies
➤ Symptoms include cough and dyspnea
➤ Spirometry usually shows a restrictive pattern of abnormalities
➤ Laboratory studies may reveal a polyclonal gammopathy or hypogammaglobulinemia

Radiologic Features
➤ Chest x-ray: patchy bilateral reticulonodular infiltrates with a predilection for the lower lobes
➤ High-resolution CT scan: areas of ground-glass opacity, often accompanied by poorly defined centrilobular and subpleural nodules; cystic spaces or lymph node enlargement may be present

Prognosis and Therapy
➤ Prognosis is variable and usually determined by the associated disease or condition
➤ Between 30% and 50% of patients die within 5 years; causes of death include infectious complications from treatment, end-stage pulmonary fibrosis, or, rarely, evolution into lymphoma
➤ Treatment consists of corticosteroids with variable results, and antiretroviral agents are used in cases associated with AIDS

LYMPHOID INTERSTITIAL PNEUMONIA (LIP)—PATHOLOGIC FEATURES

Microscopic Findings
➤ Dense, predominantly mononuclear inflammatory cell infiltrate that diffusely expands alveolar septa
➤ Infiltrate consists of lymphocytes, histiocytes, and plasma cells
➤ There may be associated germinal centers along bronchovascular bundles and interlobular septa
➤ Occasional poorly formed granulomas or multinucleated giant cells may be present
➤ Later lesions show variable amounts of fibrosis or even honeycombing

Immunohistochemistry
➤ Interstitial lymphocytes are predominantly T-cells that express CD3
➤ Germinal centers along bronchovascular bundles are predominantly B-cells and express CD20
➤ Background plasma cells show a polyclonal pattern of expression of kappa and lambda light chains

Molecular Analysis
➤ Immunoglobulin heavy chain gene rearrangement studies typically show a polyclonal pattern; occasional cases may show oligoclonal bands

Pathologic Differential Diagnosis
➤ Follicular bronchiolitis
➤ Low-grade lymphoma of BALT
➤ Pulmonary involvement by chronic lymphocytic leukemia
➤ Nodular lymphoid hyperplasia
➤ Hypersensitivity pneumonitis
➤ Nonspecific interstitial pneumonitis
➤ Usual interstitial pneumonitis

occasional foci of organizing pneumonia. Although interstitial lymphocytic infiltrates are characteristic of cellular nonspecific interstitial pneumonia, the density of the lymphoid infiltrate is less than LIP. Nonetheless, NSIP and LIP may be difficult to distinguish morphologically, and many cases of LIP in the older literature would now be reclassified as NSIP. Given their similar etiologies and associations, LIP, in fact, may be considered just a more exuberantly cellular expression of NSIP. Finally, particularly in immunocompromised patients (e.g., AIDS), infections should be considered as potential etiologies for LIP. In these patients, evidence of Epstein-Barr virus (EBV), cytomegalovirus, *Pneumocystis jiroveci*, and mycobacteria should be sought by special stains and/or molecular testing.

PROGNOSIS AND THERAPY

The prognosis of LIP is variable. There is an inconsistent response to corticosteroids and between 30% and 50% of patients die within 5 years. Antiretroviral agents may be effective in cases associated with HIV infection. Causes of death include infectious complications of treatment or advanced pulmonary fibrosis.

NODULAR LYMPHOID HYPERPLASIA

Nodular lymphoid hyperplasia is considered to represent a localized form of lymphoid hyperplasia, which presents as a discreet pulmonary mass. Perspectives on nodular lymphoid proliferations in the lung have evolved considerably. Although most nodular lymphoid proliferations in the lung were considered benign ("pseudolymphomas"), with the recognition of lymphomas of the mucosa- (bronchus-) associated lymphoid tissue, it became apparent that most of these lesions represented low-grade lymphomas. More recently, however, Abbondanzo, et al., reported 14 cases that lacked histologic features of lymphoma and did not show either light chain restriction or immunoglobulin heavy chain gene rearrangement with rigorous immunohistochemical and genetic study. Based on these results, they concluded that the entity of nodular lymphoid hyperplasia, although rare, does exist within the lung. Nodular lymphoid hyperplasia is thought to represent a reactive polyclonal expansion of BALT. The factors triggering this expansion are unknown, although they appear to be different from factors associated with other types of hyperplasia of BALT (LIP and follicular bronchiolitis). There is no association with connective tissue diseases such as Sjögren's or underlying viral infections such as HIV. Based on the presence

of acute inflammatory foci in occasional cases of nodular lymphoid hyperplasia, Abbondanzo, et al., postulated that inflammatory stimuli underlie the development of these reactive lymphoid masses.

CLINICAL FEATURES

Men and women are affected in approximately equal numbers. Median age at diagnosis is 65 (range 19-80). Pulmonary symptoms such as cough, dyspnea, and/or pleuritic chest pain are present in a minority of patients.

RADIOLOGIC FEATURES

Chest x-ray and CT scan show an isolated mass (64%) or occasionally multiple nodules (36%). Hilar or mediastinal adenopathy may be present in some patients.

PATHOLOGIC FEATURES

GROSS FINDINGS

Most lesions consist of gray, white to tan, solid, well demarcated nodules. The mean diameter is 2 cm, but they can measure up to 6 cm.

MICROSCOPIC FINDINGS

Nodular lymphoid hyperplasia is a well demarcated nodule consisting of aggregates of lymphoid follicles with reactive germinal centers and sheets of interfollicular plasma cells, most often in a subpleural location (Figure 22-7A). Plasma cells may contain Russell bodies. Foci of interfollicular fibrosis may be present and may focally efface the underlying pulmonary parenchyma. Significantly, Dutcher bodies, bronchial or pleural permeation, lymphoepithelial lesions and amyloid are absent. Resected hilar or mediastinal nodes, when present, show reactive lymphoid hyperplasia.

ANCILLARY STUDIES

IMMUNOHISTOCHEMISTRY

Immunohistochemical stains for lymphoid markers are consistent with a reactive process. Germinal centers of follicles stain for B-cell markers (CD20), while interfollicular lymphocytes consist primarily of T-cells that stain for CD3 and CD5. BCL-2 expression is absent in germinal centers, but present in the mantle zone and interfollicular T-cells. A polyclonal pattern of expression of kappa and lambda light chains is present in interfollicular plasma cells (Figure 22-7B).

MOLECULAR ANALYSIS

Polymerase chain reaction analysis for immunoglobulin heavy chain gene rearrangements shows a polyclonal pattern.

DIFFERENTIAL DIAGNOSIS

The main entity in the differential diagnosis of nodular lymphoid hyperplasia is BALT lymphoma. Other entities to be considered include LIP, follicular bronchiolitis, inflammatory pseudotumor, and plasmacytoma. Nodular lymphoid hyperplasia can usually be distinguished from BALT lymphoma by a number of findings. BALT lymphomas tend to show infiltration of pleura and bronchial cartilage, features that should not be seen with nodular lymphoid hyperplasia. Lymphangitic spread is usually prominent in BALT lymphomas, but mild and focal in nodular lymphoid hyperplasia. Lymphoepithelial lesions are absent in nodular lymphoid hyperplasia, but variably present in BALT lymphoma. Likewise, intranuclear inclusions (Dutcher bodies) are absent in nodular lymphoid hyperplasia, but variably present in BALT lymphoma. Immunohistochemical staining for kappa and lambda light chain restriction shows a polyclonal pattern in nodular lymphoid hyperplasia, but a monoclonal pattern in most cases of BALT lymphoma. In small biopsies, positive staining of lymphocytes in lymphoepithelial lesions for CD43 and CD20 is found in low-grade lymphomas of BALT, but not nodular lymphoid hyperplasia. Finally, immunoglobulin heavy chain gene rearrangements can be identified in most cases of BALT lymphoma, but are not present in nodular lymphoid hyperplasia. These criteria are summarized in Table 22-2. Recent studies have suggested that plasmacytoma is a form of BALT lymphoma. Unlike nodular lymphoid hyperplasia, it consists of a monomorphous population of plasma cells which show light chain restriction that can be detected by immunohistochemistry.

Nodular lymphoid hyperplasia is usually easily distinguished from LIP and follicular bronchiolitis. The latter two entities typically involve the lung in a diffuse manner, as opposed to the discrete mass seen in nodular lymphoid hyperplasia. Nodular lymphoid hyperplasia can be distinguished from inflammatory pseudotumor (inflammatory myofibroblastic tumor) of the lung by the absence of an associated myofibroblastic or fibrohistiocytic spindle cell proliferation.

PROGNOSIS AND THERAPY

Nodular lymphoid hyperplasia is a benign lesion, although surgical excision is usually needed to allow correct diagnosis. In Abbondanzo's study, there were no recurrences, and all patients with available follow-up (7) were alive.

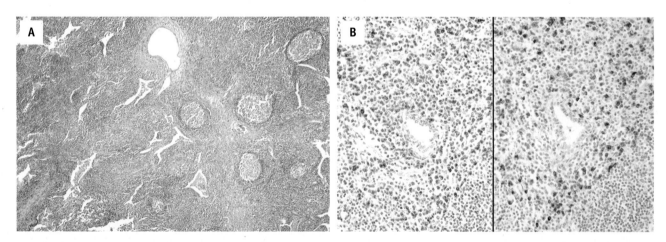

FIGURE 22-7

Nodular lymphoid hyperplasia

(A) Nodular lymphoid hyperplasia consists of a well demarcated mass containing aggregates of reactive germinal centers. **(B)** A polyclonal pattern (similar proportions of kappa and lambda light chains) is seen with immunohistochemical staining for kappa and lambda light chains (left and right images, respectively). (Photograph provided courtesy of Dr. Michael N. Koss, University of Southern California, Los Angeles, California.)

PULMONARY EXTRANODAL MARGINAL ZONE LYMPHOMA OF THE BRONCHUS-ASSOCIATED LYMPHOID TISSUE

Primary pulmonary non-Hodgkin lymphoma is rare, and accounts for about 3.6% of all extranodal lymphomas. Among lymphomas which are primary to the lung, pulmonary extranodal marginal zone lymphoma of the BALT (low-grade lymphoma of BALT) is the most common, encompassing 95% of cases of pulmonary lymphoma. Like their gastrointestinal counterparts, these lymphomas tend to remain localized and have a relatively favorable prognosis, sometimes curable by surgery alone.

Low-grade lymphomas of the BALT are post-follicular B-cell lymphomas. Like mucosa-associated lymphoid tissue (MALT) lymphomas in other organs, they are thought to arise from collections of MALT and recapitulate features of MALT histologically. MALT (BALT) is normally absent in the lung, but accumulates with chronic antigenic stimulation. Low-grade lymphomas of BALT are unique in that, unlike in other organs, a preceding chronic inflammatory process or infectious agent is not found in most cases. The origin from MALT helps to explain their tendency to remain localized, in contrast to other types of lymphomas.

The development of lymphoma from MALT has recently been associated with the acquisition of genetic mutations that alter normal cell cycle regulatory and homeostatic mechanisms. More specifically, several translocations have been identified that appear to be important in the pathogenesis of MALT lymphoma, although their frequency differs between different sites. The most common translocation identified in pulmonary low-grade lymphoma of BALT is t(11;18)(q21;q21) (53% in Streubel's study). This translocation results in the generation of a novel fusion protein, involving the apoptosis inhibitor API2 at 11q21, and a novel gene, MALT1, at 18q21. Translocations t(14;18)(q31;q21) and t(1;14)(p22;q32) have also been identified, but are much rarer. All of these translocations result in the constitutive activation of the nuclear factor kappa B (NF-kB) family of transcription factors. This family of transcription factors is important in the regulation of antigen receptor-mediated activation of lymphocytes.

TABLE 22-2
Nodular Lymphoid Hyperplasia versus MALT Lymphoma

Histology and Immunohistochemistry	Nodular Lymphoid Hyperplasia	MALT Lymphoma
Architecture	Well circumscribed lesion, usually localized	May be localized, but is infiltrative, often invading the pleura and bronchial cartilage
Lymphangitic spread	Focal, mild	Prominent
Cellularity	Reactive germinal centers with interfollicular small lymphocytes and plasma cells	Polymorphic: monocytoid B-cells, centrocyte-like (cleaved) atypical lymphocytes and plasma cells
Germinal centers	Reactive, with no follicular colonization by neoplastic cells	Reactive, with colonization by neoplastic cells
Lymphoid population	Polymorphous	Monomorphous or polymorphous
Monocytoid B-cells	Inconspicuous or absent	May be conspicuous
Plasma cells	Usually not extensive	May be extensive
Intranuclear inclusions (Dutcher bodies)	Absent	Variably present
Amyloid	Absent	May be abundant
Lymphoepithelial lesions	Absent	Variably present
Plaque-like pleural infiltration	Absent or inconspicuous	Variably present
Kappa/lambda reactivity	Polyclonal	Monoclonal in approximately 40% of cases
Bcl-2 reactivity	Negative germinal centers	Negative in the follicular center cells but positive in the colonizing neoplastic lymphocytes
Immunoglobulin heavy chain gene rearrangement	Negative	Positive in 60%

From Travis WD, Galvin JR, et al. Non-neoplastic pulmonary lymphoid lesions. *Thorax*. 2001;56:964-971, with permission.

Aneuploidy (trisomy 3 and 18) has been identified in low-grade lymphoma of BALT. Mutations of other tumor suppressor genes such as p53, Fas and p16 have also been identified and may be seen with increased frequency in those tumors with a component of large cell lymphoma.

CLINICAL FEATURES

The mean age at diagnosis is between 50 and 70 years old, although patients as young as 7 years old have been described. In most studies, females are affected slightly more often than males. Most patients are asymptomatic, and a solitary pulmonary nodule is incidentally identified on chest x-ray. Some patients may develop a cough, dyspnea, hemoptysis, or type B symptoms including weight loss, fever, and night sweats. An associated autoimmune disorder (e.g., Sjögren's syndrome, Hashimoto's thyroiditis, rheumatoid arthritis)

is present in a minority of patients (22% in Kurtin's study).

Laboratory findings are often nonspecific. The most common finding is a monoclonal immunoglobulin spike, often of IgM heavy chain type in about one third of patients. The monoclonal immunoglobulin molecules are usually low level (less than 3 g/dL) and unassociated with clinical disease. Bone marrow involvement is typically discovered in 15-20% of patients and is unassociated with the presence or absence of a monoclonal gammopathy.

RADIOLOGIC FEATURES

The most common radiographic finding is of a solitary or multiple pulmonary nodules (approximately 90% of cases) (Figure 22-8A). Occasional patients may have nodules associated with diffuse infiltrates or, rarely, infiltrates alone. Air bronchograms may be present. Hilar lymphadenopathy is rare.

PATHOLOGIC FEATURES

GROSS FINDINGS

Samples most often show a tan or white smooth-surfaced well demarcated mass or masses. Some cases have more infiltrative margins with pulmonary consolidation.

MICROSCOPIC FINDINGS

Low-grade lymphoma of BALT is characterized by a confluent proliferation of lymphocytes consisting of varying proportions of small lymphocytes, monocytoid lymphocytes, plasmacytoid lymphocytes, and plasma cells (Figure 22-8B). Occasionally, the process is not confluent but rather diffuse and interstitial, accentuated along lymphatic tracts. Despite the variety of cell types, the cytologic features are relatively monomorphous when compared to the spectrum of lymphoid hyperplasia (e.g., LIP or nodular lymphoid hyperplasia). In about half of all cases, Dutcher bodies may be identified in small lymphocytes or plasma cells. Rare isolated transformed large lymphocytes with round vesicular nuclei, prominent nucleoli, and more abundant cytoplasm, are present in most cases.

Lymphomas often involve the pleura and permeate bronchial cartilage (Figure 22-8C). Non-necrotizing infiltration of small vessels is also often present. Lymphoepithelial islands are typically observed (approximately 90% of cases), and manifest as permeation of bronchial and bronchiolar epithelia by aggregates of lymphocytes (Figure 22-8D). Reactive germinal centers are often present and may show follicular colonization by the

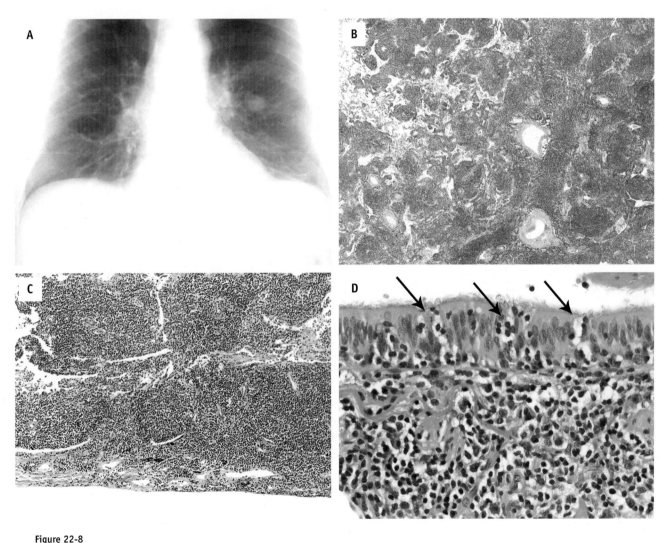

Figure 22-8

Marginal extranodal low-grade lymphoma of BALT
(A) Chest radiograph shows a solitary nodule in the left lower lobe. **(B)** Low-power view shows a nodule composed of confluent monomorphous lymphocytes. At the edges of the nodule, the lymphocytes expand alveolar septa as they spread into adjacent lung tissue. **(C)** Intermediate-power view shows involvement of pleura by the cellular lymphoid infiltrate. **(D)** Lymphoepithelial islands (arrows) are seen on this high-power view and are a characteristic feature of this disorder.

neoplastic centrocyte-like cells. In some areas, dense bands of hyalinized connective tissue may occur and partially divide the tumor. Deposits of amyloid are rare findings, and in some cases overshadow the lymphoid infiltrate. Small, ill-defined non-necrotizing granulomas are occasionally seen. In about half of all cases, involvement of mediastinal nodes is identified, and may not have been apparent in radiographic images. Involvement is usually manifested by expansion of parafollicular and paracortical zones by monocytoid or lymphoplasmacytic lymphocytes, or sometimes by marked expansion of marginal zones around atrophic follicles.

In a minority of cases (approximately 18% in Kurtin's study), areas of diffuse large-cell lymphoma exist and may be the predominant finding on the biopsy (see diffuse large B-cell lymphoma, below). These areas coexist with zones of typical BALT lymphoma, either in the same biopsy, a biopsy of a different part of the lung, or in the mediastinal nodes.

ANCILLARY STUDIES

IMMUNOHISTOCHEMISTRY/FLOW CYTOMETRY

The neoplastic cells express CD20, but not CD10, cyclin D1, and CD5 (with rare exceptions) (Table 22-3). Co-expression of CD43 by the neoplastic lymphocytes is present in approximately 70%. The neoplastic cells also typically express BCL-2. Most cases will show light chain restriction for kappa or lambda and either IgM or IgA. The pattern of light and heavy chain restriction is identical to that in the serum in patients with a monoclonal gammopathy.

MOLECULAR ANALYSIS

PCR analysis for immunoglobulin heavy chain gene rearrangements may show clonal immunoglobulin gene rearrangements, even in cases that do not show light chain restriction by immunohistochemistry. A recent study has suggested that analysis of bronchoalveolar lavage fluid for B-cell clonality by PCR is highly sensitive and specific (97%) for predicting the presence or absence of B-cell lymphoma on follow-up biopsy of patients suspected of having this disorder.

DIFFERENTIAL DIAGNOSIS

The differential diagnosis of low-grade lymphoma of BALT includes nodular lymphoid hyperplasia, LIP, and pulmonary involvement by other low-grade lymphomas. BALT lymphoma can usually be distinguished from nodular lymphoid hyperplasia by a number of findings. In contrast to nodular lymphoid hyperplasia, BALT lymphomas tend to show infiltration of pleura and bronchial cartilage. Lymphangitic spread is usually prominent in BALT lymphomas, but mild and focal in nodular lymphoid hyperplasia. Lymphoepithelial lesions are absent in nodular lymphoid hyperplasia, but only variably present in BALT lymphoma. Begueret, et al., reported that co-expression of CD43 and CD20 on lymphocytes in lymphoepithelial lesions was highly specific for lymphoma, and not present in patients with nodular lymphoid hyperplasia. Intranuclear inclusions (Dutcher bodies) are absent in nodular lymphoid hyperplasia, but variably present in BALT lymphoma. Immunohistochemical staining to detect kappa and lambda light-chain restriction shows a polyclonal pattern in nodular lymphoid hyperplasia, but usually shows a monoclonal pattern in BALT lymphoma. Finally, PCR analysis for immunoglobulin heavy chain gene rearrangement may show a monoclonal population in patients with low-grade lymphoma of BALT, but should show a polyclonal pattern in nodular lymphoid hyperplasia. These criteria are summarized in Table 22-2.

LIP may enter the differential diagnosis of cases of low-grade lymphoma of BALT, which present as a more diffuse infiltrate. In fact, many of the original cases described as LIP by Liebow are now recognized as examples of BALT lymphoma. In contrast to low-grade lymphoma of BALT, however, LIP lacks bronchial cartilage or pleural infiltration. While both LIP and lymphoma may have germinal centers, the infiltrates in low-grade lymphoma of BALT are usually more homogeneous. In difficult cases, immunohistochemical and molecular analysis may be needed. The neoplastic lymphocytes in BALT lymphomas stain predominantly as B-cells (CD20+), oftentimes with co-expression of CD43 and kappa or lambda light-chain

---

TABLE 22-3

Immunophenotypic Characteristics of Low-Grade Lymphoma of BALT and Other Entities in the Differential Diagnosis

	CD20	CD5	CD10	CD23	Cyclin D1
Low-grade lymphoma of BALT	+	−	−	−	−
Chronic lymphocytic leukemia	+	+	−	+	−
Follicular lymphoma, grade I	+	−	+	−	−
Mantle cell lymphoma	+	+	−	−	+

restriction, while the interstitial lymphocytes in LIP stain predominantly as T-cells (CD3+) without a demonstrable clonal population. PCR analysis will usually show a clonal proliferation in BALT lymphoma and a polyclonal pattern in LIP.

Pulmonary involvement by other low-grade lymphomas (e.g., chronic lymphocytic leukemia [CLL]) may be almost identical histologically to BALT lymphoma. In most cases, the diagnosis is readily apparent from the clinical history. In some cases, however, involvement of the lung precedes the development of clinically overt leukemia. In these cases, immunohistochemical stains will usually allow their distinction. CD5 is expressed by CLL/small lymphocytic lymphoma, but is typically ab-

sent in BALT lymphoma. Likewise, CD10 is expressed by most follicular lymphomas, but is absent in BALT lymphoma. These immunohistochemical differences are summarized in Table 22-3.

PROGNOSIS AND THERAPY

The prognosis of BALT lymphoma is generally favorable. Kurtin's study showed 5- and 10-year survival rates of 84.5% and 71.7%, respectively. Some patients are treated by observation or surgery alone, whereas others may receive chemotherapy and/or radiation

---

PULMONARY EXTRANODAL MARGINAL ZONE LYMPHOMA OF BRONCHUS-ASSOCIATED LYMPHOID TISSUE—FACT SHEET

Definition

▸ Post-follicular low-grade B-cell lymphoma arising from BALT; considered part of the spectrum of extranodal marginal zone lymphomas arising in association with mucosa-associated lymphoid tissue (MALT) of diverse organs (lung, gastrointestinal tract, salivary gland, thyroid)

Incidence

▸ Rare, but it is the most common type of primary pulmonary lymphoma (95%)

Gender and Age Distribution

▸ Females are affected slightly more often than males
▸ Mean age at diagnosis is 50 to 70 years old, although patients as young as age 7 have been described

Clinical Features

▸ Most patients are asymptomatic, although occasionally patients may have cough, dyspnea, or hemoptysis
▸ Bone marrow involvement occurs in 15% to 20% of patients
▸ A minority of patients (22%) have an associated autoimmune disorder (e.g., Sjögren's syndrome, Hashimoto's thyroiditis)
▸ An associated monoclonal gammopathy is present in one-third of patients

Radiologic Features

▸ Chest x-ray and CT scan usually show a single or multiple nodules
▸ Occasional cases may show diffuse infiltrates, with or without associated nodules

Prognosis and Therapy

▸ Prognosis varies with clinical stage but is generally favorable, with a 5-year survival rate of 80-90%
▸ Extrapulmonary involvement or a high-grade component is associated with a worse prognosis
▸ Recurrences, when they occur, preferentially affect the lung or other sites containing MALT
▸ Some patients are treated by observation or surgery alone, and others receive chemotherapy and/or radiation therapy

---

PULMONARY EXTRANODAL MARGINAL ZONE LYMPHOMA OF BRONCHUS-ASSOCIATED LYMPHOID TISSUE—PATHOLOGIC FEATURES

Gross Findings

▸ Well demarcated nodule or nodules, or pulmonary consolidation

Microscopic Findings

▸ Confluent proliferation of relatively monomorphous mononuclear cells
▸ Less often the process is not confluent, but rather diffuse and interstitial with a lymphangitic distribution
▸ Infiltrate consists of varying proportions of small monocytoid and plasmacytoid lymphocytes and plasma cells
▸ Dutcher bodies may be found in lymphocytes or plasma cells in 50% of cases
▸ Reactive germinal centers are often present
▸ Lymphoepithelial lesions are present in most cases (90%)
▸ Infiltration of bronchial cartilage or pleura may be present
▸ Occasional findings include dense bands of hyalinized connective tissue, deposits of amyloid and ill-defined non-necrotizing granulomas
▸ Involvement of mediastinal nodes occurs in 50% of cases

Immunohistochemistry

▸ Small lymphocytes consist of B-cells and stain for CD20, but not CD10, cyclin D1, and CD5
▸ Co-expression of CD43 is frequent (approximately 70% of cases)
▸ Most cases show a monoclonal pattern of kappa and lambda light chain expression

Molecular Analysis

▸ Immunoglobulin heavy chain gene rearrangement usually reveals a monoclonal population of B-cells

Pathologic Differential Diagnosis

▸ Nodular lymphoid hyperplasia
▸ Lymphoid interstitial pneumonia
▸ Pulmonary involvement by other low-grade lymphomas

therapy. The prognosis, however, varies with the clinical stage. The recurrence rate of BALT lymphoma localized to the lung tends to be lower than the recurrence rate when extrapulmonary involvement is present. Approximately 25% have extrapulmonary involvement at presentation. Recurrences, when they occur, preferentially affect the lung or other sites containing MALT.

LYMPHOMATOID GRANULOMATOSIS

Lymphomatoid granulomatosis (LYG) is a rare disease that typically involves the lung and often involves other organs including the central nervous system, skin, and kidneys. In the lung, it typically manifests as multiple nodules consisting of atypical angiocentric lymphoreticular infiltrates with variable amounts of associated necrosis. Most cases of LYG are T-cell rich EBV-associated B-cell lymphoproliferative disorders. This view is supported by additional colocalization studies of proliferation markers with expression of B- and T-cell antigens showing that the large atypical B-cells proliferate at a much greater rate than the background T-lymphocytes. The rate of B-cell proliferation correlates roughly with the grade of the lesion and overlaps with B-cell lymphomas in grade III lesions. Many, if not a majority, of the background population of T-cells show a cytotoxic phenotype as defined by the expression of CD3, betaF1, cytotoxic granule proteins TIA-1, and granzyme B. These findings suggest that LYG- and EBV-associated post-transplant lymphoproliferative disorders are closely related entities that arise in a background of latent EBV infection. These findings have also prompted new therapies in the management of this disease.

CLINICAL FEATURES

LYG can develop in adults and children of all ages. The median age at diagnosis is 60. Males are affected more often than females (2:1). Presenting symptoms include cough, chest pain, and dyspnea. In addition to pulmonary involvement, affected patients often have extrapulmonary manifestations in the skin (more than 40% of patients), central nervous system (30%), kidney (30%), or other organs such as the heart, liver, and adrenals. Palpable lymphadenopathy occurs in 10% of patients. Involvement of bone marrow is likewise rare. There is an increased incidence of LYG in immunocompromised patients, particularly those with AIDS. LYG cases previously reported in transplant recipients would now be reclassified as post-transplant lymphoproliferative disorders.

RADIOLOGIC FEATURES

LYG usually presents on chest x-ray as bilateral peripheral lung nodules that tend to wax and wane (Figure 22-9A). Occasional cases manifest as a solitary mass or diffuse infiltrate. Hilar lymphadenopathy is usually absent.

PATHOLOGIC FEATURES

GROSS FINDINGS

Single or multiple pulmonary nodules, often with necrotic centers, are typically observed (Figure 22-9B).

MICROSCOPIC FINDINGS

Nodules consist of atypical lymphoreticular infiltrates, and often have necrotic central regions (Figure 22-9C). A striking and characteristic feature is the angiocentricity of the lymphoreticular infiltrates. Transmural infiltration of small- and medium-sized blood vessels by lymphocytes is present, associated with angionecrosis and pulmonary infarction (Figures 22-9C,D). The lymphoreticular infiltrates contain variable numbers of cytologically atypical lymphocytes admixed with small lymphocytes and histiocytes (Figure 22-9E). In some cases of LYG, the infiltrates are more diffuse and septal rather than nodular.

LYG is subdivided into 3 grades according to the number of large Epstein-Barr virus (EBV)-infected cells present on in-situ hybridization (see below). This generally correlates with the frequency of cytologically atypical cells present. In grade I lesions, EBV-positive cells are scarce or absent (less than 5/hpf); in grade II lesions, scattered EBV-positive cells are present (between 5/hpf and 20/hpf); in grade III lesions, EBV-positive cells number greater than 20/hpf and are often present in sheets. Grade III lesions meet histologic criteria for malignant lymphoma. Patients with higher-grade lesions generally have a worse prognosis.

ANCILLARY STUDIES

IMMUNOHISTOCHEMISTRY

The cytologically atypical cells stain for B-cell markers (CD20+) (Figure 22-9F). Background reactive lymphocytes, which constitute the majority of cells, stain for T-cell markers (CD3+). These features are analogous to T-cell-rich B-cell lymphomas.

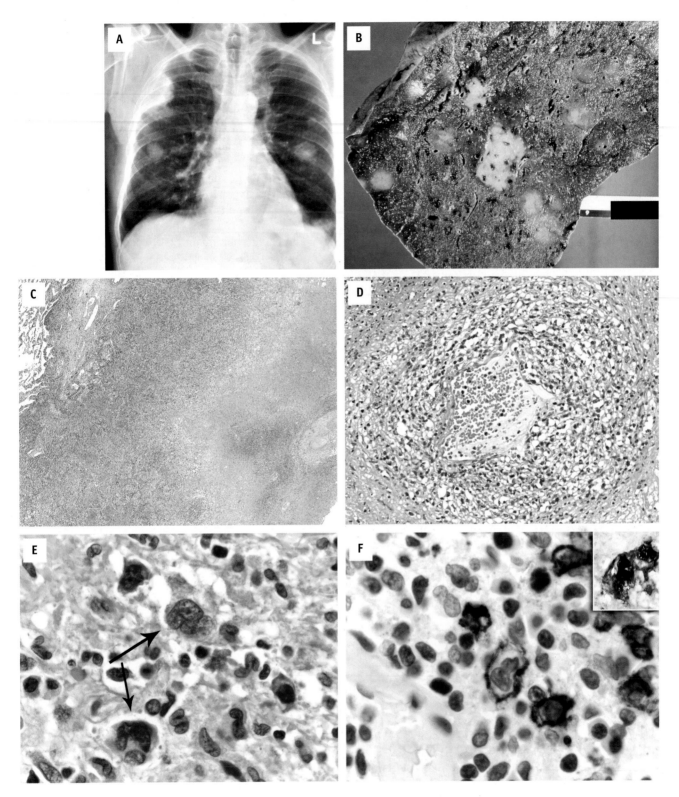

FIGURE 22-9

Lymphomatoid granulomatosis

(A) Chest radiograph shows bilateral nodules. (B) Multiple yellow-to-tan nodules are visible in this gross photograph. (C) Low-power view shows characteristic features of lymphomatoid granulomatosis, including prominent central necrosis and a surrounding polymorphous lymphoid infiltrate. A necrotic vessel is present at the right-hand edge of the image. (D) A key feature of lymphomatoid granulomatosis is the striking vascular involvement. In this image, the wall of a small artery is permeated by numerous small lymphocytes. (E) Within the infiltrate, there are scattered large atypical lymphocytes (arrows). (F) The large atypical lymphocytes stain for CD20. The inset shows a double-labeling study combining immunohistochemical staining for CD20 with in situ hybridization for EBV RNA. Immunohistochemical staining for CD20 (red cytoplasmic staining) decorates cells which are also positive for EBV by in situ hybridization (black nuclear staining). (F Inset from Guinee D, et al. *Am J Surg Pathol*. 1994;18:753-764, with permission.)

MOLECULAR ANALYSIS

In situ hybridization can be used to reveal the presence of EBV genome in the cytologically atypical B-cells (Figure 22-9F). Immunoglobulin heavy chain gene rearrangements are identified in a majority of cases.

DIFFERENTIAL DIAGNOSIS

The differential diagnosis of LYG includes Wegener's granulomatosis, post-transplant lymphoproliferative disorder (PTLD), pulmonary involvement by peripheral T-cell lymphoma, and nasal-type extranodal T/natural killer (NK)-cell lymphoma. While Wegener's granulomatosis sounds similar to LYG, it differs in its clinical and histologic features. Histologically, LYG lacks the granulomatous inflammation typically present in Wegener's granulomatosis. Likewise, large atypical EBV-positive B-cells are a cardinal feature of LYG, but should not be present in Wegener's granulomatosis.

The histologic features of PTLD in the lung overlap with LYG. However, PTLD shows angioinvasion and angiodestruction in a minority of cases, whereas these are constant features of LYG. Moreover, the background population in PTLD tends to consist of plasmacytoid B-cells with fewer T-cells. Consideration of the clinical history also usually facilitates the correct diagnosis, as PTLD occurs exclusively in the post-transplant setting.

Pulmonary involvement by extranodal T/natural killer (NK)-cell lymphoma may mimic LYG. In fact, prior to the identification of LYG as an EBV-driven B-cell proliferation, extranodal T/natural killer (NK) cell lymphoma and LYG were considered the same disease. While the cells of extranodal T/NK lymphoma harbor EBV by in situ hybridization, in contrast to LYG, most of the large atypical cells express CD3 and natural killer-associated antigens (CD56 and CD57). Scattered cytologically atypical B-cells are not identified. Clinical history is also important as extranodal T/NK-cell lymphomas usually present as aggressive destructive lesions in the nasal cavity.

Finally, in some cases histologically similar to LYG in the lung, the large atypical cells do not stain with B-cell markers but instead stain with CD3 and betaF1 (T-cell specific markers). EBV is not identified in these cases by in situ hybridization techniques. Given the differences in immunophenotype and in situ hybridization studies, these cases are best considered peripheral T-cell lymphomas. Other types of T-cell lymphoma (e.g., enteropathy-associated T-cell lymphoma) may also involve the lung and enter into the differential diagnosis.

PROGNOSIS AND THERAPY

The clinical course of LYG is variable. Up to 67% of patients die from the disease, but occasional patients (14% to 27%) may undergo spontaneous regression. Adverse prognostic factors include a higher-grade (e.g., grade II or III), involvement of the central nervous system, and age higher than 25. Death usually occurs through progressive destruction of pulmonary parenchyma. The grades of the lesions can vary over time and location, but in general, recurrences tend to progress to higher-grade lesions.

Treatment of LYG has consisted of variable combinations of chemotherapy and corticosteroids. The demonstration of LYG as an EBV-associated T-cell rich B-cell lymphoproliferative disorder has stimulated new approaches to treatment. Administration of interferon a2b as an immunologic adjuvant has been effective in causing partial or complete remission in some patients. More recent studies have reported successful treatment with anti-CD20 antibodies (rituximab).

POST-TRANSPLANT LYMPHOPROLIFERATIVE DISORDERS

Post-transplant lymphoproliferative disorders (PTLDs) refer to a spectrum of lymphoproliferative disorders arising in the setting of immunosuppression following solid organ, allogeneic bone marrow, or stem cell transplantation. Originally thought to be lymphomas, later studies showed that some of these lesions will regress with a decrease or discontinuation of immunosuppression. Historically, almost all of these cases have consisted of B-cell lymphoproliferative disorders associated with latent EBV infection. More recently, occasional cases of T-cell phenotype as well as cases unassociated with EBV have been recognized.

PTLD represents an uncontrolled proliferation of EBV-infected B-lymphocytes in a setting of exogenous immunosuppression following transplantation. In normal individuals, secondary infections with EBV from latently infected cells are controlled by activated cytotoxic T-cells. After transplantation, there is a reduction in the function or number of activated cytotoxic T-cells by immunosuppressive therapies such as cyclosporine, anti-T-lymphocyte antibodies or T-cell depletion of bone marrow allografts. Reduction in cytotoxic T-cell function or number permits uncontrolled secondary infection of B-lymphocytes (Figure 22-11). Progressive PTLD presumably results from the acquisition of additional genetic mutations. One study showed increasing numbers of mutations in *BCL-6, RAS, p53* and *c-myc* in

LYMPHOMATOID GRANULOMATOSIS—FACT SHEET

Definition

» Angiocentric T-cell rich EBV-associated B-cell lymphoproliferative disorder that usually presents as multiple necrotic pulmonary nodules

Incidence

» Rare
» Occurs at increased frequency in immunocompromised patients, particularly in a setting of AIDS

Gender and Age Distribution

» Males are affected more often than females (2:1)
» Median age at diagnosis is 60, although the disease may occur in infants as well as the elderly

Clinical Features

» Symptoms include cough, chest pain, and dyspnea
» Extrapulmonary manifestations are common in the skin, central nervous system, kidney, and other organs
» Palpable lymphadenopathy is rare

Radiologic Features

» Chest x-ray usually shows bilateral peripheral nodules that tend to wax and wane
» Occasional cases present as a solitary mass or diffuse infiltrate
» Hilar lymphadenopathy is usually absent

Prognosis and Therapy

» Clinical course is variable
» Up to 67% of patients die of the disease, usually as a consequence of progressive destruction of pulmonary parenchyma or brain involvement 14-27% undergo spontaneous regression
» Recurrences tend to progress to higher-grade lesions
» Higher lesional grade tends to correlate with worsened prognosis
» Classic treatment consists of combination chemotherapy, but more recent treatments have used interferon a2b or anti-CD20 antibodies with promising results

LYMPHOMATOID GRANULOMATOSIS—PATHOLOGIC FEATURES

Gross Findings

» Single or multiple pulmonary nodules, often with necrotic centers

Microscopic Findings

» Nodules consist of an atypical lymphoreticular infiltrate, and often have prominent central necrosis
» Cellular infiltrate demonstrates striking angiocentricity with transmural involvement of small- and medium-sized vessels by lymphocytes, associated with angionecrosis and pulmonary infarction
» Lymphoreticular infiltrate includes variable numbers of enlarged cytologically atypical lymphocytes admixed with small lymphocytes and histiocytes
» Subdivided into 3 grades (grade I, II, and III) depending upon the number of large atypical lymphocytes (EBV-positive) present
» Grade III lesions meet histologic criteria for malignant lymphoma

Immunohistochemistry

» Large atypical cells are B-cells and stain for CD20
» Majority of the reactive lymphocytes are T-cells and stain for CD3

Molecular Analysis

» EBV genome can be demonstrated by in situ hybridization in the cytologically atypical cells
» Immunoglobulin heavy chain gene rearrangements are present in a majority of cases

Pathologic Differential Diagnosis

» Wegener's granulomatosis
» Post-transplant lymphoproliferative disorder
» Pulmonary involvement by peripheral T-cell lymphoma
» Nasal-type extranodal T/NK-cell lymphoma

---

patients with monomorphic PTLD compared to polymorphic PTLD. The etiologies of T-cell PTLD or cases unassociated with EBV are not fully understood.

CLINICAL FEATURES

The incidence and type of PTLD varies with the type of organ transplanted and immunosuppressive regimen used. The overall incidence of PTLD is less than 2% among solid organ transplants, ranging from 1% in kidney transplants to 5% in heart-lung transplants. In patients with bone marrow transplants, the incidence of PTLD also varies according to the type of immunosuppression used and the use of T-cell depletion of bone marrow allografts. Males and females appear to be affected in equal numbers. PTLD can develop in extranodal sites and/or lymph nodes, and can be unifocal or multifocal. Involvement of the allograft seems to be more common in lung and heart-lung transplant recipients than in recipients of other types of transplanted organs. The time to onset of PTLD varies widely, but generally falls from months to several years following transplantation. In lung transplant recipients, the time to onset seems to be less; in one study, the median time for development of PTLD following lung transplantation was 7 months. Symptoms of PTLD are variable and reflect the organ involved. Palpable lymphadenopathy may be present.

RADIOLOGIC FEATURES

Pulmonary involvement by PTLD is characterized by single or multiple pulmonary nodules on chest x-ray and/or CT scan. On high-resolution CT scan, some nodules may be accompanied by a halo of ground-glass attenuation. Mediastinal adenopathy may be present.

PATHOLOGIC FEATURES

GROSS FINDINGS

Pulmonary nodules of PTLD have been described as white or tan, relatively well circumscribed, and often associated with prominent necrosis (Figure 22-10A).

MICROSCOPIC FINDINGS

The histologic features of PTLD involving the lung resemble those of PTLD involving other organs, and fall within a defined spectrum of lesions. The most recent 2001 World Health Organization classification system subdivides PTLD based upon the degree of monomorphism and cytologic features of the infiltrate (Table 22-4). Early lesions consist of plasmacytic hyperplasia and infectious-mononucleosis-like PTLD. These lesions predominantly affect lymph nodes, but may rarely occur in the lung or other extranodal sites. Cases involving the lung most often fall into the categories of polymorphic or monomorphic PTLD. Polymorphic PTLD lesions consist of nodules containing a spectrum of small- to medium-sized lymphocytes, large lymphocytes, and immunoblasts. These infiltrates can efface the underlying lung parenchyma. Monomorphic PTLD lesions consist of confluent sheets of large transformed atypical lymphocytes. Most cases of monomorphic PTLD are histologically similar to diffuse large B-cell lymphomas (Figure 22-10B), although a minority of cases have been classified as Burkitt/Burkitt-like lymphoma, plasma cell myeloma, or plasmacytoma-like lesions. In some cases, areas of necrosis associated with "angioinvasion" and "angiodestruction" by atypical immunoblasts are present, resembling LYG. Rare cases fall into categories of peripheral T-cell lymphoma, NK-cell type lymphomas and others. Some cases of PTLD resemble Hodgkin lymphomas and have been termed Hodgkin lymphomas and Hodgkin's disease-like PTLD.

ANCILLARY STUDIES

IMMUNOHISTOCHEMISTRY

In polymorphic PTLD, the lymphocytes usually consist of a mixture of B- and T-lymphocytes (CD20+ and CD3+, respectively). Immunoblasts often express EBV-LMP1 and EBNA2. B-cells and plasma cells may show either polyclonal or monoclonal patterns of lambda and kappa light-chain expression. Most cases, however, will show a monoclonal population on PCR analysis (see below).

In most monomorphic PTLD, the sheets of large, atypical lymphocytes are B-cells that express CD19, CD20, CD79a, and often EBV-LMP1 and EBNA2. Aberrant expression of CD43 and CD45RO may be present, and occasional cases may show expression of CD30. Cases will typically show a monoclonal pattern of kappa and lambda light-chain expression.

MOLECULAR ANALYSIS

EBV can be identified by in situ hybridization in the atypical lymphocytes in the vast majority of polymorphic and monomorphic PTLD cases. Most cases contain numerous positive cells. Although uncommonly reactive disorders may contain rare positive cells and not fulfill histologic criteria of PTLD, the finding of EBV by in situ hybridization should raise concern about PTLD, and should prompt clinical follow-up. PCR analysis of the immunoglobulin heavy chain gene will show a clonal gene rearrangement in virtually all cases of both polymorphous and monomorphous PTLD.

DIFFERENTIAL DIAGNOSIS

The differential diagnosis of pulmonary involvement by PTLD includes LYG and primary diffuse large B-cell lymphomas. As mentioned in the section on LYG, some cases of PTLD can look histologically identical to LYG. These cases are primarily distinguished by consideration of the clinical setting. Any case of an EBV-associated B-cell lymphoproliferative disorder following organ transplantation should probably be considered PTLD. Nonetheless, in the absence of clinical setting, there are some histologic differences which might help to distinguish the entities. PTLD tends to consist predominantly of B-cells, whereas the majority of cells in LYG are reactive T-cells. Angioinvasion and angiodestruction are also less constant features of PTLD than LYG. Primary pulmonary diffuse large B-cell lymphomas can usually also be distinguished by consideration of the clinical setting. Following transplantation, any diffuse large B-cell lymphoma involving the lung should probably be considered PTLD.

PROGNOSIS AND THERAPY

The prognosis of PTLD is variable. Regression may occur with reduction or elimination of immunosuppressive therapy. Progression and corresponding mortality correlate with increasing monomorphism of the infiltrate. Cytotoxic chemotherapy has been used in recalcitrant cases.

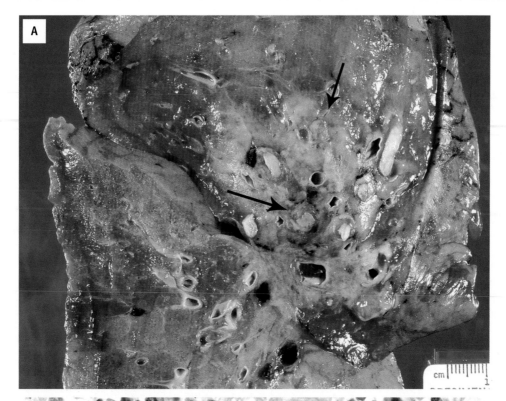

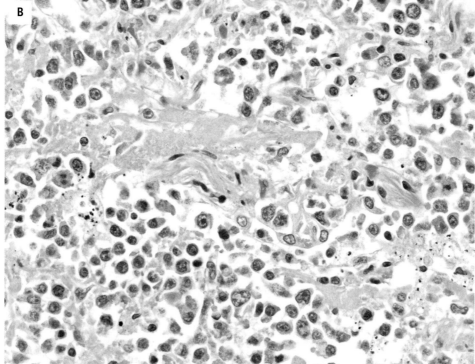

FIGURE 22-10

Post-transplant lymphoproliferative disorder
(A) Gross photograph shows 2 well demarcated pulmonary nodules (arrows) with variably necrotic centers. **(B)** PTLD—monomorphic: This example is composed of fairly monomorphic, large, cytologically atypical lymphoid cells. These cells also stained for CD20 and labeled for EBV on in situ hybridization.

TABLE 22-4

Categories of Post-Transplant Lymphoproliferative Disorders

Early lesions	Reactive plasmacytic hyperplasia	
	Infectious mononucleosis-like	
Polymorphic PTLD		
Monomorphic PTLD	B-cell neoplasms	Diffuse large B-cell lymphoma (immunoblastic, centroblastic, anaplastic)
		Burkitt/Burkitt-like lymphoma
		Plasma cell myeloma
		Plasmacytoma-like lesion
	T-cell neoplasms	Peripheral T-cell lymphoma, not otherwise specified
		Other types
Hodgkin lymphoma (HL) and Hodgkin lymphoma-like PTLD		

Data from Harris NL, Swerdlow SH, Frizzera G, et al. Post-transplant lymphoproliferative disorders. In: Jaffe ES, Harris NL, Stein H, Vardiman JW, eds. *Pathology and Genetics of Tumours of Hematopoietic and Lymphoid Tissue.* Lyon: IARC Press; 2001:264-9.

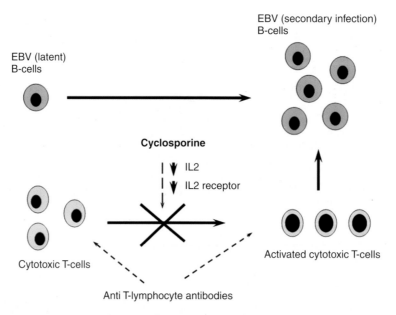

FIGURE 22-11

Schematic diagram of proposed pathogenesis of PTLD
In normal individuals with latent EBV infections, periodic secondary infections are controlled by activated cytotoxic T-cells. Immunosuppressive therapy interferes with this response by eliminating both activated and nonactivated cytotoxic T-cells (anti-T-lymphocyte antibody) or by blocking the activation of cytotoxic T-cells through a reduction in the secretion of interleukin-2 or expression of interleukin-2 receptor (cyclosporine).

More recently, anti-CD20 antibodies have been effective in some cases. Overall, PTLD is fatal in approximately 60% of patients. Patients who develop PTLD following lung transplantation appear to have a slightly worse prognosis than patients developing PTLD after transplantation of other organs.

DIFFUSE LARGE B-CELL LYMPHOMA

Diffuse large B-cell lymphoma rarely presents in the lung in the absence of involvement of lymph nodes or other sites. Diffuse large B-cell lymphoma accounts for approximately 10-20% of pulmonary lymphomas in large reported series. Approximately half of cases have coexisting areas of low-grade BALT lymphoma. Diffuse large B-cell lymphoma in the lung is thought to arise from either transformation of a preexisting BALT lymphoma or from peripheral B-lymphocytes.

CLINICAL FEATURES

In patients without HIV or AIDS, the mean age at diagnosis is approximately 60 years old (range 30-80 years). Most patients are symptomatic with fever or weight loss. Respiratory symptoms include cough, dyspnea, and hemoptysis. Large B-cell lymphoma occurs more often in immunocompromised patients (e.g., HIV infection, following organ transplant) than otherwise healthy people.

POST-TRANSPLANT LYMPHOPROLIFERATIVE DISORDER—FACT SHEET

Definition

▸ A spectrum of lymphoproliferative disorders arising in a setting of immunosuppression following solid organ or allogeneic bone marrow transplantation

▸ Most cases are EBV-associated B-cell lymphoproliferative disorders; occasional cases have a T-cell phenotype, and cases unassociated with EBV infection may also occur

Incidence

▸ Incidence varies according to the organ transplanted and type of immunosuppressive regimen used

▸ Overall incidence is less than 2% among solid organ transplant recipients, but ranges from 1% in kidney transplant recipients to 5% in heart-lung transplant patients

Mortality

▸ Fatal in 60% of patients

Gender and Age Distribution

▸ Males and females are affected in approximately equal numbers

▸ May occur at all ages

Clinical Features

▸ Clinical symptoms reflect the anatomic site of involvement, and palpable lymphadenopathy may be present

▸ Time to onset varies from months to several years following transplantation (median = 7 months)

Radiologic Features

▸ Chest x-ray and CT scan show single or multiple nodules

▸ Mediastinal lymphadenopathy may be present

Prognosis and Therapy

▸ Prognosis is variable

▸ Progression and corresponding mortality correlate with increasing monomorphism of the infiltrate

▸ Regression may occur with reduction or elimination of immunosuppressive therapy

▸ Cytotoxic therapy and anti-CD20 antibodies may be used in recalcitrant cases

---

POST-TRANSPLANT LYMPHOPROLIFERATIVE DISORDER—PATHOLOGIC FEATURES

Gross Findings

▸ White or tan, relatively well circumscribed nodules often associated with prominent necrosis

Microscopic Findings

▸ Nodules consist of an atypical lymphoreticular infiltrate, whose composition varies from polymorphic (mixture of small lymphocytes, immunoblasts, plasma cells, small cleaved and large noncleaved lymphocytes) to monomorphic (morphologically consistent with diffuse large B-cell lymphoma)

▸ Subdivided into histopathologic categories by the 2001 World Health Organization scheme (Table 22-4)

▸ Most cases involving the lung consist of either polymorphic or monomorphic PTLD

Immunohistochemistry

▸ Polymorphic PTLD: mixture of B- and T-lymphocytes (CD20+ and CD3+, respectively)

▸ Most monomorphic PTLD: sheets of large atypical lymphocytes are B-cells (CD20+, CD19+, CD79a+)

Molecular Analysis

▸ EBV can be identified by in situ hybridization in atypical lymphocytes in the vast majority of cases; most cases contain numerous positive cells

▸ Immunoglobulin heavy chain gene rearrangements are present in virtually all cases of both polymorphous and monomorphous PTLD

Pathologic Differential Diagnosis

▸ Lymphomatoid granulomatosis

▸ Reactive disorders (see text)

RADIOLOGIC FEATURES

Chest x-ray commonly shows a single or sometimes multiple opacities. Occasional patients may show a diffuse infiltrative pattern. CT scan may or may not show mediastinal adenopathy.

PATHOLOGIC FEATURES

GROSS FINDINGS

Specimens show a white to tan mass that may contain areas of necrosis (Figure 22-12A).

MICROSCOPIC FINDINGS

Histologic features are similar to those of diffuse large B-cell lymphoma involving lymph nodes. Sheets of large, blastic-appearing cells with irregularly shaped, vesicular nuclei and medium to large nucleoli are typical (Figure 22-12B). Hilar lymph nodes may be involved in some cases. Approximately half of patients have coexisting areas of low-grade BALT lymphoma.

ANCILLARY STUDIES

IMMUNOHISTOCHEMISTRY/FLOW CYTOMETRY

The neoplastic cells usually express pan-B-cell markers (CD20 and CD79a) (Figure 22-12C). A few scattered accompanying non-neoplastic CD3+ T-cells can usually be identified. Immunoglobulin light-chain restriction may be identified by flow cytometry or staining for kappa and lambda light chains.

MOLECULAR ANALYSIS

PCR analysis of the immunoglobulin heavy chain gene will show a clonal gene rearrangement in most cases.

DIFFERENTIAL DIAGNOSIS

The diagnosis of diffuse large B-cell lymphoma in the lung is usually straightforward. Principal entities in the differential diagnosis include pulmonary involvement by mediastinal large B-cell lymphoma, lymphomatoid granulomatosis (LYG), metastatic germ cell tumors, small cell carcinoma and large cell carcinoma, and anaplastic large cell lymphoma. These entities can

usually be readily distinguished by consideration of the clinical features and use of appropriate immunohistochemical stains. In contrast to primary pulmonary lymphoma, mediastinal large B-cell lymphoma presents with a mediastinal mass often in a young female. Higher-grade lesions of LYG may resemble diffuse large B-cell lymphoma. However, LYG is characterized by a strikingly angiocentric lymphoid infiltrate. In addition, the background population of T-lymphocytes is much more prominent in LYG than in diffuse B-cell lymphoma, and accounts for the majority of cells present in LYG. EBV can be identified by in situ hybridization in the large atypical cells of LYG, but is not typically present in diffuse large B-cell lymphomas when the patient is not otherwise immunocompromised. Placental-like alkaline phosphatase may be helpful in the differential diagnosis with seminoma and embryonal carcinoma. Small cell and large cell carcinomas of the lung can usually be distinguished from lymphoma by expression of cytokeratin and the lack of expression of lymphoid markers (CD45 and CD20). Expression of ALK1 and CD30 is characteristic of anaplastic large cell lymphoma, and helpful for differentiating these cases from diffuse large cell lymphoma.

PROGNOSIS AND THERAPY

The prognosis of diffuse large B-cell lymphoma is much worse than low-grade BALT lymphoma. Median survival is variably reported to range from 3 to 10 years, with much lower survival in immunocompromised patients. Treatment typically consists of combination chemotherapy.

PRIMARY PULMONARY HODGKIN LYMPHOMA

Whereas secondary involvement of the lung occurs in up to 40% of nodal-based Hodgkin lymphomas, primary presentation in the lung is rare, with less than 100 reported cases. The diagnosis of primary pulmonary Hodgkin lymphoma requires the presence of typical histologic and immunohistochemical features of the disorder and the absence of evidence of Hodgkin lymphoma at other sites, including the hilar lymph nodes. Why rare cases of Hodgkin lymphoma occur in the lung, in the absence of nodal involvement elsewhere, is unknown. Such cases may reflect initial development in an intrapulmonary or subpleural lymph node. Cases developing within BALT may explain endobronchial presentations.

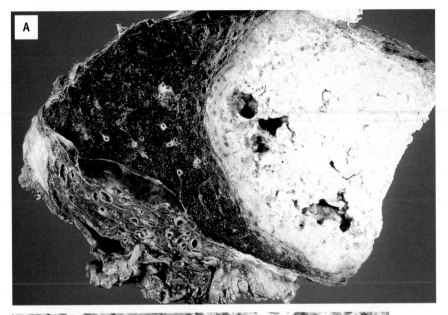

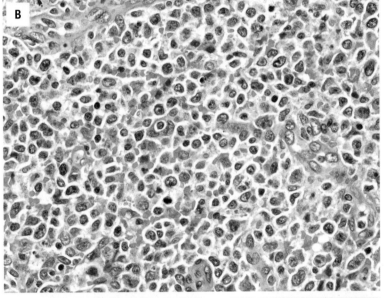

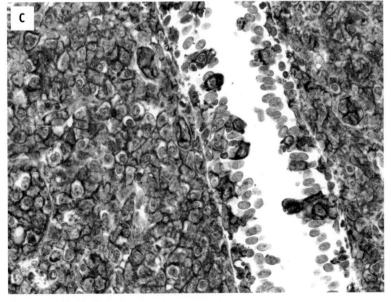

FIGURE 22-12

Diffuse large B-cell lymphoma

(A) Gross photograph shows a large, well demar-cated mass with areas of cavitation. (Photograph provided courtesy of Dr. Michael N. Koss, University of Southern California, Los Angeles, California.) **(B)** This patient presented with a large pulmonary nodule that was resected to exclude carcinoma. The nodule consists of sheets of large, cytologically atypical lymphocytes. (Case provided courtesy of Dr. David Dail, Virginia Mason Medical Center, Seattle, Washington.) **(C)** Immunohistochemical stain for CD20 decorates the large, cytologically atypical lymphocytes. The stain highlights the presence of occasional collections of lymphoid cells within the adjacent bronchial epithelium (lympho-epithelial islands) and suggests that this particular tumor may have arisen from transformation of a pre-existing low-grade lymphoma of BALT. (Case provided courtesy of Dr. David Dail, Virginia Mason Medical Center, Seattle, Washington.)

DIFFUSE LARGE B-CELL LYMPHOMA—FACT SHEET

Definition
- Primary presentation of diffuse large B-cell lymphoma in the lung, often in association with areas of low-grade BALT lymphoma

Incidence
- Approximately 10-20% of pulmonary lymphomas
- Increased incidence in immunocompromised patients (e.g., HIV infection or following organ transplantation)

Mortality
- Median survival ranges from 3-10 years (much shorter in immuno-compromised patients)

Gender and Age Distribution
- Males and females appear to be affected equally
- Mean age at diagnosis is approximately 60 years old (range 30-80) in patients without HIV or AIDS

Clinical Features
- Most patients are symptomatic, with fever and weight loss
- Respiratory symptoms include cough, dyspnea, and hemoptysis

Radiologic Features
- Chest x-ray usually shows a single or multiple opacities; occasionally patients have an infiltrative pattern
- Mediastinal lymphadenopathy may be present on CT scan

Prognosis and Therapy
- Prognosis is much worse than low-grade BALT lymphoma
- Survival is much lower in immunocompromised patients
- Treatment usually consists of combination chemotherapy

DIFFUSE LARGE B-CELL LYMPHOMA—PATHOLOGIC FEATURES

Microscopic Findings
- Similar to typical diffuse large B-cell lymphoma involving lymph nodes: sheets of blastic-appearing cells with irregularly shaped, vesicular nuclei and medium or large nucleoli
- Approximately half of cases have coexisting areas of low-grade BALT lymphoma

Immunohistochemistry
- Neoplastic cells stain for pan-B-cell markers (CD20 and CD79a)
- Monoclonal pattern of immunoglobulin light chain expression may be identified with immunohistochemical stains for kappa and lambda light chains
- Accompanying non-neoplastic T-cell stains with a pan-T-cell marker (CD3)

Molecular Analysis
- Not extensively studied (but clonal immunoglobulin heavy chain gene rearrangements are likely to be present)

Pathologic Differential Diagnosis
- Mediastinal large B-cell lymphoma
- Lymphomatoid granulomatosis
- Metastatic germ cell tumors
- Small cell carcinoma
- Large cell carcinoma
- Anaplastic large cell lymphoma

CLINICAL FEATURES

Presenting symptoms include fever, night sweats, weight loss, and dry cough. Occasional patients may be asymptomatic. Females are affected more often than males by a 2:1 margin. Affected patients have a bimodal age distribution, with peak incidences between 20 and 30 years, and 60 and 80 years.

RADIOLOGIC FEATURES

Chest x-rays and CT scans typically show a single nodule or bilateral nodules, sometimes associated with cavitation. Occasional cases may have bilateral reticulonodular infiltrates or localized pneumonic consolidation. Mediastinal lymphadenopathy is usually absent.

PATHOLOGIC FEATURES

GROSS FINDINGS

Examination reveals a grey or white mass or masses or, in some cases, consolidation of the lung. Occasional cases presenting as an occlusive endobronchial mass have been reported.

MICROSCOPIC FINDINGS

Single or multiple nodules are usually present. While these may initially appear randomly distributed, examination of the periphery of the nodules usually reveals a tendency toward a lymphatic distribution along the bronchovascular bundles, septa, and pleura. The nodules are histologically similar to Hodgkin lymphomas, in lymph nodes. Approximately two-thirds of cases are classified as nodular sclerosing Hodgkin lymphoma, and one-third are classified as mixed cellularity. Nodules consist of varying numbers of lymphocytes, plasma cells, eosinophils and Reed-Sternberg cells or their variants (Figure 22-13). Eosinophils are often prominent, and eosinophilic microabscesses may be present. Nodules may show central necrosis, sometimes with a geographic pattern. Other histopathologic features that may

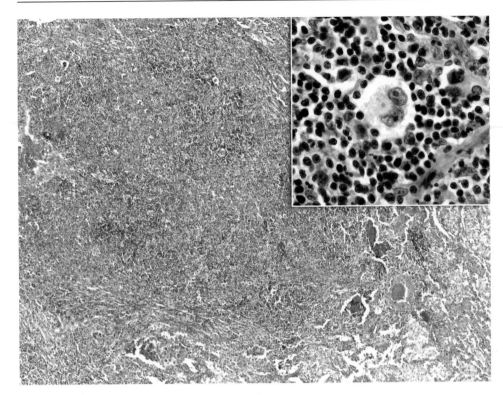

FIGURE 22-13

Pulmonary Hodgkin lymphoma
Low-power view shows a nodule composed of a polymorphous cellular infiltrate. Inset shows a classic Reed-Sternberg cell. (Case provided courtesy of Dr. David Dail, Virginia Mason Medical Center, Seattle, Washington.)

be present include involvement of the bronchial wall with destruction of cartilage plates and bronchial smooth muscle, pleural involvement, and permeation of arteries and veins by the infiltrate. Granulomatous inflammation may be present, either surrounding areas of necrosis or as associated non-necrotizing granulomas. Obstructive or acute bronchopneumonia may be present as secondary changes.

ANCILLARY STUDIES

IMMUNOHISTOCHEMISTRY

Immunohistochemical stains may be helpful for highlighting the diagnostic Reed-Sternberg cells and variants. As in typical nodal-based Hodgkin disease, Reed-Sternberg cells will almost always stain for CD30, will usually stain for CD15 (75-85%), but will not stain for CD45.

DIFFERENTIAL DIAGNOSIS

The differential diagnosis of primary pulmonary Hodgkin lymphoma includes non-Hodgkin lymphoma, LYG, Wegener's granulomatosis, granulomatous infections, and pulmonary Langerhans cell histiocytosis. Non-Hodgkin lymphomas may be distinguished by histologic, phenotypic, and molecular features indicating

the presence of a monoclonal lymphoid cell population, and a lack of Reed-Sternberg cells. LYG maybe difficult to distinguish from primary pulmonary Hodgkin lymphoma. The atypical cells in LYG, however, typically stain for CD20 and lack staining for CD15 and CD30. Although Wegener's granulomatosis and Hodgkin lymphomas may have areas of geographic necrosis, vascular involvement, granulomatous inflammation, and prominent numbers of eosinophils, they can be distinguished by the absence of typical Reed-Sternberg cells in Wegener's granulomatosis. Clinical features such as absence of nasopharyngeal and renal involvement and absence of serum c-ANCA also help to exclude Wegener's granulomatosis. Granulomatous infections occur alone or in association with Hodgkin lymphomas, and lack the typical Reed-Sternberg cells of Hodgkin lymphoma. Etiologic agents may be identified with special stains or cultures. The nodules of pulmonary Langerhans cell histiocytosis may superficially resemble Hodgkin lymphoma. This latter disease, however, is distinguished by characteristic collections of Langerhans cells which appear morphologically distinct from Reed-Sternberg cells and stain for S100 and CD1a.

PROGNOSIS AND THERAPY

Primary pulmonary Hodgkin lymphoma tends to have a less favorable prognosis than typical nodal-based Hodgkin lymphoma, with approximately 50% 2-year

---

PRIMARY PULMONARY HODGKIN LYMPHOMA—FACT SHEET

Definition
- Hodgkin lymphoma arising in the lung without evidence of involvement of hilar lymph nodes or other extrapulmonary sites

Incidence
- Extremely rare

Mortality
- 2-year survival: approximately 50% of patients

Gender and Age Distribution
- Females affected more often than males (2:1)
- Bimodal age distribution with peak incidences between 20-30 years and 60-80 years

Clinical Features
- Symptoms include fever, night sweats, weight loss, dry cough
- Occasional patients are asymptomatic

Radiologic Features
- Chest x-ray and CT scan: single or multiple nodules, sometimes associated with cavitation
- Occasional cases may have bilateral reticulonodular infiltrates or localized pneumonic consolidation
- Mediastinal lymphadenopathy is usually absent

Prognosis and Therapy
- Less favorable prognosis than nodal Hodgkin lymphoma
- Extent of disease correlates with prognosis
- Adverse prognostic factors include bilateral disease, involvement of more than one lobe, pleural involvement, cavitary disease, and type B symptoms

---

PRIMARY PULMONARY HODGKIN LYMPHOMA—PATHOLOGIC FEATURES

Gross Findings
- Single or multiple tan or white nodule(s)
- Occasional cases form an occlusive endobronchial mass

Microscopic Findings
- Nodules consist of varying mixtures of lymphocytes, plasma cells, eosinophils, and Reed-Sternberg cells or their variants
- Nodules may show central necrosis, sometimes with a geographic pattern
- Granulomatous inflammation may be present either surrounding areas of necrosis or as associated non-necrotizing granulomas

Immunohistochemistry
- Reed-Sternberg cells and variants will stain for CD30 and usually CD15 (75-85%), but not for CD45

Pathologic Differential Diagnosis
- Pulmonary involvement by non-Hodgkin lymphoma
- Lymphomatoid granulomatosis
- Wegener's granulomatosis
- Granulomatous infections
- Pulmonary Langerhans cell histiocytosis

---

differential diagnosis for patients with leukemia or lymphoma and pulmonary infiltrates, and should be evaluated for prior to concluding that leukemic or lymphomatous infiltration of the lung is the cause of the lung dysfunction. Nonetheless, involvement of the lung by some forms of leukemia (e.g., acute myelogenous leukemia) may sometimes be important in the initial presentation of disease.

survival. Extent of disease tends to influence prognosis. Adverse prognostic factors include bilateral disease, involvement of more than one lobe, pleural involvement, cavitary disease, and type B symptoms. Treatment is variable. Limited-stage disease may be treated with radiation alone. Due to its aggressive nature, however, some authors suggest combination chemotherapy and radiation therapy even with limited disease.

PULMONARY INVOLVEMENT BY LEUKEMIA/ LYMPHOMA

Pulmonary involvement by acute and chronic leukemia or non-Hodgkin B- and T-cell lymphomas is fairly common, ranging from 20 to 60% in postmortem series. Clinically significant involvement during life, however, is unusual and occurs in less than 10% of patients. Infection, drug toxicity, radiation toxicity, and pulmonary hemorrhage are frequently included in the clinical

CLINICAL FEATURES

Most of the time, but not invariably, the patient's leukemia or lymphoma will have been recognized prior to development of lung disease. Of the lymphoid leukemias, involvement by chronic lymphocytic leukemia (CLL)/small lymphocytic lymphoma is most common. Of the myelogenous leukemias, involvement by acute myelogenous leukemia (AML) occurs more frequently than involvement by chronic myelogenous leukemia (CML). Clinical symptoms of lung involvement include cough and dyspnea.

RADIOLOGIC FEATURES

Chest x-ray and CT scans show a diffuse and/or nodular infiltrate. Bronchovascular-lymphangitic, alveolar, and interstitial patterns of distribution have been described.

PATHOLOGIC FEATURES

MICROSCOPIC FINDINGS

Pulmonary involvement by leukemic or lymphomatous infiltrates tends to follow lymphatic routes. Infiltrates are most often arranged in a peribronchial or perivascular distribution or along the pleura, regardless of the histologic type (Figure 22-14A). Nodule formation with effacement of the pulmonary parenchyma can also occur, and the infiltrates can extend along alveolar septa or fill alveolar spaces. Combinations of these histologic patterns occur frequently. The cytologic features of the malignant cells reflect the type of leukemia or lymphoma (Figure 22-14B).

ANCILLARY STUDIES

SPECIAL STAINS/IMMUNOHISTOCHEMISTRY/FLOW CYTOMETRY

A wide variety of hematopoietic markers can be studied on frozen or formalin-fixed, paraffin-embedded tissue or by flow cytometric analysis. These procedures can be valuable for confirming the diagnosis of lymphoma or leukemia. Chloroacetate esterase may be helpful in cases of suspected involvement by myelogenous leukemia (Figure 22-14B).

MOLECULAR ANALYSIS

Identification of immunoglobulin heavy chain gene rearrangements by PCR analysis of lymphocytes in bronchoalveolar lavage fluid has been suggested as highly sensitive and specific (97%) for predicting the presence or absence of B-cell lymphomas on follow-up biopsies of patients with known disease. Additional studies are needed to confirm this result and to determine its utility in clinical practice.

DIFFERENTIAL DIAGNOSIS

The differential diagnosis of pulmonary involvement by leukemia/lymphoma is often broad, and correlation with the patient's history and earlier biopsies is valuable. Depending upon the clinical and histologic findings, a variety of diagnostic considerations can assume greater or lesser importance. These include differentiation of secondary involvement by lymphoma or leukemia, from primary pulmonary lymphoma (see section on pulmonary extranodal marginal zone lymphoma of BALT), and evaluation for complications of therapy including infections, drug reactions, radiation pneumonitis, alveolar proteinosis, and pulmonary veno-occlusive disease. It is also important to realize that these complications of therapy may occur concurrently with pulmonary involvement by leukemia or lymphoma. These processes may be the principal cause of the patient's symptoms and should be sought even after identification of a leukemic or lymphomatous infiltrate.

PROGNOSIS AND THERAPY

The prognosis and treatment of pulmonary involvement by leukemia or lymphoma depends upon the histologic type and therapeutic responsiveness of the primary disease.

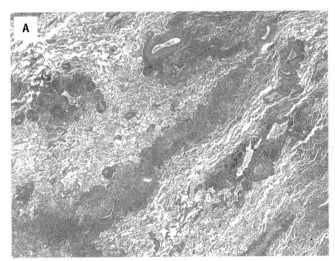
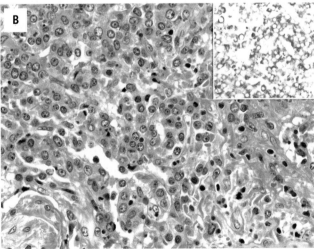

FIGURE 22-14

Pulmonary involvement by acute myelogenous leukemia
(A) Low-power view shows a cellular infiltrate with a lymphangitic distribution (following bronchovascular bundles, interlobular septa, and pleura).
(B) High-power view shows that the infiltrate is composed of monomorphous immature cells. Inset shows staining of the cells for chloroacetate esterase.

PULMONARY INVOLVEMENT BY LEUKEMIA / LYMPHOMA—FACT SHEET

Definition

›› Pulmonary involvement by acute or chronic leukemia or non-Hodgkin B- or T-cell lymphoma originating outside the lung

Incidence

›› 20-60% of patients with known leukemia or lymphoma, in some postmortem series
›› Clinically significant involvement during life is unusual, and occurs in less than 10% of patients

Clinical Features

›› Symptoms include cough and dyspnea
›› Diagnosis of malignancy will usually be established before presentation of lung involvement

Radiologic Features

›› Chest x-ray can show a diffuse or nodular infiltrate, with bronchovascular-lymphangitic, alveolar, and interstitial patterns

Prognosis and Therapy

›› Prognosis and treatment are dependent upon the type and treatment responsiveness of the disease
›› Involvement of the lung in acute leukemia and chronic lymphocytic leukemia can occasionally be important in the presentation of the disease and may precede involvement of the peripheral blood

---

PULMONARY INVOLVEMENT BY LEUKEMIA/LYMPHOMA— PATHOLOGIC FEATURES

Microscopic Findings

›› Lymphomatous and leukemic infiltrates tend to follow lymphatic routes along bronchovascular bundles and pleura
›› Neoplastic cells can also form nodules and infiltrate the lung in an interstitial or alveolar pattern
›› Cytologic features of the malignant cells are those of the specific type of leukemia or lymphoma

Immunohistochemistry, Special Stains, Flow Cytometry

›› Immunohistochemistry for lymphoid, myeloid, and monocytic antigens can be performed, as well as special stains (e.g., chloroacetate esterase) and flow cytometry, to characterize the neoplastic cells and confirm the diagnosis of leukemia or lymphoma

Molecular Analysis

›› Polymerase chain reaction studies for immunoglobulin heavy chain gene rearrangements can be performed on lymphocytes from bronchoalveolar lavage fluid specimens, and are reportedly highly sensitive and specific for detecting the presence of pulmonary involvement by lymphoma

Pathologic Differential Diagnosis

›› Primary pulmonary lymphomas
›› Infections
›› Drug reactions
›› Radiation pneumonitis
›› Alveolar proteinosis
›› Pulmonary veno-occlusive disease

INTRAVASCULAR LYMPHOMA

Intravascular lymphoma (angiotrophic large-cell lymphoma) is a type of diffuse large B-cell lymphoma in which the malignant lymphoid cells are confined to small arteries, veins, and capillaries. This disease usually presents in the skin. However, it may rarely present primarily in the lung. The neoplastic lymphoid cells are thought to lack a normal cell surface receptor necessary for migration of lymphocytes into extravascular tissues. In support of this hypothesis, a recent study has shown that the malignant cells in intravascular lymphoma lack CD29 (beta 1 integrin) and CD54 (ICAM-1), proteins which have critical roles in lymphocyte tracking and transvascular migration.

interstitial lung disease. Occasionally patients have been reported to present with pulmonary hypertension, pulmonary small vessel occlusive disease with right-sided congestive heart failure, or the adult respiratory distress syndrome. Cutaneous involvement, the most common presentation, consists of nodules or plaques. Brain involvement often manifests itself as dementia. Laboratory findings are often nonspecific, and the malignant lymphoid cells are only rarely identified on peripheral blood smear. The diagnosis of pulmonary involvement by intravascular lymphoma is often made at autopsy, but diagnosis on thoracoscopic or transbronchial biopsy has been reported.

CLINICAL FEATURES

Symptoms of pulmonary involvement include progressive dyspnea associated with fever. Based on these symptoms and diffuse interstitial infiltrates on chest x-ray, patients are often initially diagnosed with

RADIOLOGIC FEATURES

Chest x-ray may show diffuse interstitial or bilateral reticulonodular infiltrates, but may also be completely normal. Ventilation/perfusion scans may also be normal or suggest pulmonary emboli.

PATHOLOGIC FEATURES

MICROSCOPIC FINDINGS

Intravascular lymphoma consists of a proliferation of malignant lymphoid cells confined to the lumens of arteries, small veins, and capillaries (Figure 22-15A). Affected vessels may show intimal fibrosis and scarring. The malignant lymphoid cells are large, with vesicular nuclei and prominent nucleoli. Occasional apoptotic bodies or mitotic figures may be present.

ANCILLARY FEATURES

IMMUNOHISTOCHEMISTRY

The malignant cells in most cases have a B-cell phenotype and express CD20 and CD79a (Figure 22-15B). Occasional cases have been reported to have a T-cell phenotype and stain for CD3.

MOLECULAR ANALYSIS

Immunoglobulin heavy chain gene rearrangement may be identified by PCR analysis in many cases. In the rare T-cell lymphomas, rearrangement of the T-cell receptor gene may be found.

DIFFERENTIAL DIAGNOSIS

The differential diagnosis of intravascular lymphoma includes other metastatic malignancies such as metastatic carcinoma or melanoma, and involvement of the lung by other lymphomas or leukemia. These entities can usually be distinguished by use of appropriate immunohistochemical stains and consideration of other clinical and laboratory features. Metastatic carcinoma or melanoma should stain negatively for lymphoid markers and positively for either epithelial (cytokeratin) or melanocytic (S100, HMB-45) markers, respectively. Distinction from involvement by leukemia or lymphoma is usually possible on the basis of clinical features as well as examination of the peripheral blood and bone marrow. Leukemias usually have extensive bone marrow and peripheral blood involvement. Other lymphomas in the lung, either primary or secondary, usually form extravascular nodular masses.

PROGNOSIS AND THERAPY

Prognosis in intravascular lymphoma is generally poor, and the diagnosis is often made at autopsy. Occasionally patients have responded to chemotherapy.

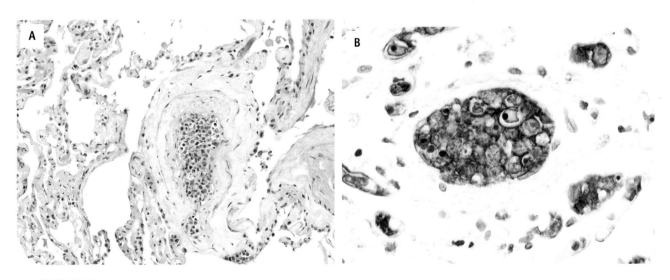

FIGURE 22-15

Intravascular lymphoma
(A) Intravascular lymphoma is characterized by collections of malignant lymphoid cells restricted to the lumens of vascular spaces. **(B)** Staining for CD20 (as shown here) and CD3 may be helpful in confirming the diagnosis, since pulmonary involvement is often subtle.

PRIMARY EFFUSION LYMPHOMA (BODY CAVITY-BASED AIDS-RELATED LYMPHOMA)

Primary effusion lymphoma is an extremely rare disease in which a lymphomatous effusion develops within a body cavity, and there is usually no associated mass lesion. Development of primary effusion lymphoma is thought to result from the oncogenic effects of latent infection of lymphocytes by human herpes virus 8 (HHV-8)/Kaposi's sarcoma herpes virus (KSHV). Most cases are associated with co-infection of EBV, suggesting a role for EBV as a cofactor in malignant transformation. Due to the expression of plasma cell differentiation markers (CD138) in most cases and identification of immunoglobulin heavy chain gene rearrangements, primary effusion lymphoma is thought to represent a high-grade lymphoma of post-germinal center B-cell origin.

CLINICAL FEATURES

Most patients have advanced AIDS. Although initially thought to be restricted to patients with AIDS, primary effusion lymphoma has been reported rarely in HIV-seronegative patients. These patients have often been immunocompromised in some other way (e.g., following organ transplantation) or have been elderly men from areas in which HHV8 is endemic. Patients most often present with a pleural, peritoneal, or pericardial effusion in the absence of clinical lymphadenopathy or organomegaly.

RADIOLOGIC FEATURES

Chest x-ray and CT scans show unilateral or bilateral pleural effusions. There may be slight thickening of the parietal pleura or pericardium. Parenchymal masses or mediastinal adenopathy are not present.

PATHOLOGIC FEATURES

CYTOLOGIC FINDINGS

Large but variably sized round or ovoid malignant lymphoid cells are present in cytologic preparations from the body fluid. These cells are sometimes multi-nucleated with very irregular and pleomorphic nuclei and multiple nucleoli (Figure 22-16). Mitotic figures are numerous.

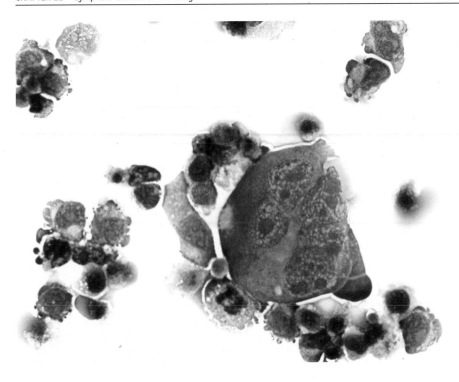

FIGURE 22-16
Pleural effusion lymphoma
Wright's and Giemsa stains show scattered, extremely pleomorphic malignant lymphoid cells.

ANCILLARY STUDIES

IMMUNOHISTOCHEMISTRY/FLOW CYTOMETRY

The neoplastic cells usually express CD45, but lack expression of pan-B-cell (CD19, CD20, CD79a) or pan-T-cell (CD3) markers on either flow cytometry or immunohistochemical stains of cell block preparations. Markers of activation (CD30) and plasma cell differentiation (CD38, CD138) are often expressed. Immunohistochemical staining for HHV8-associated latent protein is positive in nuclei of the malignant cells, and a helpful feature for diagnosis. Despite the association with coinfection by EBV, staining for EBV-LMP1 is negative.

MOLECULAR ANALYSIS

Immunoglobulin heavy chain gene rearrangements are consistently found by PCR analysis. Occasional cases may also show aberrant rearrangement of T-cell receptor genes. EBV and HHV8 are identified in the vast majority of cases by in situ hybridization, polymerase chain reaction, or Southern blot analysis.

DIFFERENTIAL DIAGNOSIS

The differential diagnosis of primary effusion lymphoma includes pleural involvement by other lymphomas as well as chronic pyothorax-associated lymphoma. Diagnosis of pleural involvement by other lymphomas is assisted by knowledge of the clinical history, which usually includes evidence of prior or concurrent overt lymph node involvement or extranodal parenchymal masses. Chronic pyothorax-associated lymphoma (see below) usually occurs in HIV-negative individuals in the setting of long-standing pleural inflammation, 20 to 40 years following therapeutic artificial pneumothorax for tuberculous pleuritis. In contrast to primary effusion lymphoma, these lymphomas are associated with a pleural-based mass in almost all cases. While they are usually associated with EBV infection, latent infection with HHV8 is not identified either on molecular or immunohistochemical analysis.

PRIMARY EFFUSION LYMPHOMA—FACT SHEET

Definition

⟶ Lymphomatous effusion developing in the pleural, peritoneal, or pericardial space, usually in a severely immunocompromised patient; an associated mass lesion is usually not present

Incidence

⟶ Extremely rare
⟶ Most patients have advanced AIDS
⟶ Rarely reported in HIV-seronegative patients who are immunocompromised in some other way (e.g., following organ transplantation) or elderly men from areas in which HHV8 is endemic

Clinical Features

⟶ Pleural, peritoneal, or pericardial effusion in the absence of lymphadenopathy or organomegaly

Radiologic Features

⟶ Chest x-ray and CT scans show unilateral or bilateral pleural effusions
⟶ There may be slight thickening of the parietal pleura or pericardium
⟶ Parenchymal masses and mediastinal lymphadenopathy are usually absent

Prognosis and Therapy

⟶ Prognosis is extremely poor, with median survival of 6 months
⟶ Response to chemotherapy is poor

PRIMARY EFFUSION LYMPHOMA—PATHOLOGIC FEATURES

Microscopic Findings

⟶ Variably sized, round or ovoid malignant cells are present on cytologic preparations
⟶ Malignant cells have irregular and pleomorphic nuclei with multiple nucleoli, and multinucleated forms may be seen
⟶ Mitotic figures are numerous

Immunohistochemistry and Flow Cytometry

⟶ Neoplastic cells express CD45 and usually lack expression of pan-B-cell (CD20, CD19, CD79a) and pan-T-cell (CD3) markers
⟶ Markers of activation and plasma cell differentiation (CD30, CD38, and CD138) are often expressed
⟶ Immunohistochemical staining for HHV8-associated latent protein is positive in nuclei of malignant cells and helpful for confirming the diagnosis
⟶ Despite the association with co-infection by EBV, staining for EBV LMP1 is negative

Molecular Analysis

⟶ Clonal immunoglobulin heavy chain gene rearrangement can usually be identified
⟶ In situ hybridization, polymerase chain reaction or Southern blot analysis will detect the presence of EBV and HHV8 in most cases

---

PROGNOSIS AND THERAPY

In AIDS patients, response to chemotherapy has been poor, with a median survival of 6 months.

PYOTHORAX-ASSOCIATED LYMPHOMA

Pyothorax-associated lymphoma occurs in HIV-negative individuals in a setting of long-standing pleural inflammation. These neoplasms typically develop 20 or more years after therapeutic artificial pneumothorax for tuberculous pleuritis. Pyothorax-associated lymphoma is thought to be derived from post-germinal center B-cells. The observation of latent infection by EBV in the majority of cases suggests a role in its development. Why this lymphoma is largely restricted to patients with tuberculosis following artificial pneumothorax is unknown.

CLINICAL FEATURES

Although a series of European cases has recently been reported, most reported cases are from Japan. Males are affected much more often than females (12:1). The most common symptoms include chest or back pain, sometimes associated with fever. Respiratory symptoms including cough, hemoptysis, and dyspnea may be present. The vast majority of patients have a history of pyothorax resulting from artificial pneumothorax for treatment of pulmonary or pleural tuberculosis. Rarely, patients have a history of pyothorax in the absence of prior tuberculous infection.

RADIOLOGIC FEATURES

Chest x-ray and CT scan commonly show a mass or masses in the pleura (80%), pleura and lung (10%), or lung near the pleura (10%).

PATHOLOGIC FEATURES

GROSS FINDINGS

Multiple pleural masses are characteristic, often with contiguous invasion of adjacent structures such as lung, liver, and diaphragm.

MICROSCOPIC FINDINGS

Histologic features of the pleural masses are those of a diffuse large B-cell lymphoma composed of highly atypical medium or large lymphoid cells with a diffuse growth pattern, round or irregular nuclei with one or more nucleoli, and moderate or abundant pale cytoplasm. Cells with features of immunoblasts or plasmacytoid differentiation may be present. Areas of necrosis are common and mitotic figures are often numerous. The adjacent pleura shows features of a chronic pleuritis.

ANCILLARY FEATURES

IMMUNOHISTOCHEMISTRY

Most cases (90%) express pan-B-cell markers (CD20, CD79a), and immunoglobulin light chain restriction can be identified in some with staining for kappa and lambda. Aberrant expression of T-cell markers (CD3) may also be noted in some cases. Immunohistochemical staining for EBV-LMP1 and EBNA2 can often be demonstrated.

MOLECULAR ANALYSIS

In situ hybridization analysis is positive for EBV in the majority (approximately 80%) of the neoplasms. Immunoglobulin heavy chain gene rearrangements can often be identified by PCR.

DIFFERENTIAL DIAGNOSIS

The differential diagnosis includes primary effusion lymphoma and secondary involvement of the pleural space by nodal-based lymphomas. These disorders are usually easily distinguished by consideration of the clinical setting and histologic and immunohistochemical features. In contrast to primary effusion lymphoma, pyothorax-associated lymphoma usually develops in immunocompetent individuals with a long history of chronic pyothorax and is associated with one or several pleural-based mass lesions. Primary effusion lymphoma is invariably associated with HHV-8, which usually cannot be demonstrated in pyothorax-associated lymphoma, either immunohistochemically or by molecular techniques. Secondary involvement of the pleura by more

---

PYOTHORAX-ASSOCIATED LYMPHOMA—FACT SHEET

Definition
➤ Pleural lymphoma occurring in HIV-negative individuals in a setting of long-standing pleural inflammation

Incidence
➤ Extremely rare
➤ Majority of patients have a long history (more than 20 years) of pyothorax after receiving therapeutic pneumothorax for tuberculosis
➤ Rare patients have a history of pyothorax in the absence of prior tuberculous infection

Gender, Race, and Age Distribution
➤ Males are affected more often than females (12:1)
➤ Most patients are older adults from Japan, although a series of European cases has also been recently reported

Clinical Features
➤ Symptoms include chest or back pain, sometimes associated with fever
➤ Respiratory symptoms include cough, hemoptysis, and dyspnea

Radiologic Features
➤ Chest x-ray and CT scan: mass or masses in the pleura (80%), pleura and lung (10%) or lung adjacent to the pleura

Prognosis and Therapy
➤ Prognosis is poor, with a median survival of 5 months
➤ Treatment with chemotherapy and radiation therapy is effective in some patients

---

PYOTHORAX-ASSOCIATED LYMPHOMA—PATHOLOGIC FEATURES

Gross Findings
➤ Mass(es) involving the pleura, with invasion of adjacent structures such as lung, liver, diaphragm, and others

Microscopic Findings
➤ Histologic appearance is similar to diffuse large B-cell lymphoma: malignant lymphoid cells have round or irregular nuclei, one or more nucleoli, and moderate or abundant pale cytoplasm
➤ Areas of necrosis are common
➤ Mitotic figures are often numerous
➤ Immunoblasts or features of plasmacytoid differentiation may be present

Immunohistochemistry
➤ Most cases (90%) express pan-B-cell markers (CD20+, CD79a+), and staining for kappa and lambda light chains may demonstrate light chain restriction in some cases
➤ Aberrant expression of T-cell markers (CD3+) is present in some cases
➤ Immunohistochemical staining for EBV LMP-1 and EBNA-2 is often positive

Molecular Analysis
➤ In situ hybridization analysis reveals the presence of EBV in most cases (80%)
➤ Immunoglobulin heavy chain gene rearrangement studies usually reveal a clonal pattern

Pathologic Differential Diagnosis
➤ Primary effusion lymphoma
➤ Secondary involvement by nodal-based lymphomas

common types of lymphomas is usually preceded by evidence of prior or concurrent overt lymph node involvement or other extranodal parenchymal masses.

PROGNOSIS AND THERAPY

Prognosis is poor, with a median survival of 5.9 months. Treatment with chemotherapy and radiation therapy is effective in some patients.

OTHER RARE LYMPHOPROLIFERATIVE DISORDERS

Extramedullary plasmacytoma occurs primarily within the upper respiratory tract. Primary presentation within the lower respiratory tract is very rare. Patients present with hilar or occasionally parenchymal masses sometimes associated with a monoclonal gammopathy. Grossly, the tumors involve a major bronchus or arise in a peribronchial location. Histologically, they are characterized by sheets of plasma cells with variable degrees of differentiation. Light chain restriction can be demonstrated by immunohistochemical staining for kappa and lambda. Occasional cases are associated with deposits of amyloid. In order to be accepted as pulmonary extramedullary plasmacytoma, the patient should not have evidence of multiple myeloma. Overall 2- and 5-year survival rates are 66% and 40%, respectively, with long-term survival of 20 years or more occasionally noted in patients. Treatment is primarily surgical excision, occasionally accompanied by chemotherapy and/or radiation therapy.

Rare examples of primary pulmonary anaplastic large cell lymphoma (ALCL) have been reported. It presents as single or multiple solid masses which obliterate the underlying pulmonary parenchyma. Endobronchial or endotracheal involvement may be present. These cases are histologically similar to cases at other extranodal sites and consist of sheets of large cells often accompanied by areas of necrosis. Individual tumor cells may be relatively monomorphic or pleomorphic, with accompanying multinucleated giant cells. The neoplastic cells stain for CD30 in a membranous and Golgi distribution. The neoplastic cells also usually stain for EMA. ALK1 expression is present in most cases of extranodal origin (either cytoplasmic and/or nuclear), although this marker has not been assessed in pulmonary cases. Although most anaplastic large cell lymphomas stain for markers of T-lymphocytes, occasional cases may not show expression due to loss of these antigens and are considered "null cell" phenotype. Nonetheless, most cases of ALCL will show T-cell receptor gene rearrange-

ments on PCR analysis, irrespective of whether they express T-cell antigens. Despite its high-grade phenotype, ALCL is usually sensitive to chemotherapy. Patients with tumors that express ALK1 have a much better prognosis (80% 5-year survival rate) than patients with ALK1-negative tumors (40% 5-year survival rate).

SUGGESTED READINGS

Intrapulmonary Lymph Node

1. Yokomise H, Mizuno H, Ike O, et al. Importance of intrapulmonary lymph nodes in the differential diagnosis of small pulmonary nodular shadows. *Chest*. 1998;113:703-6.

Follicular Bronchiolitis

2. Howling SJ, Hansell DM, Wells AU, et al. Follicular bronchiolitis: thin-section CT and histologic findings. *Radiology*. 1999; 212:637-42.
3. Nicholson AG. Reactive pulmonary lymphoid disorders. *Histopathology*. 1995;26:405-12.
4. Romero S, Barroso E, Gil J, et al. Follicular bronchiolitis: clinical and pathologic findings in six patients. *Lung*. 2003;181:309-19.
5. Yousem SA. Follicular bronchitis/bronchiolitis. *Hum Pathol*. 1985;16:700-6.

Lymphoid Interstitial Pneumonia

6. Nicholson AG. Reactive pulmonary lymphoid disorders. *Histopathology*. 1995;26:405-12.
7. Swigris JJ, Berry GJ, Raffin TA, et al. Lymphoid interstitial pneumonia: a narrative review. *Chest*. 2002;122:2150-64.
8. Travis WD, Galvin JR. Non-neoplastic pulmonary lymphoid lesions. *Thorax*. 2001, 56:964-71.

Nodular Lymphoid Hyperplasia

9. Abbondanzo SL, Rush W, Bijwaard KE, et al. Nodular lymphoid hyperplasia of the lung: a clinicopathologic study of 14 cases. *Am J Surg Pathol*. 2000;24:587-97.

Pulmonary Extranodal Marginal Zone Lymphoma of BALT

10. Begueret H, Vergier B, Parrens M, et al. Primary lung small b-cell lymphoma versus lymphoid hyperplasia: evaluation of diagnostic criteria in 26 cases. *Am J Surg Pathol*. 2002;26:76-81.
11. Ho L, Davis RE, Conne B, et al. MALT1 and the API2-MALT1 fusion act between CD40 and IKK and confer NF-kappa B-dependent proliferative advantage and resistance against FAS-induced cell death in B cells. *Blood*. 2005;105:2891-9.
12. Jaffe ES. Common threads of mucosa-associated lymphoid tissue lymphoma pathogenesis: from infection to translocation. *J Natl Cancer Inst*. 2004;96:571-3.
13. Kurtin PJ, Myers JL, Adlakha H, et al. Pathologic and clinical features of primary pulmonary extranodal marginal zone B-cell lymphoma of MALT type. *Am J Surg Pathol*. 2001;25:997-1008.
14. Okabe M, Inagaki H, Ohshima K, et al. API2-MALT1 fusion defines a distinctive clinicopathologic subtype in pulmonary extranodal marginal zone B-cell lymphoma of mucosa-associated lymphoid tissue. *Am J Pathol*. 2003;162:1113-22.
15. Zompi S, Couderc LJ, Cadranel J, et al. Clonality analysis of alveolar B lymphocytes contributes to the diagnostic strategy in clinical suspicion of pulmonary lymphoma. *Blood*. 2004;103:3208-15.

Lymphomatoid Granulomatosis

16. Guinee D Jr, Jaffe E, Kingma D, et al. Pulmonary lymphomatoid granulomatosis: evidence for a proliferation of Epstein-Barr virus infected B-lymphocytes with a prominent T-cell component and vasculitis. *Am J Surg Pathol*. 1994;18:753-64.

17. Jaffe ES, Wilson WH. Lymphomatoid granulomatosis: pathogenesis, pathology and clinical implications. *Cancer Surv*. 1997;30:233-248.
18. Zaidi A, Kampalath B, Peltier WL, et al. Successful treatment of systemic and central nervous system lymphomatoid granulomatosis with rituximab. *Leuk Lymphoma*. 2004;45:777-80.

Post-Transplant Lymphoproliferative Disorders

19. Harris NL, Swerdlow SH, Frizzera G, et al. Post-transplant lymphoproliferative disorders. In: Jaffe ES, Harris NL, Stein H, Vardiman JW, eds. *Pathology and Genetics of Tumours of Hematopoietic and Lymphoid Tissue*. Lyon: IARC Press; 2001:264-9.
20. Nalesnik MA: Clinicopathologic characteristics of post-transplant lymphoproliferative disorders. *Recent Results Cancer Res*. 2002;159:9-18.
21. Novoa-Takara L, Perkins SL, Qi D, et al. Histogenetic phenotypes of B cells in post-transplant lymphoproliferative disorders by immunohistochemical analysis correlate with transplant type: solid organ vs. hematopoietic stem cell transplantation. *Am J Clin Pathol*. 2005;123:104-12.
22. Ramalingam P, Rybicki L, Smith MD, et al. Post-transplant lymphoproliferative disorders in lung transplant patients: the Cleveland Clinic experience. *Mod Pathol*. 2002;15:647-56.

Primary Pulmonary Diffuse Large B-Cell Lymphoma

23. Cadranel J, Wislez M, Antoine M. Primary pulmonary lymphoma. *Eur Respir J*. 2002;20:750-62.
24. Fiche M, Caprons F, Berger F, et al. Primary pulmonary non-Hodgkin's lymphomas. *Histopathology*. 1995;26:529-37.
25. Nicholson AG, Harris NL. Primary pulmonary diffuse large B-cell lymphoma. Travis WD, Brambilla E, Müller-Hermelink HK, Harris CC, eds. *Pathology and Genetics of Tumours of Hematopoietic and Lymphoid Tissue*. Lyon: IARC Press; 2004:91.
26. Nicholson AG, Wotherspoon AC, Diss TC, et al. Pulmonary B-cell non-Hodgkin's lymphomas: the value of immunohistochemistry and gene analysis in diagnosis. *Histopathology*. 1995:26:395-403.

Primary Pulmonary Hodgkin Lymphoma

27. Chetty R, Slavin JL, O'Leary JJ, et al. Primary Hodgkin's disease of the lung. *Pathology*. 1995;27:111-4.
28. Yousem SA, Weiss LM, Colby TV. Primary pulmonary Hodgkin's disease. *Cancer*. 1986;57:1217-24.

Pulmonary Involvement by Leukemia/Lymphoma

29. Costa MB, Siqueira SA, Saldiva PH, et al. Histologic patterns of lung infiltration of B-cell, T-cell, and Hodgkin lymphomas. *Am J Clin Pathol*. 2004;121:718-26.
30. Hildebrand FL, Rosenow EC, Habermann TM, et al. Pulmonary complications of leukemia. *Chest*. 1990;98:1233-9.
31. Tanaka N, Matsumoto T, Miura G, et al. CT findings of leukemic pulmonary infiltration with pathologic correlation. *Eur Radiol*. 2002;12:166-74.

Intravascular Lymphoma

32. Evert M, Lehringer-Polzin M, Mobius W, et al. Angiotrophic large-cell lymphoma presenting as pulmonary small vessel occlusive disease. *Hum Pathol*. 2000;31:879-82.
33. Ponzoni M, Arrigoni G, Gould VE, et al. Lack of CD 29 (beta1 integrin) and CD 54 (ICAM-1) adhesion molecules in intravascular lymphomatosis. *Hum Pathol*. 2000;31:220-6.
34. Yousem SA, Colby TV. Intravascular lymphomatosis presenting in the lung. *Cancer*. 1990;65:349-53.

Primary Effusion Lymphoma

35. Ansari MQ, Dawson DB, Nador R, et al. Primary body cavity-based AIDS-related lymphomas. *Am J Clin Pathol*. 1996;105:221-9.
36. Carbone A, Gloghini A, Vaccher E, et al. Kaposi's sarcoma-associated herpesvirus/human herpesvirus type 8-positive solid lymphomas: a tissue-based variant of primary effusion lymphoma. *J Mol Diagn*. 2005;7:17-27.
37. Deloose ST, Smit LA, Pals FT, et al. High incidence of Kaposi sarcoma-associated herpesvirus infection in HIV-related solid immunoblastic/plasmablastic diffuse large B-cell lymphoma. *Leukemia*. 2005;19:851-5.
38. Karcher DS, Alkan S. Human herpesvirus-8-associated body cavity-based lymphoma in human immunodeficiency virus-infected patients: a unique B-cell neoplasm. *Hum Pathol*. 1997;28:801-8.

Pyothorax-Associated Lymphoma

39. Nakatsuka S, Yao M, Hoshida Y, et al. Pyothorax-associated lymphoma: a review of 106 cases. *J Clin Oncol*. 2002;20:4255-60.
40. Petitjean B, Jardin F, Joly B, et al. Pyothorax-associated lymphoma: a peculiar clinicopathologic entity derived from B-cells at late stage of differentiation and with occasional aberrant dual B- and T-cell phenotype. *Am J Surg Pathol*. 2002;26:724-32.

Extramedullary Plasmacytoma

41. Koss MN, Hochholzer L, Moran CA, et al. Pulmonary plasmacytomas: a clinicopathologic and immunohistochemical study of five cases. *Ann Diagn Pathol*. 1998;2:1-11.

Primary Anaplastic Large Cell Lymphoma

42. Rush WL, Andriko JA, Taubenberger JK, et al. Primary anaplastic large cell lymphoma of the lung: a clinicopathologic study of five patients. *Mod Pathol*. 2000;13:1285-92.

23

Uncommon Histiocytic and Dendritic Cell Proliferations

Dani S. Zander

- Introduction
- Pulmonary Langerhans Cell Histiocytosis
- Rosai-Dorfman Disease
- Erdheim-Chester Disease

INTRODUCTION

The mononuclear phagocyte system includes monocytes, macrophages/histiocytes, and dendritic cells. Macrophages/histiocytes are tissue-based cells that have an important phagocytic function and produce a variety of bioactive substances that play roles in inflammation and fibrosis. Alveolar macrophages are a normal constituent cell population in the lungs, and pulmonary histiocytic accumulations are not an uncommon finding in this location, occurring in some infections, pneumoconioses, sarcoidosis, storage diseases, lipid pneumonia, respiratory bronchiolitis, alveolar hemorrhage, drug reactions, and crystal-storing histiocytosis, disorders that are discussed elsewhere in this book. Dendritic cells present antigens to T-lymphocytes and are normally scattered throughout the airways. The most important dendritic cell proliferation involving the lung is pulmonary Langerhans cell histiocytosis (PLCH), a disease that is highly associated with tobacco smoking. PLCH is a non-neoplastic Langerhans cell proliferation that is reactive in nature, whereas the systemic form of Langerhans cell histiocytosis is a clonal, neoplastic process. Another extremely rare group of histiocytic and dendritic cell lesions arising in the lung is that of primary pulmonary histiocytic and dendritic cell neoplasms. This category includes histiocytic sarcoma, Langerhans cell sarcoma, interdigitating dendritic cell sarcoma, and follicular dendritic cell sarcoma. Finally, Rosai-Dorfman disease (RDD) and Erdheim-Chester disease must be mentioned as other disorders arising from this interesting origin. This chapter will focus upon PLCH, Rosai-Dorfman disease, and Erdheim-Chester disease.

PULMONARY LANGERHANS CELL HISTIOCYTOSIS

In 1951, the first cases of primary PLCH were described, and numerous cases have been reported since then using nomenclature including PLCH, histiocytosis X, eosinophilic granuloma, and Langerhans cell granulomatosis. PLCH is an uncommon disorder, accounting for less than 7% of interstitial lung diseases.

CLINICAL FEATURES

Most patients present with symptoms between ages 20 and 40, but a wide age range (1-69 years of age) has been reported. Individual studies have reported both male and female gender predominance. Caucasians are primarily affected, and the disease is uncommon in individuals of African or Asian descent. More than 90% of patients with PLCH are smokers versus 44% of patients with nonpulmonary Langerhans cell histiocytosis. Symptoms include dyspnea, cough, and chest pain, and constitutional symptoms (fever, weight loss, and night sweats) or hemoptysis can also occur. In approximately 10-15% of patients, pneumothorax-associated chest pain is the initial clinical presentation of the disease. Up to 25% of patients, however, are asymptomatic. Pulmonary function testing can show normal, obstructive, restrictive, or mixed patterns. Reduced diffusing capacity for carbon monoxide is common. With advanced disease, clubbing and symptoms and signs of cor pulmonale may develop.

RADIOLOGIC FEATURES

The most common chest radiographic abnormalities include ill-defined nodules and curvilinear or reticular opacities. Involvement is usually most conspicuous in the midlung zones and upper lobes and tends to be symmetrical. Over time, cystic changes tend to increase.

PULMONARY LANGERHANS CELL HISTIOCYTOSIS—FACT SHEET

Definition

» A dendritic cell disorder that presents as an interstitial lung disease primarily in smokers

Incidence

» Uncommon process, accounting for less than 7% of interstitial lung diseases

Gender, Race, and Age Distribution

» Most patients are between ages 20 and 40, but a wide age range (1-69 years of age) has been reported
» No clear gender predominance
» Caucasians are primarily affected

Clinical Features

» Symptoms include dyspnea, cough, and chest pain, and constitutional symptoms (fever, weight loss, and night sweats) or hemoptysis can also occur
» Pneumothorax is the initial clinical presentation in 10-15% of patients
» Up to 25% of patients are asymptomatic
» Pulmonary function testing can show normal, obstructive, restrictive, or mixed patterns, and reduced diffusing capacity for carbon monoxide is common
» With advanced disease, clubbing and manifestations of cor pulmonale may develop

Radiologic Features

» Chest radiograph
  » Ill-defined nodules and curvilinear or reticular opacities are most conspicuous in the midlung zones and upper lobes
  » Over time, cystic changes tend to increase
» Chest computed tomographic scans
  » Cysts are seen in 80% and nodules in 60-80% of patients, with upper and midzone predominance
  » Early cases show a centrilobular distribution of nodules, and cystic changes become more prominent with time

Prognosis and Therapy

» Clinical and radiographic stabilization occurs in up to 50% of patients, spontaneous regression in up to 25%, and progression to respiratory failure in the remaining patients
» Pulmonary hypertension is a common problem that can limit exercise tolerance
» Lung cancer, lymphoma, and myeloproliferative disorders have been reported to occur with increased frequency in patients with pulmonary Langerhans cell histiocytosis (PLCH)
» An optimum approach to therapy has not been defined
» Cessation of smoking is recommended
» Some studies have found a benefit to treatment with corticosteroids
» Chemotherapeutic agents have also been used for individual patients with rapidly progressive disease, with occasional reports of a favorable response
» Lung transplantation has also been performed for advanced disease, but PLCH has recurred after transplantation

PULMONARY LANGERHANS CELL HISTIOCYTOSIS—PATHOLOGIC FEATURES

Gross Findings

» Well-demarcated, tan-white airway-centered nodules usually less than 1 cm in diameter, often with stellate shape, particularly in the upper and middle lobes, with adjacent cysts

Microscopic Findings

» Bronchiolocentric nodules and cysts are scattered throughout the parenchyma, often accompanied by peripheral accumulations of smokers' macrophages
» Younger lesions are more cellular than older lesions and include clusters of Langerhans cells mixed with variable numbers of eosinophils, lymphocytes, plasma cells, neutrophils, and macrophages
» Langerhans cells are round or oval cells with eosinophilic cytoplasm and folded or indented nuclei that may demonstrate grooves
» As the lesions age, the Langerhans cells and other inflammatory cell populations decline and the lesions become more fibrotic, eventually evolving into stellate scars, often with radial extensions or "tentacles"
» Air spaces adjacent to the fibrotic areas become cystically enlarged

Immunohistochemical Features

» Langerhans cells express CD1a, S-100, langerin (CD207), HLA-DR, and CD4, and staining for CD45, CD68, and lysozyme is variable
» Results for CD antigens associated with B-cell and T-cell differentiation are negative, as are results for CD21, CD30, CD34, CD35, and myeloperoxidase

Ultrastructural Features

» Birbeck granules in the cytoplasm of Langerhans cells

Pathologic Differential Diagnosis

» Desquamative interstitial pneumonia
» Eosinophilic pneumonia
» Usual interstitial pneumonia
» Histiocytic and dendritic cell neoplasms
» Hodgkin lymphoma

Computed tomographic scans of the chest shows cysts in 80% and nodules in 60-80% of patients, with upper and midzone predominance. Early cases show a centrilobular distribution of nodules, and cystic changes become more prominent with time. In an adult smoker, the combination of these nodules and cysts is highly suggestive of PLCH.

PATHOLOGIC FEATURES

GROSS FINDINGS

Well-demarcated, tan-white airway-centered nodules, often with stellate shape, usually measuring less than 1 cm in diameter, are found particularly in the upper and middle lobes, with adjacent cystically enlarged air spaces.

MICROSCOPIC FINDINGS

In PLCH, bronchiolocentric nodules (Figure 23-1) are scattered throughout the parenchyma, often accompanied by peripheral accumulations of smokers' macrophages. Younger lesions tend to be more cellular than older lesions and include clusters of Langerhans cells mixed with variable numbers of eosinophils, lymphocytes, plasma cells, neutrophils, and macrophages (Figure 23-2). Langerhans cells are round or oval cells with eosinophilic cytoplasm and folded or indented nuclei that may demonstrate grooves. As the lesions age, the Langerhans cells and other inflammatory cell populations decline, and the lesions become more fibrotic, eventually evolving into stellate scars, often with radial extensions or "tentacles" (Figures 23-3 and 23-4). Air spaces adjacent to these fibrotic areas become cystically enlarged (Figure 23-4).

ANCILLARY STUDIES

IMMUNOHISTOCHEMISTRY

Langerhans cells express CD1a (Figure 23-5), S-100, langerin (CD207), HLA-DR, and CD4. Staining for CD45, CD68, and lysozyme is variable. Results for CD antigens associated with B-cell and T-cell differentiation are negative, as are results for CD21, CD30, CD34, CD35, and myeloperoxidase.

ULTRASTRUCTURAL STUDIES

Electron microscopy has been supplanted by immunohistochemistry as a diagnostic tool for PLCH, but can be useful for showing Birbeck granules in the cytoplasm of Langerhans cells.

DIFFERENTIAL DIAGNOSIS

The histologic differential diagnosis includes desquamative interstitial pneumonia (DIP), eosinophilic pneumonia (EP), usual interstitial pneumonia (UIP), histiocytic and dendritic cell neoplasms, and Hodgkin lymphoma. Identification of clusters of Langerhans cells with characteristic morphology and immunohistochemical staining reactivities should exclude these other processes; the bronchiolocentric nature of the process, cystic airspace enlargement, and accompanying mixed inflammatory infiltrates are also important for recognizing PLCH. DIP is a diffuse process, rather than a nodular process with intervening, unaffected parenchyma. The spectrum of cell types seen in PLCH is lacking in DIP, which consists predominantly of infiltrates of macrophages. EP demonstrates large numbers of eosinophils in airspaces, accompanied by variable numbers of macrophages but not clusters of Langerhans cells. An advanced, fibrotic case of PLCH can resemble UIP, but UIP affects the lower lobes more than the upper lobes, and preferentially the subpleural areas rather than the centrilobular areas

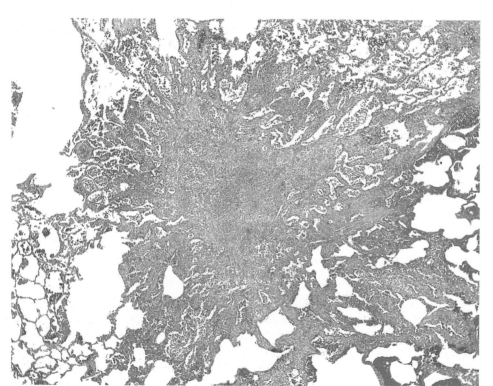

FIGURE 23-1

Pulmonary Langerhans cell histiocytosis
This stellate inflammatory and fibrotic nodule is associated with air space enlargement at its periphery.

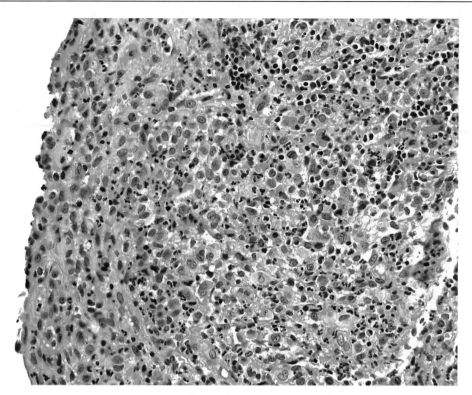

FIGURE 23-2

Pulmonary Langerhans cell histiocytosis

Numerous Langerhans cells display folded or indented nuclei and occasional nuclear grooves. Eosinophils, lymphocytes, and neutrophils accompany the Langerhans cells.

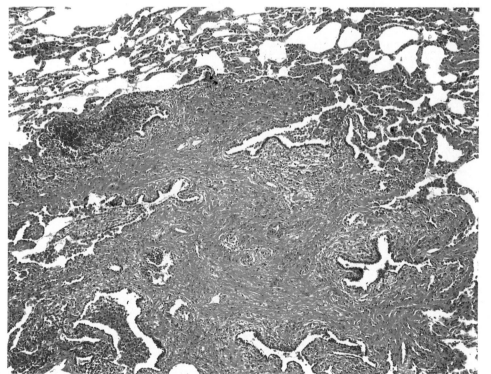

FIGURE 23-3

Pulmonary Langerhans cell histiocytosis

This older nodule has a fibrotic appearance. Pigmented smokers' macrophages fill air spaces adjacent to the edges of the nodule.

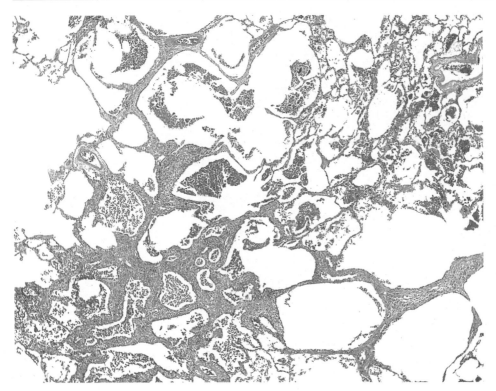

FIGURE 23-4

Pulmonary Langerhans cell histiocytosis
On the left, fibrotic "tentacles" representing the edge of a nodule are shown, with adjacent cystically expanded air spaces.

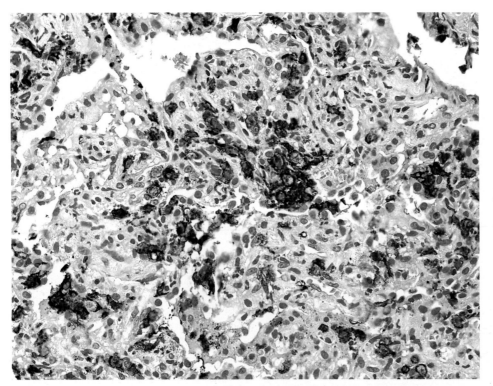

FIGURE 23-5

Pulmonary Langerhans cell histiocytosis
This immunohistochemical stain for CD1a highlights numerous Langerhans cells, singly and in clusters.

affected in PLCH. The stellate shape of the nodules is another clue to the diagnosis of PLCH rather than UIP. Histiocytic and dendritic cell neoplasms of the lung are very rare, and tumor cells usually demonstrate malignant nuclear features. Hodgkin lymphoma manifests a mixture of inflammatory cells but also includes Reed-Sternberg cells and Reed-Sternberg variants, which are lacking in PLCH.

PROGNOSIS AND THERAPY

The course of PLCH is variable and unpredictable. Up to 50% of patients will experience clinical and radiographic stabilization, spontaneous regression occurs in up to 25%, and progression to fatal respiratory failure is seen in the remaining patients. A compounding problem for many patients with PLCH is pulmonary hypertension, which can translate into limitations in exercise tolerance. Various malignancies including lung cancer, lymphoma, and myeloproliferative disorders have also been reported to develop with increased frequency in patients with PLCH.

An optimal approach to therapy has not been defined for PLCH. Cessation of smoking is recommended, and rare patients have experienced resolution of the disease after discontinuing their smoking habits. Some studies have found a benefit to treatment with corticosteroids; however, additional randomized trials are needed to evaluate the efficacy of this approach. Chemotherapeutic agents have also been used for individual patients with rapidly progressive disease, with occasional reports of a favorable response, but additional data are also needed to assess the efficacy of these agents. Finally, lung transplantation has been performed for advanced disease, but PLCH can recur after transplantation.

ROSAI-DORFMAN DISEASE

Described by Rosai and Dorfman in 1969 and 1972, RDD is a rare proliferative disorder of histiocytes involving lymph nodes and extranodal sites. Despite extensive study, no etiologic agent has been identified for RDD. The pathogenesis of this disorder has not been defined, but studies suggest that immune-mediated mechanisms and possibly dysregulation of apoptotic signaling pathways may be important. Based on studies of clonality, RDD appears to be a reactive (non-neoplastic) process. Although RDD most commonly involves lymph nodes, extranodal RDD was reported to be present in 43% of the 423 patients in the RDD Registry. In 9 of these patients, the lower respiratory tract was affected. Additional cases of pulmonary RDD have been reported since publication of

the Registry findings, but pulmonary RDD appears to be extremely rare. Lower respiratory tract involvement can take the form of endotracheal or endobronchial masses, parenchymal nodules or patchy solidification, diffuse interstitial involvement, and/or pleural involvement.

CLINICAL FEATURES

Lower respiratory tract disease has occurred more frequently in females than males, with a mean age of onset of 14 years of age according to the largest review of cases published by Foucar and colleagues. Individuals of Caucasian, African, and Asian descent have been affected. In this same series, all patients had evidence of nodal disease accompanying their lower respiratory tract disease. Symptoms can include stridor and shortness of breath.

RADIOLOGIC FEATURES

Radiologic features depend on the specific pattern of involvement. Masses, nodules, interstitial thickening, widening and nodularity of the interlobular septa and pleura, and pleural effusions have been observed.

PATHOLOGIC FEATURES

GROSS FINDINGS

Polypoid mass lesions arising from airway walls can cause airway obstruction. Parenchymal masses have been described, measuring up to 8 cm in greatest dimension. Diffuse interstitial thickening and parenchymal consolidation resembling pneumonia represent other presentations.

MICROSCOPIC FINDINGS

Mass-like or interstitial infiltrates are seen, consisting of polygonal mononuclear and multinucleated cells with mildly pleomorphic nuclei, small or absent nucleoli, and abundant cytoplasm, in a background of lymphocytes, neutrophils, macrophages, plasma cells, and eosinophils (Figure 23-6). Emperipolesis is characteristic (Figure 23-7), with lymphocytes and/or neutrophils in the cytoplasm of some of these histiocytic cells, although this may be less conspicuous than in nodal RDD. Fibroblast proliferation and collagen deposition can accompany the inflammatory cell infiltrates, and reactive type 2 pneumocyte hyperplasia may be evident. The characteristic histiocytes and foamy macrophages can also be seen in air spaces.

Ancillary Studies

Immunohistochemistry

The histiocytic cells of RDD typically stain for S100, pan-macrophage antigens (CD68, HAM56, CD14, CD15, and CD64), phagocytosis-related antigens (CD64 and IgG Fc receptor), and antigens related to lysosomal activity (lysozyme, α_1-antichymotrypsin) and immune activation (transferrin receptor and interleukin-2 receptor). CD1a-expressing cells are rare in RDD, and the histiocytes do not express the dendritic markers CD21, CD23, and CD35.

Differential Diagnosis

The differential diagnosis includes primarily PLCH, Erdheim-Chester disease, monocytic and histiocytic malignancies, T-cell lymphoma, Hodgkin lymphoma, in-

flammatory myofibroblastic tumor, sarcoidosis, histiocyte-rich infections (mycobacterial, fungal, and unusual bacterial infections), storage diseases, and aspiration pneumonia. Observation of the characteristic histiocytic cells, particularly with emperipolesis, in the mixed inflammatory background, is essential for distinguishing pulmonary RDD from these other processes. Immunohistochemical staining and histochemical staining for organisms is also helpful. PLCH includes Langerhans cells that express CD1a, whereas CD1a-expressing cells are rare in RDD. In Erdheim-Chester disease, the histiocytic cells do not show emperipolesis, and the characteristic bone lesions are present to suggest the diagnosis.

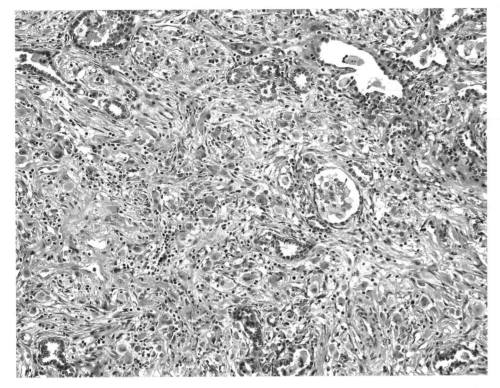

FIGURE 23-6
Rosai-Dorfman disease
The lung architecture is distorted by infiltrates of plump histiocytes with eosinophilic cytoplasm, mixed inflammatory cell infiltrates, and fibrosis. Residual air spaces are lined by reactive type 2 pneumocytes.

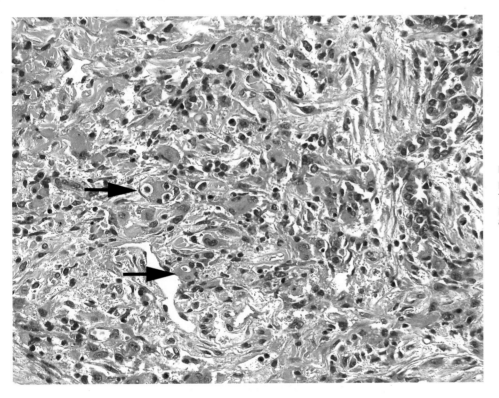

FIGURE 23-7
Rosai-Dorfman disease
Two histiocytes demonstrate emperipolesis (arrows) and lie in a fibrotic and mixed inflammatory background.

True granulomas are not seen in RDD, unlike in sarcoidosis and most histiocyte-rich infections. Patients with storage diseases usually have a history of these diseases, which assists in the classification of the pulmonary abnormalities, and histochemical stains can be helpful for highlighting the stored material in the cyto-plasm. Most malignancies will demonstrate greater degrees of nuclear atypia than those observed in RDD, and immunohistochemical staining can help to differentiate these disorders from RDD as well. Aspiration pneumonia does not manifest the S-100-expressing histiocytes of RDD and may display food particles.

PROGNOSIS AND THERAPY

In contrast to the usually benign course of nodal RDD, the prognosis of patients with lower respiratory tract disease is significantly worse, with about one-third of patients dying of the disease and more than one-third demonstrating persistent or progressive disease, according to the Registry review published by Foucar and colleagues. An optimal approach to treatment has not been defined for pulmonary RDD. Surgery and radiation were followed by persistent disease in one patient. Another patient had a good response to prednisone and chlorambucil. Tracheostomy has been performed in several patients with airway obstruction. For RDD in general, corticosteroids can reduce associated fevers and lesional size. Surgical debulking and/or radiation therapy can be performed for patients with compromise of vital organ function. High-dose chemotherapy for severe RDD has generally not been associated with a good response.

ERDHEIM-CHESTER DISEASE

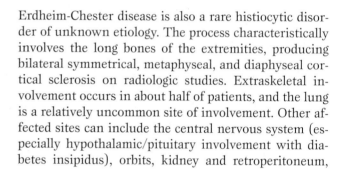

Erdheim-Chester disease is also a rare histiocytic disorder of unknown etiology. The process characteristically involves the long bones of the extremities, producing bilateral symmetrical, metaphyseal, and diaphyseal cortical sclerosis on radiologic studies. Extraskeletal involvement occurs in about half of patients, and the lung is a relatively uncommon site of involvement. Other affected sites can include the central nervous system (especially hypothalamic/pituitary involvement with diabetes insipidus), orbits, kidney and retroperitoneum,

---

ERDHEIM-CHESTER DISEASE—FACT SHEET

Definition

▸ A histiocytic disorder of unknown etiology that characteristically affects the long bones of the extremities and involves extraskeletal sites in more than half of patients

Incidence

▸ Rare disorder

Mortality

▸ The disease is fatal in about half of patients with pulmonary involvement, most commonly due to respiratory or cardiac failure

Gender and Age Distribution

▸ Usually affects middle-aged adults of both genders

Clinical Features

▸ Progressive dyspnea over a period of months to years and sometimes a dry cough
▸ Pulmonary function testing usually reveals a restrictive defect, although results can be normal, obstructive, or mixed; a reduction in diffusing capacity for carbon monoxide is often present

Radiologic Features

▸ Bilateral symmetrical metaphyseal and diaphyseal cortical sclerosis or mixed sclerotic and lytic lesions are observed in the long bones and are considered essentially pathognomonic
▸ Chest radiographs show increased interstitial markings and pleural thickening, often with an upper lobe predominance; additional findings may include bullous and cystic changes, thickening of the interlobular septa, pleural effusions, and cardiac enlargement

Prognosis and Therapy

▸ Disease is frequently progressive in patients with pulmonary involvement
▸ An optimum treatment regimen remains to be determined
▸ Results have varied with corticosteroids, chemotherapeutic agents and radiation therapy alone or in combinations, with a clinical response in a minority of patients

---

ERDHEIM-CHESTER DISEASE—PATHOLOGIC FEATURES

Microscopic Findings

▸ Histiocytic infiltrates along lymphatic routes (pleura, bronchovascular bundles, and interlobular septa) with a fibrotic background and little involvement of adjacent alveoli
▸ The histiocytes are large with round or oval nuclei and moderate or abundant eosinophilic, pale, or foamy cytoplasm
▸ Lymphocytes and plasma cells, and occasionally eosinophils, may accompany the histiocytes
▸ Multinucleated giant cells can also be seen
▸ Emperipolesis is not observed

Immunohistochemical Features

▸ The histiocytes express CD68 and factor XIIIa but not CD1a
▸ S100 staining can be present or absent, as can weak lysozyme staining
▸ Staining for Mac 387 and CD21 is negative

Ultrastructural Features

▸ Histiocytes contain phagolysosomes but not Birbeck granules

Pathologic Differential Diagnosis

▸ Usual interstitial pneumonia
▸ Pulmonary Langerhans cell histiocytosis
▸ Rosai-Dorfman disease
▸ Histiocyte-rich infections
▸ Storage diseases
▸ Monocytic and histiocytic malignancies
▸ Aspiration pneumonia

breast, skin (xanthoma-like lesions), skeletal muscle, heart, aorta, and sinonasal area.

CLINICAL FEATURES

This disorder usually affects middle-aged adults of both genders. Series of patients with lung involvement found a mean age of 53.6-57 years at the onset of symptoms, with a wide range of patient ages. Pulmonary involvement is associated with progressive dyspnea over a period of months to years and sometimes a dry cough. Pulmonary function testing usually reveals a restrictive defect, although results can be normal, obstructive, or mixed. A reduction in diffusing capacity for carbon monoxide is often present.

RADIOLOGIC FEATURES

Bilateral symmetrical metaphyseal and diaphyseal cortical sclerosis or mixed sclerotic and lytic lesions are observed in the long bones and are considered essentially pathognomonic. Chest radiographs show increased interstitial markings and pleural thickening, often with upper lobe predominance. Additional findings may include bullous and cystic changes, thickening of the interlobular septa, pleural effusions, and cardiac enlargement.

PATHOLOGIC FEATURES

MICROSCOPIC FINDINGS

Pulmonary involvement takes the form of histiocytic infiltrates along lymphatic routes (pleura, bronchovascular bundles, and interlobular septa) with a fibrotic background and little involvement of adjacent alveoli (Figure 23-8). The histiocytes are large with round or oval nuclei and moderate or abundant eosinophilic, pale, or foamy cytoplasm (Figure 23-9). Lymphocytes and plasma cells and occasionally eosinophils may accompany the histiocytes. Multinucleated giant cells can also be seen. Emperipolesis is not observed.

ANCILLARY STUDIES

IMMUNOHISTOCHEMISTRY

The characteristic histiocytes express CD68 and factor XIIIa, but not CD1a. S100 staining can be present or absent, as can weak lysozyme staining. Results for Mac

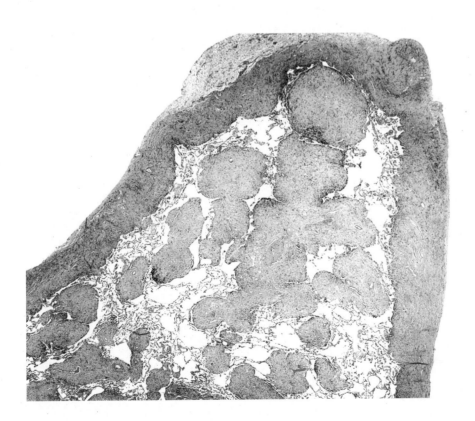

FIGURE 23-8
Erdheim-Chester disease
At low-power, there is obvious fibrotic thickening of the pleura, bronchovascular bundles, and interlobular septa. (Generously contributed by Dr. Samuel Yousem, University of Pittsburgh, Pittsburgh, Pennsylvania.)

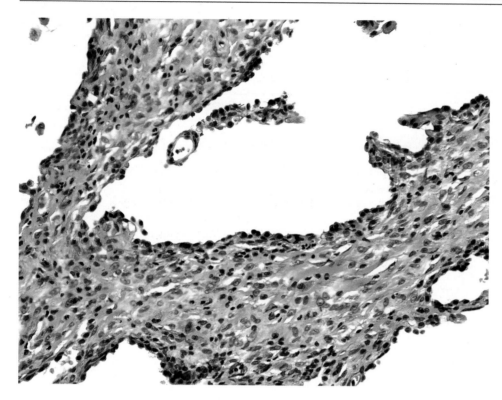

FIGURE 23- 9

Erdheim-Chester disease

Examination at higher power reveals infiltrates of histiocytes with round or oval nuclei and moderate amounts of pale cytoplasm. (Generously contributed by Dr. Samuel Yousem, University of Pittsburgh, Pittsburgh, Pennsylvania.)

387 and CD21 were negative in the small number of cases evaluated.

ULTRASTRUCTURAL STUDIES

Electron microscopic examination reveals phagolysosomes, but not Birbeck granules, in the cytoplasm of the histiocytes.

DIFFERENTIAL DIAGNOSIS

The differential diagnosis includes primarily UIP, PLCH, and RDD. UIP will not display the histiocytic infiltrates of Erdheim-Chester disease and has a more variegated histologic appearance with areas of fibrosis, normal lung, and fibroblast foci, as opposed to the more uniform appearance of the fibrosis in Erdheim-Chester disease. PLCH shows a bronchiolocentric distribution of lesions with a cellular composition that differs from Erdheim-Chester disease. PLCH will show clusters of Langerhans that stain with S100 and CD1a, whereas the histiocytic cells of Erdheim-Chester disease have a different morphology and do not stain for CD1a. In Erdheim-Chester disease, unlike RDD, emperipolesis is not observed, and RDD lacks the bony abnormalities seen in Erdheim-Chester disease. Histiocyte-rich infections caused by nontuberculous mycobacteria, fungi, *Rhodococcus equi* (malakoplakia),

or *Tropheryma whippelii* (Whipple's disease) may also be considered in the differential diagnosis, and stains and cultures for these organisms can be helpful in evaluating for these possibilities. Storage diseases represent another group of diseases that form part of the differential diagnosis. In most cases, however, the clinical history is helpful, and the radiologic findings do not fit a diagnosis of Erdheim-Chester disease. Also, the histiocytes in storage diseases demonstrate cytoplasmic accumulation of various materials, as discussed in Chapter 36. Monocytic and histiocytic malignancies may also be considered but usually demonstrate greater nuclear atypia. Aspiration pneumonia, another potential consideration, is more of an airspace disease, as opposed to Erdheim-Chester disease, which primarily involves the pleura, interlobular septa, and bronchovascular bundles.

PROGNOSIS AND THERAPY

In about half of patients with pulmonary involvement, the disease is progressive and fatal. The most common causes of death are respiratory and cardiac failure. An optimal treatment regimen remains to be determined. Results have varied with corticosteroids, chemotherapeutic agents, and radiation therapy alone or in combinations, with a clinical response in a minority of patients.

SUGGESTED READINGS

General

1. Aubry MC, Wright JL, Myers JL. The pathology of smoking-related lung diseases. *Clin Chest Med*. 2000;21:11-35.
2. McClain KL, Natkunam Y, Swerdlow SH. Atypical cellular disorders. *Hematol Am Soc Hematol Educ Program*. 2004;283-96.
3. Wang CW, Colby TV. Histiocytic lesions and proliferations in the lung. *Semin Diagn Pathol*. 2007;24:162-82.

Langerhans Cell Histiocytosis

4. Abbott GF, Rosado-de-Christenson ML, Franks TJ, Frazier AA, Galvin JR. From the archives of the AFIP: pulmonary Langerhans cell histiocytosis. *Radiographics*. 2004;24:821-41.
5. Sundar KM, Gosselin MV, Chung HL, Cahill BC. Pulmonary Langerhans cell histiocytosis: emerging concepts in pathobiology, radiology, and clinical evolution of disease. *Chest*. 2003;123:1673-83.
6. Vassallo R, Ryu JH. Pulmonary Langerhans' cell histiocytosis. *Clin Chest Med*. 2004;25:561-71.
7. Vassallo R, Ryu JH, Colby TV, Hartman T, Limper AH. Pulmonary Langerhans'-cell histiocytosis. *N Engl J Med*. 2000;342:1969-78.

Rosai-Dorfman Disease

8. Foucar E, Rosai J, Dorfman R. Sinus histiocytosis with massive lymphadenopathy (Rosai-Dorfman disease): review of the entity. *Semin Diagn Pathol*. 1990;7:19-73.

9. Paulli M, Bergamaschi G, Tonon L, et al. Evidence for a polyclonal nature of the cell infiltrate in sinus histiocytosis with massive lymphadenopathy (Rosai-Dorfman disease). *Br J Haematol*. 1995;91:415-8.
10. Rosai J, Dorfman RF. Sinus histiocytosis with massive lymphadenopathy: a newly recognized benign clinicopathological entity. *Arch Pathol*. 1969;87:63-70.
11. Rosai J, Dorfman RF. Sinus histiocytosis with massive lymphadenopathy: a pseudolymphomatous benign disorder: analysis of 34 cases. *Cancer*. 1972;30:1174-88.
12. Zander DS, Mergo PJ, Foster RA, Ohori P, Yousem S, Travis WD. Pulmonary parenchymal sinus histiocytosis with massive lymphadenopathy (Rosai-Dorfman disease): report of a case with immunohistochemical studies. *Mod Pathol*. 1997;10:174A.

Erdheim-Chester Disease

13. Bisceglia M, Cammisa M, Suster S, Colby TV. Erdheim-Chester disease: clinical and pathologic spectrum of four cases from the Arkadi M. Rywlin slide seminars. *Adv Anat Pathol*. 2003;10:160-71.
14. Bourke SC, Nicholson AG, Gibson GJ. Erdheim-Chester disease: pulmonary infiltration responding to cyclophosphamide and prednisolone. *Thorax*. 2003;58:1004-5.
15. Chung JH, Park MS, Shin DH, et al. Pulmonary involvement in Erdheim-Chester disease. *Respirology*. 2005;10:389-92.
16. Egan AJ, Boardman LA, Tazelaar HD, et al. Erdheim-Chester disease: clinical, radiologic, and histopathologic findings in five patients with interstitial lung disease. *Am J Surg Pathol*. 1999;23:17-26.
17. Rush WL, Andriko JA, Galateau-Salle F, et al. Pulmonary pathology of Erdheim-Chester disease. *Mod Pathol*. 2000;13:747-54.

24 Transplantation-Related Lung Pathology

Aliya N. Husain

COMPLICATIONS OF LUNG TRANSPLANTATION

Lung transplantation, either single, bilateral or, less often, heart-lung, has been an accepted mode of therapy for a variety of end-stage lung diseases for about 15 years. The most common indications for adults are emphysema, cystic fibrosis (CF), idiopathic pulmonary fibrosis, and primary pulmonary hypertension (PPH), and for children are CF and PPH. Advances in donor management, surgical techniques, and immunosuppressive drugs have led to improvement in the short-term survival of patients. However, in contrast to other solid organ transplants, over half of the lung transplant recipients continue to suffer and die of chronic rejection (bronchiolitis obliterans) 3 to 10 years post-transplantation. Methods of evaluation of allograft dysfunction are variable and depend on the clinical differential diagnosis, post-transplant time, and complications suspected (Table 24-1).

VASCULAR COMPLICATIONS

Post-surgical obstruction/thrombosis of the arterial or venous anastomoses, although rare, is a surgical emergency. Inflammatory cells, endothelial disruption, and recent thrombus are seen in the early post-transplant period, while organizing/organized thrombus, stenosis, and fibrosis with foreign-body giant cells are present in the intermediate to late period.

AIRWAY ANASTOMOTIC COMPLICATIONS

The anastomosis heals by formation of granulation tissue, the surface of which re-epithelializes in a few days. Occasionally, exuberant polypoid granulation tissue forms, which may need to be removed. Varying degrees of ischemic injury, manifested as coagulative necrosis of airway wall components, are commonly present. Superimposed infection may interrupt and complicate the healing process. Common organisms found on culture, endobronchial biopsy, and special stains include fungi (*Candida* and *Aspergillus* sp.) and bacteria. Fungi tend to invade necrotic cartilage. Dehiscence of the anastomosis can allow infection to spread into the mediastinum. Healing may result in fibrosis and stenosis of the airway, treatment for which includes stent placement (Figure 24-1).

ISCHEMIA-REPERFUSION INJURY

Preservation-reperfusion injury occurs in 10-20% of patients due to some combination of ischemia, reperfusion, surgical trauma, denervation, and interruption of lymphatics, resulting in endothelial injury and pulmonary edema with or without diffuse alveolar damage (Figure 24-2). On biopsy, the absence of perivascular and airway mononuclear cell infiltrates distinguishes it from acute rejection. Recovery occurs in the majority of patients in a few days to weeks with supportive therapy.

TABLE 24-1

Evaluation of Complications of Lung Transplantation

Post-Transplant Time of Onset	Complication	Method of Evaluation
Immediate (0-7 days)	Primary graft failure	Clinical
	Vascular anastomotic: bleeding, obstruction, thrombosis	Re-exploration
	Ischemia-reperfusion injury	Clinical, TBB
	Hyperacute rejection	Clinical, TBB, lymphocyte cross-match
Early (8-30 days)	Infection of lung	BAL, culture, TBB
	Airway anastomotic infection, dehiscence	Culture, EBB
	Acute rejection	TBB
Late (>30 days)	Acute rejection	TBB
	Infection of lung	BAL, culture, TBB
	Airway stenosis	Bronchoscopy, culture
	Chronic rejection	PFT, TBB, wedge biopsy
	PTLD (mass lesion)	FNAB, TBB, wedge biopsy

Abbreviations: TBB = transbronchial biopsy, BAL = bronchoalveolar lavage, EBB = endobronchial biopsy, PFT = pulmonary function tests, PTLD = post-transplant lymphoproliferative disorder, FNAB = fine needle aspiration biopsy.

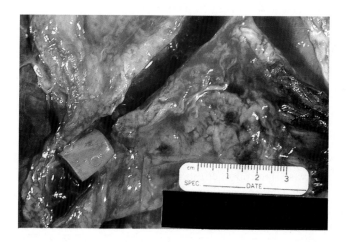

FIGURE 24-1

Stenotic bronchial anastomosis
Gross photograph of bronchial anastomosis with stenosis, status post stent placement. Careful dissection is needed to document correct placement.

REJECTION

Definite diagnosis and grading of rejection (especially acute rejection) is based on light microscopic examination of tissue obtained by transbronchial biopsy (TBB), which may be performed based on the clinical symptoms or based on a surveillance protocol. Since rejection is a patchy process, it is recommended that 5 fragments of alveolated lung tissue be examined at 3 different levels stained with hematoxylin and eosin. A working formulation for the grading of pulmonary allograft rejection, initially developed in 1990, revised in 1996 and again revised in 2007, is widely used (Table 24-2).

HYPERACUTE REJECTION

Only a few well documented cases of hyperacute (humoral or antibody-mediated) rejection of the lung have been recently reported in the literature, thus it was not included in the working formulation. Preformed antibodies bind to the endothelium and epithelium of the donor lung and activate inflammatory, complement, and coagulation cascades.

CLINICAL FEATURES

Within minutes to hours after transplantation, there is progressive respiratory failure, pulmonary edema and pleural effusion, with complete opacification of the allograft seen on radiologic examination.

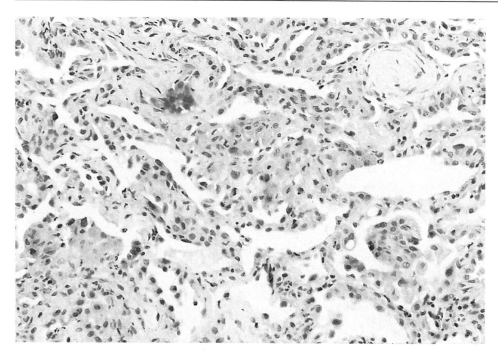

FIGURE 24-2
Ischemia-reperfusion injury
High-power photomicrograph showing edema and reactive type 2 pneumocyte hyperplasia.

TABLE 24-2

2007 Revision of the Working Formulation for the Classification and Grading of Pulmonary Allograft Rejection

A. Acute rejection	Grade 0—None
	Grade 1—Minimal
	Grade 2—Mild
	Grade 3—Moderate
	Grade 4—Severe
B. Airway inflammation—lymphocytic bronchiolitis	Grade 0—None
	Grade 1R—Low-grade
	Grade 2R—High-grade
	Grade X—Ungradeable
C. Chronic airway rejection—bronchiolitis obliterans	Grade 0—None
	Grade 1—Present
D. Chronic vascular rejection—accelerated graft vascular sclerosis	

Based on Stewart S, Fishbein MC, Snell GI, et al. Revision of the 1996 working formulation for the standardization of nomenclature in the diagnosis of lung rejection. *J Heart Lung Transplant.* 2007;26:1229-42.

PATHOLOGIC FEATURES

MICROSCOPIC FINDINGS

The histologic features of hyperacute rejection include diffuse alveolar damage (DAD), alveolar hemorrhage, interstitial neutrophilia, fibrin thrombi, and vasculitis.

ANCILLARY STUDIES

IMMUNOFLUORESCENCE

There is deposition of IgG and complement in the alveolar septa. Complement fragments C3d and C4d may also be detected.

IMMUNOHISTOCHEMISTRY

If fresh frozen tissue is not available for immunofluorescence studies, C4d deposition can be demonstrated in the vascular endothelium and/or the interstitium. Only strong staining without background should be interpreted as positive.

DIFFERENTIAL DIAGNOSIS

The main pathologic differential diagnosis is from ischemia-reperfusion injury in which there is no vasculitis and a negative lymphocyte cross-match.

PROGNOSIS AND THERAPY

Hyperacute rejection is usually fatal. Treatment approaches have included augmented immunosuppression (usually corticosteroids), plasmapheresis, and/or antibody therapy.

ACUTE REJECTION

Acute rejection is a cell-mediated process during which there is progressive infiltration of the graft by host mononuclear cells. Immune cell activation causes release of inflammatory chemokines and up-regulation of adhesion molecules. Major cellular targets include endothelial and epithelial cells.

CLINICAL FEATURES

Although acute rejection can develop as early as 3 days to many years post-transplant, most patients experience some rejection commonly around 3 months, with most episodes occurring between 2 and 9 months. Noncompliance with immunosuppressive medications is a significant cause of late episodes of acute rejection. Patients often present with low-grade fever, cough, and dyspnea and some are hypoxemic with greater than 10% decrease in pulmonary function tests. Aspiration and infection may precipitate episodes of acute rejection.

RADIOLOGIC FEATURES

On chest x-ray, there can be perihilar or lower zone alveolar or interstitial infiltrates, septal lines, subpleural edema, peribronchial cuffing, and pleural effusion.

PATHOLOGIC FEATURES

With current immunosuppressive therapy, it is rare for a lung transplant recipient to die due to acute cellular rejection. On the rare occasion that there is acute rejection seen microscopically at autopsy, there are other significant pathologic processes present which make it impossible to determine the gross findings of acute rejection.

MICROSCOPIC FINDINGS

Acute rejection is characterized by a predominantly lymphocytic infiltrate with scattered eosinophils, neutrophils, and plasma cells. The infiltrate begins in the perivascular areas and variably extends into the airways and lung parenchyma. In minimal acute rejection (grade A1), there are scattered infrequent perivascular and airway mononuclear infiltrates that are not obvious at low magnification. Blood vessels, particularly venules, are cuffed by small, round, plasmacytoid and transformed lymphocytes forming a layer of 2 to 3 cells (Figure 24-3). Mild acute rejection (grade A2) consists of greater than 3 layers of lymphocytes, with eosinophils and neutrophils around small blood vessels (Figures 24-4, 24-5). Grade A2 or higher grade acute rejection is often accompanied by lymphocytic airway inflammation (Figure 24-6). Moderate acute rejection (A3) is characterized by an extension of the inflammation into alveolar septa (Figure 24-7). In severe acute rejection (grade A4), diffuse perivascular, interstitial, and air space infiltrates associated with pneumocyte damage, macrophages, hyaline membranes, hemorrhage, and neutrophils or epithelial

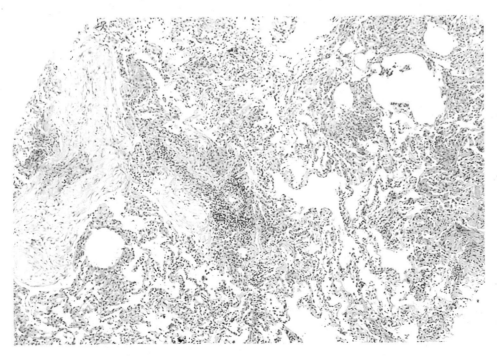

FIGURE 24-3

Minimal acute rejection

There is a minimal perivascular inflammatory infiltrate (grade A1). In addition, there is organizing pneumonia on the left, which is a nonspecific reaction to lung injury.

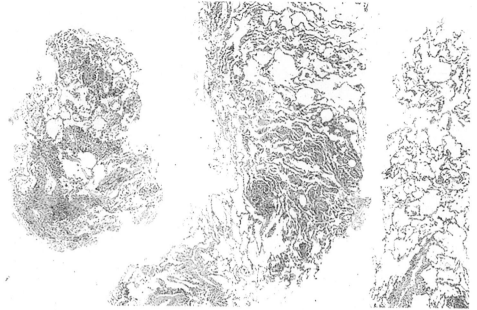

FIGURE 24-4

Mild acute rejection
Multiple foci of mild perivascular infiltrates (grade A2) are noted.

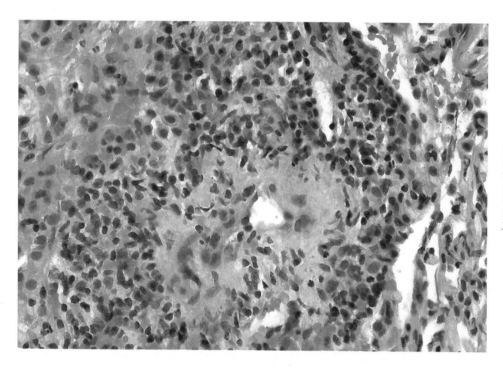

FIGURE 24-5

Mild acute rejection
There is a 4 to 5 cell-layer-thick perivascular infiltrate composed of activated lymphocytes, eosinophils, and rare plasma cells without extension into adjacent lung parenchyma (grade A2).

ulceration with fibrinopurulent exudates are seen. High-grade lymphocytic broncliolitis (grade B2R, Figure 24-8) can also be observed, and is characterized by dense bronchiolar inflammatory cell infiltrates with epithelial cell dropout, lymphocytic infiltration of the epithelium, and sometimes ulceration. The predominant inflammatory cell is the lymphocyte, but smaller numbers of neutrophils and eosinophils can accompany the lymphocytes.

ANCILLARY STUDIES

BRONCHOALVEOLAR LAVAGE (BAL)

Although the inflammatory cells, as well as mediators of inflammation, during acute rejection have been extensively studied in BAL fluid, the findings are not diagnostic. Commonly, however, lymphocytosis is present.

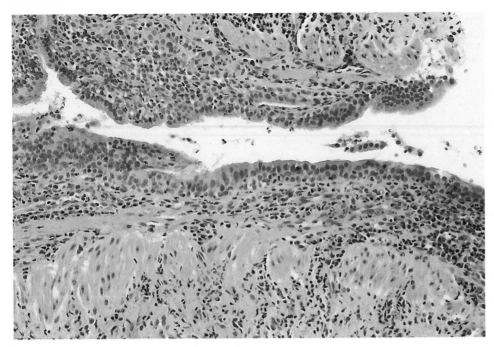

FIGURE 24-6

Low-grade lymphocytic bronchiolitis
There is a band-like inflammatory infiltrate in the bronchiolar submucosa (grade B1R).

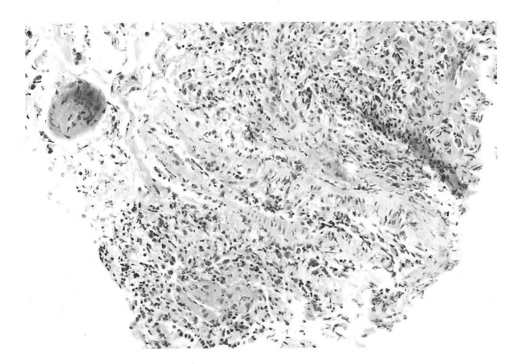

FIGURE 24-7

Moderate acute rejection
This example shows perivascular infiltration with endothelialitis (subendothelial infiltrates associated with endothelial swelling and sloughing) and extension of inflammation into adjacent alveolar septa (grade A3).

DIFFERENTIAL DIAGNOSIS

The main differential diagnosis is infection caused by bacteria, viruses, or fungi. The clinical and radiologic features are very similar to those of rejection. Microbiologic cultures and TBB are most useful. Special stains including immunohistochemistry (IHC) for CMV, Gomori methenamine silver (GMS) stain for fungus and *Pneumocystis jiroveci*, and Ziehl-Neelsen stain for acid-fast bacteria (AFB) should be performed as indicated.

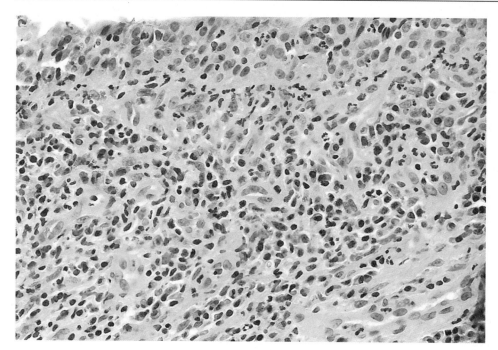

FIGURE 24-8

High-grade lymphocytic bronchiolitis
There is a moderate mixed inflammatory infiltrate in the bronchiolar submucosa, extending into the overlying
epithelium (grade B2R).

PROGNOSIS AND THERAPY

Asymptomatic minimal rejection is usually not treated.
Mild (grade A2) and higher grades of acute rejection are
treated irrespective of symptoms. Most acute rejection
episodes are effectively treated by increasing the immunosuppression (typically 3 boluses of prednisone). Persistent or repeated episodes need more aggressive therapy, which carries additional risk of infection; however,
this treatment is needed since these patients are at high
risk of developing chronic rejection.

CHRONIC REJECTION

In the lung, chronic rejection is primarily manifested as
bronchiolitis obliterans (BO).

Despite improved baseline immunosuppression and
treatment of acute rejection, BO remains the most important cause of late graft failure. Although its etiology
and pathogenesis are still not completely understood,
acute rejection certainly is one of the most important
risk factors. In general, the process of chronic rejection
is believed to occur in stages. The initial wave of
antibody-mediated response is paralleled by a cellular
infiltrate in which the monocyte/macrophage compartment plays a central role. The high antigenicity of airway epithelial cells through the up-regulated expression
of MHC, adhesion, and co-stimulatory molecules, together with the abundance of antigen-presenting cells
and circulating lymphocytes, provides an increased
propensity to damage of these structures, similar to
epithelial-lined conduits in other solid allografts (e.g.,
bile ducts, pancreatic ducts, and renal tubules). The
inflammatory mediators and growth factors produced
contribute to the fibroproliferative response of the damaged graft leading to BO.

CLINICAL FEATURES

Although the term chronic implies a late temporal process, BO can be seen as early as 3 to 6 weeks after transplantation, but primarily occurs 1 or more years later.
The onset of chronic rejection is insidious, with vague
general symptoms and nonproductive cough. There is
progressive dyspnea on exertion and irreversible decline
in pulmonary function tests not explained by other

LUNG ALLOGRAFT REJECTION—FACT SHEET

Definition

» Immune response to donor antigens in the allograft, classified according to pathogenesis and not time: hyperacute rejection is primarily humoral, acute rejection is primarily cellular, and chronic rejection is a fibrosing process

Incidence

» Hyperacute rejection is very rare and involves alveolated lung parenchyma
» 80-90% of recipients experience one or more acute rejection episodes, which involve small blood vessels and airways
» Chronic rejection develops in 50% of 3- to 5-year survivors and predominantly involves small airways

Clinical Features

» Low-grade fever, cough, and dyspnea with variable decline in pulmonary function tests

Radiologic Features

» Patchy opacities in hyperacute and acute rejection, bronchiolar wall thickening and eventually proximal bronchiectasis in chronic airway rejection

Prognosis and Therapy

» Hyperacute rejection has high mortality
» Acute rejection resolves in 80-90% with augmented immunosuppression (the remainder have repeated or persistent acute rejection)
» Chronic airway rejection leads to permanent dysfunction of the graft and is the major cause of death after 6 months post-transplantation

LUNG ALLOGRAFT REJECTION—PATHOLOGIC FEATURES

Gross Findings

» Hyperacute rejection: hyperemic and heavy lungs
» Acute rejection: unknown
» Chronic rejection: large airways with bronchiectasis; patchy consolidation, hyperinflation, and variable fibrosis of lung parenchyma

Microscopic Findings

» Hyperacute: alveolar hemorrhage, interstitial neutrophilia, diffuse alveolar damage, vasculitis
» Acute: inflammatory infiltration around blood vessels and in the bronchiolar submucosa
   » Minimal acute rejection: 2 to 3 layers of perivascular lymphocytes
   » Mild acute rejection: more than 3 layers of perivascular lymphocytes (some activated), plasma cells, eosinophils, and few neutrophils
   » Moderate acute rejection: extension of perivascular inflammatory infiltrates into adjacent alveolar septa
   » Severe acute rejection: diffuse predominantly mononuclear inflammatory cell infiltrates with hemorrhage, hyaline membranes, necrosis
» Lymphocytic bronchiolitis also represents rejection in some cases
   » Low-grade: predominantly lymphocytic infiltrates in the bronchiolar submucosa without epithelial injury
   » High-grade: predominantly lymphocytic infiltrates in the bronchiolar submucosa with epithelial injury and sometimes ulceration
» Chronic
   » Bronchiolitis obliterans (BO): patchy submucosal fibrosis resulting in partial or complete occlusion of bronchiolar lumen, with or without inflammatory infiltrates
   » Vascular: intimal fibrosis and thickening of small blood vessels

Pathologic Differential Diagnosis

» Hyperacute rejection:
   » Ischemia-reperfusion injury
   » Donor-transmitted infections
» Acute rejection:
   » Infections (bacterial, viral, or fungal)
   » Periphery of post-transplant lymphoproliferative disorder lesion
» Chronic rejection:
   » Nonspecific large airway fibrosis
» Organizing pneumonia

causes such as infection. When the decline is greater than 10% of baseline, a clinical diagnosis of bronchiolitis obliterans syndrome (BOS) is made, which does not need pathologic confirmation. BOS is graded from 1-3 based on the degree of loss of lung function. When the clinical diagnosis is not clear, a wedge biopsy is often needed, since BO is a patchy process and diagnostic yield of TBB is low.

RADIOLOGIC FEATURES

Radiology is typically non-contributory until later in the disease, when distal airway obstruction results in proximal bronchiectasis. Irregular areas of hyperinflation and consolidation may be present.

PATHOLOGIC FEATURES

GROSS FINDINGS

Early BO produces no gross changes. Progressive obstruction of small airways leads to thickening of airway walls, adjacent atelectasis and consolidation, and eventually dilatation (bronchiectasis) of proximal larger airways (Figure 24-9).

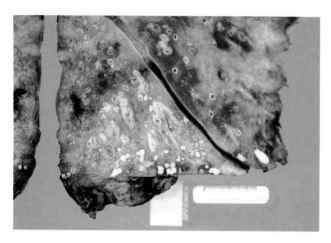

FIGURE 24-9

Chronic rejection

Gross photograph of previously transplanted lung, resected for re-transplantation, in a patient with chronic rejection manifested here as bronchiectasis, which can occur proximal to bronchiolitis obliterans. In addition, there is barium aspiration, seen as white patches at the base of the lung.

MICROSCOPIC FINDINGS

BO is patchy both in distribution and severity in individual lobes and in the same airway. There is submucosal fibrosis, which either bulges asymmetrically into the lumen and causes partial obstruction or is concentric and causes total obstruction. The histological grading of BO takes into account only the presence or absence of the lesion. Inflammation can be present (Figure 24-10A) or absent (Figure 24-10B). Secondary changes often seen are mucostasis, post-obstructive endogenous lipoid pneumonia, and foci of acute inflammation. Rarely, there can be extensive fibrosis of the entire lung, presumably due to complete atelectasis and scarring. Chronic vascular rejection (Figure 24-11) occurs much less frequently and is histologically similar to the transplant vasculopathy seen in other solid organ allografts (intimal fibrosis and vascular thickening); however, in the lung it does not usually cause significant allograft dysfunction.

DIFFERENTIAL DIAGNOSIS

The main histologic differential diagnosis is organizing pneumonia (formerly known as bronchiolitis obliterans organizing pneumonia, or BOOP), which is a healing response to various forms of lung injury and manifests as loose fibromyxoid plugs of connective tissue within alveoli and bronchioles. On the other hand, BO is dense scar tissue (mature collagen) within small airways. Masson trichrome stain is helpful for distinguishing between BO

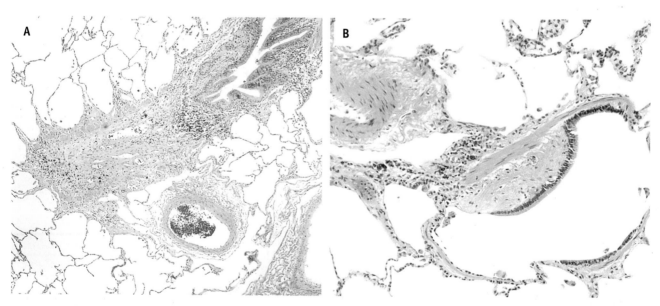

FIGURE 24-10

Chronic airway rejection (bronchiolitis obliterans)

(A) Very low-power photomicrograph of total BO seen in the middle of the picture, which is continuous with a less-involved part of the airway in the upper right. The airway smooth muscle is of approximately equal thickness all around, indicating that this is not tangential sectioning. In addition to the fibrosis, there is an inflammatory infiltrate. (B) Medium power photomicrograph of subtotal bronchiolitis obliterans (BO), with asymmetric submucosal fibrosis bulging into the bronchiolar lumen, without a cellular infiltrate.

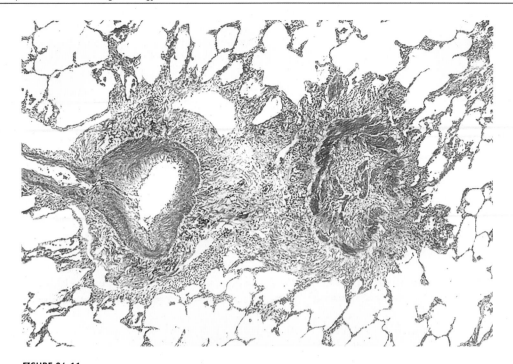

FIGURE 24-11

Chronic airway and chronic vascular rejection
Low-power photomicrograph of Masson trichrome stain, showing both BO (right) and chronic vascular rejection (left) with intimal fibrosis and medial thickening (grade C1 and D).

and organizing pneumonia. Large airway fibrosis is non-specific and should not be interpreted as BO.

PROGNOSIS AND THERAPY

Once there has been a decrease in lung function due to BO, it cannot be reversed, but aggressive immunosuppression can stabilize the disease for variable periods of time. Some patients can live with BO for a few years, but others have progressive dysfunction and complications, and die unless re-transplanted.

INFECTIONS

Like any immunocompromised patient, lung transplant recipients are at high risk of developing infections, which can be bacterial, viral, or fungal, and may cause tracheobronchitis, localized infection of the airway anastomosis, or pneumonia.

CLINICAL FEATURES

Patients present with one or more of the following: fever, cough, sputum production (often purulent in bacterial infections), dyspnea, hypoxemia, leukocytosis, and decline in spirometry. Most bacterial infections occur in the first post-transplant month, whereas viral and fungal infections tend to be seen in the 3- to 6-month period. Lung transplant patients remain susceptible to infections, since they are on immunosuppressive drugs, for the rest of their lives. Patients with BO are particularly vulnerable to development of chronic airway infections.

RADIOLOGIC FEATURES

In bacterial and fungal pneumonia, there are new or increasing patchy infiltrates, consolidation, and often pleural effusion. In viral pneumonia, there is a broad range of appearances from mild or no radiologic findings to the diffuse bilateral infiltrates of diffuse alveolar damage (DAD).

PATHOLOGIC FEATURES

GROSS FINDINGS

The airway mucosa is red, hyperemic, and boggy. Its lumen may contain mucopurulent material. Bulging granulation tissue may be present at the anastomotic site with or without mucosal ulceration. Areas of pneumonia can be identified by consolidation. Fungal pneumonia is often hemorrhagic. If DAD is present, the lungs may be dense and hyperemic, with prominent alveolar septa.

MICROSCOPIC FINDINGS

These depend on the etiology of the infection and the host response, which may be minimal. Bacterial infections usually elicit neutrophilic infiltration of airways, interstitium, and alveolar spaces. Occasionally, there is only bacterial growth and infarction with no inflammation (Figure 24-12). The most common viral infection is caused by CMV, which often infects endothelial cells and pneumocytes. This may lead to bleeding complications after diagnostic TBB (Figure 24-13). CMV is diagnosed by finding the classical single intranuclear and multiple small cytoplasmic inclusions in an enlarged cell (Figure 24-14A). Treated patients often have smudged, eosinophilic inclusions which may be difficult to identify as CMV (Figure 24-14B). Adenovirus infection is

more common in children, and scattered adult and pediatric patients develop serious pneumonias due to the other respiratory viruses (e.g., respiratory syncytial virus, parainfluenza, influenza). Fungal infections are often caused by *Aspergillus* or *Candida* sp. *Pneumocystis* pneumonia is rare due to routine prophylaxis.

ANCILLARY STUDIES

MICROBIOLOGIC CULTURES

In the symptomatic patient, culture of BAL fluid can be very helpful in identifying microbiologic organisms. Whether one or more of the agents isolated is actually the cause of a patient's disease process can only be determined by careful clinical and pathologic correlation.

SPECIAL STAINS

As indicated by clinical or biopsy findings, special stains for organisms should be performed. Many centers do GMS and AFB stains on all post-transplant biopsies.

IMMUNOHISTOCHEMISTRY

In the very early stage of CMV infection, IHC staining against immediate-early antigen may demonstrate nuclear positivity in cells lacking diagnostic cytopathic

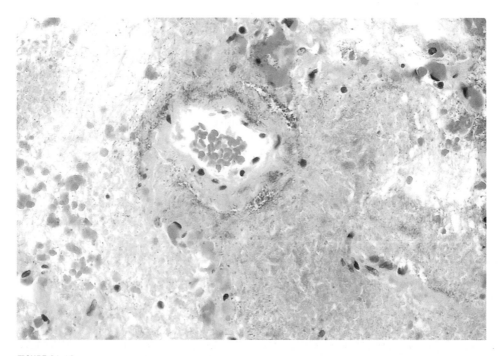

FIGURE 24-12

Bacterial pneumonia

High-power photomicrograph of lung at autopsy in a patient who died of bacterial pneumonia and sepsis 5 days post-transplant. Note bacterial colonies surrounding a blood vessel, infarction of adjacent lung, fibrinous exudate, and lack of inflammatory cells.

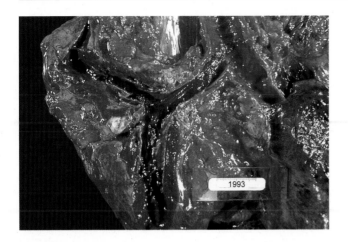

FIGURE 24-13

Cytomegalovirus pneumonia
Gross photograph of lung from a patient with CMV pneumonitis who developed massive bronchial hemorrhage after undergoing TBB (this patient had numerous CMV inclusions in endothelial cells of submucosal blood vessels).

changes. IHC is also very useful for confirming the diagnosis in patients already on treatment for CMV.

DIFFERENTIAL DIAGNOSIS

The main differential diagnosis is from acute rejection, since the symptoms are similar. Culture, biopsy, and special stains are often diagnostic.

PROGNOSIS AND THERAPY

Infection may precipitate rejection and vice versa. Infections can be very difficult to treat, with new resistant strains emerging in some patients. Prophylaxis plays an important role in preventing *Pneumocystis* and CMV pneumonias.

OTHER FORMS OF LUNG INJURY

DAD, organizing pneumonia, and interstitial fibrosis may all be seen as nonspecific responses to lung injury in the post-transplant patient. The etiologies of these responses are diverse. Alveolar proteinosis is another rare complication of transplantation.

RECURRENT DISEASES

Up to 80% of patients transplanted for sarcoidosis develop granulomas without clinical disease. Other recurrent diseases include lymphangioleiomyomatosis, bronchioloalveolar carcinoma, alveolar proteinosis, desquamative interstitial pneumonia, giant cell interstitial pneumonia, Langerhans cell histiocytosis,

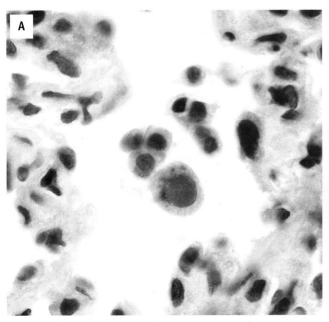
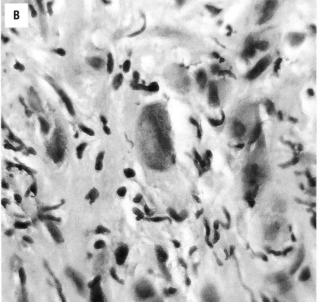

FIGURE 24-14

Cytomegalovirus pneumonia
High-power photomicrographs of **(A)** diagnostic CMV inclusions in an alveolar cell, and **(B)** post-therapy CMV inclusion showing smudging and eosinophilia.

diffuse panbronchiolitis, and idiopathic pulmonary hemosiderosis.

POST-TRANSPLANT LYMPHOPROLIFERATIVE DISORDERS

Post-transplant lymphoproliferative disorders (PTLDs) occur in 3-5% of lung transplant recipients with frequent involvement of the allograft, often as one or multiple nodules (Figure 24-15). A high index of suspicion should be maintained, and the diagnosis can be suggested on FNAB and TBB. Particularly with low-grade lesions, the need to obtain adequate tissue for complete work-up may require wedge biopsy. The histologic and molecular features are similar to those seen in any other transplant patient, as discussed in chapter 22.

PULMONARY INFECTIOUS COMPLICATIONS OF ORGAN AND BONE MARROW TRANSPLANTATION

The lung is a very common site of infection in solid organ and bone marrow transplant recipients. The spectrum of organisms and patterns of infection is generally similar to lung transplant recipients, as described above.

GRAFT-VERSUS-HOST DISEASE IN LUNG

Graft-versus-host disease (GVHD) is analogous to lung transplant rejection, since in both scenarios it is one person's bone marrow (immune competent cells) reacting to the antigens present in abundance in another person's lung.

CLINICAL FEATURES

Acute GVHD presents with low-grade fever, cough, and shortness of breath. Patients who develop chronic GVHD have progressive signs and symptoms of airway obstruction, which may be complicated by superimposed infection.

PATHOLOGIC FEATURES

MICROSCOPIC FINDINGS

In acute GVHD, there are perivascular inflammatory infiltrates (Figure 24-16) as well as airway inflammation. These can be graded from minimal to severe, similar to acute rejection grading. Bronchiolitis obliterans is the main manifestation of chronic GVHD (Figure 24-17).

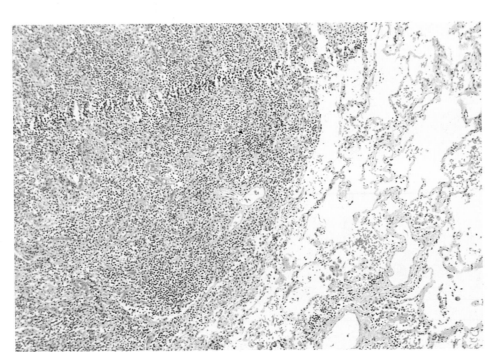

FIGURE 24-15
Post-transplant lymphoproliferative disorder
A nodular infiltrate is seen in the lung parenchyma.

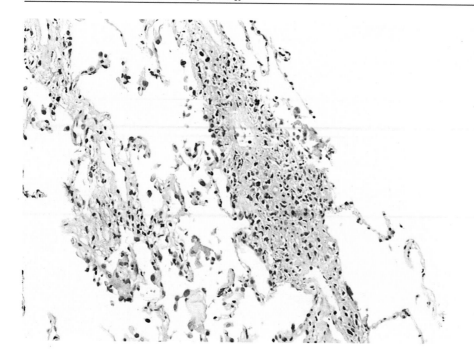

FIGURE 24-16

Acute graft-versus-host disease
The lung shows a perivascular mononuclear infiltrate in a patient with acute GVHD.

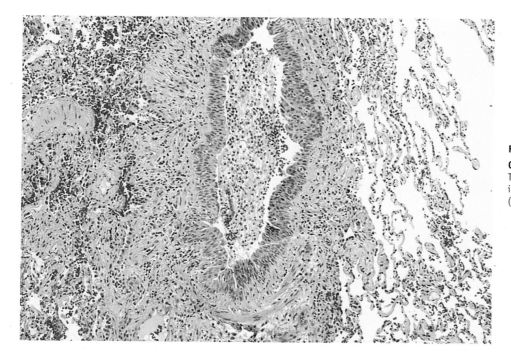

FIGURE 24-17

Chronic graft-verses-host disease
This airway shows mononuclear cell infiltrates and submucosal fibrosis (BO) in a patient with chronic GVHD.

DIFFERENTIAL DIAGNOSIS

As in lung allograft rejection, infection is the main differential diagnosis. Cultures and special stains should be performed as indicated above.

SUGGESTED READINGS

Complications of Lung Transplantation

1. Husain AN, Gaweco AS. Pathology of pulmonary allograft dysfunction. In: Norman DJ, Turka LA, eds. *Primer on Transplantation*. 2nd ed. New Jersey: American Society of Transplantation; 2001:696-704.

2. Khoor A, Yousem SA. Pathology of lung transplantation. In: Leslie KO, Wick MR, eds. *Practical Pulmonary Pathology: A Diagnostic Approach.* Philadelphia: Churchill Livingstone; 2005:401-22.

3. Lau CL, Patterson GA. Current status of lung transplantation. *Eur Respir J.* 2003;47:57s-64s.

4. Trulock EP, Christie JD, Edwards LB, et al. Registry of the International Society for Heart and Lung Transplantation: twenty-fourth official adult lung and heart-lung transplant report—2007. *J Heart Lung Transplant.* 2007;26:782-95.

Rejection

5. Colombat M, Groussard O, Lautrette A, et al. Analysis of the different histologic lesions observed in transbronchial biopsy for the diagnosis of acute rejection: clinicopathologic correlations during the first 6 months after lung transplantation. *Hum Pathol.* 2005;36:387-94.

6. Faro A, Visner G. The use of multiple transbronchial biopsies as the standard approach to evaluate lung allograft rejection. *Pediatr Transplant.* 2004;8:322-8.

7. Hopkins PM, Aboyoun CL, Chhajed PN, et al. Association of minimal rejection in lung transplant recipients with obliterative bronchiolitis. *Am J Respir Crit Care Med.* 2004;170:1022-6.

8. Slebos DJ, Postma DS, Koeter GH, Van Der Bij W, Boezen M, Kauffman HF. Bronchoalveolar lavage fluid characteristics in acute and chronic lung transplant rejection. *J Heart Lung Transplant.* 2004;23:532-40.

9. Stephenson A, Flint J, English J, et al. Interpretation of transbronchial lung biopsies from lung transplant recipients: inter- and intraobserver agreement. *Can Respir J.* 2005;2:75-7.

10. Stewart S, Fishbein MC, Snell GI, et al. Revision of the 1996 working formulation for the standardization of nomenclature in the diagnosis of lung rejection. *J Heart Lung Transplant.* 2007;26:1229-42.

11. Yousem SA, Berry GJ, Cagle PT, et al. Revision of the 1990 working formulation for the classification of pulmonary allograft rejection. Lung Rejection Study Group. *J Heart Lung Transplant.* 1996;15:1-15.

Hyperacute Rejection

12. Magro CM, Klinger DM, Adams PW, et al. Evidence that humoral allograft rejection in lung transplant patients is not histocompatibility antigen-related. *Am J Transplant.* 2003;3:1264-72.

13. Magro CM, Pope-Harman A, Klinger D, et al. Use of C4d as a diagnostic adjunct in lung allograft biopsies. *Am J Transplant.* 2003;3:1143-54.

14. Magro CM, Ross P Jr, Kelsey M, Waldman WJ, Pope-Harman A. Association of humoral immunity and bronchiolitis obliterans syndrome. *Am J Transplant.* 2003;3:1155-66.

15. Michaels PJ, Fishbein MC, Colvin RB. Humoral rejection of human organ transplants. *Springer Semin Immunopathol.* 2003;25:119-40.

16. Miller GG, Destarac L, Zeevi A, et al. Acute humoral rejection of human lung allografts and elevation of C4d in bronchoalveolar lavage fluid. *Am J Transplant.* 2004;4:1323-30.

17. Scornik JC, Zander DS, Baz MA, Donnelly W, Staples ED. Susceptibility of lung transplants to preformed donor-specific HLA antibodies as detected by flow cytometry. *Transplantation.* 1999;68:1542-46.

Acute Rejection

18. Bittmann I, Muller C, Behr J, Groetzner J, Frey L, Lohrs U. Fas/FasL and perforin/ganzyme pathway in acute rejection and diffuse alveolar damage after allogeneic lung transplantation: a human biopsy study. *Virchows Arch.* 2004;445:375-81.

19. Chakinala MM, Ritter J, Gage BF, et al. Yield of surveillance bronchoscopy for acute rejection and lymphocytic bronchitis/bronchiolitis after lung transplantation. *J Heart Lung Transplant.* 2004;23:1396-404.

Chronic Rejection

20. Bowdish ME, Arcasoy SM, Wilt JS, et al. Surrogate markers and risk factors for chronic lung allograft dysfunction. *Am J Transplant.* 2004;4:1171-78.

21. Chalermskulrat W, Neuringer IP, Schmitz JL, et al. Human leukocyte antigen mismatches predispose to the severity of bronchiolitis obliterans syndrome in lung transplantation. *Chest.* 2003;123:1824-31.

22. Chan A, Allen R. Bronchiolitis obliterans: an update. *Curr Opin Pulm Med.* 2004;10:133-41.

23. Luckraz H, Goddard M, McNeil K, et al. Microvascular changes in small airways predispose to obliterative bronchiolitis after lung transplantation. *J Heart Lung Transplant.* 2004;23:527-31.

24. Ward C, De Soyza A, Fisher AJ, Pritchard G, Forrest IA, Corris PA. Reticular basement membrane thickening in airways of lung transplant recipients is not affected by inhaled corticosteroids. *Clin Exp Allergy.* 2004;34:1905-9.

Infections

25. Chan KM, Allen SA. Infectious pulmonary complications in lung transplant recipients. *Semin Respir Infect.* 2002;17:291-302.

26. Chemaly RF, Yen-Lieberman B, Castilla EA, et al. Correlation between viral loads of cytomegalovirus in blood and bronchoalveolar lavage specimens from lung transplant recipients determined by histology and immunohistochemistry. *J Clin Microbiol.* 2004;42:2168-72.

27. Kubak BM. Fungal infection in lung transplantation. *Transpl Infect Dis.* 2002;3:24-31.

28. Nunley DR, Gal AA, Vega JD, Perlino C, Smith P, Lawrence EC. Saprophytic fungal infections and complications involving the bronchial anastomosis following human lung transplantation. *Chest.* 2002;122:1185-91.

29. Stewart S. Pulmonary infections in transplatation pathology. *Arch Pathol Lab Med.* 2007;131:1219-31.

30. Westall GP, Michaelides A, Williams TJ, Snell GI, Kotsimbos TC. Human cytomegalovirus load in plasma and bronchoalveolar lavage fluid: a longitudinal study of lung transplant recipients. *J Infect Dis.* 2004;190:1076-83.

31. Zamora MR. Cytomegalovirus and lung transplantation. *Am J Transplant.* 2004;4:1219-26.

Post-Transplant Lymphoproliferative Disorders

32. Harris NL, Swerdlow SH, Frizzera G, et al. Post-transplant lymphoproliferative disorders. In: *Pathology and Genetic of Tumours of Hematopoietic ond Lymphoid Tissue.* Lyon: IARC Press; 2001:264-9.

Pulmonary Infectious Complications of Organ and Bone Marrow Transplantation

33. Kotloff RM, Vivek N, Crawford SW. Pulmonary complications of solid organ and hematopoietic stem cell transplantation. *Am J Respir Crit Care Med.* 2004;170:22-48.

34. Stewart S. Pulmonary infections in transplantation pathology. *Arch Pathol Lab Med.* 2007;131:1219-31.

Graft-Versus-Host Disease in Lung

35. Cooke KR, Yanik G. Acute lung injury after allogeneic stem cell transplantation: is the lung a target of acute graft-versus-host disease? *Bone Marrow Transplant.* 2004;34:753-65.

36. Eikenberry M, Bartakova H, Defor T, et al. Natural history of pulmonary complications in children after bone marrow transplantation. *Biol Blood Marrow Transplant.* 2005;11:56-64.

37. Luckraz H, Zagolin M, McNeil K, Wallwork J. Graft-versus-host disease in lung transplantation: 4 case reports and literature review. *J Heart Lung Transplant.* 2003;22:691-7.

38. Nusair S, Breuer R, Shapira MY, Berkman N, Or R. Low incidence of pulmonary complications following nonmyeloablative stem cell transplantation. *Eur Respir J.* 2004;23:440-5.

39. Sakaida E, Nakaseko C, Harima A, et al. Late-onset noninfectious pulmonary complications after allogeneic stem cell transplantation are significantly associated with chronic graft-versus-host disease and with the graft-versus-leukemia effect. *Blood.* 2003;102:4236-42.

40. Wang JY, Chang YL, Lee LN, et al. Diffuse pulmonary infiltrates after bone marrow transplantation: the role of open lung biopsy. *Ann Thorac Surg.* 2004;78:267-72.

41. Wysocki CA, Panoskaltsis-Mortari A, Blazar BR, Serody JS. Leukocyte migration and graft-versus-host disease. *Blood.* 2005;105:4191-9.

42. Yen KT, Lee AS, Krowka MJ, Burger CD. Pulmonary complications in bone marrow transplantation: a practical approach to diagnosis and treatment. *Clin Chest Med.* 2004;25:189-201.

25

Other Non-Neoplastic Focal Lesions, Pseudotumors, Inclusions, and Depositions

Carol F. Farver

- Introduction
- Inflammatory Pseudotumors
- Lipoid Pneumonia
- Amyloidosis
- Pulmonary Hyalinizing Granuloma
- Minute Meningothelial-Like Lesion
- Dendriform Ossification
- Metastatic Interstitial Calcification
- Pulmonary Alveolar Microlithiasis

INTRODUCTION

This chapter addresses a variety of lung lesions that have little in common. They represent repair reactions, inclusions, deposition disorders, and masses of uncertain etiology (pseudotumors). They may present as single or multiple lesions or as infiltrative lesions. They are presented in this chapter because they do not fit well into the topics of other chapters, yet they are important to be aware of as one constructs differential diagnoses.

INFLAMMATORY PSEUDOTUMORS

Inflammatory pseudotumors (IPTs) of the lung are a group of mass-like lesions with predominantly fibroblasts and/or myofibroblasts and a combination of chronic inflammatory components including plasma cells, lymphocytes, giant cells, or foamy histiocytes. These lesions may be subdivided based on the predominant cell type, giving rise to the variety of names ascribed to them in the literature including histiocytoma, plasma cell granuloma, xanthoma, xanthogranuloma, xanthofibroma, and inflammatory myofibroblastic tumor. Although little is known regarding the pathogenesis of these lesions, it is thought that most of them may represent exaggerated tissue responses to injury. However,

some, such as the inflammatory myofibroblastic tumor found in children (chapter 6), behave more similarly to neoplasms than post-inflammatory processes. Given the confusing nomenclature and the lack of definitive evidence regarding the pathogenesis of this group of lesions, it may be best to use the term "inflammatory pseudotumor," except for the inflammatory myofibroblastic tumor in children.

CLINICAL FEATURES

IPTs occur in the lungs of people of all ages, though most are found before the age of 40, and they are the most common benign lung lesion in children. These masses are usually asymptomatic, found as incidental abnormalities on imaging studies. Patients who do present with symptoms may have a cough, chest pain, or, if the lesion is quite large, airway obstruction or dysphagia.

RADIOLOGIC FEATURES

IPTs can mimic neoplasms radiologically, usually appearing as well-defined solitary parenchymal masses, though multiple masses are seen in about 5% of cases. Cavitation or calcification is rare, but has been reported. The right lung is more commonly affected, and the size can vary from 0.5 to 36 cm. Endobronchial lesions may occur and, when present, have a broad-based polypoid configuration.

PATHOLOGIC FEATURES

GROSS FINDINGS

These lesions are not encapsulated, commonly invade into the pleura, and may extend into adjacent mediastinal structures. They commonly have a firm, white, shiny gross appearance due to the abundance of fibrous tissue present in the lesion. However, as the number of histiocytes or xanthomatous cells increases, the color becomes more yellow due to the lipid accumulation. Hemorrhagic foci may be present, causing areas of red or brown.

MICROSCOPIC FINDINGS

Microscopic appearances vary with the predominant cell type present. When spindle cells predominate, the histologic picture is one of short fascicles of myofibroblasts, sometimes with a storiform pattern with scattered lymphocytes, foamy histiocytes, and plasma cells. Multinucleated giant cells are characteristic of this variant, which is referred to as the fibrohistiocytic variant of IPT (Figure 25-1). Plasma cells predominate in the so-called plasma cell granuloma variant (Figure 25-2). These cells infiltrate among the myofibroblasts with lymphocytes and foamy histiocytes. Scattered eosinophils may be present in both variants of IPT. Finally, some IPTs consist predominantly of fibrosis and probably represent later stage sequelae of one of the other variants. In these lesions, dense collagenous-type fibrosis is present with only scattered chronic inflammatory cells.

Organizing pneumonias may present as mass-like lesions and are sometimes referred to as inflammatory pseudotumors, organizing pneumonia type. This may be an appropriate term if tissue destruction and fibrosis has occurred in the midst of the organization.

ANCILLARY STUDIES

ULTRASTRUCTURAL EXAMINATION

Ultrastructural examination of IPTs reveals the myofibroblastic or fibroblastic origins of the spindle cell population. Actin filaments may be seen in some spindle cells. The absence of intercellular junctions argues against an epithelial lesion such as a sarcomatoid carcinoma.

IMMUNOHISTOCHEMISTRY

In IPTs with a predominance of inflammatory cells, immunohistochemical studies of T and B-cell antigens and kappa and lambda light chains may help to distinguish these lesions from lymphomas by showing a lack of kappa or lambda light chain restriction. IPTs with predominant spindle cell morphology should be distinguished from sarcomatoid carcinomas. Fibroblasts and myofibroblasts of IPTs are immunoreactive to vimentin and actin and may be focally immunoreactive to desmin, but are not immunoreactive epithelial markers, such as cytokeratins, which are usually expressed by sarcomatoid carcinomas.

MOLECULAR DIAGNOSTICS

Molecular diagnostic tests may be useful in distinguishing the plasma cell granuloma type lesions from low-grade lymphomas such as marginal zone lymphomas (lymphomas of the BALT tissue) and plasmacytomas. Immunoglobulin gene rearrangements are found in plasma cell dyscrasias and most BALT-type lymphomas (chapter 22).

DIFFERENTIAL DIAGNOSIS

The differential diagnosis for IPTs of the lung differs for each variant. For the fibrohistiocytic variant, the major differential diagnosis is a sarcoma primary to the lung or a metastasis from an extrapulmonary sarcoma. Malignant fibrous histiocytomas can take origin in the lung or may present as metastases to the lung and may have overlapping morphologic features with IPTs. Histologic features that are common to MFHs and argue against IPT include high mitotic rate (greater than 3 mitoses/50 high-power fields), high-grade nuclei, and necrosis. Also, biologically aggressive behavior such as invasion into adjacent cartilage, bone, or blood vessels is more consistent with a sarcoma.

Other spindle cell lesions that may mimic this variant of IPT include sarcomatoid carcinomas, differentiated with the use of epithelial markers as described above, and inflammatory reactions to some infections. Bacteria such as non-tuberculous mycobacteria and *Actinomyces* are known to cause IPT-like reactions. Special organismal stains should always be performed on these lesions to rule out an infectious etiology.

The main differential diagnosis of a plasma cell granuloma variant of IPT is a low-grade lymphoma of BALT (marginal zone lymphoma) or a plasmacytoma. As described above, lymphomas and plasma cell dyscrasias show clonality both by immunohistochemistry and molecular studies. In addition, they usually lack the spindle cell component and giant cells that can be seen in IPTs.

PROGNOSIS AND THERAPY

IPTs are treated with complete surgical resection. The extent of the resection is controversial. Local excisions including wedge resection and segmentectomies are advocated by most, although some surgeons recommend more extensive excisions including lobectomies and pneumonectomies. After complete resection, recurrence is rare. Survival after surgery is estimated at 80-100% at 5 years, depending upon the study. Intrathoracic recurrence ranges from 5-10%, usually in the setting of an incomplete resection.

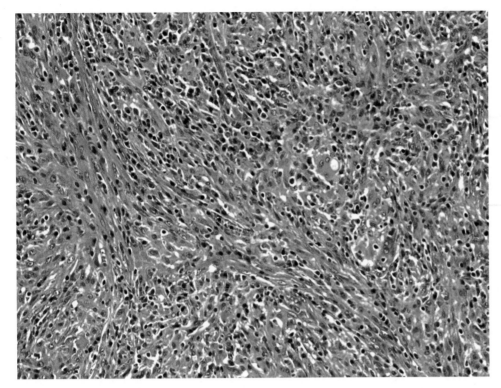

FIGURE 25-1

Inflammatory pseudotumor, fibrohis-tiocytic variant
The histologic picture includes short fascicles of myofibroblasts, sometimes with a storiform pattern, with scattered lymphocytes, plasma cells, and foamy histiocytes. Multinucleated giant cells are characteristic of this variant.

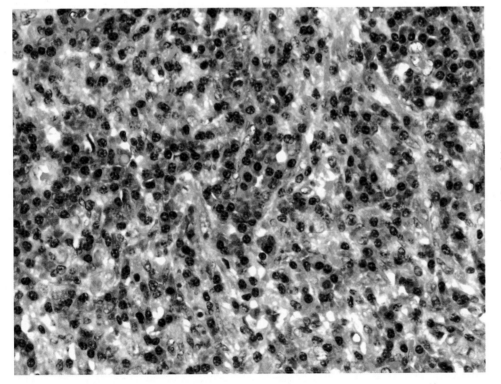

FIGURE 25-2

Inflammatory pseudotumor, plasma cell granuloma variant
Plasma cells predominate in the so-called plasma cell granuloma variant. These infiltrate among the myofibro-blasts with lymphocytes and foamy histiocytes. Scattered eosinophils may be present.

INFLAMMATORY PSEUDOTUMORS—FACT SHEET

Definition

» Mass-like lesions with fibroblasts and chronic inflammatory components including plasma cells, lymphocytes, giant cells, and foamy histiocytes

Incidence

» Uncommon

Mortality

» Survival after surgery is estimated at 80–100% at 5 years

Age Distribution

» Occur at all ages, although most are found before the age of 40 years
» Most common benign lung lesion in children

Clinical Features

» Predominantly asymptomatic; if symptoms are present, these include cough, chest pain, or with large lesions, airway obstruction or dysphagia

Radiologic Features

» Well defined, solitary parenchymal mass
» Multiple masses in 5% of cases
» Right side is more commonly affected

Prognosis and Therapy

» When treated with complete resection, recurrence of these lesions is rare

INFLAMMATORY PSEUDOTUMORS—PATHOLOGIC FEATURES

Gross Findings

» White, firm, shiny mass, ranging in size from 0.5-36 cm

Microscopic Findings

» Microscopic appearance depends upon the predominant cell type:
  » Plasma cell granuloma variant: plasma cells
  » Fibrohistiocytic variant: myofibroblasts, scattered giant cells and foamy histiocytes
  » Organizing pneumonia variant: organizing fibroblasts with scattered lymphocytes and plasma cells

Ultrastructural Features

» Spindle cell population reveals an origin from myofibroblasts or fibroblasts
» Actin filaments may be present

Immunohistochemical Features

» Polyclonal T- and B-cell populations of lymphocytes
» Spindle cells do not react with epithelial markers such as cytokeratin

Pathologic Differential Diagnosis

» Plasma cell variant: low-grade lymphoma of BALT; plasmacytoma
» Fibrohistiocytic variant: sarcoma (metastatic or primary in the lung); sarcomatoid carcinoma
» Organizing pneumonia variant: resolving bacterial pneumonia

LIPOID PNEUMONIA

Lipoid pneumonia (sometimes referred to as exogenous lipoid pneumonia) is an uncommon condition that results from chronic aspiration of animal, vegetable, or mineral lipid-containing material into the lungs. The macrophages phagocytize the lipid and cause a granuloma-like or fibrotic reaction within the area of aspiration. This produces either a dense infiltrate or mass-like lesion. Post-obstructive pneumonia commonly contains areas of foamy macrophages, a result of mucin plugging and lipid build-up from an obstructing lesion such as a tumor. This is sometimes referred to as endogenous lipoid pneumonia, an entity distinct from exogenous lipoid pneumonia.

CLINICAL FEATURES

Exogenous lipoid pneumonia usually occurs in patients with neuromuscular disorders, esophageal abnormalities such as dysphagias, and anatomic defects such as cleft palates or head and neck neoplasms.

RADIOLOGIC FEATURES

Chest x-rays usually reveal dense air space consolidation or irregular mass-like lesions, most commonly in the dependent portions of the lung. Chest CT scans reveal consolation with fat attenuation or a "crazy-paving" pattern with septal and centrilobular thickening. Traction bronchiectasis and fibrosis may be seen in severe chronic cases.

PATHOLOGIC FEATURES

GROSS FINDINGS

The lesions of lipoid pneumonia have a golden-yellow appearance due to the lipid, and they are solid and firm due to the presence of fibrosis. Superimposed infections, such as non-tuberculous mycobacterial pneumonia, can occur, which may result in cavitation.

MICROSCOPIC FINDINGS

The characteristic microscopic appearance is one of abundant intra-alveolar and interstitial foamy macrophages with variably-sized vacuoles of lipid (Figure 25-3). Giant cells and cholesterol clefts are common. Collagenous fibrosis may occur with reactive type 2 pneumocytes. Necrosis is uncommon unless infections are present.

ANCILLARY STUDIES

ULTRASTRUCTURAL EXAMINATION

Transmission electron microscopy reveals typical whorled bodies of lipid within the foamy macrophages. These consist of lamellated, concentric electron-dense lipid membranes.

FINE NEEDLE ASPIRATION BIOPSY

Large vacuolated macrophages with lipid material are found in fine needle aspirations of lipid pneumonia. Lipid histochemical stains such as Sudan black or oil red O will confirm the lipid nature of the cytoplasmic vacuoles.

DIFFERENTIAL DIAGNOSIS

Endogenous lipoid pneumonia has a similar appearance to exogenous lipoid pneumonia, except that the vacuoles of lipid are smaller and more uniform in size. Spaces representing lipid droplets that were leached out during processing are found in exogenous, but not

endogenous, lipoid pneumonia. Other foamy macrophage-rich lesions may also be considered, including storage diseases, Erdheim-Chester disease, and infections (non-tuberculous mycobacteria, *Rhodococcus equi*, and certain disseminated fungal diseases such as *H. capsulatum*). Clinical information and special stains for organisms are helpful for distinguishing these processes from lipoid pneumonia.

PROGNOSIS AND THERAPY

Therapy for lipoid pneumonia usually involves treatment of the underlying disorder that predisposed the patient to aspiration and treatment of any superimposed infections (bacterial, mycobacterial). The prognosis without infection is excellent. When infections occur, especially from aspirated non-tuberculous mycobacteria that colonize the gastric secretions, cavitary lung disease may occur, requiring surgical resection.

AMYLOIDOSIS

CLINICAL FEATURES

Amyloidosis is a spectrum of diseases in which non-branching linear fibrils of protein are deposited as insoluble fibrils in the extracellular spaces. In the lungs, four general clinical syndromes are recognized: systemic (generalized), localized, diffuse alveolar septal, and pleural.

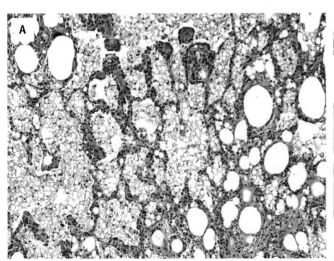
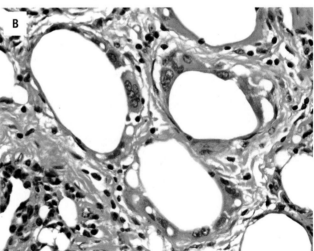

FIGURE 25-3

Lipoid pneumonia
(A) The histologic picture includes abundant intra-alveolar and interstitial foamy macrophages with variably-sized vacuoles of lipid. **(B)** Giant cells form around the lipid vacuoles. Lymphocytes infiltrate the surrounding interstitium, and significant fibrosis may occur.

LIPOID PNEUMONIA—FACT SHEET

Definition

▸▸ Chronic aspiration of animal, vegetable, or mineral lipid-containing material in the lungs producing a granuloma-like and fibrotic reaction

Age Distribution

▸▸ More commonly found in older adults who may take oil or cathartics

Clinical Features

▸▸ Usually occurs in patients with neuromuscular disorders, esophageal abnormalities such as dysphagia, or anatomic defects of the oral cavity and neoplasms of the head and neck

Radiologic Features

▸▸ Dense air space consolidation or irregular mass-like lesions in dependent portion of lungs

Prognosis and Threapy

▸▸ Excellent prognosis; may require surgery if cavitation or infection occur

---

LIPOID PNEUMONIA—PATHOLOGIC FEATURES

Gross Findings

▸▸ Golden-yellow, firm mass-like area
▸▸ Cavitation may occur if infection is present

Microscopic Findings

▸▸ Intra-alveolar and interstitial foamy macrophages with lipid vacuoles
▸▸ Giant cells and cholesterol clefts are common

Ultrastructural Features

▸▸ Lipid (whorled) bodies within macrophages consisting of electron-dense lipid membranes

Fine Needle Aspiration Biopsy Findings

▸▸ Large vacuolated macrophages; Sudan black or oil red O stain confirms the lipid material in the vacuoles

Pathologic Differential Diagnosis

▸▸ Endogenous lipid pneumonia
▸▸ Storage diseases
▸▸ Erdheim-Chester disease
▸▸ Infections: non-tuberculous mycobacteria, *Rhodococcus equi*, *H. capsulatum*

Systemic amyloidosis involves the lung 30-90% of the time, depending upon the series, and consists of primary, secondary, multiple myeloma-associated, and senile types. Primary amyloidosis is that which occurs without known cause and consists of type AL amyloid. Secondary amyloidosis, sometimes referred to as reactive, consists of type AA amyloid and is associated with systemic diseases, most often rheumatoid arthritis, chronic osteomyelitis, and malignancies. Multiple myeloma-associated amyloidosis is type AL, derived from immunoglobulin light chains, and is found in the presence of plasma cell dyscrasias. Senile amyloidosis is mild and occurs most frequently as an incidental finding in patients over the age of 80. Localized amyloidosis to the lungs is rare, but if present, usually takes the form of tracheobronchial amyloidosis (see below). Diffuse alveolar septal amyloidosis and pleural amyloidosis consist of type AL and are forms of amyloidosis limited to the lungs.

Pulmonary amyloidosis can develop at any time during adult life. The clinical presentation of amyloidosis depends upon the form the disease takes. Nodular amyloidosis usually presents as an asymptomatic nodule. When multiple nodules occur, pleuritic chest pain, dyspnea, or hemoptysis may be noted. Diffuse parenchymal amyloidosis usually presents with dyspnea or cough. Tracheobronchial amyloidosis can present with wheezing, atelectasis, or recurrent pneumonia.

as interstitial lung disease with linear or nodular densities. Tracheobronchial amyloidosis may present as airway thickening or collapse or as post-obstructive pneumonia or atelectasis.

PATHOLOGIC FEATURES

GROSS FINDINGS

Pulmonary amyloidosis takes three major forms: tracheobronchial, nodular, and diffuse parenchymal (interstitial, septal, and vascular). Tracheobronchial amyloid is usually a polypoid mass or a raised submucosal plaque (Figure 25-4A) in a major bronchus. Nodular amyloidosis takes the form of firm, waxy, gray or white nodules with well demarcated borders present within the lung parenchyma. These range from a few millimeters to 15 cm in diameter. The gross appearance of diffuse parenchymal amyloidosis has been referred to as a "uniform rubber-sponge-like appearance," which may become brittle or sandy if calcium is present.

MICROSCOPIC FINDINGS

Tracheobronchial amyloidosis presents as amyloid deposits in the submucosa. Multinucleated cells, calcification, chondrification, and ossification are commonly seen (Figure 25-4B). The nodules in nodular amyloidosis often have sharp borders and are present within the

RADIOLOGIC FEATURES

Nodular amyloidosis appears as single or multiple well circumscribed nodules on imaging studies. Cavitation is rare. Diffuse parenchymal amyloidosis usually manifests

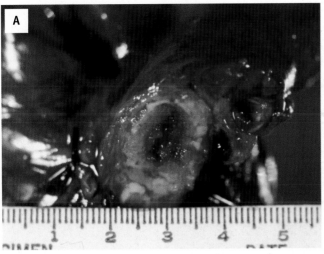

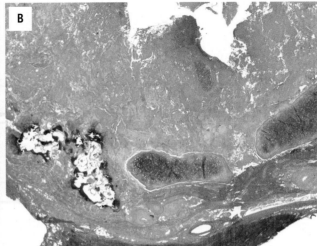

FIGURE 25-4

Tracheobronchial amyloidosis

(A) A cross-section of bronchus involved by amyloidosis has a tan, firm, transmural thickening with a markedly narrowed airway lumen. **(B)** This cross-section of a cartilaginous airway with transmural eosinophilic amyloid deposition has calcification and ossification (lower left).

pulmonary parenchyma as well-circumscribed masses (Figure 25-5). Multinucleated foreign-body-type giant cells are frequently seen "ingesting" amyloid around the edges (Figure 25-6), and plasma cells are usually present in moderate amounts. Calcification and ossification of these nodules is common. Diffuse parenchymal amyloidosis has amyloid deposition in the interstitium and within the vessels (Figure 25-7). Calcium may accompany the amyloid, and an infiltrate of lymphocytes or plasma cells is common. Giant cells are usually not seen in this form of amyloidosis.

Amyloid stains best with Congo red and has a characteristic apple-green birefringence with polarization (Figure 25-8). Amyloid presents a light to medium blue-gray color with Mallory's trichrome stain, in contrast to the more definite deep blue color of collagen. Amyloid also stains metachromatically with crystal or methyl violet, which may be useful as an initial stain for screening purposes.

ANCILLARY STUDIES

ULTRASTRUCTURAL EXAMINATION

Electron microscopy shows a tangled or felt-like mass of very long, tubular nonbranching hollow fibrils 7.5-10 nm (75-100 Å) in diameter, perhaps some 800 nm (8000 Å) long. About 10% of the components consist of a pentagonal substance (P component) that

is glycoprotein and accounts for any periodic acid-Schiff (PAS) staining.

FINE NEEDLE ASPIRATION BIOPSY FINDINGS

FNAB may be helpful in the diagnosis of nodular or tracheobronchial amyloidosis. The presence of homogeneous flocculent eosinophilic material in the aspirated sample should raise the possibility of amyloid, which must be confirmed by Congo red staining. Plasma cells, lymphocytes, and giant cells may be present, as well as deposits of calcium.

IMMUNOHISTOCHEMISTRY

Antibodies to the common types of amyloid proteins are available to biochemically type the amyloid deposited in the tissue. Antibodies for AA, Aκ, Aλ, ATTR and Aβ2M have been used to subtype the amyloid fibril proteins present, but may be less sensitive than Congo red staining with examination under polarized light.

BIOCHEMICAL ANALYSIS

Amyloid can be classified by the biochemical composition of its fibrils. The four most common types are: protein AL (amyloid light chain), derived from plasma cells and of immunoglobulin origin, usually representing the variable N-terminal end of light chains; protein AA (amyloid-associated), a unique N-terminal sequence

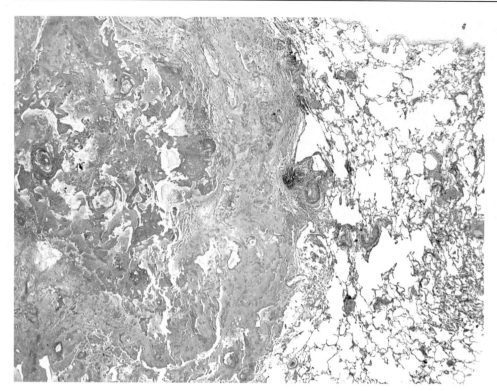

FIGURE 25-5

Nodular amyloidosis
This dense, congophilic amyloid nodule has a well circumscribed margin with adjacent normal alveoli (Congo red).

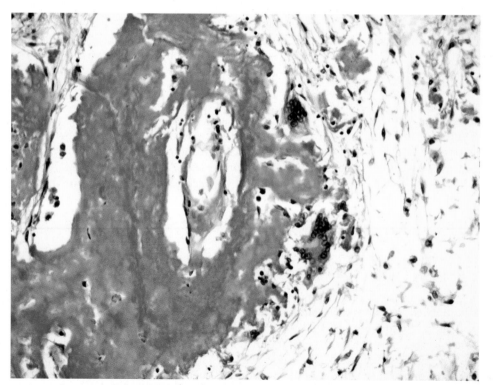

FIGURE 25-6

Nodular amyloidosis
Congophilic amyloid material may have a rim of giant cells that appear to be "ingesting" the amyloid material. Inflammatory cells, including lymphocytes and plasma cells, may be seen within and surrounding the amyloid deposits (Congo red).

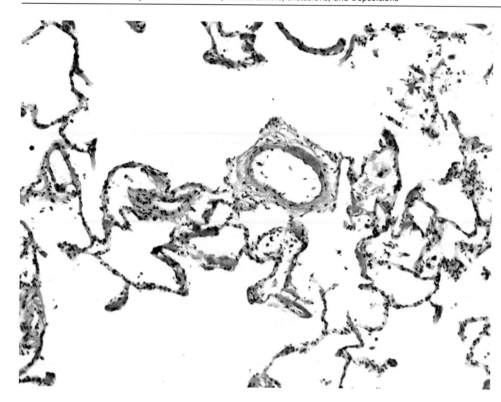

FIGURE 25-7
Diffuse parenchymal amyloidosis
Congophilic amyloid deposition is present in alveolar walls and adjacent vessels (Congo red).

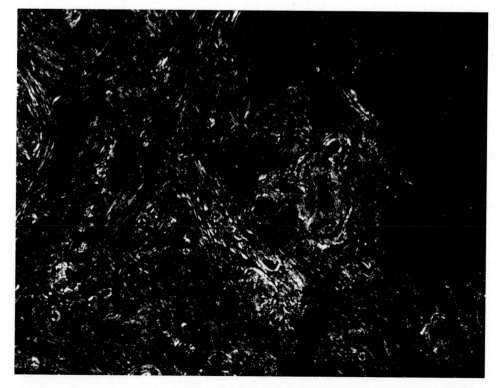

FIGURE 25-8
Nodular amyloidosis
Amyloid stains with Congo red and has characteristic apple-green birefringence under polarized light (Congo red).

AMYLOIDOSIS—FACT SHEET

Definition

» A spectrum of disease in which nonbranching linear fibrils of protein are deposited as insoluble fibrils in the extracellular spaces

Incidence

» Amyloid localized to the lung is rare, and is usually tracheobronchial or nodular

» Systemic amyloid involves the lung in 30-90% of patients, and is usually the diffuse interstitial form

Mortality

» Excellent survival with tracheobronchial and nodular forms, but the median survival is only 18–24 months with the diffuse parenchymal form

Gender, Race, and Age Distribution

» No gender or racial predilection

» Most patients are more than 40 years of age, and the senile form usually occurs at over 80 years of age

Clinical Features

» Four clinical syndromes of pulmonary amyloidosis:
  » Systemic (generalized)
  » Localized
  » Diffuse alveolar septal
  » Pleural

» Systemic amyloidosis consists of four types:
  » Primary: without known cause; consists of type AL
  » Secondary: reactive, associated with systemic diseases such as rheumatoid arthritis, chronic osteomyelitis, and malignancies; consists of type AA
  » Multiple myeloma-associated: light chain derived from plasma cells and of immunoglobulin origin; type AL
  » Senile: incidental finding in adults over 80 years old

Radiologic Features

» Nodular: single or multiple well circumscribed nodules

» Diffuse: interstitial nodular or linear densities

» Tracheobronchial: airway thickening or collapse; post-obstructive pneumonia

Prognosis and Therapy

» Nodular and tracheobronchial amyloidosis are treated with conservative excision (surgical or laser); excellent survival

» Diffuse amyloidosis has no effective treatment; poor prognosis

AMYLOIDOSIS—PATHOLOGIC FEATURES

Gross Findings

» Three forms:
  » Tracheobronchial: polypoid masses in major bronchi
  » Nodular: firm, waxy gray to white, well demarcated nodules
  » Diffuse: uniform rubber-sponge-like lung parenchyma

Microscopic Findings

» Amorphous, eosinophilic substance involving airways, vessels, and interstitium

» Tracheobronchial and nodular forms commonly have giant cells "ingesting" amyloid at edges

» Plasma cells, calcium, and bone are often present

» Amyloid stains with Congo red stains and demonstrates apple green birefringence when viewed under polarized light

» Amyloid is blue-gray with Mallory's trichrome stain, in contrast to the more definite deep blue color of collagen

» Amyloid stains metachromatically with crystal or methyl violet

Ultrastructural Features

» Tangled or felt-like mass of long, tubular nonbranching hollow fibrils 7.5-10 nm in diameter, 800 nm long

» 10% of components consist of P component, a glycoprotein

Fine Needle Aspiration Biopsy Findings

» Homogenous flocculent material that is Congo red-positive with apple-green birefringence

» Plasma cells, lymphocytes, and giant cells may be seen

Immunohistochemical Features

» Antibodies to AA, Aκ, Aλ, ATTR, and Aβ$_2$-microglobulin are available

» May be less sensitive than Congo red staining with examination under polarized light

Biochemical Features

» Four major types: AL, AA, AATR, and β$_2$-microglobulin

Pathologic Differential Diagnosis

» Light chain disease

» Pulmonary hyalinizing granuloma

» Hyalinizing fibrosis

---

non-immunoglobulin synthesized in the liver and commonly found in primary amyloidosis; protein ATTR (transthyretin) a prealbumin molecule that binds and transports thyroxine and retinol, deposited in familial amyloid polyneuropathies and senile systemic amyloidosis; and β$_2$-microglobulin, a component of the MHC class I molecules and a normal serum protein deposited in patients on long-term hemodialysis.

DIFFERENTIAL DIAGNOSIS

The differential diagnosis of pulmonary amyloidosis is primarily light chain disease. Light chain disease can take a diffuse or nodular form and has a similar histologic appearance. However, light chain disease does not show the apple green birefringence characteristic of amyloid when viewed under polarized light. Also, light chain disease will show light chain restriction, most commonly to kappa light chains, and will not have the fibrillar amyloid material by ultrastructural analysis.

Hyalinizing collagen that can be seen in some repair reactions within the lung and in hyalinizing pulmonary granulomas (see below) has similar histology, but does not stain with Congo red or show apple-green birefringence with polarization.

PROGNOSIS AND THERAPY

Nodular amyloidosis and tracheobronchial amyloidosis are treated with conservative surgical excision or laser removal. Prognosis is good for these forms. However, no treatment currently exists for diffuse parenchymal amyloidosis, and survival in these patients is poor, with the median survival period between 18 and 24 months.

PULMONARY HYALINIZING GRANULOMA

CLINICAL FEATURES

Pulmonary hyalinizing granuloma (PHG) is a nodular hyalinizing fibrotic reaction with dense, thickened collagenous bundles. Although the etiology is uncertain, there is evidence that suggests it may represent the intra-pulmonary variant of sclerosing mediastinitis, a

fibrotic response to latent *Histoplasma* infection. It can be found in association with other fibrosing diseases such as Riedel's thyroiditis, fibrosing pleuritis, retroperitoneal fibrosis, and constrictive pericarditis. Patients with this lesion are 20-80 years of age and usually present with dyspnea, chest pain, cough, or hemoptysis.

RADIOLOGIC FEATURES

Imaging studies usually reveal multiple "cotton ball"-type masses from 2 cm to 4 cm in diameter. Though cavitation and calcification can occur, they are not commonly seen.

PATHOLOGIC FEATURES

GROSS FINDINGS

The masses usually consist of firm, tan or white tissue with a shiny cut surface. They are more commonly subpleural, but may occur throughout the lung. In the majority of cases, the nodules are multiple and bilateral.

MICROSCOPIC FINDINGS

The nodules consist of thick bundles of collagen fibers organized in a whorled pattern (known as a collagen "donut"), usually around a small blood vessel (Figures 25-9A,B). Lymphocytes and plasma cells may

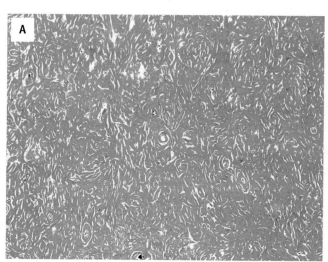
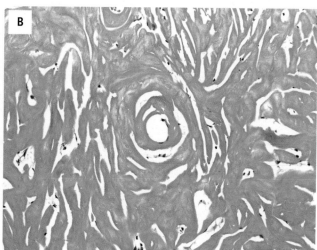

FIGURE 25-9

Pulmonary hyalinizing granuloma
(A) PHG is characterized by nodules of relatively acellular thick bundles of collagen fibers. **(B)** In some areas, these bundles of collagen whorl around small blood vessels and form a collagen "donut" type structure.

be present, but are not prominent. The name "granuloma" is a misnomer, as giant cells and macrophages are not common to the reaction and there is usually no evidence of granulomas in the surrounding lung. Organismal stains do not reveal fungi or acid fast organisms.

ANCILLARY STUDIES

ULTRASTRUCTURAL EXAMINATION

Electron microscopy reveals collagen fibrils with characteristic 640-Å periodicity with intervening electron-dense amorphous material. This material may show nonspecific staining by Congo red, but does not have the characteristic amyloid ultrastructural appearance.

IMMUNOHISTOCHEMISTRY

Lymphocytes and plasma cells within the lesions are polyclonal, and no light chain restriction for kappa or lambda is seen.

DIFFERENTIAL DIAGNOSIS

The differential diagnosis includes nodular amyloid, nodular light chain disease, and fibrotic granulomatous fungal or mycobacterial infections or sarcoidosis. Congo red stains are helpful in distinguishing hyalinizing pulmonary granuloma from nodular amyloid. The lymphatic distribution of the fibrosis in sarcoidosis (subpleural, bronchovascular areas and interlobular septae) and marked fibrosis in lymph nodes helps distinguish sarcoidosis from the random parenchymal distribution of PHG. Fibrotic granulomas from fungal or mycobacterial disease are more likely to contain residual giant cells and histiocytes from the active granulomas and do not, in general, have the whorled, concentric pattern of collagen seen in PHG.

PROGNOSIS AND THERAPY

PHG is treated with conservative surgical resection. When there is a single nodule, the clinical outcome is good, with excellent long-term survival. When multiple nodules are present and total resection is not possible, the patient may experience progressive symptoms, but deaths due to disease have not been reported.

PULMONARY HYALINIZING GRANULOMA—FACT SHEET

Definition
- ‣ Nodular hyalinizing fibrotic reaction with dense, thickened collagenous bundles

Incidence
- ‣ Rare

Mortality
- ‣ No deaths reported

Age Distribution
- ‣ Ages range from 20-80 years

Clinical Features
- ‣ Found in association with other fibrosing diseases such as Riedel's thyroiditis, fibrosing pleuritis, retroperitoneal fibrosis, and constrictive pericarditis
- ‣ Symptoms include dyspnea, chest pain, cough, and hemoptysis

Radiologic Features
- ‣ Multiple "cotton ball" masses measuring 2–4 cm

Prognosis and Therapy
- ‣ Excellent prognosis; no deaths reported
- ‣ Complete surgical excision is the treatment of choice

PULMONARY HYALINIZING GRANULOMA—PATHOLOGIC FEATURES

Gross Findings
- ‣ Firm, tan to white tissue with shiny cut surface
- ‣ Commonly subpleural

Microscopic Findings
- ‣ Thick bundles of collagen fibers organized in a whorled pattern around a blood vessel
- ‣ Plasma cells and lymphocytes may be present

Ultrastructural Features
- ‣ Collagen fibrils with 640-Å periodicity, with intervening electron-dense amorphous material

Immunohistochemical Features
- ‣ Polyclonal inflammatory cells

Pathologic Differential Diagnosis
- ‣ Nodular amyloid
- ‣ Nodular light chain disease
- ‣ Hyalinizing collagen secondary to granulomatous fungal or mycobacterial infections or sarcoidosis

MINUTE MENINGOTHELIAL-LIKE LESION

Minute meningothelial-like lesions are incidental lesions first described as small chemodectoma-like bodies. However, studies have shown that these lesions have no sensory functions and have no morphologic features of chemodectomas, but have features more similar to meningiomas, giving rise to the new nomenclature.

CLINICAL FEATURES

The lesions are incidental findings, noted in approximately 1% of autopsy lungs in patients between 12 and 90 years, and may be more common in women. Though no definite risk factors have been confirmed, studies report that the lesions may be found more commonly in lungs damaged from emphysema, congestive heart failure, thromboembolic disease, and malignancy.

RADIOLOGIC FEATURES

Single lesions are not visible on chest imaging studies. However, when multiple, the lesions may present as small nodular shadows on chest radiographs and CT scans and may have a miliary appearance.

PATHOLOGIC FEATURES

GROSS FINDINGS

Although most of these lesions are not grossly conspicuous, they are 1-3 mm in diameter, tan to yellow, and can be found in the pleura or parenchyma. They are most commonly multiple and may occur more in the right lung than in the left lung, though reports on location are not consistent.

MICROSCOPIC FINDINGS

The lesions consist of cytologically bland ovoid cells with stippled chromatin which grow in nests within the alveolar septa, usually expanding it, and they are usually found around pulmonary veins (Figure 25-10). As they expand, they may connect to each other with intervening collagen.

ANCILLARY STUDIES

ULTRASTRUCTURAL EXAMINATION

By electron microscopy, there are complex interdigitating cell processes connected by desmosomes with occasional cytoplasmic filaments. Despite its previous name of pulmonary chemodectoma, no neuroendocrine

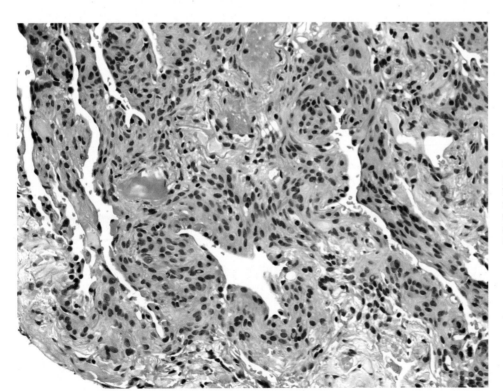

FIGURE 25-10

Minute meningothelial-like lesion
This histology consists of ovoid cells with stippled chromatin which nests within the alveolar septa, usually around pulmonary veins. Larger lesions may have a stellate-type architecture.

features are seen, and these cells most strongly resemble meningothelial cells, giving rise to the somewhat cumbersome name of minute meningothelial-like lesion.

IMMUNOHISTOCHEMISTRY

The nodules are strongly reactive for epithelial membrane antigen and vimentin, and negative for cytokeratin, S-100, neuron-specific enolase, and actin.

DIFFERENTIAL DIAGNOSIS

The differential diagnosis includes carcinoid tumorlet, granuloma, sclerosing hemangioma, primary and metastatic paraganglioma, and primary and metastatic meningioma. Carcinoid tumorlets are easily distinguishable using neuroendocrine immunohistochemical studies, which reveal strong positivity in the carcinoid cells and no immunoreactivity in the meningothelial-like lesions. Also, carcinoid tumorlets are more commonly found around airways and not pulmonary veins. Granulomas consist of histiocytes, with immunoreactivity to CD 68, and usually have a more compact form with peripheral lymphocytes and giant cells, features not seen in meningothelial-like lesions. Sclerosing hemangiomas are more commonly much larger lesions, greater than 1 cm, but when small, may be distinguished

by their immunoreactivity to thyroid transcription factor-1 (TTF-1). Primary pulmonary paragangliomas are very rare and consist of nests of epithelioid cells with a "Zellballen" pattern; these cells will stain with neuroendocrine markers, unlike the cells of minute meningothelial-like lesions. Distinction from the extremely rare primary pulmonary meningioma is based primarily upon size and demonstration of appropriate histologic features. Metastatic paraganglioma and meningioma can also be distinguished based on a clinical history of these primary tumors.

PROGNOSIS AND THERAPY

Minute meningothelial-like lesions of the lung require no treatment and have no reported effects on patient survival.

DENDRIFORM OSSIFICATION

Ossification in the lung is the presence of mature bone with or without marrow elements. It may take two forms: nodular ossification, in which lamellar bone is deposited within the alveolar space, usually secondary to pre-existing

---

MINUTE MENINGOTHELIAL-LIKE LESION—FACT SHEET

Definition
- » Incidental lesions with features most similar to meningiomas

Incidence
- » 1% of autopsy lungs

Morbidity and Mortality
- » No known morbidity or mortality

Gender and Age Distribution
- » 12-90 years of age
- » May be more common in women

Clinical Features
- » May be found in the setting of damaged lungs (emphysema, congestive heart failure, thromboembolic disease, malignancy)
- » Asymptomatic

Radiologic Features
- » Only multiple lesions may be seen (small nodular shadows)

Prognosis and Therapy
- » Excellent prognosis
- » No therapy needed

MINUTE MENINGOTHELIAL-LIKE LESION—PATHOLOGIC FEATURES

Gross Findings
- » 1-3 mm in diameter tan or yellow lesions

Microscopic Findings
- » Ovoid cells with stippled chromatin
- » Present as nests in alveolar septa and commonly found around pulmonary veins

Ultrastructural Features
- » Complex interdigitating cell processes connected by desmosomes
- » Strongly resemble meningothelial cells

Immunohistochemical Features
- » Reactive to epithelial membrane antigen and vimentin
- » No immunoreactivity to cytokeratin, S-100, neuron-specific enolase, and actin

Pathologic Differential Diagnosis
- » Carcinoid tumorlet
- » Granuloma
- » Small sclerosing hemangioma
- » Primary and metastatic paraganglioma
- » Primary and metastatic meningioma

cardiac lesions; and dendriform ossification, in which interstitial branching bone spicules and marrow protrude into the alveoli. It can be idiopathic or associated with chronic lung diseases such as idiopathic pulmonary fibrosis, sarcoidosis, adverse effects of chemotherapies such as busulfan, chronic granulomatous infections (histoplasmosis, tuberculosis), pulmonary metastases, and amyloidosis. Extra-pulmonary causes include chronic congestion due to mitral valve stenosis, chronic left-ventricular failure, hyperparathyroidism, and hypervitaminosis D.

CLINICAL FEATURES

Dendriform ossification is a rare disease with prevalence at autopsy of 0.5%. It is most commonly found in men over 60 years of age, who are asymptomatic or have minimal symptoms and have come to medical attention due to incidental changes on imaging studies. In advanced forms of the disease, a restrictive physiology may occur, and decreases in diffusing capacity can be seen.

RADIOLOGIC FEATURES

Dendriform ossification is usually not seen on chest x-rays, but, if present, usually appears as lower-lobe reticulonodular infiltrates. It may have a miliary pattern and can be confused with mycobacterial or fungal infections.

PATHOLOGIC FEATURES

GROSS FINDINGS

The lungs may be firm and gritty with fibrosis, which is thought to be the nidus for the ossification. The findings may be focal or diffuse and are more commonly found in the lower lobes and in the periphery. Progression of the lesions is central and superior.

MICROSCOPIC FINDINGS

The histopathologic picture of dendriform ossification is one of linear or dichotomous branching bone deposits within the alveolar wall, with marrow elements present (Figure 25-11). Osteoclasts and osteoblasts may be present, but are scant. As in metastatic calcification, the bone deposition gives the alveoli a rigid, expanded appearance, compared to normal alveoli. The ossification can be localized or widespread throughout the lung.

DENDRIFORM OSSIFICATION—FACT SHEET

Definition
» Calcium deposition in the lung as interstitial branching of bone spicules and marrow

Prevalence
» Prevalence at autopsy of 0.5%

Gender and Age Distribution
» More common in men over 60 years of age

Clinical Features
» Usually found in the setting of chronic lung disease
» Advanced forms of the disease may cause a restrictive physiology and decreased diffusing capacity

Radiologic Features
» Usually not seen on chest x-rays, but if present, seen as reticulonodular infiltrates
» Miliary pattern may be mistaken for fungal or mycobacterial infection

Prognosis and Therapy
» No known effective treatment
» Death due to respiratory compromise secondary to underlying lung disease is common

---

DENDRIFORM OSSIFICATION—PATHOLOGIC FEATURES

Gross Findings
» Firm and gritty lungs with fibrosis
» Lower lobe predominance

Microscopic Findings
» Linear or dichotomous branching bone deposits with marrow elements, within alveolar walls

Ultrastructural Features
» Calcium deposits within collagen fibers

Pathologic Differential Diagnosis
» Nodular pulmonary ossification
» Metastatic interstitial calcification

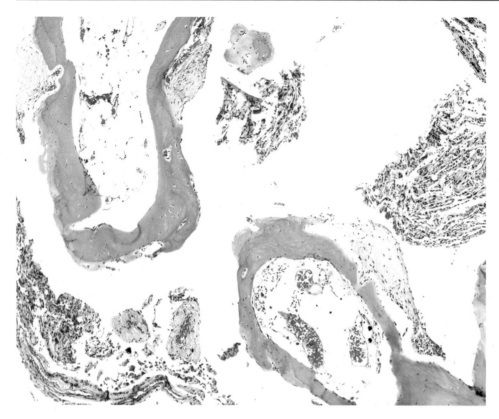

FIGURE 25-11

Dendriform ossification
These curvilinear bone deposits form within the alveolar walls, and osteoblasts are present on the internal rims of the bone.

ANCILLARY STUDIES

ULTRASTRUCTURAL EXAMINATION

Transmission electron microscopy reveals calcium deposits within collagen fibers in the area of fibrosis, a finding which is confirmed by scanning electron microscopy.

DIFFERENTIAL DIAGNOSIS

The differential diagnosis includes nodular pulmonary ossification, which is bone formation within alveolar spaces rather than within the interstitium as is seen in dendriform ossification, and has a focal, nodular distribution. Also, nodular pulmonary ossification usually develops in the setting of chronic cardiac congestion and is not found with fibrotic lung disease.

Metastatic interstitial calcification may be mistaken for dendriform ossification; however, there is no bone formation in metastatic interstitial calcification. Also, calcium is diffusely present by histochemical studies in metastatic interstitial calcification, but should be scarce or absent in histochemical stains for dendriform ossification.

PROGNOSIS AND THERAPY

There is no known effective treatment for pulmonary dendriform ossification. Corticosteroids, calcium-binding drugs, and low-calcium diets are among the therapies that have been tried, but definite benefit has not been documented. Bisphosphonates are currently employed as experimental therapy, but their benefits remain unknown.

METASTATIC INTERSTITIAL CALCIFICATION

Pulmonary calcification refers to deposition of calcium salts in the lung. Pulmonary calcifications can be divided into two types: (1) dystrophic calcification, which refers to deposition of calcium in previously injured tissue and (2) metastatic calcification, which refers to deposition of calcium in normal tissue. Deposition of calcium in the latter occurs predominantly in the interstitium and may result in interstitial changes on chest imaging studies. Thus, this should be considered in the differential diagnosis of any interstitial lung disease.

CLINICAL FEATURES

Metastatic calcification is usually the result of alterations in serum calcium and phosphorus metabolism, which have both benign and malignant causes. Benign causes include chronic renal failure, diseases of bone including osteopetrosis, Paget's disease, and hypervitaminosis D. Malignant causes include tumors that cause hypercalcemia such as parathyroid adenomas or carcinomas, multiple myeloma, leukemia, and small cell carcinoma. Patients are usually asymptomatic, but when calcium deposition is extensive, respiratory failure may occur. If death occurs, it is usually secondary to cardiac involvement.

RADIOLOGIC FEATURES

Chest x-rays may be normal in the setting of significant metastatic calcification, but usually show nonspecific infiltrates that may be mistaken for pulmonary edema or hemorrhage. Chest CT scans are more sensitive and specific for detection of calcium in the lung, which can present as multiple nodules, diffuse or patchy ground-glass opacities, or dense areas of consolidation.

PATHOLOGIC FEATURES

GROSS FINDINGS

Lungs with metastatic calcification have a firm, grainy texture and sand-like appearance. The lungs are usually heavy and maintain their architecture even when sectioned. When the pulmonary tissue is digested away in these specimens, a brittle calcium skeleton is left behind, outlining the interstitial nature of the deposition.

MICROSCOPIC FINDINGS

Calcium is deposited within the alveolar walls and vessels within the lung. In more advanced cases, deposition may occur in the airways. Alveoli with calcium have a rigid, expanded appearance when compared to adjacent normal alveoli (Figure 25-12). Foreign-body giant cells are usually seen in cases with significant calcium deposition. The calcified areas stain with von Kossa and alizarin red S stains.

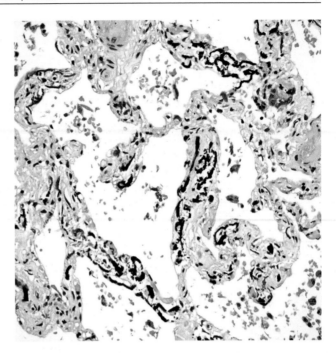

FIGURE 25-12
Metastatic interstitial calcification
Calcium is present as dark, basophilic fibrils within the alveolar walls and vessels in this lung.

ANCILLARY STUDIES

ULTRASTRUCTURAL EXAMINATION

Electron microscopy reveals both intracellular and extracellular calcium deposition, particularly within the alveolar/capillary basement membrane.

BIOCHEMICAL ANALYSIS

Biochemical analysis reveals that the calcium is usually in the form of calcium phosphate.

DIFFERENTIAL DIAGNOSIS

Metastatic calcification must be distinguished from other forms of calcium in the lung, most notably dystrophic calcium from previous injury. In general, dystrophic calcium presents as aggregates of calcium within a background of fibrosis, chronic granulomatous disease, or other repair reactions and does not present as the fine, reticular deposition of metastatic calcification.

METASTATIC INTERSTITIAL CALCIFICATION—FACT SHEET

Definition
- ‣ Deposition of calcium salts in the normal tissues of the lung
- ‣ Usually the result of serum calcium and phosphorus metabolism alternations

Incidence
- ‣ Uncommon

Morbidity and Mortality
- ‣ Morbidity and mortality are related to the underlying cause of the hypophosphatemia or hypercalcemia

Gender, Race, and Age Distribution
- ‣ No gender, race, or age predominance

Clinical Features
- ‣ Found in settings of hypophosphatemia and hypercalcemia
- ‣ Non-neoplastic causes
  - ‣ Chronic renal failure
  - ‣ Diseases of bone including osteopetrosis, Paget's disease, hypervitaminosis D
- ‣ Neoplastic causes
  - ‣ Parathyroid adenoma or carcinoma
  - ‣ Multiple myeloma
  - ‣ Leukemia
  - ‣ Small cell carcinoma

Radiologic Features
- ‣ Chest x-ray may be normal, but usually shows infiltrates with the appearance of pulmonary edema or hemorrhage

Prognosis and Therapy
- ‣ Treatment involves eliminating the underlying cause of the process
- ‣ Prognosis is related to the underlying cause

METASTATIC INTERSTITIAL CALCIFICATION—PATHOLOGIC FEATURES

Gross Findings
- ‣ Lungs have a firm, grainy texture and sand-like appearance throughout

Microscopic Findings
- ‣ Calcium deposition is seen within alveolar walls and vessels, which gives alveoli a more rigid appearance
- ‣ Foreign-body giant cells are usually present in more advanced cases
- ‣ Von Kossa and alizarin red S stains can be used to highlight the calcium

Ultrastructural Features
- ‣ Both intracellular and extracellular calcium deposition is seen
- ‣ Calcium is present within the alveolar/capillary basement membrane

Biochemical Analysis
- ‣ Calcium is in the form of calcium phosphate

Pathologic Differential Diagnosis
- ‣ Dystrophic calcification in previously injured lungs

CLINICAL FEATURES

Patients are usually 30-50 years of age and 50% have a familial history. Symptoms are absent in more than half, and dyspnea, cough, and chest pain were reported in the other cases, but usually occur late in the course. Normal or mild restrictive respiratory physiology may occur, which can progress with the disease. Most patients are stable or show little progression over many years.

RADIOLOGIC FEATURES

Chest x-rays show bilateral sand-like micronodular 1-mm densities with calcification, which represent the microliths. There is a lower lobe predominance, and the cardiac and diaphragmatic areas are usually obscured. High-resolution CT scans reveal the presence of micronodular calcifications located around the bronchovascular area and within the subpleural and perilobular areas.

PROGNOSIS AND THERAPY

Treatment of metastatic calcification involves eliminating the underlying causes of either hypophosphatemia or hypercalcemia, and may include renal transplantation or parathyroidectomy.

PULMONARY ALVEOLAR MICROLITHIASIS

Pulmonary alveolar microlithiasis (PAM) is a recessive disorder that is characterized by calcium phosphate microliths of calcospherites, filling alveoli. The etiology of the disease is still unknown, but some authors suspect that an inherited local enzymatic defect is responsible for the calcium deposition.

PATHOLOGIC FEATURES

GROSS FINDINGS

The lungs are usually quite heavy and difficult to cut due to the high content of calcium. They usually have a tan to gray appearance and a sandy texture. The microliths are from 0.02 mm to 0.5 mm and fall out of the specimen with sectioning.

MICROSCOPIC FINDINGS

The histopathologic picture is one of microliths or calcospherites, consisting of laminated calcium phosphate concretions involving the alveolar spaces (Figure 25-13). Unlike the other diseases of calcification in the lung, in PAM, the alveolar space, not the alveolar wall and interstitium, is the main area affected. There is usually no more than 1 microlith in an alveolar space. The microliths have a radial appearance and are polarizable. They stain with periodic acid-Schiff and iron stains, and ossification can occur. As the disease progresses, interstitial inflammation and fibrosis may occur.

ANCILLARY STUDIES

ULTRASTRUCTURAL EXAMINATION

Transmission electron microscopy shows radial striations and many small matrix vesicles of undetermined origin. Some report that a scale-like surface is seen by scanning electron microscopy.

FINE NEEDLE ASPIRATION BIOPSY

Microliths can be obtained by fine needle aspiration, but this finding must be correlated with imaging studies to confirm a diagnosis of PAM.

BIOCHEMICAL ANALYSIS

Biochemical analysis reveals that the microliths are composed of calcium phosphate in a hydroxyapatite crystalline arrangement. Calcium carbonate and very small amounts of magnesium and iron have also been found.

DIFFERENTIAL DIAGNOSIS

On small biopsy specimens, it may be difficult to differentiate corpora amylacea from PAM. However, the microliths of PAM do not have the black, crystalline, or core ingredients that may be present in corpora amylacea. When ossification is present, the differential diagnosis may include either an ossifying focus of metastatic calcification or pulmonary ossification (nodular or dendriform types). Unlike the latter two, the ossifications, when they occur in PAM, are present within alveolar spaces and not within the interstitium or vascular walls.

PROGNOSIS AND THERAPY

There is no known treatment to date. Corticosteroids, bronchoalveolar lavage, and chelating agents have been tried with little definitive proof of success. Lung transplantation is performed in the severest cases.

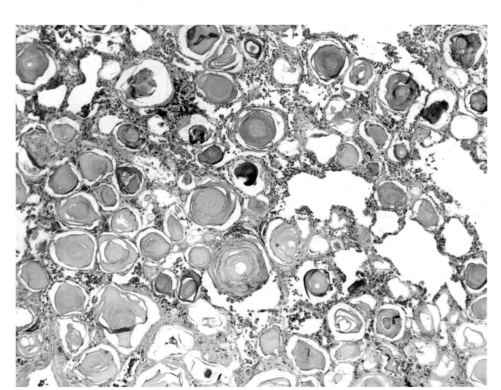

FIGURE 25-13

Pulmonary alveolar microlithiasis
Microliths or calcospherites consisting of laminated concretions fill the alveolar spaces. Note that there is only one microlith in each alveolar space and that the alveolar wall and interstitium are not involved.

PULMONARY ALVEOLAR MICROLITHIASIS—FACT SHEET

Definition
» A recessive disorder that is characterized by calcium phosphate microliths (calcospherites) filling alveoli

Incidence
» Rare

Age Distribution
» 30-50 years of age

Clinical Features
» More than half of patients have no symptoms
» When symptoms are present, they include dyspnea, cough, and chest pain
» Mild restrictive respiratory physiology may occur
» 50% have a family history of this disorder

Radiologic Features
» Chest x-ray shows sand-like micronodular 1-mm densities
» High-resolution CT reveals micronodular calcifications around bronchovascular areas, subpleural and perilobular areas

Prognosis and Therapy
» No known treatment
» Lung transplantation is performed in the most severe cases
» Most patients are stable or show little progression over many years

PULMONARY ALVEOLAR MICROLITHIASIS—PATHOLOGIC FEATURES

Gross Findings
» Heavy lungs that are difficult to cut due to high calcium content
» Tan to gray appearance with a sandy texture
» 0.02- to 0.05-mm microliths fall out of specimen upon sectioning

Microscopic Findings
» Microliths or calcospherites consisting of laminated calcium phosphate concretions are present within alveolar spaces
» Usually one microlith in an alveolar space
» Microliths are polarizable
» Microliths stain with periodic acid-Schiff and iron stains
» Ossification can occur within microliths

Ultrastructural Features
» Radial striations and small matrix vesicles of undetermined origin

Fine Needle Aspiration Biopsy Findings
» Microliths can be found by fine needle aspiration but are not specific for PAM

Biochemical Analysis
» Microliths are composed of calcium phosphate in a hydroxyapatite crystalline arrangement
» Calcium carbonate and small amounts of magnesium and iron may be found

Pathologic Differential Diagnosis
» Corpora amylacea
» Ossifying focus of metastatic calcification or pulmonary ossification

SUGGESTED REFERENCES

Inflammatory Pseudotumors

1. Anthony PP. Inflammatory pseudotumor (plasma cell granuloma) of lung, liver and other organs. *Histopathology*. 1993;23:501-3.
2. Coffin CM, Dehner LP, Meis-Kindblom JM. Inflammatory myofibroblastic tumor, inflammatory fibrosarcoma, and related lesions: an historical review with differential diagnostic considerations. *Semin Diagn Pathol*. 1998;15:102-10.
3. Cohen MC, Kaschula RO. Primary pulmonary tumors in childhood: a review of 31 years' experience and the literature. *Pediatr Pulmonol*. 1992;14:222-32.
4. Gal AA, Koss MN, McCarthy WF, Hochholzer L. Prognostic factors in pulmonary fibrohistiocytic lesions. *Cancer*. 1994;73:1817-24.
5. Hosler GA, Steinberg DM, Sheth S, Hamper UM, Erozan YS, Ali SZ. Inflammatory pseudotumor: a diagnostic dilemma in cytopathology. *Diagn Cytopathol*. 2004;31:267-70.
6. Kim TS, Han J, Kim GY, Lee KS, Kim H, Kim J. Pulmonary inflammatory pseudotumor (inflammatory myofibroblastic tumor): CT features with pathologic correlation. *J Comput Assist Tomogr*. 2005;29:633-9.
7. Matsubara O, Tan-Liu NS, Kenney RM, Mark EJ. Inflammatory pseudotumors of the lung: progression from organizing pneumonia to fibrous histiocytoma or to plasma cell granuloma in 32 cases. *Hum Pathol*. 1988;19:807-14.
8. Melloni G, Carretta A, Ciriaco P, et al. Inflammatory pseudotumor of the lung in adults. *Ann Thorac Surg*. 2005;79:426-32.
9. Pettinato G, Manivel JC, De Rosa N, Dehner LP. Inflammatory myofibroblastic tumor (plasma cell granuloma). Clinicopathologic study of 20 cases with immunohistochemical and ultrastructural observations. *Am J Clin Pathol*. 1990;94:538-46.
10. Su LD, Atayde-Perez A, Sheldon S, Fletcher JA, Weiss SW. Inflammatory myofibroblastic tumor: cytogenetic evidence supporting clonal origin. *Mod Pathol*. 1998;11:364-8.

Lipoid Pneumonia

11. Annobil SH, Morad NA, Khurana P, Kameswaran M, Ogunbiyi O, al-Malki T. Reaction of human lungs to aspirated animal fat (ghee): a clinico-pathological study. *Virchows Arch*. 1995;426:301-5.
12. Baron SE, Haramati LB, Rivera VT. Radiological and clinical findings in acute and chronic exogenous lipoid pneumonia. *J Thorac Imaging*. 2003;18:217-24.
13. Gimenez A, Franquet T, Prats R, Estrada P, Villalba J, Bague S. Unusual primary lung tumors: a radiologic-pathologic overview. *Radiographics*. 2002;22:601-19.
14. Gondouin A, Manzoni P, Ranfaing E, et al. Exogenous lipid pneumonia: a retrospective multicenter study of 44 cases in France. *Eur Respir J*. 1996;9:1463-9.
15. Ikehara K, Suzuki M, Tsuburai T, Ishigatsubo Y. Lipoid pneumonia. *Lancet*. 2002;359:1300.
16. Jouannic I, Desrues B, Lena H, Quinquenel ML, Donnio PY, Delaval P. Exogenous lipoid pneumonia complicated by *Mycobacterium fortuitum* and *Aspergillus fumigatus* infections. *Eur Respir J*. 1996;9:172-4.
17. Ohwada A, Yoshioka Y, Shimanuki Y, et al. Exogenous lipoid pneumonia following ingestion of liquid paraffin. *Intern Med*. 2002 Jun;41:483-6.
18. Gaerte SC, Meyer CA, Winer-Muram HT, Tarver RD, and Conces DJ Jr. Fat-containing lesions of the chest. *Radiographics*. 2002;Spec No:S61-78.
19. Spickard A III, Hirschmann JV. Exogenous lipoid pneumonia. *Arch Intern Med*. 1994;154:686-92.
20. Wright BA, Jeffrey PH. Lipoid pneumonia. *Semin Respir Infect*. 1990;5:314-21.

Amyloidosis

21. Chen KT. Amyloidosis presenting in the respiratory tract. *Pathol Annu*. 1989;24:253-73.
22. Dacic S, Colby TV, Yousem SA. Nodular amyloidemia and primary pulmonary lymphoma with amyloid production: a differential diagnostic problem. *Mod Pathol*. 2000;13:934-40.
23. Gillmore JD, Hawkins PN. Amyloidosis and the respiratory tract. *Thorax*. 1999;54:444-51.
24. Khoor A, Myers JL, Tazelaar HD, et al. Amyloid-like pulmonary nodules, including localized light-chain deposition: clinicopathologic analysis of three cases. *Am J Clin Pathol*. 2004;121:200-4.
25. O'Regan A, Fenlon HM, Beamis JF Jr, et al. Tracheobronchial amyloidosis: the Boston University experience from 1984 to 1999. *Medicine (Baltimore)*. 2000;79:69-9.
26. Rocken C, Sletten K. Amyloid in surgical pathology. *Virchows Arch*. 2003;443:3-16.
27. Serpell LC, Sunde M, Blake CC. The molecular basis of amyloidosis. *Cell Mol Life Sci*. 1997;53:871-7.
28. Utz JP, Swensen SJ, Gertz MA. Pulmonary amyloidosis: the Mayo Clinic experience from 1980 to 1993. *Ann Intern Med*. 1996;124:407-13.
29. Kaplan B, Martin BM, Livneh A, et al. Biochemical subtyping of amyloid in formalin-fixed tissue samples confirms and supplements immunohistological data. *Am J Clin Pathol*. 2004;121:794-800.

Pulmonary Hyalinizing Granuloma

30. Eschelman DJ, Blickman JG, Lazar HL, O'Keane JC, Schechter M. Pulmonary hyalinizing granuloma: a rare cause of a solitary pulmonary nodule. *J Thorac Imaging*. 1991;6:54-6.
31. Pinckard JK, Rosenbluth DB, Patel K, Dehner LP, Pfeifer JD. Pulmonary hyalinizing granuloma associated with Aspergillus infection. *Int J Surg Pathol*. 2003;11:39-42.
32. Yousem SA, Hochholzer L. Pulmonary hyalinizing granuloma. *Am J Clin Pathol*. 1987;87:1-6.

Minute Meningothelial-like Lesion

33. Gaffey MJ, Mills SE, Askin FB. Minute pulmonary meningothelial-like nodules: a clinicopathologic study of so-called minute pulmonary chemodectoma. *Am J Surg Pathol*. 1988;12:167-75.
34. Ionescu DN, Sasatomi E, Aldeeb D, et al. Pulmonary meningothelial-like nodules: a genotypic comparison with meningiomas. *Am J Surg Pathol*. 2004;28:207-14.
35. Kuroki M, Nakata H, Masuda T, et al. Minute pulmonary meningothelial-like nodules: high-resolution computed tomography and pathologic correlations. *J Thorac Imaging*. 2002;17:227-9.

36. Niho S, Yokose T, Nishiwaki Y, Mukai K. Immunohistochemical and clonal analysis of minute pulmonary meningothelial-like nodules. *Hum Pathol*. 1999;30:425-9.
37. Sellami D, Gotway MB, Hanks DK, Webb WR. Minute pulmonary meningothelial-like nodules: thin-section CT appearance. *J Comput Assist Tomogr*. 2001;25:311-3.

Dendriform Ossification

38. Joines RW, Roggli VL. Dendriform pulmonary ossification: report of two cases with unique findings. *Am J Clin Pathol*. 1989;91:398-402.
39. Müller KM, Friemann J, Stichnoth E. Dendriform pulmonary ossification. *Pathol Res Pract*. 1980;168:163-72.
40. Ndimbie OK, Williams CR, Lee MW. Dendriform pulmonary ossification. *Arch Pathol Lab Med*. 1987;111:1062-4.
41. Lara JF, Catroppo JF, Kim DU, da Costa D. Dendriform pulmonary ossification, a form of diffuse pulmonary ossification: report of a 26-year autopsy experience. *Arch Pathol Lab Med*. 2005. 129:348-53.

Metastatic Interstitial Calcification

42. Bonin M, Miyai K. Metastatic pulmonary calcification, morphology, chemical and x-ray microanalysis. *Lab Invest*. 1977;36:331-8.
43. Chan ED, Morales DV, Welsh CH, et al. Calcium deposition with or without bone formation in the lung. *Am J Respir Crit Care Med*. 2002;165:1654-69.
44. Kaltreider HB, Baum GL, Bogaty G, et al. So-called "metastatic" calcification of the lung. *Am J Med*. 1969;46:188-96.
45. Mulligan RM. Metastatic calcification. *Arch Pathol Lab Med*. 1947;43:177-230.

Pulmonary Alveolar Microlithiasis

46. Castellana G, Gentile M, Castellana R, et al. Pulmonary alveolar microlithiasis: clinical features, evolution of the phenotype, and review of the literature. *Am J Med Genet*. 2002;111:220-4.
47. Castellana G, Lamorgese V. Pulmonary alveolar microlithiasis: world cases and review of the literature. *Respiration*. 2003;70:549-55.
48. Mariotta S, Ricci A, Papale M, et al. Pulmonary alveolar microlithiasis: report on 576 cases published in the literature. *Sarcoidosis Vasc Diffuse Lung Dis*. 2004;21:173-81.
49. Petit MA. Pulmonary alveolar microlithiasis. *Chest*. 1991;100:290.
50. Prakash UB, Barham SS, Rosenow EC III, et al. Pulmonary alveolar microlithiasis: a review including ultrastructural and pulmonary function studies. *Mayo Clin Proc*. 1983;58:290-300.

26

Usual Lung Cancers
Dongfeng Tan • Sadir Alrawi

INTRODUCTION

Lung cancer is the third most frequent malignant neoplasm in the United States. According to the most recent data available from the Surveillance, Epidemiology, and End Results (SEER) program of the National Cancer Institute, it is estimated that over 213,000 people will be diagnosed with cancer of the lung and bronchus in 2007. Its impact is magnified by the unfortunate reality that most patients are diagnosed late in the course of their disease and die due to their tumors. SEER data estimates 160,390 deaths from lung cancer in 2007, making lung cancer the leading cause of cancer mortality in both men and women in the United States. The expected 5-year survival rate for all patients in whom lung cancer is diagnosed is approximately 15%, with substantially better rates associated with localized disease (49.1%) than with regional (15.2%) or distant (3.0%) metastasis.

Lung cancer is strongly associated with exposure to cigarette smoke. It has been shown that changes in lung cancer incidence and mortality rates parallel past trends in cigarette smoking. Tobacco smoking is believed to be responsible for close to 90% of lung cancers. The remainder are attributed to occupational exposures to carcinogens, radon exposure, air pollution, and other environmental and hereditary factors which continue

to be delineated. The association between smoking and lung cancer has been demonstrated by extensive epidemiological studies, and further supported by experimental evidence. For instance, lung cancers of smokers frequently contain G:C >T:A mutations in the TP53 gene, which are probably caused by benzopyrene, a potent carcinogen in tobacco smoke.

The World Health Organization (WHO) has recently published a detailed, updated histological classification of lung neoplasms (Table 26-1). Of particular clinical importance is the classification of most lung cancers into two major histologic categories: non-small cell lung carcinoma (NSCLC) and small cell lung carcinoma (SCLC) (small cell carcinoma is discussed in chapter 27). NSCLCs account for approximately 80% of lung cancer cases, and generally grow and spread more slowly than SCLCs. As discussed below, there are 3 main types of non-small cell lung cancers. They are named for the types of differentiation displayed by the malignant cells: adenocarcinoma, squamous cell carcinoma, and large cell carcinoma. Mixtures of these types are common, occurring in almost 50% of lung carcinomas. Significant histologic heterogeneity is also observed within the histologic categories, as will be discussed below.

Finally, lung cancers are also associated with a spectrum of local and systemic manifestations that may lead to their detection, in some cases, or may present additional complications to the care of patients with these tumors. Lung cancers originating in the large airways, primarily squamous cell and small cell carcinomas, can cause airway obstruction leading to post-obstructive pneumonia, abscesses, bronchiectasis or atelectasis. Peripheral lung cancers, usually adenocarcinomas, can invade the pleura and chest wall, leading to effusions and chest pain. Apical tumors in the superior pulmonary sulcus, known as Pancoast's tumors, invade the brachial plexus and the cervical sympathetic plexus, causing development of Horner's syndrome and pain in the shoulder and along the distribution of the ulnar nerve. Superior vena cava syndrome can result from tumor invasion or compression of the superior vena cava. Extension to other mediastinal structures can lead to dysphagia, hoarseness, diaphragmatic paralysis, and pericardial effusions. Some NSCLCs, particularly adenocarcinomas, predispose to thrombosis and embolism.

Table 26-1. Who Histological Classification of Tumors of the Lung

Malignant Epithelial Tumors

Squamous Cell Carcinoma
- Papillary
- Clear cell
- Small cell
- Basaloid

Small Cell Carcinoma
- Combined small cell carcinoma

Adenocarcinoma
- Adenocarcinoma, mixed subtype
- Acinar adenocarcinoma
- Papillary adenocarcinoma
- Bronchioloalveolar carcinoma
  - Nonmucinous
  - Mucinous
  - Mixed or indeterminate
- Solid adenocarcinoma with mucin production
  - Fetal adenocarcinoma
  - Mucinous ("colloid") carcinoma
  - Mucinous cystadenocarcinoma
  - Signet ring adenocarcinoma
  - Clear cell adenocarcinoma

Large Cell Carcinoma
- Large cell neuroendocrine carcinoma
  - Combined large cell neuroendocrine carcinoma
- Basaloid carcinoma
- Lymphoepithelioma-like carcinoma
- Clear cell carcinoma
- Large cell carcinoma with rhabdoid phenotype

Adenosquamous Carcinoma

Sarcomatoid Carcinoma
- Pleomorphic carcinoma
- Spindle cell carcinoma
- Giant cell carcinoma
- Carcinosarcoma
- Pulmonary blastoma

Carcinoid Tumor
- Typical carcinoid
- Atypical carcinoid

Salivary Gland Tumors
- Mucoepidermoid carcinoma
- Adenoid cystic carcinoma
- Epithelial-myoepithelial carcinoma

Preinvasive Lesions
- Squamous carcinoma in situ
- Atypical adenomatous hyperplasia
- Diffuse idiopathic pulmonary neuroendocrine hyperplasia

Based on Travis WD, Brambilla E, Müller-Hermelink HK, Harris CC, eds. *Pathology and Genetics of Tumours of the Lung, Pleura, Thymus and Heart.* Lyon: IARC Press; 2004:10.

GENERAL LUNG CANCER—FACT SHEET

- It is estimated that over 213,000 cases will be diagnosed in 2007 in the United States
- 80-90% of patients are active smokers
- 80% of cases are non-small cell lung cancers
- 20% of cases are small cell lung cancers
- 160,390 deaths are estimated to occur in 2007 in the United States; leading cause of cancer death
- Overall 5-year survival: 15%
- Small cell lung cancer has the most unfavorable outcome
- Bronchioloalveolar carcinoma has the most favorable outcome

Tumors are also capable of producing an array of hormones and other proteins responsible for paraneoplastic syndromes. Although a comprehensive review of these tumor-associated phenomena is outside of the scope of this chapter, familiarity with the spectrum of associated phenomena can be helpful in unraveling the diagnosis in some individuals.

NON-SMALL CELL CARCINOMAS

ADENOCARCINOMA

CLINICAL FEATURES

Adenocarcinoma is the most frequent type of lung cancer in the United States, accounting for roughly 35% of primary lung cancers, and almost half of lung cancers in some other countries. According to the World Health Organization definition, adenocarcinoma is a malignant epithelial tumor with glandular differentiation or mucin production by the tumor cells. It displays multiple growth patterns that often co-exist in individual tumors. Although adenocarcinoma is associated with cigarette smoking, the association is less strong than it is with squamous cell and small cell carcinomas. It is also the most common histologic type of lung cancer in women and non-smokers.

RADIOLOGIC FEATURES

Adenocarcinomas of the lung can present as masses, nodules or pneumonic infiltrates on chest imaging studies. They are more commonly peripheral lesions. Pleural thickening is common, and some may present with mesothelioma-like diffuse pleural space involvement.

ADENOCARCINOMA—FACT SHEET

Definition

▸ Malignant epithelial tumor with glandular differentiation or mucin production (World Health Organization)

Incidence

▸ 35% of primary lung cancers

Clinical Features

▸ Association with cigarette smoking is less than other lung cancers
▸ May be asymptomatic or associated with chest pain, cough, or constitutional symptoms

Radiologic Features

▸ Focal masses, nodular patterns, or pneumonic or diffuse forms
▸ May present as pleural thickening or with a pleural effusion

ADENOCARCINOMA—PATHOLOGIC FEATURES

Gross Findings

▸ Nodule, mass or infiltrative process, usually tan-white, with irregular or well circumscribed borders
▸ Predominantly peripheral
▸ Rarely associated with large airways
▸ Commonly associated with fibrosis or scar
▸ Necrosis may be present

Microscopic Findings

▸ Four major histologic sub-types : acinar, papillary, solid with mucin production, bronchioloalveolar
▸ Other rarer subtypes include fetal adenocarcinoma, mucinous ("colloid") carcinoma, mucinous cystadenocarcinoma, signet ring adenocarcinoma, clear cell adenocarcinoma
▸ 80% present as mixed type

Immunohistochemical Features

▸ Most are positive for TTF-1, surfactant proteins, and cytokeratin 7
▸ Most are negative for cytokeratin 20

Pathologic Differential Diagnosis

▸ Malignant mesothelioma
▸ Metastatic adenocarcinomas

PATHOLOGIC FEATURES

GROSS FINDINGS

Grossly, adenocarcinoma are usually peripheral tumors with a gray-white cut appearance (Figure 26-1). They rarely have endobronchial components and therefore do not generally cause airway obstruction with its associated symptomatology. Anthracotic pigment is com-

monly entrapped in the tumor mass. Gross necrosis is not a common feature, although it may occur in larger masses (greater than 5 cm). Adenocarcinomas may be found in association with fibrosis and pleural puckering. Penetration of the pleura, which may require elastic stains to document, is important in tumor staging (see below).

Rare adenocarcinomas with a pseudomesotheliomatous growth pattern cause a rind-like thickening of the pleura, simulating malignant mesothelioma. Immunohistochemistry (chapter 38) and electron microscopy offer approaches to distinguish these neoplasms from epithelial mesotheliomas.

MICROSCOPIC FINDINGS

Most adenocarcinomas of the lung have features indicating differentiation towards Clara cells or type 2 pneumocytes. A smaller number consist of mucinous epithelial cells, including some with goblet cell or signet ring morphology, and rare neoplasms have cells resembling fetal lung. Others demonstrate large polygonal cells with open, vesicular nuclei and large nucleoli. Histologically, four major architectural arrangements are observed: acinar, papillary, solid, and bronchioloalveolar patterns. The acinar pattern displays acini and tubules lined by cuboidal or columnar cells that may resemble bronchial epithelium,

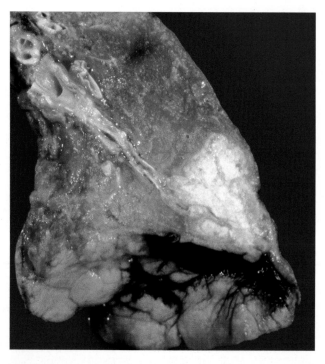

FIGURE 26-1

Adenocarcinoma

Lobectomy specimen reveals large, tan/white peripheral mass with lobulated borders adjacent to the pleura.

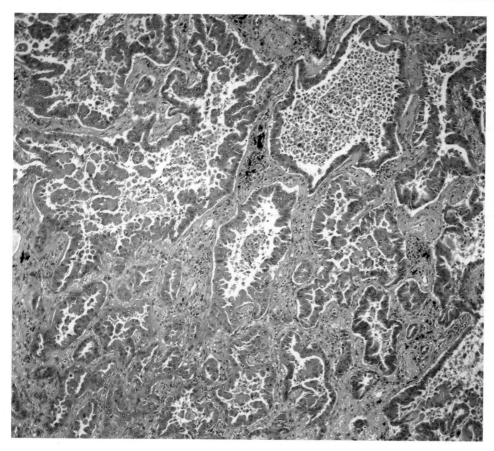

FIGURE 26-2
Adenocarcinoma
Acinar type of adenocarcinoma reveals malignant glands infiltrating through collagenous stroma.

bronchial gland cells, or Clara cells (Figure 26-2). In the papillary pattern, papillary structures with fibrovascular cores comprise the tumor (Figure 26-3). Histologic grading is performed for both acinar and papillary types and is based on the degree of gland, tubule or papillary formation; well, moderately and poorly differentiated histologic grades are used. The micropapillary pattern is less common that these four main patterns, and differs from the papillary pattern in its lack of fibrovascular cores in the papillary groups (Figure 26-4). Solid adenocarcinoma with mucin production is a common histologic subtype of adenocarcinoma and demonstrates sheets of poorly differentiated large cells that do not form acini or papillary groups, and contain stainable mucin in at least five tumor cells in two high-power fields (Figure 26-5). Most adenocarcinomas include a mixture of histologic subtypes and display cellular heterogeneity; the mixed adenocarcinoma subtype accounts for about 80% of resected adenocarcinomas. Combinations of adenocarcinoma with squamous cell carcinoma (adenosquamous carcinoma) or small cell carcinoma (combined small cell carcinoma and adenocarcinoma, considered a variant of small cell carcinoma) are also not uncommon.

ANCILLARY STUDIES

IMMUNOHISTOCHEMISTRY

Adenocarcinomas of the lung usually express thyroid transcription factor-1 (TTF-1), and cytokeratin 7. Mucinous tumors behave differently, however, and often show expression of CK7 and CK20 but not TTF-1. Adenocarcinomas of the lung also express multiple adenocarcinoma markers such as CEA, leu M1, B72.3, MOC-31, and Ber-EP4, which are helpful in differentiating them from epithelial mesotheliomas (see chapters 34 and 38).

DIFFERENTIAL DIAGNOSIS

The differential diagnosis of a malignant epithelial neoplasm in the peripheral lung or pleura frequently includes the considerations of malignant mesothelioma and metastatic adenocarcinoma. IHC is valuable for assisting in resolving the differential diagnosis, and is discussed in chapter 38. A panel approach is commonly used, including antibodies to evaluate all of the diagnostic possibilities.

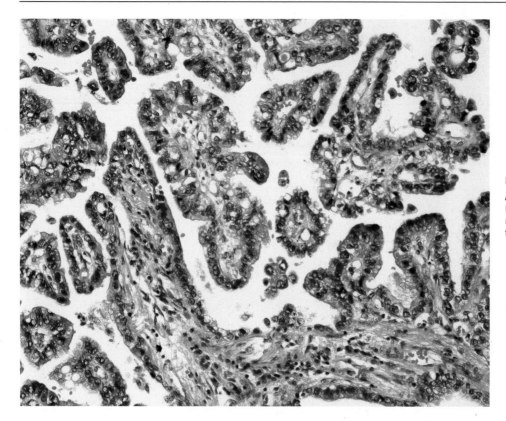

FIGURE 26-3

Adenocarcinoma
Papillary type of adenocarcinoma with neoplastic cells forming papillae with fibrovascular cores.

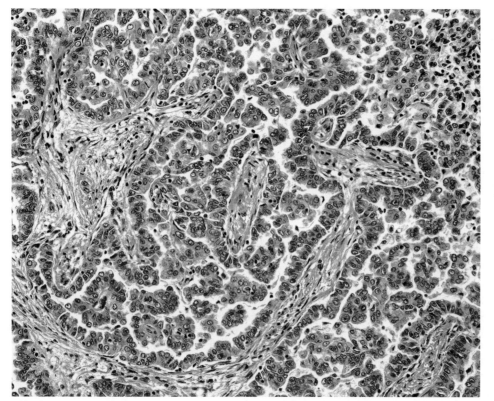

FIGURE 26-4

Adenocarcinoma
Micropapillary type of adenocarcinoma reveals small papillary clusters of neoplastic cells in glandular lumens.

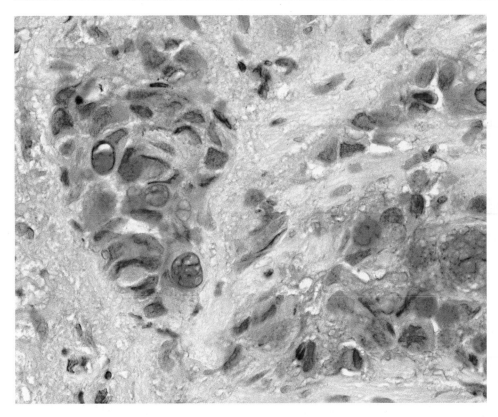

FIGURE 26-5

Adenocarcinoma
Solid type of adenocarcinoma with mucin; mucicarmine stain highlights intracellular mucin in neoplastic cells.

The results from many series suggest that calretinin, cytokeratin 5/6, and WT1 are excellent markers for identifying mesothelial differentiation, while antibodies with greater specificity for adenocarcinoma include CEA, MOC-31, Ber-EP4, and B72.3. A variety of organ-specific markers are also available that can provide information suggesting particular anatomic sites of origin for some adenocarcinomas metastatic to the lung (see chapters 29 and 38).

BRONCHIOLOALVEOLAR CARCINOMA

CLINICAL FEATURES

Bronchioloalveolar carcinoma (BAC) is a distinctive subtype of adenocarcinoma, currently defined as an *in situ* neoplasm, with a better prognosis than other NSCLCs and a weaker association with smoking. It represents less than 4% of NSCLCs.

RADIOLOGIC FEATURES

Imaging studies may demonstrate a solitary peripheral mass, multiple nodules throughout one lobe or both lungs imitating a metastatic lesion, or a pneumonic-appearing infiltrate. Mucinous BAC often has a pneumonia-like or multinodular appearance, while the nonmucinous type is more frequently a solitary mass.

PATHOLOGIC FEATURES

GROSS FINDINGS

Since BAC is, by definition, a non-invasive tumor, there is generally preservation of the outlines of the underlying architecture, although collapse and fibrosis may be present. Alveolar septa may appear thickened, and often alveolar spaces can be seen as punctate open spaces in the tan process. The mass may have irregular edges merging with the adjacent parenchyma, or may have a well demarcated nodular appearance. Satellite foci may be noted (Figure 26-6). Indentation of the pleura may be found with some BACs.

MICROSCOPIC FINDINGS

Histologically, BACs can be mucinous, nonmucinous, or a mixture of both, with the majority of cases being nonmucinous (roughly 60%). The diagnosis of BAC depends upon the observation of lepidic growth, which refers to tumor cell growth along alveolar septa. This is not an invasive growth pattern. If stromal invasion, vascular invasion, or pleural invasion is noted, then a diagnosis of BAC should not be rendered. BAC is

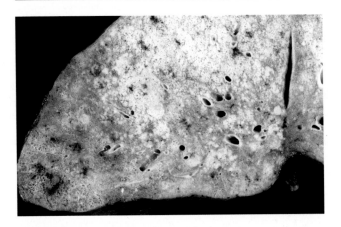

FIGURE 26-6
Bronchioloalveolar carcinoma
Lobectomy specimen with dense, grey/tan consolidation typical of bronchioloalveolar carcinoma, with satellite nodules. No necrosis is seen.

commonly seen as one pattern in an adenocarcinoma with mixed patterns. Since diagnosis of pure BAC requires exclusion of an invasive component, small biopsy specimens cannot provide this diagnosis definitively. Thorough examination of the resected cancer for foci of invasion is needed to rule out the presence of invasive tumor before a diagnosis of BAC can be established.

Cells of both mucinous and non-mucinous BAC are usually well differentiated. Nonmucinous BAC (Figure 26-7) consists of cells with features of Clara cells and/or type 2 pneumocytes growing along alveolar walls. Cells with features of Clara cells are colum-

nar or peg-shaped, with cytoplasmic snouts and eosinophilic cytoplasm. Cells with type 2 pneumocyte features are cuboidal or dome-shaped with fine cytoplasmic vacuoles, and may have an intranuclear eosinophilic inclusion. Mucinous BAC is composed of tall columnar cells with prominent cytoplasmic mucin, which typically displaces the nucleus to the base of the cell. Like non-mucinous BACs, tumor cells grow along alveolar septa, but the septa are usually thin and delicate (Figure 26-8). Alveolar spaces may contain mucin. Nuclear grade is generally low, with minimal atypia and small or absent nucleoli. This tumor is believed to have the capacity to spread aerogenously, and it often forms satellite nodules.

DIFFERENTIAL DIAGNOSIS

It is important to distinguish atypical adenomatous hyperplasia (AAH), a preinvasive lesion (see chapter 31), from nonmucinous BAC. AAH is a focal lesion usually measuring 0.5 cm or less in diameter, in which the involved alveoli and respiratory bronchioles are lined by slightly atypical cuboidal or columnar epithelial cells. In contrast to AAH, BAC typically exceeds 1 cm in size, shows stratification of cells, and displays greater degrees of cytologic atypia, nuclear pleomorphism, and crowding. Occasional lesions demonstrating features intermediate between AAH and BAC can be encountered and can be problematic. Observation of a monotonous population of atypical

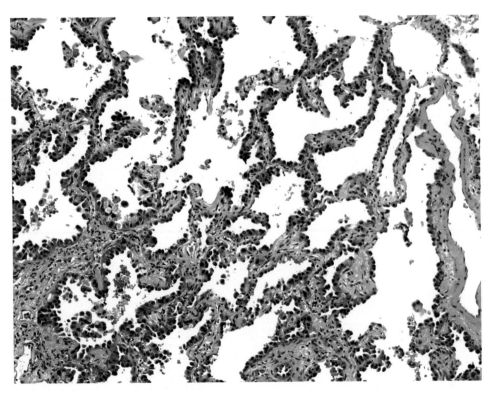

FIGURE 26-7
Bronchioloalveolar carcinoma
Non-mucinous BAC with mildly atypical cells extending along alveolar septa, with no evidence of stromal, vascular, or pleural invasion. There is preservation of the underlying pulmonary architecture.

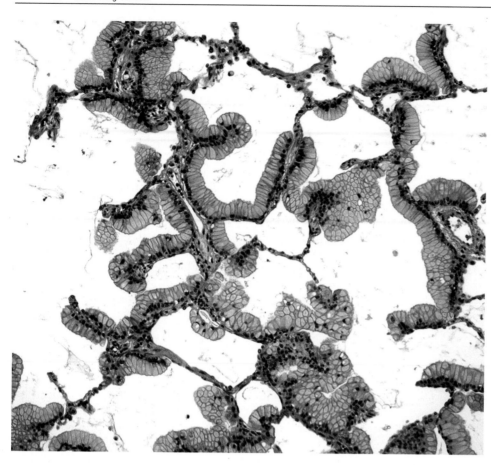

FIGURE 26-8

Bronchioloalveolar carcinoma
Mucinous BAC with tall, columnar cells with abundant mucin in cytoplasm.

BRONCHIOLOALVEOLAR CARCINOMA—FACT SHEET

Definition

▸ Distinctive type of adenocarcinoma that demonstrates lepidic growth but does not show invasion into underlying lung stroma, vasculature, or pleura (World Health Organization)

Incidence

▸ Less than 4% of NSCLCs

Clinical Features

▸ Less commonly associated with smoking than other types of NSCLC

Radiologic Features

▸ May present as a diffuse, pneumonic process, or as single or multiple nodules

---

BRONCHIOLOALVEOLAR CARCINOMA—PATHOLOGIC FEATURE

Gross Findings

▸ Single or multiple tan-white nodules or consolidation
▸ More commonly bilateral than other adenocarcinomas
▸ Mucinous type may have mucoid appearance
▸ Necrosis and hemorrhage are rare

Microscopic Findings

▸ Mucinous, non-mucinous, and mixed cell types
▸ Growth along alveolar septae (lepidic growth) is characteristic
▸ No invasion into underlying lung parenchyma, vasculature or pleura

Pathologic Differential Diagnosis

▸ Mixed adenocarcinomas with BAC components
▸ Atypical adenomatous hyperplasia
▸ Metastatic adenocarcinoma

cells favors BAC, while a heterogeneous cell population without consistent atypia favors AAH. This topic is also discussed in chapter 31.

Nonmucinous BAC must be distinguished from mixed type of adenocarcinomas . If invasion is observed in a neoplasm which also has a BAC pattern, then the diagnosis should be a mixed type of adenocarcinoma. Stromal invasion, however, can sometimes be difficult to define. A desmoplastic response with irregular glandular outlines is a helpful feature. Certainly, tumor in vascular or lymphatic spaces qualifies as evidence of invasion. Pleural invasion also requires a diagnosis of an invasive type of adenocarcinoma, as opposed to purely BAC. Solid nests of tumor which replace the normal architecture are also indicative of invasion.

Mucinous BAC may be mimicked by secondary adenocarcinoma metastatic to the lung. It is helpful to check the patient's history to reduce the likelihood of misinterpreting a metastatic adenocarcinoma as BAC.

SQUAMOUS CELL CARCINOMA

CLINICAL FEATURES

Squamous cell carcinomas (SCCs) represent approximately 30% of all NSCLCs. Their incidence has been decreasing compared to adenocarcinomas, probably due to changing smoking habits with decreasing popularity

of filterless and high-tar cigarettes. SCC is strongly linked to cigarette smoking.

RADIOLOGIC FEATURES

Most SCCs present as proximal masses in the hilum or proximal airways, and because of this proximal location, they tend to produce symptoms at an earlier stage than adenocarcinomas. Post-obstructive pneumonia is common, so patients may have symptoms of cough, hemoptysis and fever. Large tumors may produce chest pain and shortness of breath. Although SCCs may grow more quickly than other types of NSCLC, they tend to metastasize later in their course than other NSCLCs.

PATHOLOGIC FEATURES

GROSS FINDINGS

Most SCCs arise centrally from the first to third order bronchi, with fewer arising from the peripheral lung. Grossly, tumor masses are usually grayish white to yellow-tan, and necrosis and cavitation are common. The texture can be firm or gritty, and the tumor may be surrounded by areas of consolidation reflecting obstructive pneumonia. Some of the proximal tumors display an endobronchial component that may be predominant or a small part of the entire tumor (Figure 26-9). Because of their frequent central location, diagnosis is often easily accomplished by examination of sputum, bronchoalveolar lavage (BAL) fluid, bronchial brushing and washing, or endoscopic biopsy. Also, because of their central location, direct tumor invasion of adjacent hilar lymph nodes is common.

SQUAMOUS CELL CARCINOMA—FACT SHEET

Definition
➤ Epithelial tumors with squamous differentiation, manifesting varying degrees of keratinization and formation of intercellular bridges (World Health Organization)

Incidence
➤ 30% of NSCLCs
➤ Decreasing incidence compared to adenocarcinomas

Clinical Features
➤ Strong association with tobacco smoking
➤ Usually arise in the proximal airways, frequently leading to airway obstruction and development of associated complications
➤ Symptoms can include cough, hemoptysis, shortness of breath, chest pain, and constitutional symptoms
➤ Tends to metastasize later than other types of NSCLC

Radiologic Features
➤ Centrally located masses that commonly show cavitation
➤ Post-obstructive pneumonia is common

SQUAMOUS CELL CARCINOMA—PATHOLOGIC FEATURES

Gross Findings
➤ Proximal airway masses that often include an endobronchial component
➤ Gray/white to yellow/tan masses that often show necrosis and cavitation
➤ Direct extension into adjacent hilar lymph nodes is common

Microscopic Findings
➤ Keratinization and keratin pearl formation
➤ Intercellular bridges
➤ Subtypes: papillary, clear cell, small cell, basaloid

Pathologic Differential Diagnosis
➤ Small cell carcinoma
➤ Basaloid variant of large cell carcinoma
➤ Squamous cell carcinoma in situ

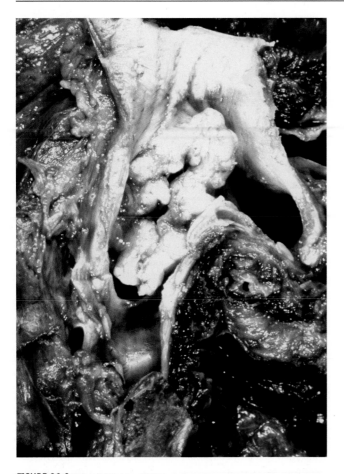

FIGURE 26-9

Squamous cell carcinoma
This tumor forms an exophytic mass that obstructs the mainstem bronchus.

MICROSCOPIC FINDINGS

SCC is a malignant epithelial tumor with features of squamous differentiation, including keratinization and/or intercellular bridges. It is graded as well differentiated if these features are prominent (Figure 26-10), moderately differentiated if they are easily seen but not extensive, and poorly differentiated if the features are focal. Keratinization can take the form of squamous pearls or individual cells with markedly eosinophilic dense cytoplasm. Squamous cell carcinoma *in situ* can be seen in airway mucosa adjacent to the invasive tumor.

Histological variants of SCC include papillary, clear cell, small cell, and basaloid variants. Papillary SCCs form exophytic lesions, usually well differentiated, that can demonstrate invasion at their bases. The clear cell variant consists primarily of cells with clear cytoplasm. The small cell variant is a poorly differentiated SCC comprised of small tumor cells with focal squamous differentiation, which lack the characteristic nuclear features of small cell carcinoma and usually have more cytoplasm. The basaloid variant has evidence of squamous differentiation and shows prominent peripheral palisading of nuclei.

DIFFERENTIAL DIAGNOSIS

Although diagnosis of SCC is usually straightforward, there are several potentially challenging scenarios. Distinction of papillary SCC from a squamous papilloma can be difficult, and may not be achievable on a small

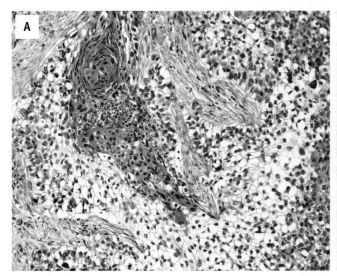
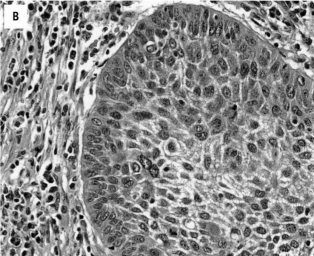

FIGURE 26-10

Squamous cell carcinoma
(A) This tumor demonstrates keratin pearl formation. (B) Intercellular bridges are present and there is peripheral palisading.

biopsy. The degree of cytologic atypia is important for making this distinction. SCC in situ can extend into bronchial glands, which can be potentially misconstrued as invasion. Small cell SCCs share the feature of small cell size and relatively scant cytoplasm with small cell carcinomas, but demonstrate differing nuclear features and immunohistochemical reactivities. Small cell carcinomas have fine chromatin and nuclear molding, features that are not characteristic of small cell SCCs. Also, many small cell SCCs stain for high molecular weight keratin and p63, but not TTF-1, while the opposite immunoreactivities are found in small cell carcinomas. The basaloid variant of large cell carcinoma may be considered in the differential diagnosis for some SCCs, but does not show squamous differentiation.

ADENOSQUAMOUS CARCINOMA

CLINICAL AND RADIOLOGIC FEATURES

Adenosquamous carcinomas account for between 0.4 and 4% of lung carcinomas and occur primarily in smokers. The WHO has defined them as carcinomas showing both squamous cell carcinoma and adenocarcinoma components, with each comprising at least 10%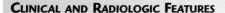

of the tumor. They usually form peripheral lung masses and may demonstrate a central scar.

PATHOLOGIC FEATURES

GROSS FINDINGS

Most adenosquamous carcinomas are firm, tan peripheral masses and some have a central scar.

MICROSCOPIC FINDINGS

According to the WHO definition, adenocarcinoma and squamous cell carcinoma must each account for at least 10% of the tumor. Microscopic features associated with adenocarcinoma and squamous cell carcinoma (Figure 26-11) are discussed in those sections of this chapter.

DIFFERENTIAL DIAGNOSIS

There are several differential diagnostic considerations. Mucoepidermoid carcinoma (chapter 28) is one entity that may occasionally present a differential diagnostic problem, since it includes cells with squamous and

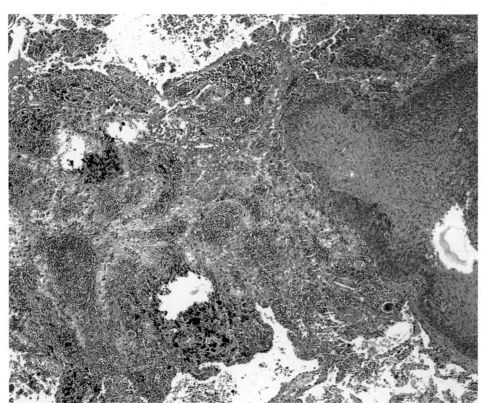

Figure 26-11
Adenosquamous carcinoma
Malignant glandular epithelium (left) and malignant squamous epithelium (right) characterize this adenosquamous carcinoma.

ADENOSQUAMOUS CARCINOMA—FACT SHEET

Definition

▸ A carcinoma in which squamous cell carcinoma and adenocarcinoma each comprise at least 10% of the tumor (World Health Organization)

Incidence

▸ Less than 4% of all lung cancers

Clinical Features

▸ Similar clinical presentation to adenocarcinoma
▸ Most patients are smokers

Radiologic Features

▸ Peripheral lung mass

ADENOSQUAMOUS CARCINOMA—PATHOLOGIC FEATURES

Gross Findings

▸ Peripheral tan-white lung mass
▸ May be associated with a scar

Microscopic Findings

▸ Squamous cell carcinoma and adenocarcinoma have features as described in these sections of this chapter

Pathologic Differential Diagnosis

▸ Mucoepidermoid carcinoma
▸ Adenocarcinoma or squamous cell carcinoma with entrapped benign cellular elements
▸ Adenocarcinoma or squamous cell carcinoma with focal squamous or glandular differentiation, respectively

---

glandular differentiation. If one observes low-grade mucoepidermoid carcinoma histology in a portion of the tumor, then it supports classifying the high-grade component as a high-grade mucoepidermoid carcinoma. Low-grade mucoepidermoid carcinoma is generally easier to separate from adenosquamous carcinoma due to its characteristic cell composition and arrangements of cells, and its usual lack of significant cytoatypia. Mucoepidermoid carcinomas are also usually centrally located, in contrast to the usually peripheral location of adenosquamous carcinoma. In addition, squamous carcinoma in situ can be found in the mucosa adjacent to some adenosquamous carcinomas, but is not observed with mucoepidermoid carcinomas.

A second situation that may be considered in the differential diagnosis of adenosquamous carcinoma is that of entrapment of benign cellular elements by the carcinoma. A squamous cell carcinoma that entraps benign bronchial glands, or an adenocarcinoma that entraps metaplastic squamous epithelium, could occasionally resemble an adenosquamous carcinoma.

The third set of considerations include adenocarcinomas with focal (< 10%) squamous differentiation and squamous cell carcinoma with focal (< 10%) glandular differentiation (gland formation or mucin-positivity). These tumors should not be classified as adenosquamous carcinomas, since they do not meet the WHO definition, but should instead by interpretated as squamous cell carcinoma or adenocarcinoma as appropriate.

LARGE CELL CARCINOMA

CLINICAL AND RADIOLOGIC FEATURES

Large cell carcinoma (LCC) is an undifferentiated carcinoma consisting of large epithelial cells lacking evidence of squamous or glandular differentiation, accounting for approximately 10% of all lung cancers in many series. It is strongly associated with cigarette smoking. The lesion tends to occur in the periphery of the lung and grows rapidly. Like most other NSCLCs, it usually presents at a late stage, resulting in a poor outcome.

On imaging studies, LCCs are typically large masses in the periphery of the lung. Basaloid carcinomas, however, tend to be more centrally located. Evidence of pleural or chest wall invasion can be found in some cases, and hilar or mediastinal lymphadenopathy can sometimes be appreciated.

PATHOLOGIC FEATURES

GROSS FINDINGS

Grossly, LCCs are often larger than 4 cm in size and have a white to gray or fish-flesh cut appearance. Gross tumor necrosis is common.

MICROSCOPIC FINDINGS

LCC is essentially a diagnosis of exclusion made based on the observation of large cells that do not show differentiation to support diagnoses of squamous cell carcinoma, adenocarcinoma, or small cell carcinoma (Figure 26-12). Small biopsy specimens are not adequate to definitively assign this diagnosis, and are usually interpreted as poorly differentiated NSCLC. Ex-amination of the subsequent resection specimen, however, allows for confident determination of the diagnosis of large cell carcinoma. In general, LCC cells display large cell size, large vesicular nuclei, prominent nucleoli, and a moderate amount of cytoplasm. They are typically arranged in sheets or large nests, frequently revealing areas of necrosis.

Several subtypes of LCC have been recognized by the WHO, including large cell neuroendocrine carcinoma

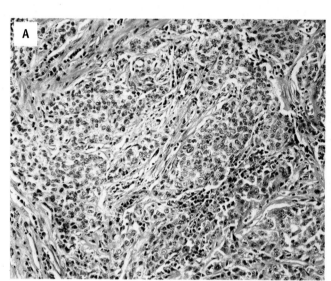 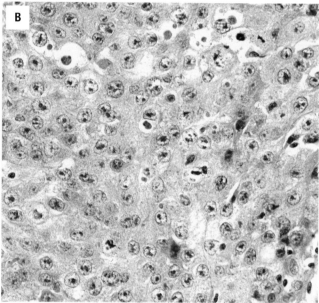

FIGURE 26-12

Large cell carcinoma
(A) This tumor consists of sheets of neoplastic cells with associated lymphocytic infiltrates. **(B)** Tumor cells are large with abundant cytoplasm and prominent nucleoli, and show no evidence of squamous or glandular differentiation.

LARGE CELL CARCINOMA—FACT SHEET

Definition
▸ Undifferentiated non-small cell carcinoma without evidence of glandular or squamous differentiation (World Health Organization)

Incidence
▸ Approximately 10% of all lung cancers

Clinical Features
▸ Similar to other NSCLCs

Radiologic Features
▸ Mass usually larger than 4 cm
▸ Most cases are peripheral lung masses
▸ Basaloid variant of LCC tends to be centrally located
▸ Mediastinal adenopathy and pneumonia may be present

LARGE CELL CARCINOMA—PATHOLOGIC FEATURES

Gross Findings
▸ Mass with white/gray or fish-flesh cut appearance
▸ Necrosis is common

Microscopic Findings
▸ Large cells with abundant cytoplasm and prominent nucleoli, in sheets or nests
▸ Variants:
  ▸ Large cell neuroendocrine carcinoma
  ▸ Basaloid carcinoma
  ▸ Lymphoepithelioma-like carcinoma
  ▸ Clear cell carcinoma
  ▸ Large cell carcinoma with rhabdoid phenotype

Pathologic Differential Diagnosis
▸ Other poorly-differentiated NSCLCs
▸ Basaloid variant of squamous cell carcinoma

(see chapter 27), basaloid carcinoma, lymphoepithelioma-like carcinoma, clear cell carcinoma, and large cell carcinoma with rhabdoid phenotype. Basaloid carcinoma is an uncommon LCC with features resembling cutaneous basal cell carcinoma. Most of these tumors develop in proximal bronchi, and an endobronchial component is often present. Morphologically, they have lobular, trabecular, or palisading growth patterns, often with foci of comedo-type necrosis (Figure 26-13). These tumors consist of small monomorphic cells with a cuboidal or fusiform shape, dense, hyperchromatic nuclei, scant cytoplasm, and a high mitotic rate. Intercellular bridges and individual cell keratinization are absent, as is nuclear molding. Other commonly observed features include rosettes, hyalin or mucoid stroma and small cystic spaces in tumor cell nests, similar again to cutaneous basal cell carcinomas.

Lymphoepithelioma-like carcinoma of the lung, a variant of LCC, resembles its nasopharyngeal counterpart, and consists of large tumor cells with vesicular nuclei and prominent nucleoli, growing in a syncytial pattern with abundant lymphocytic infiltration. Epstein-Barr virus can be found in the tumor cells by performing EBER-1 in situ hybridization. Clear cell carcinoma displays prominent clear or foamy cytoplasm that may contain glycogen. Large cell carcinoma with rhabdoid phenotype is a rare variant of LCC in which at least 10 % of tumor cells have

a rhabdoid appearance, with eosinophilic globules in the cytoplasm. The globules are intermediate filaments that may stain with vimentin or cytokeratin.

ANCILLARY STUDIES

LCCs commonly express cytokeratin, and over half may express TTF-1 and cytokeratin 7. Expression of neuroendocrine markers is usually lacking, which is helpful in distinguishing the basaloid variant of LCC from small cell carcinoma and large cell neuroendocrine carcinoma. Ultrastructural analysis of LCCs often shows squamous, glandular, or neuroendocrine features.

DIFFERENTIAL DIAGNOSIS

The differential diagnosis includes other poorly differentiated NSCLCs, but this is usually relatively easily dealt with if one applies the diagnostic criteria. Basaloid carcinoma may occasionally be difficult to distinguish from small cell carcinoma, large cell neuroendocrine carcinoma, and poorly differentiated squamous cell carcinoma, particularly the small cell variant. The presence

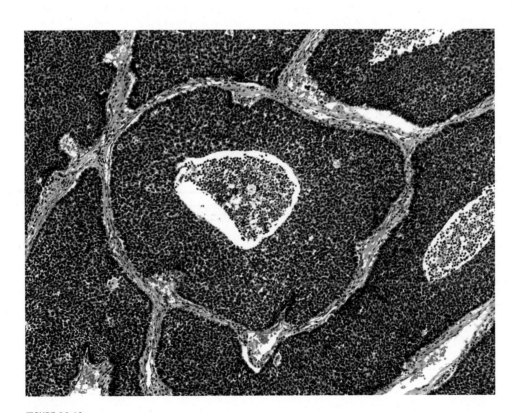

FIGURE 26-13

Basaloid carcinoma
This tumor displays nests of small cells with a palisading growth pattern, surrounding centrally located foci of comedo-type necrosis.

SARCOMATOID CARCINOMA—FACT SHEET

Definition

» A group of NSCLCs that contain a component of sarcoma or sarcoma-like differentiation (World Health Organization)

Incidence

» Uncommon or rare neoplasms, accounting for approximately 1% of lung cancers

Clinical Features

» Most commonly found in elderly patients
» Most patients have history of smoking

Radiologic Features

» Central or peripheral lung masses

SARCOMATOID CARCINOMA—PATHOLOGIC FEATURES

Gross Findings

» Tan or pink lung masses, often with necrosis or hemorrhage, that may reach a large size
» Rarely present as endobronchial polypoid masses

Microscopic Findings

» Spectrum of histologies that include a sarcoma or sarcoma-like element
» Subtypes
  » Pleomorphic carcinoma
  » Spindle cell carcinoma
  » Giant cell carcinoma
  » Carcinosarcoma
  » Pulmonary blastoma

Pathologic Differential Diagnosis

» Primary pulmonary sarcomas
» Metastatic sarcomatoid carcinomas and sarcomas

---

of fine chromatin, nuclear molding, and expression of neuroendocrine markers favor a diagnosis of small cell carcinoma over basaloid carcinoma, however. Large cell neuroendocrine carcinoma also demonstrates immunohistochemical evidence of neuroendocrine differentiation, which is helpful for separating it from basaloid carcinoma. Small cell variant of squamous cell carcinoma should show some squamous features, which will help to distinguish it from the basaloid variant of LCC.

SARCOMATOID CARCINOMA

CLINICAL FEATURES

Sarcomatoid carcinoma is defined by the World Health Organization as a category of NSCLCs with sarcoma or sarcoma-like differentiation. They are an infrequent type of NSCLC, representing approximately 1% of all lung cancers. These tumors are more common in men than women and tend to develop in older adults (mean age, 60 years), except for the pulmonary blastoma which does not show a gender predilection and affects patients

in their middle age and older years. Symptomatology is related to tumor location, with central tumors often causing development of cough, hemoptysis, and other post-obstructive pneumonia symptoms, while peripheral tumors may declare themselves with chest pain due to pleural or chest wall invasion.

RADIOLOGIC FEATURES

Tumors form central or peripheral lung masses, and may grow to very large size. Necrosis and cavitation may be noted.

PATHOLOGIC FEATURES

GROSS FINDINGS

Macroscopic features of sarcomatoid carcinomas vary. Peripheral tumors can be quite large, frequently more than 5 cm in diameter. Cut surfaces are often tan with hemorrhage and necrosis. Some examples of sarcomatoid carcinoma grow as endobronchial, polypoid masses.

MICROSCOPIC FINDINGS

These tumors encompass a spectrum of morphologies and include components of sarcoma or sarcoma-like (spindle or giant cell) neoplastic elements. Pleomorphic carcinomas have a component of NSCLC (SCC, adenocarcinoma, or large cell carcinoma) admixed with a spindle or giant cell component, the latter comprising at least 10% of the tumor. The spindle cells can have an epithelioid or mesenchymal appearance, fascicular or storiform arrangement, and fibrotic or myxoid stroma. Malignant giant cells with pleomorphic nuclei can likewise vary in their appearances, but are often dyscohesive. Spindle cell carcinoma is comprised solely of malignant spindle cells similar to those described for pleomorphic carcinoma (Figure 26-14). Inflammatory infiltrates may accompany the spindle cells in some cases. Giant cell carcinoma consists entirely of markedly pleomorphic, bizarre, often dyscohesive tumor giant cells with single or multiple hyperchromatic nuclei (Figure 26-15). Unlike pleomorphic carcinoma, a conventional NSCLC component is absent. Inflammation is frequently present, with emperipolesis. Carcinosarcoma is a biphasic tumor comprised of carcinomatous and sarcomatous elements. The former is most often a squamous cell carcinoma, and less often an adenocarcinoma or large cell carcinoma. Some cases will demonstrate features of a high-grade fetal adenocarcinoma. The sarcomatous component is a differentiated sarcoma such as a chondrosarcoma, osteosarcoma, or rhabdomyosarcoma.

Pulmonary blastoma is also a biphasic tumor in which the epithelial and mesenchymal constituents have a primitive appearance. The epithelial component may resemble well differentiated fetal adenocarcinoma, with tubules lined by cells with sub- or supranuclear vacuoles, similar to endometrial glands. The vacuoles represent glycogen accumulations that are PAS-positive. Squamoid morulae similar to those of fetal adenocarcinoma may also be present. Stromal cells are undifferentiated and blastema-like, with condensation around neoplastic glands. More mature sarcomatous elements can also be seen in some cases.

ANCILLARY STUDIES

Immunohistochemical stains for cytokeratin and EMA are usually positive in the epithelial components of the tumors, and often stain the spindle and giant cells as well. Some giant cell carcinomas will also express TTF-1 and other adenocarcinoma markers, and the fetal adenocarcinoma portion of pulmonary blastomas may also stain for neuroendocrine markers and an array of hormonal peptides. Differentiated sarcoma components usually stain as expected for the type of differentiation observed, i.e., rhabdomyosarcoma with muscle markers. The blastemal cells of blastomas general express vimentin and muscle-specific actin.

PROGNOSIS AND TREATMENT OF LUNG CARCINOMAS

Stage and performance status are the most important prognostic factors for patients with lung neoplasms, and pathologists play an important role in determining an accurate stage from resected specimens. Separate staging systems exist for non-small cell and small cell lung carcinomas.

The staging system of the American Joint Commission on Cancer (AJCC) is widely used for clinical and pathologic staging of patients with NSCLCs (Table 26-2). The "T" refers to a primary tumor that has not been previously treated, "N" refers to lymph node status, and "M" to metastatic disease status. Approximate survival for stages 1-4 NSCLC is as follows:

Stage 1: 60-80%
Stage 2: 25-50%
Stage 3: 10-40%
Stage 4: 5%

Surgical resection is recommended for most patient with Stage 1 and 2 tumors, and adjuvant chemotherapy may be given for Stage 1B and 2. Radiation therapy is an alternative treatment for patients with Stage 1 or 2 disease who are not candidates for surgery. For Stage 3A NSCLCs, neo-adjuvant chemotherapy can be given, followed by surgical resection. Stage 3B NSCLCs are treated with radiation therapy and chemotherapy, and Stage 4 disease is treated similarly with the intent of palliation. Staging and treatment of small cell carcinomas are discussed in chapter 27.

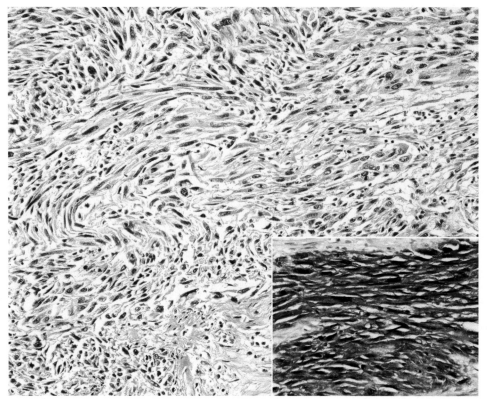

FIGURE 26-14

Spindle cell carcinoma
Spindle cell carcinoma with atypical sarcomatoid cells with immunoreactivity to pan-cytokeratin antibody (insert).

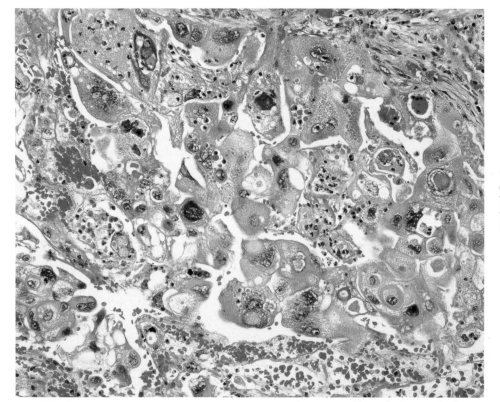

FIGURE 26-15

Giant cell carcinoma
This tumor consists of pleomorphic cells with abundant eosinophilic cytoplasm and a dyscohesive appearance.

TABLE 26-2

American Joint Commission on Cancer
Lung Cancer Staging

PRIMARY TUMOR (T)

TX	Primary tumor cannot be assessed, or tumor proven by presence of malignant cells in sputum or bronchial washings but not visualized by imaging or bronchoscopy
T0	No evidence of primary tumor
Tis	Carcinoma in situ
T1	Tumor 3 cm or less in greatest dimension, surrounded by lung or visceral pleura, without bronchoscopic evidence of invasion more proximal than the lobar bronchus (i.e., not in the main bronchus)
T2	Tumor with any of the following features of size or extent: ▸▸ More than 3 cm in greatest dimension ▸▸ Involves main bronchus, 2 cm or more distal to the carina ▸▸ Invades the visceral pleura ▸▸ Associated with atelectasis or obstructive pneumonitis that extends to the hilar region but does not involve the entire lung
T3	Tumor of any size that directly invades chest wall (including superior sulcus tumors), diaphragm, mediastinal pleura, or parietal pericardium **or** Tumor of any size in the main bronchus less than 2 cm distal to the carina but without involvement of the carina **or** Tumor of any size associated atelectasis or obstructive pneumonitis of the entire lung
T4	Tumor of any size that invades mediastinum, heart, great vessels, trachea, esophagus, vertebral body, or carina **or** Tumor of any size with separate tumor nodule(s) in same lobe **or** Tumor of any size with a malignant pleural effusion

REGIONAL LYMPH NODES (N)

NX	Regional lymph nodes cannot be assessed
N0	No regional lymph node metastasis
N1	Metastasis in ipsilateral peribronchial and/or ipsilateral hilar lymph nodes, including intrapulmonary nodes involved by direct extension of the primary tumor
N2	Metastasis in ipsilateral mediastinal and/or subcarinal lymph node(s)
N3	Metastasis in contralateral mediastinal, contralateral hilar, ipsilateral or contralateral scalene, or supraclavicular lymph node(s)

DISTANT METASTASIS (M)

MX	Distant metastasis cannot be assessed
M0	No distant metastasis
M1	Distant metastasis; includes separate tumor nodule(s) in a different lobe (ipsilateral or contralateral)

TNM STAGE GROUPINGS

Occult	TX	N0	M0
Stage 0	Tis	N0	M0
Stage IA	T1	N0	M0
Stage IB	T2	N0	M0
Stage IIA	T1	N1	M0
Stage IIB	T2	N1	M0
	T3	N0	M0
Stage IIIA	T1	N2	M0
	T2	N2	M0
	T3	N1	M0
	T3	N2	M0
Stage IIIB	Any T	N3	M0
	T4	Any N	M0
Stage IV	Any T	Any N	M1

Based on Greene FL, Page DL, Fleming ID, et al. *AJCC Cancer Staging Handbook*. Sixth edition. New York: Springer Verlag; 2002, p. 171.

SUGGESTED READINGS

1. American Cancer Society. *Cancer Facts and Figures*. Atlanta, GA: The Society, 2005.
2. Jemal A, Murray T, Samuels A, et al. Cancer statistics, 2003. *CA Cancer J Clin*. 2003;53:5-26.
3. Battafarano RJ, Meyers BF, Guthrie TJ, et al. Surgical resection of multifocal non-small cell lung cancer is associated with prolonged survival. *Ann Thorac Surg*. 2002;74:988-93.
4. Bejarano PA, Baughman RP, Biddinger PW, et al: Surfactant proteins and thyroid transcription factor-1 in pulmonary and breast carcinomas. *Mod Pathol*. 1995;9:445-52.
5. Bradley JD, Dehdashti F, Mintun MA, et al. Positron emission tomography in limited-stage small-cell lung cancer: a prospective study. *J Clin Oncol*. 2004;22:3248-54.
6. Brambilla E, Moro D, Veale D, et al. Basal cell (basaloid) carcinoma of the lung: a new morphologic and phenotypic entity with separate prognostic significance. *Hum Pathol*. 1992;23;993-1003.
7. Chapman AD, Kerr KM. The association between atypical adenomatous hyperplasia and primary lung cancer. *Br J Cancer*. 2000;83:632-6.
8. Colby TV, Koss MN, Travis WD. *Tumors of the Lower Respiratory Tract*. Atlas of tumor pathology, fasc. 13. Washington, D.C.: Armed Force Institute of Pathology , under the auspices of Universities Associated for Research and Education in Pathology, 1995.
9. Detterbeck FC, DeCamp MM Jr, Kohman LJ, et al. Lung cancer. Invasive staging: the guidelines. *Chest*. 2003;123:167S-75S.
10. Doll R, Peto R. Cigarette smoking and bronchial carcinoma: dose and time relationships among regular smokers and lifelong non-smokers. *J Epidemiol Community Health*. 1978;32:303-13.
11. Gajra A, Newman N, Gamble GP, et al. Impact of tumor size on survival in stage IA non-small cell lung cancer: a case for subdividing stage IA disease. *Lung Cancer*. 2003;42:51-7.
12. Goldstein NS, Thomas M. Mucinous and nonmucinous bronchioloalveolar adenocarcinomas have distinct staining patterns with thyroid transcription factor and cytokeratin 20 antibodies. *Am J Clin Pathol*. 2001;116:319-25.
13. Greene FL, Page DL, Fleming ID, et al. *AJCC Cancer Staging Handbook*. Sixth edition. New York: Springer Verlag; 2002.
14. Mori M, Rao SK, Popper HH, Cagle PT, Fraire AE. Atypical adenomatous hyperplasia of the lung: a probable forerunner in the development of adenocarcinoma of lung. *Mod Pathol*. 2001;14:72-84.
15. Mountain CF. Staging classification of lung cancer. A critical evaluation. *Clin Chest Med*. 2002;23:103-21.
16. Oliveira AM, Tazelaar HD, Myers FL, et al. Thyroid transcription factor-1 distinguishes metastatic pulmonary from well-differentiated neuroendocrine tumors of other sites. *Am J Surg Pathol*. 2001;25:815–9.
17. Travis WD, Brambilla E, Muller-Hermelink HK, et al., eds. *Pathology and Genetics. Tumours of the Lung, Pleura, Thymus and Heart*. World Health Organization Classification of Tumours. Lyon: IARC Press, 2004.
18. Wisnivesky JP, Yankelevitz D, Henschke CI. The effect of tumor size on curability of stage I non-small cell lung cancers. *Chest*. 2004;126:761-5.
19. Yatabe Y, Mitsudomi T, Takahashi T. TTF-1 expression in pulmonary adenocarcinomas. *Am J Surg Pathol*. 2002;26:767-73.
20. Zhang H, Liu J, Cagle PT, Allen TC, Laga AC, Zander DS. Distinction of pulmonary small cell carcinoma from poorly differentiated squamous cell carcinoma: an immunohistochemical approach. *Mod Pathol*. 2005;18:111-8.

27 Neuroendocrine Neoplasms

Elisabeth Brambilla • Sylvie Lantuejoul

- Introduction
- Small Cell Lung Carcinoma
- Carcinoid Tumors
- Large Cell Neuroendocrine Carcinoma
- Non-Small Cell Lung Carcinoma with Neuroendocrine Features

INTRODUCTION

Neuroendocrine neoplasms include a spectrum of malignant neoplasms ranging from relatively low-grade malignancies (typical carcinoid tumors) to high-grade malignancies (small cell carcinoma, large cell neuroendocrine carcinoma) that are among the most aggressive primary lung neoplasms. Over the last decade, the individual diagnostic categories have become better defined histologically; the most recent version of the World Health Organization (WHO) classification system is the current standard for histological diagnosis of these neoplasms. Areas of current and future investigation related to these neoplasms include determination of optimal therapeutic approaches and predictors of prognosis.

SMALL CELL LUNG CARCINOMA

Small cell lung carcinoma (SCLC) is defined by the World Health Organization as a "malignant epithelial tumor consisting of small cells with scant cytoplasm, ill-defined cell borders, finely granular nuclear chromatin, and absent or inconspicuous nucleoli." In 2007, an estimated 28,000 cases will occur in the U.S., representing about 12% of all lung cancers. SCLC is an aggressive lung cancer that often responds to chemotherapy and radiation therapy to extend life, but current treatment regimens do not produce a cure.

CLINICAL FEATURES

SCLC occurs in adults between 40 and 70 years of age and is highly linked to tobacco smoking. The tumor commonly presents in a central location, arising from a major bronchus. Clinical symptoms are related to the proximal location, with rapid spread to regional lymph nodes and the mediastinum. Stridor, hemoptysis, hoarseness, and vocal cord paralysis are common. SCLC is the primary cause of the superior vena cava syndrome. Metastases to distant locations occur early in the course of the disease in SCLC. Therefore, a majority of patients present with advanced stage disease. Because of this, the TNM system is less useful than the 2-stage system, which includes limited-stage disease (LD) and extensive-stage disease (ED). Limited-stage disease is usually defined as disease confined to one hemithorax, including ipsilateral and/or contralateral hilar, mediastinal and supraclavicular nodal involvement. Metastatic disease is most commonly found in the bones, bone marrow, liver and brain. Paraneoplastic syndromes are commonly associated with this neoplasm, to a greater extent than with large cell neuroendocrine carcinoma (LCNEC).

RADIOLOGIC FEATURES

Although the primary tumor is often not detected on chest radiograph, SCLC appears as a hilar or perihilar mass with mediastinal lymphadenopathy and lobar collapse on chest computed tomography (CT). A minority of cases present as peripheral masses that cannot be radiographically distinguished from other pulmonary malignancies.

PATHOLOGIC FEATURES

GROSS FINDINGS

Perihilar tumoral masses have a white-tan, soft, friable appearance and show extensive necrosis and nodal involvement. Lymphatic spread occurs along bronchovascular bundles in a sheet-like fashion and along interlobular septa, which can be grossly visible. Only 5 % of SCLCs present as peripheral coin lesions.

MICROSCOPIC FINDINGS

Sheet-like growth without a neuroendocrine (NE) architectural arrangement is the most frequent presentation, although trabeculae, peripheral palisading, and rosette formation may be seen (Figure 27-1A). Tumor cells are usually less than the size of three small lymphocytes in diameter. They have round, ovoid, or spindle-shaped nuclei. Nuclear chromatin is typically finely granular with a "salt and pepper" appearance. Nucleoli are absent or inconspicuous. The nuclear-to-cytoplasmic ratio is very high, and, there is frequent nuclear molding and undefined cell borders (Figure 27-1B). The mitotic rate is extremely high (average 60 mitoses per 10 high-power fields/2 mm²). Crush artifact is frequent due to the absence of protection by stromal tissue.

VARIANT

COMBINED SMALL CELL LUNG CARCINOMA

Combined small cell lung carcinoma is the only variant of SCLC. It presents as an admixture of SCLC with a non-small cell lung carcinoma (NSCLC) component that may be squamous cell carcinoma, adenocarcinoma, large cell carcinoma, or LCNEC (Figure 27-1C). The most frequent combination is with LCNEC, whereas an association with spindle cell or giant cell carcinoma (sarcomatoid carcinoma) is rare. For the diagnosis of combined small cell carcinoma to be assessed, at least 10 % of each SCLC and NSCLC constituent is required.

ANCILLARY STUDIES

ULTRASTRUCTURAL FEATURES

Of all NE lung carcinomas, SCLC has the lowest frequency of neurosecretory granules in the cell cytoplasm, with about 20 % having no intracytoplasmic neurosecretory granules. In both the combined variant and the pure form of SCLC, ultrastructural features of glandular and/or squamous differentiation can be seen.

IMMUNOHISTOCHEMISTRY

A vast majority of SCLCs are positive for at least one NE marker. These are, in order of frequency, CD56/NCAM, synaptophysin, and chromogranin. More than 90 % of cases, even on small biopsies, display one or several of these markers. Eighty-five percent of SCLCs express TTF-1 with a nuclear pattern of staining. The cytokeratins 1, 5, 10, and 14, recognized by the antibody CK34βE12, are not expressed in classical pure cases, but can be demonstrated as positive in the admixed NSCLC component in combined SCLC cases. Some studies have reported c-kit (CD117) expression.

FINE NEEDLE ASPIRATION BIOPSY

Fine needle aspiration biopsy and core needle biopsy can provide excellent material for diagnosis of SCLC because the diagnosis is based upon the cytological features of SCLC, while architecture is not critical for the diagnosis. Observation of a small cell proliferation, with nuclear molding, a very high nuclear-to-cytoplasmic ratio, and the "salt and pepper" quality of the chromatin are extremely useful features to rely upon to make this diagnosis on FNA. Performance of immunohistochemistry for NE markers, TTF-1, and CK34βE12 can be of aid for making the diagnosis of SCLC on FNA nspecimens.

CYTOLOGY

Other cytologic specimens are also very useful for diagnosis of SCLC (see also chapter 37). Sputum and bronchoscopic specimens show loose and irregular or syncytial clusters of small cells with nuclear molding, frequent mitoses, and the typical "salt and pepper" chromatin. Inconspicuous nucleoli are usual. Due to the fragility of the malignant nuclei, "chromatin streaks" are commonly seen in smears.

DIFFERENTIAL DIAGNOSIS

The differential diagnosis includes other NE tumors, other small cell tumors, and NSCLCs, especially when crush artifact is present that overshadows the diagnostic criteria. Lymphoid infiltrates (inflammatory or neoplastic) are distinguished by a lack of staining for cytokeratin, NE markers, and TTF-1 vs. staining for CD45 and specific cluster differentiation markers (CD 3, 5, 20). Carcinoids are rarely misdiagnosed as SCLC except on small biopsies (bronchial or FNA). This distinction is most difficult when crush artifact is present. NE

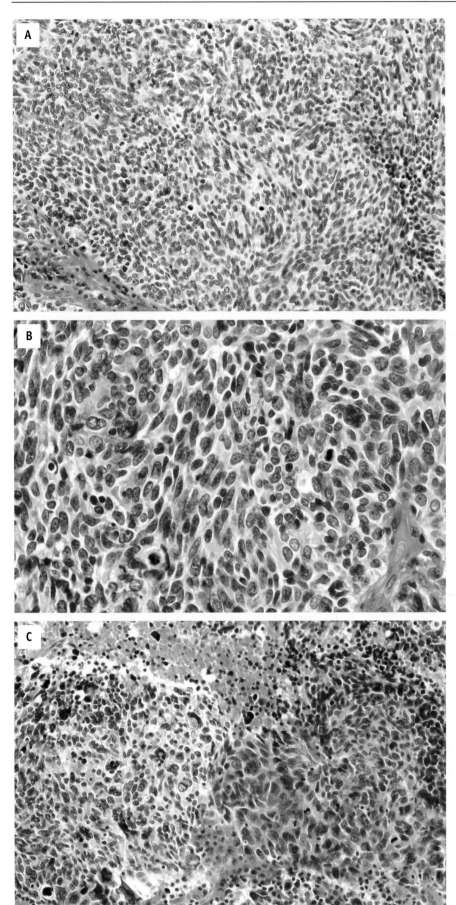

FIGURE 27-1

Small cell carcinoma

(A) Sheets of neoplastic small cells have replaced the normal lung tissue. (B) The cells have a high nuclear-to-cytoplasmic ratio, fine nuclear chromatin, no obvious nucleoli, and mitoses. (C) Small cell lung carcinoma (left) combined with large cell carcinoma (right).

markers are not helpful for distinguishing carcinoids and tumorlets from SCLC, but TTF-1 is typically negative in tumorlets and carcinoids and positive in SCLC. The presence of high mitotic activity is not compatible with the diagnosis of carcinoid, and carcinoids usually demonstrate less nuclear pleomorphism and more, better preserved cytoplasm than SCLC. Necrosis is also much more common in SCLC than carcinoid; in the latter, it is only seen in the occasional atypical carcinoid.

Primitive neuroectodermal tumors (PNETs) may also be considered in the differential diagnosis, but show larger cells, a lower nuclear-to-cytoplasmic ratio, and more loosely-arranged cells. In addition, PNETs are positive for MIC-2 (CD99). 5 % of PNETs show cytokeratin expression and TTF-1 is consistently negative.

Morphologic separation of SCLC from NSCLC is difficult in tissue preparations with small tumor representation, suboptimal tumor cell preservation, or when crush artifact is present. LCNEC is the most difficult differential diagnosis with SCLC. LCNEC is distinct from SCLC based on architectural criteria, large cell size, and vesicular nuclei with conspicuous nucleoli. LCNEC shares with SCLC the NE markers and TTF-1 positivity, large areas of necrosis, and a high mitotic count. A continuum of cell size, nuclear-to-cytoplasmic ratio, and nuclear/chromatin feature is seen in a proportion of high-grade NE tumors (about 10 %). In these cases, the diagnostic dilemma may be solved by the diagnosis of SCLC combined with a LCNEC component. Basaloid carcinoma, similar to SCLC, presents with a small, rather monomorphic cell proliferation, but display a well-defined lobular pattern (Figure 27-2A). The use of specific markers is of great help since basaloid carcinoma lacks reactivity for any NE differentiation markers and for TTF-1, but expresses the cytokeratin 1, 5, 10, 14 (recognized by

the antibody 34βE12) (Figure 27-2B). Other NSCLCs of small cell size, such as some solid adenocarcinomas and small cell variants of squamous cell carcinoma, are distinguished by absence of NE markers for the former, and presence of CK 1, 5, 10, and 14 coupled with absence of TTF-1 in the latter. Poorly differentiated squamous cell carcinomas may also stain for p63, which is not expressed by SCLC.

PROGNOSIS AND THERAPY

Overall, SCLC has a very poor prognosis, and negative prognostic factors include extensive stage, poor performance status, and elevated serum lactate dehydrogenase. No pathologic features are predictive of prognosis. The usual therapy, including etoposide and cisplatin, is effective in 50 %, followed by a partial response in 80 % of patients and complete response in 40 %. Chemosensitivity cannot be predicted based on histopathological features or markers. Recently, clinical trials have also shown a survival benefit associated with thoracic radiation therapy and prophylactic central nervous system radiation in limited-stage SCLC.

CARCINOID TUMORS

Carcinoids were first described in the digestive tract as malignant NE tumors, on the basis of their capacity to produce neurohormonal peptides similar to those secreted by neural cells. Since the first description by Arrigoni, et al., in 1972, of atypical carcinoids (ACs) of the lung, the histological criteria for the distinction

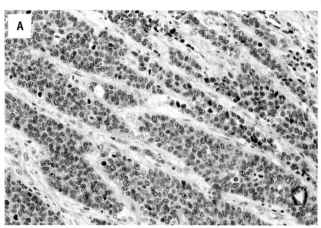
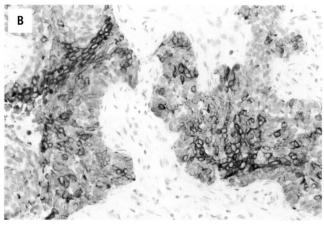

FIGURE 27-2

Basaloid carcinoma

(A) The tumor consists of relatively uniform small cells with a high mitotic rate. **(B)** There is expression of CK1, 5, 10, 14 (antibody CK 34βE12) by the majority of tumor cells.

SMALL CELL LUNG CANCER—FACT SHEET

Definition

‣ A malignant epithelial tumor consisting of small cells with scant cytoplasm, ill-defined cell borders, finely granular nuclear chromatin, and absent or inconspicuous nucleoli (World Health Organization)

Incidence

‣ Accounts for 12-18% of all lung cancers
‣ An estimated 28,000 cases will occur in the United States in 2007

Morbidity and Mortality

‣ From the time of diagnosis, the median survival intervals for limited-stage SCLC and extensive-stage SCLC are 15–20 months and 8–13 months, respectively, and 5-year survival rates are 10%–13% and 1%–2%
‣ 3-month untreated median survival
‣ Usually present at an advanced stage (extensive-stage disease)

Age Distribution

‣ Most patients are between 40 and 70 years of age

Clinical Features

‣ Stridor, hemoptysis, hoarseness, and vocal cord paralysis are common symptoms
‣ Can cause the superior vena cava syndrome and paraneoplastic syndromes
‣ Symptomatology can also be related to distant metastases
‣ The vast majority of patients are current or former tobacco smokers

Radiologic Features

‣ Chest radiographs may not show the tumor, but CT will usually reveal a hilar or perihilar mass, often with mediastinal lymphadenopathy
‣ Lobar collapse is common

Prognosis and Therapy

‣ Chemotherapy usually produces at least a partial response, and a survival advantage has also been shown for radiation therapy
‣ Surgical resection and chemotherapy is performed for localized disease in some centers
‣ Chemoresistance is common
‣ Currently, there are no histologic or immunohistochemical predictors of chemosensitivity
‣ Adverse prognostic factors include extensive stage, poor performance status, and elevated serum LDH

SMALL CELL LUNG CANCER—PATHOLOGIC FEATURES

Gross Findings

‣ Perihilar soft, white-tan masses with obvious necrosis
‣ Nodal involvement is often visible, as is spread along lymphatics in bronchovascular bundles and interlobular septa

Microscopic Findings

‣ Sheet-like growth without a neuroendocrine morphologic pattern is the most frequent architectural presentation, and trabeculae, peripheral palisading, and rosette formation may also be seen
‣ Tumor cells usually measure less than the size of three small lymphocytes in diameter, and have round, ovoid, or spindled nuclei
‣ Nuclear chromatin is typically finely granular with a "salt and pepper" appearance
‣ Nucleoli are absent or inconspicuous
‣ High nuclear-to-cytoplasmic ratio
‣ Nuclear molding
‣ Undefined cell borders
‣ High mitotic rate (average 60 mitoses per 10 high-power fields)
‣ Crush artifact is frequent
‣ Combined small cell carcinoma includes a component of NSCLC with the SCLC; each component comprises at least 10% of the tumor

Cytologic Findings

‣ Loose and irregular or syncytial clusters of small cells with nuclear molding, frequent mitoses, "salt and pepper" chromatin, and inconspicuous nucleoli
‣ Due to the fragility of the nuclei, "chromatin streaks" are commonly seen

Immunohistochemical Features

‣ More than 90% of tumors express one or more of the following neuroendocrine markers: CD56/NCAM, synaptophysin, chromogranin
‣ TTF-1 is expressed by approximately 85% of tumors
‣ CK34βE12 is not expressed by SCLC, but can be expressed by a NSCLC component of a combined SCLC

Ultrastructural Features

‣ Most tumors demonstrate some neurosecretory granules, and some will also show features of squamous or glandular differentiation

Pathologic Differential Diagnosis

‣ Lymphoma
‣ Benign lymphoid proliferations
‣ Large cell neuroendocrine carcinoma
‣ Carcinoid tumors
‣ Primitive neuroectodermal tumor
‣ Poorly differentiated non-small cell carcinomas
‣ Basaloid carcinoma

between typical and atypical carcinoids have been revised, and endorsed by the WHO.

CLINICAL FEATURES

Typical and atypical carcinoids account for 1-2% of all lung tumors. Despite their low metastatic potential, they are considered as true malignant lesions, since up to 15% of TCs and up to 50% of ACs metastasize. The age at diagnosis ranges from childhood to the ninth decade, with a mean of approximately 47 years. Although there is an equal male and female distribution, there is a slight female predominance reported in patients under the age of 50 years. However, ACs may occur in older patients with cigarette smoking as a risk factor, which is not true in TCs.

Carcinoids preferentially occur in the main bronchi, rarely in the trachea, and 16-40% are peripheral and may be multiple. Nearly 20% of cases are asymptomatic, but when central, carcinoids may present as polypoid masses invading the bronchial wall, causing hemoptysis, bronchial obstruction, cough, and wheezing. Carcinoid syndrome and Cushing syndrome are rare, and are mainly associated with metastases.

In contrast to other NE tumors of the lung, carcinoids may harbor mutations or deletions of the MEN1 gene. This gene, the locus of which is at 11p13, codes for the menin protein, and its inactivation (observed in familial pulmonary carcinoids) is responsible for the occurrence of multiple endocrine neoplasia type 1 (MEN1). MEN1 includes multiple parathyroid tumors and other NE tumors of the pancreas, duodenum, and pituitary gland. Also, sporadic mutations of the MEN1 gene may occur more often in ACs than in TCs, suggesting a more aggressive histopathological behavior for these tumors.

Carcinoids may be multiple in the context of diffuse idiopathic NE hyperplasia (DIPNECH), recognized to be a preinvasive lesion for carcinoids (see chapter 31).

RADIOLOGIC FEATURES

Carcinoid tumors present as well defined nodules, occasionally calcified or cavitated. A central, endobronchial location is more common than a peripheral location. They are PET negative.

PATHOLOGIC FEATURES

GROSS FINDINGS

Macroscopically, carcinoids are soft, tan-gray to yellow tumors, measuring from 0.5-8 cm in diameter. Many carcinoids present as polypoid endobronchial masses with smooth overlying epithelium. Others show a small endobronchial component and invade more extensively in the bronchial submucosa and adjacent lung tissue. ACs may demonstrate necrosis and hemorrhage, are frequently larger than TCs, and are more commonly peripheral.

MICROSCOPIC FINDINGS

Histologically, TCs typically exhibit an organoid pattern and are variably arranged in nest, ribbons, trabeculae, and pseudorosettes (Figures 27-3, 27-4). Other patterns include papillary, follicular, paraganglioma-like, and pseudoglandular arrangements. Tumor cells are relatively uniform in appearance, exhibiting a polygonal to fusiform shape with pale cytoplasm. Classically, pure fusiform carcinoids predominate in subpleural locations. Oncocytic features are not uncommon, in contrast to acinic cell-like, signet ring, clear cell, goblet cell, or melanocytic features. Nuclei are round to oval, with open chromatin and a small nucleolus, and classically, nucleoli

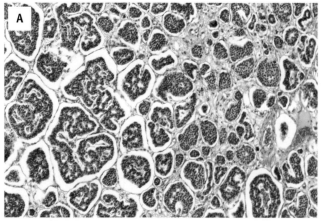 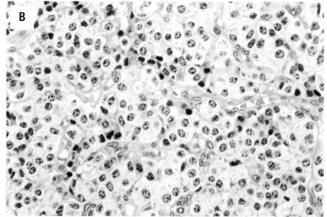

FIGURE 27-3

Carcinoid tumor

(A) Insular architecture is noted on the right, trabeculi and palisading on the left. **(B)** This carcinoid tumor is composed of clear cells with vesicular nuclei, granular chromatin, and numerous apoptotic cells and bodies.

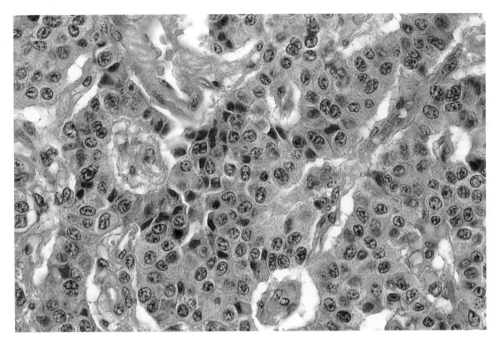

FIGURE 27-4

Typical carcinoid

This typical carcinoid displays large cells with oncocytic cytoplasm, numerous apoptotic cells, no mitoses, and a trabecular arrangement.

and pleomorphism are more conspicuous in ACs than in TCs. According to the recent WHO classification, ACs differ from TCs by the presence of punctuate coagulative necrosis and/or mitotic indices ranging from 2-10 mitoses per 10 high-power fields (one HPF = 0.2 mm^2) (Figure 27-5). In contrast, nuclear pleomorphism is not considered as a discriminating criterion for the differential diagnosis.

In both typical and atypical carcinoids, the stroma is vascular, sometimes presenting with hyaline or amyloid changes. Calcification or ossification, encountered in 10-25% of cases, is easily detected radiographically. The overlying surface epithelium frequently undergoes squamous metaplasia and may appear mildly dysplastic.

ANCILLARY STUDIES

ULTRASTRUCTURAL FEATURES

Carcinoid tumors all contain numerous dense-core neurosecretory granules, easily identifiable by electron microscopy. These tend to be smaller and fewer in atypical than in typical carcinoids.

IMMUNOHISTOCHEMISTRY

Nearly 80% of carcinoids stain for pan-cytokeratins, and as is true for other pulmonary NE tumors, they always express cytokeratins 8, 18, and 19. Expression of cytokeratins 1, 5, 10, and 14 (recognized by the antibody 34βE12) has not been observed in NE tumors of the lung, however, which is helpful in separating these

tumors from most poorly differentiated squamous cell carcinomas and adenocarcinomas.

NE markers are expressed by essentially all carcinoids. Chromogranin A is present in neurosecretory granules and synaptophysin is contained in synaptic vesicles. CD56/NCAM, which belongs to the immunoglobulin superfamily of transmembrane adhesion molecules, is widely expressed and, to date, remains the most useful immunohistochemical marker even on crushed biopsies or small specimens. In contrast, as widely reported, neuron-specific enolase (NSE) immunostaining is of little help in the diagnosis of NE tumors in general due to its lack of specificity. Varying results have been reported for TTF-1 expression, with up to one-third of TCs and ACs reportedly positive, primarily those in a peripheral location.

Staining for the proliferation antigen Ki 67 is observed in less than 10% of TC. A higher index than 4%, more frequently observed in AC, may be related to a shorter survival.

DIFFERENTIAL DIAGNOSIS

Carcinoids differ in size, but not cytologic features, from tumorlets; the latter do not exceed 5 mm in diameter. Sclerosing hemangiomas may resemble carcinoids, especially when a papillary or pseudoglandular pattern is present in the former. The demonstration of NE marker expression and absence of TTF-1 expression distinguishes carcinoids from sclerosing hemangioma. Carcinoids may be confused with paragangliomas, but paragangliomas are very rare in the

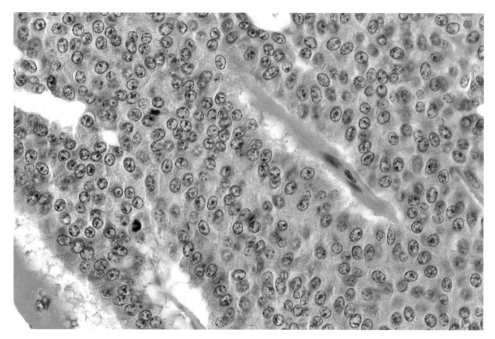

FIGURE 27-5
Atypical carcinoid
Note the presence of 2 mitoses in the same high-power field.

lung, and lack cytokeratin expression. Glomus tumors and other smooth muscle tumors can mimic carcinoids, but, unlike carcinoids, will express smooth muscle actin and will not express NE markers. Adenocarcinoma enters the differential diagnosis because a gland-like pattern can occur in carcinoids. Mucin production is not a definitive distinguishing feature since carcinoids may show mucin formation. TTF-1 expression and the absence of NE markers in adenocarcinoma are of great help. The solid-type adenoid cystic carcinoma can potentially be mistaken for carcinoid but is negative for NE markers.

PROGNOSIS AND THERAPY

At the time of diagnosis, 10-15% of TC and 40-50% of ACs present with lymph node metastases. Distant metastases are exhibited in 5-10% of TCs and 20% of ACs at presentation. The overall 5- and 10-year survival rates are 90-98% and 82-95% in TC, and only 61-72% and 35-59% in AC.

The treatment for localized TCs and ACs is complete surgical resection and lymphadenectomy. With metastatic disease, chemotherapy can be given with a cisplatin-based or streptozocin-based regimen, with moderate effectiveness.

LARGE CELL NEUROENDOCRINE CARCINOMA

Large cell neuroendocrine carcinoma (LCNEC) is a variant of large cell carcinoma. The previous synonyms of LCNEC are large cell NE tumor, NE carcinoma with intermediate differentiation, atypical endocrine tumor of the lung, and large cell carcinoma of the lung with NE differentiation. LCNEC was described in 1991 and was recognized as a distinct clinicopathological entity in the 1999 WHO classification scheme.

CLINICAL FEATURES

LCNEC accounts for about 3% of all pulmonary malignancies. Most of these tumors develop in the periphery of the lung and share symptoms and presentation with other NSCLCs. The average age at diagnosis is about 65 years of age, and most patients are male (approximately 70%) and smokers. Ectopic hormone production is extremely uncommon in LCNEC. LCNEC often presents with an advanced stage (III-IV) at the time of diagnosis.

CARCINOID TUMORS—FACT SHEET

Definition

» A tumor characterized by growth patterns that suggest neuroendocrine differentiation, with uniform cytologic features including moderate eosinophilic, finely granular cytoplasm and nuclei with a finely granular chromatin pattern (World Health Organization)
  » Typical carcinoids (TCs) display fewer than two mitoses per 2 mm^2 and lack necrosis
  » Atypical carcinoids (ACs) have 2-10 mitoses per 2 mm^2 and/or foci of necrosis

Incidence

» 1-2% of all lung tumors

Mortality

» Overall 5- and 10-year survival rates are 90-98% and 82-95% in TC, and 61-72% and 35-59% in AC

Gender and Age Distribution

» Age at diagnosis ranges from childhood to the ninth decade, with a mean of approximately 47 years
» Similar frequencies in men and women overall

Clinical Features

» Most carcinoids are central masses causing bronchial obstruction with hemoptysis, cough, and wheezing
» Symptoms associated with the carcinoid syndrome and Cushing syndrome are rare and are mainly associated with metastases
» Nearly 20% of cases are asymptomatic
» Occasional carcinoids are associated with MEN1 syndrome or diffuse idiopathic pulmonary neuroendocrine cell hyperplasia

Radiologic Features

» Well-circumscribed nodules, usually central and less often peripheral
» Post-obstructive changes are common

Prognosis and Therapy

» Up to 15% of TCs metastasize, and up to 50% of ACs metastasize
» High survival rates, despite metastasis
» The treatment for localized TCs and ACs is complete surgical resection and lymphadenectomy
» With metastatic disease, chemotherapy can be given with a cisplatin-based or streptozocin-based regimen, with moderate effectiveness

CARCINOID TUMORS—PATHOLOGIC FEATURES

Gross Findings

» Soft tan-gray to yellow masses, measuring from 0.5-8 cm in diameter
» Many carcinoids present as polypoid endobronchial masses with smooth overlying epithelium
» Others show a small endobronchial component and invade more extensively in the bronchial submucosa and adjacent lung tissue.
» Atypical carcinoids may show foci of necrosis and hemorrhage, are frequently larger than typical carcinoids, and are more commonly peripheral

Microscopic Findings

» Frequently have an organoid pattern with variable arrangement in nests, ribbons, trabeculae, and pseudorosettes; other patterns can include papillary, follicular, paraganglioma-like, and pseudoglandular architectures
» Tumor cells are relatively uniform in appearance, exhibiting a polygonal to fusiform shape with pale cytoplasm
» Oncocytic features are common, in contrast to less common acinic cell-like, signet ring, clear cell, goblet cell, or melanocytic features
» Nuclei are round to oval, with open chromatin and a small nucleolus
» Nucleoli and pleomorphism tend to be more conspicuous in atypical than in typical
» Variable mitotic rate and necrosis
  » Typical carcinoids (TCs) display fewer than two mitoses per 2 mm^2 and lack necrosis
  » Atypical carcinoids (ACs) have 2-10 mitoses per 2 mm^2 and/or foci of necrosis
» Vascular-rich stroma

Immunohistochemical Features

» Virtually all carcinoids express one or more of the following neuroendocrine markers: CD56/NCAM, synaptophysin, chromogranin
» 80% stain for pan-cytokeratin and CK 8, 18 and 19
» TTF-1 is expressed by up to one-third of tumors
» CK34βE12 is not expressed by carcinoids

Ultrastructural Features

» Numerous dense-core neurosecretory granules

Pathologic Differential Diagnosis

» Tumorlet
» Sclerosing hemangioma
» Paraganglioma
» Glomus tumors
» Adenocarcinoma
» Adenoid cystic carcinoma
» Large cell neuroendocrine carcinoma

PATHOLOGIC FEATURES

GROSS FINDINGS

LCNEC are peripheral tumors with gross characteristics similar to other NSCLCs.

MICROSCOPIC FINDINGS

LCNEC is defined histologically (Figure 27-6) as a tumor showing : (a) NE morphology (organoid nesting, trabeculae, rosettes, or palisading) (b) mitotic activity of 11 or more mitoses per 10 high-power fields (2 mm^2); (c) cytological features of NSCLC including large cell size, polygonal shape, abundant cytoplasm with low nuclear cytoplasmic ratio, and vesicular or fine nuclear chromatin with frequent conspicuous nucleoli; (d) large areas of necrosis; and (e) strong immunoreactivity for at least one NE marker (chromogranin A, synaptophysin, NCAM/CD56) (Figures 27-7, 27-8). The NE morphological pattern associated with expression of NE markers are cardinal features important for the diagnosis of LCNEC.

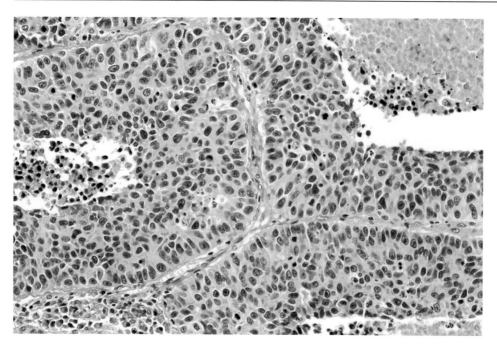

FIGURE 27-6

Large cell neuroendocrine carcinoma
Lobular architecture, peripheral palisading, rosettes, centrilobular necrosis, and a high rate of mitosis are commonly found in LCNEC.

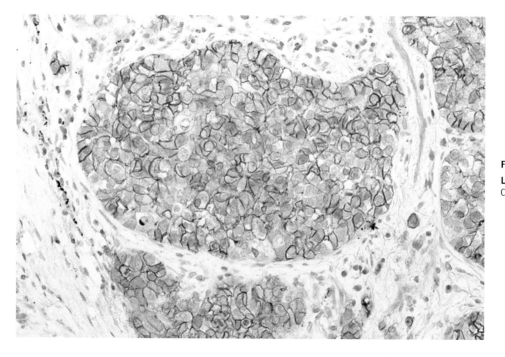

FIGURE 27-7

Large cell neuroendocrine carcinoma
CD56 (NCAM) is diffusely positive.

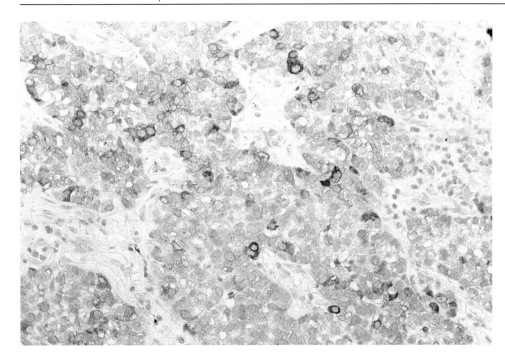

FIGURE 27-8

Large cell neuroendocrine carcinoma
Synaptophysin is expressed by this LCNEC.

VARIANT

COMBINED LARGE CELL NEUROENDOCRINE CARCINOMA

Combined large cell NE carcinoma is defined as a LCNEC associated with any NSCLC component: adenocarcinoma (Figure 27-9), squamous cell carcinoma, giant cell carcinoma, and/or spindle cell carcinoma. Importantly, a small cell carcinoma component admixed with a LCNEC is diagnosed as a combined SCLC.

ANCILLARY STUDIES

ULTRASTRUCTURAL FEATURES

Similar to other NE lung tumors, LCNEC contains neurosecretory granules in the tumor cell cytoplasm. These are often mixed in the combined cases with other differentiated features such as acinar formation with apical microvilli, tonofilaments, and desmosome-type junctions. For diagnostic purposes, the demonstration of neurosecretory granules at the ultrastructural level can replace the immunohistochemical demonstration of a NE marker.

IMMUNOHISTOCHEMISTRY

Confirmation of NE differentiation is strictly required for the diagnosis of LCNEC and can be performed with stains for chromogranin A, synaptophysin,

and NCAM/CD56. In addition, about 50% of LCNEC express TTF-1. The expression of cytokeratins 1, 5, 10, and 14, recognized by the antibody 34βE12, is constantly absent in pure LCNEC, but occurs in the admixed NSCLC component in 32% of combined LCNEC (Figure 27-10), which is helpful for confirming the diagnosis of combined LCNEC.

FINE NEEDLE ASPIRATION BIOPSY

Definitive diagnosis of LCNEC in fine needle aspiration or core needle biopsy samples is difficult due to heterogeneity of the NE morphology and NE marker expression in the tumor mass. A range of nuclear features between LCNEC and SCLC is frequent and causes difficulties in the interpretation of fine needle aspiration biopsy specimens.

DIFFERENTIAL DIAGNOSIS

The differential diagnosis of LCNEC includes basaloid carcinoma, large cell carcinoma (NOS), SCLC, and atypical carcinoid. The differential diagnosis between LCNEC and basaloid carcinoma is the most difficult based on histomorphological features alone, since one-third of basaloid carcinomas display rosettes and all are recognized with the cardinal features of lobular and trabecular architecture with peripheral palisading. Comedo-type necrosis is common to both entities. Immunohistochemical profiles, however, are important for differentiating basaloid carcinoma with rosettes and

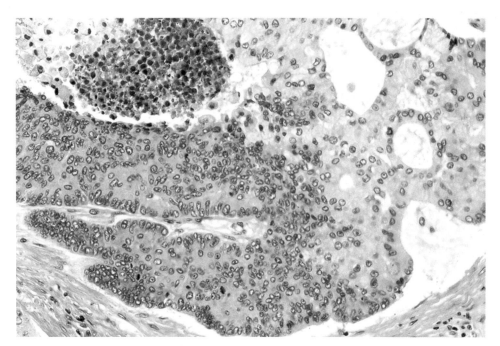

FIGURE 27-9

Combined large cell neuroendocrine carcinoma

There is a close admixture of a large cell neuroendocrine carcinoma on the left with an adenocarcinoma (mucinous) on the right.

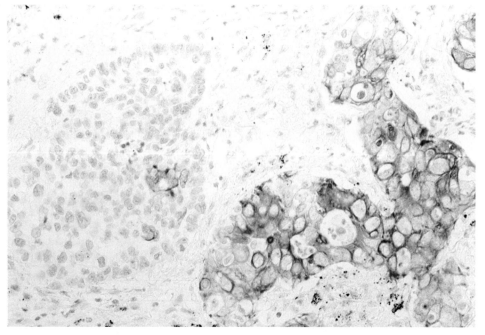

FIGURE 27-10

Combined large cell neuroendocrine carcinoma

Immunohistochemical expression of CK1, 5, 10, 14 by the squamous cell carcinoma component on the right helps to differentiate this component from the large cell neuroendocrine carcinoma component on the left, which does not stain for these cytokeratins.

palisades from LCNEC. Cytokeratin 1, 5, 10, and 14 (recognized by 34βE12 antibody) is typically negative in LCNEC and in basaloid carcinoma. In contrast, TTF-1 is expressed in 50% of LCNEC but in no cases of basaloid carcinoma (Figure 27-11). The absence of NE features needed to differentiate LCNEC from large cell carcinoma can be difficult to evaluate in small biopsies compared to larger surgical samples. In the presence of NE marker expression, the differential diagnosis between NSCLC with NE differentiation and LCNEC relies on light microscopic evidence of NE morphology.

The major differential diagnosis for LCNEC is atypical carcinoid, with which they were confused in most literature prior to the WHO classification scheme from 1999. LCNEC is distinguished from atypical carcinoid primarily by its higher mitotic index (11 or more mitoses per 2 mm²) and more extensive necrosis. There is a small proportion of LCNECs with mitotic rates between 11 and 20 mitoses per 10 high-power fields, that represent less than 20% of LCNECs. These are currently classified as LCNECs.

SCLC also enters the differential diagnosis of LCNEC. SCLC is distinguished from LCNEC by its small cell size, higher nuclear-to-cytoplasmic ratio, and nuclear chromatin that is finely granular rather than vesicular. It must be recognized that 20% of LCNECs have nuclear features similar to SCLCs, making separation of the two neoplasms more difficult. Unfortunately, there is no immunohistochemical marker that can be relied upon to distinguish between the two types of neoplasms. If a true component of SCLC can be identified, however, the diagnosis of combined SCLC is appropriate.

PROGNOSIS AND THERAPY

Since the optimal treatment for LCNEC has not been determined, it has been preferred to consider LCNEC as a subtype of large cell carcinoma in the most recent version of the WHO classification of lung tumors. Nonetheless, the majority of previous studies, with a few exceptions, have found that LCNEC has a poor survival as compared to stage-matched NSCLC, approaching the dismal outcome of SCLC. The current approach to treatment includes complete surgical resection for localized disease. Postoperative adjuvant chemotherapy and radiotherapy have generally not been successful in significantly improving survival, but continued investigations into new therapies are underway.

NON-SMALL CELL LUNG CARCINOMA WITH NEUROENDOCRINE FEATURES

In addition to the previously described NE lung tumors, NSCLCs other than LCNECs may present immunohistochemical and/or ultrastructural evidence of NE differentiation. Approximately 15% display one NE marker on a restricted percentage of tumor cells. The most frequent occurrence of NE markers without NE morphology is seen in adenocarcinoma. NSCLC with NE differentiation is not considered as a specific

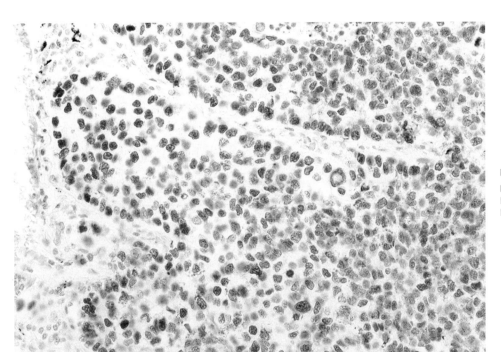

FIGURE 27-11

Large cell neuroendocrine carcinoma
Expression of TTF-1 is seen in 50% of LCNECs.

LARGE CELL NEUROENDOCRINE CARCINOMA—FACT SHEET

Definition

» A large cell carcinoma demonstrating neuroendocrine architectural features and immunohistochemical or ultrastructural evidence of neuroendocrine differentiation

Incidence

» About 3% of all lung cancers

Mortality

» Aggressive type of lung cancer with mortality similar to small cell lung carcinoma; lower survival than NSCLCs of similar stage

Gender and Age Distribution

» Average age at diagnosis is about 65 years of age
» Most patients are male

Clinical Features

» Symptoms are similar to other NSCLCs
» Most patients are smokers
» Paraneoplastic syndromes are uncommon

Radiologic Features

» Usually peripheral lung masses

Therapy

» The current approach to treatment includes complete surgical resection for localized disease
» Postoperative adjuvant chemotherapy and radiotherapy have generally not been successful in significantly improving survival

LARGE CELL NEUROENDOCRINE CARCINOMA—PATHOLOGIC FEATURES

Gross Findings

» Peripheral lung masses resembling other NSCLCs

Microscopic Findings

» Neuroendocrine morphologic features including organoid nesting, trabeculae, rosettes, or palisading
» Mitotic activity of more than 11 mitoses per 10 high-power fields
» Cytological features of NSCLC including large cell size, polygonal shape, abundant cytoplasm with low nuclear:cytoplasmic ratio, and vesicular or fine nuclear chromatin with frequent conspicuous nucleoli
» Large areas of necrosis
» Combined large cell neuroendocrine carcinoma is defined as a LCNEC associated with any NSCLC component

Immunohistochemical Features

» Immunoreactivity for at least one neuroendocrine marker (chromogranin A, synaptophysin, NCAM/CD56)
» Approximately 50% of LCNECs express TTF-1
» CK34βE12 is negative in pure LCNEC, but may be positive in the NSCLC component of combined LCNEC

Ultrastructural Features

» Dense-core neurosecretory granules are often seen in tumor cell cytoplasm
» Other features of squamous or glandular differentiation can also be observed, particularly in combined LCNEC

Pathologic Differential Diagnosis

» Basaloid carcinoma
» Large cell carcinoma (NOS)
» Small cell lung carcinoma
» Atypical carcinoid

entity, because no evidence has been provided that expression of a NE marker confers a worse or better survival and/or changes responsiveness to chemotherapy. These tumors should be referred to as NSCLCs with NE differentiation, but should not be classified as LCNEC. In contrast, they should be classified based on their type of differentiation (e.g., adenocarcinoma with NE differentiation).

SUGGESTED READINGS

Small Cell Lung Carcinoma

1. Curran WJ Jr. Therapy of limited stage small cell lung cancer. *Cancer Treat Res*. 2001;105:229-52.
2. Dy GK, Adjei AA. Novel targets for lung cancer therapy: part I. *J Clin Oncol*. 2002;20:2881-94.
3. Fletcher JA. Role of KIT and platelet-derived growth factor receptors as oncoproteins. *Semin Oncol*. 2004;31(suppl 6):4-11.
4. Gazzeri S, Brambilla E, Jacrot M, Chauvin C, Benabib AL, Brambilla C. Activation of the myc gene family in human lung carcinomas and during heterotransplantation in nude mice. *Cancer Res*. 1991;51:2566-71.
5. Halliday BE, Slagel DD, Elsheikh TE, Silverman JF. Diagnostic utility of MIC-2 immunocytochemical staining in the differential diagnosis of small blue cell tumors. *Diagn Cytopathol*. 1998;19:410-6.
6. Lally BE, Urbanic JJ, Blackstock AW, Miller AA, Perry MC. Small cell lung cancer: have we made any progress over the last 25 years? *Oncologist*. 2007;12(9):1096-104.
7. Hibi K, Takahashi T, Sekido Y, et al. Coexpression of stem cell factor and the c-kit genes in small-cell lung cancer. *Oncogene*. 1991;6:2291-6.
8. Lumadue JA, Askin FB, Perlman EJ. MIC2 analysis of small cell carcinoma. *Am J Clin Pathol*. 1994;102:692-4.
9. Osterlind K, Andersen PK. Prognostic factors in small cell lung cancer: multivariate model based on 778 patients treated with chemotherapy with or without irradiation. *Cancer Res*. 1986;46:4189-94.
10. Rygaard K, Nakamura T, Spang-Thomsen M. Expression of the protooncogenes c-met and c-kit and their ligands, hepatocyte growth factor/scatter factor and stem cell factor in SCLC cell lines and xenografts. *Br J Cancer*. 1993;67:137-46.
11. Sattler M, Salgia R. Molecular and cellular biology of small cell lung cancer. *Semin Oncol*. 2003;30:57-71.
12. Souhami RL, Bradbury I, Geddes DM, Spiro SG, Harper PG, Tobias JS. Prognostic significance of laboratory parameters measured at diagnosis in small cell carcinoma of the lung. *Cancer Res*. 1985;45:2878-82.
13. Sturm N, Rossi G, Lantuejoul S, et al. 34βE12 expression along the whole spectrum of neuroendocrine proliferations of the lung, from neuroendocrine cell hyperplasia to small cell carcinoma. *Histopathology*. 2003;42:156-66.

Carcinoid Tumors

14. Arrigoni MG, Woolner LB, Bernatz PE. Atypical carcinoid tumors of the lung. *J Thorac Cardiovasc Surg*. 1972;44:413-21.
15. Beasley MB, Thunnissen FBJM, Brambilla E, et al. Pulmonary atypical carcinoid: predictors of survival in 106 cases. *Human Pathol*. 2000;31:1255-65.

16. Bergh J, Esscher T, Steinholtz L, Nilsson K, Phalman S. Immunocytochemical demonstration of neuron-specific enolase (NSE) in human lung cancers. *Am J Clin Pathol.* 1985;84:1-7.

17. Brambilla E, Brambilla C,. Hétérogénéité des cancers bronchiques. Problèmes d'histogénèse. *Rev Mal Respir.* 1986;5:235-45.

18. Costes V, Marty-Ane C, Picot MC, et al. Typical and atypical bronchopulmonary carcinoid tumors: a clinicopathologic and KI-67-labeling study. *Hum Pathol.* 1995;26:740-5.

19. Debelenko L, Brambilla E, Agarwal SK, et al. Identification of MEN1 gene mutations in sporadic carcinoid tumors of the lung. *Hum Mol Genet.* 1997;13:2285-90.

20. Devouassoux-Shisheboran M, Hayashi T, Linnoila RI, Koss MN, Travis WD. A clinicopathologic study of 100 cases of pulmonary sclerosing hemangioma with immunohistochemical studies: TTF-1 is expressed in both round and surface cells, suggesting an origin from primitive respiratory epithelium. *Am J Surg Pathol.* 2000;24:906-16.

21. Du EZ, Goldstraw P, Zacharias J, et al. TTF-1 expression is specific for lung primary in typical and atypical carcinoids: TTF-1-positive carcinoids are predominantly in peripheral location. *Hum Pathol.* 2004;35:825-31.

22. Folpe AL, Gown AM, Lamps LW, et al. Thyroid transcription factor-1: immunohistochemical evaluation in pulmonary neuroendocrine tumors. *Mod Pathol.* 1999;12:5-8.

23. Harpole DH Jr, Feldman JM, Buchanan S, Young WG, Wolfe WG. Bronchial carcinoid tumors: a retrospective analysis of 126 patients. *Ann Thorac Surg.* 1992;54:50-5.

24. Jones MH, Virtanen C, Honjoh D, et al. Two prognostically significant subtypes of high-grade lung neuroendocrine tumours independent of small-cell and large-cell neuroendocrine carcinomas identified by gene expression profiles. *Lancet.* 2004;363:775-81.

25. Kosmidis PA. Treatment of carcinoid of the lung. *Curr Opin Oncol.* 2004;16:146-9.

26. Lantuejoul S, Moro D, Michalides RJ, Brambilla C, Brambilla E. NCAM and NCAM-PSA expression in neuroendocrine lung tumors. *Am J Surg Pathol.* 1998;22:1267-76.

27. Linnoila RI, Mushine JL, Steinberg SM, et al. Neuroendocrine differentiation in endocrine and non endocrine lung carcinoma. *Am J Clin Pathol.* 1988;90:641-52.

28. Martini N, Zaman MB, Bains MS, et al. Treatment and prognosis in bronchial carcinoid involving regional lymph nodes. *J Thorac Cardiovasc Surg.* 1994;107:1-7.

29. McCaughan BC, Martini N, Bains MS. Bronchial carcinoids. Review of 124 cases. *J Thorac Cardiovasc Surg.* 1985;89:8-17.

30. Oliveira AM, Tazelaar HD, Myers JL, Erickson LA, Lloyd RV. Thyroid transcription factor-1 distinguishes metastatic pulmonary from well-differentiated neuroendocrine tumors of other sites. *Am J Surg Pathol.* 2001;25:815-9.

31. Quaedvlieg PFHJ, Visser O, Lamers CBHW, Janssen-Heijen MLG, Taal BG. Epidemiology and survival in patients with carcinoid disease in the Netherlands. An epidemiological study with 2391 patients. *Ann Oncol.* 2001;12:1295-1300.

32. Skuladottir H, Hirsch FR, Hansen HH, Olsen JH. Pulmonary neuroendocrine tumors: incidence and prognosis of histological subtypes. A population-based study in Denmark. *Lung Cancer.* 2002;37:127-35.

33. Travis WD, Brambilla E, Muller-Hemerlink HK, Harris CC, eds. *Pathology and Genetics of Tumours of the Lung, Pleura, Thymus and Heart.* World Health Organization classification of tumours. Lyon: IARC Press; 2004.

34. Travis WD, Colby TV, Corrin B, Shimosato Y, Brambilla E. *Histological Typing of Lung and Pleural Tumours.* 3rd ed. WHO Histological Classification of Tumours. Springer-Verlag: Berlin; 1999.

35. Travis WD, Rush W, Flieder DB, et al. Survival analysis of 200 pulmonary neuroendocrine tumors with clarification of criteria for atypical carcinoid and its separation from typical carcinoid. *Am J Surg Pathol.* 1998;22:934-44.

36. Sturm N, Rossi G, Lantuejoul S, et al. Expression of thyroid transcription factor-1 (TTF-1) in the spectrum of neuroendocrine cell lung proliferations with special interest in carcinoids. *Hum Pathol.* 2002;33:175-82.

Large Cell Neuroendocrine Carcinoma and Other Non-Small Cell Carcinomas with Neuroendocrine Characteristics

37. Brambilla E, Veale D, Moro D, Morel F, Dubois F, Brambilla C. Neuroendocrine phenotype in lung cancers: comparison of immunochemistry with biochemical determination of enolase isoenzymes. *Am J Clin Pathol.* 1992;98:88-97.

38. Cerilli LA, Ritter JH, Mills SE, et al. Neuroendocrine neoplasms of the lung. *Am J Clin Pathol.* 2001;116(suppl 1):S65-96.

39. Demirer T, Ravits J, Aboulafia D. Myasthenic (Eaton-Lambert) syndrome associated with pulmonary large-cell neuroendocrine carcinoma. *South Med J.* 1994;87:1186-9.

40. Doddoli C, Barlesi F, Chetaille B, et al. Large cell neuroendocrine carcinoma of the lung: an aggressive disease potentially treatable with surgery. *Ann Thorac Surg.* 2004;77:1168-72.

41. Dresler CM, Ritter JH, Patterson AG, et al. Clinical-pathologic analysis of 40 patients with large cell neuroendocrine carcinoma of the lung. *Ann Thorac Surg.* 1997;63:180-5.

42. Fernandez FG, Battafarano RJ. Large-cell neuroendocrine carcinoma of the lung. *Cancer Control.* 2006;13:270-5.

43. Hage R, Seldenrijk K, de Bruin P, et al. Pulmonary large-cell neuroendocrine carcinoma (LCNEC). *Eur J Cardiothorac Surg.* 2003;23:457-60.

44. Iyoda A, Hiroshima K, Baba M, et al. Pulmonary large cell carcinomas with neuroendocrine features are high-grade neuroendocrine tumors. *Ann Thorac Surg.* 2002;73:1049-54.

45. Jiang SX, Kameya T, Shoji M, et al. Large cell neuroendocrine carcinoma of the lung. A histologic and immunohistochemical study of 22 cases. *Am J Surg Pathol.* 1998;22:526-37.

46. Jung KJ, Lee KS, Han J, et al. Large cell neuroendocrine carcinoma of the lung: clinical, CT, and pathologic findings in 11 patients. *J Thorac Imaging.* 2001;16:156-62.

47. Lyda MH, Weiss LM. Immunoreactivity for epithelial and neuroendocrine antibodies are useful in the differential diagnosis of lung carcinomas. *Hum Pathol.* 2000;31:980-7.

48. Mazieres J, Daste G, Molinier L, et al. Large cell neuroendocrine carcinoma of the lung: pathological study and clinical outcome of 18 resected cases. *Lung Cancer.* 2002;37:287-92.

49. Paci M, Cavazza A, Annessi V, et al. Large cell neuroendocrine carcinoma of the lung: a 10-year clinicopathologic retrospective study. *Ann Thorac Surg.* 2004;77:1163-7.

50. Sturm N, Lantuejoul S, Laverriere MH, et al. Thyroid transcription factor 1 and cytokeratins 1, 5, 10, 14 (34βE12) expression in basaloid and large-cell neuroendocrine carcinomas of the lung. *Hum Pathol.* 2001;32:918-25.

51. Takei H, Asamura H, Maeshima A, et al. Large cell neuroendocrine carcinoma of the lung: a clinicopathologic study of eighty-seven cases. *J Thorac Cardiovasc Surg.* 2002;124:285-92.

52. Travis MD, Linnoila RI, Tsokos MG, et al. Neuroendocrine tumors of the lung with proposed criteria for large-cell neuroendocrine carcinoma. An ultrastructural, immunohistochemical, and flow cytometric study of 35 cases. *Am J Surg Pathol.* 1991;15:529-53.

53. Wick MR, Berg LC, Hertz MI. Large cell carcinoma of the lung with neuroendocrine differentiation. A comparison with large cell "undifferentiated" pulmonary tumors. *Am J Clin Pathol.* 1992;97:796-805.

54. Zacharias J, Nicholson AG, Ladas GP, et al. Large cell neuroendocrine carcinoma and large cell carcinomas with neuroendocrine morphology of the lung: prognosis after complete resection and systematic nodal dissection. *Ann Thorac Surg.* 2003;75:348-52.

28 Unusual Primary Malignant Lung Neoplasms

Bruno Murer • Ulrike Gruber-Mösenbacher • Helmut H. Popper

INTRODUCTION

There are a variety of rare tumors that develop in the lung, with incidence rates of 1 in 100,000 people or lower. For this group of neoplasms, distribution patterns with respect to gender, race, or age are difficult to analyze. Most published accounts take the form of case reports or small series, and given the rare occurrence of these processes, it is likely that some examples will be classified as other, more common, types of neoplasms due to lack of familiarity with the entity, or with its potential to develop in the lungs. Nonetheless, this chapter will provide an overview of these tumors, recognizing that more information will likely become available with the growth of electronic means of communication that have facilitated the sharing of unusual cases.

SALIVARY GLAND-LIKE TUMORS

These entities represent a rare and distinctive group of neoplasms arising from the seromucous glands of the trachea and bronchi. The majority of these tumors are of low malignancy, are centrally located, and share similar histological features with their counterparts arising in the major salivary glands.

MUCOEPIDERMOID CARCINOMAS

CLINICAL FEATURES

Mucoepidermoid carcinomas are uncommon neoplasms representing less than 1% of lung tumors. There is a slight predominance in men. These tumors may be observed in any age group including children, in whom they are one of the more common bronchial tumors. In younger patients, low-grade tumors predominate, while high-grade neoplasms are more frequent in older people. Symptomatology is related to tumor size, and with smaller tumors, patients may be asymptomatic. Symptoms are due to bronchial obstruction and include cough, hemoptysis, shortness of breath, fever, and pneumonia. The majority of these tumors arise centrally in large bronchi and have endobronchial components, but there is no characteristic lobar distribution.

RADIOLOGIC FEATURES

Imaging studies reveal a well-circumscribed nodule or mass, characteristically centrally located, occasionally with calcification. Pneumonia, bronchiectasis, and atelectasis may be seen distal to the tumor.

PATHOLOGIC FEATURES

GROSS FINDINGS

Mucoepidermoid carcinomas often present as polypoid endobronchial lesions that are covered by bronchial mucosa. The mucosa can have a smooth surface or can be focally ulcerated. Tumors usually arise in the proximal bronchi, but can also take origin in the trachea. From the airways, the neoplasms can extend into the lung parenchyma as compressive masses. Tumor size ranges from 8 mm to 6 cm. The cut surfaces of the tumors have cystic and/or solid appearances, often with abundant mucus. High-grade tumors often display necrotic and hemorrhagic areas and tend to infiltrate the lung parenchyma. The pulmonary parenchyma distal to the tumor may show pneumonia, bronchiectasis, or atelectasis.

MICROSCOPIC FINDINGS

Mucoepidermoid carcinomas are subepithelial tumors arising from the bronchial submucosal glands (Figure 28-1A). They are divided into low and high-grade neoplasms based on morphologic and cytologic features. Low-grade tumors show mucus-filled cystic areas, as well as solid areas. The cysts, tubules, or glands are lined by columnar cells and low cuboidal cells with mild cytologic atypia with small, round, basally located nuclei (Figure 28-1B). The columnar cells have abundant mucin-rich cytoplasm. Mitotic figures are virtually absent, and necrosis is not observed. Lumina are typically filled with mucus, resembling thyroid follicles. Occasionally, the mucus spills into surrounding stroma, stimulating a granulomatous reaction and calcification. The solid areas are mainly composed of epidermoid and intermediate cells with minimal cytoatypia. The epidermoid cells display features of non-keratinizing squamous cells, with eosinophilic cytoplasm and distinct intercellular bridges. The intermediate cells are smaller than epidermoid cells, round or oval, with eosinophilic cytoplasm and sometimes perinuclear clearing. A clear cell appearance or oncocytic component may be seen. The stroma can be myxoid or fibrotic, sometimes with dense hyalinized collagen and calcification. A prominent lymphoplasmacytic infiltrate can be associated with the tumor.

High-grade mucoepidermoid carcinomas show a predominance of solid areas composed of intermingled epidermoid and intermediate cells, with a lesser representation of mucin-secreting cells. Tumor cells demonstrate nuclear atypia, hyperchromasia, and pleomorphism, as well as higher mitotic counts. Necrosis and perineural invasion (Figure 28-1C) may be observed.

ANCILLARY STUDIES

FINE NEEDLE ASPIRATION BIOPSY

The cytologic features of mucoepidermoid carcinomas include the presence of 3 cell types (mucinous, non-keratinizing squamoid, and intermediate cells), sometimes accompanied by extracellular mucin or cellular debris. The mucin-producing cells are round or columnar, with large amounts of vacuolated cytoplasm. The nuclei are uniform, small, and eccentrically placed. The intermediate epidermoid cells have centrally placed, round nuclei, a denser cytoplasm, and distinct cell borders. High-grade tumors contain numerous markedly atypical cells with pleomorphic nuclei and prominent nucleoli.

IMMUNOHISTOCHEMISTRY

These tumors stain with pancytokeratins and CK7 and are immunonegative for CK20 and TTF-1. The epidermoid component shows immunoreactivity for CK5/6.

DIFFERENTIAL DIAGNOSIS

Low-grade mucoepidermoid carcinomas can sometimes be difficult to differentiate from mucous gland adenomas, but the presence of intermediate cells and squamous differentiation is characteristic of mucoepidermoid carcinoma, in contrast to mucous gland adenoma. High-grade mucoepidermoid carcinomas must be differentiated from squamous cell carcinomas, which lack glandular differentiation. More problematic and controversial is the differentiation from adenosquamous carcinomas. In general, mucoepidermoid carcinomas are centrally located with an endobronchial growth pattern, and areas of low-grade mucoepidermoid carcinoma are often present, unlike adenosquamous carcinomas. They lack an associated in situ carcinoma of the surface bronchial epithelium, which may be present in adenosquamous carcinoma. Prominent keratinization and keratin pearl formation is more typical of adenosquamous carcinoma than high-grade mucoepidermoid carcinoma. Metastasis from a mucoepidermoid carcinoma arising in the head and neck should also be excluded prior to classifying a mucoepidermoid carcinoma as a primary pulmonary neoplasm.

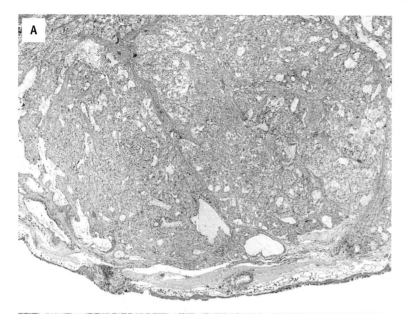

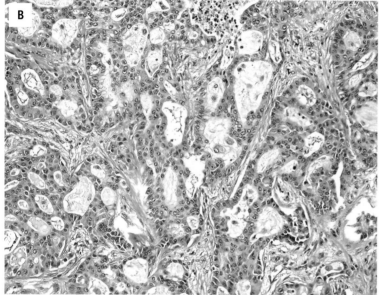

FIGURE 28-1

Mucoepidermoid carcinoma
(A) This tumor forms a subepithelial mass in this bronchus.
(B) Tumor cells form glands with microcystic spaces that are lined by cuboidal or columnar cells, and smaller numbers of squamoid cells are seen. **(C)** Perineural invasion occurs in some of these neoplasms, as well as in adenoid cystic carcinomas.

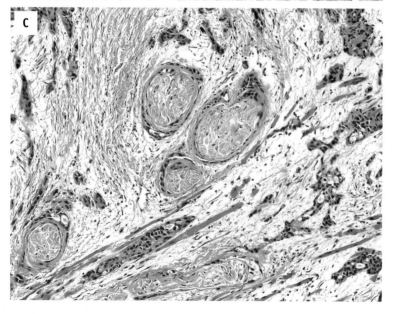

MUCOEPIDERMOID CARCINOMA—FACT SHEET

Definition

▸ A malignant tumor composed of nonkeratinizing squamous cells, mucin-producing cells, and cells of intermediate type, similar to its counterpart arising in the major salivary glands

Incidence

▸ Less than 1% of lung neoplasms

Morbidity and Mortality

▸ Bronchial obstruction by the tumor can lead to pneumonia, bronchiectasis, and atelectasis
▸ Low-grade tumors are associated with low mortality
▸ For high-grade tumors, survival is similar to non-small cell lung carcinomas

Gender, Race, and Age Distribution

▸ Slight predominance in men
▸ Occurs at any age from childhood to late adulthood
▸ Low-grade tumors predominate in younger people
▸ High-grade tumors predominate in older people
▸ More frequent in Caucasians

Clinical Features

▸ Symptoms include cough, hemoptysis, shortness of breath, and fever

Radiologic Features

▸ Well-circumscribed nodule or mass, often within an airway
▸ Pneumonia, bronchiectasis, or atelectasis distal to the tumor

Prognosis and Therapy

▸ Sleeve resection or laser therapy is used for low-grade tumors, surgical resection and post-operative radiotherapy for high-grade tumors
▸ Low-grade tumors rarely metastasize to lymph nodes, while high-grade tumors can metastasize to bone, liver, adrenals, and brain
▸ Survival is related to grade, with low mortality and long survival associated with low-grade tumors, and mortality similar to non-small cell carcinomas associated with high-grade tumors

MUCOEPIDERMOID CARCINOMA—PATHOLOGIC FEATURES

Gross Findings

▸ Polypoid endobronchial mass usually originating in a lobar or segmental bronchus
▸ Cystic and/or solid appearance with mucus
▸ Infiltrative margins with necrosis and hemorrhage in high-grade tumors
▸ Post-obstructive pneumonia, bronchiectasis, and atelectasis may be seen

Microscopic Findings

Low-grade tumors

▸ Mucus-filled cysts, tubules, or glands, and solid areas
▸ The columnar and cuboidal cells lining the cysts show mild atypia, round, basally located nuclei, and apical mucin-rich cytoplasm
▸ Solid areas are composed of epidermoid and intermediate cells
▸ The stroma may be dense or hyalinized with calcification

High-grade tumors

▸ A solid, epidermoid, and/or intermediate component usually predominates, with less evidence of cyst or gland formation
▸ Marked nuclear atypia and pleomorphism, and high mitotic activity are typical
▸ Necrosis and hemorrhage can be present

Fine Needle Aspiration Biopsy

▸ Three types of cells: mucinous, nonkeratinizing squamoid, and intermediate cells
▸ Mucinous cells have vacuolated cytoplasm and small nuclei
▸ Epidermoid cells have round, central nuclei and dense cytoplasm
▸ Atypical cells with pleomorphic nuclei and prominent nucleoli are present in high-grade tumors

Immunohistochemical Features

▸ Tumor cells are positive for pancytokeratins and CK7
▸ Epidermoid cells express CK5/6
▸ Usually immunonegative for CK20 and TTF-1

Pathologic Differential Diagnosis

▸ Mucous gland adenoma
▸ Adenosquamous carcinoma

PROGNOSIS AND THERAPY

The treatment and prognosis of these tumors are related to the histologic grade. Low-grade tumors generally have an excellent prognosis, particularly in children. Metastasis to regional lymph nodes occurs in less than 5% of low-grade tumors, and most patients have long survival. Central lesions are treated by sleeve resection or laser therapy. High-grade mucoepidermoid carcinomas behave more aggressively, and prognosis is related to the clinical stage at the time of diagnosis. Metastasis to liver, bone, and brain is not uncommon, and survival is similar to non-small cell carcinomas of the lung. High-grade tumors are treated with surgical resection and post-operative radiotherapy.

ADENOID CYSTIC CARCINOMA

CLINICAL FEATURES

Adenoid cystic carcinomas are the most common tumors of the tracheobronchial glands. They are more commonly seen in the trachea, where they account for approximately 40% of malignant tumors. Less frequently (less than 1%), they arise from the mainstem or lobar bronchi, and exceptionally they may arise from more distal bronchi. They are most often diagnosed in the fifth decade of life, and there is no apparent gender or racial predilection. Symptomatology is related to bronchial obstruction and its sequelae, and

consists of cough, hemoptysis, wheezing, and shortness of breath.

RADIOLOGIC FEATURES

A central mass is characteristically present, and post-
obstructive pneumonia, bronchiectasis, or atelectasis
may be visible.

PATHOLOGIC FEATURES

GROSS FINDINGS

Most adenoid cystic carcinomas present as endobronchial polypoid, soft, and well-circumscribed masses.
Less often, they develop as annular, gray, poorly circumscribed lesions producing thickening of the airway
wall. Tumors range in size from 1 to 4 cm in greatest
dimension.

MICROSCOPIC FINDINGS

The architectural patterns observed in adenoid
cystic carcinomas include cribriform, tubular, and solid
arrangements. The cribriform pattern is the most
common, and is characterized by nests of cells arranged around spaces filled with PAS-positive hyaline
material or basophilic mucoid material, having an appearance resembling "Swiss cheese" (Figure 28-2A).
Luminal cells can be flat, cuboidal, or columnar, and
surrounding cells are usually small and uniform in size
and shape, with round nuclei and pale eosinophilic
cytoplasm. Supporting connective tissue stroma separates the islands of tumor cells. Some adenoid cystic
carcinomas have a predominantly tubular pattern in
which the cells are arranged in a circular pattern
around eosinophilic or basophilic material. In the solid
pattern, the cells form irregular islands in which cyst-
like spaces are absent or sparse (Figure 28-2B). Mitotic
figures are generally rare or absent. Perineural invasion and infiltration along the bronchial wall are relatively common.

ANCILLARY STUDIES

FINE NEEDLE ASPIRATION BIOPSY

Smears from adenoid cystic carcinoma contain clusters of cohesive, small, uniform epithelial cells with
ovoid nuclei and inconspicuous nucleoli (Figure 28-2C).
The cytoplasm is scant, delicate, and nonvacuolated.

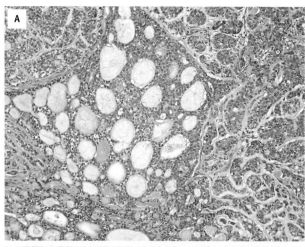

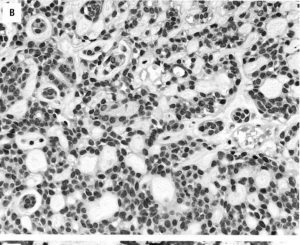

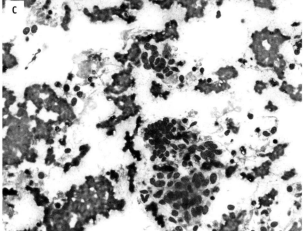

FIGURE 28-2

Adenoid cystic carcinoma

(A) This tumor displays cribriform and solid patterns. Mucohyaline and mucoid material is noted in the microcystic spaces, and stromal hyalinization is present between some of the solid nests. **(B)** Cytologically bland tumor cells form strands separated by hyaline matrix. **(C)** Crowded, monomorphic groups of tumor cells were noted in this fine needle aspiration specimen.

Neoplastic clusters may include central, acellular spheres of dense, homogeneous material.

Immunohistochemistry

The luminal cells show positive staining with cytokeratins, CEA, EMA, and occasionally with alpha-1-antichymotrypsin. The cells around the pseudocysts demonstrate staining reactivities of myoepithelial cells, with positivity for vimentin, smooth muscle actin, S100 protein, p63, and variable staining for cytokeratins and GFAP. The extracellular, eosinophilic material stains for type IV collagen, laminin, heparin sulfate proteoglycan, and entactin.

Differential Diagnosis

The differential diagnosis of adenoid cystic carcinoma includes conventional adenocarcinomas of the lung manifesting trabecular or cribriform patterns, and basaloid carcinoma. Immunohistochemical stains to demonstrate the presence of myoepithelial cells and intraluminal basement membrane material are useful to differentiate adenoid cystic carcinoma from other types of non-small cell lung carcinomas. In biopsy samples, adenoid cystic carcinoma may also be difficult to differentiate from small cell carcinoma. The characteristic chromatin pattern, nuclear molding, and expression of neuroendocrine markers favor a diagnosis of small cell carcinoma, while demonstration of myoepithelial differentiation supports a diagnosis of adenoid cystic carcinoma. The differential diagnosis from a metastatic adenoid cystic carcinoma of head and neck origin requires careful clinical correlation.

Prognosis and Therapy

Adenoid cystic carcinomas are generally characterized by long survival, but patients may have multiple local recurrences and late metastases. Lymph node metastases occur in about 20% of cases. More aggressive behavior is observed in tumors with a solid growth pattern, and

---

ADENOID CYSTIC CARCINOMA—FACT SHEET

Definition
- Malignant epithelial tumor demonstrating ductal and myoepithelial differentiation, similar to its counterpart arising in the major salivary glands

Incidence
- Uncommon pulmonary neoplasm, accounting for less than 1% of malignant tumors of the lung
- More frequent in the trachea than in bronchi

Morbidity and Mortality
- In advanced stages, death is due to widespread metastases
- Post-obstructive pneumonia is a frequent complication

Gender, Race, and Age Distribution
- Most frequently diagnosed in the fifth decade
- Equal gender distribution
- No apparent racial predilection

Clinical Features
- Symptoms are usually related to bronchial obstruction (cough, hemoptysis, wheezing)

Radiologic Features
- Central mass, commonly accompanied by post-obstructive pneumonia, bronchiectasis, or atelectasis

Prognosis and Therapy
- Prognosis depends on the clinical stage at presentation
- Complete surgical resection is the treatment of choice, and radiation therapy is also commonly used

---

ADENOID CYSTIC CARCINOMA—PATHOLOGIC FEATURES

Gross Findings
- Typically grow as polypoid endobronchial masses
- Less often, present as annular lesions with thickening of the airway walls
- Size ranges from 1-4 cm

Microscopic Findings
- Three main architectural patterns: cribriform, tubular, solid
- Uniform epithelial cells with round nuclei and pale eosinophilic cytoplasm, low mitotic rate
- Perineural invasion is common

Fine Needle Aspiration Biopsy
- Clusters of small epithelial cells with ovoid nuclei, inconspicuous nucleoli, and scant cytoplasm
- Acellular spheres of homogeneous material often surrounded by tumor cells

Immunohistochemical Features
- Luminal cells express cytokeratins, CEA, and EMA
- Cells around pseudocysts stain with vimentin, S-100, p63, and actin
- Extracellular material is immunoreactive for type IV collagen, laminin, heparin sulfate proteoglycan, and entactin

Pathologic Differential Diagnosis
- Conventional adenocarcinoma
- Basaloid carcinoma

with neoplasms that are diagnosed at an advanced stage. Well-demarcated endobronchial neoplasms are associated with long survival, up to 15 years. The treatment of choice is complete resection, usually requiring lobectomy or pneumonectomy, with radiation therapy. It may be difficult to achieve complete resection since the tumor can be more widely infiltrative than is appreciated from imaging studies and bronchoscopy, and frozen sections may be needed to produce a clear surgical margin. Bronchoplastic surgical procedures and laser therapy have been used for palliation.

ACINIC CELL CARCINOMA

CLINICAL FEATURES

This is a very rare tumor, presenting as a parenchymal or endobronchial mass. Although most patients are adults, it has also been reported in a 4-year-old child. Symptoms are related to the location of the tumor; obstructive manifestations are common when tumors occur in the bronchus, while peripheral lesions may be asymptomatic.

RADIOLOGIC FEATURES

A nodule or mass is usually seen.

PATHOLOGIC FEATURES

GROSS FINDINGS

Tumors are well circumscribed, varying in size from 1 to 4 cm, with a homogeneous cut surface.

MICROSCOPIC FINDINGS

Acinic cell carcinomas resemble their salivary gland counterparts, showing a predominantly homogeneous solid growth pattern with cohesive sheets (Figure 28-3), acinar structures, and papillocystic areas. In some cases, fibrous septa divide the tumor into lobules, giving an organoid appearance. The tumor cells are cytologically bland, with rounded, hyperchromatic, or vesicular nuclei that are centrally or eccentrically placed. Large amounts of PAS- and mucicarmine-positive cytoplasm or PAS-negative clear cytoplasm are present. Cellular pleomorphism, mitoses, and necrosis are absent. Extremely rare reports describe tumors combining acinic cell carcinoma and carcinoid.

ANCILLARY STUDIES

IMMUNOHISTOCHEMISTRY

Immunohistochemical staining shows a strong positive reaction for cytokeratins and EMA and weak staining for amylase and alpha-1-antichymotrypsin.

ULTRASTRUCTURAL FEATURES

Zymogen granules are characteristic.

DIFFERENTIAL DIAGNOSIS

The differential diagnosis includes oncocytic carcinoid, sugar tumor, and bronchial granular cell tumor. These entities are distinguished from acinic cell carcinoma by histologic appearance supported by a panel of immunohistochemical stains. Carcinoids display a positive reaction for neuroendocrine markers, which are typically not expressed by acinic cell carcinoma (NCAM and CGA). Sugar tumors show a negative reaction for cytokeratins but are immunopositive for HMB45. Granular cell tumors stain with S100 protein, which is not expressed by acinic cell carcinomas. Primary clear cell adenocarcinoma of the lung and metastatic renal cell carcinoma and other clear cell neoplasms may also be included in the differential diagnosis. These tumors are distinguished from acinic cell carcinoma primarily based on morphologic features including greater nuclear pleomorphism, higher mitotic rate, and necrosis in the carcinomas.

PROGNOSIS AND THERAPY

These tumors appear to have an indolent behavior, even although they can metastasize to the lymph nodes and can recur. Complete surgical resection is the treatment of choice.

EPITHELIAL-MYOEPITHELIAL CARCINOMA

CLINICAL FEATURES

Primary pulmonary epithelial-myoepithelial carcinomas are very rare and occur in middle-aged patients (mean age of 50 years) of both genders. Presenting symptoms include dyspnea, cough, and recurrent

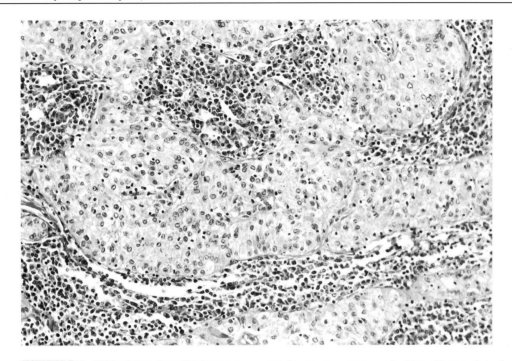

FIGURE 28-3

Acinic cell carcinoma
Polygonal cells with abundant pale eosinophilic cytoplasm and uniform round nuclei form sheets, and are accompanied by an intense inflammatory infiltrate.

ACINIC CELL CARCINOMA—FACT SHEET

Definition
» Malignant epithelial neoplasm arising from bronchial glands, with differentiation toward serous acinar cells, similar to its lesional counterpart in the major salivary glands

Incidence
» Very rare

Morbidity
» Bronchial obstruction can lead to pneumonia

Gender, Race, and Age Distribution
» Usually occur in adults, but can occur in children
» No characteristic gender or racial predilection

Clinical Features
» Symptoms are related to bronchial obstruction (cough, wheezing, shortness of breath) by centrally located tumors
» Usually asymptomatic when peripherally located

Radiologic Features
» Nodule or mass lesion

Prognosis and Therapy
» Generally good prognosis due to indolent behavior
» Complete surgical resection is the treatment of choice
» Tumors can metastasize to lymph nodes and can recur

ACINIC CELL CARCINOMA—PATHOLOGIC FEATURES

Gross Findings
» Polypoid endobronchial lesion or well-circumscribed nodule in lung parenchyma

Microscopic Findings
» Uniform, round cells with abundant granular or clear cytoplasm
» Nuclei are small and hyperchromatic or large and vesicular
» Cells are organized in sheets, nests, or small glands, or have an organoid pattern due to fibrous septa
» Cellular pleomorphism, mitoses, and necrosis are absent

Immunohistochemical Features
» Immunopositive for cytokeratins and EMA
» Weak staining for amylase and alpha-1-antichymotrypsin

Ultrastructural Features
» Zymogen granules

Pathologic Differential Diagnosis
» Oncocytic carcinoid
» Sugar tumor
» Granular cell tumor
» Primary clear cell adenocarcinoma of the lung
» Metastatic renal cell carcinoma or other clear cell neoplasms

pulmonary infections. Rarely, these tumors may be asymptomatic.

RADIOLOGIC FEATURES

A nodule or mass is visible, usually centrally located.

PATHOLOGIC FEATURES

GROSS FINDINGS

Epithelial-myoepithelial carcinomas usually present as well demarcated, polypoid, endobronchial masses. Tumor size ranges from 1 to 5 cm.

MICROSCOPIC FINDINGS

Histologically, the tumor shows pushing margins and is composed of glands and sheets of spindle cells (Figure 28-4). The glands are filled by colloid-like material and lined by two types of cells. The inner layer consists of cuboidal cells with acidophilic cytoplasm,

and the outer layer of myoepithelial cells with pale, often clear cytoplasm. Solid areas of spindle cells with acidophilic cytoplasm are also seen. The mitotic rate and degree of cytoatypia are generally low.

ANCILLARY STUDIES

IMMUNOHISTOCHEMISTRY

The myoepithelial cells are strongly immunopositive for S100 and smooth muscle actin; they can also stain for CD10, calponin, and p63. The inner lining cells of the glands are positive for keratins and EMA. A positive reaction to p27/kip-1 has been observed in both spindle (cytoplasmic) and glandular cells (nuclear and cytoplasmic).

DIFFERENTIAL DIAGNOSIS

The differential diagnosis is broad and principally includes other biphasic tumors arising in the bronchi. Pleomorphic adenoma usually contains a myoepithelial

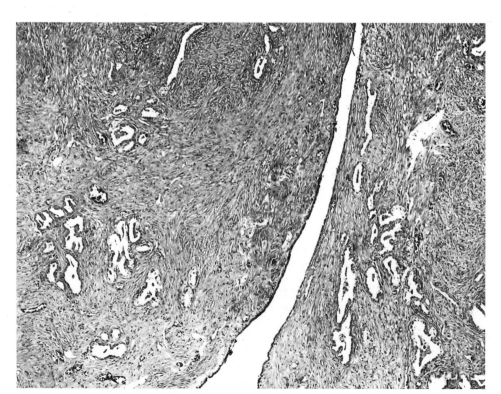

FIGURE 28-4
Epithelial-myoepithelial carcinoma
Glands are separated by spindle cells and collagen.

component, but also a myxochondroid or chondroid component is present. Cribriform and infiltrative growth patterns are characteristic of adenoid cystic carcinoma and are not seen in epithelial-myoepithelial carcinoma. Metastatic epithelial-myoepithelial carcinoma usually presents as multiple peripheral nodules, but should be excluded prior to classifying the tumor as a lung primary. When clear cells predominate, clear cell tumors of the lung or a metastatic clear cell carcinoma should be considered in the differential diagnosis. The absence of a biphasic pattern in these tumors and the immunophenotype of the neoplastic cells can help to distinguish it from these other entities. Clear cell carcinoid can be excluded on the basis of negative stains for neuroendocrine markers.

PROGNOSIS AND THERAPY

Complete surgical resection usually produces a cure, although late recurrence has been reported.

FETAL ADENOCARCINOMA

CLINICAL FEATURES

Fetal adenocarcinoma is a relatively indolent tumor, most prevalent in the fourth decade and having a slight female predominance. Symptomatology is generally related to the location of the neoplasm. Tumors involving the bronchi can cause a cough and hemoptysis. Since many of these tumors are asymptomatic, however, they are often discovered incidentally on routine chest radiographs. Although about 80% of these tumors develop in smokers, there is not a clear association with smoking.

RADIOLOGIC FEATURES

A solitary nodule with lobulated margins is typical.

EPITHELIAL-MYOEPITHELIAL CARCINOMA—FACT SHEET

Definition
➤ Tumor composed of myoepithelial cells with varied morphologies and ductal epithelial cells, forming glands, ducts, and sheets, similar to its counterpart in the major salivary glands

Incidence
➤ Very rare

Morbidity and Mortality
➤ Recurrent airway infections are common due to airway obstruction
➤ No deaths related to the neoplasm

Gender and Age Distribution
➤ Occur primarily in middle-aged patients
➤ Slight female predominance

Clinical Features
➤ Symptoms include cough and dyspnea due to airway obstruction

Radiologic Features
➤ Nodule or mass, usually centrally located

Prognosis and Therapy
➤ Complete surgical resection is the treatment of choice and usually produces a cure
➤ Late recurrence has been described

EPITHELIAL-MYOEPITHELIAL CARCINOMA—PATHOLOGIC FEATURES

Gross Findings
➤ Well demarcated, solid, polypoid endobronchial mass, 1-5 cm in size

Microscopic Findings
➤ Biphasic growth pattern consisting of spindle cells and glands lined by 2 types of cells (epithelial and myoepithelial cells)
➤ Generally low mitotic rate

Immunohistochemical Features
➤ Myoepithelial cells stain with S100, smooth muscle actin, CD10
➤ Inner layer of epithelial cells in glands stain with cytokeratins and EMA

Pathologic Differential Diagnosis
➤ Pleomorphic adenoma of the bronchus
➤ Adenoid cystic carcinoma
➤ Clear cell carcinoid
➤ Other primary pulmonary and metastatic clear cell neoplasms
➤ Metastatic epithelial-myoepithelial carcinoma

PATHOLOGIC FEATURES

GROSS FINDINGS

Fetal adenocarcinomas generally occur in peripheral or mid-lung locations and present as sharply circumscribed nodules ranging from 1-5 cm in greatest dimension. Presentation in a central location as a polypoid intrabronchial mass has also been described. The cut surface is solid and whitish-yellow or tan. Hemorrhage and necrosis may be evident in larger masses, but invasion of the visceral pleura or chest wall is not characteristic of this tumor.

MICROSCOPIC FINDINGS

The characteristic histopathologic features of fetal adenocarcinoma include distinctive glandular structures and morule formation. The rather uniform glandular component is composed of complex branching tubular structures resembling fetal lung (Figure 28-5A). A single layer of columnar cells lines the glands. These cells have clear cytoplasm with supranuclear and/or subnuclear vacuoles containing glycogen, giving the cells a resemblance to endometrial cells (Figure 28-5B). The nuclei are round or oval with a small to medium size, and for the most part have a low-grade appearance with little pleomorphism or atypia. The morular component represents solid aggregates of cells with eosinophilic cytoplasm and a squamous appearance (Figure 28-5B). No intercellular bridges or keratin formation is present in the morules. Necrosis and nuclear pleomorphism are rarely seen, and mitotic figures are rarely found in the glandular component. The stroma in fetal adenocarcinoma is characteristically inconspicuous, sometimes

fibromyxomatous, and with scattered inflammatory cells. A sarcomatous or immature blastemal stroma should not be seen; if this type of stroma is present, then the tumor should be classified as a pulmonary blastoma.

Nakatani and colleagues also described a higher grade form of fetal adenocarcinoma that they distinguished from the low-grade form by the following criteria: presence of disorganized glands, large vesicular nuclei, prominent nucleoli, pronounced anisonucleosis, absence of morules, transition to conventional adenocarcinoma, broad areas of necrosis, desmoplastic stroma, over-expression of p53 protein, and production of alpha-fetoprotein.

ANCILLARY STUDIES

IMMUNOHISTOCHEMISTRY

The cells of the glandular and morular components express keratin, CEA, EMA, surfactant apoprotein A, and secretory component. Nuclear staining for TTF-1 can be observed in many glandular cells, and focal immunoreactivity for alpha-fetoprotein is occasionally seen in glandular cells. Morular cells often show immunoreactivity for Clara cell protein CC10 and GATA-6, and can demonstrate focal expression of neuroendocrine markers. The nuclei of morular cells also react intensely with biotin.

HISTOCHEMISTRY

Periodic acid-Schiff (PAS) staining is helpful to demonstrate the presence of intracytoplasmic glycogen in glandular lining cells. Mucicarmine stains highlight

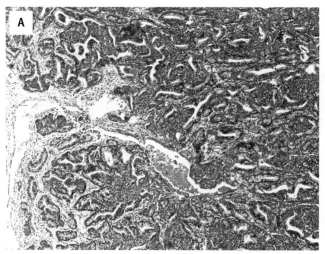
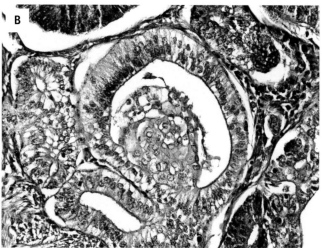

FIGURE 28-5

Fetal adenocarcinoma

(A) This tumor is composed of closely packed, branching glands with little intervening stroma. **(B)** A morule occupies the center of a gland, which is lined by columnar cells with clear cytoplasm and nuclei with little atypia.

mucin, which may be present in small amounts within some glandular lumina.

ULTRASTRUCTURAL FEATURES

The glandular cells show well-developed junctional complexes, short microvilli, and basal bodies. Abundant intracytoplasmic glycogen granules are characteristically found in many epithelial cells. The morular cells have distinct basal lamina and cytoplasmic interdigitations. Some of them have osmiophilic lamellar bodies, clusters of spherical bodies, and vacuoles in the cytoplasm. The nuclei show fine filaments replacing the central nuclear area. Tumor cells can also occasionally possess characteristics of neuroendocrine cells.

DIFFERENTIAL DIAGNOSIS

The main differential diagnosis of fetal adenocarcinoma includes conventional adenocarcinoma, pulmonary blastoma, and metastatic endometrial carcinoma. Histologic characteristics distinguish fetal adenocarcinoma from conventional adenocarcinoma and blastoma. The distinctive glycogen vacuoles and morules help to differentiate fetal adenocarcinoma from conventional adenocarcinoma. Pulmonary blastomas will have a sarcomatous or immature blastemal stroma in addition to a glandular component resembling fetal adenocarcinoma. Obtaining clinical history and performing TTF-1 staining are helpful for differentiating fetal adenocarcinoma from metastatic endometrial carcinoma.

PROGNOSIS AND THERAPY

Fetal adenocarcinomas tend to be relatively indolent and usually present at clinical stage I. The tumor-associated mortality rate is 10%, and survival is generally long (mean follow-up of 70 months). Tumors

---

FETAL ADENOCARCINOMA—FACT SHEET

Definition

→ Histologically distinctive type of adenocarcinoma resembling fetal lung

Incidence

→ Account for approximately 0.3% of malignant lung tumors

Mortality

→ Tumor-associated mortality rate is 10%

Gender, Race, and Age Distribution

→ Slight female predominance
→ Most prevalent in fourth decade
→ No apparent racial predilection

Clinical Features

→ Often asymptomatic
→ Cough and hemoptysis when bronchi are involved
→ 80% observed in smokers

Radiologic Features

→ Solitary nodule with lobulated margins

Prognosis and Therapy

→ Long survival
→ Tumors with features of conventional adenocarcinoma are associated with more aggressive behavior
→ Complete surgical resection is the preferred therapy
→ Chemotherapy and radiotherapy do not appear to improve survival

---

FETAL ADENOCARCINOMA—PATHOLOGIC FEATURES

Gross Findings

→ Sharply circumscribed, solid nodule or mass, ranging in size from 1 to 5 cm
→ Cut surface is whitish, with hemorrhagic areas and necrosis in larger lesions

Microscopic Findings

→ Branching glandular structures resembling fetal lung
→ Glandular lining cells have supranuclear and subnuclear vacuoles containing glycogen, resembling endometrial cells
→ Morules consisting of squamoid cells
→ Most cases have low-grade nuclear features, with little pleomorphism or atypia

Immunohistochemical Features

→ Keratins, CEA, EMA, surfactant apoprotein A and secretory component are expressed in both glandular epithelial and morular cells
→ TTF-1 can be expressed in glandular cells
→ Expression of Clara cell protein (CC10) and neuroendocrine markers can be observed in morular cells

Ultrastructural Features

→ Glandular cells show well-developed junctional complexes, short microvilli. and basal bodies
→ Glycogen granules are typically seen in glandular epithelial cells
→ Morular cells have distinct basal lamina and cytoplasmic interdigitations
→ Tumor cells may show neuroendocrine differentiation

Pathologic Differential Diagnosis

→ Conventional adenocarcinoma
→ Pulmonary blastoma
→ Metastatic endometrial carcinoma

having features of conventional adenocarcinoma, more widespread neuroendocrine differentiation, and extensive alpha-fetoprotein production can show more aggressive behavior. In addition, over-expression of p53 and a high Ki67 labeling index appear to be associated with a worse prognosis. Complete surgical resection is currently the primary treatment. Chemotherapy and radiation have been used without any significant improvement in survival.

MUCINOUS (COLLOID) CARCINOMA

CLINICAL FEATURES

Mucinous carcinomas (MCs) of the lung account for approximately 0.24% of all pulmonary neoplasms. Most patients are between 33 and 81 years (median 60 years) and there is a slightly higher prevalence in men. Although many patients are asymptomatic, presenting symptoms can include cough, hemoptysis, and chest pain.

RADIOLOGIC FEATURES

Imaging studies reveal a solitary nodule or mass, usually in the periphery of the lung, or a more diffuse infiltrate. There is a slight predilection for the upper lobes.

PATHOLOGIC FEATURES

GROSS FINDINGS

Tumors are described as well circumscribed, unencapsulated masses, varying in size from 0.5 to 10 cm in greatest dimension. They have a characteristic gray-white, glistening, soft, gelatinous cut surface.

MICROSCOPIC FINDINGS

Histologically, the tumors are relatively paucicellular and consist of large pools of mucin filling the alveolar spaces and dissecting through stroma, with tumor cells floating in the mucin (Figure 28-6A,B). Tall columnar, mucin-secreting epithelial cells line alveolar septa, and are often not very abundant (Figure28-6B,C). Some of these cells can have features of goblet cells. There may be small epithelial tufts or micropapillae. Tumor cells are usually well differentiated and demonstrate basally

located nuclei, sometimes with prominent nucleoli. Cytological atypia may be seen, but it is usually slight, and mitotic activity is absent or minimal.

ANCILLARY STUDIES

IMMUNOHISTOCHEMISTRY

The neoplastic columnar cells of MC express CK7 and CK20, TTF-1, CDX-2, and MUC-2.

HISTOCHEMISTRY

The extracellular mucin is strongly positive with mucicarmine stain and predigested PAS stains. PAS positivity is also observed on the luminal aspects of the goblet cells.

DIFFERENTIAL DIAGNOSIS

The most important issue lies in determining whether a tumor represents a primary lung cancer or a metastasis from another primary site. For this purpose, the expression of TTF-1 and CK7 can be useful for supporting a pulmonary origin. Nevertheless, clinical and radiographic correlation is mandatory for definitive diagnosis. Mucinous bronchioloalveolar carcinoma (m-BAC) is another entity that must be considered in the differential diagnosis. M-BAC has a different radiographic and macroscopic pattern, often presenting as lobar or sublobar consolidation. M-BAC is more cellular than MC, with a characteristic lepidic growth pattern of mucin-producing cells. The expression of CDX-2 and MUC-2 may be helpful in such a setting to support an interpretation of MC, since m-BAC does not stain with CDX-2/MUC-2. Signet ring carcinomas lack the abundant extracellular mucin characteristic of MCs, and consist of nests of signet ring cells. Lung cysts and mucus plugs may also be considered in the differential diagnosis, but should also not show individual tumor cells and nests of tumor cells floating in mucin, as is seen in MC, and should not demonstrate atypical columnar cells lining alveolar septa.

PROGNOSIS AND THERAPY

The majority of MCs present at stage I (A or B) and are generally associated with long survival (more than 5 years) without disease. Metastases to bone or brain can occur, however. Complete surgical resection is the treatment of choice.

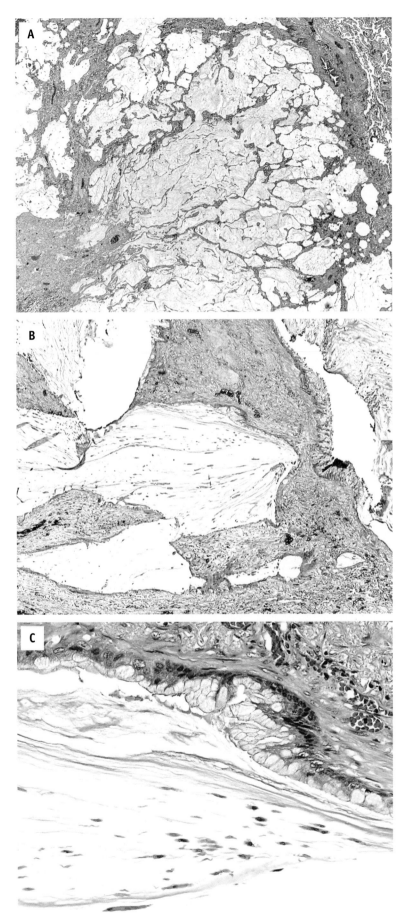

FIGURE 28-6

Mucinous carcinoma

(A) Mucin fills most of the air spaces in this view. **(B)** Portions of the septa are lined by neoplastic columnar cells with mucinous cytoplasm. Abundant extracellular mucin is present. **(C)** This high-power view shows mucinous columnar cells with mildly atypical basally oriented nuclei.

MUCINOUS CYSTADENOCARCINOMA

This is a very rare tumor that has been reported in adults of both genders. Tumors are well circumscribed and typically display fibrous capsules that may not be complete. They have mucoid cut surfaces. Microscopic features include central cystic mucin accumulation and neoplastic columnar cells with atypia lining the walls of the cystic lesion. Small numbers of neoplastic cells can be found in the mucin. It is recognized, however, that there can be histologic overlap of these features with mucinous carcinomas, and some have advocated classifying these tumors with other mucinous neoplasms as "mucin-rich tumors of the lung."

SIGNET RING ADENOCARCINOMA

CLINICAL FEATURES

Signet ring adenocarcinomas (SRAs) account for 0.14-0.19% of lung cancers. This pattern, however, can also be a focal finding associated with other histologic types of adenocarcinoma. SRAs develop in both genders, with a slight male predominance, and occur in patients ranging in age from 30 to 75 years (mean of 52 years). Presenting symptoms are weight loss, shortness of breath, hemoptysis, nausea, chest pain, and pneumonia. A relationship to smoking has not been established.

RADIOLOGIC FEATURES

Imaging studies show a solid mass, usually peripheral.

PATHOLOGIC FEATURES

GROSS FINDINGS

Tumors usually present as single masses measuring between 2.0 and 8.0 cm in diameter. They are soft, glistening and gray. They can have a peripheral or sometimes a central location.

MICROSCOPIC FINDINGS

Tumors can display acinar or diffuse patterns, the latter demonstrating sheets or cords of tumor cells. The neoplastic cells have vacuolated cytoplasm with displacement of the nuclei to the periphery, giving them a signet ring appearance (Figure 28-7). The cells

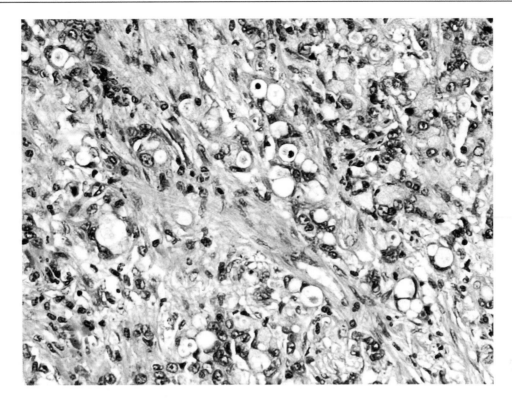

FIGURE 28-7

Signet ring adenocarcinoma

Tumor cells display characteristic signet ring morphology, with a single large mucin vacuole that displaces the nucleus to the periphery of the cell.

have distinct borders without marked atypia or an elevated mitotic count. The interposed stroma is scant and generally composed of connective tissue, but sometimes it may be more prominent and desmoplastic. A dense inflammatory reaction can occasionally be seen. Necrosis is often observed. Areas of conventional adenocarcinoma generally accompany the signet ring pattern.

ANCILLARY STUDIES

IMMUNOHISTOCHEMISTRY

These tumors show strong immunopositivity for CEA and pan-cytokeratins. In addition, over 90% of SRAs express a cytokeratin profile of CK7+/CK20−, and most are immunopositive for TTF-1. Villin reactivity has been demonstrated in about 30% of cases. All the tumors are negative for CDX-2.

HISTOCHEMISTRY

The intracellular mucin of SRAs stains with PAS with and without diastase, Alcian blue at pH 2.7, and mucicarmine. Less intense staining is observed using Alcian blue at pH 0.9.

DIFFERENTIAL DIAGNOSIS

Primary pulmonary SRAs must be distinguished from metastatic carcinomas from the gastrointestinal tract, breast, pancreas, and ovary. The differentiation of a primary tumor from a metastatic process is particularly important on biopsy material to plan treatment. In the appropriate clinical setting, the use of immunohistochemical stains may facilitate the diagnosis. An immunostaining profile of CK7+/CK20−/TTF-1+ favors a lung primary. Staining for estrogen and progesterone receptors favors a breast primary, while staining for CK20 and CDX-2 favors colonic primary. Finally, an immunohistochemical profile of CK7+/CK20+/TTF-1− is more suggestive of a pancreatic or ovarian primary. The differential diagnosis may also encompass other primary lung tumors, including mucinous bronchioloalveolar carcinoma, mucinous carcinoma, and acinic cell carcinoma. Mucinous bronchioloalveolar carcinomas are characterized by a lepidic growth pattern of mucinous epithelial cells along alveolar septa. Mucinous carcinomas show extensive pools of extracellular mucin with the neoplastic cells floating in the mucus. In addition, the neoplastic cells express CK7 and CK 20, CDX-2 and MUC-2, the latter not seen in SRA. Acinic cell carcinomas lack the signet ring morphology, and their cells are mucicarmine-negative.

SIGNET RING ADENOCARCINOMA—FACT SHEET

Definition
▸ Malignant epithelial tumor with a distinctive "signet ring" appearance due to abundant intracellular mucin production

Incidence
▸ 0.14-0.19% of lung cancers

Mortality
▸ High mortality rate with disseminated disease

Gender, Race, and Age Distribution
▸ Slight male predominance
▸ Age range from 30 to 75 years (median 60 years)
▸ No recognized racial predilection

Clinical Features
▸ Symptoms include weight loss, shortness of breath, hemoptysis, and pneumonia
▸ Relationship to smoking is not well established

Radiologic Features
▸ Solid mass, usually peripheral

Prognosis and Therapy
▸ Aggressive behavior with frequent metastasis
▸ Surgery, chemotherapy, radiotherapy, or a combination of these modalities can be used for therapy

---

SIGNET RING ADENOCARCINOMA—PATHOLOGIC FEATURES

Gross Findings
▸ Soft, glistening gray mass, ranging in size from 2 to 8 cm

Microscopic Findings
▸ Signet ring cell morphology with acinar and diffuse growth patterns
▸ Conventional adenocarcinoma patterns frequently accompany the SRA pattern

Immunohistochemical Features
▸ Strong positivity for CEA, cytokeratins, and TTF-1
▸ CK7+/CK20− profile expressed in over 90% of cases
▸ Negative for CK20 and CDX-2

Pathologic Differential Diagnosis
▸ Metastatic adenocarcinomas
▸ Mucinous bronchioloalveolar carcinoma
▸ Mucinous carcinoma
▸ Acinic cell carcinoma, primary or metastatic

PROGNOSIS AND THERAPY

SRAs display aggressive behavior with widespread metastases, sometimes present at clinical presentation. Therapy includes surgical resection, radiation, chemotherapy, or a combination of these modalities. For patients whose tumors include more than 50% SRA, the 5-year survival rate is reported to be less than 30%.

PULMONARY BLASTOMA

CLINICAL FEATURES

Pulmonary blastoma is a very rare entity that accounts for 0.5% of all malignant lung neoplasms. In the most recent version of the World Health Organization classification system, it is classified under the heading of sarcomatoid carcinoma. It occurs largely in adults, with an average age at diagnosis in the fourth decade of life, with an equal distribution between men and women. More than 80% of patients are tobacco smokers. Symptoms arise secondary to bronchial or pleural involvement and include cough, dyspnea, hemoptysis, and chest pain. Other clinical manifestations, such as weight loss, fever, pneumonia, and pneumothorax are less frequent. Approximately 40% of patients are asymptomatic at the time of diagnosis.

RADIOLOGIC FEATURES

Chest radiographs usually show a well-defined mass lesion, which may be large enough to completely opacify the hemithorax and cause mediastinal shift. Computed tomography reveals a mixed solid and cystic lesion with variable contrast enhancement and a necrotic center, and pleural effusion may be present.

PATHOLOGIC FEATURES

GROSS FINDINGS

Tumors usually present as well-demarcated masses, sometimes with satellite nodules. A polypoid endobronchial growth pattern is very rare. The tumors range in diameter from 1 to 28 cm (median, 6 cm). Their cut surfaces are typically variegated and soft, frequently with necrotic areas in central locations.

MICROSCOPIC FINDINGS

Pulmonary blastoma is a biphasic tumor consisting of primitive, malignant glandular and mesenchymal elements (Figure 28-8A). The glandular elements usually resemble those of fetal adenocarcinoma, and are reminiscent of fetal bronchioles between 10 and 16 weeks' gestation (pseudoglandular stage) or endometrial glands (Figure 28-8B). They consist of branching tubular structures lined by non-ciliated columnar epithelium, often with clear cytoplasm and subnuclear or supranuclear vacuoles. Variable degrees of nuclear atypia are observed in the epithelial cells. The epithelial cells can also be arranged in solid cords or nests with a basaloid pattern or as undifferentiated sheets of cells. Rosette-like formation may be occasionally seen. Morules are present in about 50% of cases. The mesenchymal component consists of embryonal elements, and can also include sarcomatous adult elements. The undifferentiated, primitive stroma is composed of densely packed, hyperchromatic, fusiform or stellate cells, in a myxoid background, which can be arranged around the neoplastic glands. Occasionally, the primitive stroma can differentiate into cartilage, bone, or striated muscle, creating an element of adult-type sarcoma (chondrosarcoma, osteosarcoma, rhabdomyosar-

coma). Areas of necrosis are frequent, and mitotic activity is prominent in both mesenchymal and epithelial components.

ANCILLARY STUDIES

IMMUNOHISTOCHEMISTRY

The epithelial component of pulmonary blastoma demonstrates staining for keratins (AE1-AE3, CAM5.2), CEA, EMA, pulmonary surfactant, Clara cell antigen, and often markers of neuroendocrine differentiation (chromogranin A and individual hormones). Vimentin and actin are usually expressed in mesenchymal cells, which can also express desmin and myoglobin if differentiating towards muscle, or S-100 protein in foci of chondroid differentiation. Interestingly, both epithelial and mesenchymal components may show strong cytoplasmic reactivity for CD117, and more than 50% of cases show over-expression of p53 with mutation of the p53 gene. Aberrant nuclear and cytoplasmic expression of beta-catenin is present in both epithelial and stroma cells.

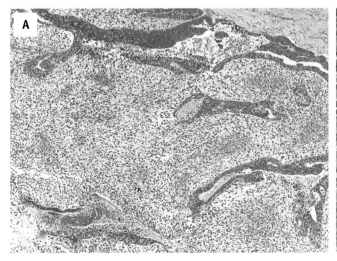 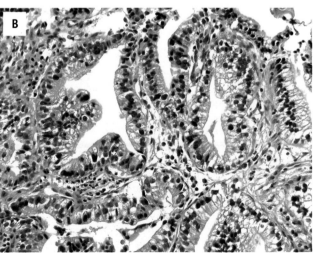

FIGURE 28-8

Pulmonary blastoma
(A) This biphasic tumor is composed of malignant epithelial elements (glands) and undifferentiated mesenchymal elements. **(B)** The glandular element typically resembles fetal adenocarcinoma.

HISTOCHEMISTRY

PAS staining highlights the intracellular glycogen in the glandular cells of pulmonary blastoma. Focal mucin may be observed in glandular lumens.

DIFFERENTIAL DIAGNOSIS

Pulmonary blastoma must be differentiated from fetal adenocarcinoma, which replicates the epithelial component of pulmonary blastoma but lacks the malignant mesenchymal component. Pulmonary blastoma may be confused with pleuropulmonary blastoma, which is essentially a pediatric neoplasm lacking the malignant epithelial component observed in pulmonary blastoma. The distinctive morphologic features of pulmonary blastomas, particularly the embryonic type of epithelium and morules, permit differentiation from carcinosarcomas. Metastatic endometrioid carcinomas may be diffi-

cult to differentiate from pulmonary blastoma without clinical information, but generally lack the malignant stromal component of pulmonary blastoma. Metastatic sarcomas can also be considered in the differential diagnosis, but lack the distinctive epithelial component of pulmonary blastoma.

PROGNOSIS AND THERAPY

The prognosis of pulmonary blastoma is poor, with a 5-year survival of approximately 16-20% despite frequent presentation at early clinical stages, and a mortality rate of approximately 75% within 2 years. The preferred treatment is complete surgical resection, usually requiring lobectomy or pneumonectomy. Combination chemotherapy in inoperable tumors and adjuvant therapy do not appear to significantly improve the survival rate. The efficacy of local radiotherapy has been debated.

PULMONARY BLASTOMA—FACT SHEET

Definition
➤ Biphasic tumor with distinctive malignant epithelial and mesenchymal components, resembling fetal lung

Incidence
➤ 0.5% of malignant lung neoplasms

Morbidity and Mortality
➤ High mortality rate (approximately 75%) within 2 years
➤ Chest pain due to pleural involvement in more than 50% of cases

Gender, Race, and Age Distribution
➤ Equal gender distribution
➤ Affects adults with an average age at diagnosis in the fourth decade of life
➤ No apparent racial predilection

Clinical Features
➤ Cough, dyspnea, hemoptysis, and chest pain are common symptoms, but 40% are asymptomatic
➤ More than 80% of patients are smokers

Radiologic Features
➤ Well-defined solitary mass lesion, characteristically solid and cystic with variable contrast enhancement and a necrotic center on computed tomography scan
➤ Pleural effusion may be present

Prognosis and Therapy
➤ Poor prognosis, with a 5-year survival rate of approximately 20%
➤ Complete surgical resection is the preferred treatment
➤ Chemotherapy has been used in advanced stages

PULMONARY BLASTOMA—PATHOLOGIC FEATURES

Gross Findings
➤ Well-demarcated mass, measuring up to 28 cm
➤ Satellite nodules may be present
➤ Polypoid endobronchial growth is very rare
➤ Cut surface is variegated, and necrosis is common

Microscopic Findings
➤ Biphasic proliferation of malignant epithelial and mesenchymal elements
➤ Epithelial component resembles fetal airway epithelium or endometrioid glands and typically consists of branching tubular structures lined by nonciliated columnar epithelia with clear cytoplasm; morules are present in approximately 50% of cases
➤ Mesenchymal component includes undifferentiated stellate or fusiform cells in a myxoid background and can include a component of conventional sarcoma (chondrosarcoma, osteosarcoma, rhabdomyosarcoma)
➤ Necrosis and hemorrhage are frequent

Immunohistochemical Features
➤ Epithelial component cells stain with keratins, CEA, EMA, pulmonary surfactant, Clara cell antigen, and sometimes neuroendocrine markers
➤ Mesenchymal component stains with vimentin and actin; desmin and myoglobin, or S-100 protein, can be positive in areas of muscle or cartilaginous differentiation, respectively

Pathologic Differential Diagnosis
➤ Fetal adenocarcinoma
➤ Pleuropulmonary blastoma
➤ Carcinosarcoma
➤ Metastatic endometrioid carcinoma
➤ Metastatic Wilms' tumor
➤ Metastatic sarcomas

BASALOID CARCINOMA

CLINICAL FEATURES

Basaloid carcinomas are included in the large cell carcinoma category of lung carcinomas. They are usually found in men with a mean age of approximately 60 years. The presenting symptoms are similar (cough, hemoptysis, chest pain) to other non-small cell carcinomas.

RADIOLOGIC FEATURES

Imaging studies reveal a solitary mass, more frequently central than mid-lung or peripheral.

PATHOLOGIC FEATURES

GROSS FINDINGS

Basaloid carcinomas usually present as central masses of variable size (1-6 cm), often with endobronchial growth and infiltrative margins. Less often, they can be found in peripheral locations. The cut surfaces are white, and lymph node metastases are frequent.

MICROSCOPIC FINDINGS

Basaloid carcinoma has an infiltrative, solid lobular or trabecular growth pattern with peripheral palisading (Figure 28-9). The tumor is composed of small cuboidal or fusiform cells with hyperchromatic nuclei and very scant cytoplasm, but nuclear molding is not observed. Nucleoli are generally absent or inconspicuous. Mitotic count is very high (more than 15 mitoses per 10 HPF). Necrosis is often observed in the centers of the solid nests, and small cystic spaces with mucoid material, hyalinosis, mucoid degeneration of the stroma, and rosette formation are other features that can be noted in this tumor. No squamous differentiation is present.

ANCILLARY STUDIES

IMMUNOHISTOCHEMISTRY

Tumor cells are immunopositive for pankeratins and high molecular weight keratins, such as cytokeratins 1, 5, 10, and 14 (34βE12), but are negative for TTF-1. Focal expression of neuroendocrine markers, particularly synaptophysin and NCAM, occurs in about 10% of tumors.

DIFFERENTIAL DIAGNOSIS

The main differential diagnoses include poorly differentiated squamous cell carcinoma, small cell carcinoma, and large cell neuroendocrine carcinoma. The presence of peripheral palisading, absence of intercellular bridges and keratinization, and the high rate of mitosis favor a diagnosis of basaloid carcinoma over poorly differentiated squamous cell carcinoma. More difficult is the differential diagnosis from small cell carcinoma and large cell neuroendocrine carcinoma. The lack of nuclear molding, presence of vesicular rather than "salt and pepper" nuclear chromatin, lack of immunoreactivity for TTF-1, and positive staining for 34βE12 keratin supports a diagnosis of basaloid carcinoma over small cell carcinoma. Large cell neuroendocrine carcinoma generally consists of larger cells with greater amounts of cytoplasm and frequent prominent nucleoli. It should show neuroendocrine architectural arrangements, immunoreactivity for neuroendocrine markers, or ultrastructural evidence of neurosecretory granules, and, unlike basaloid carcinoma, does not show small cystic spaces with mucoid material, hyalinosis or mucoid degeneration of the stroma.

PROGNOSIS AND THERAPY

Some studies have reported a poorer prognosis (5-year survival of 10-15%) for basaloid carcinomas as compared to poorly differentiated squamous cell carcinomas, while other studies have not found a significant difference in prognosis (actuarial 5-year survival rate of 40.6% in patients with poorly differentiated squamous cell carcinoma and 36.5% in those with basaloid carcinoma). Surgical resection is the main therapeutic approach for these tumors.

TERATOMA

CLINICAL FEATURES

Primary teratomas of the lung are extremely rare neoplasms that are thought to originate from derivatives of the third pharyngeal pouch. They generally present with non-specific symptoms including chest pain, cough, hemoptysis, bronchiectasis, and pneumonia. A more

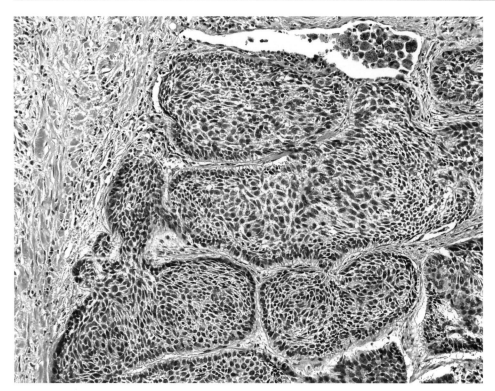

FIGURE 28-9
Basaloid carcinoma
Closely approximated tumor cell nests contain cuboidal and fusiform tumor cells with peripheral palisading.

BASALOID CARCINOMA—FACT SHEET

Definition
▸ A subset of large cell carcinomas resembling basal cell carcinoma of the skin

Incidence
▸ Less than 1% of lung cancers

Morbidity and Mortality
▸ Reported 5-year survival rates vary from 10-15% to 36.5%

Gender, Race, and Age Distribution
▸ More common in men
▸ Mean age of approximately 60 years
▸ No apparent racial predilection

Clinical Features
▸ Common symptoms include cough, hemoptysis, and chest pain

Radiologic Features
▸ Mass, usually central or in the mid-lung zones, less often peripheral

Prognosis and Therapy
▸ Prognosis varies with individual reports
▸ Surgical resection is the preferred therapy

BASALOID CARCINOMA—PATHOLOGIC FEATURES

Gross Findings
▸ Mass lesion, more frequently central than peripheral
▸ Lymph node metastasis may be observed

Microscopic Findings
▸ Solid, lobular, or trabecular patterns with peripheral palisading
▸ Small cuboidal or fusiform cells, no nuclear molding
▸ High mitotic rate
▸ Comedo-like necrosis is often observed in the centers of the solid nests
▸ Other common features include small cystic spaces with mucoid material in cell nests, hyalinosis, mucoid degeneration of the stroma, and rosette formation
▸ No squamous differentiation is present

Immunohistochemical Features
▸ Immunoreactivity for pankeratins and high molecular weight keratins
▸ Lack of immunoreactivity for TTF-1
▸ Infrequent immunoreactivity for neuroendocrine markers

Pathologic Differential Diagnosis
▸ Poorly differentiated squamous carcinoma
▸ Small cell carcinoma
▸ Large cell neuroendocrine carcinoma

specific symptom is trichoptysis, which may be accompanied by the bronchoscopic finding of hair in the bronchial lumen. These tumors occur in adults and children (from 10 months to 68 years) and are most often diagnosed in the first or second decades of life. Some reports indicate that they are slightly more common in women than in men.

RADIOLOGIC FEATURES

Imaging studies reveal lobulated cystic masses, often perihilar, more commonly in the upper lobes. Calcification within the lesion, cavitation, peripheral translucent areas (air from a bronchial communication), or areas of high fat content can be visualized radiographically. Radiographic evidence of post-obstructive pneumonia or bronchiectasis may accompany the tumor.

PATHOLOGIC FEATURES

GROSS FINDINGS

Teratomas are well-circumscribed mass lesions measuring up to 30 cm in greatest dimension. A dominant cyst or, more often, multilocular cysts with a spectrum of sizes, are seen on the cut surface. Some cysts are filled with yellow-white semisolid keratinous material or mucoid secretions. Bone and cartilage may be recognizable. Solid areas can be present and sometimes predominate over cystic regions. Hemorrhagic and necrotic areas may indicate the presence of malignant foci. Connection with the bronchial tree is a relatively common finding.

MICROSCOPIC FINDINGS

One or more representative tissue components from each of the embryonic germ cell layers of ectoderm, endoderm, and mesoderm are present in varying proportions. Mature teratomas of the lung are characterized in most cases by cysts lined by keratinizing squamous epithelium with cutaneous appendages in their walls (Figure 28-10A). Small cysts lined by a gastroenteric mucosa, and solid components consisting of other mature tissues such as pancreas, islands of hepatocytes, and neuroepithelium are also present. Bone, cartilage, fat, and muscle are the typical tissues of mesodermal origin (Figure 28-10B). Foreign-body granulomatous inflammation is sometimes present in teratomas or in the adjacent lung parenchyma, and bronchiectasis may develop due to airway obstruction. The presence of immature epithelial, mesenchymal, or neural elements defines the immature teratoma. Very rarely, high-grade sarcoma, carcinoma, embryonal carcinoma, or chorio-

carcinoma may occur in mature or immature teratomas of the lung.

ANCILLARY STUDIES

IMMUNOHISTOCHEMISTRY

Immunoreactivities depend upon the particular tissue types represented. Placental-like alkaline phosphatase (PLAP), alpha fetoprotein (AFP), and human chorionic gonadotropin (HCG) may be useful in cases with malignant foci to evaluate for the presence of malignant germ cell tumor constituents.

DIFFERENTIAL DIAGNOSIS

Determination that a teratoma is primary in the lung, rather than metastatic, depends upon clinical investigation to exclude the presence of other extrapulmonary primary sites. Other lesions that can be considered in the differential diagnosis are the bronchogenic cyst, which consists of a cyst lined by respiratory epithelium with small islands of underlying mature cartilage, and the hamartoma, which is composed of fibrous tissue, adipose tissue, and cartilage. Cystic adenomatoid malformation may also be considered, but is generally discovered in the neonatal period or in childhood and is composed of malformed but recognizable pulmonary tissue.

PROGNOSIS AND THERAPY

The prognosis is excellent in mature teratomas, and surgical resection is usually curative. Prognostic uncertainty arises in teratomas with immature tissues, although many cases are associated with favorable behavior. Teratomas with overtly malignant components are generally associated with short survival.

OTHER GERM CELL TUMORS

Pulmonary origin for other types of germ cell tumors is extremely rare, and requires exclusion of extrapulmonary primary neoplasms. Choriocarcinoma can occur in pure form or in combination with other more common types of lung cancer, and is usually rapidly fatal. Rare reports also exist of endodermal sinus tumors and mixed germ cell tumors of the lung. It is important to note, however, that conventional lung cancers can also

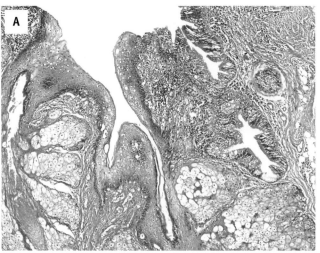
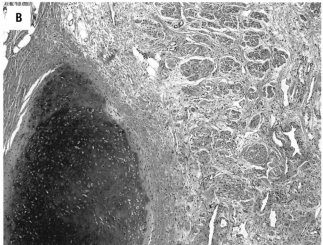

FIGURE 28-10

Teratoma
(A) Skin with cutaneous appendages is a common component of pulmonary teratomas, and is accompanied in this case by respiratory epithelium.
(B) Cartilage, smooth muscle, and occasional adipocytes were also found in this case.

produce human chorionic gonadotropin, alpha fetoprotein, and human placental lactogen. Therefore, immunohistochemical staining for one or more of these substances should not be construed as sufficient to diagnose a germ cell tumor; appropriate histology must also be present.

LEIOMYOSARCOMA, METASTASIZING LEIOMYOMA

CLINICAL FEATURES

Much of the literature on primary pulmonary leiomyosarcomas is based on morphologically diagnosed tumors that antedate the widespread use of immunohistochemistry. Leiomyosarcomas can occur at any age. Differing gender predominance data have been presented in different reports, some noting higher frequencies in men and others in women. They usually grow as endobronchial tumors and obstruct the lumens of airways. Airway obstruction can lead to development of pneumonia and other post-obstructive changes, which may produce signs that trigger detection of the tumor.

In contrast, metastasizing leiomyoma of the lung is usually located peripherally and rarely produces symptoms. Unifocal and multifocal lesions have been described. It is usually diagnosed in elderly women with a

previous history of a uterine smooth muscle tumor, and is believed to represent metastatic leiomyosarcoma in many cases.

RADIOLOGIC FEATURES

These lesions typically present as lung masses. Leiomyosarcomas tend to be central, whereas metastasizing leiomyomas tend to be peripheral. In the case of metastasizing leiomyoma, patients sometimes have multiple nodules.

PATHOLOGIC FEATURES

GROSS FINDINGS

Leiomyosarcoma is usually a well-circumscribed tumor arising from the bronchial wall, with a predominantly endobronchial growth pattern. Invasive growth can be seen. Metastasizing leiomyoma is located in the lung periphery and can present as multiple or single nodules, but is otherwise not different in its gross appearance from other mesenchymal tumors. The cut surfaces of both appear gray-white and glistening, and sometimes a whorled pattern can be discerned. In high-grade leiomyosarcoma, there can be necrosis and hemorrhage in the tumor.

TERATOMA—FACT SHEET

Definition

▸ Teratomas are germ cell tumors consisting of tissues derived from the 3 embryonic germ cell layers; extrapulmonary origin must be excluded before concluding that a teratoma originated in the lung

Incidence

▸ Rare neoplasms

Morbidity and Mortality

▸ Bronchiectasis and pneumonia are common due to airway obstruction by the tumor
▸ Tumor-associated mortality, usually within 6 months, has been observed in malignant teratomas

Gender and Age Distribution

▸ Prevalence in women is higher according to some reports
▸ Broad age range from neonates to adults, but most often diagnosed in the first and second decades of life

Clinical Features

▸ Symptoms include chest pain, hemoptysis, cough, and fever due to pneumonia
▸ Trichoptysis is a specific symptom

Radiologic Features

▸ Lobulated cystic masses, often perihilar, more commonly in the upper lobes
▸ Calcification within the lesion, cavitation, peripheral translucent areas (air from a bronchial communication), or areas of high fat content can be seen
▸ Post-obstructive pneumonia or bronchiectasis may accompany the tumor

Prognosis and Therapy

▸ Mature teratomas have an excellent prognosis and can be cured by surgical resection
▸ Completely resected immature teratomas generally have a good prognosis
▸ Poor prognostic indicators include malignant epithelial or sarcomatous components and other types of germ cell malignancy

TERATOMA—PATHOLOGIC FEATURES

Gross Findings

▸ Well-circumscribed mass measuring up to 30 cm in greatest dimension
▸ Multilocular cysts and/or solid areas are seen on cut surface
▸ Cysts are filled with yellow-white semisolid keratinous material or mucoid secretions
▸ Bone and cartilage may be noted
▸ Hemorrhagic and necrotic areas may indicate the presence of malignant foci
▸ Connection with the bronchial tree is common

Microscopic Findings

▸ Heterogeneous elements commonly include keratinizing squamous epithelial-lined cysts with cutaneous appendages, islands of neuroglia, pancreas, hepatocytes, gastroenteric mucosa, bone, cartilage, fat, and muscle
▸ Immature neuroepithelium, fetal cartilage, and embryonic mesenchyme are features of immature teratoma
▸ High-grade soft tissue sarcomas, carcinomas, and germ cell malignancy may be seen

Pathologic Differential Diagnosis

▸ Metastatic teratoma
▸ Bronchogenic cyst
▸ Hamartoma
▸ Congenital cystic adenomatoid malformation

ANCILLARY STUDIES

IMMUNOHISTOCHEMISTRY

Smooth muscle differentiation can be confirmed by immunohistochemical stains for smooth muscle actin, muscle-specific actin, desmin, and other myogenic markers. Keratin can also be expressed by some leiomyosarcomas. Expression of estrogen and progesterone receptors has been noted in metastasizing leiomyoma.

DIFFERENTIAL DIAGNOSIS

MICROSCOPIC FINDINGS

Both tumors are composed of plump spindle cells with elongated, cigar-shaped nuclei (Figures 28-11, 28-12). Nucleoli are slightly enlarged in low-grade leiomyosarcomas, but prominent in high-grade leiomyosarcomas. Chromatin is granular in metastasizing leiomyomas and coarse in leiomyosarcoma. Perinuclear glycogen vacuoles can be present, and can be highlighted by a PAS stain. Collagen fibers are scarce. At least 5 mitoses per 2 mm^2 are observed in leiomyosarcomas, and leiomyosarcomas may show blood vessel invasion. In metastasizing leiomyomas, mitoses are rare. Leiomyosarcomas show variable degrees of pleomorphism and may show hemorrhage and necrosis (Figure 28-11).

Other primary and metastatic sarcomas enter into the differential diagnosis for primary pulmonary leiomyosarcoma, and knowledge of the clinical history is important for excluding metastatic leiomyosarcoma. Primary pulmonary fibrosarcoma, malignant peripheral nerve sheath tumor (MPNST), malignant fibrous histiocytoma, synovial sarcoma, spindle cell carcinoma, and sarcomatoid melanoma can be considered in the differential diagnosis, but can be differentiated based upon histology and immunohistochemical staining properties. Fibrosarcomas are characterized by abundant collagen fiber deposition. In addition, they have a more monomorphic appearance and often show a herringbone pattern. MPNSTs can usually

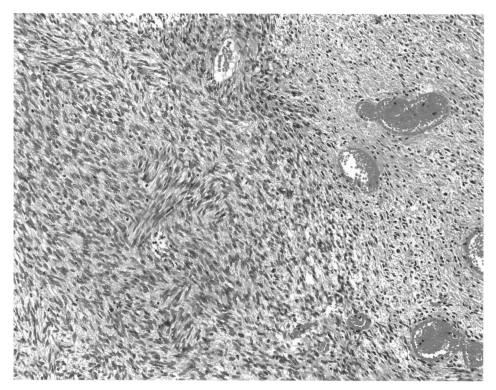

FIGURE 28-11

Leiomyosarcoma
A dense proliferation of spindle cells forms fascicles and displays necrosis (right).

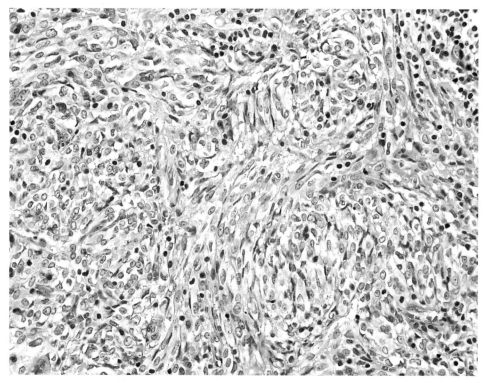

FIGURE 28-12

Metastasizing leiomyoma
Tumor cells show minimal nuclear atypia, no mitoses, and form fascicles.

be differentiated from leiomyomatous tumors by their typical wavy or comma-shaped nuclei. S100 staining and lack of expression of muscle markers are helpful for supporting a diagnosis of MPNST. Malignant fibrous histiocytomas can be difficult to separate from high-grade leiomyosarcomas, but strong and diffuse expression of muscle

markers, fascicle formation, and identification of a lower grade component can be helpful for supporting an interpretation of leiomyosarcoma. Synovial sarcoma characteristically shows focal keratin and/or EMA expression, as well as Bcl-2 and CD99 staining, and glandular components can stain with BER-EP4 and CEA; smooth muscle actin and desmin are usually negative, unlike leiomyosarcoma. Spindle cell carcinoma often demonstrates expression of keratin and EMA, but some cases may not stain with these antibodies and can be difficult to distinguish from sarcomas. Expression of S100 and lack of expression of muscle markers assists in distinguishing sarcomatoid melanomas from leiomyosarcomas.

Metastasizing leiomyomas have provoked a debate about their origin for decades. In many cases, they represent metastases from uterine low-grade leiomyosarcomas removed years earlier by hysterectomy. The time elapsed between the primary tumor in the uterus and development of the metastasizing leiomyomas in the

---

LEIOMYOSARCOMA, METASTASIZING LEIOMYOMA—FACT SHEET

Definition

» Metastasizing leiomyoma is a low-grade malignant smooth muscle neoplasm that probably represents metastatic leiomyosarcoma of uterine origin in the majority of patients
» Leiomyosarcoma is an aggressive sarcoma demonstrating smooth muscle differentiation

Incidence

» Uncommon neoplasms

Morbidity and Mortality

» Metastasizing leiomyoma can rarely be a cause of death
» High mortality rate with high-grade leiomyosarcoma, much lower with low-grade tumors
» Morbidity can be associated with metastases in high-grade leiomyosarcoma

Gender, Race, and Age Distribution

» Leiomyosarcomas can occur at any age, and reports vary regarding gender predominance
» Predominance of elderly females in metastasizing leiomyoma
» No apparent racial predilection

Clinical Features

» Metastasizing leiomyoma is usually asymptomatic and is usually diagnosed in women with a previous history of a uterine smooth muscle tumor
» For leiomyosarcomas, symptoms are related to airway obstruction with frequent development of pneumonia and other post-obstructive changes

Radiologic Features

» Metastasizing leiomyoma: single or multiple nodules, often peripheral
» Leiomyosarcoma: lung nodule or mass, usually in a central location

Prognosis and Therapy

For metastasizing leiomyoma:

» Slowly growing tumor with a benign clinical course
» Surgical resection is the usual treatment

For primary pulmonary leiomyosarcoma:

» An overall 5-year survival rate of 45% was reported in one study, and another study found a strong association between mortality rate and tumor grade
» Other important prognostic variables include the presence or absence of metastasis and tumor size
» Surgical excision is the treatment of choice
» Chemotherapy and/or radiotherapy may be used in high-grade leiomyosarcoma

---

LEIOMYOSARCOMA, METASTASIZING LEIOMYOMA—PATHOLOGIC FEATURES

Gross Findings

» Leiomyosarcoma is a firm, tan endobronchial tumor without a capsule, which may show invasive growth
» Metastasizing leiomyoma has well-circumscribed borders and a firm, tan appearance, and is usually peripheral
» Cut surfaces of both appear gray-white and glistening, and sometimes a whorled pattern is apparent
» In high-grade leiomyosarcomas, tumor necrosis and hemorrhage can be seen

Microscopic Findings

» Spindle cells with elongated cigar-shaped nuclei and eosinophilic cytoplasm that may contain perinuclear glycogen vacuoles
» Variable degrees of nuclear enlargement and pleomorphism in leiomyosarcomas, with higher degrees in high-grade tumors
» Nucleoli can be prominent in high-grade leiomyosarcomas
» Mitotic figures are rare in metastasizing leiomyoma, but can be abundant in leiomyosarcoma, depending on the grade
» Hemorrhage and necrosis may be seen in high-grade leiomyosarcomas

Immunohistochemical Features

» Stains for smooth muscle actin, muscle-specific actin, desmin, and other myogenic markers are usually positive
» Keratin can also be expressed by some leiomyosarcomas
» Expression of estrogen and progesterone receptors has been noted in metastasizing leiomyoma

Pathologic Differential Diagnosis

For primary pulmonary leiomyosarcoma:

» Metastatic extrapulmonary leiomyosarcoma
» Primary and metastatic fibrosarcoma, malignant peripheral nerve sheath tumor, malignant fibrous histiocytoma, synovial sarcoma, spindle cell carcinoma, and sarcomatoid melanoma

For metastasizing leiomyoma:

» Inflammatory myofibroblastic tumor

lung can be up to 20 years. In certain cases, retrospective review reveals features of a low-grade leiomyosarcoma, while in others, the malignant nature of the primary uterine smooth muscle tumor may not have been apparent due to sampling error. However, in other patients, no other primary tumor can be found, so a primary pulmonary origin is presumed. The differential diagnosis includes inflammatory myofibroblastic tumor. However, a mixture of histiocytes, lymphocytes, and plasma cells typically accompanies the myofibroblastic proliferation in the inflammatory myofibroblastic tumor, and is not a prominent feature of metastasizing leiomyoma.

PROGNOSIS AND THERAPY

Metastasizing leiomyoma is a slowly growing tumor with a benign course, and surgical removal is adequate treatment. Leiomyosarcoma of the lung is treated by surgical resection. Depending on the grade, chemotherapy and/or radiotherapy may be added. A 5-year survival rate of 45% was been reported in one study for leiomyosarcomas overall. In another study, 6 patients with low- or intermediate-grade pulmonary leiomyosarcomas were reported to be alive and well from 2 to 12 years after diagnosis, while 8 of 9 patients with follow-up for high-grade leiomyosarcoma died due to the neoplasms with extensive metastases from 1 to 24 months after diagnosis (median survival time, 5 months). Important prognostic variables include grade, the presence or absence of metastasis, and tumor size. The prognosis of these tumors in children has been reported to be superior to that in adults.

MALIGNANT FIBROUS HISTIOCYTOMA

CLINICAL FEATURES

Primary pulmonary malignant fibrous histiocytoma (MFH) presents as a rapidly growing mass lesion usually arising in older individuals. It can rarely occur in children. Symptoms are similar to those of other types of lung neoplasms, and can include cough, chest pain, hemoptysis, and fever.

RADIOLOGIC FEATURES

MFH is usually a single mass located in the lung periphery, with ill-defined borders. Chest wall invasion may be noted. Necrosis is common.

PATHOLOGIC FEATURES

GROSS FINDINGS

On cut surface, this tumor is typically variegated and shows a mixture of soft gray-yellow-red areas corresponding to cell-rich zones, collagen-rich white-yellow regions, and hemorrhagic and necrotic areas.

MICROSCOPIC FINDINGS

MFH demonstrates storiform and pleomorphic components (Figure 28-13). In storiform areas, the cells look like fibroblasts, but are more polymorphic, and mitoses are abundant. Collagen is deposited in short interweaving bundles. In pleomorphic areas, there are many tumor giant cells, sometimes multinucleated and discohesive, with scarce matrix between the cells. Chromatin is coarse and nucleoli are often seen. Mitotic rates are high, and atypical mitotic figures are often numerous. Vascular invasion can be observed.

ANCILLARY STUDIES

Immunohistochemistry reveals expression of vimentin by tumor cells. Staining for muscle markers (actin, desmin), CD68, and alpha-1-antichymotrypsin has also been noted. Rarely, single cells can show a weak reaction for pancytokeratin antibodies. S100 and CD34 are negative.

DIFFERENTIAL DIAGNOSIS

In the differential diagnosis, primary pulmonary spindle cell and giant cell carcinomas, fibrosarcoma, leiomyosarcoma, MPNST, sarcomatoid mesothelioma, malignant solitary fibrous tumor, inflammatory myofibroblastic tumor (IMT), and metastatic sarcomas, sarcomatoid carcinomas, and sarcomatoid melanoma may be considered. Spindle cell and giant cell carcinomas are usually cytokeratin-positive, and collagen deposition is usually absent in giant cell carcinomas. In fibrosarcoma, cells and collagen are arranged into long bundles, often with a herringbone pattern. Leiomyosarcomas may demonstrate a fascicular arrangement and consist of spindle and sometimes pleomorphic cells, so they can resemble MFH. Leiomyosarcomas usually express muscle markers, and the cytomorphology resembles smooth muscle cells rather than myofibroblasts (in MFH), assisting in the differential diagnosis, but some cases can be difficult to separate. MPNSTs are frequently S100-positive and produce little collagen; tumor cell nuclei may also have a wavy or comma-shaped appearance. Sarcomatoid mesothelioma may be hard to

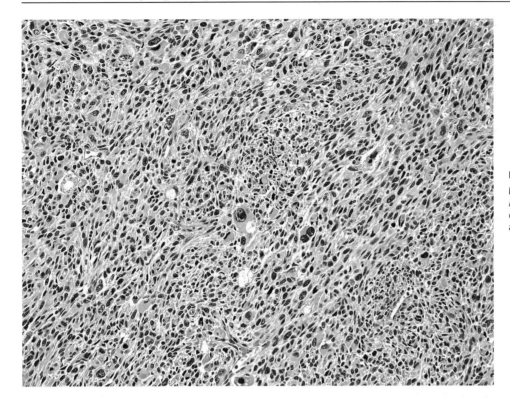

FIGURE 28-13
Malignant fibrous histiocytoma
A polymorphous population of spindle cells and pleomorphic giant cells characterizes this neoplasm.

MALIGNANT FIBROUS HISTIOCYTOMA—FACT SHEET

Definition

▸ A high-grade sarcoma characterized by storiform and pleomorphic patterns, consisting of cells with fibroblastic, myofibroblastic, and anaplastic cytomorphologies

Incidence

▸ Rare neoplasms

Morbidity and Mortality

▸ High mortality rate
▸ Morbidity secondary to local spread in the lung and to the chest wall, and to metastasis

Gender and Age Distribution

▸ Primarily develop in older adults, rarely in children, of both genders

Clinical Features

▸ Symptoms are similar to those of other types of lung neoplasms, and can include cough, chest pain, hemoptysis, and fever

Radiologic Features

▸ Single mass located in the lung periphery, with ill-defined borders, often with necrosis
▸ Chest wall invasion may be noted

Prognosis and Therapy

▸ The tumor is associated with a high recurrence rate and mortality rate
▸ Surgical resection is the usual treatment approach
▸ The roles of chemotherapy and radiation therapy remain to be defined

---

MALIGNANT FIBROUS HISTIOCYTOMA—PATHOLOGIC FEATURES

Gross Findings

▸ Variegated cut surface including a mixture of soft gray-yellow-red areas corresponding to cell-rich zones, collagen-rich white-yellow regions, and hemorrhagic and necrotic areas

Microscopic Findings

▸ Storiform and pleomorphic components are typical
▸ In storiform areas, the cells look like fibroblasts, but are more polymorphic, and mitoses are abundant; collagen is deposited in short interweaving bundles
▸ In pleomorphic areas, there are many tumor giant cells, sometimes multinucleated, discohesive, with numerous mitoses including atypical mitotic figures
▸ Vascular invasion may be observed

Immunohistochemical Features

▸ Vimentin is widely expressed by tumor cells
▸ Staining for muscle markers (actin, desmin), CD68 and alpha-1-antichymotrypsin may be present
▸ Rarely, single cells can show weak reactivity with pan-cytokeratin antibodies
▸ S100 and CD34 are negative

Pathologic Differential Diagnosis

▸ Primary pulmonary spindle cell and giant cell carcinomas, fibrosarcoma, leiomyosarcoma, malignant peripheral nerve sheath tumor, sarcomatoid mesothelioma, malignant solitary fibrous tumor, and inflammatory myofibroblastic tumor
▸ Metastatic sarcomas, sarcomatoid carcinomas, and sarcomatoid melanoma

differentiate from MFH on purely morphologic grounds, but it usually expresses cytokeratin and may express some of the mesothelioma markers, such as thrombomodulin and calretinin. Another difference is that the cell polymorphism of MFH is quite characteristic, as opposed to the relative monotony of tumor cells seen in sarcomatoid mesothelioma. Malignant solitary fibrous tumor should not cause a problem in the differential diagnosis due to the lower number of mitoses, the lesser degree of cellular polymorphism, and the expression of CD34 in most cases. Differentiation from IMT is based on the lower degree of nuclear pleomorphism in IMT and the prominent inflammatory infiltrates in IMT, as well as expression of ALK-1 in IMT. Metastatic neoplasms include a very broad spectrum of histologies and immunoreactivities, and obtaining history is important in directing evaluation for the specific differential diagnostic considerations.

PROGNOSIS AND THERAPY

The prognosis of MFH is usually poor and the mortality rate is high. The tumor is typically rapidly growing, although in our experience it metastasizes quite late in its course. Complete resection is usually attempted, but the recurrence rate is high. The roles of chemotherapy and radiation therapy remain to be defined.

EPITHELIOID HEMANGIOENDOTHELIOMA, ANGIOSARCOMA

CLINICAL FEATURES

Pulmonary epithelioid hemangioendothelioma (PEH) usually occurs in adults, but can arise occasionally in children and adolescents. The mean age is approximately 40 years, and the range extends from 7 to 72 years of age. PEH shows a strong predilection for women (80%), and most patients are Caucasian. Patients are frequently asymptomatic or can complain of pleuritic chest pain, dyspnea, cough, and hemoptysis. Involvement of the liver may also be present in patients with PEH. Primary pulmonary angiosarcoma is extremely rare and occurs in adults.

RADIOLOGIC FEATURES

Imaging studies typically show multiple bilateral nodules in PEH, although a solitary mass appearance has also been described. In the multinodular presentation, diagnoses of metastatic disease or disseminated infection are often contemplated. Angiosarcoma is more frequently a single mass.

PATHOLOGIC FEATURES

GROSS FINDINGS

PEH nodules are characteristically well circumscribed, grayish-tan, and firm. Calcification may be noted. Pleural involvement may become diffuse and raise a suspicion of mesothelioma. Angiosarcomas form firm, gray-tan masses with invasive edges and variable degrees of hemorrhage.

MICROSCOPIC FINDINGS

PEH lesions show a variety of features. There is often abundant hyaline, myxohyaline, or mucoid matrix in which infiltrative tumor cells are found (Figure 28-14A). The matrix is particularly conspicuous and sclerotic (Figure 28-14B) in the centers of the nodules, which may also be necrotic, calcified, or ossified. Tumor cells are generally small and round or oval; a key diagnostic feature is the presence of intracytoplasmic vacuoles representing capillary lumen formation in some of these cells (Figure 28-14C). Red cells can occasionally be seen in some of these structures. Spread of tumor into adjacent airways can occur through formation of small polypoid structures. Mitoses are only occasionally seen. Lymphangitic spread can be observed in some cases, whereas intravascular growth is commonly seen.

Angiosarcomas demonstrate greater cellularity, more cytoatypia and mitoses, and less matrix than PEH. Infiltrative growth into alveolar septa along preexisting capillaries is quite characteristic (Figure 28-15). Mitotic counts are in the range of 1-2 per high-power field. Cells have an epithelioid appearance with prominent nucleoli and vesicular chromatin. Tumors can demonstrate variable degrees of blood vessel formation.

ANCILLARY STUDIES

IMMUNOHISTOCHEMISTRY

PEH and angiosarcoma cells characteristically express endothelial markers (CD31, CD34, factor VIII, Fli1) and vimentin. In PEH cells, the intracytoplasmic lumens may be highlighted by staining with factor VIII. Focal cytokeratin expression can also be observed in up to 30% of PEH and angiosarcoma cases.

EPITHELIOID HEMANGIOENDOTHELIOMA, ANGIOSARCOMA—FACT SHEET

Definition

» PEH and angiosarcoma are malignant vascular neoplasms of low- or intermediate-grade (PEH) or high-grade (angiosarcoma)

Incidence

» PEH is rare, and primary pulmonary angiosarcoma is extremely rare

Morbidity and Mortality

» The 5-year survival rate for PEH is 47-71%
» High mortality rate is associated with angiosarcoma
» PEH is slowly growing, with distant metastasis usually relatively late in its course
» Angiosarcoma is a rapidly growing tumor, which often gives rise to distant metastasis early in its course

Gender, Race, and Age Distribution

» For PEH, the mean age is approximately 40 years, and the range 7-72 years
» PEH shows a strong predilection for women (80%), and most patients are Caucasian
» Angiosarcoma occurs in adults

Clinical Features

» In PEH, patients are frequently asymptomatic or can complain of pleuritic chest pain, dyspnea, cough, or hemoptysis
» Angiosarcoma presents with similar symptoms
» Liver involvement can be present in PEH

Radiologic Features

» Multiple bilateral nodules are typical of PEH, although a solitary mass appearance has also been described
» PEH can also involve the pleura in a manner resembling malignant mesothelioma
» Angiosarcoma is usually a single mass

Therapy

» If feasible, surgical removal is the best treatment for PEH and angiosarcoma, and systemic chemotherapy has also been used

EPITHELIOID HEMANGIOENDOTHELIOMA, ANGIOSARCOMA— PATHOLOGIC FEATURES

Gross Findings

» PEH nodules are characteristically well circumscribed, grayish-tan and firm; calcification may be noted; pleural involvement may become diffuse and resemble mesothelioma
» Angiosarcomas form firm, gray-tan masses with invasive edges and variable degrees of hemorrhage

Microscopic Findings

In PEH:

» Nodules contain abundant bluish myxohyaline or mucoid matrix with infiltrative tumor cells
» Nodules are centrally sclerotic and may be necrotic, calcified, or ossified
» Tumor cells are generally small and round or oval
» A key diagnostic feature is the presence of intracytoplasmic vacuoles representing capillary lumen formation in some of these cells; red cells can occasionally be seen in some of these structures
» Spread of tumor into adjacent airways can occur through formation of small polypoid structures
» Mitoses are only occasionally seen
» Lymphangitic spread can be observed

In angiosarcoma:

» Angiosarcomas demonstrate greater cellularity, more cytoatypia and mitoses, and less matrix than PEH
» Cells have an epithelioid appearance with prominent nucleoli and vesicular chromatin
» Variable degrees of blood vessel formation

Immunohistochemical Features

» PEH and angiosarcoma cells characteristically express endothelial markers (CD31, CD34, factor VIII, Fli1) and vimentin
» In PEH cells, the intracytoplasmic lumens may be highlighted by staining with factor VIII
» Focal cytokeratin expression can be observed in up to 30% of PEH and angiosarcoma cases

Ultrastructural Features

» Tumor cells demonstrate tight junctions, cytoplasmic filaments, pinocytotic vesicles, and Weibel-Palade bodies
» Basement membrane material may surround tumor cells
» Intracytoplasmic lumens are characteristic of PEH

Pathologic Differential Diagnosis

» Differentiation between PEH and epithelioid angiosarcoma is based on grade
» For PEH, the differential diagnosis includes sclerosing hemangioma, malignant mesothelioma, adenocarcinoma, organizing infarcts, nodular amyloidosis, and a variety of metastatic neoplasms
» For primary pulmonary angiosarcoma, the differential diagnosis includes metastatic angiosarcoma; other types of sarcomas, both primary and metastatic; and sarcomatoid carcinomas, mesotheliomas, and melanomas may also be considered

ULTRASTRUCTURAL FEATURES

Tumor cells demonstrate tight junctions, cytofilaments, pinocytotic vesicles, and Weibel-Palade bodies. Basement membrane material can surround tumor cells. Intracytoplasmic lumens are characteristic of PEH.

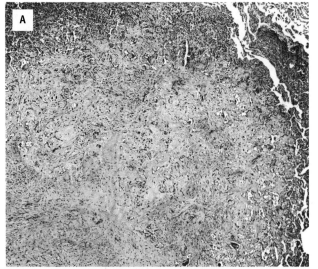

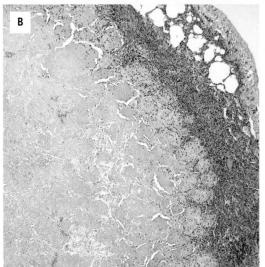

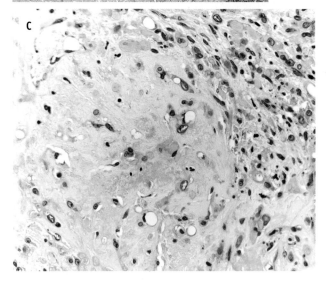

FIGURE 28-14

Epithelioid hemangioendothelioma
(A) Infiltrative tumor cells are associated with a dense hyaline background.
(B) This nodule has a sclerotic background and shows polypoid extensions of
tumor into adjacent alveoli at its periphery. **(C)** Tumor cells are small with
hyperchromatic nuclei, and lie in abundant matrix. Several tumor cells display
intracytoplasmic lumens.

DIFFERENTIAL DIAGNOSIS

For PEH, the differential diagnosis includes sclerosing
hemangioma, malignant mesothelioma, adenocarcinoma,
organizing infarcts, nodular amyloidosis, and a variety of
metastatic neoplasms. The distinctive histologic features
and the immunoreactivity of the tumor cells for endothelial markers should allow for differentiation of PEH from
these other entities. Differentiation between PEH and
epithelioid angiosarcoma is based on grade. PEH is a low-
or intermediate-grade tumor, and angiosarcoma a high-
grade sarcoma. The distinction is based primarily upon
cytoatypia and mitotic rate. Cellularity is also higher in
angiosarcoma than PEH, and more matrix is present in
PEH than angiosarcoma. For primary pulmonary angiosarcoma, the most important differential diagnosis lies
with metastatic angiosarcoma. In fact, questions have
been raised about the site of origin in some cases reported
as primary pulmonary angiosarcomas, without complete
exclusion of an extrapulmonary lesion. The differential
diagnosis also includes other types of sarcomas, both primary and metastatic. Sarcomatoid carcinomas, mesotheliomas, and melanomas may also be considered. Observation of blood vessel formation, myxohyaline matrix, and
expression of endothelial markers supports a diagnosis of
angiosarcoma.

PROGNOSIS AND THERAPY

If feasible, surgical removal is the best treatment for PEH
and angiosarcoma, and systemic chemotherapy has also
been used. The 5-year survival rate for PEH is 47-71%.
Hemorrhagic symptoms (hemoptysis, pleural effusion)
were adverse prognostic factors for PEH on multivariate
analysis. Prognosis is very poor for angiosarcoma.

SARCOMAS OF LARGE PULMONARY BLOOD VESSELS

CLINICAL FEATURES

Sarcomas arising from the large pulmonary blood vessels are rare tumors, particularly the sarcomas of venous
origin. Pulmonary vein sarcomas seem to be more common in women, while pulmonary artery sarcomas were
reported to show no gender predilection in some studies, and a slight female predominance in others. Pulmonary artery and vein sarcomas arise in patients with a
mean age of 49-50 years (range, 23-74 years for pulmonary vein sarcomas, 13-81 for pulmonary artery

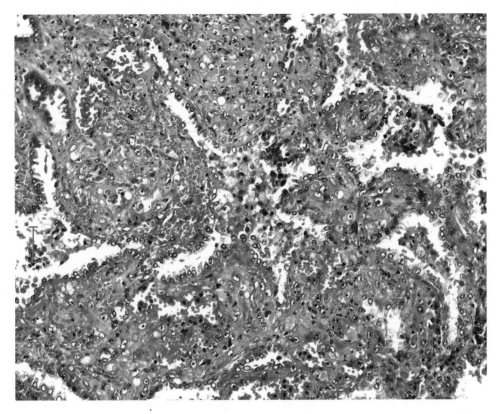

FIGURE 28-15
Epithelioid angiosarcoma
Tumor cells infiltrate alveolar septa and demonstrate vesicular nuclei, prominent nucleoli, and eosinophilic cytoplasm.

sarcomas). The diagnosis of sarcoma of a large pulmonary artery or vein is most often made at autopsy. Patients present with symptoms of acute pulmonary embolism or myocardial infarction, including dyspnea and chest pain. Hemoptysis, cough, or systemic symptoms of fever, weight loss, and malaise may also be noted. Physical signs can likewise mimic those of pulmonary embolism, myocardial infarction, or heart failure and can include cardiac murmurs, cyanosis, peripheral edema, jugular venous distention, and hepatomegaly.

RADIOLOGIC FEATURES

For pulmonary artery sarcomas, findings resemble those of thromboembolism, but have some distinguishing features. Expansion of large pulmonary vessels with a solid or heterogeneous density, unilateral distribution of involvement, and smooth vascular tapering without abrupt narrowings and cut-offs can be observed. If associated with pulmonary nodules, cardiac enlargement, and decreased vascularity, the findings should cause consideration of a diagnosis of pulmonary artery sarcoma. The intraluminal masses can also be detected by pulmonary angiography, which can show smooth tapering of pulmonary arteries and "to-and-fro" motion of pedunculated or lobulated lesions. Recently, intravascular ultrasound study and fluorine-18-2-fluoro-2 deoxy-D-glucose positron emission tomographic tumor imaging have

been reported as helpful ancillary techniques in the evaluation of potential pulmonary artery sarcomas. For pulmonary venous sarcomas, presentation as a lung, hilar, or left atrial mass has been described.

PATHOLOGIC FEATURES

GROSS FINDINGS

Pulmonary artery intimal sarcomas characteristically form mucoid or gelatinous masses that may have a focally gritty or chondroid consistency, with variable degrees of hemorrhage and necrosis. They tend to grow intraluminally in a polypoid manner, extend distally into smaller artery branches with a smooth tapering pattern, and occlude the lumens of the vessels. Invasion of the vascular wall and adjacent hilar and lung parenchymal tissues can be seen in advanced cases. Reported sites of tumor origin include the pulmonary trunk (85%), right pulmonary artery (71%), left pulmonary artery (65%), pulmonary valve (32%), and right ventricular outflow tract (10%). For leiomyosarcomas of the pulmonary vein, the site of origin is more frequently on the right than the left, and the tumors on the left tend to enter the left atrium. They are fleshy masses that demonstrate mural involvement of the vein and can occlude the lumens of the involved vessels. Pulmonary parenchymal invasion can be seen.

MICROSCOPIC FINDINGS

Pulmonary artery sarcomas include intimal sarcomas and mural sarcomas. Although very rare, intimal sarcomas are more common than mural sarcomas. Intimal sarcomas occupy and expand the intimal region of the blood vessel (Figure 28-16A) and can extend through the vessel wall into adjacent tissues. They tend to be poorly differentiated, but show some degree of fibroblastic or myofibroblastic differentiation, and consist of spindle cells in a myxoid background with areas of more prominent collagen deposition (Figure 28-16B). Foci of osteosarcoma, chondrosarcoma, or rhabdomyosarcoma may be present, in which case the tumor can be diagnosed as "intimal sarcoma with focal osteosarcoma," for example. Grading of pulmonary artery sarcomas can be approached using the grading systems used for soft tissue sarcomas (NCI and FNCLCC systems), which are based on assessment of tumor differentiation, mitotic count, and tumor necrosis. It is also common to see recanalized thrombotic material admixed with the intravascular tumor (Figure 28-16B). Mural sarcomas are classified according to histologic type (leiomyosarcoma, osteosarcoma, chondrosarcoma, rhabdomyosarcoma, pleomorphic sarcoma). Most sarcomas of pulmonary venous origin are intermediate- or high-grade leiomyosarcomas, with a histologic appearance similar to that described earlier in this chapter for other leiomyosarcomas.

ANCILLARY STUDIES

IMMUNOHISTOCHEMISTRY

For pulmonary artery sarcomas, immunohistochemistry is usually not necessary because of the unique location of the tumor and the characteristic gross and microscopic appearance. Nonetheless, intimal sarcomas usually express vimentin and demonstrate variable staining for smooth muscle actin and desmin. Endothelial markers (CD31, CD34, and factor VIII) are typically negative. Other types of sarcomas display staining reactivities similar to those observed in the same histologic types of soft tissue sarcomas. For pulmonary venous sarcomas, tumor cells express smooth muscle actin, muscle-specific actin, desmin, and vimentin, but do not stain for epithelial membrane antigen, S100 protein, or factor VIII-related antigen. Focal keratin staining may be observed in some cases.

DIFFERENTIAL DIAGNOSIS

The differential diagnosis includes metastatic sarcomas and other sarcomatoid malignancies, direct extension into a pulmonary vessel by a lung parenchymal or mediastinal sarcoma, and a cellular organizing thrombus.

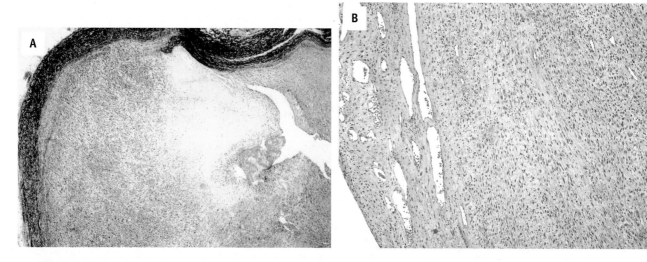

FIGURE 28-16

Pulmonary artery intimal sarcoma

(A) The tumor almost completely fills the arterial lumen (elastic van Gieson stain). **(B)** This poorly differentiated intimal sarcoma (middle and right) is associated with recanalized thrombus (left).

SARCOMAS OF LARGE PULMONARY BLOOD VESSELS—FACT SHEET

Definition

» Sarcomas arising in the large pulmonary arteries and veins

Incidence

» Rare neoplasms, but pulmonary artery intimal sarcoma is the most common

Morbidity and Mortality

» High mortality rates
» Morbidity secondary to vascular obstruction and development of heart failure

Gender and Age Distribution

» Female predominance for pulmonary vein sarcomas
» Pulmonary artery sarcomas reported to show no gender predilection in some studies, and a slight female predominance in others
» Mean age of 49-50 years for pulmonary artery and vein sarcomas (range, 23-74 years for pulmonary vein sarcomas, 13-81 for pulmonary artery sarcomas)

Clinical Features

» Symptoms can resemble acute pulmonary embolism or myocardial infarction, with dyspnea and chest pain
» Hemoptysis, cough, or systemic symptoms of fever, weight loss, and malaise may be noted
» Physical signs can mimic those of pulmonary embolism, myocardial infarction or heart failure, including cardiac murmurs, cyanosis, peripheral edema, jugular venous distention, and hepatomegaly

Radiologic Features

For pulmonary artery sarcomas:

» Expansion of large pulmonary vessels with a solid or heterogeneous density, unilateral distribution of involvement, and smooth vascular tapering without abrupt narrowings and cut-offs
» Pulmonary angiography can highlight the intraluminal masses with smooth tapering of pulmonary arteries and "to-and-fro" motion of pedunculated or lobulated lesions

For pulmonary vein sarcomas:

» Presentation as a lung, hilar, or left atrial mass has been described

Prognosis and Therapy

For pulmonary artery sarcomas:

» Tumors often metastasize to the lung and mediastinum (50%), but less often (16%) to extrathoracic sites
» Surgical resection is the preferred treatment approach
» Adjuvant radiotherapy or chemotherapy may have a role in treatment
» Overall, the mean survival for pulmonary artery sarcomas ranges from 14 to 18 months

For pulmonary vein sarcomas:

» Local or mediastinal recurrence develops in about one third of patients
» Metastases to the liver, scalp, and axillary lymph nodes have been described
» Complete surgical resection is usually attempted if feasible
» Little responsiveness to chemotherapy and radiation
» Postoperative survival at 6 months and 1, 2, 3, and 5 years reported to be 75%, 73%, 50%, 33%, and 20%, respectively

SARCOMAS OF LARGE PULMONARY BLOOD VESSELS—PATHOLOGIC FEATURES

Gross Findings

For pulmonary artery sarcomas:

» Origin in pulmonary trunk or main pulmonary arteries is most common
» Mucoid or gelatinous masses that may have a focally gritty or chondroid consistency, with variable hemorrhage and necrosis
» Polypoid intraluminal growth with distal extension into smaller artery branches with a smooth tapering pattern, causing luminal obstruction
» Invasion of the vascular wall and adjacent hilar and lung parenchymal tissues can be seen in advanced cases

For pulmonary vein sarcomas:

» Fleshy masses that demonstrate mural involvement of the vein and can occlude the lumens of the involved vessels
» Pulmonary parenchymal invasion can be seen

Microscopic Findings

For pulmonary artery sarcomas:

» Intimal sarcomas tend to been poorly differentiated, show some degree of fibroblastic or myofibroblastic differentiation, and consist of spindle cells in a myxoid background with areas of more prominent collagen deposition; foci of osteosarcoma, chondrosarcoma, or rhabdomyosarcomas may be present
» Grading can be performed using the grading systems for soft tissue sarcomas (NCI and FNCLCC systems)
» Common to see recanalized thrombotic material admixed with the intravascular tumor
» Mural sarcomas are classified according to histologic type (leiomyosarcoma, osteosarcoma, chondrosarcoma, rhabdomyosarcoma, pleomorphic sarcoma)

For pulmonary vein sarcomas:

» Most are intermediate- or high-grade leiomyosarcomas

Immunohistochemical Features

» Pulmonary artery intimal sarcomas usually express vimentin and demonstrate variable staining for smooth muscle actin and desmin; endothelial markers (CD31, CD34, and factor VIII) are typically negative
» Other types of arterial sarcomas display staining reactivities similar to those observed in the corresponding histologic types of soft tissue sarcomas
» For pulmonary vein sarcomas, tumor cells express smooth muscle actin, muscle-specific actin, desmin, and vimentin, but do not stain for epithelial membrane antigen, S100 protein, or factor VIII–related antigen; focal keratin staining may be observed in some cases

Pathologic Differential Diagnosis

» Metastatic sarcomas and other sarcomatoid malignancies
» Direct extension into a pulmonary vessel by a lung parenchymal or mediastinal sarcoma
» Cellular organizing thrombus

PROGNOSIS AND THERAPY

For pulmonary artery intimal sarcomas, the prognosis is poor. These tumors often metastasize to the lung and mediastinum (50%), but less often (16%) to extrathoracic sites. Surgical resection is the preferred treatment approach and has been performed by pneumonectomy, local excision, and endarterectomy. Adjuvant radiotherapy or chemotherapy has been reported to improve 1- and 2-year survival, and may have a role in treatment. Overall, the mean survival for pulmonary artery sarcomas ranges from 14 to 18 months. Long term survival, however, has been reported in 2 cases of mural sarcoma and 1 case of low-grade intimal sarcoma.

For pulmonary vein sarcomas, local or mediastinal recurrence develops in about one third of patients, and metastases to the liver, scalp, and axillary lymph nodes have been described. Complete surgical resection is usually attempted if feasible, but there is little responsiveness to chemotherapy and radiation. The mortality rate appears to be high. Postoperative survival rates at 6 months and 1, 2, 3, and 5 years were reported to be 75%, 73%, 50%, 33%, and 20%, respectively.

OTHER SARCOMAS

A wide variety of other sarcomas can arise in the lungs, but remain rare lesions in this anatomic site. Primary pulmonary synovial sarcomas, osteosarcomas, chondrosarcomas, liposarcomas, rhabdomyosarcomas, malignant peripheral nerve sheath tumors, and glomangiosarcomas generally demonstrate histologic appearances and immunoreactivities similar to those described in these neoplasms in other locations. Although most occur in adults, rhabdomyosarcomas also develop in children, sometimes in association with cystic adenomatoid malformations. For the most part, the primary treatment is surgical resection. Before diagnosing a tumor as a primary pulmonary sarcoma, however, it is important to rule out the possibility that the pulmonary neoplasm is a metastasis from an extrapulmonary primary sarcoma.

Primary pulmonary synovial sarcomas have been increasingly diagnosed in recent years. These tumors arise in adults of both genders, with a median age of 50. Tumor size ranges from 2 to 15.5 cm (mean, 9 cm). Tumor histology is most frequently the monophasic fibrous type, and less frequently poorly differentiated (Figure 28-17). Immunohistochemical staining for AE1/AE3, CAM5.2 and/or EMA is usually at least focally present, vimentin is usually positive, and Bcl-2, CD99, and calretinin staining have also been described. Detection of the characteristic SYT-SSX1 or SYT-SSX2 fusion gene transcripts represents an important aid to diagnosis. The mortality rate due to the neoplasm is 50%, with deaths occurring

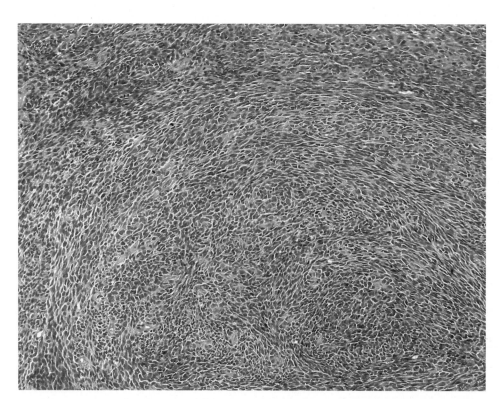

FIGURE 28-17
Synovial sarcoma
The tumor consists of a dense proliferation of uniform spindle cells with little cytoplasm.

1 to 9 years after surgery. A 30% local recurrence rate and a 40% rate of distant metastasis have been reported.

CONGENITAL PERIBRONCHIAL MYOFIBROBLASTIC TUMOR

CLINICAL FEATURES

This congenital tumor is extremely rare and usually presents as a mass lesion shortly after birth. Polyhydramnios and non-immune hydrops fetalis may complicate the pregnancy.

RADIOLOGIC FEATURES

Imaging studies reveal a well-circumscribed heterogeneous mass.

PATHOLOGIC FEATURES

GROSS FINDINGS

The tumor is typically well circumscribed and unencapsulated, with a smooth or multinodular surface, and can measure up to 10 cm in diameter. The cut surface is fleshy and yellow-tan or tan-gray. The tumor shows a peribronchial growth pattern, and invasion, distortion, or occlusion of the associated bronchus is common.

MICROSCOPIC FINDINGS

The tumor extends along bronchovascular bundles (Figure 28-18A) and invades the bronchial wall. Invasion of lung parenchyma and pleura can occur. The tumor cells are spindle-shaped and arranged in fascicles (Figure 28-18B), and may have a herringbone pattern. Nuclei are elongated or round, chromatin is finely dispersed, and there is no pleomorphism or anaplasia. Mitotic activity varies, but atypical mitoses are not observed. Hemorrhage and cyst formation may be present.

ANCILLARY STUDIES

IMMUNOHISTOCHEMISTRY

Tumor cells express vimentin, while reactivity for smooth muscle actin, muscle-specific actin, desmin, and other muscle markers is lacking or focal. Calponin staining has also been described.

DIFFERENTIAL DIAGNOSIS

Given patient age, presentation, and pathologic features, the differential diagnosis is essentially limited to this disorder.

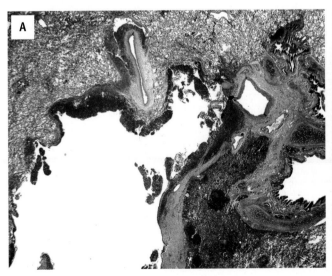
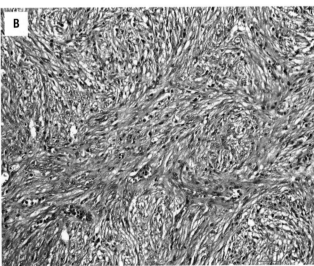

FIGURE 28-18

Congenital peribronchial myofibroblastic tumor
(A) The tumor infiltrates along a bronchovascular bundle. **(B)** The neoplastic spindle cells demonstrate no mitoses or atypia and form fascicular arrangements.

CONGENITAL PERIBRONCHIAL MYOFIBROBLASTIC TUMOR—FACT SHEET

Definition
- A congenital peribronchovascular proliferation of uniform spindle cells with fibroblastic/myofibroblastic differentiation

Incidence
- Extremely rare neoplasm

Mortality
- Mortality can be associated with fetal hydrops associated with the tumor

Gender, Race, and Age Distribution
- A congenital tumor in neonates and fetuses of both genders
- No apparent racial predilection

Clinical Features
- Respiratory compromise due to the mass lesion
- Polyhydramnios and fetal hydrops may be related to the tumor

Radiologic Features
- A mass primarily involving peribronchovascular structures, but also capable of invading lung parenchyma, interlobular septa, and pleura

Prognosis and Therapy
- Surgical removal can produce a cure

CONGENITAL PERIBRONCHIAL MYOFIBROBLASTIC TUMOR—PATHOLOGIC FEATURES

Gross Findings
- Well-circumscribed and unencapsulated mass with a smooth or multi-nodular surface, measuring up to 10 cm in diameter
- Tumor involves peribronchovascular structures, commonly distorts or occludes the associated bronchus, and can invade lung parenchyma or pleura
- Fleshy yellow-tan or tan-gray cut surface

Microscopic Findings
- Tumor cells are spindle-shaped and arranged in fascicles, and may have a herringbone pattern
- Elongated or round nuclei with fine chromatin and no pleomorphism or anaplasia
- Mitotic activity varies, but atypical mitoses are not observed
- Hemorrhage and cyst formation may be present

Immunohistochemical Features
- Tumor cells express vimentin, while reactivity for smooth muscle actin, muscle-specific actin, desmin, and other muscle markers is lacking or focal
- Calponin staining has also been described

Pathologic Differential Diagnosis
- There is no other entity in the differential diagnosis, given patients' ages, the tumor presentation, and the histology

---

PROGNOSIS AND THERAPY

Surgical resection is the preferred treatment. If no other complications are present, this should be curative. If present, however, fetal hydrops is associated with its own morbidity and mortality.

PARAGANGLIOMA

CLINICAL FEATURES

Primary paragangliomas of the lung are extremely rare tumors arising in adults of both genders. As is true of many endocrine neoplasms, there are no clear-cut features that predict biological behavior. Paragangliomas can induce clinical symptoms related to paroxysmal increases in blood pressure, but more often they are asymptomatic.

RADIOLOGIC FEATURES

Radiologic studies reveal a well-circumscribed nodule or mass.

PATHOLOGIC FEATURES

GROSS FINDINGS

Paragangliomas are usually well-circumscribed, gray-red nodules measuring up to several centimeters in diameter.

MICROSCOPIC FINDINGS

As in any other location, paragangliomas consist of epithelioid cell nests with a Zellballen pattern surrounded by a fine fibrovascular stroma with sustentacular cells (Figure 28-19). The tumor cells are round or ovoid, with abundant cytoplasm, round or oval nuclei with fine or speckled chromatin, and occasional nucleoli.

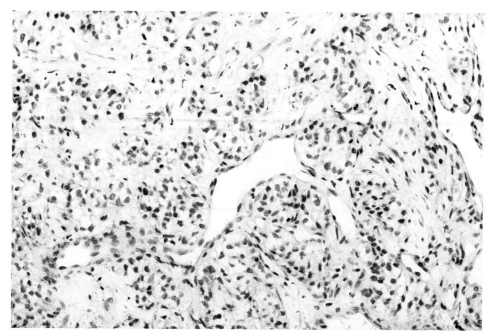

FIGURE 28-19
Paraganglioma
Cytologically bland tumor cells are arranged in a Zellballen pattern, and a prominent vascular supply is noted.

ANCILLARY STUDIES

IMMUNOHISTOCHEMISTRY

Paragangliomas express neuroendocrine markers (chromogranin A, synaptophysin, CD56) and neurofilament protein, but do not stain for cytokeratins and EMA. Sustentacular cells stain for S100 protein.

ULTRASTRUCTURAL FEATURES

Tumor cells contain abundant dense core granules with eccentric halos (norepinephrine-type granules).

DIFFERENTIAL DIAGNOSIS

The differential diagnosis includes metastatic paraganglioma, carcinoid, acinic cell tumor, sugar tumor, and glomus tumor. Information from the clinical history can help to evaluate the likelihood of metastatic paraganglioma, but since the extrapulmonary lesions may not have been discovered at the time of pulmonary evaluation, they cannot always be ruled out. Carcinoids usually express cytokeratin as well as neuroendocrine markers. In addition, although scattered S100-positive Langerhans cells are sometimes seen in carcinoids, numerous S100-positive sustentacular cells will be seen in paragangliomas. Expression of neuroendocrine markers is very helpful for distinguishing paraganglioma from the other entities in the differential diagnosis, because it is not observed in acinic cell tumors, sugar tumors, and glomus tumors.

PROGNOSIS AND THERAPY

Currently, there are no established criteria for predicting the biological behavior of primary paraganglioma of the lung. Although most tumors seem to have a benign clinical course, invasive behavior with hilar and mediastinal lymph node metastasis has been described in rare patients. Surgical resection is the main treatment approach.

MALIGNANT MELANOMA

CLINICAL FEATURES

Primary pulmonary malignant melanoma is a very rare neoplasm that can be diagnosed only in patients without an extrapulmonary primary melanoma. The tumors arise in adults, with a mean age of 51 years, and a range of 29-80 years. A gender predilection has not been observed. Symptoms of cough, hemoptysis, and lobar collapse are explained by the frequent endobronchial location of the tumor. Tracheal origin has also been described.

PARAGANGLIOMA—FACT SHEET

Definition

» A tumor arising from autonomic nerve structures within the lung, morphologically identical to paragangliomas arising in other sites

Incidence

» Extremely rare neoplasm

Mortality

» Little data is available, but the mortality rate appears low or nonexistent

Gender and Age Distribution

» This tumor arises in adults of both genders

Clinical Features

» Most often an incidental finding unassociated with symptoms
» Rare cases are associated with hypertension

Radiologic Features

» Well-circumscribed nodule or mass

Prognosis and Therapy

» Most often have a benign clinical course
» No established criteria for assessing prognosis
» Complete surgical resection is the treatment of choice

PARAGANGLIOMA—PATHOLOGIC FEATURES

Gross Findings

» Usually a well-circumscribed, gray-red nodule measuring up to several centimeters in diameter

Microscopic Findings

» Epithelioid cell nests in a Zellballen pattern surrounded by a fine fibrovascular stroma with sustentacular cells
» Tumor cells are round or ovoid, with abundant cytoplasm, round or oval nuclei with fine or speckled chromatin, and occasional nucleoli

Immunohistochemical Features

» Usually express neuroendocrine markers (chromogranin A, synaptophysin, CD56) and neurofilament protein, but do not stain for cytokeratins and EMA
» Sustentacular cells stain for S100 protein

Ultrastructural Features

» Tumor cells contain abundant dense core granules with eccentric haloes ("norepinephrine-type granules")

Pathologic Differential Diagnosis

» Metastatic paraganglioma is the most important differential diagnosis, which cannot be resolved with histology
» Carcinoid
» Acinic cell tumor
» Sugar tumor
» Glomus tumor

RADIOLOGIC FEATURES

Imaging studies typically show a nodule or mass.

PATHOLOGIC FEATURES

GROSS FINDINGS

These tumors arise from the bronchial mucosa and often have a polypoid appearance. The tumor is usually soft, gray-white, and may show pigmentation. Adjacent to the tumor, brown-pigmented foci can sometimes be seen in the mucosa.

MICROSCOPIC FINDINGS

Tumor histology is similar to that of melanoma arising in other sites (Figure 28-20). Pagetoid spread can be observed in adjacent bronchial mucosa. The tumor may also be accompanied by nevus-like lesions in the adjacent mucosa.

ANCILLARY STUDIES

IMMUNOHISTOCHEMISTRY

Staining for S100 and HMB45 is characteristic. Cytokeratin can be focally positive, and neuroendocrine stains are negative.

ULTRASTRUCTURAL FEATURES

Melanosomes can be seen in the cytoplasm of tumor cells.

DIFFERENTIAL DIAGNOSIS

The major differential diagnosis lies with metastatic melanoma. Careful scrutiny of the medical history can often be helpful in this regard. In addition, observation of an associated nevus-like lesion in the adjacent bronchial mucosa is helpful for supporting the diagnosis of primary pulmonary melanoma. Peripherally

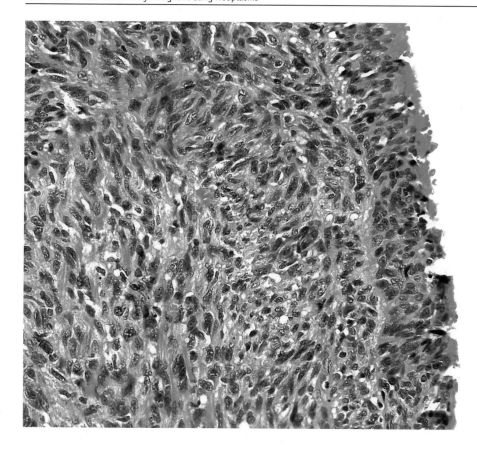

FIGURE 28-20
Malignant melanoma
The tumor replaces the subepithelial tissues of this bronchus and has an intra-epithelial component as well.

MALIGNANT MELANOMA—FACT SHEET

Definition

▸▸ A malignant tumor presumably derived from melanocytes, arising in patients without an extrapulmonary primary melanoma

Incidence

▸▸ Extremely rare neoplasm

Morbidity and Mortality

▸▸ High mortality rate
▸▸ Tumors often cause airway obstruction and its complications

Gender and Age Distribution

▸▸ Arise in adults with a mean age of 51 years and a range of 29-80 years
▸▸ No apparent gender predilection

Clinical Features

▸▸ Symptoms of cough, hemoptysis, and lobar collapse are explained by the frequent endobronchial location of the tumor

Radiologic Features

▸▸ Imaging studies typically show a nodule or mass and may show post-obstructive pneumonia or bronchiectasis

Prognosis and Therapy

▸▸ The prognosis is usually poor
▸▸ Surgical resection is the main treatment approach
▸▸ Some patients have been treated with aggressive chemotherapy

MALIGNANT MELANOMA—PATHOLOGIC FEATURES

Gross Findings

▸▸ Soft, gray-white, and variably pigmented polypoid masses arising from the bronchial or tracheal mucosa
▸▸ "Flat" lesions have been described less frequently
▸▸ Adjacent to the tumor, brown-pigmented foci can sometimes be seen in the mucosa

Microscopic Findings

▸▸ Tumor histology is similar to that of melanoma arising in other sites
▸▸ Pagetoid spread can be observed in adjacent bronchial mucosa
▸▸ Nevus-like lesions can sometimes be seen in the adjacent mucosa

Immunohistochemical Features

▸▸ Staining for S100 and HMB45 is characteristic
▸▸ Cytokeratin can be very focally positive, and neuroendocrine stains are negative

Ultrastructural Features

▸▸ Melanosomes are seen in the cytoplasm of tumor cells

Pathologic Differential Diagnosis

▸▸ Metastatic melanoma
▸▸ Carcinoid
▸▸ Peripheral nerve sheath neoplasms (schwannoma, neurofibroma, malignant peripheral nerve sheath tumor)

located lesions of melanoma are generally metastatic. Carcinoids, both pigmented and not, may also be considered in the differential diagnosis, but demonstrate expression of neuroendocrine markers and cytokeratin. Peripheral nerve sheath neoplasms (schwannoma, neurofibroma, malignant peripheral nerve sheath tumor) also express S100, but differ histologically from melanoma and do not typically express melanocytic markers.

PROGNOSIS AND THERAPY

The prognosis of primary pulmonary malignant melanoma is usually poor. As is true for other mucosal melanomas, these tumors tend to be detected late, sometimes after metastatic disease has been diagnosed. Surgical resection is the main treatment approach, and some patients have been treated with aggressive chemotherapy.

SUGGESTED READINGS

Mucoepidermoid Carcinoma

1. Segletes LA, Steffe CH, Geisinger KR. Cytology of primary pulmonary mucoepidermoid and adenoid cystic carcinoma. A report of four cases. *Acta Cytol.* 1999;43:1091-7.
2. Shilo K, Foss R, Franks TJ, DePeralta-Venturina M, Travis WD. Pulmonary mucoepidermoid carcinoma with prominent tumor-associated lymphoid proliferation. *Am J Surg Pathol.* 2005;29:407-11.
3. Shimizu J, Watanabe Y, Oda M, Morita K, Tsunezuka Y, Nonomura A. Clinicopathologic study of mucoepidermoid carcinoma of the lung. *Int Surg.* 1988;83:1-3.
4. Yousem SA, Hochholzer L. Mucoepidermoid tumors of the lung. *Cancer.* 1987;60:1346-52.

Adenoid Cystic Carcinoma.

5. Bennett AK, Mills SE, Wick MR. Adenoid cystic carcinoma of the lung. Pathology case review. *Pathol Case Rev.* 2004;9:253-8.
6. Moran CA, Suster S, Askin FB. Benign and malignant salivary gland-type tumors of the lung: clinicopathologic and immunohistochemical study of eight cases. *Cancer.* 1994;73:2481-90.
7. Moran CA, Suster S, Koss MN. Primary adenoid cystic carcinoma of the lung: a clinicopathologic and immunohistochemical study of 16 cases. *Cancer.* 1994;73:1390-7.
8. Yousem SA, Nicholson AG. Adenoid cystic carcinoma. In: Travis WD, Brambilla E, Muller-Hermelink HK, Harris CC, eds. *Pathology and Genetics. Tumours of the Lung, Pleura, Thymus and Heart.* Lyon: IARC Press; 2004: 65-6.

Acinic Cell Carcinoma

9. Chuah KL, Yap WM, Tan HW, Koong HN. Recurrence of pulmonary acinic cell carcinoma. *Arch Pathol Lab Med.* 2006;130:932-3.
10. Fechner RE, Bentinck BR, Askew IB. Acinic cell tumor of the lung. A histologic and ultrastructural study. *Cancer.* 1972;29:501-8.
11. Katz DR, Bubis JJ. Acinic cell tumor of the bronchus. *Cancer.* 1976;38:830-2.
12. Lee HY, Mancer K, Koong HN. Primary acinic cell carcinoma of the lung with lymph node metastasis. *Arch Pathol Lab Med.* 2003;127:e216-9.
13. Lee HY, Mancer K, Koong HN. Primary acinic cell carcinoma of the lung with lymph node metastasis. *Arch Pathol Lab Med.* 2006;130:932-3.
14. Moran CA, Suster S, Koss MN. Acinic cell carcinoma of the lung ("Fechner tumor"): a clinicopathologic, immunohistochemical and ultrastructural study of five cases. *Am J Surg Pathol.* 1992;16:1039-50.

15. Rodriguez J, Diment J, Lombardi L, Dominoni F, Tench W, Rosai J. Combined typical carcinoid and acinic cell tumor of the lung: a heretofore unreported occurrence. *Hum Pathol.* 2003;34:1061-5.
16. Sabaratnam RM, Anunathan R, Govender D. Acinic cell carcinoma: an unusual cause of bronchial obstruction in a child. *Pediatr Devel Pathol.* 2004;7:521-6.
17. Ukoha OO, Quartararo P, Carter D, Kashgarian M, Ponn RB. Acinic cell carcinoma of the lung with metastasis to lymph nodes. *Chest.* 1999;115:591-5.

Epithelial-Myoepithelial Carcinoma

18. Doganay L, Bilgi S, Ozdil A, Yoruk Y, Altaner S, Kutlu K. Epithelial-myoepithelial carcinoma of the lung. A case report and review of the literature. *Arch Pathol Lab Med.* 2003;127:e177-80.
19. Fulford LG, Kamata Y, Okudera K, et al. Epithelial-myoepithelial carcinomas of the bronchus. *Am J Surg Pathol.* 2001;25:1508-14.
20. Nistal M, Garcia-Viera M, Martinez-Garcia C, Paniagua R. Epithelial-myoepithelial tumor of the bronchus. *Am J Surg Pathol.* 1994;18:421-5.
21. Pelosi G, Fraggetta F, Maffini F, Solli P, Cavallon A, Viale G. Pulmonary epithelial-myoepithelial tumor of unproven malignant potential: report of a case and review of the literature. *Mod Pathol.* 2001;14:521-6.
22. Wilson RW, Moran CA. Epithelial-myoepithelial carcinoma of the lung: immunohistochemical and ultrastructural observations and review of the literature. *Hum Pathol.* 1997;28:631-5.
23. Yousem SA, Nicholson AG. Epithelial-myoepithelial carcinoma. In: Travis WD, Brambilla E, Muller-Hermelink HK, Harris CC, eds. *Pathology and Genetics. Tumours of the Lung, Pleura, Thymus and Heart.* Lyon: IARC Press; 2004:67.

Fetal Adenocarcinoma

24. Colby TV, Koss MN, Travis WD. Mixed epithelial and mesenchymal tumors. In: Colby TV, Koss MN, Travis WD. *Tumors of the Lower Respiratory Tract.* Atlas of tumor pathology, fasc. 13. Washington, DC: Armed Forces Institute of Pathology, under the auspices of Universities Associated for Research and Education in Pathology; 1995. 395-417.
25. Babycos PB, Daroca PJ. Polypoid pulmonary endodermal tumor resembling fetal lung: report of a case. *Mod Pathol.* 1995;8:303-6.
26. Nakatani Y, Dickersin RG, Mark EJ. Pulmonary endodermal tumor resembling fetal lung: a clinicopathologic study of five cases with immunohistochemical and ultrastructural characterization. *Hum Pathol.* 1990;21:1097-107.
27. Nakatani Y, Kitamura H, Inayama Y, et al. Pulmonary adenocarcinoma of fetal lung type. A clinicopathologic study indicating differences in histology, epidemiology, and natural history of low-grade and high-grade forms. *Am J Surg Pathol.* 1998;22:399-411.
28. Yamazaki K. Pulmonary well-differentiated fetal adenocarcinoma expressing lineage-specific transcription factors (TTF-1 and GATA-6) to respiratory epithelial differentiation: an immunohistochemical and ultrastructural study. *Virchows Arch.* 2003;442:393-9.

Mucinous Tumors

29. Butnor KJ, Sporn TA, Dodd LG. Fine needle aspiration cytology of mucinous cystadenocarcinoma of the lung: report of a case with radiographic and histologic correlation. *Acta Cytol.* 2001;45:779-83.
30. Graeme-Cook F, Mark EJ. Pulmonary mucinous cystic tumors of borderline malignancy. *Hum Pathol.* 1991;22:185-90.
31. Higashiyama M, Doi O, Kodama K, Yokouchi H, Tateishi R. Cystic mucinous adenocarcinoma of the lung. Two cases of cystic variant of mucus-producing lung adenocarcinoma. *Chest.* 1992;101:763-6.
32. Ishibashi H, Moriya T, Matsuda Y, et al. Pulmonary mucinous cystadenocarcinoma: report of a case and review of the literature. *Ann Thorac Surg.* 2003;76:1738-40.
33. Moran CA. Mucin-rich tumors of the lung. *Adv Anat Pathol.* 1995;2:299-305.
34. Moran CA. Pulmonary adenocarcinoma: the expanding spectrum of histologic variants. *Arch Pathol Lab Med.* 2006;130:958-62.
35. Rossi G, Murer B, Cavazza A, et al. Primary mucinous (so-called colloid) carcinomas of the lung. A clinicopathologic and immunohistochemical study with special reference to CDX-2 homebox gene and MUC-2 expression. *Am J Surg Pathol.* 2004;28:442-52.

36. Roux FJ, Lantuèjoul S, Brambilla E, Brambilla C. Mucinous cystadenoma of the lung. *Cancer*. 1995;76:1540-4.

Signet Ring Adenocarcinoma

37. Castro CY, Moran CA, Flieder DG, Suster S. Primary signet-ring cell adenocarcinomas of the lung: a clinicopathologic study of 15 cases. *Histopathology*. 2001;39:397-401.
38. Kish JK, Ro JY, Ayala AG, McMurtrey MJ. Primary mucinous adenocarcinoma of the lung with signet-ring cells: a histochemical comparison with signet-ring cell carcinomas of other sites. *Hum Pathol*. 1989;20:1097-102.
39. Merchant SH, Amin MB, Tamboli P, et al. Primary signet-ring cell carcinoma of the lung. Immunohistochemical study and comparison with non-pulmonary signet-ring cell carcinomas. *Am J Surg Pathol*. 2001;25:1515-9.
40. Tsuta K, Ishii G, Yoh K, et al. Primary lung carcinoma with signet-ring cell carcinoma components: clinicopathological analysis of 39 cases. *Am J Surg Pathol*. 2004;28:868-74.

Pulmonary Blastoma

41. Chejfec G, Cosnow I, Gould NS, Husain AN, Gould VE. Pulmonary blastoma with neuroendocrine differentiation in cell morules resembling neuroepithelial bodies. *Histopathology*. 1990;17:353-8.
42. Corrin B, Chang YL, Rossi G, et al. Sarcomatoid carcinoma. In: Travis WD, Brambilla E, Muller-Hermelink HK, Harris CC, eds. *Pathology and Genetics. Tumours of the Lung, Pleura, Thymus and Heart*. Lyon: IARC Press; 2004:53-8.
43. Koss MN, Hochholzer L, O'Leary T. Pulmonary blastomas. *Cancer*. 1991;67:2368-81.
44. Walker RI, Suvarna K, Matthews S. Case report: pulmonary blastoma: presentation of two atypical cases and review of the literature. *Br J Radiol*. 2005;78:437-40.
45. Wick MR, Ritter JH, Humphrey PA. Sarcomatoid carcinomas of the lung. A clinicopathologic review. *Am J Clin Pathol*. 1997;108:40-53.
46. Yousem SA, Wick MR, Randhawa P, Manivel JC. Pulmonary blastoma. An immunohistochemical analysis with comparison with fetal lung in its pseudoglandular stage. *Am J Clin Pathol*. 1990;93:167-75.

Basaloid Carcinoma

47. Brambilla E, Moro D, Veale D, et al. Basal cell (basaloid) carcinoma of the lung: a new morphologic and phenotypic entity with separate prognostic significance. *Hum Pathol*. 1992;23:993-1003.
48. Kim DJ, Kim KD, Shin DH, Ro JY, Chung KY. Basaloid carcinoma of the lung: a really dismal histologic variant? *Ann Thorac Surg*. 2003;76:1833-7.
49. Moro D, Brichon PY, Brambilla E, Veale D, Labat D, Brambilla C. Basaloid bronchial carcinoma. A histologic group with a poor prognosis. *Cancer*. 1994;73:2734-9.
50. Sturm N, Lantuejoul S, Laverriere MH, et al. Thyroid transcription factor 1 and cytokeratins 1, 5, 10, 14 (34betaE12) expression in basaloid and large-cell neuroendocrine carcinomas of the lung. *Hum Pathol*. 2001;32:918-25.

Teratoma

51. Asano S, Hoshikawa Y, Yamane Y, Ikeda M, Wakasa H. An intrapulmonary teratoma associated with bronchiectasia containing various kinds of primordium: a case report and review of the literature. *Virchows Arch*. 2000;436;384-8.
52. Iwasaki T, Iuchi K, Matsumura A, Sueki H, Yamamoto S, Mori T. Intrapulmonary mature teratoma. *Jpn J Thorac Cardiovasc Surg*. 2000;48: 468-72.
53. Morgan DE, Sanders C, McElvein RB, Nath H, Alexander CB. Intrapulmonary teratoma: a case report and review of the literature. *J Thorac Imaging*. 1992;7:70-7.
54. Nicholson AG. Teratoma. In: Travis WD, Brambilla E, Muller-Hermelink HK, Harris CC, eds. *Pathology and Genetics. Tumours of the Lung, Pleura, Thymus and Heart*. Lyon: IARC Press; 2004:119.
55. Zenker D, Aleksic I. Intrapulmonary cystic benign teratoma: a case report and review of the literature. *Ann Thorac Cardiovasc Surg*. 2004;10:290-2.

Leiomyosarcoma and Metastasizing Leiomyoma

56. Abramson S, Gilkeson RC, Goldstein JD, Woodard PK, Eisenberg R, Abramson N. Benign metastasizing leiomyoma: clinical, imaging, and pathologic correlation. *AJR Am J Roentgenol*. 2001;176:1409-13.
57. Esteban J-M, Allen W-M, Schaerf R-H. Benign metastasizing leiomyoma of the uterus: histologic and immunohistochemical characterization of primary and metastatic lesions. *Arch Pathol Lab Med*. 1999;123:960-2.
58. Etienne-Mastroianni B, Falchero L, Chalabreysse L, et al. Primary sarcomas of the lung: a clinicopathologic study of 12 cases. *Lung Cancer*. 2002;38: 283-9.
59. Guccion JG, Rosen SH. Bronchopulmonary leiomyosarcoma and fibrosarcoma. A study of 32 cases and review of the literature. *Cancer*. 1972;30: 836-47.
60. Jautzke G, Muller-Ruchholtz E, Thalmann U. Immunohistological detection of estrogen and progesterone receptors in multiple and well differentiated leiomyomatous lung tumors in women with uterine leiomyomas (so-called benign metastasizing leiomyomas). A report on 5 cases. *Pathol Res Pract*. 1996;192:215-23.
61. Jimenez JF, Uthman EO, Townsend JW, Gloster ES, Seibert JJ. Primary bronchopulmonary leiomyosarcoma in childhood. *Arch Pathol Lab Med*. 1986;110:348-51.
62. Moran CA, Suster S, Abbondanzo SL, Koss MN: Primary leiomyosarcomas of the lung: a clinicopathologic and immunohistochemical study of 18 cases. *Mod Pathol*. 1997;10:121-8.
63. Patton KT, Cheng L, Papavero V, et al. Benign metastasizing leiomyoma: clonality, telomere length and clinicopathologic analysis. *Mod Pathol*. 2006;19:130-40.
64. Tietze L, Gunther K, Horbe A, et al. Benign metastasizing leiomyoma: a cytogenetically balanced but clonal disease. *Hum Pathol*. 2000;31: 126-8.
65. Wick MR, Scheithauer BW, Piehler JM, Pairolero PC. Primary pulmonary leiomyosarcomas. A light and electron microscopic study. *Arch Pathol Lab Med*. 1982;106:510-4.
66. Yellin A, Rosenman Y, Lieberman Y. Review of smooth muscle tumours of the lower respiratory tract. *Br J Dis Chest*. 1984;78:337-51.

Malignant Fibrous Histiocytoma

67. Aoe K, Hiraki A, Maeda T, et al. Malignant fibrous histiocytoma of the lung. *Anticancer Res*. 2003;23:3469-74.
68. Derre J, Lagace R, Nicolas A, et al. Leiomyosarcomas and most malignant fibrous histiocytomas share very similar comparative genomic hybridization imbalances: an analysis of a series of 27 leiomyosarcomas. *Lab Invest*. 2001;81:211-5.
69. Gal AA, Koss MN, McCarthy WF, Hochholzer L. Prognostic factors in pulmonary fibrohistiocytic lesions. *Cancer*. 1994;73:1817-24.
70. Halyard MY, Camoriano JK, Culligan JA, et al. Malignant fibrous histiocytoma of the lung. Report of four cases and review of the literature. *Cancer*. 1996;78:2492-7.
71. Herrmann BL, Saller B, Kiess W, et al. Primary malignant fibrous histiocytoma of the lung: IGF-II producing tumor induces fasting hypoglycemia. *Exp Clin Endocrinol Diabetes*. 2000;108:515-8.
72. Nistal M, Jimenez-Heffernan JA, Hardisson D, Viguer JM, Bueno J, Garcia-Miguel P. Malignant fibrous histiocytoma of the lung in a child. An unusual neoplasm that can mimick inflammatory pseudotumour. *Eur J Pediatr*. 1997;156:107-9.
73. Shah SJ, Craver RD, Yu LC. Primary malignant fibrous histiocytoma of the lung in a child: a case report and review of literature. *Pediatr Hematol Oncol*. 1996;13:531-8.
74. Yousem SA, Hochholzer L. Malignant fibrous histiocytoma of the lung. *Cancer*. 1987;60:2532-41.

Epithelioid Hemangioendothelioma and Angiosarcoma

75. Bagan P, Hassan M, Le Pimpec Barthes F, et al. Prognostic factors and surgical indications of pulmonary epithelioid hemangioendothelioma: a review of the literature. *Ann Thorac Surg*. 2006;82:2010-13.
76. Chen TM, Donington J, Mak G, et al. Recurrence of pulmonary intravascular bronchoalveolar tumor with mediastinal metastasis 20 years later. *Respir Med*. 2006;100:367-70.
77. Cronin P, Arenberg D. Pulmonary epithelioid hemangioendothelioma: an unusual case and a review of the literature. *Chest*. 2004;125:789-93.
78. Duck L, Baurain JF, Machiels JP. Treatment of a primary pulmonary angiosarcoma, *Chest*. 2004;126:317-8.

79. Kitaichi M, Nagai S, Nishimura K, et al. Pulmonary epithelioid haemangioendothelioma in 21 patients, including three with partial spontaneous regression. *Eur Respir J.* 1998;12:89-96.

80. Kojima K, Okamoto I, Ushijima S, et al. Successful treatment of primary pulmonary angiosarcoma. *Chest.* 2003;124:2397-2400.

81. Kpodonu J, Tshibaka C, Massad MG. The importance of clinical registries for pulmonary epithelioid hemangioendothelioma. *Chest.* 2005;127:1870-71.

82. Ledson MJ, Convery R, Carty A, Evans CC. Epithelioid haemangioendothelioma. *Thorax.* 1999;54:560-1.

83. Palvio DH, Paulsen SM, Henneberg EW. Primary angiosarcoma of the lung presenting as intractable hemoptysis. *Thorac Cardiovasc Surg.* 1987;35:105-7.

84. Pandit SA, Fiedler PN, Westcott JL. Primary angiosarcoma of the lung. *Ann Diagn Pathol.* 2005;9:302-4.

85. Rock MJ, Kaufman RA, Lobe TE, Hensley SD, Moss ML. Epithelioid hemangioendothelioma of the lung (intravascular bronchioloalveolar tumor) in a young girl. *Pediatr Pulmonol.* 1991;11:181-6.

86. Sheppard MN, Hansell DM, Du Bois RM, Nicholson AG. Primary epithelioid angiosarcoma of the lung presenting as pulmonary hemorrhage. *Hum Pathol.* 1997;28:383-5.

87. Spragg RG, Wolf PL, Haghighi P, Abraham JL, Astarita RW. Angiosarcoma of the lung with fatal pulmonary hemorrhage. *Am J Med.* 1983;74:1072-6.

88. Travis WD, Tazelaar HD, Miettinen M. Epithelioid haemangioendothelioma/angiosarcoma. In: Travis WD, Brambilla E, Muller-Hermelink HK, Harris CC, eds. *Pathology and Genetics. Tumours of the Lung, Pleura, Thymus and Heart.* IARC Press; 2004:97-8.

89. Weiss SW, Ishak KG, Dail DH, Sweet DE, Enzinger FM. Epithelioid hemangioendothelioma and related lesions. *Semin Diagn Pathol.* 1986;3:259-87.

90. Yousem SA. Angiosarcoma presenting in the lung. *Arch Pathol Lab Med.* 1986;110:112-5.

Sarcomas of Large Pulmonary Blood Vessels

91. Anderson MB, Kriett JM, Kapelanski DP, Tarazi R, Jamieson SW. Primary pulmonary artery sarcoma: a report of six cases. *Ann Thorac Surg.* 1995;59:1487-90.

92. Babatasi G, Massetti M, Galateau F, Khayat A. Leiomyosarcoma of the pulmonary veins extending into the left atrium or left atrial leiomyosarcoma: multimodality therapy. *J Thorac Cardiovasc Surg.* 1998;116:665-7.

93. Cox JE, Chiles C, Aquino SL, Savage P, Oaks T. Pulmonary artery sarcomas: a review of clinical and radiographic features. *J Comput Assist Tomogr.* 1997;21:750-5.

94. Johansson L, Carlen B. Sarcoma of the pulmonary artery: report of four cases with electron microscopic and immunohistochemical examinations, and review of the literature, *Virchows Arch.* 1994;424:217-24.

95. Kruger I, Borowski A, Horst M, de Vivie ER, Theissen P, Gross-Fengels W. Symptoms, diagnosis, and therapy of primary sarcomas of the pulmonary artery. *Thorac Cardiovasc Surg.* 1990;38:91-5.

96. Laroia ST, Potti A, Rabbani M, Mehdi SA, Koch M. Unusual pulmonary lesions: case 3. Pulmonary vein leiomyosarcoma presenting as a left atrial mass. *J Clin Oncol.* 2002;20:2749-51.

97. McGlennen RC, Manivel JC, Stanley SJ, Slater DL, Wick MR, Dehner LP. Pulmonary artery trunk sarcoma: a clinicopathologic, ultrastructural, and immunohistochemical study of four cases. *Mod Pathol.* 1989;2:486-94.

98. Okuno T, Matsuda K, Ueyama K, et al. Leiomyosarcoma of the pulmonary vein. *Pathol Int.* 2000;50:839-46.

99. Tanaka H, Hasegawa S, Egi K, Tachou H, Saitoh F, Sunamori M. Successful radical resection of a leiomyosarcoma of the pulmonary trunk. *J Thorac Cardiovasc Surg.* 2001;122:1039-40.

100. Tazelaar HD, Flieder DB. Pulmonary vein sarcoma. In: Travis WD, Brambilla E, Muller-Hermelink HK, Harris CC, eds. *Pathology and Genetics. Tumours of the Lung, Pleura, Thymus and Heart.* Lyon: IARC Press; 2004:108.

101. Tsunezuka Y, Oda M, Takahashi M, Minato H, Watanabe G. Primary chondromatous osteosarcoma of the pulmonary artery. *Ann Thorac Surg.* 2004;77:331-34.

102. Yi ES. Tumors of the pulmonary vasculature. *Cardiol Clin.* 2004;22:431-440, vi-vii.

103. Yi JE, Tazelaar HD, Burke A, Manabe T. Pulmonary artery sarcoma. In: Travis WD, Brambilla E, Muller-Hermelink HK, Harris CC, eds. *Pathology and Genetics. Tumours of the Lung, Pleura, Thymus and Heart.* Lyon: IARC Press; 2004:109-10.

Other Sarcomas

104. Chapman AD, Pritchard SC, Yap WW, et al. Primary pulmonary osteosarcoma: case report and molecular analysis. *Cancer.* 2001;91:779-84.

105. Cohen M, Emms M, Kaschula RO. Childhood pulmonary blastoma: a pleuropulmonary variant of the adult-type pulmonary blastoma. *Pediatr Pathol.* 1991;11:737-49.

106. Comin CE, Santucci M, Novelli L, Dini S. Primary pulmonary rhabdomyosarcoma: report of a case in an adult and review of the literature. *Ultrastruct Pathol.* 2001;25:269-73.

107. Dennison S, Weppler E, Giacoppe G. Primary pulmonary synovial sarcoma: a case report and review of current diagnostic and therapeutic standards. *Oncologist.* 2004;9:339-42.

108. Doladzas T, Arvelakis A, Karavokyros IG, et al. Primary rhabdomyosarcoma of the lung arising over cystic pulmonary adenomatoid malformation. *Pediatr Hematol Oncol.* 2005;22:525-9.

109. Etienne-Mastroianni B, Falchero L, Chalabreysse L, et al. Primary sarcomas of the lung: a clinicopathologic study of 12 cases. *Lung Cancer.* 2002;38:283-9.

110. Gaertner EM, Steinberg DM, Huber M, et al. Pulmonary and mediastinal glomus tumors—report of five cases including a pulmonary glomangiosarcoma: a clinicopathologic study with literature review, *Am J Surg Pathol.* 2000;24:1105-14.

111. Hayashi T, Tsuda N, Iseki M, Kishikawa M, Shinozaki T, Hasumoto M. Primary chondrosarcoma of the lung. A clinicopathologic study. *Cancer.* 1993;72:69-74.

112. Kadowaki T, Hamada H, Yokoyama A, et al. Two cases of primary pulmonary osteosarcoma. *Intern Med.* 2005;44:632-7.

113. Keel SB, Bacha E, Mark EJ, Nielsen GP, Rosenberg AE. Primary pulmonary sarcoma: a clinicopathologic study of 26 cases. *Mod Pathol.* 1999;12:1124-31.

114. Krygier G, Amado A, Salisbury S, Fernandez I, Maedo N, Vazquez T. Primary lung liposarcoma. *Lung Cancer.* 1997;17:271-5.

115. Loddenkemper C, Perez-Canto A, Leschber G, Stein H. Primary dedifferentiated liposarcoma of the lung. *Histopathology.* 2005;46:710-2.

116. McCluggage WG, Bharucha H. Primary pulmonary tumours of nerve sheath origin. *Histopathology.* 1995;26:247-4.

117. Mikami Y, Nakajima M, Hashimoto H, Kuwabara K, Sasao Y, Manabe T. Primary poorly differentiated monophasic synovial sarcoma of the lung. A case report with immunohistochemical and genetic studies. *Pathol Res Pract.* 2003;199:827-33.

118. Muwakkit SA, Rodriguez-Galindo C, El Samra AI, et al Primary malignant peripheral nerve sheath tumor of the lung in a young child without neurofibromatosis type 1. *Pediatr Blood Cancer.* 2006;47:636-8.

119. Okamoto S, Hisaoka M, Daa T, Hatakeyama K, Iwamasa T, Hashimoto H. Primary pulmonary synovial sarcoma: a clinicopathologic, immunohistochemical, and molecular study of 11 cases. *Hum Pathol.* 2004;35:850-6.

120. Ozcan C, Celik A, Ural Z, Veral A, Kandiloglu G, Balik E. Primary pulmonary rhabdomyosarcoma arising within cystic adenomatoid malformation: a case report and review of the literature. *J Pediatr Surg.* 2001;36:1062-5.

121. Przygodzki RM, Moran CA, Suster S, Koss MN. Primary pulmonary rhabdomyosarcomas: a clinicopathologic and immunohistochemical study of three cases. *Mod Pathol.* 1995;8:658-61.

122. Said M, Migaw H, Hafsa C, et al. Imaging features of primary pulmonary liposarcoma. *Australas Radiol.* 2003;47:313-7.

123. Yellin A, Schwartz L, Hersho E, Lieberman Y. Chondrosarcoma of the bronchus. *Chest.* 1983;84:224-6.

Congenital Peribronchial Myofibroblastic Tumor

124. Alobeid B, Beneck D, Sreekantaiah C, Abbi RK, Slim MS. Congenital pulmonary myofibroblastic tumor: a case report with cytogenetic analysis and review of the literature. *Am J Surg Pathol.* 1997;21:610-4.

125. Horikoshi T, Kikuchi A, Matsumoto Y, et al. Fetal hydrops associated with congenital pulmonary myofibroblastic tumor. *J Obstet Gynaecol Res.* 2005;31:552-5.

126. McGinnis M, Jacobs G, el-Naggar A, Redline RW. Congenital peribronchial myofibroblastic tumor (so-called "congenital leiomyosarcoma"). A distinct neonatal lung lesion associated with nonimmune hydrops fetalis. *Mod Pathol*. 1993;6:487-92.

127. Travis WD, Dehner LP, Manabe T, Tazelaar HD. Congenital peribronchial myofibroblastic tumour. In: Travis WD, Brambilla E, Muller-Hermelink HK, Harris CC, eds. *Pathology and Genetics. Tumours of the Lung, Pleura, Thymus and Heart*. Lyon: IARC Press; 2004:102-3.

Paraganglioma

128. Aubertine CL, Flieder DB. Primary paraganglioma of the lung. *Ann Diagn Pathol*. 2004;8:237-41.

129. da Silva RA, Gross JL, Haddad FJ, Toledo CA, Younes RN. Primary pulmonary paraganglioma: case report and literature review. *Clinics*. 2006;61:83-6.

130. deLuise VP, Holman CW, Gray GF. Primary pulmonary paraganglioma. *N Y State J Med*. 1977;77:2270-1.

131. Gosney JR, Denley H, Resl M. Sustentacular cells in pulmonary neuroendocrine tumors. *Histopathology*. 1999;34:211-5.

132. Hangartner JR, Loosemore TM, Burke M, Pepper JR. Malignant primary pulmonary paraganglioma. *Thorax*. 1989;44:154-6.

133. Hsu LH, Tsou MH, You DL, Hsu WH. Primary pulmonary paraganglioma. *Zhonghua Yi Xue Za Zhi (Taipei)*. 2002;65:446-9.

134. Lemonick DM, Pai PB, Hines GL. Malignant primary pulmonary paraganglioma with hilar metastasis. *J Thorac Cardiovasc Surg*. 1990;99: 563-4.

135. Miller DL, Allen MS. Rare pulmonary neoplasms. *Mayo Clin Proc*. 1993;68:492-8.

136. Shibahara J, Goto A, Niki T, Tanaka M, Nakajima J, Fukayama M. Primary pulmonary paraganglioma: report of a functioning case with immunohistochemical and ultrastructural study. *Am J Surg Pathol*. 2004;28: 825-9.

137. Singh G, Lee RE, Brooks DH. Primary pulmonary paraganglioma: report of a case and review of the literature. *Cancer*. 1977;40:2286-9.

Malignant Melanoma

138. Bagwell SP, Flynn SD, Cox PM, Davison JA. Primary malignant melanoma of the lung. *Am Rev Respir Dis*. 1989;139:1543-7.

139. Dountsis A, Zisis C, Karagianni E, Dahabreh J. Primary malignant melanoma of the lung: A case report. *World J Surg Oncol*. 2003;1:26.

140. Lie CH, Chao TY, Chung YH, Lin MC. Primary pulmonary malignant melanoma presenting with haemoptysis. *Melanoma Res*. 2005;15:219-21.

141. Nicholson AG. Melanoma. In: Travis WD, Brambilla E, Muller-Hermelink HK, Harris CC, eds. *Pathology and Genetics. Tumours of the Lung, Pleura, Thymus and Heart*. Lyon: IARC Press; 2004:121.

142. Ost D, Joseph C, Sogoloff H, Menezes G. Primary pulmonary melanoma: case report and literature review. *Mayo Clin Proc*. 1999;74:62-6.

143. Wockel W, Morresi-Hauf A. Primary bronchial malignant melanoma. *Pathologe*. 1998;19:299-304.

29 Pulmonary Involvement by Extrapulmonary Neoplasms

Marie Christine Aubry

- **Introduction**
- **Metastatic Carcinoma, Sarcoma, Melanoma**
  Parenchymal Nodules
  Interstitial Thickening
  Pulmonary Hypertension and Infarct
  Airway Obstruction
  Pleural Effusion
  Diffuse Pulmonary Hemorrhage
- **Secondary Pulmonary Lymphoma**
- **Secondary Pulmonary Leukemia**

INTRODUCTION

Metastases to the lung are the most common malignancy of the lung, with an incidence ranging from 30 to 55% in various series. This is not surprising since the entire cardiac output and lymphatic fluid produced by the body flow through the pulmonary vascular system. If direct invasion of lung and trachea is included, then the incidence is even higher. In autopsy series, the most common primary sites with pulmonary metastases include breast, colon, kidney, uterus, and head and neck (Table 29-1). With improved survival of patients with malignancies, and increasing numbers of palliative surgeries, metastatic disease to the lung in bronchial and surgical specimens is growing. With the advent of novel therapies, distinguishing metastasis from primary lung tumors will become increasingly important.

PATHOGENESIS

Metastatic disease of the lungs can occur by different mechanisms (Table 29-2), and each route is usually associated with characteristic clinical, radiologic, and pathologic features, although overlap is frequent

(Tables 29-3 and 29-4). Direct extension of tumor usually occurs from a contiguous neoplasm or from direct intravascular involvement. This mechanism is less common than true metastasis and is associated primarily with primary thymic, esophageal, or thyroid neoplasms invading directly into lung or trachea. Rarely, direct extension to the lung occurs from the vasculature. Renal cell carcinoma and germ cell tumors can invade the inferior vena cava and enter the right heart, then extend into pulmonary arteries.

True metastases can be defined as viable tumor can cells transported from one site to another. They occur due to tumor spread via the vasculature, commonly the pulmonary arteries, and also the lymphatic vessels and bronchial arteries. Metastasis is itself a very complex multistep process, in which cells must acquire the capability of invading into and migrating through extracellular matrix into the vasculature, then disseminate through the vessels, avoiding destruction by the immune system, and form secondary deposits. Therefore, few metastases are produced, despite million of cells being released into circulation. In the lung, this process usually results in tumor emboli. Although some emboli may be large, the majority are small, involving the small arteries and arterioles. The fate of the embolized tumor cells is variable, but occasionally growth through the vasculature into the surrounding lung parenchyma, with formation of a nodule, occurs. In some instances, the tumor cells remain confined to the vasculature and spread diffusely through the vascular channels, including lymphatic vessels. This

---

OVERVIEW—FACT SHEET

Incidence
- ‣ Metastasis is the most common malignancy in the lung
- ‣ Incidence varies between 30% and 55%

Pathogenesis of Metastasis
- ‣ Direct extension
- ‣ Vascular and lymphatic invasion
- ‣ Pleural space seeding
- ‣ Airway dissemination

TABLE 29-1

Frequency of Various Tumors Metastatic to the Lung at Presentation and at Autopsy

Tumor Type		Frequency at Presentation	Frequency at Autopsy
Urologic	Kidney	5-30%	50-75%
	Bladder	5-10%	25-30%
	Prostate	5-25%	15-55%
Gynecologic	Uterine/Cervix	15%	20-30%
	Endometrium	2-5%	30-40%
	Ovary	5%	45%
Gastrointestinal	Colorectal	5%	10-30%
	Gastric		20-30%
Head and neck		5%	10-40%
Breast		5%	60%
Thyroid		4-10%	65%
Melanoma		5%	65-80%
Choriocarcinoma		60%	70-100%
Osteosarcoma		10%	75%
Lymphoma	Hodgkin	9%	22-62%
	Non-Hodgkin	5%	25%

Data taken from Libshitz HI, North LB, *Radiol Clin North Am*. 1982;20:437-51.

TABLE 29-2

Mechanisms of Metastatic Spread

Direct Extension	
Vascular:	Pulmonary arteries
	Bronchial arteries
	Lymphatic vessels
Pleural space	
Airways	

TABLE 29-3

Metastatic Patterns

Common	Uncommon	
Parenchymal nodules ("cannon balls")	Nodules:	Solitary
Pleural effusion		Miliary
		Cavitary
		Calcified
		Cystic with spontaneous pneumothorax
	Lymphangitic carcinomatosis with interstitial thickening	
	Pulmonary hypertension and infarcts	
	Airway obstruction with obstructive pneumonia or atelectasis	
	Alveolar hemorrhage syndrome	

METASTATIC CARCINOMA, SARCOMA, MELANOMA

PARENCHYMAL NODULES

CLINICAL FEATURES

The most common manifestation of metastatic disease to the lung consists of multiple nodules, usually derived from small tumor emboli with secondary extension into the adjacent lung parenchyma. Of patients with multiple metastases, 80-90% have a previous history of malignancy or are diagnosed with a synchronous primary. Patients are usually asymptomatic (75-90%). Symptoms are related to the growth and location of the nodules and include cough, hemoptysis, and wheezing. Extension into pleura and chest wall can lead to chest pain or Pancoast's syndrome. Spontaneous pneumothorax is an uncommon presentation of pulmonary metastasis, accounting for less than 1% of patients with spontaneous pneumothorax in one large series, and most commonly recognized in patients with osteosarcoma, soft tissue sarcoma, and endometrial stromal sarcoma. Some patients may have predominantly cystic lesions without developing pneumothoraces. Although uncommon, multiple pulmonary cysts or spontaneous pneumothorax may be the first manifestation of metastatic disease in patients with known malignancy.

RADIOLOGIC FEATURES

The most sensitive image modality currently available to evaluate patients with multiple lung nodules is the computed tomography (CT) scan, and helical CT scan is

can be followed by dissemination to hilar and mediastinal lymph nodes. Metastases via bronchial arteries are thought to be much less common and perhaps result in endobronchial metastasis. Tumor dissemination through the airways is poorly understood and probably rare, thought to occur primarily with bronchioloalveolar carcinoma.

Table 29-4
Pathologic Presentations and Associated Neoplasms

Cystic nodules	Endometrial stromal sarcoma Leiomyosarcoma
Miliary nodules	Thyroid (medullary) carcinoma Prostatic carcinoma Pancreatic carcinoma Melanoma
Cavitary nodules	Colonic carcinoma Head and neck carcinomas Cervical carcinoma Osteosarcoma
Calcified nodules	Thyroid (papillary) carcinoma Colonic carcinoma Osteosarcoma Chondrosarcoma
Solitary nodule	Renal cell carcinoma Breast carcinoma Colonic carcinoma Urothelial carcinoma Melanoma Osteosarcoma
Lymphangitic carcinomatosis	Breast carcinoma Gastric carcinoma Pancreatic carcinoma Prostatic carcinoma Lymphoma
Tumor emboli	Renal cell carcinoma Gastric carcinoma Hepatocellular carcinoma Breast carcinoma Sarcoma (origin from large vessels) Choriocarcinoma
Endobronchial masses	Breast carcinoma Renal cell carcinoma Colonic carcinoma Melanoma Sarcoma
Pleural effusion/ metastasis	Breast carcinoma Ovarian carcinoma Gastric carcinoma Lymphoma
Diffuse pulmonary hemorrhage	Angiosarcoma Choriocarcinoma

perhaps more sensitive than high-resolution CT scan, in particular for lesions less than 0.6 cm. Despite its sensitivity, since up to 60% of metastases are reported as 0.5 cm or less, CT scan can underestimate the burden of metastatic disease. Also, CT scan is not specific since nodules can consist of granulomas or other benign processes.

Metastatic tumor nodules are multiple in the majority of cases, ranging in size from hardly visible to large growths capable of occupying an entire lung, with an average size of 1.0-2.0 cm. Mediastinal and hilar nodes are usually not enlarged. Pulmonary metastases are most commonly found in the outer third, subpleural regions of the lower lung zones (lower lobes affected in 37% vs. upper lobes in 21%). Rarely, the deposits are so minute and numerous as to suggest miliary tuberculosis. This miliary pattern has been described with medullary carcinoma of the thyroid, malignant melanoma, and prostatic carcinoma, amongst others. Cavitation has been reported in 4% of metastases and occurs less commonly than with primary lung cancer. It has been described in metastatic squamous cell carcinoma, mainly from the head and neck or cervix, adenocarcinoma of the colon, and osteosarcoma. Calcification of metastatic lesions is rare and occurs in neoplasms with matrix production such as osteosarcoma or chondrosarcoma. It has also been described in neoplasms with psammoma bodies such as papillary carcinoma of the thyroid, or through dystrophic calcification of mucin in mucinous adenocarcinomas from the colon or other primary site. When calcified metastatic lesions are small, they can mimic benign lesions such as calcified granulomas.

Metastatic neoplasms presenting as solitary nodules are uncommon, accounting for 1-5% of all lung metastases and 2-10% of solitary pulmonary nodules. Neoplasms most likely to result in solitary metastases are carcinomas of the colon, kidney, and breast; sarcomas, particularly osteosarcoma; and malignant melanoma.

PATHOLOGIC FEATURES

Parenchymal nodules are usually well circumscribed and of variable size (Figure 29-1). Occasionally, they can be approximately of equal size, thought to reflect a single embolic shower. The size of the cavities in cavitary metastasis is often variable, ranging from less than 1.0 cm to over 6.0 cm, and the walls are shaggy and thick, measuring between 0.3 to 2.5 cm. Blood, necrotic material, and, rarely, a fungus ball can be identified. Communication with the adjacent bronchial tree is occasionally present. In cystic metastasis, the wall is usually very thin, less than 0.3 cm, and smooth, and the cavity filled with air.

Parenchymal nodules are usually located adjacent to pulmonary arteries and arterioles. Small tumor emboli can sometimes be identified, and parenchymal growth is usually destructive, forming a relatively well-circumscribed nodule, comprised of variable proportions of viable and necrotic tumor and reactive stroma. Rarely, the growth pattern is lepidic, along intact lung architecture, mimicking bronchioloalveolar carcinomas (Figure 29-2). This growth pattern is seen mainly in carcinomas of the colon and pancreaticobiliary system. In cavitary lesions, vascular invasion in the vicinity of the metastasis is a common finding. The walls of the cavitary or cystic lesions are also comprised of a mixture of tumor and stroma, and occasionally, the tumor can be difficult to identify.

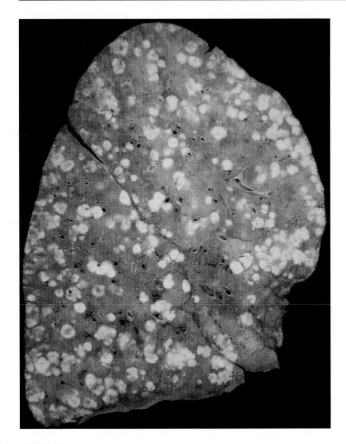

FIGURE 29-1

Multinodular metastasis
Fixed autopsy lung of metastatic squamous cell carcinoma of the cervix resulting in numerous well-circumscribed nodules of variable size, ranging between 0.1 and 1.3 cm.

INTERSTITIAL THICKENING

CLINICAL AND RADIOLOGIC FEATURES

Lymphangitic carcinomatosis is an uncommon pattern of tumor spread, occurring in less than 10% of pulmonary metastases. It can mimic interstitial lung disease clinically and radiologically. It usually occurs as a result of hematogenous spread with involvement of the interstitial space and then the lymphatic vessels. Although it can be seen in any metastatic neoplasm, the most common primaries include carcinomas of the breast, stomach, pancreas, and prostate. Dyspnea typically develops with an insidious onset yet rapid progression over weeks. The CT scan appearance is characterized by smooth to nodular thickening of the interlobular septa and peribronchovascular interstitium, usually with preservation of the underlying lung parenchyma. The thickening is usually asymmetrical. Associated pleural effusion is present in up to 30% of patients and hilar or mediastinal enlargement in up to 40%.

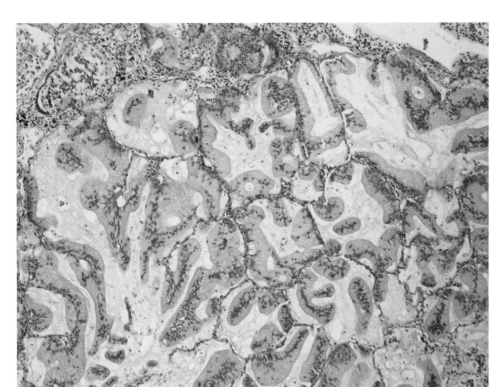

FIGURE 29-2

Metastasis mimicking mucinous bronchioloalveolar carcinoma
Patient with pancreatic adenocarcinoma who developed multiple lung nodules. Several of the nodules were composed of mucinous cells lining intact alveolar septa, although a few glands were also seen.

PATHOLOGIC FEATURES

GROSS FINDINGS

Lymphangitic carcinomatosis is characterized by thickening of the interlobular septa and peribronchovascular and subpleural connective tissue. The thickening can be linear or nodular and is variable, from slight to obvious thickening up to 1 cm (Figure 29-3).

MICROSCOPIC FINDINGS

In lymphangitic carcinomatosis, the neoplastic cells are usually easily identified within the lymphatic spaces (Figure 29-4), but also form cords and clusters within the interstitium, usually associated with a desmoplastic reaction. Occasionally, the desmoplastic reaction is so prominent as to conceal the neoplastic cells, and the clue is the growth pattern along the lymphatic pathways (Figure 29-5). The tumor growth can result in spread of the neoplasm outside the interstitium, resulting in the formation of parenchymal nodules, altering the typical pattern.

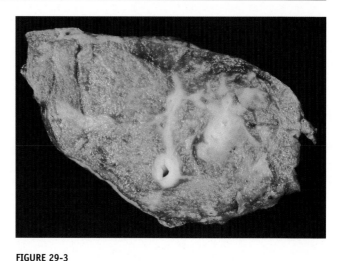

FIGURE 29-3
Lymphangitic metastasis
Metastatic leiomyosarcoma from a retroperitoneal primary causes thickening of the bronchovascular bundles and interlobular septa.

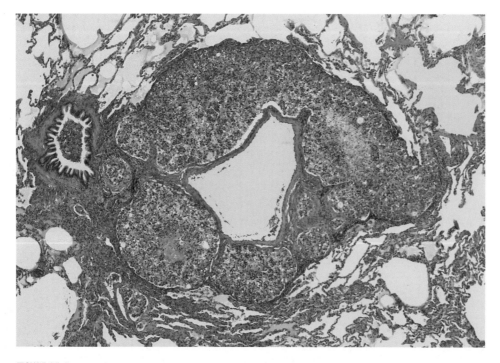

FIGURE 29-4
Lymphangitic metastasis
Nests of tumor cells are easily identified within periarterial lymphatic vessels, as illustrated here. They are also present in peribronchiolar and perivenous lymphatic vessels.

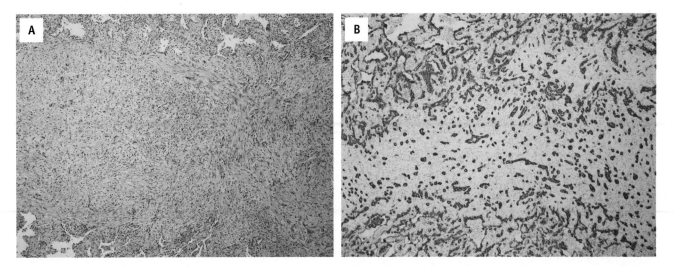

FIGURE 29-5

Lymphangitic metastasis
(A) The interlobular septum is thickened by dense reactive fibrosis, rendering the neoplastic cells inconspicuous. **(B)** The keratin stain highlights numerous tumor cells (keratin AE1/AE3).

PULMONARY HYPERTENSION AND INFARCT

CLINICAL FEATURES

Tumor involvement of pulmonary vessels has been reported in up to 41% of patients at autopsy, and is considered the main cause of death in 14-25%. The most common primary neoplasms include carcinomas of the stomach, pancreas, breast, liver, and choriocarcinoma. This pattern of metastasis often overlaps with other patterns, mostly lymphangitic, which results in overlapping clinical and radiologic manifestations. If it is the sole manifestation of metastatic disease, then patients will often be asymptomatic. The most common symptom, when present, is dyspnea. Patients may develop pulmonary hypertension with signs of cor pulmonale. If the tumor emboli have resulted in infarcts, pleuritic chest pain, hemoptysis, or even sudden death can occur.

RADIOLOGIC FEATURES

Radiologically, these lesions are difficult to diagnose. Indirect findings of pulmonary hypertension such as dilatation of the central pulmonary arteries and right ventricle can be identified, as well as infarcts. A ventilation-perfusion scan or CT scan with contrast may be helpful in identifying large tumor emboli.

PATHOLOGIC FEATURES

GROSS FINDINGS

Tumor emboli are usually not visible grossly unless larger, segmental arteries are involved. The appearance of tumor emboli can be different from thromboemboli, with tumor emboli displaying a more solid, gritty, or myxoid texture with white-beige color (Figure 29-6). Tumor emboli may be associated with infarcts.

MICROSCOPIC FINDINGS

Tumor emboli are most often identified only histologically, with small arteries and arterioles usually affected. Rarely, diffuse alveolar septal capillary involvement is present. The tumor cells form small clusters with or without associated recent or organized thrombus within vascular spaces (Figure 29-7).

AIRWAY OBSTRUCTION

Although neoplastic infiltration of the tracheal and main bronchial walls is a common finding at autopsy (19-51%), usually as the result of direct extension from parenchymal tumor or nodal metastasis, metastasis presenting as a distinct, usually solitary, endobronchial mass is uncommon, occurring in between 2 and 4% of

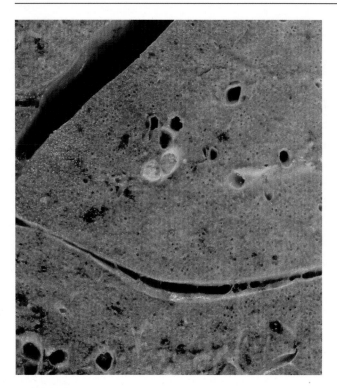

FIGURE 29-6
Tumor embolus
Fixed autopsy lung showing tumor embolus from breast carcinoma. Note the pale beige color of the embolus.

cases. The most common neoplasms resulting in endobronchial masses are melanoma, sarcomas, and carcinomas of the breast and kidney. Symptoms can consist of dyspnea, wheezing, persistent cough, and hemoptysis. Occasionally, expectoration of tumor fragments can occur. Radiologic findings are those of partial or complete airway obstruction with air trapping, atelectasis, or obstructive pneumonia.

PATHOLOGIC FEATURES

GROSS FINDINGS

Endobronchial metastasis can result in concentric narrowing of the airway or formation of a polypoid endobronchial mass.

MICROSCOPIC FINDINGS

With endobronchial metastases, the tumor cells are often present within the submucosal lymphatics, and infiltration of the bronchial wall with mucosal replacement from a contiguous mass is commonly seen.

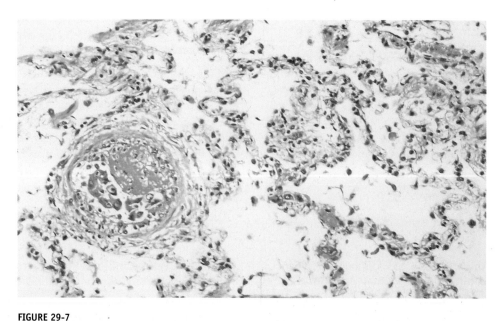

FIGURE 29-7

Metastatic renal cell carcinoma in a patient with acute cor pulmonale
At autopsy, diffuse alveolar septal capillary involvement and numerous tumor emboli in small arterioles were identified.

PLEURAL EFFUSION

Pleural involvement by extrapleural neoplasms is discussed in chapter 34.

DIFFUSE PULMONARY HEMORRHAGE

CLINICAL AND RADIOLOGIC FEATURES

Diffuse pulmonary hemorrhage (DPH) is an uncommon manifestation of neoplasia. Indeed, when patients are diagnosed with DPH, common causes investigated include Wegener's granulomatosis and other types of vasculitis, connective tissue diseases such as systemic lupus erythematosus, and Goodpasture's syndrome. Metastatic angiosarcoma is the most common neoplasm responsible for DPH, with at least 19 patients reported in the literature. Other neoplasms reported to cause DPH include other vascular neoplasms, such as Kaposi sarcoma and epithelioid hemangioendothelioma, and metastatic choriocarcinoma.

Symptoms and signs of hemoptysis, anemia, and pulmonary alveolar infiltrates are found in all patients, although in patients with neoplasms, radiologic infiltrates will often be described as nodular, surrounded by ground-glass infiltrates.

PATHOLOGIC FEATURES

GROSS FINDINGS

The gross appearance of neoplasms presenting as DPH can vary with tumor type. In cases of metastatic angiosarcoma or Kaposi sarcoma, multiple subpleural and parenchymal hemorrhagic, often blue, nodules are typically seen.

MICROSCOPIC FINDINGS

In this clinical setting, transbronchial biopsy is commonly nondiagnostic, showing nonspecific findings of hemorrhage. The diagnosis of neoplasm is usually made on wedge biopsy or, in some cases, at autopsy (Figure 29-8).

DIFFERENTIAL DIAGNOSIS

Although recognizing pulmonary metastasis is usually straightforward in patients with a known history of malignancy, presenting with multiple nodules, difficulty in diagnosing pulmonary metastasis can arise due to uncommon clinical, radiologic, and histologic manifestations (Table 29-5). Clinicians and/or pathologists may be unaware of a prior diagnosis of malignancy, especially when the malignancy occurred years or decades previously. This is well recognized in tumors with a

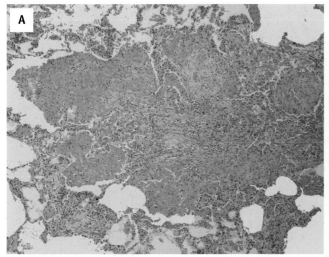 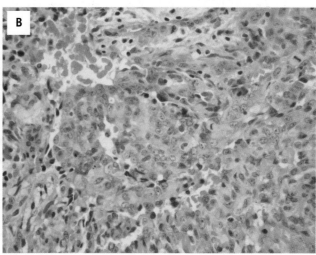

FIGURE 29-8

Metastatic angiosarcoma presenting as diffuse pulmonary hemorrhage
(A) There is acute and organizing alveolar hemorrhage associated with nodular thickening around a bronchiole. **(B)** Atypical cells form vascular channels.

TABLE 29-5

Challenges in Recognizing Pulmonary Metastasis

1. Long interval between occurrence of primary and metastasis
2. No known primary neoplasm
3. Misdiagnosis on previous surgical specimen
4. Unusual clinical presentation
5. Resemblance to lung primary
6. Change in phenotype from primary

good prognosis such as endometrial stromal sarcoma or stage I carcinoma of the colon or kidney.

Prior misdiagnosis can also be misleading, emphasizing the need to review previous surgical specimens, even those of apparently benign tumors. The metastasis can be the first manifestation of an unrecognized primary, and the difficulty may be compounded if the presentation is unusual, such as spontaneous pneumothorax with cystic lesions, pulmonary hypertension, or diffuse pulmonary hemorrhage. Challenges also arise when a metastasis mimics a known lung disease. For example, cystic endometrial stromal sarcoma can resemble lymphangioleiomyomatosis (Figure 29-9). The key to identifying a potential metastasis in these unusual circumstances is to think about the possibility of metastatic disease and always include it in the differential diagnosis.

There are no reliable clinical or radiologic features to separate a solitary metastasis from a new primary pulmonary carcinoma. In general, the probability of a new lung primary or unrelated lesion is greater than that of a solitary metastasis. Indeed, in one study, 36% of patients with a previous history of malignancy and a solitary nodule proved to have an unrelated pulmonary or mediastinal tumor, and 18% had a benign lesion. Although metastases are usually well circumscribed with smooth borders, in another study, up to 50% were described with poorly defined, irregular margins. Determination of histologic tumor type can also be helpful for assessing the likelihood of primary versus metastatic neoplasia. For example,

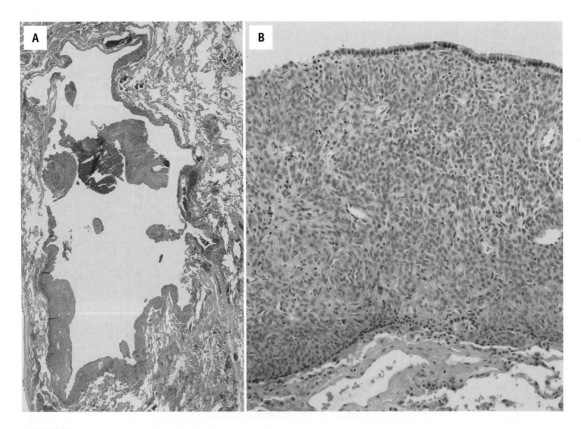

FIGURE 29-9

Metastatic endometrial stromal sarcoma mimicking lymphangioleiomyomatosis
(A) Low-power photomicrograph of a thin-walled cystic lesion. **(B)** Intermediate-power photomicrograph of the wall of the cyst. The short spindle cells are associated with small thick-walled arterioles. The cells were negative for smooth muscle actin and HMB-45 and showed strong immunoreactivity for estrogen receptor protein. The patient had a hysterectomy for endometrial stromal sarcoma 15 years prior.

melanoma and sarcoma are more often metastatic than primary. Diagnosis of primary pulmonary melanoma or sarcoma is made only when thorough clinical history, review of previous surgical material, and clinical and radiologic evaluation has ruled out any possibility of an extrapulmonary primary site.

For common histologic types of carcinomas, such as adenocarcinoma and squamous cell carcinoma, the separation between primary and metastasis can be very difficult; however, some carcinomas may have distinct features. Colonic adenocarcinomas characteristically display a cribriform pattern with nuclear pseudostratification and dirty necrosis. The presence of clear cells or colloid raises the diagnosis of renal clear cell or thyroid carcinoma. The presence of in situ carcinoma, particularly in association with squamous cell carcinoma, supports an interpretation of primary lung carcinoma. The presence of lepidic growth can also be misleading, since some metastases can exhibit lepidic growth, imitating bronchioloalveolar carcinoma. Metastases with lepidic growth can often be recognized, however, by their greater degree of cytologic atypia and other features such as a cribriform pattern, necrosis, or angiolymphatic invasion. These features are helpful but not specific for a metastatic origin, though.

Comparing the morphologic features of a potential metastasis to a known primary can be valuable for confirming the diagnosis of metastatic disease or determining that the tumor represents a new primary; however, the morphologic appearance of a metastasis may differ from the primary tumor, making proper identification of the lesion difficult. For example, metastatic malignant melanoma is often amelanotic or can assume a spindle cell growth pattern (Figure 29-10), experience stromal hyalinization, or contain osteoclast-like giant cells. Some tumors undergo what is called the "maturation effect," either as an inherent property of the tumor, result of host-tissue interaction, or treatment effect. This is common in sarcomas, germ cell tumors, and childhood malignancies such as Wilms' tumor or neuroblastoma. Metastatic osteosarcoma can become heavily collagenized, resulting in a paucicellular nodule resembling a scar. Metastatic germ cell tumors often take the form of mature teratomas. Finally, some other metastases display histologic features not well demonstrated in the primary tumors, such as sex-cord like differentiation in endometrial stromal sarcoma or sarcomatoid differentiation in renal cell carcinoma.

ANCILLARY STUDIES

IMMUNOHISTOCHEMISTRY

Immunohistochemistry can be a useful tool in separating metastasis from primary (Table 29-6), and is also discussed in chapter 38. Lung adenocarcinoma exhibits nuclear immunoreactivity for thyroid transcription factor 1 (TTF-1) in approximately 80% of cases. It is also seen in thyroid neoplasms, but is absent in other adenocarcinomas. Since thyroglobulin is commonly expressed

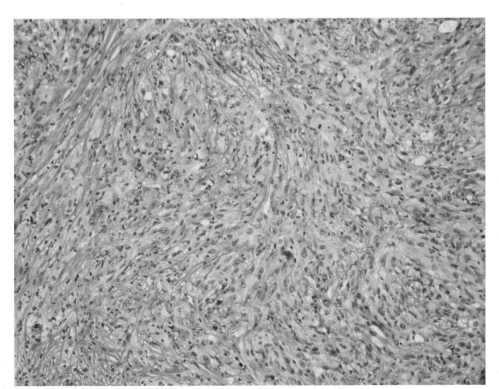

FIGURE 29-10

Metastatic malignant melanoma
This metastatic malignant melanoma was composed of amelanotic spindle cells. The original cutaneous melanoma showed epithelioid cells, some of which contain melanin pigment.

TABLE 29-6

Immunohistochemical Studies Useful for Separating Primary from Metastatic Lung Neoplasms

Features	Tumors		Immunohistochemical Studies
Epithelioid features	Carcinomas:	Lung adenocarcinoma	CK7+, TTF-1+, MOC 31+, pCEA+
		Lung adenocarcinoma, mucinous	CK7+/−, CK20+/−, TTF-1+/−, Cdx2+/−
		Thyroid neoplasms (papillary)	TTF-1+, thyroglobulin+
		Colorectal carcinoma	CK7−, CK20+, TTF-1−, cdx2+
		Breast carcinoma	CK7+, TTF-1−, ER+, S100 prot+, GCDFP15+, mammaglobin+
		Renal cell carcinoma	Vimentin+, CK7−/+, RCC+
		Prostate carcinoma	CK7−/+, PSA+, PAP+
		Ovarian carcinoma	CK7+, CA125+, ER+
		Hepatocellular carcinoma	CK7−, HepPar 1+
	Malignant mesothelioma		CK5/6+, calretinin+, MOC31−, pCEA−
	Melanoma		S100 prot+, HMB45+, Melan-A+, tyrosinase+, keratin−
	Germ cell tumors		Keratin+/−, PLAP+/−, c-kit (CD117)+/−
Spindle cell features	Carcinoma		Keratins−/+, Actin SM−/+, S100 prot−, CD31−
	Melanoma		S100 prot+, HMB45−/+, Melan-A−/+, tyrosinase−/+,
	Sarcomas:	Leiomyosarcoma	Actin SM+, keratin−/+, S100 prot−
		Synovial sarcoma	Keratin+/−, S100 prot−/+, actin SM−
		Endometrial stromal sarcomas	ER+, PR+, actin AM−/+, keratin−/+, S100 prot−
		Angiosarcoma	CD31+, CD34+, keratin +, actin SM−/+, S100 prot−

For the purpose of simplification, "+" implies immunoreactivity in > 80% of cases and "-" immunoreactivity in < 15% of cases.
TTF-1 = thyroid transcription factor; pCEA = polyclonal carcinoembryonic antigen; ER = estrogen receptor; GCDFP15 = gross cystic disease fluid protein-15; RCC = renal cell carcinoma marker; PSA = prostate-specific antigen; PAP = prostatic acid phosphatase; HepPar 1 = hepatocyte paraffin 1; PLAP = placental alkaline phosphatase; actin SM = smooth muscle actin; PR = progesterone receptor protein.

in thyroid neoplasms but negative in lung carcinomas, it is useful to distinguish both tumor types.

The combination of cytokeratin 7 and 20, TTF-1, and Cdx2 can be useful in separating pulmonary adenocarcinoma from metastatic colorectal carcinoma. Colorectal carcinomas are uniformly positive for CK20 and Cdx2, and negative for CK7 and TTF-1. Primary adenocarcinomas usually exhibit CK7 and TTF-1 immunoreactivity; however, mucinous tumors of the lung may express a variable profile, including expression of CK20 and Cdx2 and loss of TTF-1 expression. Breast primaries can express S-100 protein, gross cystic disease fluid protein-15 (GCDFP-15) and estrogen receptor protein (ER), findings usually absent in lung primaries. Renal cell carcinoma (RCC) usually co-expresses vimentin and keratin AE1/AE3, but expresses CK7 in less than 30% of cases. Immunoreactivity for RCC marker is also characteristic of many renal cell carcinomas. In cases of metastatic adenocarcinoma mimicking epithelial malignant mesothelioma, a panel comprised of keratin CK5/6, calretinin, MOC31, and polyclonal CEA seems to offer excellent specificity and sensitivity in

distinguishing between these entities. Although spindle cell carcinomas of the lung are often only focally positive for keratins, if at all, they are also usually negative for markers used in identifying sarcomas or spindle cell melanoma.

MOLECULAR TECHNIQUES

Although molecular techniques offer promise for assisting in resolving questions of primary versus metastatic origin, few molecular genetic markers today are sufficiently specific to a single tumor to be useful as a diagnostic tool. One useful marker, however, is the SYT-SSX fusion transcript in synovial sarcoma.

PROGNOSIS AND THERAPY

Treatment and prognosis will vary depending on tumor type and extent of metastatic disease (i.e. widespread versus limited to the lung), and a detailed discussion for each tumor type is beyond the scope of this chapter. Pulmonary metastases are usually, in up to 85% of patients, a manifestation of widespread disease, and thus are not amenable to surgery. Therefore palliative therapy, in the form of chemotherapy, radiation, laser ablation, talc pleurodesis, or other therapies, depending on tumor site, will often be considered in symptomatic patients. Metastasectomy, usually with video-assisted thoracoscopy, is increasingly performed for certain tumors but several guidelines are followed. The procedure should be considered curative and thus is reserved for metastasis that is limited to the lung and completely resectable. Malignancy needs to be ruled out in any pleural or pericardial effusions. Since cytology alone may be falsely negative (up to 60% of cases in some series), a negative result warrants a biopsy. The primary tumor should be controlled before considering curative resection of metastasis. The patient must be able to tolerate the surgery without any significant increase in short- and long-term morbidity and mortality due to associated co-morbid factors. And finally, any alternative therapy superior to surgery should considered, for example, chemotherapy for non-seminomatous germ cell tumors. When these guidelines are followed, survival rates as high as 60% have been reported following metastasectomy.

SECONDARY PULMONARY LYMPHOMA

Secondary pulmonary involvement in patients with malignant lymphoma occurs more frequently than primary lymphoma of the lung, and the lung is a common site of extranodal involvement. Although some autopsy series report a higher frequency of secondary lung involvement by Hodgkin lymphoma (HL) (39-62%), compared to non-Hodgkin lymphomas (NHL) (about 25%), other series show similar frequencies. HL involvement of the lung usually occurs with extensive, stage III and IV, extrathoracic disease. Secondary lung involvement by NHL occurs more frequently in patients with intermediate-or high-grade lymphomas as compared to patients with low-grade lymphomas. In one large series, excluding HLs and T-cell lymphomas, 74% of secondary lymphomas were classified as intermediate- or high-grade tumors, in contrast to only 41% of primary pulmonary lymphomas. Pleural infiltration by lymphoma is present in up to 20% of patients, usually at presentation, or in the course of the disease. Pleural effusion will occur more commonly with nodular sclerosis HL or large cell lymphoma.

CLINICAL FEATURES

Pulmonary symptoms are uncommon in patients with secondary pulmonary involvement, and pulmonary disease is usually discovered incidentally during evaluation of patients with presumed or established diagnoses of lymphoma. The clinical presentation is usually related to the lymphoma per se with diffuse lymphadenopathy or systemic symptoms of fever, night sweats, and weight loss. When present, pulmonary symptoms include dry cough, dyspnea, hemoptysis, or pneumonia.

SECONDARY PULMONARY LYMPHOMAS—FACT SHEET

Overview

▸ Secondary pulmonary involvement by lymphoma is more common than primary pulmonary lymphoma

▸ Reported frequency varies between 25 and 60% for Hodgkin's lymphoma (HL) and 25% for non-Hodgkin's lymphoma (NHL), usually intermediate- to high-grade

Clinical Features

▸ Usually no pulmonary symptoms with incidental discovery during staging of lymphoma

▸ Symptoms usually related to lymphoma

Radiologic Features

▸ Parenchymal disease present at diagnosis in 9% of HL and 5% of NHL

▸ Commonly associated with mediastinal lymphadenopathy

▸ Common patterns are nodules, bronchovascular-lymphangitic, and pneumonic infiltrates

Prognosis and Therapy

▸ Treatment is usually chemotherapy, with or without radiation

▸ Involvement of the lung in advanced stage HL does not affect overall prognosis

▸ Pleural effusion, particularly with positive cytology, is an adverse factor

---

SECONDARY PULMONARY LYMPHOMAS—PATHOLOGIC FEATURES

▸ Usually peribronchial and perivascular infiltrates, with or without nodules

▸ Interstitial infiltrates seen mostly with T-cell lymphoma

▸ Pleural infiltrates common in B-cell lymphomas

▸ Common subtypes are diffuse large B-cell lymphoma, followed by small lymphocytic lymphoma/chronic lymphocytic leukemia

RADIOLOGIC FEATURES

Chest X-ray is as sensitive as CT scan to detect the presence of lymphoma, but CT scans better assess the extent of disease. Radiologic evidence of parenchymal disease is present at the time of diagnosis in 9% of patients with HL and 5% with NHL. Associated mediastinal lymphadenopathy is a common finding in patients with HL, while, in contrast, NHL involvement of the lung frequently occurs in the absence of mediastinal disease. Three radiologic patterns of lung involvement are described, often overlapping in the same patients. The most common pattern is the formation of nodules, usually single and unilateral, with ill-defined borders. Occasionally, lymphomas can form endobronchial masses. The other patterns consist of bronchovascular-lymphangitic and pneumonic alveolar infiltrates.

PATHOLOGIC FEATURES

Histologically, several infiltration patterns can be seen with lymphoma, and as with radiologic patterns, there are often multiple patterns within the same patient. They are similar to other types of metastatic disease. There seems to be, in some cases, an association between the patterns of infiltrations and lymphoma subtypes. In a recent autopsy series, the most common pattern consisted of peribronchial and perivascular infiltrates, both in HL and NHL. However, nodular infiltrates were twice as frequent in HL as NHL (Figure 29-11). Other patterns

described included alveolar and interstitial patterns. Interstitial infiltrates were preferentially associated with T-cell lymphomas. Finally, pleural infiltrates were common, seen in 76% of B-cell lymphomas. Frequently reported sub-types of B-cell lymphoma metastatic to the lung include diffuse large B-cell lymphoma and small lymphocytic lymphoma/chronic lymphocytic leukemia, comprising over 75% of B-cell lymphomas involving the lung. Burkitt, follicular, and mantle cell lymphomas have also been described. Their morphology and immunophenotype are similar to their nodal counterparts. The frequency of T-cell lymphoma involving the lung is approximately half of that of B-cell lymphoma, and the most common subtype is peripheral T-cell lymphoma, not otherwise characterized. Other described subtypes are extranodal NK/T-cell lymphoma, mycosis fungoides, and anaplastic T-cell lymphoma.

PROGNOSIS AND THERAPY

In general, lymphomas involving the lung are treated with chemotherapy, with or without radiation. The prognosis of patients with advanced-stage HL is not altered by the coexistence of pulmonary involvement. If the disease is limited to the chest, recurrence is more frequent in the presence of bilateral lung disease. Overall, for HL limited to the chest, 5-year survival of 81% has been reported. The prognosis of patients with secondary NHL varies with the histologic type, with reported 5-year survival rates of 33-88%. The presence of a pleural effusion, especially with a positive cytology, worsens the prognosis.

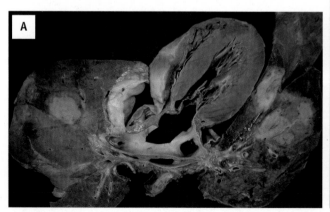

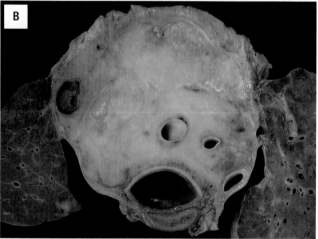

FIGURE 29-11

Hodgkin lymphoma involving the lung
(A) Gross photograph shows multiple bilateral nodules. **(B)** Extensive mediastinal involvement was also present.

SECONDARY PULMONARY LEUKEMIA

Leukemias of myeloid and lymphocytic differentiation also can involve the lung. Leukemic infiltrates are a common finding at autopsy; however, clinically significant pulmonary involvement is uncommon. Indeed, leukemic infiltrates can be seen in combination with other abnormalities, particularly pulmonary infections, and do not always represent the more important pathological finding.

Leukemic infiltrates show a prominent lymphangitic and vasocentric distribution, involving small arteries and arterioles, alveolar septal capillaries, and veins. The infiltrates are often patchy and can be very subtle in specimens (Figure 29-12). Microvascular occlusion by aggregates of leukemic cells in patients with increased numbers of leukocytes and blasts, a condition referred to as leukostasis, can lead to acute respiratory failure. Acute respiratory failure can also occur in these patients within 48 hours of initiating chemotherapy, a reaction termed leukemic cell lysis pneumonopathy. In this condition, intravascular leukemic aggregates are associated with small infarcts, perivascular hemorrhage, and edema. Localized leukemic masses (granulocytic sarcoma, chloroma) are uncommon in patients with myeloid leukemias. Chronic lymphocytic leukemia (CLL) can involve the lung in a manner indistinguishable from small lymphocytic lymphoma. In some patients, CLL will display a distinctive predilection for large and/or small airways. Bronchocentric or bronchiolocentric disease can lead to bronchial obstruction and severe respiratory symptoms in some patients.

SECONDARY PULMONARY LEUKEMIA—FACT SHEET

» Common finding at autopsy, but rarely clinically significant
» Lymphangitic and vasocentric distribution
» Acute respiratory failure can be caused by leukostasis or leukemic cell lysis pneumonopathy

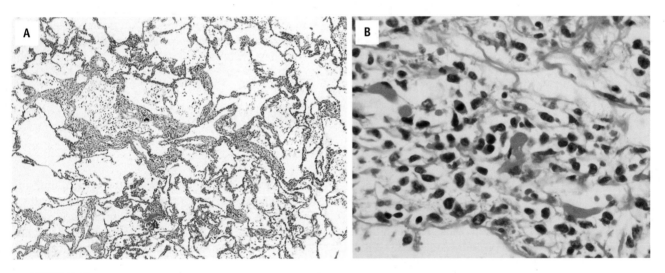

FIGURE 29-12

Acute myelomonocytic leukemia involving the lung
(A) Low-power photomicrograph showing patchy mild alveolar septal thickening. This finding is quite subtle and easily missed. **(B)** High-power photomicrograph show the septal thickening to be the result of atypical hematopoietic cells.

Suggested Readings

1. Avdalovic M, Chan A. Thoracic manifestations of common nonpulmonary malignancies of women. *Clin Chest Med.* 2004;25:379-90.
2. Berkman N, Breuer R, Kramer MR, Polliack A. Pulmonary involvement in lymphoma. *Leuk Lymphoma.* 1996;20:229-37.
3. Fraser RS, Muller NL, Colman N, Pare PD. Secondary neoplasms. In: *Fraser and Pare's Diagnosis of Diseases of the Chest.* Philadelphia: W.B. Saunders Company; 1999:1381-418.
4. Greelish JP, Friedberg JS. Secondary pulmonary malignancy. *Surg Clin North Am.* 2000;80:633-57.
5. Myers JL, Kurtin P. Lymphoproliferative disorders of the lung. In: Thurlbeck W, Churg A, eds. *Pathology of the Lung.* New York: Thieme Medical Publishers, Inc.; 1995:553-88.
6. Seo JB, Im JG, Goo JM, Chung MJ, Kim MY. Atypical pulmonary metastases: spectrum of radiologic findings. *Radiographics.* 2001;21:403-17.
7. Suster S, Moran CA. Unusual manifestations of metastatic tumors to the lungs. *Semin Diagn Pathol.* 1995;12:193-206.

30 Pulmonary Processes of Indeterminate Malignant Potential

Anna E. Sienko

- Introduction
- Intrathoracic Desmoid Tumor
- Pulmonary and Pleural Thymomas
- Pulmonary Inflammatory Myofibroblastic Tumor
- Primary Pulmonary Meningioma

INTRODUCTION

The lung serves as a primary site for several processes of "indeterminate malignant potential," disorders whose behavior cannot currently be predicted from their histologic characteristics. Since all of these entities are uncommon or rare, they can be difficult to recognize and may be confused with other more common processes. This chapter will present their distinctive features and provide information to assist in their diagnosis.

INTRATHORACIC DESMOID TUMORS

Desmoid tumors, also referred to as aggressive fibromatosis, are locally invasive proliferations of fibroblasts and myofibroblasts that are usually thought to arise from the fascia and connective tissue (aponeurosis) of skeletal muscle. Although common in the abdomen, intrathoracic desmoid tumors arising from the lung or pleura are very rare. Desmoid tumors are clonal proliferations and often have mutations in the *APC* gene or β-*catenin* gene.

CLINICAL FEATURES

The age distribution of patients with intrathoracic desmoid tumors is broad and ranges from 2.5 to 66 years of age. No gender predilection is recognized. Most patients

present with a mass and symptoms of dyspnea and chest pain if there is nerve involvement. Asymptomatic cases have been reported, however, with the tumor discovered as an incidental finding on a chest X-ray performed for another reason. Some patients have a prior history of either thoracic surgery or chest trauma. In females, chest wall desmoids have been reported after mastectomy and silicone breast implants.

RADIOLOGIC FEATURES

Chest radiographs usually demonstrate a mass without necrosis or calcifications. Chest wall origin is more common than primary pleural or pulmonary origin, and pleural involvement may occur in a tumor originating in the chest wall.

PATHOLOGIC FEATURES

GROSS FINDINGS

Tumor size can range from 3.0 cm to 21.0 cm, and weight can be up to 21.0 kg. Desmoid tumors form masses that can be contiguous with visceral or parietal pleura or chest wall, or can lie in the lung parenchyma. They are well demarcated, but have infiltrative edges. The cut surface is firm, dense, and white, often with a "glistening" appearance.

MICROSCOPIC FINDINGS

Histologically, there are variations in cellularity from region to region, with some areas having a hypocellular, highly collagenized appearance (Figure 30-1), while others are more cellular (Figure 30-2), and a myxoid appearance may be present (Figure 30-3). The cells have features of fibroblasts and myofibroblasts, and are often arranged in long fascicles with slit-like blood vessels. No significant inflammatory component is seen, with only focal collections of lymphocytes in a perivascular distribution. Mitoses are rare, and cytological atypia is absent or minimal.

636

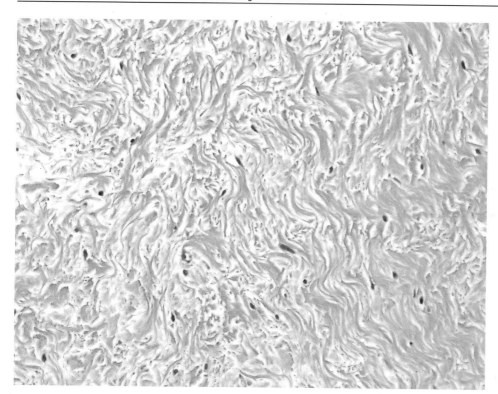

FIGURE 30-1

Desmoid tumor
This field is hypocellular and highly collagenous. (Courtesy of Dr. Dani Zander, Penn State Hershey Medical Center, Hershey, Pennsylvania.)

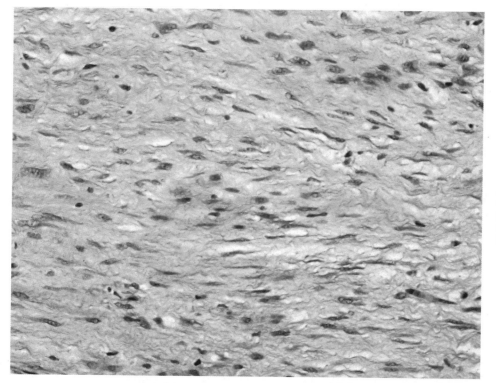

FIGURE 30-2

Desmoid tumor
Other regions show a more dense proliferation of bland spindle cells with features of fibroblasts and myofibroblasts. (Courtesy of Dr. Dani Zander, Penn State Hershey Medical Center, Hershey, Pennsylvania.)

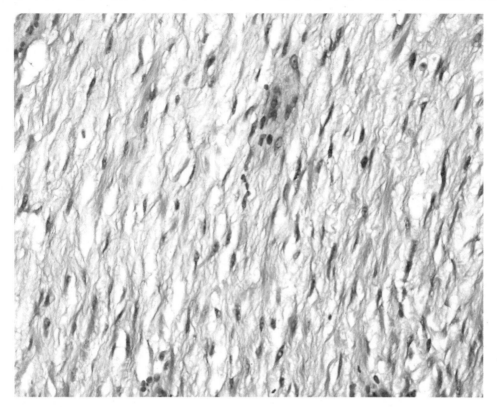

FIGURE 30-3
Desmoid tumor
A myxoid appearance is shown. (Courtesy of Dr. Dani Zander, Penn State Hershey Medical Center, Hershey, Pennsylvania.)

ANCILLARY STUDIES

Immunohistochemical staining typically demonstrates immunoreactivity with vimentin and muscle markers (particularly smooth muscle actin and muscle-specific actin, and less often desmin), but generally does not reveal expression of S-100, CD34, BCL-2, or epithelial membrane antigen (EMA). Some desmoid tumors have been shown to express estrogen and progesterone receptors. Desmoid tumors also characteristically demonstrate overexpression of β-catenin with nuclear and cytoplasmic staining.

DIFFERENTIAL DIAGNOSIS

The differential diagnosis includes solitary fibrous tumor (SFT), neurofibroma, and sarcomatoid malignancies including sarcomas (particularly fibrosarcoma and malignant fibrous histiocytoma), sarcomatoid carcinomas, sarcomatoid melanoma, and sarcomatoid malignant mesothelioma. Attention to histological features

and use of immunohistochemical stains will usually allow for differentiation of desmoid tumors from these other entities. Like desmoid tumors, SFTs typically show regional variation in cellularity and collagenization, and the more cellular areas in SFTs may show fascicular, storiform, hemangiopericytic, or "patternless" growth patterns. Desmoid tumors characteristically stain for vimentin and smooth muscle actin, but show no staining with CD34 or BCL-2 in contrast to SFTs, which usually express these substances. Increased mitoses, necrosis, and cytological atypia in a spindle cell lesion favor a diagnosis of sarcoma, sarcomatoid carcinoma, sarcomatoid melanoma, or sarcomatoid mesothelioma over desmoid tumor, which is cytologically bland with scant or absent mitoses. Mesotheliomas may be the most difficult to separate, since the degree of atypia can be minimal in desmoplastic variants. However, most mesotheliomas stain for pancytokeratin, while desmoid tumors do not. Mesotheliomas also frequently stain for cytokeratin 5/6, calretinin, and EMA, while desmoid tumors do not show immunoreactivity for these markers. Neurofibromas are S-100-positive and show wavy nuclear contours, while desmoid tumors are immunonegative for S-100 and usually lack the wavy nuclear characteristics.

PROGNOSIS AND THERAPY

Intrathoracic desmoid tumors generally behave in a similar fashion to desmoid tumors in other anatomic sites. Although they have no propensity to metastasize, there is a relatively high rate of recurrence. In reported series, the overall 5-year survival rate was 93%, but the recurrence rate for intrathoracic desmoid tumors was 60%. The treatment of choice is complete surgical resection with wide margins. Radiation therapy has been recommended when a wide local excision cannot be performed. Some desmoid tumors have been shown to express estrogen and progesterone receptors, and anti-estrogen therapy has been administered, with reported tumor regression. Cases of tumor regression have also been reported with use of non-steroidal anti-inflammatory drugs (NSAIDs), presumably due to blockage of prostaglandin synthesis. Chemotherapy has been used in patients with inoperable desmoid tumors with reports of tumor stability and partial regression.

PULMONARY AND PLEURAL THYMOMAS

Although thymomas are usually located in the anterior mediastinum, they can occasionally develop in other sites such as the lower neck, thyroid, pericardium, lung, and pleura. The derivation of these unusual tumors is unknown, but origin from an embryologic hyperdescent of thymic tissue has been proposed, and derivation from uncommitted germinative cells has been suggested.

CLINICAL FEATURES

Primary intrapulmonary and pleural thymomas are rare. These neoplasms occur in adults with a reported age range of 20-80 years, mean age of 55 years, and slight female predominance. Although most patients have no history of a thymoma-related paraneoplastic

---

INTRATHORACIC DESMOID TUMORS—FACT SHEET

Definition

▸ Locally invasive proliferations of fibroblasts and myofibroblasts that can arise from the lung or pleura, or extend into these structures from the chest wall

Incidence

▸ Intrathoracic desmoids are rare, and intrapulmonary tumors are extremely rare

Gender and Age Distribution

▸ Age range of 2.5 to 66 yrs., no apparent gender predilection

Morbidity and Mortality

▸ Behavior is similar to abdominal and intra-abdominal desmoids
▸ 60% recurrence rate
▸ 93% 5-year survival rate

Clinical Features

▸ Palpable mass or incidental finding on routine chest radiograph
▸ Dyspnea may be present
▸ Some patients have a history of prior chest trauma or thoracic surgery

Radiologic Features

▸ Pleural-based or lung parenchymal mass, or mass extending intrathoracically from the chest wall
▸ Involvement of ribs may be seen

Prognosis and Therapy

▸ Do not metastasize
▸ Complete surgical resection is the treatment of choice
▸ Reported cases of tumor regression with use of anti-estrogen treatment or nonsteroidal anti-inflammatory agents
▸ Tumor stability and partial regression reported with chemotherapy in inoperable cases

---

INTRATHORACIC DESMOID TUMORS—PATHOLOGIC FEATURES

Gross Findings

▸ Mass of variable size, reported range 3-21 cm, with firm, white cut surface

Microscopic Findings

▸ Hypocellular to moderately cellular infiltrate of fibroblasts and myofibroblasts
▸ Long fascicular arrangement in bland collagenous or myxoid background
▸ Mild or absent inflammation
▸ Few or absent mitoses and minimal or absent cytological atypia

Immunohistochemical Features

▸ Immunoreactivity for vimentin, smooth muscle actin, muscle-specific actin, and, less often, desmin
▸ No staining with S-100, CD34, Bcl-2, or EMA
▸ Some stain for estrogen and progesterone receptors

Pathologic Differential Diagnosis

▸ Solitary fibrous tumor
▸ Neurofibroma
▸ Sarcomatoid malignancies:
  ▸ Sarcomas
  ▸ Sarcomatoid carcinoma
  ▸ Sarcomatoid melanoma
  ▸ Sarcomatoid malignant mesothelioma

syndrome, occasional tumors are associated with myasthenia gravis, pure red cell aplasia, or acquired hypogammaglobulinemia. Patients may note symptoms of fever, weakness, cough, hemoptysis, chest pain, or dyspnea, but most are asymptomatic.

RADIOLOGIC FEATURES

Diagnostic imaging usually reveals a mass in the lung parenchyma or on the pleural surface, and occasionally as a process that appears to encase the lung. Intrapulmonary tumors can be centrally located, subpleural, or rarely endobronchial, and very rare reports of multiple concurrent intrapulmonary thymomas exist. Pleural thymomas develop as solitary lesions on the pleural surface, or may grow circumferentially around the lung, mimicking mesothelioma or metastatic tumor.

PATHOLOGIC FEATURES

Intrapulmonary and pleural thymomas display a spectrum of gross and histological features similar to those of mediastinal thymomas.

GROSS FINDINGS

The tumor may appear well circumscribed or infiltrative, and size ranges from 0.5 cm to 10.0 cm. Fibrous encapsulation may or may not be recognized. The cut surface is generally tan-red, and internal septations may divide the mass into angulated compartments.

MICROSCOPIC FINDINGS

The histological picture can range from a lymphocyte-predominant lesion to epithelioid-predominant to the usual "classic" biphasic admixture of small, round lymphocytes and epithelial cells (Figure 30-4). The lymphocytes and epithelial cells are usually arranged in a lobular pattern, separated by fibrous bands and septa. Foci of necrosis, hemorrhage (stromal blood lakes), cyst formation, and prominent perivascular spaces with serum accumulation can also be seen, as well as dystrophic calcification. The epithelial cells vary cytologically from cells with indistinct cellular borders, oval regular nuclei, and inconspicuous nucleoli to cells demonstrating irregular hyperchromatic nuclei with promi-nent nucleoli. Pseudoglandular arrays or pseudorosette formation by the epithelial cells has been described. Some thymomas demonstrate a predominantly spindle cell morphology with bland regular nuclei, and can have an associated

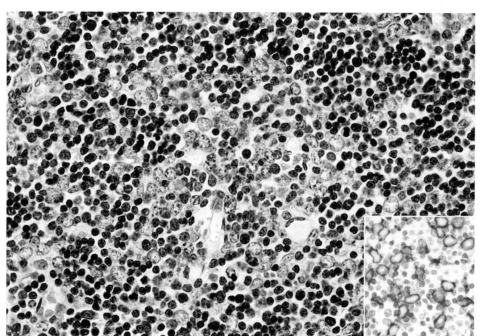

FIGURE 30-4
Pulmonary thymoma
This view shows a population of epithelial cells with pale-staining nuclei, and a large number of small lymphocytes. The epithelial cells are highlighted by a pancytokeratin stain (inset). (Courtesy of Dr. Dani S. Zander, Penn State Hershey Medical Center, Hershey, Pennsylvania.)

prominent network of blood vessels with a "staghorn" pattern similar to hemangiopericytomas. Mitotic activity is variable. Hassall's corpuscles are rarely seen.

Intra-pulmonary and pleural thymomas have been classified based on morphology and component of lymphocytes using classification systems for mediastinal thymomas. The descriptive scheme of Bernatz *et al.* classified thymomas as predominantly spindle cell, predominantly lymphocytic, predominantly epithelial, and predominantly mixed. The WHO classification system is based on cell shape and nuclear features (Type A: oval/spindle shape; Type B: dendritic/plump "epithelioid" shape). Type B is subdivided based on the proportion of lymphocytes and the degree of atypia of the epithelioid cells into types B1, B2, and B3.

ANCILLARY STUDIES

The epithelial component stains with pancytokeratin (Figure 30-4) and p63, and often with CK 5/6 and HBME-1, the latter potentially representing a source of confusion with malignant mesothelioma. Unlike mesothelioma, however, WT-1 and thrombomodulin are typically negative. The lymphoid cells ("true thymocytes") express CD3, CD1a, TdT, and CD99.

DIFFERENTIAL DIAGNOSIS

The differential diagnosis includes other primary pulmonary or pleural tumors and metastatic neoplasms, particularly metastatic thymoma from a mediastinal primary. The possibility of a mediastinal primary should be excluded prior to making a diagnosis of primary intrapulmonary or pleural thymoma. For differentiating thymomas from the other histologic types of neoplasms in the differential diagnosis, the presence of a prominent lymphoid component in the tumor, and usual lack of nuclear atypia in the epithelioid cell component are helpful clues to distinguish thymomas from other histological tumor types. Diffuse malignant mesothelioma represents a differential diagnostic consideration, particularly in a case that grows circumferentially around the lung. Immunoreactivities of mesothelioma overlap with those of thymomas (frequent reactivity with CK5/6 and HBME-1), but the lack of staining with WT-1 and thrombomodulin may help differentiate these neoplasms in difficult cases. A variety of metastatic carcinomas can resemble thymomas, but usually show more cytologic atypia and a scant or mild lymphoid cell infiltrate. Depending upon the morphologic features of the process, a panel of immunohistochemical stains can be constructed to help evaluate for a metastatic carcinoma. Spindle cell and epithelioid sarcomas may also enter into the differ-

ential diagnosis, but usually demonstrate more cytologic atypia and mitoses. SFT shows more architectural variegation, may demonstrate a "patternless" or storiform pattern, does not usually contain a significant lymphoid cell infiltrate, and often stains with CD34 and BCL-2, while thymomas are typically immunonegative for CD34, and only approximately one third of cases express BCL-2.

PROGNOSIS AND THERAPY

Intrapulmonary and pleural thymomas are slowly growing tumors that are optimally treated with complete surgical resection. Tumors that are found to be encapsulated, well circumscribed, and completely resectable have a very good prognosis. Thymomas showing an infiltrative pattern or pleural encasement are associated with a more aggressive course. Radiation therapy has been recommended for inoperable tumors.

PULMONARY INFLAMMATORY MYOFIBROBLASTIC TUMOR

Inflammatory myofibroblastic tumor (IMT) is an important cause of lung masses in children and young adults, but also occurs in adults. It has been referred to under the heading of "inflammatory pseudotumor," although this terminology has been applied to a histologic spectrum of entities. "Plasma cell granuloma" has also been used for this lesion, and lesions that have been classified as inflammatory fibrosarcoma and fibrous histiocytoma also show overlapping histologic features. The origin of IMT is uncertain, and its identity as a neoplasm or non-neoplastic reaction to lung injury has been debated. The aggressive behavior of some IMTs, however, has indicated a neoplastic proliferation in at least some cases. A subset of cases is preceded by a pulmonary infection, and recently, human herpesvirus-8 gene sequences were found in several cases of IMT.

CLINICAL FEATURES

IMT is a rare entity reported to represent 0.04-1% of all lung tumors. It is a common pulmonary neoplasm in childhood and young adulthood, but also develops in adults, with ages ranging to 84. No gender predilection is seen. IMTs are frequently detected as incidental findings on routine chest radiograph in asymptomatic patients or in patients with nonspecific symptoms such as cough, chest pain, dyspnea, and hemoptysis. Some patients also manifest features of a paraneoplastic syndrome, with fever, anemia, weight loss, elevated erythrocyte sedimentation rate, hyperglobulinemia, and leukothrombocytosis, and these abnormalities may abate when the mass is removed.

RADIOLOGIC FEATURES

Most often, IMT presents as a solitary lung nodule or mass, but cases of multifocal and bilateral pulmonary involvement have been reported. IMTs usually appear well demarcated and demonstrate internal heterogeneity and occasionally calcifications. Although they generally measure less than 5.0 cm in size, rare cases can exceed 10.0 cm in size. Tumors can occur in central and peripheral locations, and can invade the pleura and mediastinum.

PATHOLOGIC FEATURES

GROSS FINDINGS

IMTs form masses without true capsules and demonstrate gray-white rubbery cut surfaces. Size is usually less than 5.0 cm. The edges of the lesions are relatively well demarcated. Gross hemorrhage and necrosis are not characteristic, but calcifications can be present. Polypoid endotracheal or endobronchial presentations have been described, as have central and peripheral lung masses.

MICROSCOPIC FINDINGS

Microscopically, the tumor typically shows a prominent component of non-neoplastic inflammatory cells, particularly including plasma cells and lymphocytes, and in some cases foamy macrophages, superimposed upon a proliferation of spindle cells (Figures 30-5, 30-6). The spindle cells are usually cytologically bland and arranged in fascicles or in a storiform pattern, and have features of fibroblasts and myofibroblasts. A minority of cases, however, display increased cytologic atypia, ganglion-like cells, or necrosis. Mitotic activity can vary from low to brisk. Areas of dense fibrosis and sclerosis can also be observed. At its edge, "tongues" of the tumor often extend into adjacent lung parenchyma. A breakdown of IMTs into types, based on histological features, has been suggested: (a) an organizing pneumonia pattern with foamy macrophages, fibroblasts, and inflammatory cells; (b) a fibrous histicytoma pattern, the most common pattern, composed of bland myofibroblasts and variable numbers of inflammatory cells; and (c) the less common lymphohistiocytic pattern.

ANCILLARY STUDIES

The spindle cells characteristically stain for vimentin, smooth muscle actin, muscle-specific actin, calponin, and caldesmon. Desmin and anaplastic lymphoma kinase (ALK) staining is observed in about half of the cases, and p80 expression is also frequent. Lesions are usually immunonegative for CD34, S-100, and epithelial membrane antigen (EMA), but some degree of cytokeratin staining is observed in approximately one third of cases. Translocations involving the ALK locus at 2p23 are found in many cases. Flow cytometry reveals aneuploidy in some cases, but most cases appear to be diploid.

DIFFERENTIAL DIAGNOSIS

The differential diagnosis includes true organizing pneumonia, inflammatory sarcomatoid carcinoma, inflammatory malignant fibrous histiocytoma (IMFH),

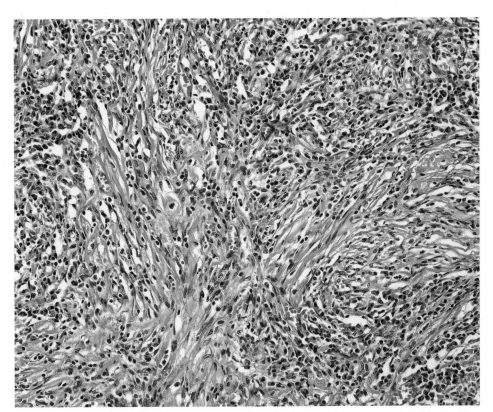

FIGURE 30-5

Inflammatory myofibroblastic tumor
This case shows numerous inflammatory cells, particularly plasma cells, admixed with bland spindle cells. (Courtesy of Dr. Dani S. Zander, Penn State Hershey Medical Center, Hershey, Pennsylvania.)

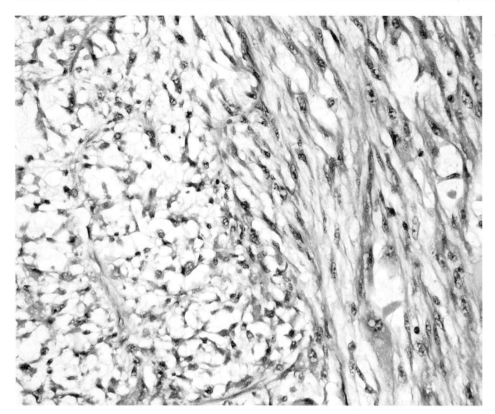

FIGURE 30-6
Inflammatory myofibroblastic tumor
This example displays numerous foamy macrophages (left) adjacent to the myofibroblasts (right). (Courtesy of Dr. Alberto Ayala, The Methodist Hospital, Houston, Texas.)

other spindle cell sarcomas, desmoid tumor, and solitary fibrous tumor (SFT). True organizing pneumonia shows alveolar filling by fibroblastic "plugs" and does not grow in an infiltrative manner. Inflammatory sarcomatoid carcinoma shows staining with cytokeratins and EMA, but not typically with muscle markers and ALK, as does IMT. IMFH characteristically shows a greater degree of pleomorphism, and although some examples will stain for muscle markers, the frequency is lower than for IMTs. IMTs are also more likely to express ALK-1 and p80 than IMFHs. Desmoid tumors are composed of cells with myofibroblastic characteristics and variable amounts of collagen, but typically show less inflammation than IMTs and do not typically stain for ALK, although muscle markers are expressed by both processes. SFTs show less inflammation, and the spindle cell population usually stains for CD34 and not muscle markers.

PROGNOSIS AND THERAPY

Complete surgical resection is the treatment of choice, with the extent of the surgery depending on the size and location of the tumor. The roles of corticosteroids, cyclooxygenase 2 inhibitors, chemotherapy, and radiotherapy are not well defined. If complete excision is possible, the outcome is usually excellent, and no further intervention is advocated. For incompletely

resected cases, recurrence is not uncommon. Metastasis is rare, and malignant transformation has been reported to occur in a small number of cases. Rare examples of spontaneous regression have also been reported. Fatal IMTs usually show extensive involvement of adjacent structures including the pleura, mediastinum, large airways, or diaphragm, with or without distant metastasis.

PRIMARY PULMONARY MENINGIOMA

Meningiomas are the most common benign neoplasms of the neural axis and are thought to arise from meningocytes that surround or "cap" arachnoid villi. Meningiomas have been reported in extracranial locations in the head and neck area, mediastinum, lungs, retroperitoneum, and, rarely, in mature adult teratomas. Primary pulmonary meningiomas are very rare, and the diagnosis can be made only after complete exclusion of metastatic primary intracranial or spinal meningioma. The origin of primary pulmonary meningiomas is unknown, but theories include origination from intrathoracic heterotopic proliferations of meningocytes or arachnoid cells that form the meningothelial-like nodules occasionally found in the lung parenchyma. Meningothelial-like nodules and concurrent primary pulmonary meningioma have been reported.

PULMONARY INFLAMMATORY MYOFIBROBLASTIC TUMOR—FACT SHEET

Definition

▸▸ Infiltrative proliferation of myofibroblasts and fibroblasts, usually accompanied by plasma cells, lymphocytes, and other inflammatory cells, with a wide spectrum of clinical behavior

Incidence

▸▸ 0.04-1% of all lung tumors

Morbidity and Mortality

▸▸ Morbidity and mortality is associated with invasion of adjacent structures (mediastinum, pleura, diaphragm) or metastasis

Gender, Race, and Age Distribution

▸▸ Relatively frequent neoplasm of childhood and young adulthood
▸▸ Also develop in adults, with ages ranging to 84 years
▸▸ No gender or racial predilection

Clinical Features

▸▸ Often an incidental finding in an asymptomatic patient
▸▸ Can be associated with cough, dyspnea, hemoptysis, or chest pain
▸▸ Subset of cases preceded by symptoms of pulmonary infection
▸▸ Can be associated with a paraneoplastic syndrome including fever, weight loss, elevated erythrocyte sedimentation rate, hyperglobulin-emia, and leukothrombocytosis

Radiologic Features

▸▸ Usually a solitary well-demarcated central or peripheral lung nodule or mass, generally measuring less than 5.0 cm in diameter, with internal heterogeneity and occasional calcifications
▸▸ Occasionally multifocal and bilateral
▸▸ Can invade the pleura or mediastinum

Prognosis and Therapy

▸▸ Complete surgical resection is the treatment of choice, and if achieved, is associated with an excellent prognosis
▸▸ Incomplete resection is associated with a higher risk of recurrence
▸▸ Roles of corticosteroids, cyclooxygenase 2 inhibitors, chemotherapy, and radiotherapy are not well defined
▸▸ Metastasis is rare, and malignant transformation has been reported to occur in a small number of cases
▸▸ Rare reports of spontaneous regression
▸▸ Fatal cases usually show extensive involvement of adjacent structures (pleura, mediastinum, diaphragm), with or without metastasis

PULMONARY INFLAMMATORY MYOFIBROBLASTIC TUMOR—PATHOLOGIC FEATURES

Gross Findings

▸▸ Mass with a gray-white cut surface, usually less than 5 cm, without hemorrhage or necrosis

Microscopic Findings

▸▸ Varied histology, including a background population of bland spindle cells arranged in fascicles or in a storiform pattern, accompanied by variable numbers and types of inflammatory cells, often particularly rich in plasma cells and lymphocytes
▸▸ Infiltrative edges
▸▸ Variable mitotic activity
▸▸ Increased cytoatypia, ganglion-like cells, or necrosis in a subset of cases
▸▸ Areas of dense fibrosis can be present

Immunohistochemical Features

▸▸ Spindle cells are immunopositive for vimentin, smooth muscle actin, muscle-specific actin, calponin, and caldesmon; desmin staining is present in about half of cases
▸▸ Anaplastic lymphoma kinase (ALK) and p80 expression are common
▸▸ Cytokeratin staining is observed in approximately one third of cases
▸▸ Usually immunonegative for CD34, S-100, and EMA

Cytogenetics

▸▸ Frequently manifest translocations involving the ALK locus at 2p23

Flow Cytometry

▸▸ Some cases are aneuploid, but most are diploid

Pathologic Differential Diagnosis

▸▸ Organizing pneumonia
▸▸ Inflammatory sarcomatoid carcinoma
▸▸ Inflammatory malignant fibrous histiocytoma
▸▸ Other spindle cell sarcomas
▸▸ Desmoid tumor
▸▸ Solitary fibrous tumor

CLINICAL FEATURES

Most cases of pulmonary meningioma are asymptomatic solitary nodules that are discovered incidentally on routine chest radiograph. Rarely, patients complain of cough. Pulmonary meningiomas are found in both men and women with a wide age distribution ranging from 24 to 74 years of age (average of 55 years), with a slightly higher occurrence noted in older women.

RADIOLOGIC FEATURES

The lesions are well-circumscribed solitary nodules or "coin lesions," usually measuring between 4 mm and 12 cm. Both lungs can harbor these tumors, although one series noted a higher prevalence in the left lung. On positron emission tomography scan, intrapulmonary meningioma can cause a false-positive interpretation of malignancy due to increased F-18-fluorodeoxyglucose uptake.

PATHOLOGIC FEATURES

GROSS FINDINGS

Intrapulmonary meningiomas are most often received in a wedge resection of lung or on occasion as a mass "shelled" out from surrounding lung parenchyma. Usually, there is no bronchial or pleural attachment or involvement. Grossly, most lesions are well demarcated, loosely attached to surrounding lung parenchyma, round, and firm with a brown/gray to white/yellow/gray cut surface without hemorrhage or necrosis. Malignant examples have an infiltrative appearance and can involve pleura and other adjacent structures.

MICROSCOPIC FINDINGS

Most pulmonary meningiomas have histologic appearances resembling syncytial or transitional intracranial meningiomas, with smaller numbers of fibrous-type tumors. A case of chordoid pulmonary meningioma has also been reported. Most tumors are well demarcated from adjacent lung parenchyma. The cells of meningioma are round, oval, or spindle shaped, and arranged in syncytial sheets, fascicles, or whorls. Some pulmonary meningiomas have tumor cells concentrically arranged around blood vessels. Variable amounts of collagen and blood vessels with hyaline degenerative changes may be present. Tumor cells demonstrate bland monomorphic nuclei, moderate amounts of eosinophilic cytoplasm, and indistinct cell borders. Mitoses are rare and cytologic atypia is usually lacking. Psammoma bodies can also be seen. Increased mitotic activity, nuclear pleomorphism, necrosis, and prominent nucleoli are features that should raise concern about the possibility of aggressive clinical behavior.

ANCILLARY STUDIES

Like intracranial meningioma, pulmonary meningioma typically displays diffuse immunohistochemical staining for vimentin and epithelial membrane antigen (EMA). Some cases show variable staining for S-100, CD34, and actin. Cytokeratin staining in primary pulmonary meningiomas is negative, whereas intracranial meningiomas usually stain positive. Ultrastructural findings include interdigitating cell membranes and desmosomes, with no evidence of basal lamina, neurosecretory granules, or microvilli. In intracranial meningiomas, genetic alterations in chromosome 22 appear to develop early in the process, and other genetic changes include deletions of 1p and 14q, but the frequencies of these abnormalities in pulmonary meningioma is unknown.

DIFFERENTIAL DIAGNOSIS

Before classifying a meningioma in the lung as a primary pulmonary neoplasm, metastasis from a primary lesion in the central nervous system must be excluded. Pulmonary meningiomas must be differentiated from primary or metastatic carcinomas of the lung, solitary fibrous tumor (SFT), inflammatory myofibroblastic tumor (IMT), hemangiopericytoma, spindle cell myoepithelioma, schwannoma, and melanoma. Histologic features that are particularly helpful for the recognition of meningioma include the characteristic "whorls" and psammoma bodies, in combination with bland cytological features and very low mitotic activity. Most carcinomas will display malignant cytologic characteristics, and immunohistochemical staining for more site-specific substances (TTF-1, PSA, uroplakin, and others, as discussed in Chapter 38) would support the diagnosis of carcinoma. SFT and IMT may be considered in the differential diagnosis of fibrous meningioma, but have differing histologic features, as discussed earlier in this chapter and in Chapter 33. SFT is usually immunopositive for CD34 and Bcl-2, while fibrous meningioma expresses these antigens less frequently. IMTs typically stain with smooth muscle actin and muscle-specific actin. EMA is characteristically negative in SFT and IMT. Similarly, hemangiopericytomas also do not stain with EMA, but do stain with smooth muscle actin, whereas pulmonary meningiomas show the opposite pattern of immunoreactivity. Spindle cell myoepithelioma demonstrates epithelial and muscle differentiation, with expression of keratins and muscle markers. Schwannomas stain with S-100 and CD56, but not EMA. S-100, HMB-45 and Mart-1 stains are often positive in melanomas and typically negative in meningioma, and cytoatypia, increased mitotic rate, and necrosis are commonly seen in melanoma.

PROGNOSIS AND THERAPY

For primary pulmonary meningiomas, the treatment of choice is complete surgical resection. Almost all primary pulmonary meningiomas are benign lesions that are cured by complete resection. Follow-up of these cases up to 7 years after surgical treatment revealed no recurrences or additional morbidity. Two primary malignant pulmonary meningiomas have been reported in patients without nervous system lesions. One case was associated with recurrence 5 months after surgical resection, and lymph node and diaphragmatic metastasis. In the other case, the patient had a liver mass that was suspected to represent a metastasis, but had not undergone biopsy.

PRIMARY PULMONARY MENINGIOMA—FACT SHEET

Definition

» Primary tumor of lung with features similar to meningiomas of the neural axis

Incidence

» Very rare

Gender, Race, and Age Distribution

» Age distribution from 24 to 74 years, mean of 55 yrs.
» Occur in both genders, but with a slightly higher frequency in older women
» No apparent racial predilection

Clinical Features

» Usually an incidental finding on a routine chest radiograph in an asymptomatic patient
» Rarely associated with a cough

Radiologic Features

» Well circumscribed solitary nodule or "coin lesion," usually measuring between 4 mm and 12 cm

Prognosis and Therapy

» Complete surgical resection is the treatment of choice, and is curative for patients with benign lesions
» Two primary malignant pulmonary meningiomas associated with recurrence and metastasis

---

PULMONARY MENINGIOMA—PATHOLOGIC FEATURES

Gross Findings

» Well-demarcated lung nodules or masses, ranging in size from 4 mm to 12 cm, usually loosely attached to the surrounding lung parenchyma
» Firm, with a brown/gray to white/yellow/gray cut surface, without hemorrhage or necrosis
» Malignant examples have an infiltrative appearance and can involve pleura and other adjacent structures

Microscopic Findings

» Spectrum of histologic appearances similar to intracranial meningiomas
» Syncytial and transitional types are most common
» Round, oval, or spindle cells arranged in sheets, fascicles, or whorls
» Cells usually have bland nuclei, moderate amounts of eosinophilic cytoplasm, and indistinct cell borders
» Mitoses are rare, and cytologic atypia is usually lacking
» Psammoma bodies may be present
» Increased mitotic activity, nuclear pleomorphism, necrosis, and prominent nucleoli are features that should raise concern about the possibility of aggressive clinical behavior

Immunohistochemical Features

» Immunopositive for vimentin and EMA
» Variable staining with S-100, CD34, and actin
» Cytokeratin staining is usually lacking

Pathologic Differential Diagnosis

» Metastatic meningioma from a central nervous system primary
» Non-small cell lung carcinoma
» Pulmonary metastases from extrapulmonary carcinomas
» Solitary fibrous tumor
» Inflammatory myofibroblastic tumor
» Hemangiopericytoma
» Spindle cell myoepithelioma
» Schwannoma
» Metastatic melanoma

SUGGESTED READINGS

Intrathoracic Desmoid Tumor

1. Abbas AE, Deschamps C, Cassivi SD, et al. Chest wall desmoid tumors: results of surgical intervention. *Ann Thorac Surg*. 2004;78:1219-23.
2. Andino L, Cagle PT, Murer B, et al. Pleuropulmonary desmoid tumors: immunohistochemical comparison with solitary fibrous tumors and assessment of β-catenin and cyclin D1 expression. *Arch Pathol Lab Med*. 2006;130:1503-9.
3. Enzinger FM, Weiss SW. Fibromatoses. In: *Soft Tissue Tumors*. 3rd ed. New York: Mosby; 1995:210-23.
4. Iqbal M, Rossoff LJ, Kahn L, Lackner RP. Intrathoracic desmoid tumor mimicking primary lung neoplasm. *Ann Thorac Surg*. 2001;71:1698-1700.
5. Peled N, Babyn PS, Manson D, Nanassy J. Aggressive fibromatosis simulating congenital lung malformation. *Can Assoc Radiol J*. 1993;44:221-2.
6. Privette A, Fenton SJ, Mone MC, Kennedy AM, Nelson EW. Desmoid tumor: a case of mistaken identity. *Breast J*. 2005;11:60-4.
7. Shimizu J, Kawaura Y, Tatsuzawa Y, Maeda K, Oda M, Kawashima A. Desmoid tumor of the chest wall following chest surgery: report of a case. *Surg Today*. 1999;29:945-7.
8. Takeshima Y, Nakayori F, Nakano T, et al. Extra-abdominal desmoid tumor presenting as an intrathoracic tumor: case report and literature review. *Pathol Int*. 2001;51:824-8.

9. Varghese TK, Gupta R, Yeldani AV, Sundaresan SR. Desmoid tumor of the chest wall with pleural involvement. *Ann Thorac Surg*. 2003;76:937-9.
10. Wilson RW, Gallateau-Salle F, Moran CA. Desmoid tumors of the pleura: a clinicopathological mimic of localized fibrous tumor. *Mod Pathol*. 1999;12:9-14.

Pulmonary and Pleural Thymomas

11. Cagle PT, Allen TC, Barrios R, et al. *Color Atlas and Text of Pulmonary Pathology*. 1st ed, New York: Lippincott Williams & Wilkins; 2005.
12. Fushimi H, Tanio Y, Kotoh K. Ectopic thymoma mimicking diffuse pleural mesothelioma: A case report. *Hum Pathol*. 1998;29:409-10.
13. Leslie KO, Wick MR. *Practical Pulmonary Pathology, A Diagnostic Approach*. 1st ed, New York: Churchill Livingstone; 2005.
14. Moran SA, Suster S, Fishback NF, Koss MN. Primary intrapulmonary thymoma. A clinicopathologic and immunohistochemical study of eight cases. *Am J Surg Pathol*. 1995;19:304-12.
15. Pan C-C, Chen PC, Chou T-y, Chiang H. Expression of calretinin and other mesothelioma-related markers in thymic carcinoma and thymoma. *Hum Pathol*. 2003;34:1155-62.
16. Pomplun S, Wotherspoon AC, Shah G, Goldstraw P, Ladas G, Nicholson AG. Immunohistochemical markers in the differentiation of thymic and pulmonary neoplasms. *Histopathology*. 2002;40:152-8.

17. Sakuraba M, Sagara Y, Tamura A, Park Z, Hebisawa A, Komatsu H. A case of invasive thymoma with endobronchial growth. *Ann Thorac Cardiovasc Surg*. 2005:11:114-6.

18. Veynovich B, Masetti P, Kaplan PD, Jasnosz KM, Yousem SA, Landreneau RJ. Primary pulmonary thymoma. *Ann Thorac Surg*. 1997;64:1471-3.

Inflammatory Myofibroblastic Tumor

19. Amir R, Danahey D, Ferrer K, Maffee M. Inflammatory myofibroblastic tumor presenting with tracheal obstruction in a pregnant woman. *Am J Otolaryngol*. 2002;23:362-7.

20. Bousnina S, Racil H, Marniche K, et al. Inflammatory pseudo-tumor of the lung. A pathology clinical study of one case. *Rev Pneumol Clin*. 2004;60:55-7.

21. Chan PWK, Omar KZ, Ramanujam. Successful treatment of unresectable inflammatory pseudotumor of the lung with COX-2 inhibitor. *Pediatr Pulmonol*. 2003;36:167-9.

22. Chun YS, Wang L, Nascimento AG, Moir CR, Rodeberg DA. Pediatric inflammatory myofibroblastic tumor: anaplastic lymphoma kinase (ALK) expression and prognosis. *Pediatr Blood Cancer*. 2005;44:1-6.

23. Coffin CM, Dehner LP, Meis-Kindblom JM. Inflammatory myofibroblastic tumor, inflammatory fibrosarcoma, and related lesions; an historical review with differential diagnostic considerations. *Semin Diagn Pathol*. 1998;15:102-10.

24. Debelenko LV, Arthur DC, Pack SD, Helman LJ, Schrump DS, Tsokos M. Identification of CARS-ALK fusion in primary and metastatic lesions of an inflammatory myofibroblastic tumor. *Lab Invest*. 2003;83:1255-65.

25. Das Narla L, Newman B, Spottswood SS, Narla S, Kolli R. Inflammatory pseudotumor. *Radiographics*. 2003;23:719-29.

26. Hussain SF, Salahuddin N, Khan A, Memon SSJ, Fatimi SH, Ahmed R. The insidious onset of dyspnea and right lung collapse in a 35-year-old man. *Chest*. 2005;127:1844-7.

27. Priebe-Richter C, Ivanyi P, Buer J, et al. Inflammatory pseudotumor of the lung following invasive aspergillosis in a patient with chronic graft-vs.-host disease. *Eur J Haematol*. 2005;75:68-72.

28. Sakurai H, Hasegawa T, Watanabe S, Suzuki K, Asamura H, Tsuchiya R. Inflammatory myofibroblastic tumor of the lung. *Eur J Cardiothorac Surg*. 2004;25:155-9.

Primary Pulmonary Meningioma

29. Cesario A, Galetta D, Margaritora S, Granone P. Unsuspected primary pulmonary meningioma. *Eur J Cardiothorac Surg*. 2002;21:553-5.

30. Cura M, Smoak W, Dala R. Pulmonary meningioma: false-positive positron emission tomography for malignant pulmonary nodules. *Clin Nucl Med*. 2002 27:701-4.

31. Kaleem Z, Fitzpatrick MM, Ritter JH. Primary pulmonary meningioma. Report of a case and review of the literature. *Arch Pathol Lab Med*. 1997;121:631-6.

32. Lockett L, Chiang V, Scully N. Primary pulmonary meningioma: report of a case and review of the literature. *Am J Surg Pathol*. 1997;21:453-60.

33. Michal M. Meningeal nodules in teratoma of the testis. *Virchows Arch*. 2001;438:198-200.

34. Moran CA, Hochholzer L, Rush W, Koss MN. Primary intrapulmonary meningiomas: clinicopathologic and immunohistochemical study of 10 cases. *Cancer*. 1998;78:2328-33.

35. Picquet J, Valo I, Jousset Y, Enon B. Primary pulmonary meningioma first suspected of being a lung metastasis. *Ann Thorac Surg*. 2005;79: 1407-9.

36. Prayson R, Farver CF. Primary pulmonary malignant meningioma. *Am J Surg Pathol*. 1999;23:722-6.

37. Rowsell C, Sirbovan J, Rosenblum MK, Perez-Ordonez B. Primary chordoid meningioma of lung. *Virchows Arch*. 2005;446:333-7.

38. Spinelli M, Claren R, Colombi R, Sironi M. Primary pulmonary meningioma may arise from meningothelial-like nodules. *Adv Clin Path*. 2000;4: 35-9.

39. Van der Meij JJ, Boomars KA, van den Bosch JM, van Boven WJ, de Bruin PC, Seldenrijk CA. Primary pulmonary malignant meningioma. *Ann Thorac Surg*. 2005;80:1523-5.

40. Wick MR, Nappi O. Ectopic neural and neuroendocrine neoplasms. *Semin Diagn Pathol*. 2003;20:305-23.

31 Precursors of Malignancy

Keith M. Kerr

- Introduction
- Squamous Dysplasia/Carcinoma-in-situ
- Atypical Adenomatous Hyperplasia
- Diffuse Idiopathic Pulmonary Neuroendocrine Cell Hyperplasia

INTRODUCTION

There are several pulmonary diseases discussed elsewhere in this book that, among the many effects they have upon the patient, convey a recognized predisposition to lung cancer development. These diseases include many forms of diffuse pulmonary fibrosis (idiopathic pulmonary fibrosis, connective tissue disease–associated pulmonary fibrosis, asbestosis), congenital adenomatoid malformations, juvenile tracheobronchial squamous papillomatosis, and other acquired and congenital cystic lung lesions. Readers are referred to the suggested reading at the end of this chapter for further information.

The 2004 World Health Organization (WHO) classification of lung tumors describes three entities which are regarded primarily as precursors of malignancy in the lung: squamous dysplasia/carcinoma in situ (SD/CIS), atypical adenomatous hyperplasia (AAH) and diffuse idiopathic pulmonary neuroendocrine cell hyperplasia (DIPNECH). It is believed that SD/CIS and AAH precede a large proportion of lung cancers and certainly define two separate pathways of lung tumor development: SD/CIS, the essential part of central bronchial carcinogenesis, leading to squamous cell and perhaps some other carcinomas, and AAH, the basis of peripheral lung adenocarcinogenesis. DIPNECH is, by a considerable margin, the least common and least important of the three lesions and is included in the WHO classification due to its association with peripheral carcinoid tumors.

SQUAMOUS DYSPLASIA/ CARCINOMA-IN-SITU

Bronchial SD/CIS incorporates a range of recognized entities, all of which show cytologic atypia within a squamous-type epithelium lining conducting airways in the lung. Mild, moderate, and severe dysplasia and carcinoma-in-situ represent a biologic continuum and should be considered together with changes in respiratory epithelium that may precede their formation, namely, basal cell hyperplasia (BCH) (Figure 31-1) and squamous metaplasia (SM) (Figure 31-2). Goblet cell hyperplasia (GCH) is included for completeness though its role as a precursor of malignancy is controversial. This spectrum of change is the likely precursor of most "bronchogenic" carcinomas, primarily central squamous cell carcinomas but possibly others, including small cell lung cancers.

CLINICAL FEATURES

While basal hyperplasia, goblet cell hyperplasia, and squamous metaplasia are essentially reactive, adaptive changes seen in a variety of chronic irritative situations (tobacco smoking, asthma, chronic infection, irradiation, vitamin A deficiency, air pollution), the presence of dysplasia and CIS is strongly associated with heavy tobacco use or, in many fewer people, radiation exposure. With the exception of goblet cell hyperplasia, which is responsible for the disease-defining mucous expectoration of chronic bronchitis, the other changes are asymptomatic, which partly explains why early lung cancer is so difficult to detect. The strong association with carcinogen exposure mentioned above allows identification of populations at risk for developing SD/CIS, a key factor in creating strategies for lung cancer screening. Past smoking demographics probably account for SD/CIS being more commonly described in males, and both the length and intensity of the smoking history correlate with the frequency of squamous metaplasia and the extent and degree of atypia in SD/CIS. Good data are rare, but

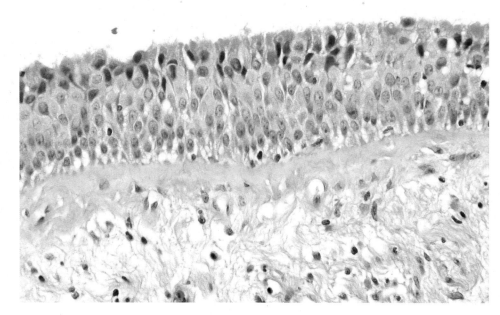

FIGURE 31-1

Basal cell hyperplasia
Regular basaloid cells lacking atypia occupy three or more rows at the base of the epithelium while differentiated columnar cells remain on the surface. This basaloid zone may undergo squamous differentiation (not shown here).

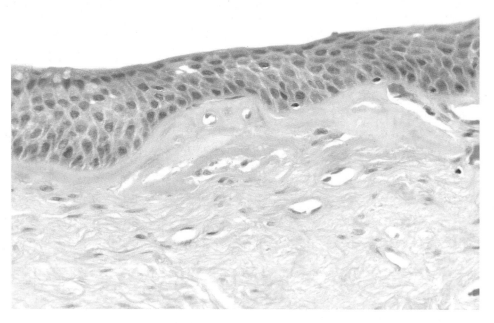

FIGURE 31-2

Squamous metaplasia
Occasional residual surface columnar cells may be seen on the left.

approximately 40% of heavy smokers will have SD/CIS, most will have BCH or SM, and SD/CIS is more frequent in lungs where invasive squamous cell carcinoma has already developed.

There is a considerable literature on the genetic changes that can be detected not only in SD/CIS but also in BCH, SM, and even in morphologically normal respiratory epithelium of chronic tobacco smokers. There is evidence that various genetic losses (loss of tumor suppressor genes), gene mutation and hypermethylation, and gene upregulation occur in a non-random and sequential manner, which correlates with and perhaps determines the morphologic changes that appear as SD/CIS evolves and invasive cancer supervenes. Among the changes that occur are hyperproliferation, changes to promote neovascularization, losses at chromosome loci 3p, 9p, 8p, 17p, 13q, and 5q (perhaps in that order), *P53* mutation, loss of p16 expression through hypermethylation of *P16,* and upregulation of cyclin D1. Many other alterations are also described. Some appear earlier than others but none is obligatory, and there may be many potential pathways at a genomic level, through which invasive disease may develop. There is some evidence to suggest that disruption of the p16 ^{INK4A}-cyclin D1-CDK4-RB pathway is important in bronchial carcinogenesis and that pathway dysfunction through hypermethylation of the P16 promoter and upregulation of cyclin D1 is characteristic of squamous carcinogenesis, whereas in SCLC development this pathway tends to be disrupted by RB loss. It has been suggested that these genetic lesions may in part determine the cell type of the tumor, which develops from the bronchial epithelial precursor.

RADIOLOGIC FEATURES

SD/CIS cannot be detected radiologically, another reason why early lung cancer detection is so problematic. Rarely, a circumferential non-obstructive lesion may compromise airway drainage through loss of mucociliary function, leading to distal pneumonia.

PATHOLOGIC FEATURES

GROSS FINDINGS

In surgically resected lung or at autopsy examination, the vast majority of SD/CIS lesions are invisible on gross examination. Carcinoma-in-situ is not infrequently found on the spurs of carinae, occasionally giving the mucosa a pale, granular, opaque character with loss of the mucosal rugae and pits. It is believed that the genetic changes, which drive this disease, occur in clonal patches, which are widespread in the bronchial mucosa, a so-called field effect. Such patches of morphologically normal mucosa contain several tens of thousands of basal epithelial cells and measure approximately 1 mm². Studies have shown that patches of CIS range from approximately 4 to 12 mm in diameter and 2 to 4 mm in thickness. Studies using autofluorescence bronchoscopy (see below) have shown dysplastic lesions of 1 to 3 mm diameter. There are also descriptions in the literature of exophytic papillary non-invasive squamous tumors with atypia sufficient to consider them papillary carcinoma-in-situ. Contemporary experience and opinion, however, has placed these lesions in the category of papillary squamous cell carcinoma in the WHO classification since most, though not all, of these lesions will show even limited invasion.

The lack of gross features means that most SD/CIS lesions are also invisible at standard so-called white-light bronchoscopy (WLB). About 30% to 40% of CIS lesions may be visible to an experienced bronchoscopist as flattened or, less often, nodular patches of mucosa lacking normal luster, perhaps granular, red, and with an abnormal vascular pattern. Abnormal bronchial mucosa loses green autofluorescence when viewed under blue light using special sensors. Autofluorescence bronchoscopy (AFB) dramatically increases the detection rate, by a factor of approximately 6, for all grades of SD/CIS lesions, but is rather nonspecific since many lesions detected at AFB show hyperplastic changes, inflammation, or no significant pathology at biopsy.

MICROSCOPIC FINDINGS

The major revision of the WHO lung tumor classification published in 1999 included, for the first time, descriptions of and criteria for the diagnosis of mild, moderate, and severe bronchial dysplasia and carcinoma-in-situ. Previously some rather complex systems of classification were proposed based on either histologic material from autopsy examination or cytologic preparations. The new classification assumes a full-thickness squamous epithelium and uses criteria similar to those for grading dysplasia in other sites such as the cervix, considering a range of cytologic and architectural changes distributed in the lower, middle, and upper thirds of the epithelium. It is, however, recognized that this is a biologic system, and this division into different grades is artificial. Within the bronchial tree of any person with SD/CIS, the degree of atypia will vary even within a single high-power microscopy field, and all the proposed defining criteria for a particular grade of disease will not necessarily be present. Table 31-1 shows a modified version of the criteria presented in the 2004 revision of the WHO classification.

Mild dysplasia is difficult to recognize (Figure 31-3). Expansion of the basal cell zone into, but not beyond, the lower third of the epithelium is probably the best criterion. Cytologic atypia is minimal, and rare mitotic figures should be basal.

Moderate dysplasia may show the basal cell expansion with vertically orientated nuclei extending no further than the middle third of the epithelium. More atypia is allowed, and mitoses can occur off the basal layer but are confined to the lower third of the epithelium (Figure 31-4).

Severe dysplasia shows a marked increase in atypia, cell crowding extends into the upper third of the epithelium,

TABLE 31-1

Microscopic Features of Squamous Dysplasia and Carcinoma-in-situ

	Mild Dysplasia	Moderate Dysplasia	Severe Dysplasia	Carcinoma-in-situ
Epithelial Cytology	• Mild increase in cell size, minimal pleomorphism • Mild variation of N/C ratio • Finely granular chromatin, minimal nuclear angulation, nucleoli inconspicuous or absent • Vertically oriented nuclei in lower third • Mitoses absent or very rare	• Mild increase in cell size, pleomorphism moderate • Moderate variation of N/C ratio • Finely granular chromatin; nuclear angulations, grooves and lobulations present, nucleoli inconspicuous or absent • Vertically oriented nuclei in lower two thirds • Mitotic figures in lower third	• Marked increase in cell size and pleomorphism • N/C ratio often high and variable • Chromatin uneven and coarse, prominent nuclear angulations and folds, nucleoli frequent and conspicuous • Vertically oriented nuclei in lower two thirds • Mitotic figures in lower two thirds	• Marked increase in cell size and pleomorphism • N/C ratio often high and variable • Chromatin uneven and coarse, prominent nuclear angulations and folds, nucleoli variable. • Nuclei haphazardly oriented relative to epithelial surface • Mitotic figures throughout epithelium
Epithelial Architecture	• Mild increase in epithelial thickness • Complete epithelial maturation • Superficial flattening of epithelial cells • Intermediate cell zone often present • Basilar zone expanded into lower third	• Moderate increase in epithelial thickness • Partial epithelial maturation • Superficial flattening of epithelial cells • Intermediate cells confined to upper third of epithelium • Basilar zone expanded into lower two thirds	• Marked increase in epithelial thickness • Little epithelial maturation • Superficial flattening of epithelial cells • Intermediate cell zone rare • Basilar zone expanded well into upper third	• Epithelium ranges from greatly thickened to thinner than normal • No maturation; epithelium would be same inverted • Superficial flattening minimal or absent • Intermediate cell zone absent • Cellular crowding throughout epithelium

(Modified and abridged from Franklin WA, Wistuba II, Geisinger K et al. Squamous dysplasia and carcinoma in situ. In: Travis WD, Brambilla E, Müller-Hermelink HK, et al, eds. *World Health Organization Classification of Tumours. Pathology and Genetics of Tumours of the Lung, Pleura, Thymus and Heart.* Lyon: IARC Press; 2004:68-72.)

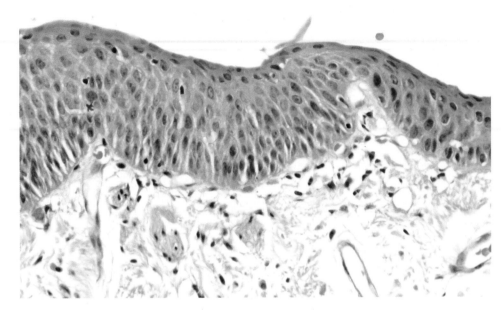

FIGURE 31-3
Mild dysplasia
Mild dysplasia is characterized by minimal atypia involving the lower third of the epithelium only.

A   **B**

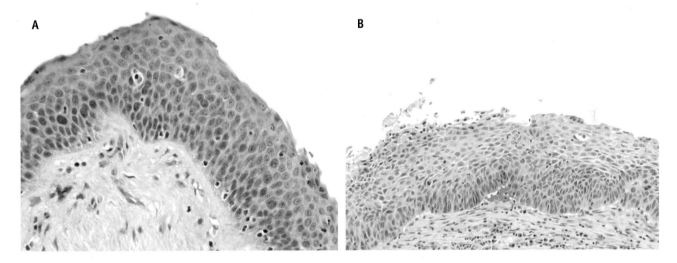

FIGURE 31-4

Moderate dysplasia

Notable cytologic atypia extending upwards to involve the middle third of the epithelium, sufficient for moderate dysplasia, even in the absence of mitoses **(A)**. The extent of the basaloid zone seems less, but a mitotic figure is present well off the base of the epithelium **(B)**.

yet there is evidence of flattening; the epithelium clearly has a "top." Mitoses extend into, but not beyond, the middle third of the epithelium (Figure 31-5).

The best way to think of carcinoma-in-situ in this classification is "chaos." The malignant-looking squamous epithelium has no "top." Inverted, it would look more or less the same, with atypia and mitoses throughout (Figure 31-6).

Occasionally a localized epithelial lesion with a papillary structure, derived from sprouts of subepithelial capillaries invaginating into the overlying epithelium, may be found in airway mucosa. Although these lesions are sometimes covered by respiratory-type epithelium, most show a squamous epithelium with varying degrees of cytologic atypia, hence their classification as angiogenic squamous dysplasia (ASD) (Figure 31-7).

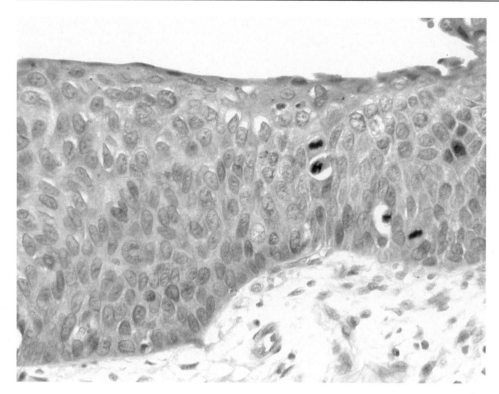

FIGURE 31-5
Severe dysplasia
Enlarged atypical cells at all levels
with minimal surface maturation.
Mitotic figures in the lower and middle
thirds of the epithelium.

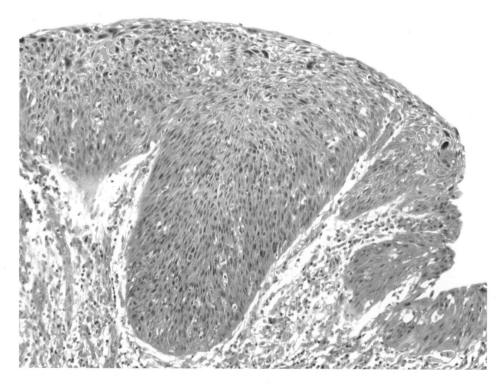

FIGURE 31-6
Carcinoma in situ
Severe pleomorphism at all levels and
a lack of maturation or organization
in the epithelium characterize carcinoma-in-situ. In this example, the epithelium is also very thick.

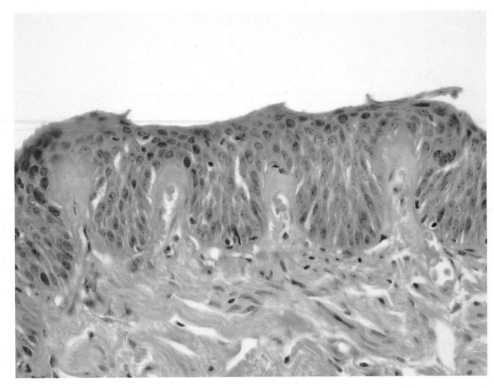

FIGURE 31-7

Squamous dysplasia, angiogenic
This example of angiogenic squamous dysplasia shows cytologic atypia as well as the characteristic vascular sprouts, covered by a thickened basement membrane, protruding upwards into the epithelium.

ANCILLARY STUDIES

Ultrastructural studies have nothing to offer in terms of diagnosis. Immunohistochemistry is equally unhelpful. There is plentiful literature on a range of markers, but none is of any proven diagnostic benefit.

Squamous atypia may be recognized in sputum cytology specimens and in exfoliated cells obtained at bronchoscopic examination. Classification systems exist, based upon cellular and nuclear characteristics similar to those described in Table 31-1 for tissue biopsy samples. While squamous metaplasia may show up as sheets of cells, dysplasias usually manifest as single cells with changes in tinctorial characteristics of the cytoplasm (basophilia and eosinophilia) and increasing nuclear aberration (increasing size, N/C ratio, coarse chromatin, irregular chromatin distribution, and irregularity of the nuclear outline).

DIFFERENTIAL DIAGNOSIS

Although the advent of published criteria for SD/CIS is most welcome and will improve diagnostic reproducibility, there are many problems with the diagnosis. The criteria are based upon a full-thickness squamous epithelium with a sufficient number of cell layers present to allow its separation into thirds. It is the author's view that, relatively speaking, true full-thickness keratinizing

squamous metaplasia as a basis for supervening dysplasia is less common. More often, squamous change with prickle cells develops in a background of basal cell hyperplasia, and dysplasia of even high grade may supervene within this basal cell population while columnar cells persist on the epithelial surface (Figure 31-8). Basal cell hyperplasia, which is all but full thickness, may be confused with severe dysplasia or CIS by the unwary. BCH shows a regular cell population with no atypia. Not infrequently atypical epithelium may be very thin or may have shed its superficial cells during tissue processing, making grading extremely difficult. In all situations where strict application of the WHO criteria is inappropriate or impossible, a more pragmatic approach, assessing those characteristics of the lesion that can be recognized, is best. In these situations going no further than classifying lesions as low- or high-grade is reasonable. Some studies have considered moderate and severe dysplasia together as "high-grade" dysplasia, and there is some molecular evidence to justify this practice.

Squamous metaplasia may occur in the lung in other diseases, and where inflammation is prominent, a degree of reactive atypia is common (Figure 31-9). In bronchiectasis or tuberculous cavities there may be squamous metaplasia with atypia, and atypical squamous metaplasia is not uncommon in the regenerating hyperplastic epithelium of the proliferative phase of diffuse alveolar damage (DAD). The context in which such atypical squamous epithelium is found is important is reaching the correct diagnosis. Physicians must be cautious of making a diagnosis of SD/CIS without the context of

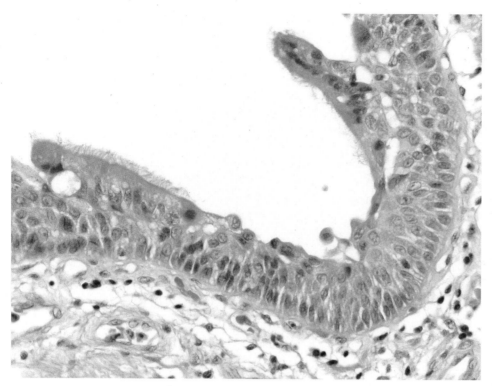

FIGURE 31-8

Squamous atypia

Strips of ciliated respiratory epithelium remain, overlying a zone of squamous epithelial cells exhibiting high-grade atypia. It may be that squamous metaplasia and dysplasia develop in the basaloid zone without a full-thickness squamous epithelium ever being present. Later the residual columnar epithelial cells are shed, leaving dysplastic squamous epithelium, which is often thin and difficult to grade.

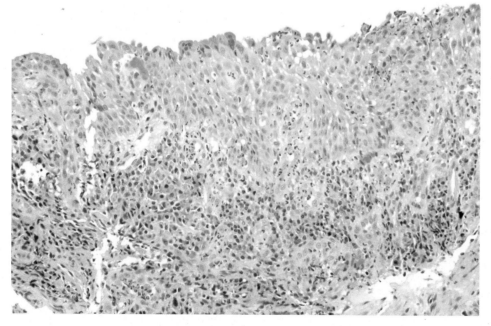

FIGURE 31-9

Squamous metaplasia with reactive atypia

This irregular metaplastic squamous epithelium is associated with marked bronchial mucosal inflammation. The mild cytologic atypia is considered reactive. The airway that was biopsied drained a zone of long-standing infection with a lung abscess.

epithelium lining an intrinsically normal bronchus. There are pitfalls even in this situation. Mucosa around areas of chronic ulceration, or in airways draining an area of chronic infection, may show atypical squamous metaplasia but also marked mucosal inflammation and should not be classified SD/CIS. Chemo/irradiation injury and viral infection can give bizarre epithelial atypia. Chemo/radiotherapy may also affect bronchial gland cells, and viral changes may be very focal, involving single cells or small groups.

In diagnostic bronchial biopsy specimens with CIS, care must be taken not to miss evidence of bronchial mucosal invasion. Isolated nests or small groups of severely atypical squamous cells (particularly with a fibrotic stromal response), necrosis, irregular outlines to sheets of malignant-looking squamous epithelium, and vascularization of such epithelium, all favor invasive disease. Basement membranes may be very hard to identify, and even in CIS it may be variably thickened or thin. Knowledge of the bronchoscopic findings may help: was there a tumor mass seen and biopsied, or was the biopsy from a vague area of mucosal irregularity? Sometimes, when invasion cannot be ruled out, a diagnosis of "at least carcinoma-in-situ" is appropriate. SD/CIS may extend from the bronchial surface into

bronchial gland ducts and even replace the glands themselves. A misdiagnosis of invasive carcinoma may be avoided by appreciating the retained lobular architecture of the glands.

PROGNOSIS AND THERAPY

Predicting the likelihood of SD/CIS progressing to invasive disease has become an area of considerable interest, particularly with renewed interest in lung cancer screening and improved detection of SD/CIS using AFB. Proper longitudinal studies of SD/CIS in humans are almost impossible, even with the improved disease localization afforded by AFB surveillance. Follow-up studies of patients with squamous atypia in sputum have found that up to almost 50% of patients eventually develop invasive carcinoma. Relatively speaking, fewer patients have been followed up by repeated AFB and biopsy, but such studies are increasingly reported. Results have so far been highly variable, and there are many confounding factors at work. Some generalizations may be drawn from the data already published:

- Progression of SD/CIS is certainly not inevitable, and lesions may wax and wane or completely

---

SQUAMOUS DYSPLASIA/CARCINOMA-IN-SITU—FACT SHEET

Definition
- Lesions characterized by cytologic and architectural atypia of squamous epithelium, occurring as single or multiple foci within tracheobronchial epithelium, and which are the precursors of bronchogenic (squamous cell) carcinoma

Incidence
- Occurs in approximately 40% of heavy tobacco smokers
- More common in lungs also bearing squamous cell carcinoma

Mortality
- Generally none

Gender, Race, and Age Distribution
- More common in males than females
- No apparent racial predilection
- Disease of adults

Clinical Features
- No specific features

Radiologic Features
- Not radiologically detectable

Prognosis and Therapy
- Risk factor for invasive carcinoma but no data to enumerate risk
- Progression not inevitable but more likely with higher grade disease
- Smoking cessation is recommended
- Treatments are under investigation

SQUAMOUS DYSPLASIA/CARCINOMA-IN-SITU—PATHOLOGIC FEATURES

Gross Findings
- Usually none but may appear as ill-defined areas of roughened mucosa
- Occur in central cartilaginous airways, often on the spur of bifurcations
- Autofluorescence bronchoscopy will demonstrate lesions more easily

Microscopic Findings
- By definition, this lesion occurs in a squamous-type epithelium
- Graded as mild, moderate, or severe dysplasia or carcinoma-in-situ
- Grading based upon distribution of basaloid and/or atypical squamous cells and mitoses within the epithelium
- Carcinoma-in-situ is characterized by the most marked cytological atypia and lack of maturation in a chaotic epithelium
- Some dysplastic lesions retain a layer of differentiated columnar epithelial cells on the surface

Cytologic Features
- Atypical squamous cells may be found in samples taken at bronchoscopy or in sputum
- Grading based upon the degree of nuclear structural abnormality and cytoplasmic tinctorial characteristics
- Distinction between in-situ and invasive carcinoma is difficult

Pathologic Differential Diagnosis
- Basal cell hyperplasia
- Squamous metaplasia
- Chemo-/irradiation-induced epithelial cell injury
- Invasive carcinoma in small samples

regress. Smoking cessation may hasten, but does not guarantee, regression.

- If disease does progress to invasion, this probably takes years rather than months.
- Each stage of SD/CIS may persist for many months or years, but more advanced disease progresses faster and is less likely to regress.

There is a body of work reporting on molecular biologic markers that may predict outcome in SD/CIS. Although there are data to suggest that abnormal expression of p53, p16INKA, BAX, bcl2, Fhit, and cyclins D1 and E, as well as some genetic abnormalities, may have a predictive role, none of these can, so far, be used to reliably predict outcome for a single patient.

Detection of SD/CIS poses problems for those caring for patients with this disease, especially when prediction of outcome is so uncertain. "Watch and wait" may be appropriate in many situations, as chemoprevention strategies are still the subject of early trials. Field cancerization and problems localizing SD/CIS makes surgical resection an infrequent option, but some data suggests that photodynamic therapy may have a role in some cases.

ATYPICAL ADENOMATOUS HYPERPLASIA

AAH is found in the alveolated part of the lung, often in a centriacinar location. Much evidence now exists, based on morphology, morphometry, cytofluorimetry, and both cell and molecular biologic studies, in support of the hypothesis that these small, localized lesions represent the earliest morphologic change in the stepwise development of peripheral adenocarcinoma.

It is believed that there is a progression of disease whereby AAH lesions become larger, more cellular, and atypical, eventually developing into localized nonmucinous bronchioloalveolar carcinoma (BAC). As currently defined, this form of BAC may be considered the stage of adenocarcinoma-in-situ, and further events involving collapse of the alveolar framework and fibrogenesis appear to herald the onset of invasion within the lesion. Thus AAH can be considered the adenoma in an adenoma-carcinoma sequence of adenocarcinogenesis in the lung periphery.

CLINICAL FEATURES

AAH lesions are asymptomatic. They are thus, for all practical purposes, incidental findings during the histopathologic examination of alveolated lung tissue. The prevalence of AAH in the general population is unknown. Prospective autopsy-based studies in non-cancer-bearing subjects have found AAH in 2% to 4% of cases. AAH is more likely to be found in lungs bearing primary carcinoma and adenocarcinoma in particular. The best prospective studies have found AAH in 9.3% to 49% (average 22%) of lung specimens surgically resected for primary carcinoma. AAH lesions are most likely to be found in resected lung bearing adenocarcinoma (mean prevalence approximately 28%) and less often in those with large cell undifferentiated carcinoma (13%) and squamous cell carcinoma (9%). Reported data vary widely, at least in part due to variation in techniques used for detecting the lesions.

Few studies have reported prevalence data sorted by sex of patient; one study in Caucasian patients found AAH more common in females (19%) versus males (9%) with resected primary lung cancer and more common still in females (30%) versus males (19%) with resected adenocarcinoma. Two Japanese studies are inconclusive on this point.

Data on other demographic factors associated with AAH are minimal and often contradictory. The volume of literature on AAH emanating from Japan compared to elsewhere, combined with the long history of adenocarcinoma as the dominant prevalent lung cancer type in this part of the world, raises the possibility that Asian genotypes may predispose to this disease. Some studies suggest Japanese patients who presently have or have had any cancer, not only lung cancer, have more AAH while a family history of excess cancers was not so associated. Caucasian patients have shown the opposite. Data on smoking history and AAH prevalence are also few and inconclusive; in the United States and the United Kingdom there probably is an association—in Japan perhaps not.

Less is known about the genetic alterations that occur in AAH, when compared to SD/CIS. Many of the same genes and chromosome loci appear to be involved. Abnormal p53 protein expression is frequent, yet *P53* mutations are rare in AAH. Unlike in SD/CIS, *K-RAS* mutations appear to be important in the evolution of adenocarcinoma from AAH. These data have been reviewed in some relevant literature listed at the end of this chapter.

RADIOLOGIC FEATURES

There are no characteristic radiologic features for AAH: most of the lesions are completely invisible, even on high-resolution CT scans. It is worth noting, however, that, largely in the context of detailed lung cancer screening trials in Japan, a proportion of small, so-called pure ground-glass nodules detected on fine-section spiral CT scans prove to be AAH after surgical excision. This appearance is not, however, specific; some of these nodules are BAC, a few even show invasive carcinoma, and many prove to be benign, inflammatory foci.

PATHOLOGIC FEATURES

GROSS FINDINGS

The vast majority of AAH lesions are incidental findings on microscopic examination of lung tissue. It is possible, however, to visualize some AAH lesions macroscopically on the cut surface of the lung. Optimum specimen preparation, sectioning, and viewing are required for success. Lung resection specimens should be inflated per-bronchially with fixative (the author uses 10% neutral buffered formalin, but Bouin's fluid has also been advocated), allowed to fix for 24 hours and carefully sectioned in thin slices. Parallel parasagittal 1-cm thick slices are then cut and viewed under bright light and running water (Figure 31-10). Lesions cannot be visualized if the background lung is affected by fibrosis, emphysema, or pneumonia. Lesions may appear as pale cream, gray, or yellowish foci with an indistinct margin. Their surfaces may be stippled with a few depressions representing the alveolar spaces in the lesion. Sampling any such lesions will increase the chance of detecting lesions, but many such gross foci will not be AAH, instead representing non-specific fibrotic or inflammatory foci. Random sampling of peripheral lung, which is grossly normal, may still reveal AAH.

MICROSCOPIC FINDINGS

The 2004 WHO classification defines AAH as "a localized proliferation of mild to moderately atypical cells lining involved alveoli and, sometimes, respiratory bronchioles, resulting in focal lesions in peripheral alveolated lung, usually less than 5 mm in diameter and generally in the absence of underlying interstitial inflammation and fibrosis" (Figure 31-11).

Generally speaking, these lesions stand out against the normal background lung because of mild to moderate thickening of the alveolar walls, which are expanded by a variable degrees of collagenization, fibroplasia, and occasionally, elastosis. Lymphocytes are usually few but may be numerous and may occasionally aggregate into follicles. This fibrosis and inflammation do not extend beyond the limits of the lesion as defined by the epithelial cell population lining the alveolar walls. Lesions often lie close to, or may appear contiguous with, respiratory bronchioles. In some cases the alveolar spaces appear dilated and some lesions have a cystic appearance. Many lesions show an excess of macrophages in their alveolar lumina.

Alveolar walls in AAH are lined by a variable, heterogeneous mixture of round, cuboidal, or low columnar cells. "Peg" cells with apical snouts are not uncommon, large round cells with double nuclei may be present, and sometimes these have a narrow base and an expanded apex containing the nuclei. Most lesions have these cells admixed in a discontinuous layer around involved alveoli (Figure 31-12). Part or all of some lesions can show a more complete cellular layer with fewer gaps and a tendency for cells to be more columnar. Occasional tufts of cells may protrude into the alveolar spaces, but true papillae are not seen. Marked cell crowding, overlapping, and multilayering suggest a diagnosis of bronchioloalveolar carcinoma (BAC; see below under differential diagnosis). Ciliated and mucous cells are not seen in AAH.

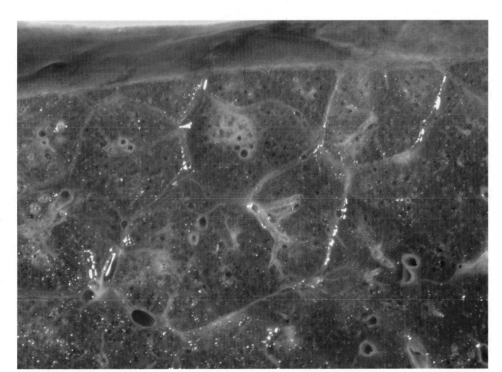

FIGURE 31-10

Atypical adenomatous hyperplasia
Occasionally millimeter-sized foci of AAH may be visible on the cut surface of well-prepared lung. The alveolar spaces can be clearly seen within this sub pleural lesion, as can the adjacent bronchiole.

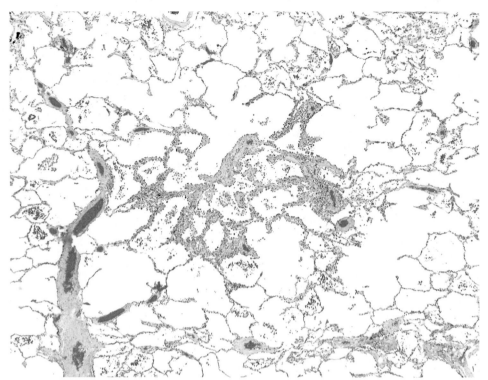

FIGURE 31-11
Atypical adenomatous hyperplasia
This tiny lesion shows thickened alveolar walls studded by plump alveolar lining cells. The surrounding lung is unremarkable.

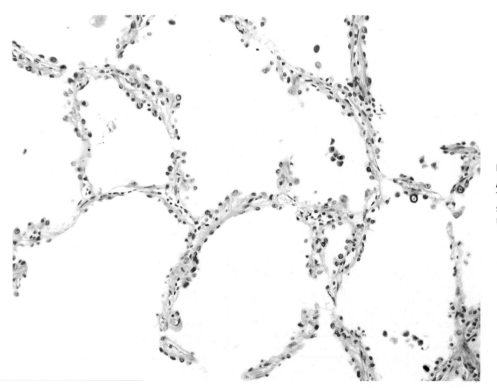

FIGURE 31-12
Atypical adenomatous hyperplasia
This relatively low-grade AAH lesion shows clear gaps between the rounded alveolar lining cells.

Nuclei are generally round to oval and regular with a homogeneous chromatin pattern that may occasionally be quite hyperchromatic. Large and mild to moderately atypical nuclei may be scattered in the lesions. Nuclear inclusions are common (Figure 31-13). Mitotic figures are very rare.

There is no doubt that within the range of appearances acceptable as AAH, some lesions are more cellular and atypical than others (Figure 31-14), and some authors have attempted to separate AAH into high- and low-grade lesions. Although recognizing that this range of appearances exists, that multiple lesions from the same lung may show different "grades," and that individual lesions vary, there are to date no agreed-upon criteria for grading AAH, and the 2004 WHO panel did not recommend this practice.

In the 1999 WHO lung cancer classification, AAH was considered to be less than 5 mm in size, and some authors have proposed that lesions exceeding this dimension be regarded as BAC. In the 2004 classification, however, this 5-mm limit was dropped, recognizing that, while 65% to 75% of AAH lesions are less than 3 mm, 10% to 20% measure over 5 mm; lesions in excess of 10 mm are found by most authors with extensive experience of AAH. Larger lesions have a tendency to be more cellular, though this is by no means always the case.

Whether AAH lesions are noted on gross inspection of the lung tissue or are found incidentally at microscopy, it is safe to assume that they are generally present as multiple foci. While some patients may yield only a single focus despite extensive tissue sampling, it is a fact that the more assiduously these lesions are sought, the more often they are found. A minority of patients have very large numbers of AAH lesions detectable even in single lobectomies; these are universally resections for peripheral adenocarcinomas, and the lung frequently shows, as well as dozens of AAH lesions, foci of localized non-mucinous BAC, and occasionally, additional synchronous primary adenocarcinomas.

ANCILLARY STUDIES

Ancillary studies have little role to play in the diagnosis of AAH.

Ultrastructural studies have shown that AAH foci show some cells with features of Clara cells and others that are type II pneumocytes.

This is further supported by immunohistochemical studies that show many AAH cells express the surfactant marker SPA and some express the Clara cell marker UP1. AAH strongly expresses TTF-1, which probably acts, in this context, as a lineage marker for peripheral airway epithelium. Some AAH lesions, especially "higher grade" lesions, express CEA. Studies using markers of proliferative/cell cycle activity show low indices, approximately 1%. Many other immunohistochemical

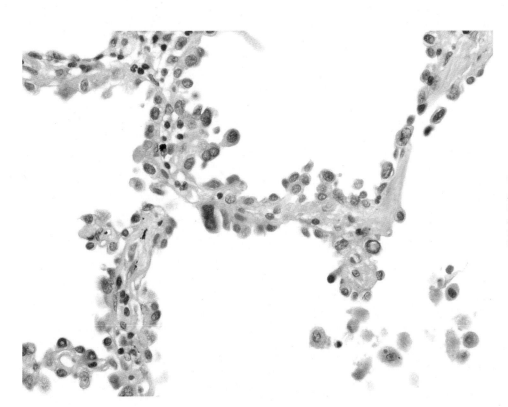

FIGURE 31-13

Atypical adenomatous hyperplasia
Nuclear inclusions are not unusual in AAH. Columnar "peg" cells with apical nuclei may be seen, as may double nuclei.

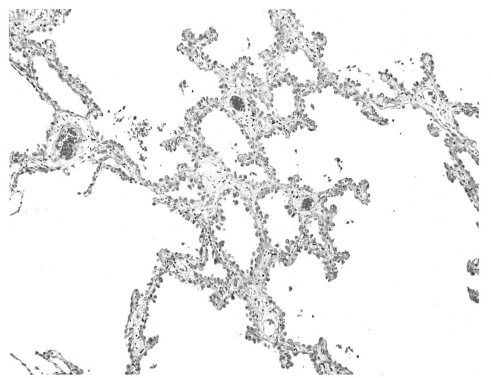

FIGURE 31-14
Atypical adenomatous hyperplasia
This is a more cellular AAH lesion. Cell density and atypia are less than expected in BAC.

studies on AAH are reported, and are included in the reading list at the end of this chapter.

Cytology has no role to play in the diagnosis of AAH. Some have recommended the use of the term atypical bronchioloalveolar cell proliferation as the best "diagnosis" when features fall short of those required for a diagnosis of adenocarcinoma, and the differential diagnosis includes AAH and bronchioloalveolar carcinoma.

DIFFERENTIAL DIAGNOSIS

Primarily AAH must, on the one hand, be distinguished from reactive bronchioloalveolar cell hyperplasia, and on the other, from the lesion that may evolve from AAH: localized non-mucinous bronchioloalveolar carcinoma (BAC). A few other localized peripheral lung lesions also enter the differential diagnosis of AAH.

In distinguishing AAH from reactive bronchioloalveolar cell hyperplasia, a sense of context and perspective is essential. Whenever there is a background process such as pneumonia, IPF/UIP, NSIP, DAD, or other form of pneumonitis, a diagnosis of AAH cannot really be entertained. All these diseases are associated with reactive hyperplasia as part of the generalized fibroin-

flammatory picture. AAH is best recognized when it occurs on a background of essentially normal lung. It is even difficult to recognize in the presence of emphysema. As mentioned above, a degree of fibrosis and/or inflammation is acceptable in the interstitium of AAH, but this generally does not extend beyond the limits of the lesion. Although most common in tumor-bearing lungs, AAH may be difficult to identify with certainty if there is obstructive pneumonia distal to the tumor. In contrast to the heterogeneous cell population in AAH, reactive lesions in some circumstances show a more monotonous and continuous population of regular cuboidal cells, frequently adjacent to coarse scars, septa, or the pleura. Of course some examples of reactive type II pneumocyte hyperplasia may show atypia, but the context is important in reaching the correct diagnosis.

Bronchiolar respiratory epithelial metaplasia/ hyperplasia occurs in a number of circumstances. Centriacinar peribronchiolar metaplasia (Lambertosis) adjacent to respiratory bronchioles may cause confusion but is easily separated from AAH by recognizing the crisp delineation of alveoli contiguous with a frequently scarred respiratory bronchiole, surrounded by some fibrosis and lined by a regular population of bronchiolar cells, including easily identifiable ciliated cells. Honeycomb lung will never be confused with AAH.

The distinction between AAH and localized non-mucinous BAC is a contentious issue. Since one probably progresses into the other, the point at which BAC "exists" is somewhat arbitrary. Both AAH and BAC are lesions of alveolated lung in which the alveolar framework is essentially preserved, the lesion being defined by the cell population lining the alveolar walls. Size is not a reliable criterion for making the distinction, though most lesions of this type below 5 mm are viewed as AAH and most over 10 mm are viewed as BAC. Morphometric studies have provided thresholds for mean cell size and nuclear area that correlate with the H&E classification of lesions but are not practically useful in the usual diagnostic setting. It is proposed that most AAH will rarely show more than ONE of the following criteria while localized non-mucinous BAC will fulfill THREE OR MORE. These criteria are:

- High cell density with overlapping nuclei
- Marked cell stratification

- True papillae or cells showing a "picket-fence" pattern
- Definite columnar cell shape with cell height exceeding that of the columnar cells of adjacent terminal bronchioles
- Coarse nuclear chromatin and prominent nucleoli

BAC generally shows a more homogeneous cell population than AAH and also shows a continuous lining of cells around alveoli, with a transition to adjacent alveolar lining cells. Commensurate with the hypothesis that AAH progresses into BAC, transitional lesions will be encountered that show some areas fulfilling the above criteria for BAC, while other areas fall short, retaining an AAH-like appearance. In such circumstances, the diagnosis of BAC should prevail.

Papillary adenoma of type II pneumocytes is a rare benign lesion in which the high-power microscopic features may look similar to a more cellular AAH. There are, however, several important differences. Papillary adenoma has true papillae with fibrovascular

---

ATYPICAL ADENOMATOUS HYPERPLASIA—FACT SHEET

Definition

- A focal lesion usually <5 mm diameter due to proliferation of atypical bronchioloalveolar cells lining centriacinar alveoli, occurring in the absence of background lung fibrosis

Incidence

- Background incidence uncertain, possibly 2% to 4%
- More common in cancer-bearing lungs; found in association with about 28% of adenocarcinomas and 9% of squamous cell carcinomas

Morbidity and Mortality

- None directly attributable to the lesions

Gender, Race, and Age Distribution

- May be more common in females
- Anecdotally more frequent in Asian (Japanese) subjects
- Age distribution that of cancer-bearing population (>50 yr); otherwise unknown

Clinical Features

- No specific features

Radiologic Features

- May be visible on thin-section high-resolution CT scan as tiny foci of so-called ground-glass opacification of lung parenchyma, but features are not specific for AAH

Prognosis and Therapy

- No evidence that presence of lesion(s) influences outcome of cancer-bearers with AAH
- No data on actual risk or rate of progression of AAH to BAC and invasive adenocarcinoma
- Usually incidental findings in lungs resected for cancer

ATYPICAL ADENOMATOUS HYPERPLASIA—PATHOLOGIC FEATURES

Gross Findings

- Most lesions are grossly invisible but may appear as pale gray, yellow, or white lesions, usually <5 mm diameter, on the cut surface
- Most common in the upper lobes and subpleurally

Microscopic Findings

- Mild/moderately atypical round or cuboidal cells lining alveolar walls
- "Peg" or "hobnail" cells common; columnar cells uncommon
- Cytologic heterogeneity frequent
- Cell population makes discontinuous layer on alveolar walls
- Alveolar walls are mildly thickened and occasionally inflamed

Ultrastructural Features

- Most lesions include cells with features of Clara cells and type II pneumocytes

Cytologic Features

- AAH cannot be diagnosed on cytologic specimens

Immunohistochemical Features

- None to help with diagnosis

Pathologic Differential Diagnosis

- Bronchioloalveolar carcinoma
- Reactive pneumocyte hyperplasia
- Peribronchiolar metaplasia
- Micronodular pneumocyte hyperplasia of tuberous sclerosis

cores, the lesions may be encapsulated, are generally 1 to 4 cm in diameter and may contain ciliated cells. Although alveolar adenoma contains "alveolar" spaces lined by a variable population of flattened, cuboidal, and "hobnail" cells, this is a well-circumscribed, discrete yet unencapsulated lesion that has a myxoid and collagenous stroma surrounding the cystic spaces, which are obviously not native alveolar spaces. Although lesions less than 1 cm in diameter have been described, lesions are commonly larger and can measure up to 6 cm.

Micronodular pneumocyte hyperplasia (MNPH) may bear an extremely close similarity with cellular forms of AAH and, indeed, also to small BAC lesions. These lesions are most often seen in patients with tuberous sclerosis complex and most occur in combination with pulmonary lymphangioleiomyomatosis. The lesions themselves are approximately the same size as AAH but tend to be more homogeneously cellular and have continuous runs of bland plump type II pneumocytes lining small distorted or collapsed alveolar spaces whose walls show irregular thickening with prominent reticulin. Immunohistochemical stains for tuberin are positive in MNPH. The cellularity of the lesions is further emphasized by abundant airspace macrophage accumulation.

PROGNOSIS AND THERAPY

Although there is good evidence to support the notion that AAH is a precursor of BAC and therefore of lung adenocarcinoma, there are no longitudinal studies showing progression of disease. It is not known what the risk or rate of progression might be, and studies have shown that the outcome for patients with lung cancer and AAH is no worse than for those with lung cancer alone. Anecdotally, however, the author has seen several cases of second metachronous adenocarcinomas presenting in patients who were successfully treated and apparently cured of their first AAH-associated lung cancer. As more patients are subjected to screening using spiral CT scanning, it is possible that some patients with multifocal AAH/BAC may be detected and some longitudinal observation may then be possible.

There are also no data on appropriate treatments for AAH. In most cases the treatment is determined by the associated lesions for which the surgery was performed. In circumstances where AAH is serendipitously discovered, however, the pathologist may be faced with the question of what to advise, working on the principle that other lesions may remain in the patient's lungs. In such circumstances, intervention is inappropriate, and a baseline high-resolution CT scan with follow-up may be the most appropriate choice.

DIFFUSE IDIOPATHIC PULMONARY NEUROENDOCRINE CELL HYPERPLASIA

This condition, usually referred to as DIPNECH, is extremely rare and is included in the WHO classification of pre-invasive lung lesions since it is associated with the development of carcinoid tumors. As the name implies, it is characterized by the diffuse widespread hyperplasia of pulmonary neuroendocrine cells (PNCs) in the airway epithelium, generally in the absence of those fibroinflammatory lung diseases that are known to be associated with PNC hyperplasia. This hyperplasia leads to the development of carcinoid tumorlets and, in some cases, lesions large enough to be considered peripheral spindle cell carcinoid tumors.

CLINICAL FEATURES

Described cases of DIPNECH have been seen in patients of wide age range, though most have been between 40 and 60 years old, and there is a female preponderance. Most patients present with several years of slowly progressive breathlessness and nonproductive cough that may be mistaken for asthma. Pulmonary function testing may show reduced gas transfer and obstructive or mixed obstructive/restrictive changes. Physical examination is unrevealing. It is likely that cases with similar pathology but less widespread small airway narrowing, and subsequently no symptoms referable to any such change, do exist as a sub-clinical form of DIPNECH.

RADIOLOGIC FEATURES

In cases where there are well-developed carcinoid tumorlets and carcinoid tumors, lung nodules may be seen on CT scans or even on the plain chest radiograph if large enough. Variable signs of air trapping may be evident in cases with marked small airway narrowing.

PATHOLOGIC FEATURES

GROSS FINDINGS

In cases where there are well-developed carcinoid tumorlets or tumors, nodules may be visible on the cut surface of the lung as white or grey-white foci (Figure 31-15). Carcinoid tumors may have a homogeneous granular cut surface.

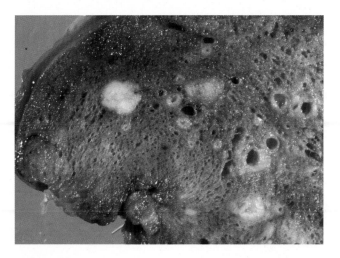

FIGURE 31-15

Carcinoids in a case with tumorlets and pulmonary neuroendocrine cell hyperplasia
This patient had a wedge resection for carcinoid tumor. As well as the main tumor, the specimen showed several other carcinoid tumors (three visible in this image), many carcinoid tumorlets, and extensive PNC hyperplasia.

MICROSCOPIC FINDINGS

Hyperplasia of neuroendocrine cells in the lung is manifested by an increase in single cells, small groups, and linear runs of basal PNCs in airway epithelium (Figure 31-16). These changes are widespread. Nodules of cells, covered by columnar respiratory epithelium and contained by the epithelial basement membrane, may protrude into and apparently obstruct small airways (Figure 31-17). Accompanying fibrosis may contribute

to this obstructive lesion. The airway obstruction may lead to distal bronchiolar dilatation. These changes, in the correct context and in the absence of those fibroinflammatory conditions known to be associated with PNC hyperplasia, are sufficient for a diagnosis of DIPNECH. Not infrequently, however, the hyperplastic changes present are more pronounced, taking the form of so-called carcinoid tumorlets (Figure 31-18). Tumorlets are characterized by the extension of PNCs outside the epithelial basement membrane and usually beyond the limits of the airway wall leading to, in association with a variable amount of fibrosis, the formation of small nodules of up to 5 mm in diameter. Any nodule of PNCs measuring over 5 mm is considered, by definition, a carcinoid tumor, and some patients with DIPNECH may have multiple such tumors—peripheral (spindle cell) carcinoid tumors.

ANCILLARY STUDIES

It is standard practice to confirm the neuroendocrine nature of these cellular aggregates by immunohistochemistry. Although a number of neuroendocrine markers such as synaptophysin and CD56 may be employed, the most specific and effective in this condition is chromogranin. As well as confirming the neuroendocrine nature of the nodular lesions, the immunohistochemistry preparations facilitate recognition of the subtle widespread intraepithelial hyperplasia of PNCs.

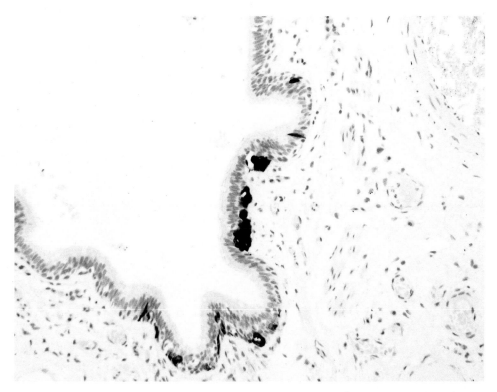

FIGURE 31-16

Diffuse idiopathic pulmonary neuroendocrine cell hyperplasia
Chromogranin immunohistochemistry identifies clusters of PNCs in the basal layer of an otherwise normal bronchiole.

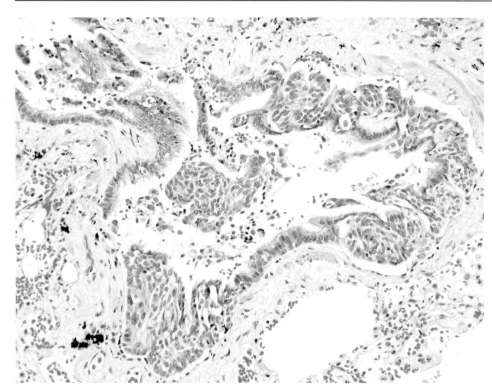

FIGURE 31-17

Diffuse idiopathic pulmonary neuro-endocrine cell hyperplasia
This airway is distorted by nodules of PNCs protruding into the lumen.

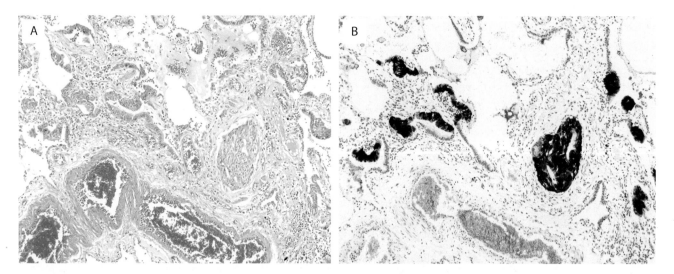

FIGURE 31-18

Tumorlet and pulmonary neuroendocrine cell hyperplasia
This small tumorlet has obliterated the associated bronchiole (right center), the pulmonary arteriole remaining below **(A)**. A degree of peribronchiolar metaplasia has resulted. The extent of the PNC hyperplasia is better appreciated on the chromogranin-stained adjacent section **(B)**.

DIFFERENTIAL DIAGNOSIS

As already mentioned, PNC hyperplasia may be seen in a number of fibroinflammatory conditions in the lung, in particular in bronchiectasis, but also described in bronchopulmonary dysplasia, cystic fibrosis, diffuse panbronchiolitis, COPD, Langerhans cell histiocytosis, and intralobar sequestration. Thus, the diagnosis of DIPNECH would require the absence of these associated conditions. It is worth noting that carcinoid tumors are not described in these contexts.

Evidence of widespread PNC hyperplasia may be seen in lungs resected for carcinoid tumors, especially of the peripheral spindle cell type. It is uncertain whether this is a reactive phenomenon secondary to the tumor or a localized (or even generalized)

DIPNECH-like proliferation that has not caused sufficient airway obstruction to be of functional significance. Similar PNC hyperplasia may be seen in lung tissue resected for other reasons, such as primary carcinoma, but again, the relationship between this change and DIPNECH is unclear.

PROGNOSIS AND THERAPY

DIPNECH leads to a slow deterioration in pulmonary function. Such is the rarity of the disease that there is little published experience with therapy. There is a reported case treated by single lung transplantation. The carcinoid tumors that occur are low-grade, and atypical tumors are not found.

DIFFUSE IDIOPATHIC PULMONARY NEUROENDOCRINE CELL HYPERPLASIA—FACT SHEET

Definition
- A diffuse and widespread proliferation of pulmonary neuroendocrine cells, in the absence of background fibroinflammatory disease and often associated with airflow limitation

Incidence
- Very rare condition, probably fewer than 20 cases reported

Morbidity and Mortality
- Reported cases have progressed to respiratory failure

Gender, Race, and Age Distribution
- Female preponderance, no data on race distribution, most reported cases between 40 and 60 years of age

Clinical Features
- May present with a long history of cough and asthma-like features
- Patients show airflow limitation consistent with small airway obstruction

Radiologic Features
- Small nodules may be visible on chest radiograph and CT scan

Therapy
- Anecdotal report of a case treated by lung transplantation
- Carcinoid tumors may require surgical treatment

DIFFUSE IDIOPATHIC PULMONARY NEUROENDOCRINE CELL HYPERPLASIA—PATHOLOGIC FEATURES

Gross Findings
- Carcinoid tumors and tumorlets may be visible as solid nodules

Microscopic Findings
- Excess PNCs present as single cells, linear runs, and small clusters in the respiratory epithelium; the cell nodules may protrude into the airway lumens
- Widespread airway involvement
- Tumorlets are common and may obliterate small airways
- Spindle cell carcinoid tumors are frequent

Ultrastructural Features
- Neuroendocrine cells with neurosecretory granules

Cytologic Features
- No role in diagnosis

Immunohistochemical Features
- Neuroendocrine markers are useful to confirm the nature of the abnormal cells and demonstrate their distribution

Pathologic Differential Diagnosis
- Tumorlets associated with bronchiectasis and other conditions
- PNC hyperplasia ± carcinoid tumors, without evidence of airflow limitation

SUGGESTED READINGS

General References

1. Kerr KM. Morphology and genetics of preinvasive pulmonary disease. *Curr Diag Pathol*. 2004;10:259-68.
2. Kerr KM. Pulmonary preinvasive neoplasia. *J Clin Pathol*. 2001;54:257-71.
3. Kerr KM, Fraire, A. Preinvasive diseases. In: Tomashefski J, Farver C, Cagle P, Fraire A, eds. *Dail and Hammer's Pulmonary Pathology*. 3rd ed. Springer (In press).
4. Ma Y, Seneviratne CK, Koss M. Idiopathic pulmonary fibrosis and malignancy. *Curr Opin Pulm Med*. 2001;7:278-82.
5. Samet JM. Does idiopathic pulmonary fibrosis increase lung cancer risk? *Am J Respir Crit Care Med*. 2000;161:1-2.
6. Travis WD. Lung. In: Henson DE, Albores-Saavedra J, eds. *Pathology of Incipient Neoplasia*. New York: Oxford University Press; 2001:295-316.
7. Yang Y, Fujita J, Tokuda M, et al. Lung cancer associated with several connective tissue diseases: with a review of literature. *Rheumatol Int*. 2001;21:106-11.

Squamous Dysplasia/Carcinoma-in-situ

8. Bota S, Auliac J-B, Paris C, et al. Follow-up of bronchial precancerous lesions and carcinoma in situ using fluorescence endoscopy. *Am J Respir Crit Care Med*. 2001;164:1688-93.
9. Franklin WA, Wistuba II, Geisinger K, et al. Squamous dysplasia and carcinoma in situ. In: Travis WD, Brambilla E, Müller-Hermelink HK, et al, eds. *World Health Organization Classification of Tumours. Pathology and Genetics of Tumours of the Lung, Pleura, Thymus and Heart*. Lyon: IARC Press; 2004:68-72.
10. Lam S, MacAulay C, LeRiche JC, et al. Detection and localization of early lung cancer by fluorescence bronchoscopy. *Cancer*. 2000;89:2468-73.
11. Nagamoto N, Saito Y, Sato M, et al. Clinicopathological analysis of 19 cases of isolated carcinoma in situ of the bronchus. *Am J Surg Pathol*. 1993;17:1234-43.
12. Wistuba II, Mao L, Gazdar AF. Smoking molecular damage in bronchial epithelium. *Oncogene*. 2002;21:7298-06.

Atypical Adenomatous Hyperplasia

13. Aoyagi Y, Yokose T, Minami Y, et al. Accumulation of losses of heterozygosity and multistep carcinogenesis in pulmonary adenocarcinoma. *Cancer Res*. 2001;61:7950-4.

14. Chapman AD, Kerr KM. The association between atypical adenomatous hyperplasia and primary lung cancer. *Br J Cancer*. 2000;83:632-6.
15. Kerr KM, Fraire AE, Pugatch B, et al. Atypical adenomatous hyperplasia. In: Travis WD, Brambilla E, Müller-Hermelink HK, et al, eds. *World Health Organization Classification of Tumours. Pathology and Genetics of Tumours of the Lung, Pleura, Thymus and Heart*. Lyon: IARC Press; 2004:73-5.
16. Kitamura H, Kameda Y, Ito T, et al. Atypical adenomatous hyperplasia of the lung. Implications for the pathogenesis of peripheral lung adenocarcinoma. *Am J Clin Pathol*. 1999;111:610-22.
17. Miller RR, Nelems B, Evans KG, et al. Glandular neoplasia of the lung. A proposed analogy to colonic tumours. *Cancer*. 1988;61:1009-14.
18. Noguchi M, Morokawa A, Kawasaki M, et al. Small adenocarcinoma of the lung. Histologic characteristics and prognosis. *Cancer*. 1995;75:2844-52.

Diffuse Idiopathic Pulmonary Neuroendocrine Cell Hyperplasia

19. Aguayo SM, Miller YE, Waldron JA, et al. Idiopathic diffuse hyperplasia of pulmonary neuroendocrine cells and airway disease. *N Engl J Med*. 1992;327:1285-8.
20. Churg A, Warnock ML. Pulmonary tumourlet. A form of peripheral carcinoid. *Cancer*. 1976;37:1469-77.
21. Gosney JR, Travis WD. Diffuse Idiopathic Pulmonary Neuroendocrine Cell Hyperplasia. In: Travis WD, Brambilla E, Müller-Hermelink HK, et al, eds. *World Health Organization Classification of Tumours. Pathology and Genetics of Tumours of the Lung, Pleura, Thymus and Heart*. Lyon: IARC Press; 2004:76-7.
22. Miller MA, Mark GJ, Kanarek D. Multiple peripheral pulmonary carcinoids and tumourlets of carcinoid type, with restrictive and obstructive lung disease. *Am J Med*. 1978;65:373-8.
23. Miller RR, Muller NL. Neuroendocrine cell hyperplasia and obliterative bronchiolitis in patients with peripheral carcinoid tumours. *Am J Surg Pathol*. 1995;19:653-8.

32 Benign Neoplasms of the Lungs
Douglas B. Flieder

- Benign Mesenchymal Neoplasms
- Hamartoma
- Benign Salivary Gland-Type Neoplasms
- Mucous Gland Adenoma
- Mucinous Cystadenoma
- Alveolar Adenoma
- Papillary Adenoma
- Solitary Papillomas
- Sclerosing Hemangioma
- Clear Cell Tumor
- Granular Cell Tumor

BENIGN MESENCHYMAL NEOPLASMS

Not surprisingly, the lung is a source of virtually all described mesenchymal tumors. While leiomyomas, schwannomas, lipomas, neurofibromas, hemangiomas, and lymphangiomas can originate in the lung, one should be certain that such lesions are not metastatic low-grade sarcomas, especially the smooth muscle tumors. Pulmonary hamartomas are the most common benign lung tumors and warrant further discussion. Chondromas are discussed within the differential diagnosis of hamartomas.

HAMARTOMA

CLINICAL FEATURES

Pulmonary hamartomas are defined as neoplastic mixtures of mature mesenchymal tissue elements normally found within the lung, often with one element predominating. The World Health Organization prefers the nosologically incorrect term hamartoma, and

synonyms include chondroid hamartoma, benign mesenchymoma, and hamartochondroma. The incidence of this lesion is 0.32%, and a two- to four-fold male predominance is observed. The peak incidence is in the sixth or seventh decade of life, yet rare cases have been reported in children as young as 9 years old. Genetic mutations of the high-mobility group (HMG) proteins, and in the regions 6p21 and 12q13-15, confirm the neoplastic rather than hamartomatous nature of the lesion. Most patients with hamartomas are asymptomatic since tumors are often peripheral coin lesions, and almost all are incidentally discovered on chest radiographs. Approximately 10% are endobronchial, and these may present with cough, hemoptysis, or obstructive pneumonia. Hamartomas are rarely multiple. Associations with other pulmonary diseases, including lung cancer or malignant transformation, have not been convincingly demonstrated.

RADIOLOGIC FEATURES

Pulmonary hamartomas are usually well-circumscribed, smoothly marginated solitary peripheral nodules measuring less than 4.0 cm. They represent up to 14% of so-called coin lesions. A small percentage demonstrate radiographic calcifications including so-called diagnostic popcorn calcifications.

PATHOLOGIC FEATURES

GROSS FINDINGS

Well-circumscribed and lobulated peripheral hamartomas are surrounded by compressed lung parenchyma. These bulging tumors can often be shelled out from the adjacent lung tissue and usually are not connected to airways. Cut surfaces range from semi-firm white and pearly in tumors with large amounts of cartilage to tan and gelatinous in cartilage-poor lesions (Figure 32-1A). Gritty specks are also appreciated in those with calcification. Focal cystic

669

HAMARTOMA—FACT SHEET

Definition

» Benign neoplasm composed of varying proportions of mesenchymal tissues combined with entrapped respiratory epithelium (World Health Organization)

Incidence

» The incidence is 0.32%

Gender and Age Distribution

» Two- to four-fold male predominance
» Peak incidence is in the sixth or seventh decade of life
» Rare cases have been reported in children as young as 9 years old

Clinical Features

» Usually asymptomatic
» Endobronchial lesions may present with cough, hemoptysis, or obstructive pneumonia

Radiologic Features

» Usually well-circumscribed, smoothly marginated solitary peripheral nodules measuring less than 4.0 cm
» A small percentage demonstrates radiographic calcifications including so-called diagnostic popcorn calcifications
» Rarely multiple lesions

Prognosis and Therapy

» Hamartomas are slow-growing benign neoplasms amenable to conservative surgical resection
» Sleeve excision or lobectomy may be required depending on the size and/or location of the tumor and peritumoral findings
» Sarcomatous transformation of and adenocarcinomas arising in hamartomas are exceedingly rare events

---

HAMARTOMA—PATHOLOGIC FEATURES

Gross Findings

» Parenchymal tumors are multilobulated, semifirm, white or gray
» Endobronchial tumors are polypoid and usually soft yellow
» Tumors are usually less than 4.0 cm

Microscopic Findings

» Lobulated masses of mature hyaline cartilage surrounded by fat, smooth muscle, bone, or fibrovascular tissue
» Punctate calcifications
» Peripheral clefts lined by respiratory-type epithelium
» Endobronchial tumors are more lipomatous with shallow or absent epithelial invaginations

Fine Needle Aspiration Biopsy Findings

» Biphasic smears with epithelial and mesenchymal tissues
» Cartilage and fibromyxoid tissue prominent on Diff-Quik smears
» Epithelium can be abundant and reactive
» Background without blood, necrosis, or inflammation
» Cell block highlights benign mesenchymal and epithelial tissues

Pathologic Differential Diagnosis

» Monomorphic benign soft tissue tumors, especially chondroma
» Chondrosarcoma

---

change is often seen, while rare tumors may be largely cystic with interspersed solid areas. Endobronchial lesions are often fleshy, yellow, and glistening owing to the large amount of adipose tissue in the tumor. These tumors are usually found in the large central airways and are broad-based polyps.

MICROSCOPIC FINDINGS

Hamartomas are composed of varying proportions of benign mesenchyme including cartilage, adipose tissue, smooth muscle, bone, and fibrovascular tissue (Figure 32-1B). In most peripheral lesions, one sees lobulated masses of mature cartilage surrounded by strands or islands of fibromyxoid connective tissue, fat, bone, and smooth muscle (Figure 32-1C). The edges of the lesion feature cleft like-spaces or invaginations of respiratory-type epithelium (Figure 32-1D). Rare peripheral hamartomas without cartilage must demonstrate at least two mesenchymal elements, such as adi-

pose tissue, smooth muscle, or primitive fibromyxoid tissue, in order to diagnose this entity. Up to 15% of tumors feature calcification.

Endobronchial lesions differ from parenchymal lesions in several respects. These polypoid tumors often feature large amounts of mature adipose tissue surrounded by a compressed layer of myxoid tissue while smooth muscle and seromucinous glands may be admixed. Cartilage is either absent or present in very small amounts. Rarely, the cartilage shows increased cellularity and/or nuclear pleomorphism but certainly not malignant features. While attached to the bronchial wall, these central lesions are not continuous with bronchial cartilage plates. Epithelial invaginations, if present, are shallow, and surface epithelium is intact.

ANCILLARY STUDIES

FINE NEEDLE ASPIRATION BIOPSY

In theory, fine needle aspiration biopsy diagnosis of pulmonary hamartoma is quite simple, as one need only to recognize non-organized epithelial and mesenchymal tissues on smears and/or cell blocks (Figure 32-2). However, many pitfalls exist (evidenced by a false positive rate of over 20%) and extreme caution in addition to radiographic correlation is recommended in each case. While Diff-Quik-stained smears highlight

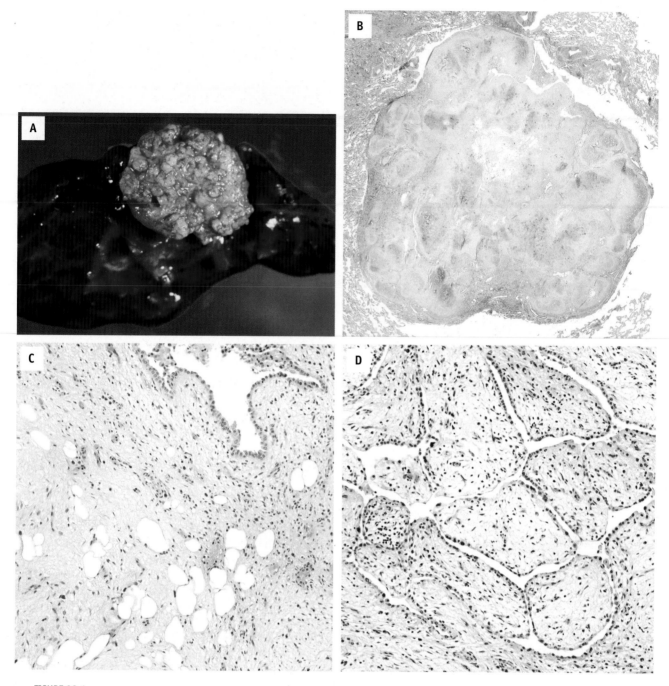

FIGURE 32-1

Hamartoma

(A) Hamartoma protruding from cut surface of lung with characteristic white, lobulated surface. **(B)** At low magnification, the multilobulated cartilaginous nature of the tumor is obvious. Note how the tumor tears away from surrounding lung tissue allowing easy removal by the surgeon. **(C)** Non-cartilaginous areas feature benign adipocytes admixed with myxoid fibrovascular tissue and entrapped respiratory epithelium. **(D)** The edges of the tumor contain non-neoplastic entrapped respiratory-type epithelium. This finding outlines the lesion but should not be mistaken for an epithelial tumor component.

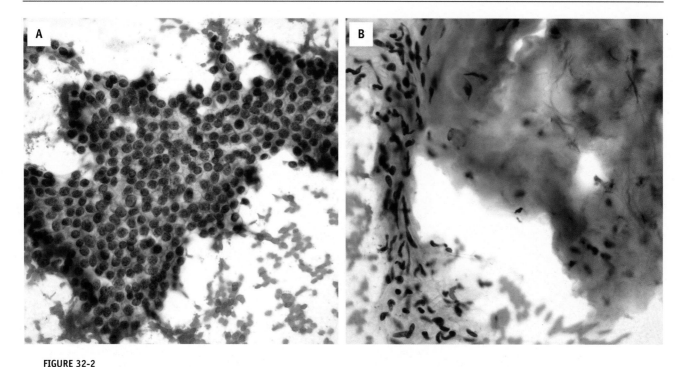

FIGURE 32-2

Hamartoma

Fine needle aspiration biopsy diagnosis of hamartoma should include sheets of benign respiratory-type epithelium **(A)** and mesenchymal elements such as cartilage or spindle cells in a myxoid matrix **(B)** (Papanicolaou stain).

the cartilaginous/fibromyxoid material, these elements may be subtle on Papanicolaou-stained smears. Also, the invaginated epithelium accompanying lesions can be plentiful and reactive and thus easily mistaken for adenocarcinoma or even carcinoid tumor. The absence of background necrosis, blood, and inflammation should aid in avoiding a diagnosis of malignancy while a cell block should highlight the mesenchymal elements and non-neoplastic nature of the epithelium.

DIFFERENTIAL DIAGNOSIS

Pulmonary hamartoma should be distinguished from monomorphic soft tissue tumors including bronchial chondroma and chondrosarcoma. Chondromas occur in young patients, primarily women, in the setting of Carney triad (pulmonary chondromas, gastrointestinal stromal tumors and extra-adrenal paragangliomas) but can also occur sporadically. Chondromas, unlike hamartomas, arise from and lie in continuity with bronchial cartilage, lack invaginated respiratory epithelium, and never contain other mesenchymal elements (Figure 32-3). While central hamartomas may feature increased chondrocyte cellularity and cytologic atypia, features diagnostic of chondrosarcoma in other anatomic locations, such findings are not indicative of malignancy as long as one correctly identifies another mesenchymal element in the tumor.

PROGNOSIS AND THERAPY

Pulmonary hamartomas are slow-growing benign neoplasms amenable to conservative surgical resection. In some instances sleeve excision or lobectomy may be required depending on the size and/or location of the tumor and peritumoral findings. Sarcomatous transformation of and adenocarcinomas arising in hamartomas are exceedingly rare events such that many radiographically detected and FNAB-proven hamartomas are followed rather than resected. Although it has been suggested that patients with hamartomas are at increased risk for subsequent lung cancer, supportive epidemiologic or pathologic evidence is lacking.

BENIGN SALIVARY GLAND-TYPE NEOPLASMS

Seromucinous glands within the walls of large bronchi can give rise to virtually any of the recognized benign salivary gland-type neoplasms. Pleomorphic adenomas, monomorphic adenomas, oncocytomas, myoepitheliomas, and adenomyoepitheliomas are extremely rare primary lung tumors. Of note, primary endobronchial or peripheral pleomorphic adenomas are less likely to feature either

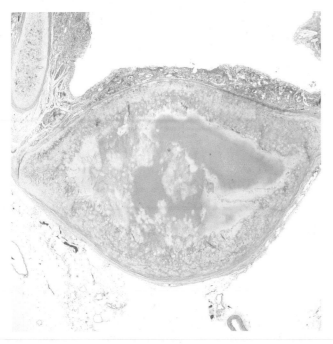

FIGURE 32-3
Chondroma
In distinction from hamartoma, this chondroma arises from the bronchial cartilage and lacks other mesenchymal components and epithelial invaginations.

a prominent glandular component or chondroid stroma than their salivary gland counterparts and rather resemble "cellular mixed tumor" with sheets or islands of epithelial and/or myoepithelial cells and a myxoid matrix.

MUCOUS GLAND ADENOMA

CLINICAL AND RADIOLOGIC FEATURES

This rare endobronchial tumor has been reported in children and the elderly with a mean age of 52 years. Thought to arise from bronchial mucus glands, most tumors are central, but peripheral lesions also have been described. In the largest series, women outnumbered men by 2.5 to 1. Individuals present with obstructive symptoms and radiographic studies may demonstrate a coin lesion or endobronchial mass in lobar or segmental bronchi with distal parenchymal consolidation.

MUCOUS GLAND ADENOMA—FACT SHEET

Definition
- Benign, predominantly exophytic tumor of the tracheobronchial seromucinous glands and ducts, composed of mucus-filled cysts, tubules, glands, and papillary formations lined by a spectrum of benign epithelium (World Health Organization)

Incidence
- Rare

Gender and Age Distribution
- In the largest series, women outnumbered men by 2.5 to 1
- Reported in children and the elderly with a mean age of 52 years

Clinical Features
- Obstructive symptoms

Radiologic Features
- Coin lesion or endobronchial mass in lobar or segmental bronchi with distal parenchymal consolidation

Prognosis and Therapy
- Should be conservatively resected via bronchoscopic extirpation or sleeve resection
- Lobectomy may be required if the peripheral lung is extensively damaged

---

MUCOUS GLAND ADENOMA—PATHOLOGIC FEATURES

Gross Findings
- Endobronchial tumors are white to tan with solid and cystic gelatinous surfaces

Microscopic Findings
- Well-circumscribed non-invasive tumors located internal to the bronchial cartilage
- Mucin-filled cysts may resemble colloid
- Epithelium may be tubulocystic or papillocystic
- Columnar, cuboidal, or flattened mucus-secreting cells line cysts
- Stroma is fibrous or hyalinized

Immunohistochemical Features
- Epithelial component positive for cytokeratin, EMA, and CEA
- Stromal component focally positive for smooth muscle actin and S-100 protein

Pathologic Differential Diagnosis
- Mucoepidermoid carcinoma
- Adenocarcinoma

PATHOLOGIC FEATURES

GROSS FINDINGS

Tumors range in size from 0.7 to 7.5 cm with a mean diameter of 2.3 cm. The white-pink to tan, smooth and shiny tumors have solid and cystic gelatinous cut surfaces.

MICROSCOPIC FINDINGS

Mucous gland adenomas are well-circumscribed and non-invasive exophytic masses located internal to the cartilage plates of the bronchial wall. Numerous neutral and acid mucin-filled cystic spaces protrude into bronchial lumens with an intact overlying respiratory epithelium (Figure 32-4A). Tubulocystic and papillocystic appearances are also common. Cysts are lined by cytologically bland columnar, cuboidal, or flattened mucus-secreting cells (Figure 32-4B). Oncocytic and clear cell changes are often observed. Intervening stroma is usually fibrous or hyalinized, and cyst contents may resemble colloid. Hyperchromasia, pleomorphism, and mitoses are not seen.

ANCILLARY STUDIES

IMMUNOHISTOCHEMISTRY

Epithelial cells stain for cytokeratin, EMA, and CEA while stromal cells are focally positive for smooth muscle actin and S-100 protein.

DIFFERENTIAL DIAGNOSIS

Mucoepidermoid carcinoma and adenocarcinoma comprise the morphologic differential diagnosis. Low-grade mucoepidermoid carcinoma may be predominantly glandular with dilated cysts, and distinction on endobronchial biopsy is probably not possible. Despite the architectural similarities, squamous and intermediate cells are only seen in mucoepidermoid carcinoma. Adenocarcinomas are rarely entirely exophytic without underlying invasion and feature cytologic atypia, mitoses, and necrosis.

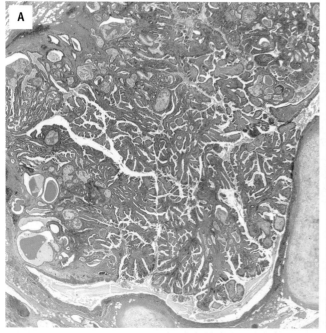
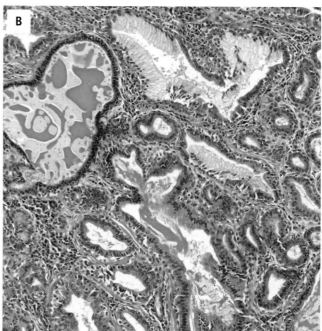

FIGURE 32-4

Mucous gland adenoma

(A) This complex endobronchial tumor features tubulocystic and papillocystic growth patterns. Mucin fills many spaces, and invasion of bronchial wall is not seen. **(B)** The glandular epithelium may be cuboidal, columnar, or mucinous. Stromal is often inflamed or hyalinized. Cytologic atypia is not seen.

PROGNOSIS AND THERAPY

These benign tumors should be conservatively resected via bronchoscopic extirpation or sleeve resection. Lobectomy may be required if the peripheral lung is extensively damaged.

MUCINOUS CYSTADENOMA

CLINICAL AND RADIOLOGIC FEATURES

Mucinous cystic neoplasms of the lung encompass a histologic spectrum of rare tumors ranging from mucinous cystadenoma to mucinous cystadenocarcinoma. While the former lesion is benign, mucinous cystadenocarcinoma is malignant but may have a slightly better prognosis than usual lung adenocarcinoma (see chapter 26). Of note, WHO does not recognize the existence of so-called pulmonary mucinous cystic tumors of borderline malignancy. Mucinous cystadenoma is a tumor of adults in their sixth and seventh decades of life. Most cases have been reported in tobacco smokers, yet an etiologic link has not been established. Patients are asymptomatic, and the tumor presents as an incidental

rounded well-demarcated mass without calcification on x-ray and CT scans. Since minimally invasive diagnostic procedures may yield mucin or clusters of goblet cells, surgical excision and complete histologic sampling are required for diagnosis.

PATHOLOGIC FEATURES

GROSS FINDINGS

Unilocular glistening gray mucus-filled cysts measure from 0.8 to 5.0 cm and lack mural nodules.

MICROSCOPIC FINDINGS

The simple unilocular cyst is filled with mucus, and the fibrous tissue wall is lined by a discontinuous layer of low cuboidal to tall columnar cells with considerable cytoplasmic mucin (Figure 32-5A, B). Nuclei are basally located, but focal pseudostratification can be seen. Nuclei are round or flattened, and nucleoli are inconspicuous. Distortion may suggest papillary fronds, but true papillae, necrosis, and cytologic atypia are not seen. Non-epithelialized segments of the cyst wall usually feature foreign-body giant cell reaction and lymphoplasmacytic infiltrates. Surrounding lung is often inflamed and atelectatic.

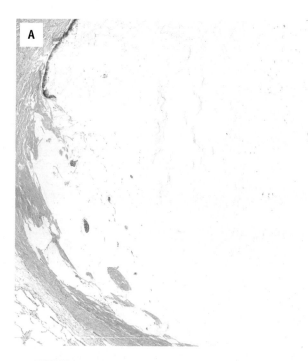

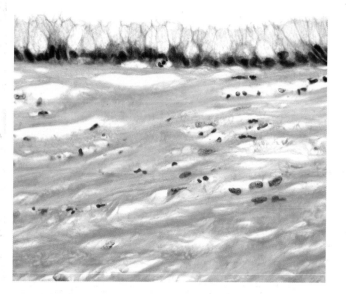

FIGURE 32-5

Mucinous cystadenoma

(A) This unilocular mucus-filled cyst is only focally lined with epithelium. The remainder of the cyst wall is fibrotic. **(B)** Cuboidal to columnar mucin-rich epithelial cells line the cyst wall. While all of the nuclei in this example have basal orientation, focal cellular stratification may be seen.

MUCINOUS CYSTADENOMA—FACT SHEET

Definition

▸ Benign localized cystic mass filled with mucin and surrounded by a fibrous wall lined by well-differentiated columnar mucinous epithelium (World Health Organization)

Incidence

▸ Rare

Age Distribution

▸ Adults in their sixth and seventh decades

Clinical Features

▸ Usually asymptomatic

Radiologic Features

▸ Rounded well-demarcated mass without calcification

Prognosis and Therapy

▸ Benign tumors that are almost always cured by complete excision

---

MUCINOUS CYSTADENOMA—PATHOLOGIC FEATURES

Gross Findings

▸ Unilocular cyst filled with gelatinous mucin, measuring up to 5.0 cm
▸ No mural nodules

Microscopic Findings

▸ Mucus-filled cyst with fibrous wall partially lined by epithelium
▸ Discontinuous epithelial layer of cuboidal to columnar cells with cytoplasmic mucin
▸ Nuclei basally located with minimal crowding
▸ Foreign-body giant cell reaction and stromal inflammation prominent

Immunohistochemical Features

▸ Mucinous epithelium is cytokeratin- and CK7-positive

Pathologic Differential Diagnosis

▸ Mucinous cystadenocarcinoma
▸ Primary or metastatic mucinous "colloid" adenocarcinoma
▸ Intrapulmonary bronchogenic cyst

ANCILLARY STUDIES

IMMUNOHISTOCHEMISTRY

The mucinous epithelium is cytokeratin- and CK7-positive and usually CK20- and TTF-1-negative.

DIFFERENTIAL DIAGNOSIS

Mucinous cystadenoma should be differentiated from overt malignancies, including mucinous cystadenocarcinoma and mucinous "colloid" adenocarcinoma, as well as developmental and post-infectious lesions. Primary lung and metastatic mucinous carcinomas may not feature overt malignant cytologic features, yet mucus extravasation and tumor cells floating in mucin are seen. CK7 positivity can aid in discerning a primary lung from metastatic colon tumor. Mucinous bronchioloalveolar carcinoma may line emphysematous parenchyma and appear cystic, but it always features lepidic growth. Intrapulmonary bronchogenic cysts are at least in part lined by ciliated columnar epithelium. The fibrous tissue wall also features cartilage and/or seromucinous glands.

PROGNOSIS AND THERAPY

Mucinous cystadenomas are benign tumors. With only one documented local recurrence, it appears that complete excision is curative.

ALVEOLAR ADENOMA

CLINICAL FEATURES

Alveolar adenomas are rare benign peripheral lung tumors, probably representing a combined proliferation of pneumocytes and septal mesenchyme. A slight female predominance and a mean presenting age of 53 years are noted. Virtually all tumors are peripheral, usually subpleural, and almost always incidental radiographic findings. Neither morbidity nor mortality associated with this tumor has been reported.

RADIOLOGIC FEATURES

Chest x-ray and CT appearances are those of a well-circumscribed homogenous noncalcified mass, while contrast enhancement on CT and MRI displays cystic spaces with central fluid and rim enhancement.

ALVEOLAR ADENOMA—FACT SHEET

Definition

▸ Benign peripheral lung tumor consisting of low cuboidal epithelium lining a network of spaces separated by a variably thin to thick spindle cell-rich stroma (World Health Organization)

Incidence

▸ Rare

Gender and Age Distribution

▸ Slight female predominance
▸ Mean presenting age of 53 years

Clinical Features

▸ Usually asymptomatic

Radiologic Features

▸ Well-circumscribed homogenous non-calcified peripheral lung mass
▸ Contrast enhancement on CT and MRI displays cystic spaces with central fluid and rim enhancement

Prognosis and Therapy

▸ Conservative surgical excision is curative

ALVEOLAR ADENOMA—PATHOLOGIC FEATURES

Gross Findings

▸ Well demarcated and multicystic with yellow to tan cut surfaces

Microscopic Findings

▸ Multicystic with spaces filled with eosinophilic granular debris
▸ Central cysts larger than peripheral spaces
▸ Cysts lined by bland cuboidal and hobnail cells
▸ Interstitium is myxoid and collagenous with bland spindle cells

Immunohistochemical Features

▸ Epithelial component positive for cytokeratin and TTF-1
▸ Stromal component focally positive for actins

Pathologic Differential Diagnosis

▸ Lymphangioma
▸ Sclerosing hemangioma
▸ Bronchioloalveolar carcinoma

PATHOLOGIC FEATURES

GROSS FINDINGS

Tumors measure from 0.7 to 6.0 cm and appear well demarcated, lobulated, and multicystic with soft to firm pale yellow to tan cut surfaces.

MICROSCOPIC FINDINGS

Alveolar adenomas are well-circumscribed unencapsulated multicystic biphasic tumors with ectatic spaces filled with eosinophilic granular material (Figures 32-6A, B). Spaces are lined by cytologically bland cuboidal and hobnail cells (Figure 32-6C). The interstitium is myxoid and collagenous with bland spindle cells. Cystic spaces are larger in the center of the lesion, and foci of squamous metaplasia can be seen. Mitoses and necrosis are absent.

ANCILLARY STUDIES

IMMUNOHISTOCHEMISTRY

Epithelial lining cells stain for cytokeratin, TTF-1, and surfactant apoproteins, indicating a type II pneumocyte phenotype, while stromal cells are focally positive for smooth muscle and muscle-specific actin.

DIFFERENTIAL DIAGNOSIS

The differential diagnosis includes lymphangioma, sclerosing hemangioma, and adenocarcinoma, bronchioloalveolar subtype. Lining cell positivity for cytokeratin confidently excludes lymphangioma from consideration, while the single growth pattern, absence of blood lakes, and stromal cell negativity for TTF-1 distinguish alveolar adenoma from sclerosing hemangioma (see below). Bronchioloalveolar carcinoma is never well circumscribed, lacks a stromal component, and features cellular crowding with at least mild cytologic atypia.

PROGNOSIS AND THERAPY

Conservative surgical excision is curative.

PAPILLARY ADENOMA

CLINICAL FEATURES

A very rare neoplasm, fewer than 20 papillary adenomas have been reported. Males appear to predominate, and the tumor has been documented in individuals from age 7 to 60 years. The peripheral parenchymal lesion does not involve airways and comes to clinical attention as an incidental radiographic finding. The tumor is thought to arise from a bronchoalveolar stem

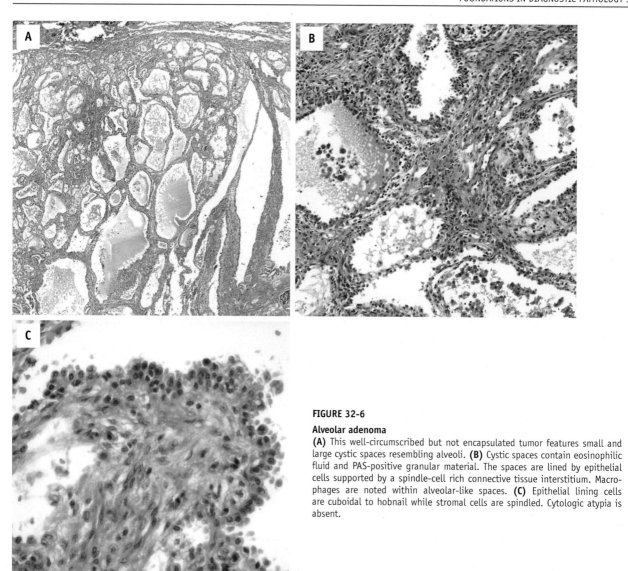

FIGURE 32-6

Alveolar adenoma

(A) This well-circumscribed but not encapsulated tumor features small and large cystic spaces resembling alveoli. **(B)** Cystic spaces contain eosinophilic fluid and PAS-positive granular material. The spaces are lined by epithelial cells supported by a spindle-cell rich connective tissue interstitium. Macrophages are noted within alveolar-like spaces. **(C)** Epithelial lining cells are cuboidal to hobnail while stromal cells are spindled. Cytologic atypia is absent.

PAPILLARY ADENOMA—FACT SHEET

Definition

➤ Benign circumscribed papillary neoplasm composed of cytologically bland epithelial cells lining fibrovascular cores (World Health Organization)

Incidence

➤ Rare

Gender and Age Distribution

➤ Males appear to predominate
➤ Patient ages between 7 and 60 years

Clinical Features

➤ Asymptomatic

Radiologic Features

➤ Peripheral parenchymal lesion

Prognosis and Therapy

➤ Surgical excision is curative

PAPILLARY ADENOMA—PATHOLOGIC FEATURES

Gross Findings

➤ Well circumscribed up to 4.0 cm in diameter
➤ Tan brown and spongy cut surfaces

Microscopic Findings

➤ Complex fibrovascular cores may be inflamed
➤ Epithelium is cuboidal to columnar with smooth eosinophilic cytoplasm
➤ Eosinophilic intranuclear inclusions can be seen
➤ Atypia, mitoses, and necrosis are absent

Immunohistochemical Features

➤ Epithelial component positive for cytokeratin, TTF-1, Clara cell protein

Pathologic Differential Diagnosis

➤ Sclerosing hemangioma
➤ Papillary adenocarcinoma
➤ Papillary carcinoid tumor

cell that can differentiate towards type II pneumocytes, ciliated respiratory epithelium, or Clara cells.

PATHOLOGIC FEATURES

GROSS FINDINGS

Usually well circumscribed, 1.0- to 4.0-cm tumors, with a tan, brown spongy cut surface.

MICROSCOPIC FINDINGS

Most examples lack infiltrative growth, and tumors are composed of fibrovascular cores lined by cuboidal to columnar epithelial cells with smooth eosinophilic cytoplasm (Figures 32-7A, B). Ciliated and oncocytic cells can be seen, and nuclei are round to oval with occasional eosinophilic intranuclear inclusions. Atypia and mitoses are rare to absent, and necrosis is not seen.

ANCILLARY STUDIES

IMMUNOHISTOCHEMISTRY

Papillary adenomas stain for cytokeratin, Clara cell protein, TTF-1, and surfactant apoproteins, but not chromogranin or synaptophysin.

DIFFERENTIAL DIAGNOSIS

One is more likely to be dealing with a sclerosing hemangioma, papillary adenocarcinoma, or papillary carcinoid tumor and should consider these lesions before diagnosing a papillary adenoma. Sclerosing hemangioma features several architectural patterns and both "surface" and "stromal" cells stain for TTF-1. Primary lung papillary adenocarcinoma and metastatic papillary thyroid carcinoma have infiltrative growth patterns in addition to crowded fibrovascular cores and nuclear atypia. Eosinophilic intranuclear inclusions are not a discerning feature. Papillary carcinoid tumor has granular cytoplasm and finely granular chromatin as well as neuroendocrine marker staining.

PROGNOSIS AND THERAPY

Surgical excision is curative.

SOLITARY PAPILLOMAS

CLINICAL FEATURES

Solitary papillomas are rare endobronchial tumors. Most papillomas feature a squamous epithelial surface. Solitary squamous cell papillomas are seen predominantly

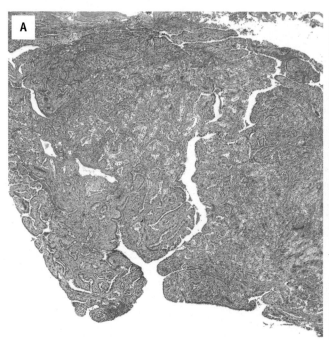
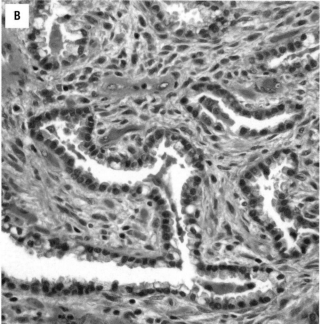

FIGURE 32-7

Papillary adenoma

(A) This well-circumscribed benign neoplasm is composed of epithelial-lined fibrovascular cores. **(B)** Cuboidal and columnar epithelium features clear and granular cytoplasm resembling Clara cells. Nuclei are round and regular and no atypia or mitotic activity are seen. The stroma is vascular and often inflamed.

SOLITARY PAPILLOMAS—FACT SHEET

Definition

▸ Papillary tumors consisting of delicate connective tissue fronds with squamous, glandular, or mixed epithelial surfaces (World Health Organization)

Incidence

▸ Rare

Gender and Age Distribution

▸ Solitary squamous cell papillomas occur predominantly in men with a median age of 54 years

Clinical Features

▸ Obstructive symptoms

Radiologic Features

▸ CT scans demonstrate small endobronchial protuberances or nodular airway thickening
▸ Distal nodular opacities and bronchiectasis may be seen

Prognosis and Therapy

▸ Complete surgical excision is recommended
▸ Incomplete excision may be followed by recurrence

SOLITARY PAPILLOMAS—PATHOLOGIC FEATURES

Gross Findings

▸ Range from 0.2 to 9.0 cm
▸ Arise from mainstem bronchi or major segmental bronchi
▸ Tan white soft to tan semi-firm endobronchial excrescences

Microscopic Findings

▸ Loose fibrovascular cores covered with either stratified squamous single layer or pseudostratified layer of glandular epithelium, or a combination of the two
▸ Squamous cell papillomas can be exophytic or inverted
▸ Squamous lesions feature orderly squamous maturation ending with keratinized surface cells
▸ Squamous lesions may feature HPV cytopathic effect or dysplasia related to HPV infection
▸ Glandular lesions can be lined by any cell type seen in respiratory epithelium
▸ Mixed lesions require 30% of the minor component

Pathologic Differential Diagnosis

▸ Inflammatory polyps
▸ Squamous cell carcinoma
▸ Adenocarcinoma
▸ Papillary adenoma

in men with a median age of 54 years, and juvenile and adult laryngotracheal papillomatosis rarely involves the lower respiratory tract. Although more than half of patients are tobacco smokers, an etiologic role has not been established. However, an association with human papilloma virus (HPV) subtypes 6/11 and 16/18 suggests a possible pathogenetic role for the virus. HPV has not been identified in either glandular or mixed squamous cell or glandular papillomas. Most patients present with obstructive symptoms. HPV subtyping of squamous lesions may be prognostically useful, but all papillomas have a benign clinical course when completely excised.

RADIOLOGIC FEATURES

Computed tomography scans demonstrate small endobronchial protuberances or nodular airway thickening. Distal nodular opacities and bronchiectasis may be seen.

PATHOLOGIC FEATURES

GROSS FINDINGS

Solitary papillomas usually arise from the walls of large caliber bronchi. Lesions can be white to tan-red and semi-firm with either a papillary or solid appearance. Tumors range from 0.2 to 9.0 cm with a median size of 1.5 cm.

MICROSCOPIC FINDINGS

Exophytic squamous cell papillomas are composed of a loose fibrovascular core covered by stratified squamous epithelium (Figure 32-8A). Maturation from the basal layer to the surface is seen, and hyperkeratosis may be present. Over 20% of these tumors feature clumped keratohyaline and eosinophilic cytoplasmic inclusions as well as koilocytic change (Figure 32-8B). Dysplasia may be encountered. Interestingly, HPV 6/11 is noted in uncomplicated cases, whereas those with dysplasia are more often associated with HPV 16/18.

Inverted lesions have both exophytic and random invaginations of squamous epithelium. Basal lamina invests the endophytic nests. Involvement of bronchial wall seromucinous glands can be prominent.

Glandular papillomas feature non-inflamed thick arborizing stromal stalks lined by pseudostratified or columnar epithelium without micropapillary fronds (Figure 32-9). Epithelium may be ciliated or non-ciliated, cuboidal or columnar, and goblet cells may be interspersed. The cytoplasm may be clear or eosinophilic, and nuclei are bland without atypia or mitotic activity. No necrosis is noted.

Mixed squamous cell and glandular papillomas feature both squamous and glandular epithelium (Figure 32-10). The World Health Organization stipulates that at least

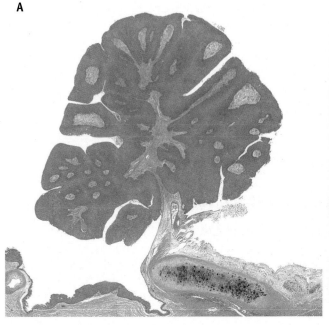

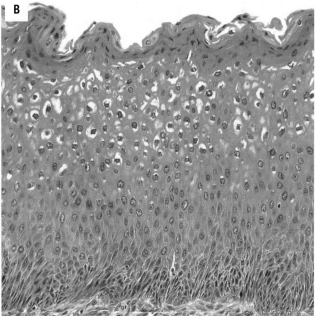

FIGURE 32-8

Squamous cell papilloma

(A) This exophytic papilloma is attached to the bronchial wall by a stalk and features bulbous epithelial-rich papillae. **(B)** Approximately 20% of squamous cell papillomas feature wrinkled nuclei, binucleate forms, and perinuclear halos indicative of HPV infection. Parakeratosis is also a common finding.

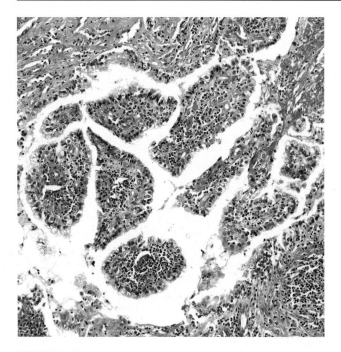

FIGURE 32-9

Glandular papilloma

Inflamed fibrovascular cores are lined by columnar epithelium with focal clear cell change. Cellular crowding, cytologic atypia, and mitoses are absent. Unlike papillary adenomas, glandular papillomas are endobronchial tumors.

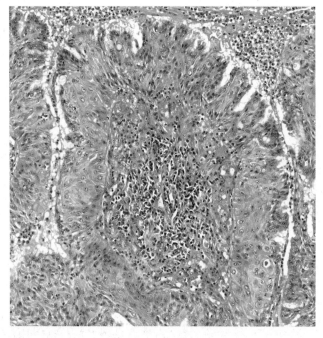

FIGURE 32-10

Mixed squamous cell and glandular papilloma

Inflamed fibrovascular cores are lined by both glandular-respiratory-type and non-keratinizing squamous epithelium. The squamous component may feature dysplasia, but unlike squamous cell papillomas, viral cytopathic change has not been reported. Glandular atypia and necrosis are not seen.

30% of the epithelium should be of the second epithelial type. Squamous atypia can be seen but glandular atypia or tumoral necrosis should not be present.

DIFFERENTIAL DIAGNOSIS

Squamous cell papillomas should be distinguished from inflammatory polyps and squamous cell carcinoma. Inflammatory endobronchial polyps may show focal squamous metaplasia but are usually composed of voluminous granulation tissue-like stroma and subepithelial dense lymphoplasmacytic infiltrates. Surface epithelium is not commonly proliferative. Well-differentiated squamous cell carcinoma can be papillary and endobronchial but usually demonstrates malignant cytologic features in addition to irregular infiltrating nests of cells within desmoplastic stroma. Entrapped glands within the stalk of the papilloma should not be mistaken for invasion. Inverted squamous cell papillomas with mild cytologic atypia may be indistinguishable from invasive squamous cell carcinoma. Features supporting a diagnosis of carcinoma include parenchymal destruction, cellular pleomorphism, loss of maturation, prominent dyskeratosis, and hyperkeratosis.

Glandular papillomas should not be misdiagnosed as adenocarcinoma and can be distinguished from other rare lesions, including papillary adenomas and the papillary variant of mucus gland adenoma. Carcinoma features epithelial crowding, malignant cytology, and usually bronchial wall invasion. Papillary adenomas are parenchymal lesions without airway wall attachment, while the papillary variant of mucus gland adenoma lacks large fibrovascular stromal cores.

Of note, bronchoscopic cytologic specimens and endobronchial biopsies can only suggest a diagnosis of papilloma, but complete excision is required for a definitive diagnosis.

PROGNOSIS AND THERAPY

Solitary squamous cell papillomas are considered benign tumors, but the focal presence of cytologic atypia, occasional presence of HPV subtypes 6, 11, 16, and 18, and reports of squamous cell carcinoma arising at prior papilloma excision sites all emphasize the need for complete removal. It has been suggested that papillomas with HPV 16/18 have a higher risk of carcinomatous transformation. Progression to papillomatosis is very rare and may be related to electrical or laser fulguration. Glandular and mixed papillomas are also benign but may recur if incompletely excised.

SCLEROSING HEMANGIOMA

CLINICAL FEATURES

Described in the United States almost 50 years ago, sclerosing hemangioma (SH) is still of great academic interest. Although never considered a vascular lesion, it was named such on account of the frequent hemorrhage and hemosiderin within the tumor. Although this misnomer resonates with pathologists, a reasonable alternative designation is pneumocytoma since current evidence suggests a primitive undifferentiated respiratory epithelial cell origin. Interestingly, the two different types of neoplastic cells comprising the tumor feature the same monoclonal pattern. Also, one of the tumor cells, the so-called stromal cell, has no normal counterpart in human lung. Sclerosing hemangioma is quite rare in Western countries but has an incidence comparable to carcinoid tumor in Japan. Cases have been reported in all age groups including children, but the median age of patients is 46 years. Eighty percent of tumors arise in women, and approximately 20% of patients present with respiratory complaints such as cough, hemoptysis, or chest pain. Tumors can involve any lobe, but there are few reports of endobronchial, pleural, and mediastinal locations. Most lesions are solitary, but 4% are multifocal. Hilar and mediastinal lymph node metastases were reported in less than 1% of cases of this benign or very low-grade neoplasm.

RADIOLOGIC FEATURES

Chest x-rays demonstrate well-defined homogeneous round tumors with occasional cystic changes and rare calcification. CT findings show marked contrast enhancement with foci of low attenuation, indicating cystic change.

PATHOLOGIC FEATURES

GROSS FINDINGS

Sclerosing hemangiomas range in size from 0.3 to 10 cm, but most are less than 3.0 cm in greatest dimension. Tumors are sharply circumscribed with solid gray to tan and yellow smooth or mottled cut surfaces. Intratumoral hemorrhage may be focal or extensive, and cysts or calcification may be observed.

MICROSCOPIC FINDINGS

Tumor histology features four distinct architectural patterns and two neoplastic cell types (Figures 32-11A, B). The majority of tumors demonstrate papillary, sclerotic, solid, and hemorrhagic growth patterns; more than one third feature three of the patterns. The remainder contain only two patterns, and only rare cases have a single architectural pattern (which some might not consider a SH but rather an adenoma). The papillary pattern is the most plentiful but may merge with sclerotic areas, as foci of hyaline collagen can expand papillary stalks as well as form solid sheets. The solid pattern may contain small tubules, and the hemorrhagic areas feature large blood-filled spaces lined by tumor cells.

Cuboidal tumor cells (also called surface cells), line papillae and, cysts, and form tubules, whereas round cells (so-called stromal cells) fill the papillary cores and form the sheets in solid areas. The "surface cells" are cuboidal with voluminous eosinophilic cytoplasm and prominent nuclei. Intranuclear inclusions and multinucleation are often observed (Figures 32-11C, D). The "stromal cells" are slightly smaller than the "surface cells" and are typically described as having well-defined borders, clear to eosinophilic cytoplasm, a central location, round to oval nuclei with fine dispersed chromatin, and usually indiscernible nucleoli. However, oftentimes these cells are indistinguishable from the "surface cells." Cytoplasmic vacuoles may even resemble signet-ring cells. Focal nuclear atypia can be seen in either cell type, and mitotic indices are low with reports of no more than 1 per 10 high-power (×40) fields.

Associated histologic findings include xanthoma cells, cholesterol clefts, hemosiderin, and calcification, as well as laminated whorls, granulomas, necrosis, mature adipose tissue, and numerous mast cells. Nests of neuroendocrine cells can also be seen, and on very rare occasions, sclerosing hemangioma may be combined with a typical carcinoid tumor.

ANCILLARY STUDIES

ULTRASTRUCTURAL FEATURES

Both types of epithelial cells demonstrate type II pneumocytic features including cytoplasmic lamellar bodies.

IMMUNOHISTOCHEMISTRY

"Surface cells" express pancytokeratin, cytokeratin 7 (CK7), epithelial membrane antigen (EMA), thyroid transcription factor-1 (TTF-1), and surfactant apoprotein A. "Stromal cells" are usually pancytokeratin negative but EMA and TTF-1 positive. Interestingly they are

---

SCLEROSING HEMANGIOMA—FACT SHEET

Definition

» Rare benign neoplasm with a distinctive variety of histologic patterns, lined by and filled with two distinctive types of epithelial cells (World Health Organization)

Incidence and Location

» Rare in Western countries but more common in Japan

Gender and Age Distribution

» Reported in all age groups including children; the median age of patients is 46 years
» 80% occur in women

Clinical Features

» 20% of patients have respiratory complaints such as cough, hemoptysis, or chest pain

Radiologic Features

» Most lesions are solitary, but 4% are multifocal, and any lobe can be affected
» Chest x-rays show well-defined homogeneous round tumors with occasional cystic change and rare calcification
» CT demonstrates marked contrast enhancement with foci of low attenuation, indicating cystic change

Prognosis and Therapy

» Hilar and mediastinal lymph node metastases are rare
» Complete surgical excision is curative
» No reported recurrences or tumor-related deaths

SCLEROSING HEMANGIOMA—PATHOLOGIC FEATURES

Gross Findings

» Mostly solitary and peripheral
» Sharply circumscribed with solid gray to tan cut surfaces with hemorrhage and cystic spaces usually seen

Microscopic Findings

» Tumors usually feature papillary, sclerotic, solid, and hemorrhagic growth types; more than 30% feature three of these four patterns
» Papillary pattern most frequent
» "Surface cells" line papillae, cysts, and form tubules; "stromal cells" fill the papillae and solid areas
» "Surface cells" are cuboidal with eosinophilic cytoplasm and large nuclei, intranuclear inclusions, and occasional multinucleation
» "Stromal cells" are round with well-defined borders and central round nuclei with fine chromatin with rare signet-ring forms
» Secondary findings include xanthoma cells, cholesterol clefts, hemosiderin, calcification, and adipose tissue

Immunohistochemical Features

» "Surface cells" express cytokeratin, CK7, EMA, and TTF-1
» "Stromal cells" express EMA and TTF-1 but rarely cytokeratin or CK7

Fine Needle Aspiration Biopsy Findings

» Moderately cellular with both epithelial types arranged in tight papillary clusters or flat sheets
» Xanthoma cells, hemosiderin, and red blood cells are often seen

Pathologic Differential Diagnosis

» Papillary adenocarcinoma of the lung, thyroid, and salivary gland
» Typical carcinoid tumor
» Clear cell tumors

---

also CK7 and surfactant apoprotein A and B negative (Figure 32-12). Progesterone receptor expression is observed in more than half of "stromal cells," suggesting a role for female sex hormones in the development of this female-predominant tumor.

FINE NEEDLE ASPIRATION BIOPSY

While the cytomorphologic features of SH have been described, one should exercise great caution before making a definitive diagnosis given the great similarities to lung adenocarcinoma and carcinoid tumor. Good samples are moderately cellular and feature both epithelial cell types arranged in tight papillary clusters or flat sheets. The round to polygonal or even spindled "surface cells" with clear chromatin and intranuclear inclusions and round "stromal cells" with clear to eosinophilic cytoplasm and indistinct nucleoli may be accompanied by xanthoma cells, binucleate cells, hemosiderin-laden macrophages, red blood cells, and lamellar concretions, but necrosis, pleomorphism, and atypia are not seen.

DIFFERENTIAL DIAGNOSIS

The differential diagnosis includes both primary lung and metastatic tumors. Since carcinomas can have pure papillary or mixed papillary and solid architecture with bland nuclei, intranuclear inclusions, and multinucleated tumor cells (as seen in bronchioloalveolar carcinoma), one should predicate a diagnosis of SH on the presence of at least two architectural patterns in addition to identifying the two cell populations. Both metastatic papillary thyroid carcinoma and the papillary variant of low-grade mucoepidermoid carcinoma lack additional architectural patterns, and the latter features an intimate admixture of squamous and mucinous cells. TTF-1-positivity in papillary thyroid carcinoma should not lead to an erroneous diagnosis of SH. Typical carcinoid tumor (TC), including the papillary subtype, lacks architectural variety and features only one cell type. Round regular nuclei with finely granular chromatin also characterize typical

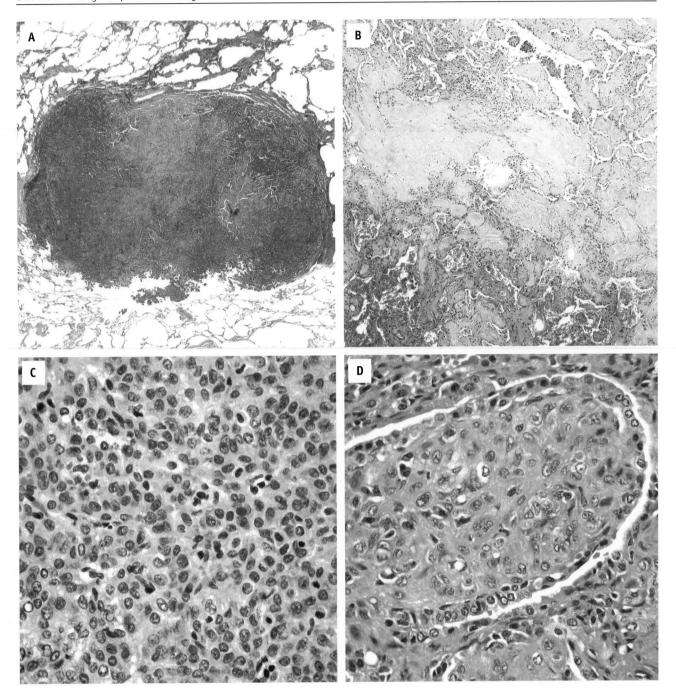

FIGURE 32-11

Sclerosing hemangioma

(A) This well-circumscribed tumor features papillary, solid, hemorrhagic, and sclerotic growth patterns at low magnification. **(B)** At higher magnification, one appreciates the merging of different growth patterns. Sclerotic papillary cores merge to form expansive areas of fibrosis. **(C)** Solid areas are composed of stromal cells. While classically described as having well-defined borders, round nuclei with fine chromatin, and rare nucleoli, morphologic variability can be observed. **(D)** Surface cells are cuboidal with eosinophilic cytoplasm and occasional intranuclear inclusions. The stromal cells are irregular in size and shape.

carcinoid tumor. Strong staining with chromogranin and/or synaptophysin also discriminates TC from SH. Clear cell lesions including clear cell "sugar" tumor of lung and metastatic renal cell carcinoma may be considered in the broad differential diagnosis owing to clear cytoplasm and tumor vascularity, but the sinusoidal vascular patterns of these tumors differ greatly

from the blood lakes observed in SH, and neither of these lesions has the distinct varied architectural patterns, two cell populations without cytologic atypia, or immunohistochemical profile of SH.

A particularly difficult diagnostic dilemma can arise when a small coin lesion arrives in the frozen section laboratory. A diagnosis of carcinoma or carcinoid tumor

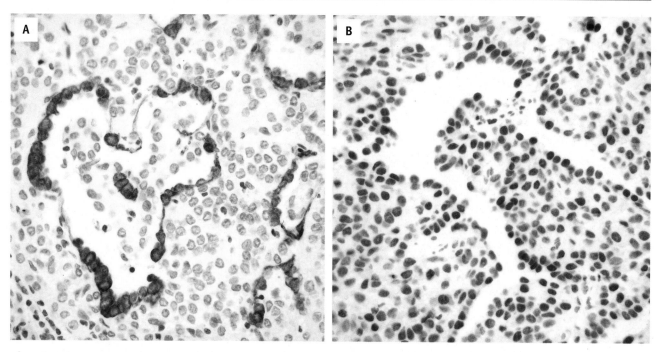

FIGURE 32-12

Sclerosing hemangioma

Only surface cells react with anti-cytokeratin antibodies. The stromal cells are negative **(A)**. Interestingly, both cell types are positive for TTF-1 **(B)**.

results in a thoracotomy and lobectomy, whereas a diagnosis of SH requires no further treatment. Most cases of SH are diagnosable at frozen section if one recognizes tumor circumscription at the macro- and microscopic levels and various histologic growth patterns. Cytologic atypia or the predominance of a single architectural pattern should increase the possibility of a carcinoma, and a definitive diagnosis should be deferred.

PROGNOSIS AND THERAPY

Sclerosing hemangioma is a clinically benign tumor. No recurrences or tumor-related deaths have been reported, even in the rare instances of multifocal tumors or intrathoracic lymph node metastases. Surgical excision alone is curative.

CLEAR CELL TUMOR

CLINICAL FEATURES

Clear cell tumor of the lung (CCTL) is an extremely rare usually benign neoplasm which, until recently, was of uncertain histogenesis. However, an association

with the tuberous sclerosis-associated lesions angiomyolipoma, lymphangioleiomyomatosis, and micronodular pneumocyte hyperplasia led investigators to conclude that the tumor originates from perivascular epithelioid cells (PEC), and belongs to a body-wide collection of clear cell tumors termed PEComas. Interestingly, diffuse pulmonary interstitial involvement with similar tumor-like cells has been reported. Alternate designations include "sugar" tumor and epithelioid myomelanocytoma. The tumor is usually seen in adults, but cases in children and the elderly have been reported. There is a slight female predominance. Most lesions arise in peripheral lung, but endobronchial and tracheal lesions also have been documented. A lobar predilection is not recognized. The peripheral lesions do not produce symptoms, whereas the central lesions present with dyspnea, cough, or hemoptysis.

PATHOLOGIC FEATURES

GROSS FINDINGS

Clear cell tumors range from a few millimeters to 6.5 cm in size, with a median of 2.0 cm. The well-circumscribed tumors shell out from surrounding lung parenchyma and feature a red-tan uniform cut surface. Necrosis and hemorrhage are almost never seen.

ANCILLARY STUDIES

ULTRASTRUCTURAL FEATURES

Electron microscopy indicates that tumor cells contain abundant free and membrane-bound glycogen as well as premelanosomes. Interdigitating cellular processes, pericellular basal lamina, and plasmalemmal pinocytosis have also been described.

IMMUNOHISTOCHEMISTRY

Tumor cells are consistently positive for vimentin, HMB-45, and MART-1, and negative for epithelial markers. CD117 and collagen type IV also stain tumor cells, while S-100 protein, CD34, and muscle-specific actin are often at least focally positive.

DIFFERENTIAL DIAGNOSIS

The differential diagnosis includes epithelial and nonepithelial tumors. Clear cell carcinomas or carcinomas with clear cells originating in the lung or metastatic from renal, breast, or salivary gland primaries may have bland cytology, rare mitoses, and cytoplasmic glycogen, but all stain for epithelial markers such as cytokeratins or EMA. Unlike CCTL, carcinomas are also HMB-45 negative. Metastatic clear cell sarcoma and malignant

MICROSCOPIC FINDINGS

The unencapsulated but well-circumscribed tumor features sheets or vague nests of neoplastic cells surrounded or compartmentalized by thin-walled vascular channels lacking a muscular wall and focal hyaline stroma that may become calcified (Figure 32-13A). Entrapped respiratory epithelium is often seen around the edges of the tumor. Tumor cells are round to oval with occasional spindled forms. Cells have distinct cell borders and abundant clear to lightly eosinophilic granular cytoplasm. Nuclei vary in size and shape but are usually oval with finely granular chromatin and occasional nucleoli (Figure 32-13B). Multinucleated cells are seen in most tumors and may be prominent. Occasional large cells with granules radiating from the nucleus in a linear fashion are called spider cells, while rare cells with acidophilic cytoplasm are called neuroid cells. Finely granular brown lipochrome pigment can be seen but should not be mistaken for melanin pigment. Mitoses are virtually absent. Since tumor cells are filled with glycogen, strong PAS positivity is noted along with diastase sensitivity (Figures. 32-13C, D).

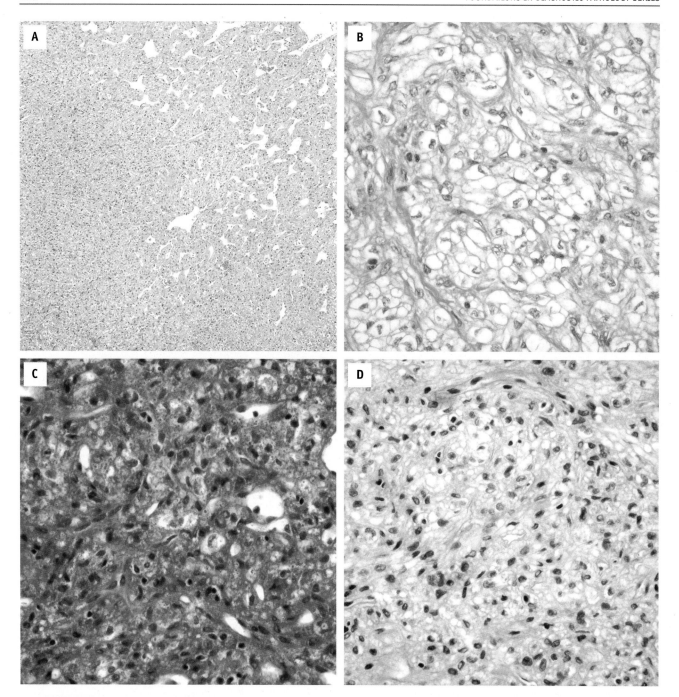

FIGURE 32-13

Clear cell tumor

(A) This rare tumor features sheets or nests of cells separated by thin-walled vascular channels lacking a muscular layer. Necrosis and hemorrhage are absent. (B) High magnification demonstrates nests of oval tumor cells with distinct cell borders and abundant clear cytoplasm. There is variation in nuclear size, and nucleoli may be prominent. Abundant cytoplasmic glycogen is demonstrated with a periodic acid-Schiff (PAS) stain (C), and the glycogen is removed after diastase digestion (D).

melanoma, especially the "balloon cell" variant, differ only in their light microscopic morphologies. These malignancies invariably feature cytologic atypia and mitotic activity and lack the ectatic vascular spaces without a muscle layer seen in CCTL. The clear cell variant of typical carcinoid tumor lacks cytoplasmic glycogen and is cytokeratin positive. A granular cell tumor may share morphologic features with CCTL as well as S-100 protein positivity, but this lesion lacks cytoplasmic glycogen and is HMB-45 negative. Lastly, a diagnosis of CCTL should not be made on cytologic or frozen section specimens.

PROGNOSIS AND THERAPY

While most of the case reports and small series report a benign clinical course, two tumors did metastasize and one was deadly. Nevertheless, conservative surgical resection is considered curative.

GRANULAR CELL TUMOR

CLINICAL FEATURES

Granular cell tumors (GCT) are usually benign neoplasms found in many anatomic locations throughout the body. While most are located in the tongue, skin, and breast, a small percentage (no more than 6%) are seen in the bronchial tree or lung. Though originally thought to be of skeletal muscle derivation, late 20th century studies suggest a peripheral nerve sheath and probably Schwann cell origin. Older terms include granular cell myoblas-

toma and Abrikossoff tumor in honor of the original descriptor. Tumors have been reported in all ages, but the median age is 40 years and men and women are equally affected. A slight predilection for individuals of African descent has been reported. Most tumors are endobronchial, often located near bifurcations, and thus the majority of patients present with cough, recurrent obstructive pneumonia, asthma, or hemoptysis. Most tumors are solitary, but multifocal endobronchial or both endobronchial and parenchymal tumors occur in 10% of patients. Rare individuals present with bronchopulmonary and cutaneous GCTs. Interestingly, approximately 10% of patients with GCT also have coexistent malignant neoplasms arising from the lung, kidney, or esophagus.

RADIOLOGIC FEATURES

Although x-rays may show atelectasis or pneumonia, endobronchial or peripheral coin lesions may be identified. Computed tomography may show an infiltrative border in central lesions and a spiculated appearance in peripheral tumors, suggesting a diagnosis of malignancy. Multifocal tumors raise the possibility of metastatic disease.

GRANULAR CELL TUMOR—FACT SHEET

Definition
- Benign neural tumor characterized by large granular-appearing eosinophilic cells (World Health Organization)

Incidence
- Uncommon pulmonary neoplasm

Gender and Age Distribution
- Reported in all ages, but the median age is 40 years
- No gender predominance
- Slight predilection for individuals of African descent

Clinical Features
- Symptoms include cough, recurrent obstructive pneumonia, asthma, and hemoptysis
- Rare individuals present with bronchopulmonary and cutaneous GCTs, and about 10% have coexistent malignant neoplasms arising from the lung, kidney, or esophagus

Radiologic Features
- Endobronchial or peripheral coin lesions that may have an infiltrative border or a spiculated appearance

Prognosis and Therapy
- The clinical course is benign
- Conservative surgical resection, bronchoscopic extirpation, laser therapy, or sleeve resection can be performed
- Some asymptomatic small endobronchial tumors are followed
- Tumors that have caused extensive destruction of distal lung parenchyma may require lobectomy or pneumonectomy

---

GRANULAR CELL TUMOR—PATHOLOGIC FEATURES

Gross Findings
- Endobronchial lesions may cause mucosal distortion
- Peripheral lesions may be spiculated with solid, pale yellow-tan to gray, and gritty cut surfaces

Microscopic Findings
- Nests of cells infiltrate bronchial wall structures
- Sheets of uniform round to spindled cells with abundant eosinophilic granular cytoplasm
- Granules can be coarse or fine (PAS-positive but diastase-resistant)
- Nuclei are small and round; chromatin is slightly granular
- Perineural invasion can be conspicuous

Immunohistochemical Features
- Tumor cells positive for vimentin, S-100 protein, CD56, CD57, and CD68
- Tumor cells negative for epithelial markers

Fine Needle Aspiration Biopsy Findings
- Single and loose three-dimensional clusters
- Elongated spindled or oval cells with abundant cytoplasm
- Giemsa stain may suggest a granulomatous process

Pathologic Differential Diagnosis
- Oncocytic carcinoid tumor
- Acinic cell carcinoma
- Metastatic renal cell carcinoma
- Histiocytic processes, especially malakoplakia

PATHOLOGIC FEATURES

GROSS FINDINGS

Tumors can range from 0.3 to 6.5 cm in diameter, but most measure approximately 1.0 cm at the time of diagnosis. Endobronchial tumors distort the overlying mucosa and may even produce a papillary mucosal appearance. Most GCTs are infiltrative with extension into peribronchial tissues. Peripheral lesions may be spiculated. Cut surfaces are solid, pale yellow-tan to gray, and oftentimes gritty. Necrosis and hemorrhage are not seen.

MICROSCOPIC FINDINGS

Nests and large aggregates of tumor cells with scant interspersed fibrous tissue infiltrate and splay most bronchial wall structures but do not invade adjacent lung parenchyma (Figure 32-14A). Direct extension into lymph nodes may be observed. Sheets of uniform round, oval, or spindled neoplastic cells contain abundant eosinophilic or amphophilic granular cytoplasm. The granules are usually fine, but coarse irregular granules may resemble Michaelis-Gutmann bodies. Tumor cytoplasm is PAS-positive but diastase-resistant. Nuclei are small, round and either centrally or paracentrally

located, whereas chromatin may be slightly granular and nucleoli are usually inconspicuous (Figure 32-14B). Rare large nuclei with irregular contours and nucleoli or signet ring morphology can be seen. Perineural invasion may be conspicuous, yet mitotic figures, necrosis, and vascular invasion are not seen. Overlying respiratory mucosa often features squamous metaplasia and occasionally hyperplasia, but pseudoepitheliomatous hyperplasia is not a common finding. A thickened hyalinized basement membrane separates tumor from mucosa.

ANCILLARY STUDIES

ULTRASTRUCTURAL FEATURES

Tumor cells are filled with small cytoplasmic osmiophilic membrane-limited granules and larger lamellated granules, (secondary and tertiary lysosomes).

IMMUNOHISTOCHEMISTRY

GCT reacts with antibodies to vimentin and S-100 protein as well as CD56, CD57, and CD68. Tumor cells are also positive for myelin basic protein, calretinin, and alpha-inhibin. Epithelial markers are negative.

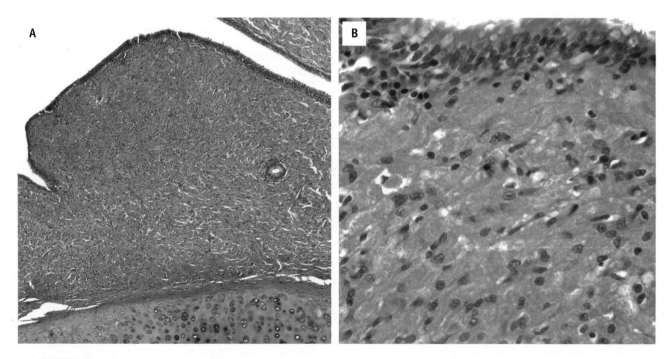

FIGURE 32-14

Granular cell tumor

(A) Tumors usually expand bronchial wall submucosa; in this example, the tumor chokes seromucinous glands and overruns other submucosal structures. At bronchoscopy, an endobronchial polypoid appearance was appreciated. (B) Sheets of large cells feature voluminous finely to coarsely granular eosinophilic cytoplasm with small oval nuclei, granular chromatin, and occasionally prominent nucleoli.

Fine Needle Aspiration Biopsy

Although the submucosal tumor does not usually spontaneously exfoliate cells, bronchial brushings and washings, in addition to FNAB samples, can yield a diagnosis. Single and loose three-dimensional clusters of elongated spindled or oval cells feature abundant cytoplasm distended with eosinophilic granules. Nuclei are usually small and bland but may be large with vesicular chromatin and atypia. Of note, on Giemsa staining an epithelioid granulomatous, rather than a neoplastic process, may be suspected.

Differential Diagnosis

The histologic differential diagnosis includes oncocytic carcinoid tumor, bronchial acinic cell carcinoma, as well as metastatic renal cell carcinoma and histiocytic processes, most notably malakoplakia. Oncocytic carcinoid tumor features an organoid growth pattern and larger nuclei with finely granular chromatin as well as cytokeratin, chromogranin, and synaptophysin immunoreactivity. Carcinomas with granular cytoplasm, including acinic cell carcinoma and metastatic renal cell and breast carcinoma, often feature larger nuclei with more atypia than that appreciated in GCT and always react with epithelial antibodies. Renal cell carcinoma is also loosely cohesive on cytologic specimens. Be aware that S-100 protein staining may be seen in acinic cell carcinomas. While the histiocytes in malakoplakia may contain coarse granules, dense inflammatory infiltrates, bone fide Michaelis-Gutmann bodies, and S-100 negativity differentiate the processes.

Lastly, although pseudoepitheliomatous hyperplasia is not a common finding in endobronchial GCT, overlying squamous metaplasia or hyperplasia should not be overinterpreted as neoplastic. In fact, these findings should lead to a thorough examination of submucosal tissue in such biopsies.

Prognosis and Therapy

Whereas soft tissue GCTs can be benign, atypical, or malignant, pulmonary tumors are benign. Treatment depends on the location and size of the lesion. Peripheral tumors can be conservatively excised, and small central tumors can be managed with bronchoscopic extirpation (if less than 0.8 cm), laser therapy, or sleeve resection. Tumors that have caused extensive destruction of distal lung parenchyma may require lobectomy or pneumonectomy depending on the location of the tumor. Individuals with multiple asymptomatic small endobronchial tumors can be followed.

SUGGESTED READINGS

Hamartoma

1. Fletcher JA, Longtine J, Wallace K, et al. Cytogenetic and histologic findings in 17 pulmonary chondroid hamartomas: evidence for a pathogenetic relationship with lipomas and leiomyomas. *Genes Chromosomes Cancer.* 1995;12:220-3.
2. Gjevre JA, Myers JL, Prakash UB. Pulmonary hamartomas. *Mayo Clin Proc.* 1996;71:14-20.
3. Hughes JH, Young NA, Wilbur DC, et al. Fine-needle aspiration of pulmonary hamartoma. A common source of false-positive diagnoses in the College of American Pathologists interlaboratory comparison program in nongynecologic cytology. *Arch Pathol Lab Med.* 2005;129:19-22.
4. Kazmierczak B, Meyer-Bolte K, Tran KH, et al. A high frequency of tumors with rearrangements of genes of the HMGI(Y) family in a series of 191 pulmonary chondroid hamartomas. *Genes Chromosomes Cancer.* 1999;26:125-33.
5. Tomashefski JF Jr. Benign endobronchial mesenchymal tumors: their relationship to parenchymal pulmonary hamartomas. *Am J Surg Pathol.* 1982;6:531-40.

Benign Salivary Gland Tumors

6. England DM, Hochholzer L. Truly benign "bronchial adenoma." Report of 10 cases of mucus gland adenoma with immunohistochemical and ultrastructural findings. *Am J Surg Pathol.* 1995;19:887-99.
7. Moran CA, Suster S, Askin FB, Koss MN. Benign and malignant salivary gland-type mixed tumors of the lung. Clinicopathologic and immunohistochemical study of eight cases. *Cancer.* 1994;73:2481-90.
8. Tsuji N, Tateishi R, Ishiguro S, et al. Adenomyoepithelioma of the lung. *Am J Surg Pathol.* 1995;19:956-62.

Mucinous Cystadenoma

9. Gao ZH, Urbanski SJ. The spectrum of pulmonary mucinous cystic neoplasia. *Am J Clin Pathol.* 2005;124:62-70.
10. Graeme-Cook F, Mark EJ. Pulmonary mucinous cystic tumors of borderline malignancy. *Hum Pathol.* 1991;22:185-90.
11. Kragel PJ, Devaney KO, Meth BM, et al. Mucinous cystadenoma of the lung. A report of two cases with immunohistochemical and ultrastructural analysis. *Arch Pathol Lab Med.* 1990;114:1053-6.
12. Matsuo T, Kimura NY, Takamori S, Shirouzu K. A case of recurrent pulmonary mucinous cystadenoma. *Eur J Cardiothorac Surg.* 2005;28:176-7.

Alveolar Adenoma

13. Burke LM, Rush WI, Khoor A, et al. Alveolar adenoma: A histochemical, immunohistochemical, and ultrastructural analysis of 17 cases. *Hum Pathol.* 1999;30:158-67.
14. Yousem SA, Hochholzer L. Alveolar adenoma. *Hum Pathol.* 1986;17:1066-71.

Papillary Adenoma

15. Dessy E, Braidotti P, Del Curto B, et al. Peripheral papillary tumor of type-II pneumocytes: a rare neoplasm of undetermined malignant potential. *Virchow Arch.* 2000;436:289-95.
16. Fukuda T, Ohnishi Y, Kanai I, et al. Papillary adenoma of the lung. Histological and ultrastructural findings in two cases. *Acta Pathol Jpn.* 1992;42:56-61.
17. Sheppard MN, Burke L, Kennedy M. TTF-1 is useful in the diagnosis of pulmonary papillary adenoma. *Histopathology.* 2003;43:404-5.

Solitary Papillomas

18. Flieder DB, Koss MN, Nicholson A, et al. Solitary pulmonary papillomas in adults. A clinicopathologic and in situ hybridization study of 14 cases combined with 27 cases in the literature. *Am J Surg Pathol.* 1998;22:1328-42.
19. Popper HH, Wirnsberger G, Juettner-Smolle FM, et al. The predictive value of human papilloma virus (HPV) typing in the prognosis of bronchial squamous cell papillomas. *Histopathology.* 1992;21:323-30.

Sclerosing Hemangioma

20. Chan ACL, Chan JKC. Can pulmonary sclerosing haemangioma be accurately diagnosed by intra-operative frozen section? *Histopathology.* 2002;41:392-403.
21. Dacic S, Sasatomi E, Swalsky PA, et al. Loss of heterozygosity patterns of sclerosing hemangioma of the lung and bronchioloalveolar carcinoma indicate a similar molecular pathogenesis. *Arch Pathol Lab Med.* 2004;128:880-4.
22. Devouassoux-Shisheboran M, Hayashi T, Linnoila RI, et al. A clinicopathologic study of 100 cases of pulmonary sclerosing hemangioma with immunohistochemical studies. TTF-1 is expressed in both round and surface cells, suggesting an origin from primitive respiratory epithelium. *Am J Surg Pathol.* 2000;24:906-16.
23. Gal AA, Nassar VH, Miller JI. Cytologic diagnosis of pulmonary sclerosing hemangioma. *Diagn Cytopathol.* 2002;26:163-6.
24. Nicholson AG, Magkou C, Snead D, et al. Unusual sclerosing haemangiomas and sclerosing haemangioma-like lesions, and the value of TTF-1 in making the diagnosis. *Histopathology.* 2002;41:404-13.

Clear Cell Tumor

25. Bonetti F, Martignoni G, Doglioni C, et al. Clear cell ("sugar") tumor of the lung is a lesion strictly related to angiomyolipoma-the concept of a family of lesions characterized by the presence of the perivascular epithelioid cells (PEC). *Pathology.* 1994;26:230-6.
26. Flieder DB, Travis WD. Clear cell "sugar" tumor of the lung: association with lymphangioleiomyomatosis and multifocal micronodular pneumocyte hyperplasia in a patient with tuberous sclerosis. *Am J Surg Pathol.* 1997;21:1242-7.

27. Gaffey MJ, Mills ME, Askin FB, et al. Clear cell tumor of the lung. A clinicopathologic, immunohistochemical, and ultrastructural study of eight cases. *Am J Surg Pathol.* 1990;14:248-59.
28. Lantuejoul S, Isaac S, Pinel N, et al. Clear cell tumor of the lung: An immunohistochemical and ultrastructural study supporting a pericytic differentiation. *Mod Pathol.* 1997;10:1001-8.
29. Pileri SA, Cavazza A, Schiavina M, et al. Clear-cell proliferation of the lung with lymphangioleiomyomatosis-like change. *Histopathology.* 2004;44:156-63.
30. Sale GE, Kulander BG. "Benign" clear-cell tumor (sugar tumor) of the lung with hepatic metastases ten years after resection of pulmonary primary tumor. *Arch Pathol Lab Med.* 1988;112:1177-8.

Granular Cell Tumor

31. Deavers M, Guinee D, Koss MN, Travis WD. Granular cell tumors of the lung. Clinicopathologic study of 20 cases. *Am J Surg Pathol.* 1995;19:627-35.
32. Elmberger PG, Skold CM, Collins BT. Fine needle aspiration biopsy of intrabronchial granular cell tumor. *Acta Cytol.* 2005;49:223-4.
33. Nappi O, Ferrara G, Wick MR. Neoplasms composed of eosinophilic polygonal cells: an overview with consideration of different cytomorphologic patterns. *Semin Diagn Pathol.* 1999;16:82-90.
34. Ordonez NG, Mackay B. Granular cell tumor: a review of the pathology and histogenesis. *Ultrastruct Pathol.* 1999;23:207-22.

33 Primary Pleural Neoplasms

Thomas Sporn

- Introduction
- Malignant Pleural Mesothelioma
- Solitary Fibrous Tumor
- Synovial Sarcoma and Other Primary Pleural Sarcomas
- Desmoid Tumor
- Primitive Neuroectodermal Tumor and Desmoplastic Small Round Cell Tumor
- Neoplasms Metastatic to the Pleura

INTRODUCTION

In contrast to the common pleural metastases from pulmonary and extrapulmonary malignancies, primary tumors of the pleura constitute a relatively rare group of benign and malignant neoplasms, with different pathways of differentiation and histogenesis reflecting the complexity of the serosal membrane lining the thoracic cavity. The pleura contains not only a mesothelial lining but also a subjacent matrix of elastic fibro-connective tissue containing lymphovasculature, blood vessels, and scattered submesothelial mesenchymal cells. Tumors arising from the pleura manifest differentiation reflecting each of its constituent cell types. Despite different pathways of histogenesis, primary pleural neoplasms often resemble one another as well as metastatic tumors, closely, sharing common gross distributions and histologic patterns. Accordingly, the pathologist's task to render a proper diagnosis for these tumors can be laborious and may require the use of several ancillary studies, as well as familiarity with pertinent clinical and radiographic features. The malignant tumors of the pleura share the common features of diagnosis at typically late stage, difficult clinical management, and aggressive behavior, whereas the resectability of the benign lesions frequently predicts biologic behavior and prognosis.

MALIGNANT PLEURAL MESOTHELIOMA

Malignant mesotheliomas constitute the group of aggressive malignant epithelial neoplasms arising from the serosal membranes lining the pleural and peritoneal cavities as well as the pericardium. These cavities are lined by a single layer of flattened to cuboidal cells of mesodermal origin constituting the mesothelium, but it remains uncertain whether mesotheliomas result from transformation of the differentiated mesothelial cell, progenitor submesothelial mesenchymal cells, or both. Mesothelioma develops most frequently in the pleura, but its counterparts in the pericardium, peritoneum, and tunica vaginalis of the testis are also well recognized.

CLINICAL FEATURES

A historically rare neoplasm, mesothelioma in North America has an incidence of 15 to 20 cases per million persons per year for men and a much lower incidence in women. It remains a signal malignancy, an epidemiologic marker for exposure to asbestos, with which it is most highly associated. The peak incidence for mesothelioma in North America is likely on the wane, but the tumor's incidence in Europe, Australia, and Japan as well as developing countries may not peak for several more decades, in the latter instances owing to a more contemporaneous usage of asbestos in those societies relative to the Western world. Malignant pleural mesothelioma has an overwhelming male predominance, reflecting the predominance of men in occupations most commonly associated with asbestos exposure. Exposure to commercial amphibole asbestos remains the major cause of pleural mesothelioma, yet it remains uncertain why, among the millions of individuals so exposed, so few develop mesothelioma, and the search for co-carcinogens remains ongoing. Typical of asbestos-associated diseases in general, a prolonged latent interval, that period of time between exposure and the development of clinical disease, is characteristic and, in the case of mesothelioma, is usually measured in decades. Owing to its potential for clinically silent growth, the presentation of mesothelioma is all too often at late stage and is usually characterized by dyspnea and pleural effusion and may be accompanied by chest pain stemming from chest wall invasion. Distant metastases are often discovered at autopsy but are rarely of clinical significance premortem and may remain undetected during life. Invasive procedures such as thoracoscopy may lead to development of subcutaneous tumor nodules.

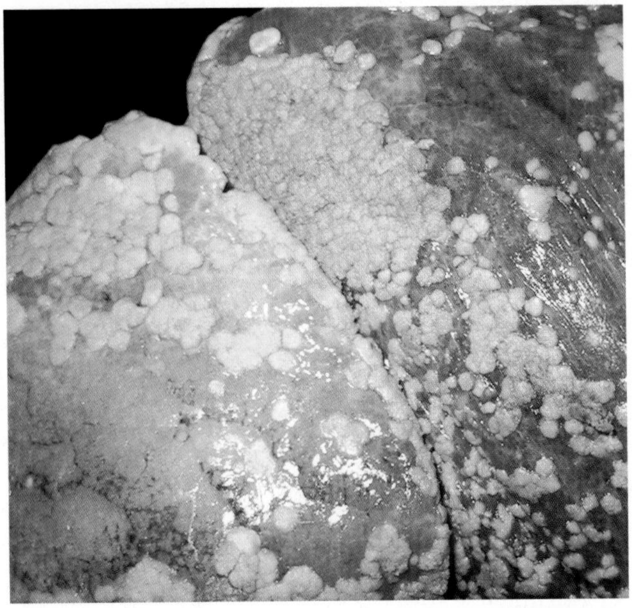

RADIOLOGIC FEATURES

Plain chest radiographs typically show pleural effusions and often pleural-based tumor masses. Radiographically demonstrable pleural plaques indicative of asbestos exposure are observed in 20% of cases. Locally advanced tumor is often evident, with circumferential encasement of the lung by a lobulated rind of tumor, with extension into fissures and interlobular septa. In rare cases, a single dominant tumor mass may be demonstrable. Computed tomography (CT) and magnetic resonance imaging (MRI) may aid in demonstrating chest wall or diaphragmatic invasion and are useful in preoperative assessment of resectability.

FIGURE 33-1
Pleural mesothelioma, early stage
This mesothelioma presents as multiple and focally coalescent nodules on the visceral pleura of the lung.

PATHOLOGIC FEATURES

GROSS FINDINGS

The typical gross features in early disease consist of small nodules in the parietal pleura, although the visceral pleura may give rise to mesothelioma as well. Subsequent growth leads to coalescence of these nodules, with extensive involvement of the pleural surfaces (Figure 33-1). The circumferential rind of tumor at late stage is typically lobulated, firm, and white (Figure 33-2). Tumor growth follows the distribution of the pleural surface with invasion into mediastinum, chest wall, and diaphragm. The tumor tracks along the pleural reflections into the lung fissures, and finger-like extensions into interlobular septa are common. Metastases to mediastinal and hilar lymph nodes, as well as the parenchyma of the lung, are usually evident in late-stage disease. Rare instances of localized invasive mesothelioma without diffuse pleural spread have been reported.

MICROSCOPIC FINDINGS

Malignant mesothelioma is characterized by a broad range of microscopic appearances, often within an individual tumor. The World Health Organization recog-

nizes four basic histologic variants: epithelial (epithelioid), sarcomatoid, and biphasic mesotheliomas, as well as a separate category including those tumors with heterologous elements. The most common variant is epithelial, featuring tubulopapillary, pseudoacinar, microglandular, trabecular, or sheet-like growth patterns, or combinations thereof (Figure 33-3). The tumor cells are typically cuboidal, with moderate amounts of cytoplasm and paracentric nuclei. Cytologic atypia is typically modest in comparison to adenocarcinoma, the principal member of its differential diagnosis, although pleomorphic mesothelioma with characteristic high-grade cytologic features is recognized, as is the unusual deciduoid subtype. The deciduoid variant, initially reported as a peritoneal tumor in young women, also occurs within the pleura and has cytologic features reminiscent of the decidual reaction with round or polygonal cells and abundant cytoplasm (Figure 33-4). The well-differentiated papillary subtype, originally described as an indolent neoplasm involving the peritoneum of young women, demonstrates prominent fibrovascular cores lined by a single layer of cuboidal cells with minimal nuclear atypia and only focal stromal invasion (Figures 33-5, 33-6). The sarcomatoid variant is the least common and features architectural complexity with storiform and fascicular

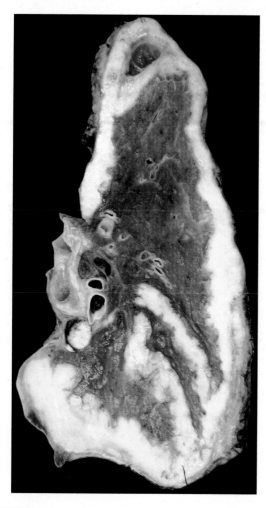

FIGURE 33-2

Pleural mesothelioma, late stage

This advanced mesothelioma demonstrates diffuse pleural growth, circumferential encasement of lung, extension along fissures, and hilar lymph node metastases.

growth patterns with spindled cellularity of high nuclear grade (Figure 33-7). The tumor may incorporate giant cells, mimicking malignant fibrous histiocytoma, or have heterologous elements composed of osteosarcomatous or chondrosarcomatous foci (Figure 33-8). The desmoplastic variant of sarcomatoid mesothelioma is particularly deceptive, composed largely of hyalinized collagen, challenging the pathologist to demonstrate frankly sarcomatoid foci or invasion into subpleural tissues that help permit its distinction from the benign fibrosing pleural reactions it may resemble (Figure 33-9). The biphasic variant of malignant mesothelioma exhibits one or more of the many epithelial patterns as well as areas of sarcomatoid tumor.

ANCILLARY STUDIES

CYTOLOGY

Some 90% of malignant mesotheliomas are associated with pleural effusions. The presence of diagnostically useful cells in effusion cytology may be affected by histologic subtype, with sarcomatoid and desmoplastic variants resulting in more paucicellular effusions than epithelial neoplasms (Figure 33-10). Given the difficult distinction between the reactive and malignant mesothelial phenotype, even aided by immunohistochemistry, the diagnosis of mesothelioma based solely on cytologic grounds is hazardous, and effusion cytology is best used as a screening test and precursor to more definitive studies such as thoracoscopic or percutaneous core needle biopsy. Cytologic examination of pleural fluid is also valuable for diagnosis

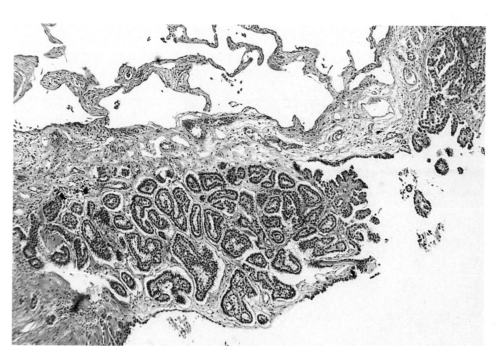

FIGURE 33-3

Epithelial mesothelioma

This tumor shows invasive pseudoacinar architecture at the pleural surface.

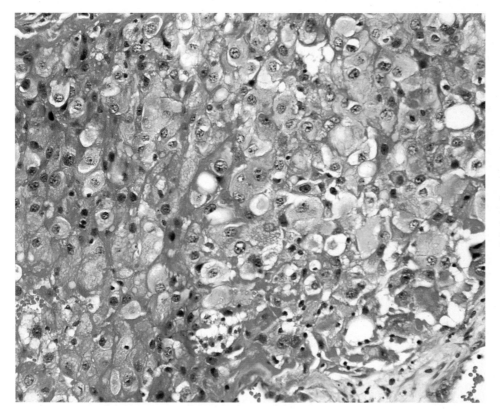

FIGURE 33-4

Malignant mesothelioma, epithelial variant (deciduoid subtype)
Sheets of large, round cells with abundant cytoplasm, paracentric nuclei, and prominent nucleoli are typical of this tumor.

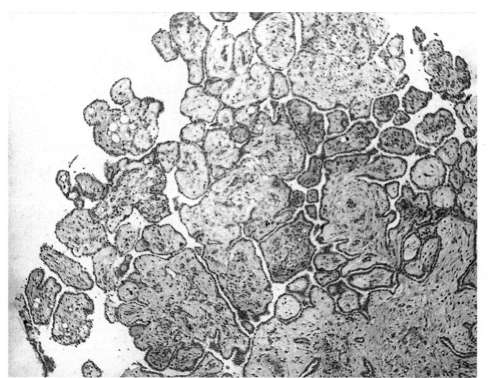

FIGURE 33-5

Well-differentiated papillary mesothelioma
This tumor displays exophytic growth and no stromal invasion.

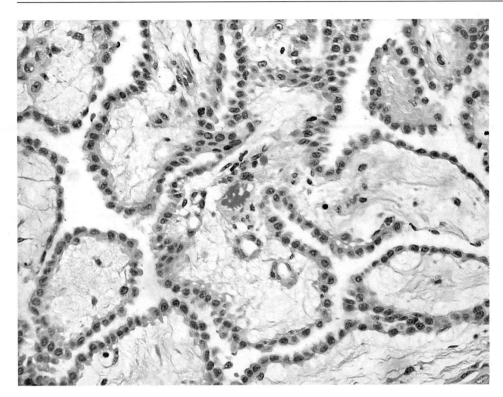

FIGURE 33-6
Well-differentiated papillary meso-thelioma
Well-developed fibrovascular cores are lined by a single layer of low-grade cuboidal tumor cells.

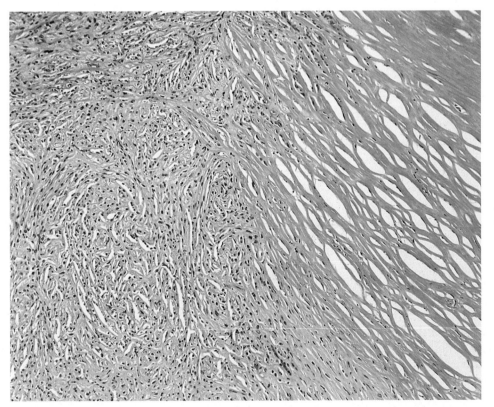

FIGURE 33-7

Sarcomatoid mesothelioma
The sarcomatous spindle cell proliferation invades a local pleural plaque.

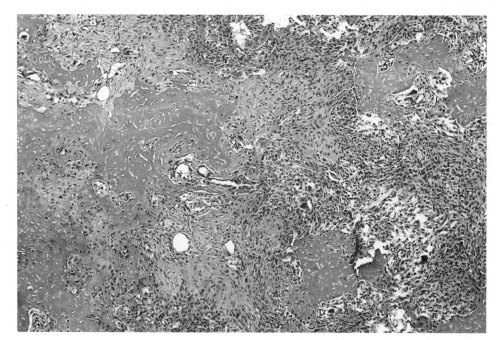

FIGURE 33-8
Sarcomatoid mesothelioma with osteosarcomatous heterologous differentiation
Osteoid production by tumor cells is conspicuous in this view.

of metastatic neoplasms, particularly adenocarcinomas, which may clinically and radiographically resemble mesothelioma.

HISTOCHEMISTRY

Histochemical staining for neutral mucins and hyaluronic acid may occasionally be useful in distinguishing adenocarcinoma metastatic to the pleura from epithelial mesothelioma, but it has largely been supplanted by immunohistochemistry. Mucin production is typical of adenocarcinoma and can be detected with a periodic acid-Schiff (PAS) stain, with mucin specificity enhanced by diastase predigestion. Mucicarmine staining also frequently highlights cellular mucin in adenocarcinomas, but staining has also been described in a subset of mesotheliomas. Hyaluronic acid production is more typical of mesothelioma, and this can be highlighted with alcian blue or colloidal iron stains, reversible with hyaluronidase pretreatment.

IMMUNOHISTOCHEMISTRY

Immunohistochemistry is chiefly used for distinguishing epithelial mesothelioma from adenocarcinoma. A panel approach is usually taken, with the panel composed of antibodies with high sensitivity and specificity for mesothelioma and adenocarcinoma. Epithelial mesothelioma generally demonstrates positive immunoreactivity for calretinin, cytokeratin 5/6, Wilms Tumor 1 (WT-1), and D2-40 (Figure 33-11) and stains negatively for carcinoembryonic antigen (CEA), thyroid transcrip-

tion factor-1 (TTF-1), Ber-Ep4, B72.3, and CD15 (also see chapter 38). A converse immunophenotype is typically observed for adenocarcinoma involving the pleura. Numerous other antibodies have also been evaluated, with variable reproducibility. Immunoreactivity with pan-keratin antibodies does not distinguish between mesothelioma and adenocarcinoma but is valuable for supporting diagnoses of sarcomatoid and desmoplastic mesotheliomas. Unfortunately, reactive stromal proliferations can also show immunostaining for pan-keratin, so a positive result should not be construed as providing definitive evidence of malignancy, and histologic criteria for malignancy must still be fulfilled. Furthermore, cytokeratin immunoreactivity is observed in synovial sarcoma, as well as some angiosarcomas, and constitutes a potential source of confusion in the evaluation of sarcomatoid or biphasic tumors. As is generally true, immunohistochemical staining results must be interpreted in the context of the histopathology, and use of a panel approach to evaluation of pleural neoplasms can often provide a greater degree of security than reliance upon one or two stains (also see chapter 38).

ULTRASTRUCTURAL EXAMINATION

Equivocal histochemical or immunohistochemical findings in cases of suspected epithelial mesothelioma may be clarified using transmission electron microscopy. Although no single ultrastructural feature is unique to mesothelioma, the combination of long, slender surface microvilli, abundant intermediate filaments, and tonofibrillar bundles is characteristic.

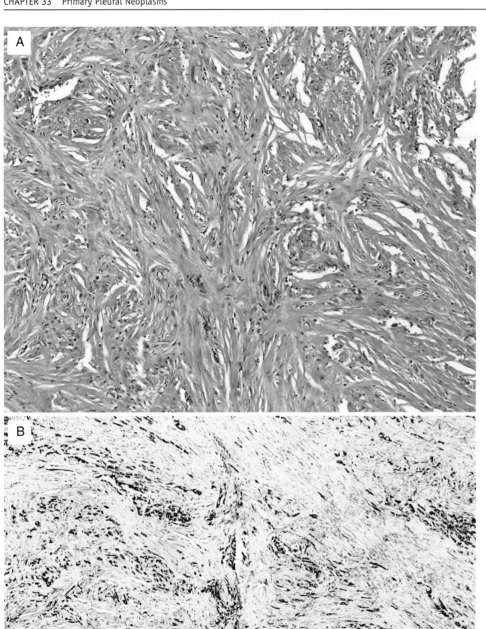

FIGURE 33-9

Desmoplastic mesothelioma
The "patternless" growth pattern of
these cytologically bland tumor cells in
hyalinized stroma is characteristic of
this neoplasm **(A)**, as is immunoreactivity with anti-cytokeratin **(B)**.

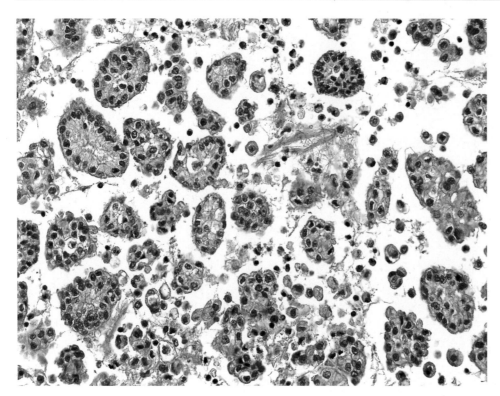

FIGURE 33-10

Malignant mesothelioma, epithelial, in pleural fluid

This fluid contains a mixture of papillary groups, clusters and individual polygonal cells with relatively mild cytologic atypia.

DIFFERENTIAL DIAGNOSIS

Malignant mesothelioma must be distinguished from reactive conditions leading to mesothelial hyperplasia and benign fibrosing pleural conditions. The demonstration of stromal, subpleural, or chest wall invasion is invaluable for differentiating between mesothelioma and reactive processes. Another helpful finding is necrosis, which favors malignancy. Also, with spindle cell proliferations, an evolution from hypocellular fibrinous exudate to granulation tissue to fibrosis, as one moves from the luminal surface deeper, is more in keeping with an organizing pleural effusion (also see chapter 35). Other malignant tumors that may be considered in the differential diagnosis include a broad spectrum of carcinomas and sarcomas metastatic to the pleura, as well as the uncommon sarcomas arising primarily in the pleura (also see chapter 34). Immunohistochemistry facilitates differentiation between these entities and malignant mesothelioma (see earlier discussion and chapter 38).

PROGNOSIS AND THERAPY

With presentation typically at a late clinical stage, the median survival of malignant mesothelioma from time of diagnosis is 12 months, and the tumor almost invariably causes death within a few years of diagnosis. A survival benefit for a highly selected patient population treated with radical surgery and postoperative combined modality therapy has been shown, but debulking surgery in the forms of pneumonectomy or pleurectomy with adjuvant chemo-radiotherapy is typically directed with palliative intent. The well-differentiated papillary subtype, however, usually behaves differently than other histologic variants of malignant mesothelioma and typically is associated with a more indolent course. In patients with the well-differentiated papillary subtype, a recent study found an average survival of 74 months as compared with 9.89 months for 1248 paired patients with diffuse malignant mesothelioma, and a 10-year survival rate of 30.8%.

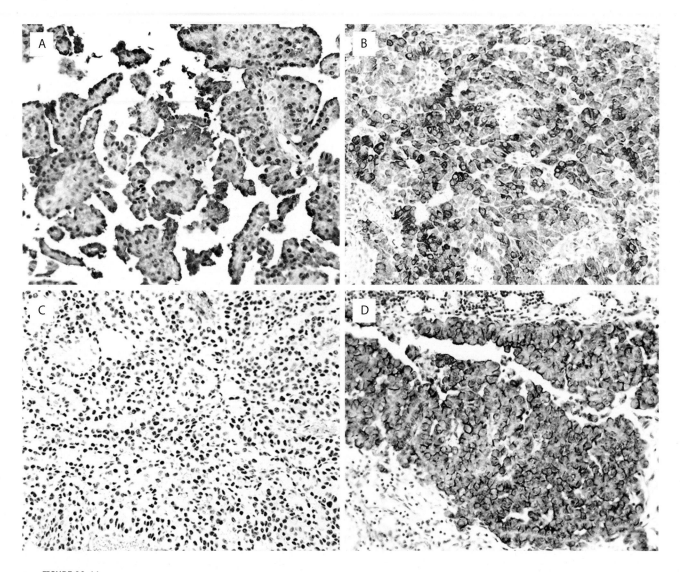

FIGURE 33-11

Malignant mesothelioma
Shown are representative examples of immunohistochemistry for **(A)** calretinin, **(B)** cytokeratin 5/6, **(C)** Wilms tumor-1, and **(D)** D2-40.

MALIGNANT PLEURAL MESOTHELIOMA—FACT SHEET

Definition
» Group of histologically diverse, clinically aggressive malignant epithelial neoplasms arising primarily in the serosal membranes of the pleural cavity and peritoneum and demonstrating mesothelial differentiation

Incidence and Epidemiology
» Rare tumors, with an estimated incidence of 15 to 20 cases per million
» Higher frequency in men
» Typically associated with occupational or paraoccupational exposure to amphibole asbestos
» Long latency period following exposure and peak incidence in late adulthood

Clinical Features
» Typical presentation at late stage with bulky pleural/chest wall tumors and accompanying large effusions, dyspnea, and chest pain

Radiologic Features
» Usually large pleural-based mass(es) or circumferential encasement of lung by the tumor, which appears as thickened pleura
» Tumor growth into diaphragm, pericardium, and chest wall is often observed
» Pleural effusion

Prognosis and Therapy
» Highly aggressive tumors with dismal prognosis related to typical presentation at late stage
» Death often within 1 year following diagnosis
» Survival benefit for radical surgery and adjuvant chemo-radiotherapy in select group of patients, but for most patients therapies are palliative

MALIGNANT PLEURAL MESOTHELIOMA—PATHOLOGIC FEATURES

Gross Findings
» Early lesions consist of multiple pleural nodules
» Late-stage tumors encase the lung in a confluent rind of tumor with growth down fissures and interlobular septa and into diaphragm, pericardium, and chest wall
» Hilar and mediastinal lymph node metastases frequently develop with advancing disease

Microscopic Findings
» Epithelial (epithelioid), sarcomatoid, and biphasic variants and a separate category of tumors showing the presence of heterologous elements
» Spectrum of histologic appearances within each of the above variants (described in text)

Histochemical Features
» Mesotheliomas can produce acid mucopolysaccharides/hyaluronic acid and are Alcian blue/colloidal iron positive, sensitive to hyaluronidase pretreatment
» Mesotheliomas characteristically do not produce mucins (although rare cases may show focal staining)
» (+) PAS reaction due to cytoplasmic glycogen is reversed with diastase pretreatment

Immunohistochemical Features
» Epithelial mesotheliomas are generally positive for cytokeratins including cytokeratin 5/6, calretinin, WT1, and D2-40 and usually stain negatively for CEA, CD15, Ber EP4, B72.3, MOC31, and TTF-1
» Cytokeratin and vimentin immunoreactivity is typical of sarcomatoid and desmoplastic variants, while other "mesothelial-specific" antibodies are less likely to be positive than in epithelial mesotheliomas
» Cytokeratin immunostains are useful in desmoplastic mesotheliomas for demonstrating subpleural soft tissue invasion

Ultrastructural Features
» Classic features of epithelial mesothelioma tumor cells include long, slender surface microvilli with aspect ratios in excess of 10 to 1, abundant intermediate filaments, and tonofibrillar bundles

Pathologic Differential Diagnosis
» Epithelial mesothelioma
  » Reactive conditions with mesothelial hyperplasia
  » Adenocarcinoma metastatic to pleura
  » Epithelioid angiosarcoma
  » Epithelioid metastases of non-epithelial malignancies (e.g., malignant melanoma)
» Sarcomatoid mesothelioma
  » Solitary fibrous tumor
  » Primary and metastatic sarcomas of the pleura
  » Sarcomatoid carcinomas of the lung and elsewhere (metastatic)
  » Sarcomatoid metastases of non-epithelial malignancies (e.g. malignant melanoma)
» Desmoplastic mesothelioma
  » Solitary fibrous tumor
  » Desmoid tumor
  » Fibrosing pleuritis (fibrous pleurisy)

SOLITARY FIBROUS TUMOR

Historically bearing the misleading name benign meso-thelioma or benign fibrous mesothelioma, solitary (or localized) fibrous tumor is the most common mesenchy-mal pleural neoplasm. Unlike mesothelioma, solitary fibrous tumor (SFT) has no association with asbestos exposure and has been shown on the basis of immuno-histochemical and ultrastructural studies to be derived from submesothelial mesenchymal elements. These tu-mors can also arise less frequently in the parenchyma of the lung as well as numerous other locations throughout the body.

CLINICAL FEATURES

Typically occurring in middle age, SFT has been de-scribed in childhood and in all life stages and with ap-proximately equal gender distribution. Often clinically occult, a large percentage of these tumors are detected incidentally. Common clinical complaints include dys-pnea, chest pain, and cough, accompanied by pulmonary osteoarthropathy, digital clubbing, and pleural effusion. The common laboratory finding of hypoglycemia is be-lieved to be related to the tumor's elaboration of an insu-lin-like growth factor and has been reported more fre-quently in women.

RADIOLOGIC FEATURES

SFTs show no predilection for laterality and are typically located in the inferior zones of the chest. Ranging in size from 1 cm to occupying the entirety of the pleural cavity, these sharply circumscribed and lobulated masses are of uniform density, and the obtuse angle formed by the tu-mor at its intersection with mediastinum or chest wall suggests an extrapulmonary location. Occasionally, these tumors may lie in or adjacent to a fissure or intraparen-chymally. Calcification is seen in fewer than 10% of cases. A reported increase in attenuation following con-trast reflects the tumor's vascularity.

PATHOLOGIC FEATURES

GROSS FINDINGS

Most SFTs arise from the visceral pleura and are often attached to it by a vascularized pedicle (Figure 33-12). Other tumors may have a sessile appearance or appear inverted into the parenchyma of the lung. Although most neoplasms appear well circumscribed, a small number demonstrate infiltrative margins that may make complete resection more difficult. Occasionally reaching great size, these tumors are often 5 to 6 cm in greatest dimension. Firm and rubbery, the cut surface of the tumor is usually gray-white and whorled and may show superficial vascu-lature and hemorrhage.

MICROSCOPIC FINDINGS

A variable pattern of spindled cellularity and hyalin-ized collagen is characteristic, with variegation in growth patterns in the cellular areas, which causes confusion with other mesenchymal neoplasms or mesothelioma (Figure 33-13). Sclerotic and acellular areas may feature wiry, "keloidal" collagen fibers, as well as myxoid or degenerative foci (Figure 33-14). There frequently is abrupt transition from cellular to acellular zones, and areas of spindled cellularity may show fascicular, stori-form, hemangiopericytic, or "patternless" growth pat-terns (Figure 33-15). The nuclear features are typically low-grade and uniform. Generally considered a benign neoplasm, histologic criteria predictive of malignancy have been proposed, including high cellularity, mitotic activity in excess of 4 figures per 10 high-power fields, increased pleomorphism, and necrosis. These features may be observed in clinically indolent tumors, though, or may be absent in infiltrative or poorly resectable tumors.

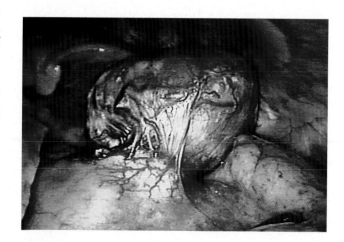

FIGURE 33-12

Solitary fibrous tumor

This intraoperative view shows a vascularized and pedunculated attachment of the tumor to the visceral pleura of the lung. (Courtesy of S. Balderson PA-C and T. A. D'Amico MD, Division of Thoracic Surgery, Duke University Medical Center, Durham, North Carolina.)

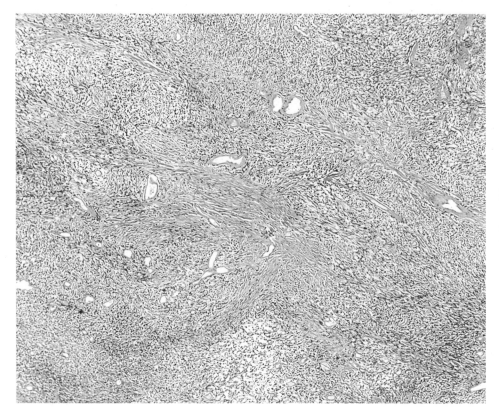

FIGURE 33-13
Solitary fibrous tumor
This scanning magnification image highlights the variations in pattern of the spindled tumor cells and a central area of fibrosis and paucicellularity.

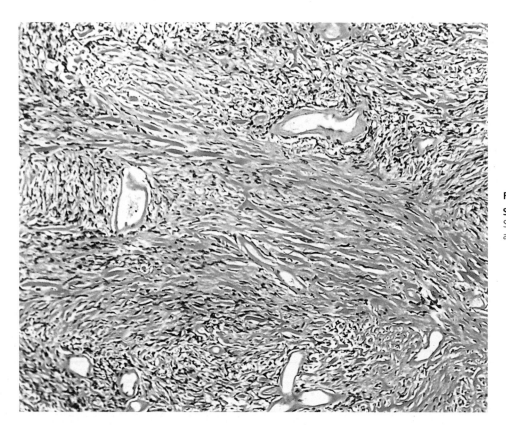

FIGURE 33-14
Solitary fibrous tumor
Sclerosis and wiry "keloidal" collagen are common features of this neoplasm.

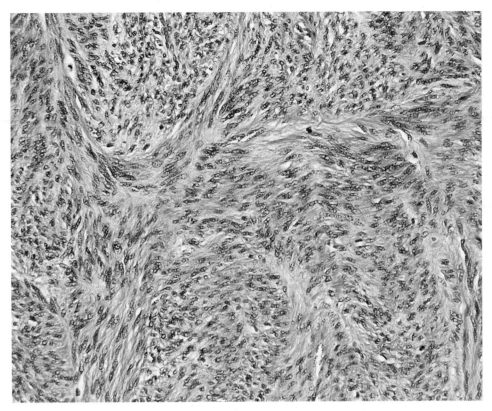

FIGURE 33-15

Solitary fibrous tumor

Fascicular and storiform cellular growth patterns, as well as mild cytoatypia, are evident in this view and fall within the spectrum of histology seen in solitary fibrous tumors.

ANCILLARY STUDIES

Immunohistochemistry is a useful adjunct to exclude epithelial/mesothelial differentiation or alternate types of mesenchymal differentiation. The tumor cells are uniformly non-reactive to anti-cytokeratins, epithelial membrane antigen, desmin, S-100, and calretinin. Although not specific for this entity, positive immunoreactivity for vimentin and CD34 is typical, and the tumor may also express BCL-2. Examination of tumor ultrastructure shows fibroblastic features and is of limited value.

DIFFERENTIAL DIAGNOSIS

The differential diagnosis of SFT is that of sarcomatoid neoplasms, chiefly synovial sarcoma and the sarcomatoid and desmoplastic variants of malignant pleural mesothelioma, as well as pleural desmoid tumor. Familiarity with the gross and radiographic features should alert the pathologist to the likelihood of SFT and direct further workup. The observation of a pedicle is very suggestive of this entity. Immunohistochemistry as described above is usually helpful for supporting the diagnosis of SFT and eliminating other diagnostic considerations (see also chapter 38).

PROGNOSIS AND THERAPY

Biologic behavior and prognosis appear to be linked to resectability. Because SFT is typically a benign tumor, complete excision is usually curative, even in a high percentage of cases with histologic features suggesting a malignant phenotype. The tumor's pedicle may facilitate its resection and is considered a favorable prognostic indicator. In the setting of malignant microscopic features and incomplete resection, this tumor retains the potential for local recurrence, intrathoracic spread, and metastasis, but tumor-associated death is very uncommon.

SOLITARY FIBROUS TUMOR OF THE PLEURA—FACT SHEET

Definition

▸▸ Mesenchymal tumor derived from submesothelial connective tissues, usually behaving in a benign fashion and occasionally more aggressively

Incidence

▸▸ Uncommon

Morbidity and Mortality

▸▸ Although most tumors are indolent, a subset is locally invasive
▸▸ Local recurrence can occur with incomplete resection
▸▸ Metastasis is uncommon, and death is rare

Epidemiology

▸▸ Typically diagnosed in individuals in the sixth and seventh decades of life but have been reported in all age groups
▸▸ No gender predilection
▸▸ No association with exposure to asbestos

Clinical Features

▸▸ Often clinically occult and detected incidentally
▸▸ Larger tumors may cause symptoms of dyspnea and cough
▸▸ Rare association with hypoglycemia, a finding reported more frequently in women
▸▸ May be associated with digital clubbing, pulmonary hypertrophic osteoarthropathy

Radiologic Features

▸▸ Sharply circumscribed and of uniform density
▸▸ Increased attenuation following contrast administration reflects vascularity
▸▸ Rarely calcified
▸▸ May cause pleural effusion

Prognosis and Therapy

▸▸ Resectability is the major predictor of clinical behavior, and complete resection is usually associated with an excellent prognosis
▸▸ Invasive and incompletely resected tumors can recur and have the potential for intrathoracic spread and distant metastasis
▸▸ Malignant histologic features have been recognized in a subset of neoplasms, and negative associations with recurrence-free and metastasis-free survival have been reported
▸▸ No role for chemotherapy or radiation therapy

SOLITARY FIBROUS TUMOR OF THE PLEURA—PATHOLOGIC FEATURES

Gross Findings

▸▸ Typically 5 to 6 cm, may be extremely large and occupy entire pleural cavity
▸▸ Often attached to the pleural surface by a vascular pedicle
▸▸ Usually smooth and encapsulated
▸▸ Whorled gray-white tumor surface on cut section
▸▸ Can also arise within the parenchyma of the lung

Microscopic Findings

▸▸ Usually bland fibroblastic proliferation, typically features zonation with cellular areas and collagenization, sometimes wiry "keloidal" collagen
▸▸ Fascicular, storiform, hemangiopericytic, and "patternless" growth patterns
▸▸ Proposed histologic criteria for malignancy include mitotic activity in excess of 4 per 10 HPF, increased pleomorphism, and necrosis

Immunohistochemical Features

▸▸ Positive vimentin, CD34, and BCL-2 immunoreactivity
▸▸ Negative cytokeratin, epithelial membrane antigen, calretinin, S-100, desmin, and actin immunoreactivity

Pathologic Differential Diagnosis

▸▸ Sarcomatoid and desmoplastic mesothelioma
▸▸ Desmoid tumor
▸▸ Monophasic synovial sarcoma
▸▸ Other spindle cell sarcomas

SYNOVIAL SARCOMA AND OTHER PRIMARY PLEURAL SARCOMAS

Primary sarcomas of the pleura represent an extremely uncommon group of tumors. The majority of sarcomatoid malignancies occurring in this site are more likely to be sarcomatoid carcinomas with secondary pleural involvement or the sarcomatoid variant of malignant pleural mesothelioma. Rare examples across the spectrum of malignant mesenchymal neoplasia have been described as case reports or anecdotally. The more clinically relevant forms include synovial sarcoma, vascular sarcomas (angiosarcoma, Kaposi's sarcoma), and pleuropulmonary blastoma (see chapter 6). Malignant peripheral nerve sheath tumors, osteosarcomas, and chondrosarcomas have also been reported to arise in the pleura, but it is possible that some reports of osteosarcomas and chondrosarcomas of the pleura represent cases of mesothelioma with heterologous differentiation. Primitive neuroectodermal tumor and desmoplastic round cell tumor are sarcomatous malignancies discussed elsewhere in this chapter.

CLINICAL FEATURES

Pleural sarcomas have been described in all age groups. The pleuropulmonary blastomas of childhood typically are diagnosed in the first four years of life but have been reported later in childhood and in young adulthood as well. The uncommon cases of synovial sarcoma in the pleura have also been described in a generally younger subset of patients than those afflicted with mesothelioma or vascular sarcomas. These sarcomas as a group share the common features of a large pleural-based mass or pleural thickening, which may mimic the gross presentation of mesothelioma, and accompanying pleural effusions, leading to the non-specific complaints of chest pain and dyspnea. The common course of these tumors presenting at late stage is resistance to therapy and poor prognosis, with death often in the initial years following diagnosis.

RADIOLOGIC FEATURES

These tumors lack a distinctive set of radiologic features and are considered as ancillary members of the differential diagnosis of pleural-based masses from the standpoint of the radiologist. These neoplasms are typically large and infiltrative and may feature diffuse pleural spread and growth along fissures, encasing the lung in a pattern reminiscent of mesothelioma.

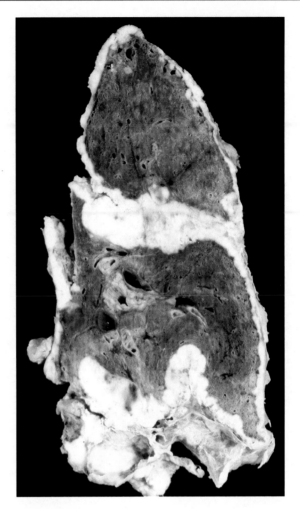

FIGURE 33-16

Epithelioid hemangioendothelioma of the pleura, late stage
Circumferential encasement of lung and pleurotropic growth produces a resemblance to malignant mesothelioma.

PATHOLOGIC FEATURES

GROSS FINDINGS

Sarcomatous tumors of the pleura generally present as mass lesions or nodular pleural thickening and may be accompanied by effusions, which may be grossly bloody. These tumors can be localized or have a gross appearance and distribution akin to malignant mesothelioma (Figure 33-16). Pleural synovial sarcomas may feature a pedicle. The cut surfaces of these fleshy tumors are typically gray-white and can be hemorrhagic. Pleuropulmonary blastomas may be cystic, solid, or have both cystic and solid components.

MICROSCOPIC FINDINGS

The histologic features of pleural sarcomas recapitulate those of their soft tissue or skeletal counterparts. Synovial sarcomas are usually monophasic fibrous or poorly differentiated. The spindle cell component shows compact, dense, and fibrosarcomatous growth, with

round-oval nuclei (Figure 33-17). Epithelioid foci may have pseudoglandular or tubulopapillary features, with cuboidal cells containing moderate amounts of cytoplasm, large nuclei, and occasional prominent nucleoli. Sarcomas with vascular differentiation occur as both epithelioid angiosarcoma and hemangioendothelioma and, despite differences in histologic features, are high-grade and aggressive tumors, with behavior akin to the mesotheliomas they grossly resemble. Epithelioid angiosarcomas are cellular tumors with tubulopapillary features or sheet-like growth, often associated with a bloody tumor diathesis. The tumor cells are usually round-polygonal with moderate amounts of eosinophilic cytoplasm and hyperchromatic nuclei (Figure 33-18). By contrast,

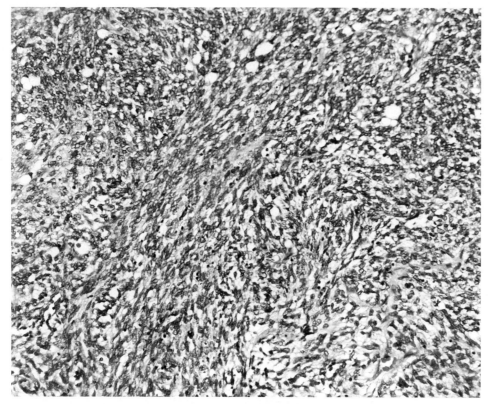

FIGURE 33-17
Synovial sarcoma
The predominant spindle cell component of this biphasic tumor demonstrates formation of fascicles.

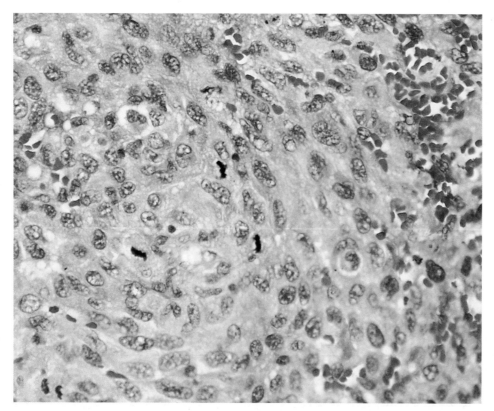

FIGURE 33-18
Epithelioid angiosarcoma
This tumor is composed of sheets of
plump spindled and epithelioid tumor
cells with high-grade nuclear features
and conspicuous mitoses in a bloody
background.

epithelioid hemangioendothelioma is less cellular, with infiltrative and lobular growth of clusters or short strands of tumor cells within a hyaline stroma (Figure 33-19). The tumor cells often contain cytoplasmic vacuoles corresponding to intracytoplasmic lumina, which may contain erythrocytes or their fragmented remnants. Pleuropulmonary blastomas typically have biphasic microscopic features: small elongate blastemal cells with hyperchromatic nuclei and undifferentiated mesenchymal cells, although the histologic spectrum is quite broad (discussed more extensively in chapter 6).

ANCILLARY STUDIES

IMMUNOHISTOCHEMISTRY

The principal diagnostic adjunct in the evaluation of sarcomatoid pleural malignancies is immunohistochemistry. The strong and diffuse expression of cytokeratins is generally exclusionary of mesenchymal differentiation and more typical of sarcomatoid carcinoma or mesothelioma. The tendency of synovial sarcomas to express cytokeratins or epithelial membrane antigen at least focally, in all reported pleural cases, constitutes a potential source of diagnostic confusion with mesothelioma. This potential pitfall is heightened by the frequent expression of calretinin and HBME-1 by synovial sarcoma. The expression of Ber-EP4 by synovial sarcoma results in additional mimicry of carcinoma. Epithelioid angiosarcoma and hemangioendothelioma may show focal cytokeratin immunoreactivity but are characterized by the expression of the vascular endothelial markers CD31, CD34, and factor VIII, as well as vimentin (Figure 33-20). Pleuropulmonary blastomas typically express vimentin and desmin, as well as other mesenchymal markers, with keratin expression limited to entrapped epithelium or mesothelium.

ULTRASTRUCTURAL STUDIES

Electron microscopy can be helpful in cases of epithelioid angiosarcoma, demonstrating the well-developed basal lamina, pinocytotic vesicles, numerous intermediate filaments, and Weibel-Palade bodies typical of vascular differentiation.

CYTOGENETIC AND MOLECULAR DIAGNOSTIC STUDIES

The histology and immunophenotype of synovial sarcoma, particularly in its monophasic form, may present significant problems in its distinction from mesothelioma or SFT. To that end, RT-PCR and in situ hybridization techniques can be used to show the SYT-SSX1 or SYT-SSX2 fusion transcripts resulting from the t(X;18)(p11.2;q11.2) translocation that is present in at least 90% of cases of synovial sarcoma.

PROGNOSIS AND THERAPY

Primary pleural synovial sarcoma is an aggressive neoplasm that commonly recurs and metastasizes. Median and 5-year disease-specific survival was reported to be 50 months and 31.6% respectively, and median and 5-year disease-free survival was 24 months and 20.9%. Death is often due to uncontrolled local disease. Pleural

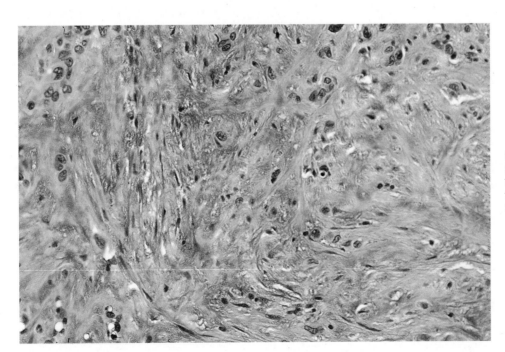

FIGURE 33-19

Epithelioid hemangioendothelioma
This paucicellular tumor features clusters of vacuolated cells in a hyaline and myxoid stroma.

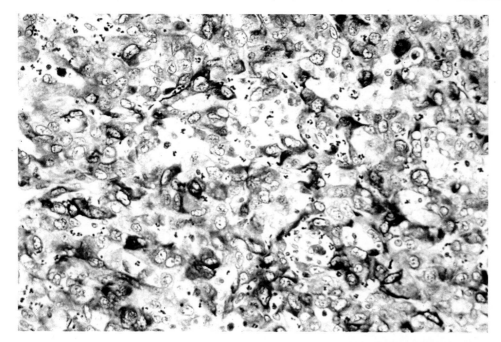

FIGURE 33-20
Epithelioid angiosarcoma
This tumor displays CD31 immunoreactivity.

SYNOVIAL SARCOMA AND OTHER PRIMARY PLEURAL SARCOMAS—FACT SHEET

Definition
▸ Malignant mesenchymal neoplasms arising primarily in the pleura

Incidence and Epidemiology
▸ Rare tumors, much less common than soft tissue sarcomas metastatic to the pleura
▸ Synovial sarcomas tend to occur in young or middle-aged adults
▸ Vascular tumors are more common in the elderly or middle-aged adults
▸ No apparent gender predilection

Morbidity and Mortality
▸ Extremely aggressive tumors that often recur and metastasize following resection and adjuvant chemo-radiotherapy
▸ Death often occurs within several years of diagnosis

Clinical Features
▸ Symptoms may include chest pain, dyspnea, hemoptysis, and constitutional symptoms

Radiologic Features
▸ Bulky pleural-based tumors or pleural thickening mimicking mesothelioma

Prognosis and Therapy
▸ Typical presentation is at late clinical stage
▸ Generally poor response to therapy, occasional long-term survivors

---

SYNOVIAL SARCOMA AND OTHER PRIMARY PLEURAL SARCOMAS—PATHOLOGIC FEATURES

Gross Findings
▸ Bulky gray-white tumor masses often with hemorrhage and necrosis, or pleural thickening with nodularity

Microscopic Findings
▸ Generally resemble soft tissue sarcoma counterparts
▸ Synovial sarcoma is usually monophasic fibrous or poorly differentiated but can also be biphasic
▸ Angiosarcoma is often epithelioid, resembling epithelial mesothelioma

Immunohistochemical Features
▸ Synovial sarcoma
  ▸ Generally positive for cytokeratins, epithelial membrane antigen, vimentin, bcl-2
  ▸ Frequently positive for CD56, Ber Ep4, calretinin, CD99
  ▸ Generally negative for CD34, actins, desmin, WT-1
▸ Angiosarcoma
  ▸ Generally positive for vascular markers CD31, CD34, and Factor VIII
  ▸ May be focally positive for cytokeratin

Ultrastructural Features
▸ In vascular tumors, features may include well-developed basal lamina, pinocytotic vesicles, numerous intermediate filaments, and Weibel-Palade bodies

Molecular Studies
▸ Synovial sarcoma carries a characteristic t(X;18)(p11;q11) translocation, resulting in SYT-SSX gene fusion

Pathologic Differential Diagnosis
▸ Metastatic sarcomas
▸ Malignant solitary fibrous tumor
▸ Malignant mesothelioma
▸ Metastatic sarcomatoid carcinoma
▸ Metastatic sarcomatoid melanoma

angiosarcomas generally have a poor prognosis, but occasional long-term survivors have been reported.

DESMOID TUMOR

Desmoid tumors constitute a group of benign clonal neoplasms of fibroblastic or myofibroblastic origin that are locally invasive. Historically, desmoid tumor has been classified according to its gross distribution, with the recognition of abdominal, intraabdominal, and extraabdominal subtypes. The extraabdominal tumors are typically located within the musculature of shoulder and chest wall presenting as palpable masses, with only rare examples of an intrathoracic variant. In this location, they have been reported to arise in both visceral and parietal pleura, where they are apt to be confused with other more common spindle cell proliferations, particularly SFT.

CLINICAL FEATURES

These uncommon tumors have been reported in adolescence through middle age, with mean occurrence in the fifth decade. A history of antecedent trauma may be elicited, and the clinical presentation of chest pain and dyspnea is non-specific.

RADIOLOGIC FEATURES

Intrathoracic desmoid tumors tend to be large and nonpedunculated masses, 5 to 16 cm in greatest dimension, based in either visceral or parietal pleura, with sharp circumscription and rounded borders, unaccompanied by pleural effusion. Involvement of bilateral chest cavities by a single posterior tumor, with mediastinal shift and compression of both lungs, has been reported.

PATHOLOGIC FEATURES

GROSS FINDINGS

Broad-based pleural attachment is typical, with smooth surface. The cut section is firm, gray-white and bosselated, without hemorrhage or necrosis.

MICROSCOPIC FINDINGS

Histologically, desmoid tumors have the typical features shared by these neoplasms in other anatomic locations, which include a variably cellular proliferation of bland spindle cells in a collagenous or myxoid stromal matrix (Figures 33-21, 33-22). Areas of wiry, "keloidal" collagen are not usually observed but may be present, and an infiltrative peripheral border is characteristic.

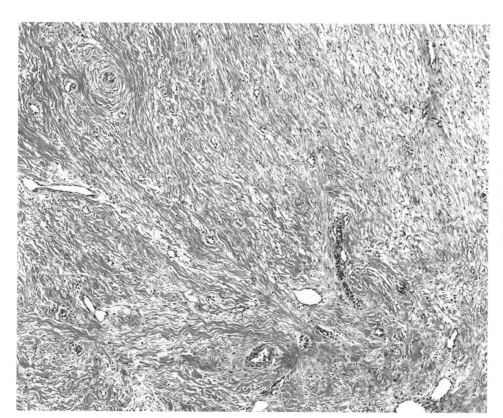

FIGURE 33-21

Desmoid tumor
This example shows prominent collagenization, bland spindle cells, and focal myxoid change. (Courtesy of Dani Zander, MD, Penn State Hershey Medical Center, Hershey, Pennsylvania.)

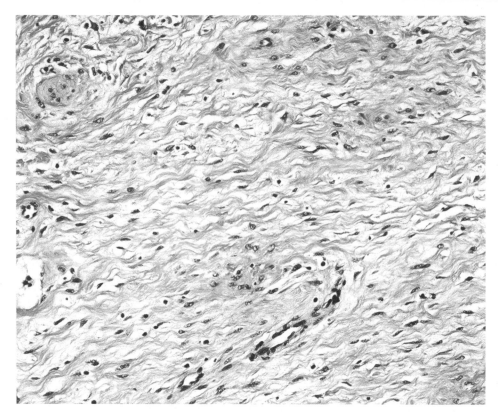

FIGURE 33-22
Desmoid tumor
Spindle cells have features of fibroblasts, without cytoatypia, and lie in a collagenized background. (Courtesy of Dani Zander, MD, Penn State Hershey Medical Center, Hershey, Pennsylvania.)

Hemangiopericytomatous or storiform growth patterns are not observed. The nuclear features are characteristically low-grade, and mitoses are rare.

ANCILLARY STUDIES

IMMUNOHISTOCHEMISTRY

Typical of desmoid tumor's fibroblastic/myofibroblastic differentiation, characteristic spindle cell expression of vimentin and both smooth muscle and muscle-specific actins is observed. Expression of desmin is less common. Negative staining for anti-cytokeratins, S-100, and CD34 is characteristic.

DIFFERENTIAL DIAGNOSIS

Desmoid tumor must be distinguished from other pleural-based, low-grade spindle cell proliferations, particularly SFT. This may be especially difficult on small thoracoscopic forceps or needle biopsy specimens. Nonetheless, immunohistochemistry for muscle markers and CD34 is useful for assisting in correct classification, as discussed above. SFT will usually show an opposite pattern of reactivity, with staining for CD34 and a lack of staining for muscle markers. Desmoid tumor typically contains neither the patternless or storiform patterns of compact cellular fascicles nor the hemangiopericytomatous foci characteristic of SFT and often has a more fibrillar or myxoid stromal matrix lacking strands of keloidal collagen. An absence of wavy nuclei aids in its distinction from benign neural tumors such as neurofibroma or schwannoma, which are also usually immunoreactive for S100. Other spindle cell sarcomas may also be considered in the differential diagnosis but usually manifest more nuclear pleomorphism, mitotic activity, and sometimes necrosis or characteristics reflecting specific types of differentiation. Sarcomatoid and desmoplastic mesotheliomas represent other diagnostic considerations, but will usually be immunoreactive for cytokeratin.

PROGNOSIS AND THERAPY

Similar to its extrapleural counterparts, desmoid tumor shares a high incidence of local recurrence following incomplete resection, but no instances of distant metastases or death have been reported. Proper diagnosis and distinction from SFT is essential for the planning of desmoid tumor resection, as its growth beyond grossly visible borders mandates wide resection, with en bloc excision of ribs and chest wall soft tissues if these areas are involved. In the few reported cases of pleural desmoid tumor, residual or recurrent disease following resection has been reported, and there may be at least a palliative role for postoperative radiation.

PRIMITIVE NEUROECTODERMAL TUMOR AND DESMOPLASTIC SMALL ROUND CELL TUMOR

Primitive neuroectodermal tumors (PNETs) number among the small round cell neoplasms affecting the young, sharing many clinical and pathologic features with Ewing's sarcoma. These tumors uncommonly arise in the pleura or chest wall, where they have also been termed Askin tumor and malignant small cell tumor of the thoracopulmonary region. Desmoplastic small round cell tumor (DSRCT), which has been more commonly reported in the peritoneum, is a related but distinct neoplasm, which may also uncommonly occur in the pleura.

CLINICAL FEATURES

Thoracopulmonary PNET and DSRCT are both typically tumors of young adulthood, but have been reported in all age groups, and are slightly more common in males. Often associated with pleural effusions, these tumors form masses that may be apparent in the chest wall. Symptoms can include non-specific complaints of dyspnea and chest pain.

RADIOLOGIC FEATURES

Thoracic imaging studies typically reveal a large pleural-based mass or chest wall soft tissue tumor that may involve the pleura or lung secondarily. Pleural effusion is commonly observed.

PATHOLOGIC FEATURES

GROSS FINDINGS

Thoracopulmonary PNET is a soft, pale, and fleshy tumor, with hemorrhage and necrosis apparent on cut section. Large size, with tumor bulk in excess of 10 cm, is common. Similarly, DSRCT presents with nodular masses that may be associated with pleural effusion.

MICROSCOPIC FINDINGS

In PNET, a dense, uniform population of small round blue cells is typical, which may feature formation of rosettes (Figure 33-23). Scant cytoplasm is evident, and PAS-positivity may be observed. The nuclei are usually uniform and round with indistinct nucleoli. DSRCT has similar cytologic features, with a background of dense fibrosis. Focal rhabdoid features and necrosis may be seen.

ANCILLARY STUDIES

IMMUNOHISTOCHEMISTRY

PNET demonstrates characteristic immunoreactivity for CD99, typically in a diffuse and membranous pattern (Figure 33-24), and similar expression is observed in a minority of cases of DSRCT. Immunohistochemical evidence for neuroectodermal differentiation is suggested by variable expression of neuron-specific enolase, neurofilament protein, and synaptophysin. Both DSRCT and PNET may focally express cytokeratins. DSRCT expresses cytokeratins with higher frequency, as well as Wilms' tumor antigen (WT1) and vimentin, and typically shows dot-like positivity for desmin. Recently, PNET was also shown to express tight junction structural and linker proteins, suggesting partial epithelial differentiation.

CYTOGENETIC STUDIES

The PNET family is characterized by the t(11;22)(q24;q12) reciprocal translocation as well as rearrangements of the EWS gene, with the formation of EWS-FLI1 fusion transcript. DSRCT features a similar translocation t(11;22)(p13;q12) associated with the EWS-WT1 fusion transcript.

ULTRASTRUCTURAL STUDIES

In DSRCT, perinuclear aggregates of intermediate filaments may be seen by transmission electron microscopy. Intracytoplasmic neolumina, with short microvilli characteristic of submesothelial cells, have also been reported.

DIFFERENTIAL DIAGNOSIS

The differential diagnosis for small round cell tumors in this location includes PNET and DSRCT, as well as lymphoma, rhabdomyosarcoma, neuroblastoma, and small cell carcinoma. Immunohistochemistry, cytogenetic studies, and clinical and radiologic data can be helpful for assisting in differentiation between these entities.

PROGNOSIS AND THERAPY

The prognosis of PNETs is related to clinical stage, which in turn is affected by tumor size and resectability. Long-term survival can be achieved in early-stage tumors, defined as less than 5 cm in size and grossly resectable by excision, which are also treated with adjuvant combined modality therapy. A subset of survivors is at risk for the development of treatment-related sarcomas and leukemia. Overall survival is reportedly between 30% and 40%. DSRCTs of pleura are usually fatal within a few years of diagnosis.

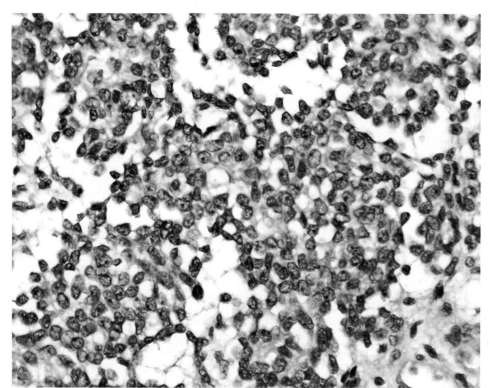

FIGURE 33-23
Primitive neuroectodermal tumor
This small round blue cell tumor shows characteristic dense growth. Tumor cells contain minimal cytoplasm, with round nuclei and indistinct nucleoli.

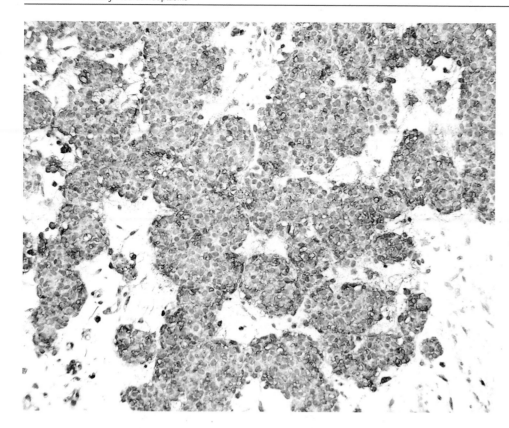

FIGURE 33-24
Primitive neuroectodermal tumor
Diffuse and membranous CD99 immuno-reactivity, as shown here, is commonly observed.

PRIMITIVE NEUROECTODERMAL TUMOR—FACT SHEET

Definition

▸ Soft tissue sarcoma grouped among small round cell tumors of childhood and young adulthood, sharing significant clinical and pathologic overlap with the Ewing's sarcoma family of tumors

Incidence

▸ Uncommon presentation of an uncommon tumor

Gender, Race, and Age Distribution

▸ Described in all age groups, most common between the ages of 10 and 30
▸ Equal incidence among the genders
▸ Strong predilection for Caucasians

Clinical Features

▸ Painful, rapidly growing pleural-based or chest wall mass
▸ No elevation in urinary catecholamines helps distinguish from neuroblastoma

Prognosis and Therapy

▸ Complete resection with chemotherapy is usually the preferred thera-peutic approach, and radiation therapy may be added for individual patients
▸ Completely resected small early stage lesions (< 5 cm) treated with chemotherapy and radiation therapy may be curable in some cases
▸ Overall survival is reportedly 30% to 40%

PRIMITIVE NEUROECTODERMAL TUMOR—PATHOLOGIC FEATURES

Gross Findings

▸ Pale, soft, and fleshy tumor with necrosis and hemorrhage on cut section
▸ Can involve pleura or chest wall

Microscopic Findings

▸ Small round cells growing in sheets and nests with rosette formation
▸ Nuclei are round and hyperchromatic
▸ Cytoplasm is scant

Immunohistochemical Features

▸ Characteristic expression of CD99, often with coexpression of neuron-specific enolase, chromogranin, synaptophysin, and neurofilament protein, and occasionally cytokeratins and desmin

Cytogenetic Features

▸ t(11;22)(q24;q12), EWS-FLI-1 fusion transcript

Pathologic Differential Diagnosis

▸ Desmoplastic small round cell tumor
▸ Small cell carcinoma of the lung (older individuals)
▸ Lymphoma
▸ Rhabdomyosarcoma
▸ Neuroblastoma

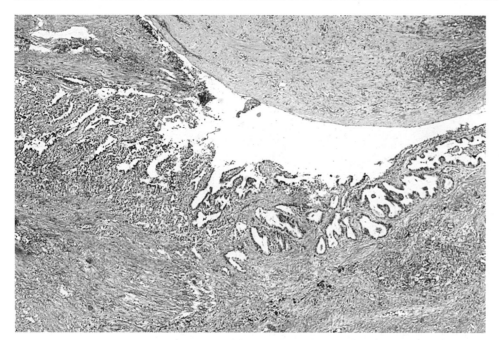

FIGURE 33-25

Pseudomesotheliomatous adenocarcinoma
Pleurotropic spread of tumor cells is evident in this view.

DESMOPLASTIC SMALL ROUND CELL TUMOR—FACT SHEET

Definition
- ▸▸ A small round cell tumor of young adulthood

Incidence
- ▸▸ Rare pleural neoplasm, more common in the peritoneum

Age and Gender Distribution
- ▸▸ Occur in young adults of both genders

Clinical Features
- ▸▸ Chest pain

Prognosis
- ▸▸ Death usually occurs within several years of diagnosis

DESMOPLASTIC SMALL ROUND CELL TUMOR—PATHOLOGIC FEATURES

Gross Findings
- ▸▸ Pleural-basaed masses or encasement of the lung
- ▸▸ Often involve the mediastinum

Microscopic Findings
- ▸▸ Sheets and nests of small round cells in a desmoplastic stromal backround

Immunohistochemical Features
- ▸▸ Tumors express cytokeratins, EMA, WT1, vimentin, and sometimes CD15
- ▸▸ Dot-like positivily for desmin is characteristic

Cytogenetic Features
- ▸▸ +(11;22) (p13;q12), EWS-WT1 gene fusion

Pathologic Differential Diagnosis
- ▸▸ Peripheral neuroectodermal tumor
- ▸▸ Lymphoma
- ▸▸ Rhabdomyosarcoma
- ▸▸ Neuroblastoma

NEOPLASMS METASTATIC TO THE PLEURA

Metastases to the pleura are far more common than any of the primary pleural tumors discussed above and are covered in more detail in chapter 34. Carcinomas are most apt to develop pleural metastases following direct extension or lymphatic spread. Carcinoma of the lung is the most common form of pleural metastatic disease and may occur as a diffuse process or as pleurotropic growth of an underlying primary peripheral carcinoma ("pseudomesotheliomatous" carcinoma). Carcinomas of the breast,

gastrointestinal tract, ovary, pancreas, and kidney also commonly metastasize to the pleura (Figure 33-25). Pleural metastases from prostatic carcinoma have been described in at least 20% of autopsied cases. Less commonly, thymic epithelial tumors may spread to the pleura with growth patterns resembling mesothelioma. Malignant lymphoma and leukemia may permeate the pleural lymphatics and result in effusions.

SELECTED READINGS

Malignant Pleural Mesothelioma

1. Allen TC, Cagle PT, Churg AM, et al. Localized malignant mesothelioma. *Am J Surg Pathol.* 2005;29:866-73.
2. Butnor KJ, Sporn TA, Hammar SP, Roggli VL. Well-differentiated papillary mesothelioma. *Am J Surg Pathol.* 2001;25:1304-9.
3. Cagle PT, Churg A. Differential diagnosis of benign and malignant mesothelial proliferations on pleural biopsies. *Arch Pathol Lab Med.* 2005;129:1421-7.
4. Churg A, Colby TV, Cagle PT, et al. The separation of benign and malignant mesothelial proliferations. *Am J Surg Pathol.* 2000;24:1183-2000.
5. Galateau-Sallé F, Vignaud JM, Burke L, et al. Well-differentiated papillary mesothelioma of the pleura: a series of 24 cases. *Am J Surg Pathol.* 2004;28:534-40.
6. Mangano WE, Cagle PT, Churg A, Vollmer RT, Roggli VL. The diagnosis of desmoplastic malignant mesothelioma and its distinction from fibrous pleurisy: a histologic and immunohistochemical analysis of 31 cases including p53 immunostaining. *Am J Clin Pathol.* 1998;110:191-9.
7. Ordonez NG. Immunohistochemical diagnosis of epithelioid mesothelioma: an update. *Arch Pathol Lab Med.* 2005;129:1407-14.
8. Robinson BWS, Lake RA. Advances in malignant mesothelioma. *N Engl J Med.* 2005;353:1591-603.
9. Roggli VL, Sharma A, Butnor KJ, Sporn T, Vollmer RT. Malignant mesothelioma and occupational exposure to asbestos: a clinicopathologic correlation of 1445 cases. *Ultrastruct Pathol.* 2002;26:1-11.
10. Rusch VW. A proposed new international TNM staging system for malignant pleural mesothelioma from the International Mesothelioma Interest Group. *Lung Cancer.* 1996;14:1-12.
11. Sporn TA, Roggli VL. Mesothelioma. In: Roggli VL, Oury TD, Sporn TA, eds. *Pathology of Asbestos-Associated Diseases.* New York: Springer, 2004. pp. 104-67.
12. Wang ZJ, Reddy GP, Gotway MB, et al. Malignant pleural mesothelioma: evaluation with CT, MR imaging and PET. *Radiographics.* 2004;9:105-19.

Solitary Fibrous Tumor

13. Cardillo G, Facciolo F, Cavazzana AO, Capece G, Gasparri R, Martelli M. Localized (solitary) fibrous tumors of the pleura: an analysis of 55 patients. *Ann Thorac Surg.* 2000;70:1808-12.
14. England DM, Hochholzer L, McCarthy MJ. Localized benign and malignant fibrous tumors of the pleura. *Am J Surg Pathol.* 1989;13:640-58.
15. Granville L, Laga AC, Allen TC, et al. Review and update of uncommon primary pleural tumors: a practical approach to diagnosis. *Arch Pathol Lab Med.* 2005;129:1428-43.
16. Hanau CA, Miettinen M. Solitary fibrous tumor: histological and immunohistochemical spectrum of benign and malignant variants presenting at different sites. *Hum Pathol.* 1995;26:440-9.
17. Kanthan R, Torkian R. Recurrent solitary fibrous tumor of the pleura with malignant transformation. *Arch Pathol Lab Med.* 2004;18:460-2.
18. Moran CA, Suster S, Koss MN. The spectrum of histologic growth patterns in benign and malignant fibrous tumors of the pleura. *Semin Diagn Pathol.* 1992;9:169-80.
19. Sung SH, Chang JW, Kim J, Lee KS, Han J, Park SI. Solitary fibrous tumors of the pleura: surgical outcome and clinical course. *Ann Thorac Surg.* 2005;79:303-7.

Synovial Sarcomas and Other Primary Sarcomas

20. Aubry MC, Bridge JA, Wickert R, Tazelaar HD. Primary monophasic synovial sarcoma of the pleura: five cases confirmed by the presence of the SYT-SSX fusion transcript. *Am J Surg Pathol.* 2001;25:776-81.
21. Begueret H, Galateau-Sallé F, Guillou L, et al. Primary intrathoracic synovial sarcoma: a clinicopathologic study of 40 t(X;18)-positive cases from the French Sarcoma Group and the Mesopath Group. *Am J Surg Pathol.* 2005;29:339-46.
22. Crotty EJ, McAdams HP, Erasmus JJ, Sporn TA, Roggli VL. Epithelioid hemangioendothelioma of the pleura: clinical and radiologic features. *Am J Roentgenol.* 2000;175:1545-9.
23. Essary LR, Vargas SO, Fletcher CD. Primary pleuropulmonary synovial sarcoma: reappraisal of a recently described anatomic subset. *Cancer.* 2002;94:459-69.

24. Falconieri G, Bussani R, Mirra M, Zanella M. Pseudomesotheliomatous angiosarcoma: a pleuropulmonary lesion simulating malignant mesothelioma. *Histopathology.* 1997;30:429-34.
25. Gaertner E, Zeren EH, Fleming MV, Colby TV, Travis WD. Biphasic synovial sarcomas arising in the pleural cavity: a clinicopathologic study of five cases. *Am J Surg Pathol.* 1996;20:36-45.
26. Lin BT, Colby T, Gown AM, et al. Malignant vascular tumors of the serous membranes mimicking mesothelioma: a report of 14 cases. *Am J Surg Pathol.* 1996;20:1431-9.
27. Miettinen M, Limon J, Niezabitowski A, Lasota J. Calretinin and other mesothelioma markers in synovial sarcoma: analysis of antigenic similarities and differences with malignant mesothelioma. *Am J Surg Pathol.* 2001;25:610-7.
28. Nicholson AG, Goldstraw P, Fisher C. Synovial sarcoma of the pleura and its differentiation from other primary pleural tumors: a clinicopathological and immunohistochemical review of three cases. *Histopathology.* 1998;33:508-13.
29. Okby NT, Travis WD. Liposarcoma of the pleural cavity: clinical and pathological features of 4 cases with a review of the literature. *Arch Pathol Lab Med.* 2000;124:699-703.
30. Pramesh CS, Madur BP, Raina S, Desai SB, Mistry RC. Angiosarcoma of the pleura. *Ann Thorac Cardiovasc Surg.* 2004;10:187-90.
31. Zhang PJ, Livolsi VA, Brooks JJ. Malignant epithelioid vascular tumors of the pleura: report of a series and literature review. *Hum Pathol.* 2000;31:29-34.

Desmoid Tumor

32. Andino L, Cagle PT, Murer BT, et al. Pleuropulmonary desmoid tumors: immunohistochemical comparison with solitary fibrous tumors and assessment of beta-catenin and cyclin D1 expression. *Arch Pathol Lab Med.* 2006;130:1503-9.
33. Brunneman RB, Ro JY, Ordonez NG. Mooney J, El-Naggar AK, Ayala AG. Extrapleural solitary fibrous tumor. A clinicopathologic study of 24 cases. *Mod Pathol.* 1999;51:1034-42.
34. Takeshima Y, Nakayori F, Nakano T, et al. Extraabdominal desmoid tumor presenting as an intrathoracic tumor: case report and literature review. *Pathol Internat.* 2001;51:824-8.
35. Wilson RW, Gallateau-Sallé F, Moran CA. Desmoid tumors of the pleura: a clinicopathologic mimic of localized fibrous tumor. *Mod Pathol.* 1999;12:9-14.

Primitive Neuroectodermal Tumor and Desmoplastic Small Round Cell Tumor

36. Christiansen S, Semik M, Dockhorn-Dworniczak B, et al. Diagnosis, treatment and outcome of patients with Askin tumors. *Thorac Cardiovasc Surg.* 2000;48:311-5.
37. Folpe AL, Goldblum JR , Rubin BP, et al. Morphologic and immunophenotypic diversity in Ewing family tumors: a study of 66 genetically confirmed cases. *Am J Surg Pathol.* 2005;29:1025-33.
38. O'Sullivan MJ, Perlman EJ, Furman J, Humphrey PA, Dehner LP, Pfeifer JD. Visceral peripheral neuroectodermal tumors: a clinicopathologic and molecular study. *Hum Pathol.* 2001;32:1109-15.
39. Parkash V, Gerald WL, Parma A, Miettinen M, Rosai J. Desmoplastic small round cell tumor of the pleura. *Am J Surg Pathol.* 1995;19:659-65.
40. Sapi Z, Szentirmay Z, Orosz Z. Desmoplastic small round cell tumour of the pleura: a case report with further cytogenetic and ultrastructural evidence of "mesothelioblastemic" origin. *Eur J Surg Oncol.* 1999;25:633-4.
41. Syed S, Haque AK, Hawkins HK, Sorensen PH, Cowan DF. Desmoplastic small round cell tumor of the lung. *Arch Pathol Lab Med.* 2002;126:1226-8.
42. Travis WD, Churg A, Aubry MC, et al. Mesenchymal tumours. In:Trawis WD, Brambilla E, Müller-Hermelink HK, Harris CC, eds. *Pathology and Genetics: Tumours of the Lung, Pleura, Thymus and Heart.* Lyon: IARC Press, 2004, p.144.

34 Pleural Involvement by Extrapleural Neoplasms

Kelly J. Butnor

INTRODUCTION

Over 150,000 malignant pleural effusions occur each year in the United States, the majority of which result from pleural metastases of extrapleural malignancies. While pleural involvement generally occurs at an advanced stage of disease, in some cases symptoms related to pleural involvement are the presenting manifestation. Occasionally, it is difficult to determine the site of origin of pleural metastases; in as many as 10% of malignant pleural effusions, no primary site is found. Metastases can grow along the pleura in a "pseudomesotheliomatous" fashion, simulating the appearance of malignant mesothelioma.

Extrapleural malignancies can gain access to the pleural space from pleural lymphatics that connect with mediastinal and transdiaphragmatic chest wall lymphatics. Other mechanisms by which tumors involve the pleura include direct extension from an adjacent site, such as the lung, or through hematogenous spread. Tumors that metastasize to the pleura by lymphohematogenous dissemination have a tendency to involve the inferior aspects of the pleura, which are the most dependent regions of the pleura, often bilaterally.

While pleural involvement has been described for neoplasms originating in nearly every anatomic site, the most common extrapleural neoplasm to involve the pleura is lung carcinoma. Breast carcinoma is second in frequency, which in large part accounts for the 1.5 to 2 times higher incidence of malignant pleural effusions in women.

This chapter focuses on the most common extrapleural neoplasms to involve the pleura and reviews the features that distinguish these neoplasms from malignant pleural mesothelioma. The most common presenting symptom of pleural involvement by extrapleural neoplasms is dyspnea secondary to the pleural effusion. However, an identical presentation may also occur with malignant mesothelioma. Pathologic evaluation is necessary to distinguish between these entities.

LUNG CARCINOMA METASTATIC TO THE PLEURA

Lung carcinoma is the most frequent cause of malignant pleural effusions in the United States. Between 7% and 15% of all lung carcinomas are accompanied by malignant pleural effusions. Although malignant pleural effusions are observed in all histologic types of lung carcinoma, they are most commonly associated with adenocarcinoma. The frequency of malignant pleural effusion in adenocarcinoma is almost certainly related to the propensity for adenocarcinoma to arise in the periphery of the lung, where it can directly invade the visceral pleura and gain access to the pleural lymphatics.

CLINICAL FEATURES

Lung carcinoma should be strongly suspected if dyspnea is accompanied by hemoptysis.

RADIOLOGIC FEATURES

Lung carcinoma metastatic to the pleura often manifests radiographically as a pleural effusion. Occasionally, an effusion may be so voluminous as to obscure a pulmonary mass, requiring drainage to facilitate detection. An intrapulmonary site of origin is radiographically evident in most cases but is sometimes difficult to discern. Intrapulmonary tumors may extend directly into the pleura. Alternatively, the pleura can be studded by multiple small nodules or become irregularly thickened by larger nodules (Figure 34-1). In rare cases, the pleura appears diffusely thickened. This last pattern can mimic malignant mesothelioma, particularly in cases where a discrete intrapulmonary mass is not apparent.

PATHOLOGIC FEATURES

GROSS FINDINGS

Malignant pleural effusions from lung carcinomas are typically exudative and appear somewhat cloudy. Occasionally, they are grossly bloody. Depending on the extent of involvement, lung carcinomas that directly invade the pleura may produce puckering and slight granularity of the visceral pleura surface. In more advanced cases, they can form a white to tan firm nodular pleural mass (Figure 34-2A). Pulmonary carcinomas that reach the pleura through lymphohematogenous dissemination may give rise to multiple firm white to tan nodules of variable size (Figure 34-2B). Rarely, metastatic tumor diffusely plugs pleural lymphatic channels, forming a finely reticulated pattern over the pleural surfaces without generating a pleural mass or nodule (Figure 34-2C). An uncommon pattern of pleural involvement, so-called pseudomesotheliomatous carcinoma, can cause considerable confusion with malignant mesothelioma. Pseudomesotheliomatous carcinomas are characterized by firm, white to tan rind-like diffuse pleural thickening that may encase

the underlying lung (Figures 34-2D, 34-3). In some cases of pseudomesotheliomatous carcinoma, an intrapulmonary source may not be grossly evident, making the diagnosis more challenging.

MICROSCOPIC FINDINGS

The overall configuration of metastatic tumor to the pleura is often best appreciated at scanning magnification (Figure 34-4 A, B). Whether it is an adenocarcinoma or one of the other types of lung carcinoma, the histologic features recapitulate those seen in the primary tumor (Figure 34-5). Pulmonary adenocarcinoma metastatic to the pleura can exhibit an array of patterns, including acinar, glandular, tubulopapillary, micropapillary, and solid growth (Figures 34-5C-E). In some cases, tumor consists of only sparse glands in a desmoplastic stroma (Figure 34-5F). In other cases, particularly those in which there is confluent growth of tubulopapillary formations or solid sheets of tumor, distinction from malignant pleural mesothelioma becomes particularly important.

The cells in pulmonary adenocarcinoma tend to exhibit more eccentric nuclei, more prominent nucleoli, and greater pleomorphism than those of malignant mesothelioma. A careful search may disclose intracytoplasmic vacuoles in some pulmonary adenocarcinomas. However, the degree of overlap between the histologic features of pulmonary carcinoma—in particular, adenocarcinoma but also malignant mesothelioma—necessitates correlation with the clinical and radiographic features and, in most cases, the use of ancillary techniques.

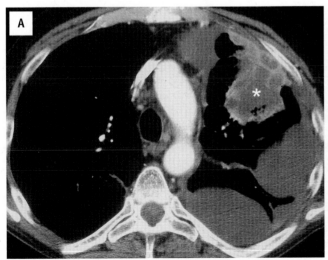
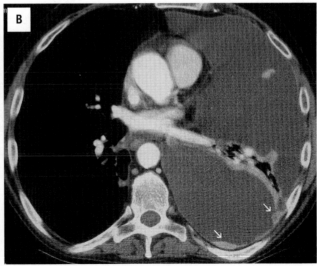

FIGURE 34-1

Lung carcinoma metastatic to the pleura
(A) On this chest CT scan, a peripheral lung adenocarcinoma (*) directly invades the pleura. **(B)** Additional metastases separate from the primary tumor appear as pleural nodules (arrows). (Courtesy of Jeffrey Klein, M.D. Burlington, Vermont.)

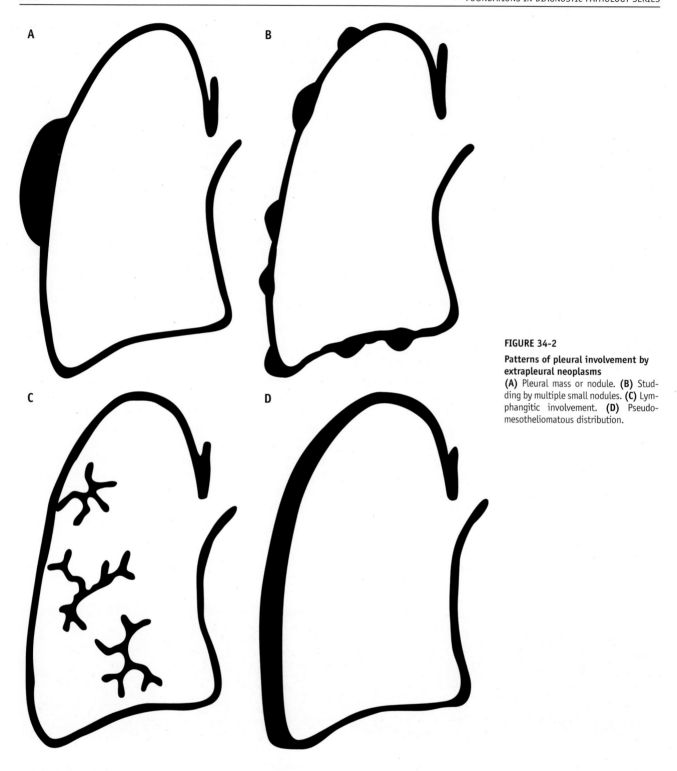

FIGURE 34-2

Patterns of pleural involvement by extrapleural neoplasms

(A) Pleural mass or nodule. **(B)** Studding by multiple small nodules. **(C)** Lymphangitic involvement. **(D)** Pseudomesotheliomatous distribution.

ANCILLARY STUDIES

PLEURAL EFFUSION CYTOLOGY/FINE NEEDLE ASPIRATION BIOPSY

Transthoracic fine needle aspiration biopsy of a pleural mass is often a satisfactory method for diagnosing pleural involvement by carcinoma of the lung. In tumors that produce a malignant pleural effusion, diagnosis can often be achieved by cytologic examination of pleural fluid. The cytologic features of pulmonary carcinomas metastatic to the pleura resemble those of the primary tumor. For metastatic pulmonary adenocarcinoma, tumor cells typically have a high nuclear-to-cytoplasmic ratio, irregular nuclear contours, and one or more nucleoli (Figure 34-6). Neoplastic cells may appear individually or as sheets, acini, papillary formations, or three-dimensional clusters. Three-dimensional clusters

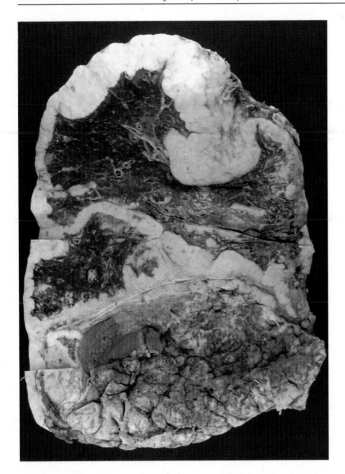

FIGURE 34-3

Lung carcinoma metastatic to the pleura

Gross photograph of surgically resected pseudomesotheliomatous pulmonary carcinoma metastatic to the pleura. Rind-like encasement of the lung mimics the pattern of growth seen with malignant pleural mesothelioma. (Courtesy of Prof. Richard Attanoos, Cardiff, United Kingdom.)

in adenocarcinoma typically have smooth community borders. As mentioned previously, intracytoplasmic vacuoles may be seen in cases. Mitotic figures, especially atypical forms, are also a helpful feature.

Malignant mesothelioma can also appear as papillary clusters in cytologic preparations. However, in contrast to pulmonary adenocarcinomas, tumor cell clusters in malignant mesothelioma typically have knobby rather than smooth outlines. The cell borders of malignant mesothelioma are lacy rather than sharply demarcated, and intercellular "windows" are often seen. Although they may demonstrate degenerative intracytoplasmic vacuoles, the rounded secretory-type vacuoles observed in some adenocarcinomas are not a feature of malignant mesothelioma. Despite these differences, it can be difficult to separate metastatic carcinoma of the lung from malignant pleural mesothelioma on the basis of cytologic features alone, a distinction that can be aided by histochemical and immunohistochemical techniques.

HISTOCHEMISTRY AND IMMUNOHISTOCHEMISTRY

Just as there is no single entirely sensitive and specific histochemical or immunohistochemical marker for malignant mesothelioma, so too is the case for lung carcinoma metastatic to the pleura. A panel of stains is typically used to distinguish between these entities.

Mucin stains are effective and inexpensive tools for separating metastatic pulmonary adenocarcinoma from malignant mesothelioma. Although rare cases of mucin-producing malignant mesothelioma have been reported, intense staining of intracytoplasmic vacuoles and/or glandular lumens by periodic acid-Schiff following diastase pretreatment (PAS-D) strongly favors a diagnosis of adenocarcinoma (Figure 34-7A). Diastase pretreatment is essential to abolish staining of glycogen, an abundant component of most malignant mesotheliomas. Alcian blue following hyaluronidase pretreatment is another method for highlighting mucin in pulmonary adenocarcinomas (Figure 34-7B). With rare exception, alcian blue with hyaluronidase is negative in malignant mesothelioma. Malignant mesotheliomas are often rich in hyaluronic acid, the staining of which is abolished by hyaluronidase pretreatment. As Mayer's mucicarmine stains both mucin and hyaluronic acid, it is not recommended for distinguishing metastatic pulmonary adenocarcinoma from malignant pleural mesothelioma.

As for immunohistochemistry, pulmonary adenocarcinomas metastatic to the pleura are typically positive for TTF-1, CEA, LeuM1 (CD15), and BerEP4 (Figures 34-8A, B). Of these, the most specific marker for metastatic carcinoma of pulmonary origin is TTF-1. For other histologic types of lung carcinoma, the immunohistochemical profile of the metastatic tumor usually matches the primary tumor. Markers that are typically positive in malignant mesothelioma, such as calretinin, thrombomodulin, podoplanin (D2-40), and CK 5/6, are negative in the overwhelming majority of metastatic pulmonary adenocarcinomas (Figure 34-8C). However, care must be taken with interpreting thrombomodulin and CK 5/6 staining, which are positive in the majority of pulmonary squamous cell carcinomas as well as malignant mesotheliomas.

ULTRASTRUCTURAL EXAMINATION

With the array of immunohistochemical markers available, electron microscopy is not as frequently employed as it once was in the distinction between malignant mesothelioma and lung carcinoma metastatic to the pleura. Nevertheless, in equivocal cases, ultrastructural examination can be a valuable tool. In contrast to the abundant, long, slender microvilli of malignant mesothelioma, pulmonary adenocarcinoma have microvilli that are short and stubby (Figure 34-9). Adenocarcinomas may contain secretory granules. Such structures are lacking in mesothelioma, as are terminal bars, which are found near the glandular lumens in adenocarcinoma.

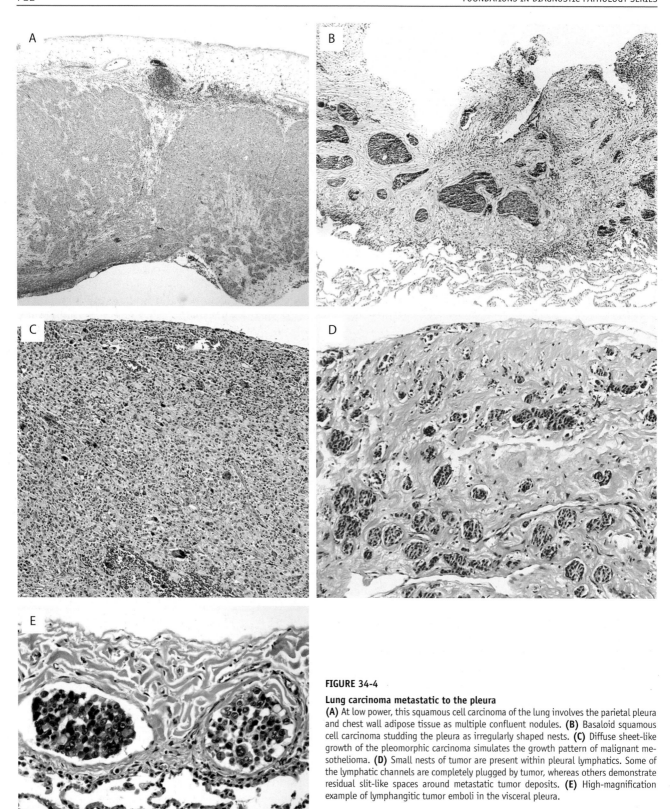

FIGURE 34-4

Lung carcinoma metastatic to the pleura
(A) At low power, this squamous cell carcinoma of the lung involves the parietal pleura and chest wall adipose tissue as multiple confluent nodules. (B) Basaloid squamous cell carcinoma studding the pleura as irregularly shaped nests. (C) Diffuse sheet-like growth of the pleomorphic carcinoma simulates the growth pattern of malignant mesothelioma. (D) Small nests of tumor are present within pleural lymphatics. Some of the lymphatic channels are completely plugged by tumor, whereas others demonstrate residual slit-like spaces around metastatic tumor deposits. (E) High-magnification example of lymphangitic tumor emboli in the visceral pleura.

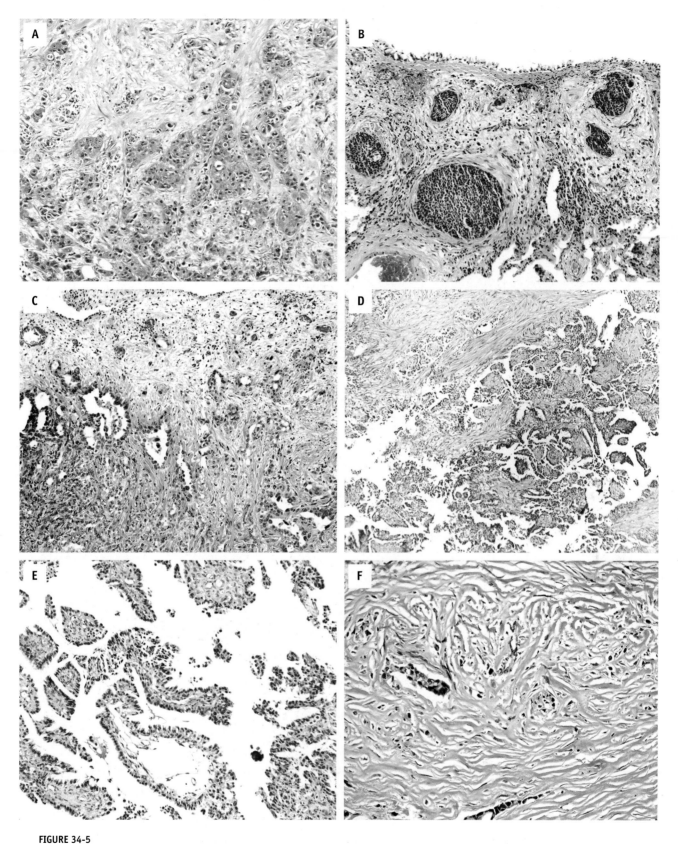

FIGURE 34-5

Lung carcinoma metastatic to the pleura

(A) In this metastatic squamous cell carcinoma, tumor infiltrates the pleura as nests and small cords. **(B)** This medium-power photomicrograph of the case shows small nodules and irregular nests of hyperchromatic tumor cells with scant cytoplasm. A reactive mesothelial lining is present on the surface of the visceral pleura. The differential diagnosis would include metastatic small cell carcinoma. The morphologic features were similar to the patient's primary lung tumor. **(C)** At medium power, this adenocarcinoma metastatic to the visceral pleura grows as acini and tubules. **(D)** This example exhibits a papillary configuration with arborizing fibrovascular cores and marked desmoplasia. **(E)** At high power, epithelial tufting and psammoma body formation is seen. Psammoma bodies can be seen in carcinomas with a papillary configuration from a variety of sites. Differential considerations would include metastatic ovarian carcinoma and malignant mesothelioma with a papillary growth pattern. **(F)** Neoplastic glands can be quite sparse in tumors that infiltrate fibrotic pleura, making detection difficult, particularly in small samples. Metastatic tumors associated with marked desmoplasia can exhibit a similar growth pattern.

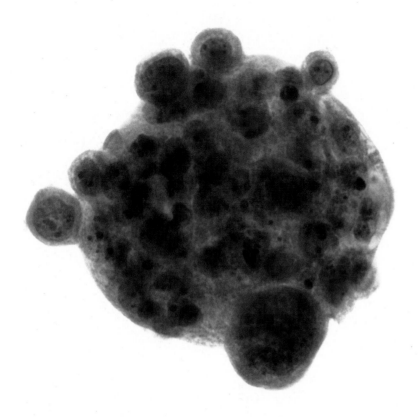

FIGURE 34-6

Lung carcinoma in pleural effusion
Pleural fluid from a patient with pulmonary adenocarcinoma showing a three-dimensional cluster of tumor cells, which features relatively smooth community borders, high nuclear-to-cytoplasmic ratios, moderate anisocytosis, occasional nucleoli, hyperchromasia, and irregular nuclear membranes (Papanicolaou).

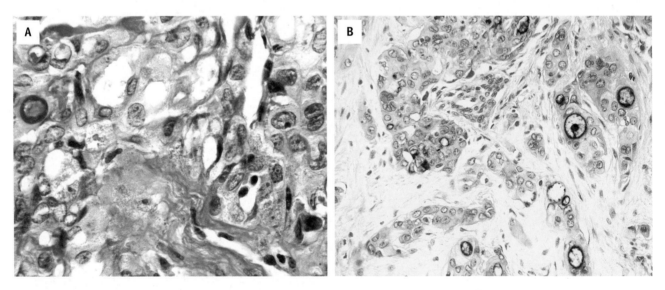

FIGURE 34-7

Lung carcinoma metastatic to the pleura
In mucin-producing adenocarcinomas, pretreatment with diastase or hyaluronidase does not diminish staining of intracytoplasmic mucin droplets. This contrasts with malignant mesotheliomas, the majority of which do not contain mucin. **(A)** Periodic acid-Schiff with diastase (PAS-D). **(B)** Alcian blue with hyaluronidase.

DIFFERENTIAL DIAGNOSIS

Malignant mesothelioma is the principal entity to consider in the differential diagnosis of pulmonary carcinoma metastatic to the pleura. Reactive mesothelial hyperplasia in the setting of pleuritis is also a consideration, as it is sometimes so exuberant as to simulate malignancy. Distinction between these entities demands the integration of clinical, radiographic, and, in many cases, immunohistochemical data. It is important to remember that not all pleural effusions that arise in the setting of lung cancer are malignant.

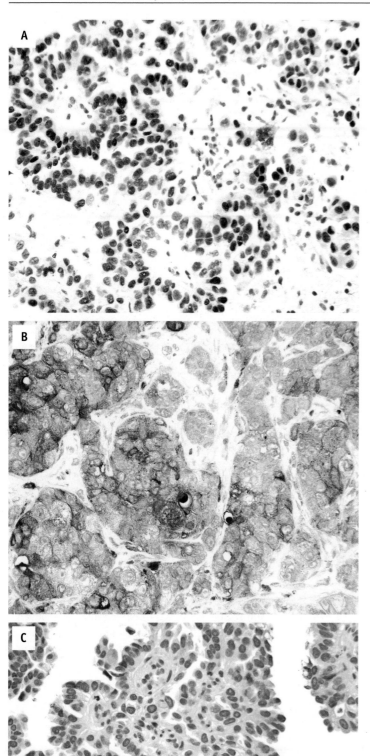

FIGURE 34-8

Lung carcinoma metastatic to the pleura
(A) TTF-1 strongly decorates tumor cells in a nuclear distribution.
(B) This metastatic carcinoma demonstrates cytoplasmic staining for
CEA with variable membrane accentuation. **(C)** Calretinin staining is
absent in this metastatic adenocarcinoma of the lung. Most carcinomas of pulmonary origin are negative for this mesothelium-associated
marker.

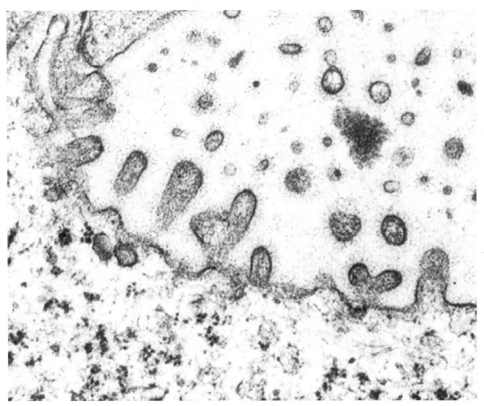

FIGURE 34-9
Lung carcinoma metastatic to the pleura
In contrast to malignant mesothelioma, the microvilli of pulmonary adenocarcinoma are short and stubby. (Courtesy of Victor Roggli, M.D., Durham, North Carolina, and Samuel Hammar, M.D., Bremerton, Washington.)

Cytologic examination to assess for the presence of neoplastic cells is necessary to distinguish paramalignant from malignant pleural effusions.

PROGNOSIS AND THERAPY

The prognosis of patients with lung carcinoma involving the pleura is very poor, with only 15% of patients surviving longer than 6 months after the development of malignant pleural effusion. Drainage of malignant pleural effusions may provide temporary symptomatic relief.

PLEURAL METASTASES FROM NON-PULMONARY EPITHELIAL NEOPLASMS

A variety of epithelial neoplasms originating in sites other than the lung metastasize to the pleura. The most common of these is breast carcinoma, and other common primary sites include the thyroid, ovary, gastrointestinal tract, pancreas, and kidney.

CLINICAL FEATURES

Symptoms related to pleural involvement are generally a late manifestation of disease in patients who already have an established diagnosis of carcinoma. One notable exception is renal cell carcinoma, which has a propensity to manifest early in its course to distant sites.

PATHOLOGIC FEATURES

GROSS FINDINGS

The spectrum of gross features is similar to that of metastatic lung carcinoma.

MICROSCOPIC AND CYTOLOGIC FINDINGS

The histologic and cytologic features of non-pulmonary carcinomas metastatic to the pleura are similar to their primary counterparts. For patients who have a known diagnosis of carcinoma, comparison of the pleural tumor morphology with the primary neoplasm can often obviate

---

LUNG CARCINOMA METASTATIC TO THE PLEURA—FACT SHEET

Incidence

‣ Accounts for about 60,000 malignant pleural effusions each year in the United States, which equals 40 times the number of malignant pleural effusions due to malignant mesothelioma

Clinical Features

‣ Dyspnea secondary to pleural effusion is the predominant symptom

Radiologic Features

‣ Pleural effusion
‣ Multiple small nodules, irregular thickening by larger nodules, or rarely, diffuse thickening of the pleura
‣ Intrapulmonary component usually evident but may be difficult to detect in some cases

Prognosis

‣ Signifies advanced stage of disease
‣ Only 15% of lung cancer patients survive more than 6 months after development of malignant pleural effusion

---

the need for ancillary stains. Examples of several types of metastatic carcinoma are shown (Figure 34-10A-D). In tumors that demonstrate a papillary growth pattern, such as papillary thyroid carcinomas and some ovarian serous carcinomas, psammoma bodies may be seen in pleural metastases. Metastatic colon carcinoma may exhibit foci of so-called dirty necrosis (Figure 34-10E).

HISTOCHEMISTRY AND IMMUNOHISTOCHEMISTRY

Like some pulmonary adenocarcinomas metastatic to the pleura, mucin production can be demonstrated in some metastatic carcinomas of non-pulmonary origin by PAS or alcian blue pretreated with diastase or hyaluronidase, respectively. In contrast to lung adenocarcinoma, breast carcinoma metastatic to the pleura is negative for TTF-1. Other immunohistochemical markers that may aid in this distinction are the recently developed relatively specific marker mammaglobin, which stains about 85% of breast carcinomas, and gross cystic disease fluid protein (GDFDP)-15, although the latter stains only about 50% of breast carcinomas. Staining for estrogen and progesterone receptors can be somewhat helpful in evaluating breast carcinoma metastases to the pleura in patients for whom the estrogen and progesterone receptor status of the original tumor is known. However, it is important to remember that a minority of lung adenocarcinomas (5%-10%) also exhibit weak to moderate estrogen receptor immunoreactivity.

As is true for most metastatic lung adenocarcinomas, follicular and papillary thyroid carcinomas metastatic to the pleura stain positively for TTF-1. Fortunately, however, metastatic follicular and papillary thyroid carcinomas are also usually immunoreactive for thyroglobulin,

---

LUNG CARCINOMA METASTATIC TO THE PLEURA—PATHOLOGIC FEATURES

Gross Findings

‣ White to tan, firm pleural nodules or masses
‣ Occasionally, in cases of lymphangitic spread, finely reticulated pattern over the pleural surfaces
‣ Uncommonly, white to tan, rind-like diffuse pleural thickening with encasement of the underlying lung; so-called pseudomesotheliomatous growth pattern

Microscopic Findings

‣ Morphology usually similar to primary tumor
‣ Array of patterns in adenocarcinoma includes acinar, glandular, tubulopapillary, micropapillary, and solid patterns
‣ Intracytoplasmic mucin vacuoles in most adenocarcinomas
‣ Adenocarcinoma cells often have eccentric nuclei, prominent nucleoli, and greater pleomorphism than cells of malignant mesothelioma
‣ Desmoplastic stroma is common

Fine Needle Aspiration Biopsy/Pleural Effusion Cytology Findings

‣ Cells have high nuclear-to-cytoplasmic ratio, irregular nuclear contours, and one or more nucleoli
‣ Cells arranged in sheets, acini, papillary formations, or three-dimensional clusters
‣ Three-dimensional clusters usually have smooth community borders

Histochemical and Immunohistochemical Features

‣ In mucin-producing tumors, intracytoplasmic vacuoles are positive for PAS and alcian blue; staining is not abolished by pretreatment with diastase (PAS-D) or hyaluronidase in the case of alcian blue
‣ Adenocarcinomas of the lung are generally positive for TTF-1, CEA, LeuM1 (CD15), and/or Ber-EP4
‣ Squamous cell carcinoma may be negative for TTF-1 and positive for CK5/6

Ultrastructural Features

‣ Adenocarcinomas usually demonstrate short stubby microvilli, may contain secretory granules, and may show terminal bars adjacent to gland lumens

Pathologic Differential Diagnosis

‣ Malignant mesothelioma
‣ Metastatic carcinoma of non-pulmonary origin
‣ Reactive mesothelial hyperplasia

---

a marker that is negative in metastatic pulmonary adenocarcinoma. Carcinoembryonic antigen (CEA) staining, a frequent feature of metastatic pulmonary adenocarcinoma, is distinctly uncommon in metastatic follicular and papillary thyroid carcinoma. It must be kept in mind that the immunoprofile of metastatic medullary carcinoma of the thyroid differs from follicular and papillary carcinoma. Medullary carcinoma typically shows strong immunostaining for CEA but is negative for TTF-1 and thyroglobulin.

Metastatic renal cell carcinoma presents a diagnostic challenge, as it may not stain with traditional glycoprotein-associated markers, such as CEA. Antibodies such as CD10 and RCC marker (RCC Ma) may be of some utility

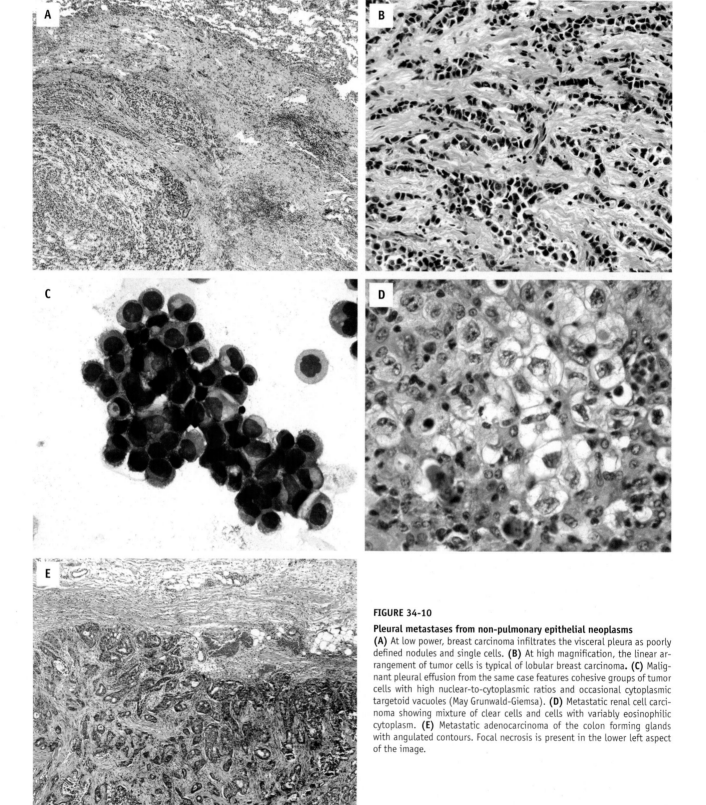

FIGURE 34-10

Pleural metastases from non-pulmonary epithelial neoplasms
(A) At low power, breast carcinoma infiltrates the visceral pleura as poorly defined nodules and single cells. **(B)** At high magnification, the linear arrangement of tumor cells is typical of lobular breast carcinoma. **(C)** Malignant pleural effusion from the same case features cohesive groups of tumor cells with high nuclear-to-cytoplasmic ratios and occasional cytoplasmic targetoid vacuoles (May Grunwald-Giemsa). **(D)** Metastatic renal cell carcinoma showing mixture of clear cells and cells with variably eosinophilic cytoplasm. **(E)** Metastatic adenocarcinoma of the colon forming glands with angulated contours. Focal necrosis is present in the lower left aspect of the image.

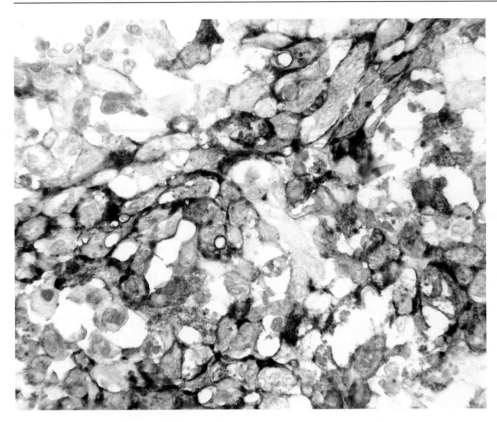

FIGURE 34-11

Pleural metastasis from renal cell carcinoma

Metastatic renal cell carcinoma demonstrating strong immunoreactivity for CD10.

(Figure 34-11). Strong diffuse staining for these markers suggests metastatic renal cell carcinoma. The stains must be interpreted cautiously, as malignant mesothelioma can also stain for these markers, although staining is generally patchy and less intense. In contrast to mesothelioma, metastatic renal cell carcinoma is typically negative for calretinin and CK 5/6 and is sometimes positive for CD15 and MOC-31.

CA19-9 is relatively specific for metastatic pancreatic adenocarcinoma. Metastatic ovarian carcinoma is positive for WT1 and negative for CEA in the majority of cases. In contrast to metastatic lung carcinoma, which is positive for CK7 and negative for CK20, metastatic colon carcinoma typically shows the opposite immunoprofile and, unlike lung carcinoma, is usually positive for CDX2. However, some cases of mucinous pulmonary adenocarcinoma may also show CK20 positivity.

DIFFERENTIAL DIAGNOSIS

Carcinomas of non-pulmonary origin metastatic to the pleura must be differentiated from metastatic lung carcinoma and the epithelial variant of malignant mesothelioma. Tumors with cytoplasmic clearing should raise the possibility of not only metastatic conventional (clear cell) renal cell carcinoma but also malignant mesothelioma, as rare cases of clear cell mesothelioma have been described. Metastatic carcinomas with a papillary architecture can also be mimicked by malignant mesothelioma, which occasionally can exhibit a strikingly papillary architecture.

PROGNOSIS AND THERAPY

The prognosis of patients with non-pulmonary carcinoma involving the pleura is poor, like patients with pulmonary carcinoma metastatic to the pleura. Pleural involvement usually represents a late complication of disease.

METASTATIC SARCOMAS TO THE PLEURA

Sarcomas occasionally involve the pleura secondarily, often through hematogenous dissemination from a distant site or by direct extension from the chest wall or mediastinum. Pleura involvement is typically a late manifestation of disease, and in most cases a diagnosis of sarcoma has already been established. A variety of sarcomas are reported to metastasize to the pleura, including osteosarcoma and liposarcoma (Figure 34-12).

NON-PULMONARY NEOPLASMS INVOLVING THE PLEURA—FACT SHEET

Incidence

➤ Breast carcinoma is the second most common extrapleural neoplasm to involve the pleura

➤ Lymphoma is the third most common cause of malignant pleural effusion

Clinical Features

➤ Dyspnea secondary to pleural effusion

➤ Pleurodynia

Prognosis

➤ Generally poor outcome as pleural involvement usually occurs at a late stage of disease

---

NON-PULMONARY NEOPLASMS INVOLVING THE PLEURA—PATHOLOGIC FEATURES

Gross Findings

➤ Gross appearance and distribution patterns similar to lung carcinoma involving the pleura

➤ Sarcomas with chondroid differentiation may have a bluish cast

➤ Malignant melanoma metastatic to the pleura may or may not be pigmented

Microscopic Findings

➤ Usually similar to primary tumor

➤ Papillary structures with or without psammoma bodies in papillary carcinoma of the thyroid and ovarian carcinomas

➤ Metastatic colon carcinoma may exhibit "dirty" necrosis

Fine Needle Aspiration Biopsy/Pleural Effusion Cytology Findings

➤ Usually similar to features of primary tumor

➤ Exfoliative cytology and aspiration specimens of sarcomas are often low in cellularity

Immunohistochemical Features (Selected Neoplasms)

➤ Adenocarcinomas are generally positive for CEA and LeuM1 (CD15) and are generally negative for markers that are typically positive in mesothelioma such as calretinin

➤ Specific markers can be useful depending on the presumed or known site of origin

   ➤ Breast carcinoma: Gross cystic fluid disease protein (GCFDP-15) and mammaglobulin

   ➤ Thyroid carcinoma: TTF-1 and thyroglobulin

   ➤ Renal cell carcinoma: CD10 and RCC Ma

   ➤ Leiomyosarcoma: Smooth muscle actin (SMA)

   ➤ Tumors of peripheral nerve sheath origin (e.g., schwannoma): S100

   ➤ Malignant melanoma: HMB45, S100, MART-1

   ➤ Lymphoma: Leukocyte common antigen (CD45) and other lymphoid antigens

   ➤ Leukemia: CD34, myeloperoxidase (MPO)

   ➤ Thymoma: CD5

Pathologic Differential Diagnosis

➤ Lung carcinoma involving the pleura

➤ Malignant mesothelioma

   ➤ Epithelial variant (for carcinomas)

   ➤ Sarcomatoid and biphasic variants (for sarcomas or sarcomatoid carcinomas involving the pleura)

➤ Reactive mesothelial hyperplasia

Myxoid liposarcoma appears to be the most common variant of liposarcoma to involve the pleura.

DIFFERENTIAL DIAGNOSIS

For sarcomas metastatic to the pleura, differential diagnostic considerations are broad and include primary pleural sarcomas, sarcomatoid malignant mesothelioma, sarcomatoid carcinomas, and other poorly differentiated malignancies, such as melanoma and high-grade lymphomas. The accurate diagnosis of metastatic sarcoma requires the integration of clinical and radiographic information. When possible, the histopathologic features of the pleural tumor should be compared with those of the primary tumor. Immunohistochemical stains should be interpreted with caution, particularly in small biopsies, as cytokeratin staining has been reported in some sarcomas. Conversely, the lack of immunoreactivity for cytokeratins does not exclude sarcomatoid carcinoma or malignant mesothelioma, as these tumors may show focal or absent staining. In difficult cases, particularly when a prior history of sarcoma is lacking, ultrastructural examination may be useful.

HEMATOLOGIC MALIGNANCIES INVOLVING THE PLEURA

Hematologic malignancies commonly involve the pleura secondarily, in contrast to the low frequency of primary effusion lymphomas. Lymphoma is the most common hematologic malignancy to involve the pleura and is the most common cause of chylous pleura effusion. About 40,000 malignant pleural effusions each year result from lymphoma, making it the third most common category of tumor to cause malignant pleura effusions.

Both Hodgkin and non-Hodgkin lymphomas can involve the pleura (Figure 34-13A,B). Up to 30% of patients with lymphoma develop pleural effusions. Although pleural infiltration is believed to be the most common cause, a substantial proportion of pleural effusions in patients with lymphoma are paramalignant and result from obstructed lymphatic drainage caused by enlarged hilar or mediastinal nodes. Leukemic pleural infiltrates develop in about to 5% of cases of leukemia, and multiple myeloma involves the pleura in less than 1%

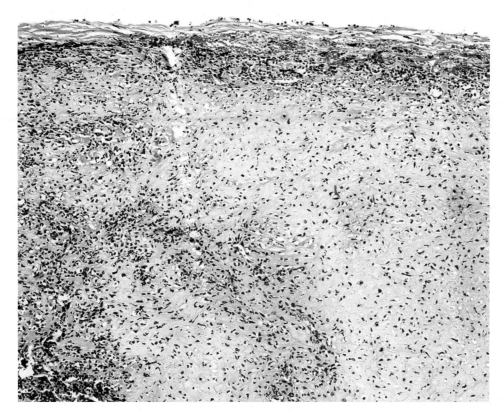

FIGURE 34-12

Metastatic chondrosarcoma involving of the pleura
Chondroid differentiation is evident in the right half of the photomicrograph.

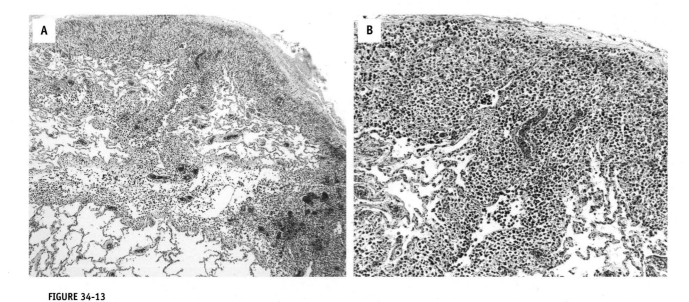

FIGURE 34-13

Hematologic malignancies involving the pleura
(A) At low power, this diffuse large B-cell lymphoma diffusely involves the visceral pleura and subpleural interlobular septa. (B) At higher magnification, a sheet of monomorphous lymphocytes obliterates the pleuropulmonary interface.

of cases. Pleural involvement by other hematologic neoplasms is rare.

DIFFERENTIAL DIAGNOSIS

The main differential diagnostic considerations are poorly differentiated/undifferentiated carcinoma, lymphohistiocytoid mesothelioma, and thymic carcinoma. Immunostaining for pancytokeratin can be helpful in disclosing an epithelial component that is overshadowed by a reactive lymphoid infiltrate on routine stains. Lymphohistiocytoid mesotheliomas should also stain for mesothelium-associated immunomarkers and exhibit histiocytes within the inflammatory infiltrate. Depending on the histologic type, thymomas can be rich in lymphocytes but should retain an overall lobulated architecture. Immunostaining for CD5 will highlight the epithelial component in most thymic carcinomas.

OTHER METASTATIC NEOPLASMS OF THE PLEURA

A variety of other neoplasms metastasizing to the pleura have been reported, including melanoma, ependymoma, meningioma, and thymoma. In the majority of cases, the diagnosis of an extrapleural neoplasm has already been established, as pleural involvement typically occurs at an advanced stage of disease.

As with other types of tumors metastatic to the pleura, establishing a history of an extrapleural neoplasm, comparing the morphology of the pleural tumor with the original tumor, and selectively employing immunostains are essential to defining the diagnosis.

SUGGESTED READINGS

Lung Carcinoma Metastatic to the Pleura

1. Attanoos RL, Gibbs AR. "Pseudomesotheliomatous" carcinomas of the pleura: a 10-year analysis of cases from the Environmental Lung Disease Research Group, Cardiff. *Histopathology.* 2003;43:44-52.
2. Comin CE, Novelli L, Boddi V, et al. Calretinin, thrombomodulin, CEA, and CD15: a useful combination of immunohistochemical markers for differentiating pleural epithelial mesothelioma from peripheral pulmonary adenocarcinoma. *Hum Pathol.* 2001;32:529-36.

Pleural Metastases from Non-Pulmonary Epithelial Neoplasms

3. Ciampa A, Fanger G, Khan A, et al. Mammaglobin and CRxA-01 in pleural effusion cytology: potential utility of distinguishing metastatic breast carcinoma from other cytokeratin 7-positive/cytokeratin 20-negative carcinomas. *Cancer.* 2004;102:368-72.
4. Ordonez NG. The diagnostic utility of immunohistochemistry in distinguishing between mesothelioma and renal cell carcinoma: a comparative study. *Hum Pathol.* 2004;35:697-710.

Metastatic Sarcomas to the Pleura

5. Pearlstone DB, Pisters PW, Bold RJ, et al. Patterns of recurrence in extremity liposarcoma: implications for staging and follow-up. *Cancer.* 1999;85:85-92.

Hematologic Malignancies Involving the Pleura

6. Alexandrakis MG, Passam FH, Kyriakou DS, et al. Pleural effusions in hematologic malignancies. *Chest.* 2004;125:1546-55.

Other Metastatic Neoplasms of the Pleura

7. Beaty MW, Fetsch P, Wilder AM, et al. Effusion cytology of malignant melanoma. A morphologic and immunocytochemical analysis including application of the MART-1 antibody. *Cancer.* 1997;25:57-63.

35

Inflammatory and Fibrosing Pleural Processes

Joanne L. Wright

- Organization of Pleural Effusion
- Acute Bacterial Pleuritis (Empyema)
- Eosinophilic Pleuritis
- Tuberculous Pleuritis
- Rheumatoid Pleuritis
- Apical Cap
- Pleural Plaque
- Rounded Atelectasis

ORGANIZATION OF PLEURAL EFFUSION

Organization of pleural effusion is a nonspecific repair reaction of an exudative or bloody effusion stemming from a variety of causes. Whereas the majority of exudative effusions are named according to their etiology (i.e., postradiation effusion), any pleural effusion that is associated with an acute inflammatory condition in the adjacent lung is termed a parapneumonic effusion. The term complicated parapneumonic effusion refers to a parapneumonic effusion that does not resolve with antibiotic therapy and requires tube thoracostomy for resolution.

CLINICAL FEATURES

Effusions can develop at any age and are associated with a multiplicity of diseases and treatments. Parapneumonic effusions are quite common and are found in up to 40% of patients with bacterial pneumonia. Symptoms may be related to the primary disease or the presence of the fluid, and include cough, chest pain, sputum production, and varying degrees of shortness of breath. Chest radiographs are necessary for diagnosis.

PATHOLOGIC FEATURES

Grossly, a layer of gray or tan material may coat the pleura. The histologic changes can be divided into exudative, fibrinous, and organizing stages. In the exudative stage, the pleural capillaries are dilated, and there are reactive changes with enlargement of mesothelial cells, which remain in a single layer; small deposits of fibrin can be found adherent to the pleura. The fibrinous stage is characterized by layered fibrin deposition, granulation tissue, and mesothelial reaction (Figure 35-1A). The mesothelial cells may be cytologically atypical, but the atypia is confined to the area of the organizing effusion, and mesothelial cells are never found in the underlying adipose tissue. The organizing stage is characterized by progressive fibrosis and a chronic inflammatory cell infiltrate (Figure 35-1B). The fibrous tissue is most dense adjacent to the chest wall.

DIFFERENTIAL DIAGNOSIS

Active organizing pleurisy may be confused with malignant mesothelioma, particularly in small biopsy specimens. Important differential diagnostic points include the layered appearance of the reactive process compared to the diffuse cellularity, or deep cellularity, of malignant mesothelioma. Mesotheliomas will invade underlying adipose tissue, whereas invasive mesothelial cell proliferation is absent in reactive processes.

PROGNOSIS AND THERAPY

The course of the effusion depends upon its etiology and the responsiveness of the underlying condition to therapy. Many effusions require drainage, and some will require surgical intervention. Diagnostic thoracentesis is appropriate in cases of significant parapneumonic effusions to differentiate infected, complicated effusions

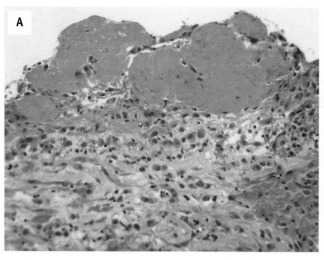

FIGURE 35-1

Organization of pleural effusion
(A) There is a layer of fibrin with intermingled proliferating mesothelial cells on the pleural surface. **(B)** This organizing effusion demonstrates zonation, i.e., layering of fibrin, granulation tissue, and fibrosis.

from uncomplicated effusions, the former requiring tube thoracostomy. In effusions complicating other diseases, drainage is initiated on a case-by-case basis. Decortication is reserved for those patients who have inadequate drainage after tube thoracostomy and for those patients with persistent pleural thickening and significant pulmonary function deficits.

ORGANIZATION OF PLEURAL EFFUSION—FACT SHEET

Definition
➤ Nonspecific repair reaction of an exudative or bloody pleural effusion

Clinical Features
➤ Symptoms are related to the primary disease or the presence of fluid and include cough, chest pain, sputum production, and varying degrees of shortness of breath

Prognosis and Therapy
➤ The course of the effusion depends upon its etiology and the responsiveness of the underlying condition to therapy
➤ Many effusions require drainage
➤ Diagnostic thoracentesis can be performed in cases of significant parapneumonic effusions to differentiate infected, complicated effusions from uncomplicated effusions
➤ Tube thoracostomy is necessary for treatment of complicated parapneumonic effusions
➤ Decortication is reserved for cases with inadequate drainage or persistent pleural thickening with associated pulmonary function deficits

---

ACUTE BACTERIAL PLEURITIS (EMPYEMA)

An empyema is defined as pus in the pleural space; as the exact definition for pus is more difficult, some authors require identification of organisms, either directly or by culture.

CLINICAL FEATURES

Approximately 60% of empyemas evolve from parapneumonic effusions. At the present time, anaerobic organisms are more commonly isolated than aerobic organisms, with most patients having more than one organism identified. Postsurgical (pneumonectomy) empyemas are

---

ORGANIZATION OF PLEURAL EFFUSION—PATHOLOGIC FEATURES

Microscopic Findings
➤ Exudative phase: Dilated pleural capillaries, foci of fibrin, mesothelial cell enlargement
➤ Fibrinous phase: Layered fibrin, granulation tissue, mesothelial cell proliferation
➤ Organizing phase: Progressive fibrosis, chronic inflammatory cell infiltrate

Pathologic Differential Diagnosis
➤ Malignant mesothelioma

an important clinical problem, and empyemas uncommonly follow thoracentesis. Empyema is infrequently found as a complication of pleural rheumatoid nodules, probably because of the formation of bronchopleural fistulas with necrosis of the nodules.

Symptoms (cough, sputum production) may be those of the adjacent pneumonic process, when empyema complicates a parapneumonic effusion. Other symptoms and signs include fever and leukocytosis, expectoration of pleural fluid (if a bronchopleural fistula is present), air-fluid levels in the pleural space, or drainage of purulent material from an incision or needle tract.

PATHOLOGIC FEATURES

Grossly, the pleura is usually coated with a layer of tan or yellow-green material (Figure 35-2A). Microscopically, empyemas progress through the same general stages as uncomplicated effusions, but the fibrinous

stage is characterized by a thick layer of neutrophils (Figure 35-2B).

ANCILLARY STUDIES

Cultures and special stains for bacteria and fungi can be performed. Organisms may or may not be identified, depending upon the specific agent and the success of antibiotic therapy.

DIFFERENTIAL DIAGNOSIS

An empyema must be differentiated from a necrotic tumor. If possible, the organism(s) responsible should be identified. Histochemical stains for bacteria and fungi should be performed. Culture may be more sensitive and specific than histochemical staining, however.

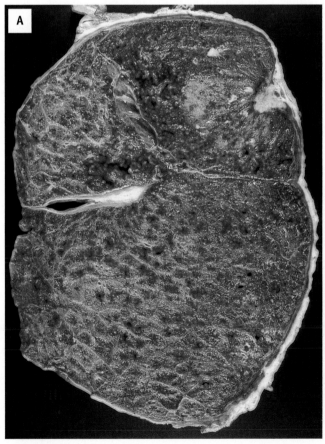

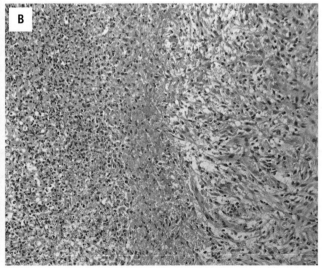

FIGURE 35-2

Empyema

(A) The pleural exudate lies immediately adjacent to the pneumonic consolidation but also extends along the pleural surfaces and into the interlobar fissure. **(B)** This high-power view shows dense acute inflammatory exudate on the left and granulation tissue on the right.

ACUTE BACTERIAL PLEURITIS (EMPYEMA)—FACT SHEET

Definition
▸ Pus in the pleural space

Clinical Features
▸ Symptoms (cough, sputum production) are often related to an adjacent pneumonic process, and signs of sepsis (fever and leukocytosis) are commonly present

Therapy
▸ Treatment includes tube thoracostomy and antimicrobial therapy
▸ Decortication is performed if pleural sepsis is not controlled by drainage
▸ Bronchopleural fistula is an important potential complication

---

ACUTE BACTERIAL PLEURITIS (EMPYEMA)—PATHOLOGIC FEATURES

Microscopic Findings
▸ Exudative stage: Dilated pleural capillaries, foci of fibrin, mesothelial cell enlargement
▸ Fibrinous stage: Layered fibrin with a massive infiltrate of neutrophils, granulation tissue, mesothelial cell proliferation
▸ Organizing stage: Progressive fibrosis, chronic inflammatory cell infiltrate

Ancillary Studies
▸ Cultures and special stains for bacteria and fungi may reveal an etiologic agent

Pathologic Differential Diagnosis
▸ Necrotic neoplasms

PROGNOSIS AND THERAPY

Tube thoracostomy combined with antibiotic therapy represents the usual primary therapy; multiple tubes may be required if more than one locule is present. Decortication may be necessary if pleural sepsis is not controlled by the tube thoracostomies. Development of a bronchopleural fistula is an important complication; if the infected pleural fluid is not drained exteriorly, it is likely to drain interiorly and produce a severe bronchopneumonia. Chest CT scans will be helpful, but not entirely infallible, in distinguishing an air-fluid level secondary to a bronchopleural fistula from one related to a lung abscess.

EOSINOPHILIC PLEURITIS

Eosinophilic pleuritis is a reactive pleural process characterized by the presence of numerous eosinophils.

CLINICAL FEATURES

Eosinophilic pleuritis is classically induced by pneumothorax and is often seen in resected bullae. It can, however, also be found as a consequence of a pleural effusion or hemothorax, or in settings of infections with parasites (hydatid disease, amebiasis, ascariasis) or fungi.

PATHOLOGIC FEATURES

Numerous eosinophils infiltrate the pleura, and are often accompanied by macrophages, giant cells, and other inflammatory cells (Figure 35-3). Reactive mesothelial cell proliferation may also be present.

DIFFERENTIAL DIAGNOSIS

Langerhans cell histiocytosis (eosinophilic granuloma) may be considered in the differential diagnosis, but it is a lung parenchymal disease rather than a pleural disease and consists of stellate nodular aggregates of S-100- or CD-1a-positive Langerhans cells accompanied by other inflammatory cells and variable degrees of fibrosis. A chest radiograph should identify the diffuse pulmonary parenchymal nature of this disease.

PROGNOSIS AND THERAPY

Infective eosinophilic pleuritis must be treated with antimicrobial agents and drainage. Simple reactive eosinophilic pleuritis due to pneumothorax has no consequence, whereas those cases secondary to hemothorax may require drainage or decortication.

TUBERCULOUS PLEURITIS

Tuberculous pleuritis is defined as a pleural effusion and pleuritis secondary to infection by *Mycobacterium tuberculosis*. In most cases, tuberculous pleuritis is believed to stem from either rupture of a subpleural granuloma into the pleural space or dissemination of the mycobacteria via the pleural lymphatics. Delayed type hypersensitivity appears to play a large role in the development of effusions.

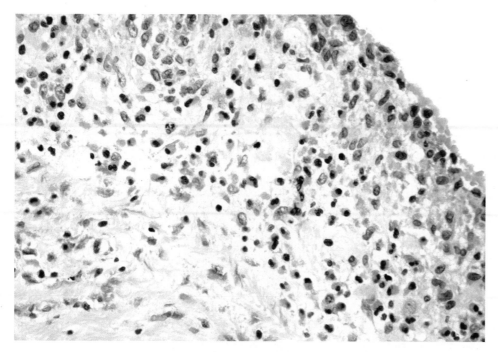

FIGURE 35-3

Eosinophilic pleuritis, post-pneumothorax
Note the prominent eosinophil infiltrates in the pleura and the thin layer of proliferating mesothelial cells.

EOSINOPHILIC PLEURITIS—FACT SHEET

Definition

▸ Reactive pleural process characterized by pleural infiltration by numerous eosinophils

Clinical Features

▸ Eosinophilic pleuritis is most commonly induced by pneumothorax but is also found with some effusions, hemothorax, and infections with parasites and fungi

Therapy

▸ Infective processes are treated with antimicrobial agents and drainage
▸ Lesions secondary to pneumothorax require no treatment

EOSINOPHILIC PLEURITIS—PATHOLOGIC FEATURES

Microscopic Findings

▸ Numerous eosinophils infiltrating the pleura, accompanied by reactive mesothelial cells, macrophages, and other inflammatory cells

Pathologic Differential Diagnosis

▸ Langerhans cell histiocytosis

CLINICAL FEATURES

Pleural effusions secondary to *M. tuberculosis* occur in 3% to 4% of newly diagnosed cases of tuberculosis in North America but are more common in other areas of the world. Clinically, the disease presents with fever, chest pain, and dyspnea, with little sputum or cough.

PATHOLOGIC FEATURES

Pleural granulomas (Figure 35-4) are highly suggestive of tuberculous pleuritis, even in the absence of caseation or stainable acid-fast bacteria. Less-organized

aggregates of macrophages can be found in infections in immunocompromised patients. A combination of culture and histology can establish the diagnosis in approximately 90% of cases.

ANCILLARY STUDIES

Acid fast staining may demonstrate the organism.

DIFFERENTIAL DIAGNOSIS

Infections with *M. avium intracellulare* and fungi can induce similar pleural reactions, as can sarcoidosis. Rheumatoid nodules may also be considered in the differential diagnosis.

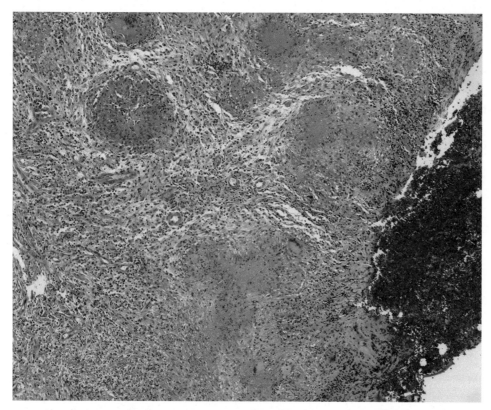

FIGURE 35-4
Tuberculous pleuritis
The thickened pleura demonstrates multiple necrotizing granulomas.

PROGNOSIS AND THERAPY

Goals of therapy include prevention of active tuberculosis, relief of symptoms, and prevention of fibrothorax. Antimicrobial agents are given, and serial thoracenteses are performed not as a primary treatment but to relieve symptoms. Pleural thickening decreases with treatment, so decortication is not usually considered unless there is little response to therapy. Bronchopleural fistula is a potential complication and requires insertion of a chest tube.

RHEUMATOID PLEURITIS

Rheumatoid pleuritis is defined as a pleural reaction or rheumatoid nodule(s) in a patient with rheumatoid arthritis.

CLINICAL FEATURES

Pleural disease may occur in as many as 40% of patients with rheumatoid arthritis and usually consists of pleuritis or pleural effusions. Effusions can alternate from side to side, resolve and recur on the same side, and are bilateral

---

TUBERCULOUS PLEURITIS—FACT SHEET

Definition
▸ Pleural effusion and pleuritis secondary to infection by *Mycobacterium tuberculosis*

Clinical Features
▸ Symptoms: fever, chest pain, dyspnea, with little sputum or cough

Prognosis and Therapy
▸ Antituberculous agents to prevent active tuberculosis
▸ Serial thoracenteses to relieve symptoms
▸ Decortication is reserved for persistent fibrosis
▸ Bronchopleural fistula occurs as potential complication and requires drainage

---

TUBERCULOUS PLEURITIS—PATHOLOGIC FEATURES

Microscopic Findings
▸ Granulomas with or without caseation
▸ Sheets of macrophages, especially in patients who are immunocompromised

Pathologic Differential Diagnosis
▸ Non-tuberculous mycobacterial and fungal infections
▸ Sarcoidosis
▸ Rheumatoid pleuritis

in approximately one fourth of patients. Symptoms include chest pain, fever, and dyspnea. Rheumatoid nodules are uncommon lesions but may be resected as a result of evaluation of a pleural or parenchymal mass lesion.

PATHOLOGIC FEATURES

Reactive pleuritis is nonspecific with exudative, fibrinous, and organizing components as described above (Figure 35-5A). Rheumatoid nodules are necrobiotic nodules similar to those found in the soft tissue (Figure 35-5B). There is a central zone of necrotic eosinophilic material that is surrounded by fibroblasts, collagen, and macrophages. Although giant cells can be identified, they are not as common as would be expected in an infective granuloma. Characteristic cytologic findings in pleural fluids include elongated and multinucleated histiocytes and necrotic debris that often has a granular appearance (Figure 35-5C). Other inflammatory cells may accompany these histiocytes and may show degenerative changes. Cellular degeneration can also lead to cholesterol crystals in the shape of flat, rhomboidal plates.

DIFFERENTIAL DIAGNOSIS

Infective granulomas, particularly tuberculous and fungal in origin, must be considered in the differential diagnosis. Evaluation includes appropriate special stains.

PROGNOSIS AND THERAPY

Although pleural effusions may resolve spontaneously, therapy is directed to prevent progressive pleural fibrosis. Drainage is often performed. Decortication is restricted to treatment of patients with thickened pleura associated with dyspnea.

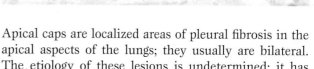

APICAL CAPS

Apical caps are localized areas of pleural fibrosis in the apical aspects of the lungs; they usually are bilateral. The etiology of these lesions is undetermined; it has been suggested that apical caps represent the residua of infection, that they are secondary to ischemia, or that they are the residua of ruptured blebs or bullae.

CLINICAL FEATURES

There are no symptoms associated with these abnormalities.

PATHOLOGIC FEATURES

Grossly, apical caps appear as apical zones of tan or gray fibrous tissue (Figure 35-6). Microscopically, dense fibrous tissue without significant mesothelial proliferation is observed in the lung apex. There may be aggregates of pigment or calcifications.

RHEUMATOID PLEURITIS—FACT SHEET

Definition
- Nonspecific pleuritis, pleural effusion, and/or necrobiotic nodules in patients with rheumatoid arthritis

Clinical Features
- Found in up to 40% of patients with rheumatoid arthritis
- Symptoms: chest pain, fever, and dyspnea

Prognosis and Therapy
- May resolve spontaneously
- Therapy is directed towards prevention of progressive pleural fibrosis

---

RHEUMATOID PLEURITIS—PATHOLOGIC FEATURES

Microscopic Findings
- Reactive pleuritis (exudative, fibrinous, and organizing pleuritis)
- Rheumatoid necrobiotic nodule

Cytologic Findings
- Elongated histiocytes
- Multinucleated histiocytes
- Necrotic debris, often granular
- Mixed inflammatory cells with variable degrees of cellular degeneration
- Flat, rhomboidal cholesterol crystals may be present

Pathologic Differential Diagnosis
- Infective granulomas (mycobacterial, fungal)

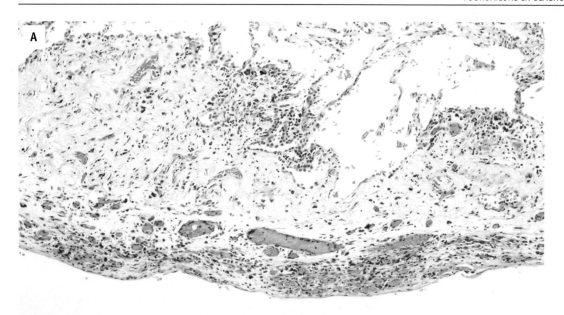

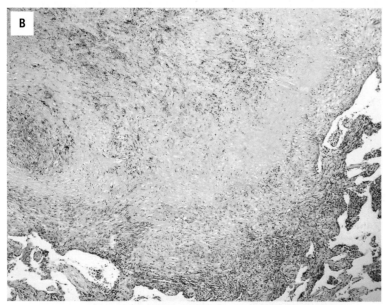

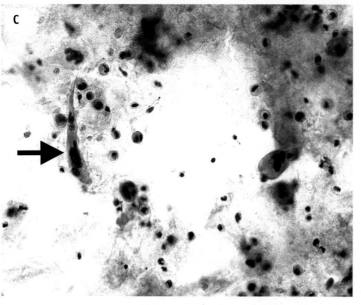

FIGURE 35-5

Rheumatoid pleural disease

(A) Organizing pleuritis. The pleura overlying the rheumatoid nod-ule demonstrates an early organizing pleuritis with increased colla-gen and chronic inflammatory cells. **(B)** Subpleural rheumatoid nodule. Note the central dense fibrous tissue with peripheral fibro-blastic proliferation. **(C)** Rheumatoid pleural effusion. Key cytologic findings represented include elongated (arrow) and multinucleated histiocytes and necrotic debris. Other inflammatory cells are also present.

APICAL CAPS—FACT SHEET

Definition

▸ Localized areas of pleural fibrosis in the apical aspects of the lungs

Clinical Features

▸ Common lesions
▸ No clinical symptoms

Prognosis and Therapy

▸ No required therapy
▸ No associated morbidity or mortality

APICAL CAPS—PATHOLOGIC FEATURES

Gross Findings

▸ Apical zones of dense tan or gray fibrous tissue, usually bilateral

Microscopic Findings

▸ Dense fibrous tissue without significant mesothelial proliferation or granulomas

Pathologic Differential Diagnosis

▸ Scarred infective lesions, especially tuberculosis

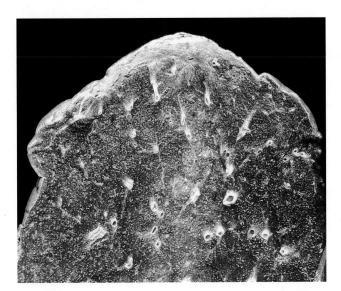

FIGURE 35-6
Apical cap
The lung apex is distorted by a thick fibrous rim.

PLEURAL PLAQUES

Pleural plaques are discrete pleural lesions composed of dense collagenous plaques, which are usually associated with asbestos exposure, and can occasionally be a result of trauma or organized localized effusion/empyema.

CLINICAL FEATURES

Patients are asymptomatic. Plaques are usually discovered incidentally on chest radiographs or during surgery.

PATHOLOGIC FEATURES

Grossly, pleural plaques consist of raised, well-demarcated, smooth or knobbed white or tan plaques that are most commonly found on the parietal pleura between the rib margins or on the diaphragmatic surfaces (Figure 35-7A). Microscopy shows layered collagen in a "basket weave" pattern (Figure 35-7B). There may be areas of calcification or metaplastic bone. Asbestos fibers are not present within the plaque.

PROGNOSIS AND THERAPY

Apical caps are usually of no clinical consequence and require no treatment. However, if the fibrosis extends into the lung parenchyma, there is a small increase in incidence of lung carcinoma arising in association with the scar.

DIFFERENTIAL DIAGNOSIS

Scarred infective lesions such as tuberculosis may have similar appearances, but granulomas are not generally found in apical caps.

DIFFERENTIAL DIAGNOSIS

Desmoplastic malignant mesothelioma can be considered in the differential diagnosis but is a more diffuse process that is invasive, is more cellular, and shows some degree of cytoatypia.

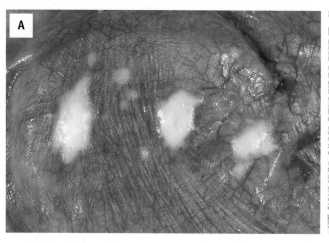

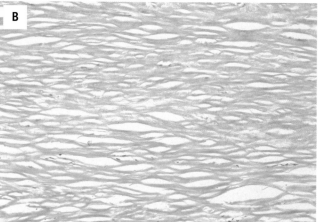

FIGURE 35-7

Pleural plaques

(A) The lesions are raised, are well demarcated, and have smooth surfaces. **(B)** The collagen has a basket weave appearance.

PLEURAL PLAQUE—FACT SHEET

Definition

» Discrete raised collagenous plaque

Clinical Features

» Patients are asymptomatic
» Classically associated with asbestos exposure
» May be associated with rounded atelectasis

Prognosis and Therapy

» Incidental abnormality with no prognostic implications
» No therapy needed

PLEURAL PLAQUES—PATHOLOGIC FEATURES

Gross Findings

» Dense white or gray plaques, usually on the parietal pleura or diaphragm

Microscopic Findings

» Layered collagen in a basket weave pattern
» May have focal areas of calcification or metaplastic bone
» No asbestos bodies or mesothelial proliferation

Pathologic Differential Diagnosis

» Desmoplastic malignant mesothelioma

PROGNOSIS AND THERAPY

Pleural plaques are generally only indicative of asbestos exposure and have no prognostic significance and no relationship to the development of other asbestos-induced diseases, such as asbestosis or malignant mesothelioma. If present on the visceral pleura, they may be associated with rounded atelectasis. No therapy is needed.

ROUNDED ATELECTASIS

Rounded atelectasis refers to entrapment of a portion of the subpleural lung caused by adhesions of the overlying fibrotic pleura or pleural plaque. This condition is

also known as folded lung, shrinking atelectasis, and Blesovsky's syndrome. Although the majority of lesions are related to asbestos exposure, they have also been reported to be induced by trauma, infection, or localized organized effusion.

CLINICAL FEATURES

Patients are usually asymptomatic and the lesions are detected as incidental opacities on chest radiograph. The fibrotic pleural reaction pulls and twists the underlying lung parenchyma to form a "pseudo" mass lesion. Characteristically, the "tumor" disappears when the surgeon incises the overlying fibrotic pleura.

ROUNDED (SHRINKING) ATELECTASIS—FACT SHEET

Definition

▸▸ Entrapment of subpleural lung caused by overlying fibrosis or pleural plaque

Clinical Features

▸▸ Patients are usually asymptomatic
▸▸ Incidental finding that is resected due to concern about malignancy or infection

Prognosis and Therapy

▸▸ For most patients, the lesion has no prognostic implications and no therapy is needed.
▸▸ Rare patients require pleurectomy to relieve respiratory failure caused by atelectasis.

ROUNDED (SHRINKING) ATELECTASIS-PATHOLOGIC FEATURES

Microscopic Findings

▸▸ Dense pleural fibrosis with underlying chronic atelectasis

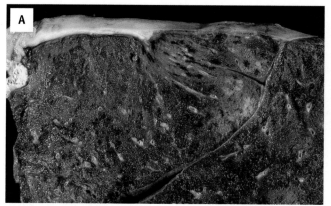

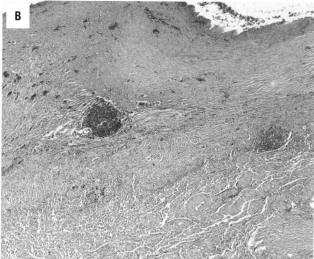

FIGURE 35-8

Rounded atelectasis
(A) The thickened fibrotic pleura has distorted the underlying lung parenchyma to form a pseudo-mass lesion. **(B)** The lung parenchyma is atelectatic adjacent to the fibrotically thickened pleura. (Figure 35-8A From Churg A, Green FHY. *Pathology of Occupational Lung Disease*. 2nd ed. Baltimore: Williams & Wilkins; 1998, with permission.)

PATHOLOGIC FEATURES

Lesions are found in the visceral pleura and consist of non-specific pleural fibrosis with changes of chronic atelectasis in the underlying lung (Figure 35-8A,B). The latter include alveolar macrophage accumulation with or without parenchymal fibrosis. There may be asbestos fibers in the underlying lung, since these lesions can be associated with asbestos exposure.

DIFFERENTIAL DIAGNOSIS

The pathologic findings are distinctive. Clinical and radiographic differential diagnoses usually include malignancies and infections.

Prognosis and Therapy

Although these lesions are generally excised to rule out carcinoma, rounded atelectasis itself does not usually require treatment. Only large lesions that have induced respiratory compromise require pleurectomy to untether the lung parenchyma.

SUGGESTED READINGS

1. Askin FB, McCann BG, Kuhn C. Reactive eosinophilic pleuritis. *Arch Pathol Lab Med*. 1977;101:187-92.
2. Chapman SJ, Davies RJ. Recent advances in parapneumonic effusion and empyema. *Curr Opin Pulm Med*. 2004;10:299-304.
3. Churg A, Colby TV, Cagle P, et al. The separation of benign and malignant mesothelial proliferations. *Am J Surg Pathol*. 2000;24:1183-1200.
4. Krausz T, Barker F. Reactive effusions. In Gray W, McKee GT, eds. *Diagnostic Cytopathology*. 2nd ed. Philadelphia: Elsevier Science Limited, 2003; 145-7.
5. Light RW. *Pleural diseases*. 4th ed. Baltimore: Lippincott, Williams & Wilkins; 2001.

36 Pulmonary Manifestations of Systemic Diseases

Omar R. Chughtai • Dani S. Zander

INTRODUCTION

Many systemic diseases are associated with lung or pleural injury, either as a component of the disease or as a consequence of other types of injury induced by the disease or its treatment. This chapter focuses upon systemic diseases that can involve the lung or pleura as a direct component of the disorder. Secondary lung disease can develop as an immunologic or inflammatory reaction to a wide variety of drugs or radiation, or by predisposition to infections, as is the case with immuno-suppressive agents used for therapy. Secondary lung disease can also arise from conditions (i.e., scleroderma) that lead to aspiration and its pulmonary sequelae.

CONNECTIVE TISSUE DISEASES

Connective tissue diseases are associated with a diverse spectrum of pulmonary and pleural pathology. Interstitial lung diseases, inflammatory airway lesions, pleural disorders, vascular abnormalities, and focal lesions (such as rheumatoid nodules) fall within the array of changes described in association with specific connective tissue diseases. These abnormalities can occur as isolated findings or, in some cases, can coexist. Although, for the most part, the existence of a collagen vascular disease will be recognized before a lung biopsy is obtained, in a smaller number of patients the lung disease may precede development of more classical manifestations of the specific connective tissue disease. In this group of patients, the role of the connective tissue disease in the genesis of the lung disorder may be recognized only with hindsight. Also, opportunistic infections and drug reactions represent other potential differential diagnostic considerations in these patients, since many individuals are treated with immunosuppressive agents and other drugs known to trigger reactions. D-penicillamine, gold, and methotrexate are recognized to cause a variety of patterns of pulmonary injury, which are catalogued on *www.pneumotox.com*, but any agent can potentially serve as the stimulus for a reaction.

RHEUMATOID ARTHRITIS

Pulmonary and pleural disease is common in patients with rheumatoid arthritis (RA) and can manifest itself in a wide range of forms. The clinical presentation and radiographic findings depend upon the nature of the pathology present in the individual patient, and coexistence of more than one manifestation is a frequent event. At autopsy, histologic pleural disease is found in up to 40% of patients with RA. Pleural effusion is the most common

---

PLEUROPULMONARY MANIFESTATIONS OF RHEUMATOID ARTHRITIS—FACT SHEET

Pleural Disease

- ▸ Pleural effusion
- ▸ Pleuritis
- ▸ Pneumothorax
- ▸ Empyema

Interstitial Lung Disease

- ▸ Usual interstitial pneumonia
- ▸ Nonspecific interstitial pneumonia
- ▸ Lymphoid interstitial pneumonia
- ▸ Desquamative interstitial pneumonia
- ▸ Organizing pneumonia

Airway Disease

- ▸ Lymphocytic and follicular bronchitis and bronchiolitis
- ▸ Constrictive bronchiolitis (bronchiolitis obliterans)
- ▸ Bronchiectasis

Rheumatoid Nodules (Pleural or Pulmonary)

Caplan's Syndrome

Apical Fibrobullous Disease

Vascular Disease

- ▸ Pulmonary hypertension
- ▸ Pulmonary hemorrhage due to small vessel vasculitis

Amyloidosis

---

pleuropulmonary manifestation of RA and may be clinically silent or associated with chest pain. Most effusions are small, exudative effusions. The pleural surfaces typically show deposition of a hypocellular layer of fibrinous material that can organize over time. Multinucleated giant cells and elongate macrophages can be seen in pleural fluid cytology specimens. Rheumatoid nodules can also develop, primarily in visceral pleura. Rupture of a rheumatoid nodule has been postulated to account for pneumothoraces and empyemas developing in patients with rheumatoid pleural disease.

Interstitial lung disease is the most frequent pulmonary manifestation of RA. Interstitial changes are noted in up to 50% of lung computed tomography (CT) scans performed in patients with RA, with the most common findings being ground-glass opacities and reticulation. On pulmonary function testing, decreased carbon monoxide diffusing capacity is observed in up to 40% of RA patients. Bronchoalveolar lavage fluid can demonstrate a lymphocytic or neutrophilic alveolitis. Patterns of nonspecific interstitial pneumonia (NSIP) and usual interstitial pneumonia (UIP) are most characteristic, and individuals have symptomatology and radiographic abnormalities

similar to patients with the idiopathic forms of these interstitial pneumonias. Histologically, as well, these processes resemble idiopathic examples of NSIP and UIP (Chapter 16). In brief, the NSIP pattern consists of a temporally homogeneous interstitial mononuclear inflammatory cell infiltrate, interstitial fibrosis, or a combination of both, without honeycombing. Cellular, fibrotic, and mixed subtypes are recognized. The UIP pattern, in contrast, consists of a temporally heterogeneous combination of interstitial fibrosis, honeycombing, fibroblast foci, and variable degrees of inflammation with a predominant subpleural distribution (Figure 36-1). Follicular bronchiolitis and organizing pneumonia are commonly found as minor patterns in patients with a predominant NSIP or UIP pattern. Lymphoid interstitial pneumonia and desquamative interstitial pneumonia have been reported less frequently than NSIP and UIP in patients with RA. The prognosis of RA-associated interstitial lung disease is probably related to the pattern(s) of lung disease represented. In general, patterns of UIP and fibrotic NSIP are associated with poorer survival than cellular NSIP. Among patients with the UIP pattern and a collagen vascular disease (not specifically RA), the UIP pattern appears to be associated with longer survival than idiopathic UIP. Treatment of RA-associated interstitial lung disease may include corticosteroids alone or in combination with azathioprine, cyclophosphamide, methotrexate, cyclosporine, or other agents.

Physiologic evidence of chronic airway obstruction is found in 16% to 38% of patients with RA. Airway lesions associated with RA include chronic and follicular bronchitis and bronchiolitis, constrictive (obliterative) bronchiolitis, and bronchiectasis. Chronic airway inflammation refers to lymphoplasmacytic inflammation in the walls of airways. When accompanied by lymphoid aggregates with germinal centers, the terms follicular bronchitis and bronchiolitis are used. Follicular bronchiolitis can be a cause of airflow obstruction in patients with RA and not uncommonly occurs in association with interstitial lung disease in these patients. Cough is a common symptom. Chest radiographs can show small nodules, which are seen to lie in centrilobular locations on high-resolution computed tomography (HRCT). Histologically, there is hyperplasia of the bronchial-associated lymphoid tissue, which forms peribronchiolar lymphoid follicles, often containing germinal centers, and can produce compression of the bronchiolar lumen. Corticosteroids are the primary treatment, but in refractory cases, a cytotoxic agent may be added. Erythromycin has also been reported to be effective.

Constrictive bronchiolitis occurs more commonly in women than in men with RA and was earlier thought to be a complication of penicillamine or gold therapy. Its onset is insidious, with productive cough followed by dyspnea as a common presentation. Chest radiographs appear normal or hyperinflated, and HRCT typically shows expiratory air trapping. Histologically,

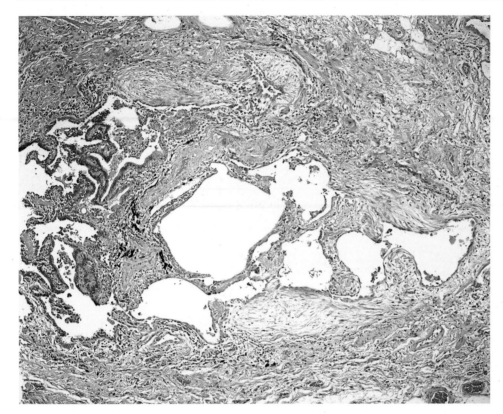

FIGURE 36-1

Usual interstitial pneumonia pattern
This example displays dense interstitial fibrosis with fibroblast foci, mild interstitial mononuclear infiltrates, metaplastic epithelium, and honeycomb change.

subepithelial deposition of mature collagen in bronchioles is characteristic (Figure 36-2). Variable degrees and types of inflammation may accompany the collagen deposition, and there may be loss or obliteration of the bronchiolar smooth muscle layer by the fibrosing process. Luminal narrowing or complete fibrotic obstruction results. Constrictive bronchiolitis usually follows a progressive clinical course and generally has a poor response to therapies.

Bronchiectasis has been reported in 5% to 12% of patients with RA, according to autopsy studies, but the frequency of clinically significant bronchiectasis is much lower (1%-5%). Why patients with RA are more likely to develop bronchiectasis is unclear, but the answer may be related to an increased susceptibility to airway infections possibly related to a defect in humoral immunity.

Organizing pneumonia can accompany these other airway and interstitial lesions, or it can occur as an isolated finding. As in other settings, it consists of connective tissue that fills alveoli and bronchioles, accompanied by variable degrees of chronic inflammation. It is typically responsive to corticosteroids. Apical fibrobullous disease, similar to that of ankylosing spondylitis, can develop in occasional patients with RA. Amyloidosis is another uncommon potential complication. Pulmonary vascular abnormalities associated with RA include pulmonary hypertension and, rarely, diffuse pulmonary hemorrhage secondary to small vessel vasculitis.

Rheumatoid nodules can also develop in patients with RA, usually as incidental findings in the lungs or pleura. These lesions are histologically identical to subcutaneous rheumatoid nodules and consist of a focus of acellular necrosis, surrounded by a rim of palisaded epithelioid histiocytes, surrounded again by a zone of lymphocytes, plasma cells, and fibroblasts (Figure 36-3). Caplan's syndrome (rheumatoid pneumoconiosis) was originally described in coal workers with RA, in whom large necrobiotic nodules resembling rheumatoid nodules developed in the lungs. Patients with exposure to inhaled silica can develop a similar picture. The nodules can measure up to 5 cm and characteristically demonstrate circumferential bands of dust within the necrobiotic zone of the nodule. The differential diagnosis includes tuberculosis and progressive massive fibrosis with ischemic necrosis.

SYSTEMIC LUPUS ERYTHEMATOSUS

Pleuropulmonary manifestations of systemic lupus erythematosus (SLE) are reported to develop in 50% to 70% of affected individuals. Pleural involvement (pleural effusion, pleuritis) is the most common intrathoracic presentation of SLE and may be the first indication of the disorder. It occurs in 45% to 60% of patients and can present with pleuritic pain, dyspnea, cough, and fever. Pericarditis

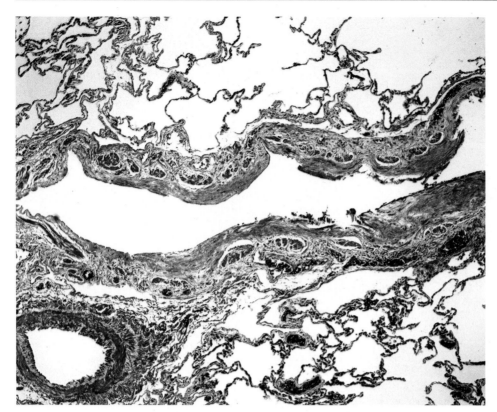

FIGURE 36-2

Constrictive (obliterative) bronchiolitis
Dense subepithelial collagen deposition produces narrowing of the airway lumen (Masson trichrome stain).

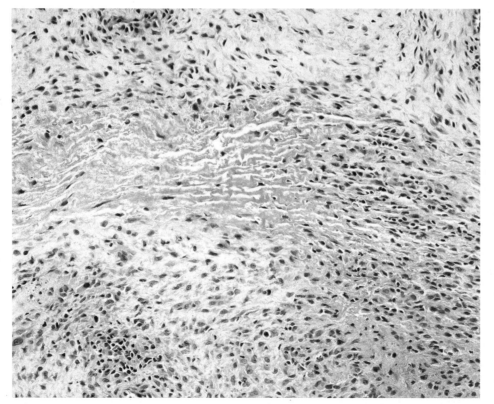

FIGURE 36-3

Rheumatoid nodule
A central zone of necrobiotic collagen is surrounded by histiocytes and then partially rimmed by lymphocytes.

PLEUROPULMONARY MANIFESTATIONS OF SYSTEMIC LUPUS ERYTHEMATOSUS—FACT SHEET

» Pleuritis and pleural effusion
» Acute lupus pneumonitis
» Diffuse alveolar hemorrhage with small vessel vasculitis
» Thromboembolic disease
» Catastrophic antiphospholipid syndrome
» Pulmonary hypertension
» Chronic interstitial lung disease
  » Usual interstitial pneumonia
  » Nonspecific interstitial pneumonia
  » Lymphoid interstitial pneumonia
  » Organizing pneumonia
» Chronic, follicular, and constrictive bronchiolitis
» Shrinking lung syndrome
» Amyloidosis

can be associated. The effusion is usually a serous or sero-sanguineous sterile exudate with a predominance of neutrophils or mononuclear cells. Lupus erythematosus cells can be found among the cells in the effusion. Pleural biopsy typically reveals lymphocytic and plasma cell infiltration of the pleura with fibrinous exudate and variable degrees of organization and fibrosis. In most patients, the effusion will either resolve spontaneously or will respond to corticosteroid therapy, usually within a period of days.

Acute lupus pneumonitis refers to an acute pulmonary syndrome associated with diffuse pulmonary infiltrates on chest radiograph. It occurs in 1% to 4% of SLE patients. In some patients, it represents the first manifestation of SLE, whereas in others it develops during the course of the disease. Symptoms are nonspecific and include cough, dyspnea, fever, and occasionally hemoptysis; also, hypoxemia is often present. Chest radiographs and CT scans show unilateral or bilateral alveolar infiltrates, particularly involving the lower lobes, and small pleural effusions. The histologic findings include diffuse alveolar damage, cellular interstitial pneumonitis, and organizing pneumonia. The most important differential diagnosis is that of a pulmonary infection with bacteria, viruses, or fungi, and evidence of infection should be aggressively sought. The treatment of acute lupus pneumonitis includes high doses of corticosteroids, combined in some cases with other immunosuppressive or cytotoxic agents or plasmapheresis. The process has a 50% mortality rate and a tendency to recur. There may be some overlap with SLE-associated diffuse alveolar hemorrhage.

Diffuse alveolar hemorrhage is a catastrophic complication that develops in less than 2% of patients with SLE. Most cases occur in women, and the median age is mid to late 20s. Symptoms of dyspnea, hemoptysis, and fever develop over a period of days and are accompanied by a decreasing hematocrit. Although most patients have

an established diagnosis of SLE, in some patients diffuse alveolar hemorrhage is a presenting manifestation of the disorder. Bronchoalveolar lavage will produce a hemorrhagic fluid sample, and lung biopsy will usually show a small vessel vasculitis (Figure 36-4). Immune complexes can be detected by immunofluorescence or electron microscopy in some cases. The differential diagnosis includes infections with bacteria, viruses, or fungi, as well as other causes of small vessel vasculitis (Chapter 8). Unfortunately, a consistently successful treatment approach for SLE-associated diffuse alveolar hemorrhage has not been determined. High-dose corticosteroid therapy by itself does not appear to be very effective, and cyclophosphamide and plasmapheresis have been added for some patients, with variable results.

Other pulmonary vascular abnormalities found in patients with SLE include thromboembolic disease and pulmonary hypertension. Antiphospholipid and anti-cardiolipin antibodies are frequently found in patients with SLE and predispose to thrombosis and embolism. Catastrophic antiphospholipid syndrome develops in rare individuals with SLE, as well as individuals possessing antiphospholipid antibodies without SLE. The syndrome presents with rapidly developing multiorgan failure due to occlusive vascular disease. The lung manifests features of the acute respiratory distress syndrome (diffuse alveolar damage), pulmonary embolism and thrombosis, and/or alveolar hemorrhage. The mortality rate is 50%, in most due to cardiac problems. Many patients are treated with a combination of anticoagulation, corticosteroids, and plasmapheresis or intravenous gammaglobulins, with recovery reported in 70% of patients in one review. Pulmonary hypertension develops in 5% to 14% of patients with SLE. Pathologic features are identical to those of other causes of pulmonary hypertension, and rarely pulmonary veno-occlusive disease can be responsible. The pathophysiology is not well understood, and antiphospholipid antibodies, anti-endothelial cell antibodies, vasculitis, vasospasm, and inflammation may contribute to the development of pulmonary hypertension.

Although CT reveals interstitial changes in 30% to 38% of patients with SLE, clinically significant interstitial pneumonia occurs far less often, in 3% to 13% of patients, and is rarely severe. Interstitial lung disease develops insidiously, sometimes with mild exacerbations. Histologic patterns include UIP, NSIP, and lymphoid interstitial pneumonia and may be accompanied by follicular bronchiolitis and organizing pneumonia. Treatment with corticosteroids usually produces improvement, and methotrexate has also been used successfully.

Airway involvement can take the forms of chronic, follicular, or constrictive bronchiolitis. Amyloidosis is another extremely unusual problem that can arise in patients with SLE. The "shrinking lung syndrome," another rare complication of SLE, refers to basilar

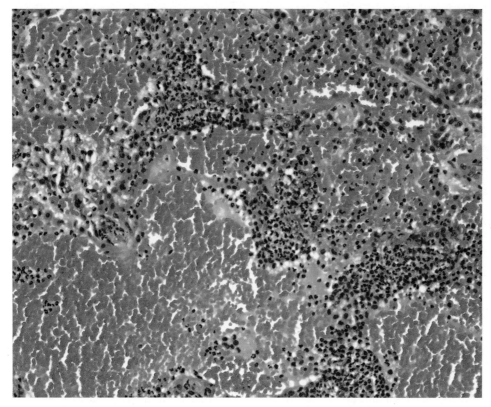

FIGURE 36-4
Small vessel vasculitis
In a background of hemorrhage, alveolar septa are densely permeated by neutrophils, with patchy septal necrosis.

atelectasis, diaphragmatic elevation, and consequent small lung volumes. Dyspnea is the main presenting symptom, and respiratory muscles can show myopathic changes. The pathophysiology of this syndrome is poorly understood, but administration of corticosteroids may produce some improvement.

SCLERODERMA

Lung involvement is found in 40% to 60% of patients with scleroderma and represents the most common cause of death in patients with this condition. Although lung disease usually makes its appearance within several years of diagnosis, it can develop later in some patients. Interstitial lung disease with progressive fibrosis is the most common form of pulmonary disease, with about 25% of scleroderma patients developing clinically significant interstitial lung disease. NSIP (Figure 36-5) is the most common histologic pattern seen in patients with scleroderma, and UIP is much less common. Fibrotic NSIP exceeds cellular NSIP by a factor of approximately 3 to 1. Ground-glass opacities are the predominant radiographic change, particularly in the basal and subpleural regions of the lungs, and honeycombing may also be apparent. Treatment usually includes cyclophosphamide and corticosteroids, which can often stabilize or improve lung function tests and HRCT changes. Other treatments are under evaluation.

A spectrum of other pulmonary complications can arise in patients with scleroderma. Pulmonary hypertension occurs in 5% to 33% of scleroderma patients, and clinically severe pulmonary hypertension affects 9% of patients with scleroderma. It tends to occur late, often 7 to 9 years after diagnosis. It is associated with a high mortality rate (56% 3-year survival after diagnosis). Histologic changes are identical to primary pulmonary hypertension. Lung cancer incidence is increased between four- and 16-fold in patients with scleroderma compared with the general population. Tumors arise primarily in patients with pulmonary fibrosis and are most frequently adenocarcinomas (often bronchioloalveolar carcinomas); other histologic types can also occur. Other reported pulmonary pathology in scleroderma includes organizing pneumonia, small airway disease, alveolar hemorrhage, and pleural fibrosis. Aspiration, predisposed to by esophageal dysfunction, represents another source of lung injury that may contribute to the pulmonary fibrosis in some individuals.

SJÖGREN'S SYNDROME

Sjögren's syndrome (SS) is a common autoimmune disease characterized by the infiltration of organs by T-lymphocytes. Lacrimal and salivary glands are the most frequently involved sites, and typical symptoms include xerostomia (dry mouth), xerophthalmia (dry

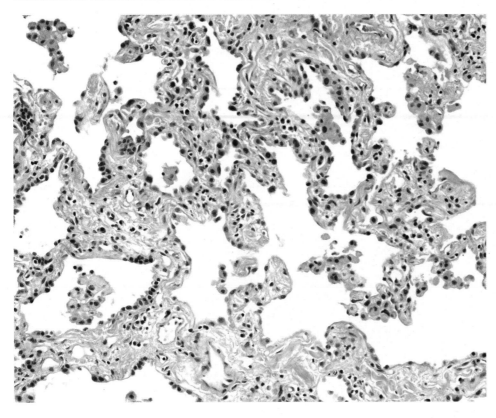

FIGURE 36-5

Nonspecific interstitial pneumonia
Alveolar septa are fibrotically thickened, with minimal mononuclear inflammatory cell infiltrates. Reactive pneumocytes, including some with mild nuclear atypia, line the septa.

eyes), and arthritis. Primary SS occurs as an isolated disorder, whereas secondary SS occurs in association with a separate connective tissue disease, primarily RA. Lung involvement tends to be more common and significant in secondary SS than in primary SS. Although HRCT changes are found in 34% to 65% of SS patients, clinically significant pulmonary disease seems to affect fewer than 10% of SS patients. Airway manifestations include bronchial lymphocytic infiltration, particularly in submucosal glands, leading to atrophy; chronic, follicular, and constrictive bronchiolitis; and bronchiectasis. The persistent chronic inflammatory state is believed to lead to desiccation (xerobronchitis) and impairment of mucociliary clearance. Many affected patients develop a dry irritating

cough and recurrent airway infections. HRCT studies can reveal bronchial thickening, bronchiolar nodules, bronchiectasis, and air trapping.

Interstitial lung disease affects 8% to 45% of patients with primary SS. Patients present with dyspnea and cough, and HRCT reveals a spectrum of abnormalities including ground-glass, consolidation, reticular, and nodular opacities. Histopathologic patterns include NSIP, UIP, and lymphoid interstitial pneumonia (Figure 36-6).

PLEUROPULMONARY MANIFESTATIONS OF SCLERODERMA—FACT SHEET

- ⇥ Interstitial lung disease
  - ⇥ Nonspecific interstitial pneumonia
  - ⇥ Usual interstitial pneumonia
  - ⇥ Organizing pneumonia
- ⇥ Small airway disease
- ⇥ Pulmonary hypertension
- ⇥ Alveolar hemorrhage
- ⇥ Pleural fibrosis
- ⇥ Lung cancer, most frequently adenocarcinoma
- ⇥ Aspiration pneumonia

PLEUROPULMONARY MANIFESTATIONS OF SJÖGREN'S SYNDROME—FACT SHEET

- ⇥ Airway disease
  - ⇥ Bronchial lymphocytic infiltration, particularly in submucosal glands, and glandular atrophy
  - ⇥ Chronic, follicular, and constrictive bronchiolitis
  - ⇥ Bronchiectasis
- ⇥ Interstitial lung disease
  - ⇥ Nonspecific interstitial pneumonia
  - ⇥ Usual interstitial pneumonia
  - ⇥ Lymphoid interstitial pneumonia
  - ⇥ Organizing pneumonia
- ⇥ Primary pulmonary lymphoma
- ⇥ Amyloidosis
- ⇥ Lung cysts
- ⇥ Pulmonary hypertension
- ⇥ Cryoglobulinemia with pulmonary hemorrhage
- ⇥ Pleuritis

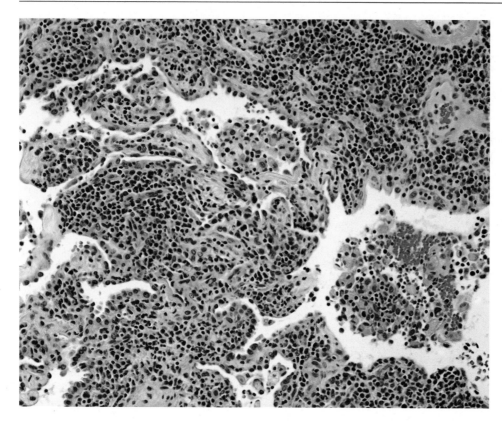

FIGURE 36-6
Lymphoid interstitial pneumonia
Dense infiltrates of lymphocytes and plasma cells expand alveolar septa and also populate some alveolar sacs.

Organizing pneumonia and bronchiolitis can accompany these patterns. Treatment with corticosteroids, with or without another immunosuppressive agent, appears to produce improvement or stabilization of the interstitial lung disease in most patients, although those with UIP may be more likely to progress.

Other pulmonary pathology reported in patients with SS includes lung cysts, primary pulmonary lymphoma, diffuse interstitial amyloidosis, pulmonary hypertension, and cryoglobulinemia with pulmonary hemorrhage. Pulmonary lymphoma develops in 1% to 2% of all patients with SS, and secondary pulmonary involvement by lymphoma arising in an extrapulmonary location also occurs in some patients with SS-associated lymphoma. Pleural disease is not common in SS, but pleuritis has been reported.

POLYMYOSITIS AND DERMATOMYOSITIS

Polymyositis (PM) and dermatomyositis (DM) are associated with a range of pulmonary manifestations that can arise during the course of the disease or precede other more typical features. The spectrum of pulmonary manifestations includes interstitial lung disease, lung cancer (small cell and non-small cell carcinomas), aspiration pneumonia (predisposed to by respiratory muscle weakness), pulmonary hypertension, vasculitis with pulmonary hemorrhage, and pleuritis. These complica-

tions represent common causes of death in patients with PM and DM. Patients with the antisynthetase syndrome have a particularly high frequency of lung disease; this syndrome includes PM or DM (63%-100%), interstitial lung disease (40%-100%), Raynaud's phenomenon (25%-100%), thick cracked skin over the tips and sides of the fingers, and the presence of one of the seven antisynthetase antibodies.

Interstitial lung disease affects 20% to 30% of PM and DM patients and is associated with a poor prognosis, leading to death in 30% to 66% of patients. Both acute and chronic forms are recognized. The acute form most often has the clinical, radiographic, and pathologic features of the acute respiratory distress syndrome/ diffuse alveolar damage. The prognosis is usually poor, despite treatment with corticosteroids and immunosuppressive agents. A better response to corticosteroids is found with cases displaying patterns of NSIP and organizing pneumonia. Pulmonary hemorrhage with small vessel vasculitis has also been reported. More chronic presentations are associated with the histologic patterns of NSIP (usually the fibrotic or mixed type), UIP, or organizing pneumonia. These patterns can be combined, and alveolar proteinosis has been described in association with an example of NSIP. CT scans generally show reticular and/or ground-glass opacities with or without consolidation. Corticosteroids with or without cyclophosphamide, cyclosporine, and tacrolimus are often used for treatment, and for milder disease, azathioprine or methotrexate can be used.

PLEUROPULMONARY MANIFESTATIONS OF POLYMYOSITIS AND DERMATOMYOSITIS—FACT SHEET

- ⇥ Interstitial lung disease
  - ⇥ Nonspecific interstitial pneumonia
  - ⇥ Usual interstitial pneumonia
  - ⇥ Organizing pneumonia
  - ⇥ Diffuse alveolar damage
- ⇥ Pulmonary hypertension
- ⇥ Alveolar hemorrhage with small vessel vasculitis
- ⇥ Lung cancer
- ⇥ Aspiration pneumonia
- ⇥ Pleuritis

MIXED CONNECTIVE TISSUE DISEASE

Patients with mixed connective tissue disease have features of SLE, scleroderma, RA, and PM-DM and have high titers of antibodies against uridine-rich RNA-small nuclear ribonucleoprotein (anti-RNP). Many of these patients evolve into a single connective tissue disease, usually scleroderma, during the first five years after diagnosis. Although pleuropulmonary disease is common in patients with mixed connective tissue disease, it often is subclinical. Manifestations resemble those of SLE, scleroderma, and PM-DM. More frequent pleuropulmonary abnormalities include interstitial lung disease, pleural effusion and pleuritis, and pulmonary hypertension, and less frequently reported features include vasculitis and hemorrhage, pulmonary thromboembolism, aspiration pneumonia, pulmonary nodules, and pulmonary cysts.

ANKYLOSING SPONDYLITIS

HRCT abnormalities appear to be very common (range 50%-85%) in ankylosing spondylitis, even in patients with early disease. These changes include apical fibrobullous disease (most common), interstitial lung disease, emphysema, bronchiectasis, and pleural thickening. Most of the published studies, however, are limited by a lack of matched control subjects.

RELAPSING POLYCHONDRITIS

Pulmonary involvement can be focal or more diffuse throughout the airways. Inflammatory airway injury leads to destruction of bronchial cartilage, followed by scarring and contractive distortion of the tracheobronchial anatomy. Airway obstruction can result and can lead to accumulation of secretions and increased risk of pulmonary infections.

INHERITED CONNECTIVE TISSUE DISORDERS

MARFAN'S SYNDROME

Marfan's syndrome is an autosomal dominant disorder caused by a defective gene involved with fibrillin production. About 10% of patients develop pulmonary abnormalities, particularly spontaneous pneumothorax and emphysema. Bilateral bullae, or blebs, can be seen radiographically in the upper lung zones. Obstructive sleep apnea is also common in individuals with this syndrome.

EHLERS-DANLOS SYNDROME

Ehlers-Danlos syndrome is a group of inherited disorders characterized by articular hypermobility, skin extensibility, and tissue fragility. Hemoptysis occurs in patients with Ehlers-Danlos syndrome, probably due to mucosal fragility, and can be triggered by forced expiration in physical exercise, coughing, or shouting. Tracheobronchomegaly (dilatation of both the trachea and bronchi) and bullae have been reported in patients with Ehlers-Danlos syndrome.

INFLAMMATORY BOWEL DISEASE

Although primarily affecting the gastrointestinal tract, Crohn's disease and ulcerative colitis are recognized as well for their extraintestinal manifestations. Lung and pleural pathology appears to be more common in patients with these disorders than may be generally appreciated. Although clear explanations are not available for the propensity of these disorders to involve the respiratory system, common embryologic origin of gastrointestinal and respiratory epithelia from the foregut, common cell types (goblet cells, submucosal glands, submucosal lymphoid tissue), and shared participation in host mucosal defense may be related. Respiratory symptoms appear to be more common in patients with inflammatory bowel disease (IBD) than in the general population, and 25% to 53% of IBD patients display abnormalities on HRCT including air trapping, ground-glass opacification, peripheral reticular opacities, diffuse infiltrates, nodular infiltrates, masses, and cysts. The age of onset varies widely, but often patients are in the fifth decade of life. Females are more frequently affected than males, and patients with ulcerative colitis outnumber those with Crohn's disease. Although the onset of lung disease usually follows the diagnosis of the gastro-intestinal disorder, some individuals develop lung disease before other more typical manifestations of IBD. Corticosteroids represent the main treatment modality, and responsiveness varies, at least in part depending upon the pathology present.

Published series indicate that the large airways are the most common location of IBD involvement. Bronchiectasis is the classic manifestation (Figure 36-7). Other large airway changes can include chronic inflammation, suppurative large airway disease without airway dilation, and acute bronchitis. Small airway and alveolar abnormalities include chronic bronchiolitis, acute bronchiolitis with bronchopneumonia-like features and suppuration/abscess, NSIP, organizing pneumonia, and eosinophilic pneumonia. Giant cells or non-necrotizing granulomas may be present in patients with Crohn's disease, and necrobiotic nodules have been reported in rare patients with ulcerative colitis. Rare reports exist of pulmonary vasculitis, pleuritis, and pleural effusion in patients with IBD. Asthma, sarcoidosis, and thromboembolism also appear to be more common in individuals with IBD than in the general population. In some patients receiving mesalamine, the differential diagnosis for the bronchiolitis, granulomatous inflammation, and/or interstitial pneumonia includes a reaction to mesalamine.

PRIMARY BILIARY CIRRHOSIS

Pulmonary pathology reported in association with primary biliary cirrhosis includes lymphocytic bronchitis and bronchiolitis, organizing pneumonia, and chronic interstitial pneumonia. Rare reports have also appeared describing pulmonary hemorrhage and glomerulonephritis, or microscopic polyangiitis, in individuals with primary biliary cirrhosis.

TUBEROUS SCLEROSIS COMPLEX

Tuberous sclerosis complex (TSC) is an autosomal-dominant disorder caused by inactivating mutations in TSC1 or TSC2. Individuals manifest mental retardation, seizures, and central nervous system and visceral hamartomas. Pulmonary manifestations include lymphangioleiomyomatosis (LAM), which occurs in up to 34% of women with TSC, micronodular pneumocyte hyperplasia (MNPH), clear cell (sugar) tumor of the lung, and the rare pulmonary angiomyolipoma. LAM and the clear cell (sugar) tumor are discussed more fully

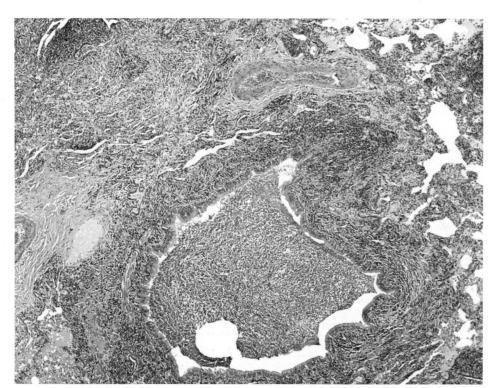

FIGURE 36-7
Bronchiectasis
This dilated, inflamed bronchus is filled with inflammatory exudate. Adjacent parenchyma demonstrates features of a chronic pneumonia. (Generously contributed by Dr. Samuel Yousem, University of Pittsburgh, Pittsburgh, Pennsylvania.)

in other sections of this book, so only brief descriptions are provided here. Pulmonary LAM is a progressive cystic lung disease usually diagnosed in young or middle-aged women. Approximately 15% of women with LAM have TSC. LAM is characterized by infiltration of atypical smooth muscle-like cells around airways, blood vessels, and lymphatics, with formation of enlarged cystic air spaces (Figure 36-8). The LAM cells express muscle markers, HMB45 (Figure 36-9), and estrogen and progesterone receptors.

MNPH is found in TSC patients of either gender. The lesions may be seen with or without accompanying LAM and occur in young or middle-aged individuals. They are well-demarcated nodules usually measuring 1 to 3 mm in diameter. Histologically, they consist of a proliferation of enlarged cytologically benign type 2 pneumocytes, with an associated increase in alveolar macrophages and interstitial reticulin (Figure 36-10). The pneumocytes stain for cytokeratin, epithelial membrane antigen, BER-EP4, and often surfactant apoprotein B. MNPH is considered to be a benign hamartomatous process.

Clear cell (sugar) tumors are rare lesions probably derived from perivascular epithelioid cells, arising in individuals across a wide age range. They are usually discovered incidentally, and rare cases are associated with TSC. They consist of round or ovoid cells with distinct cell borders and abundant clear or eosinophilic cytoplasm. Mitoses are usually absent, necrosis

is extremely rare, and nuclear atypia is mild or minimal. Tumor cells stain for HMB45 and demonstrate strong diastase-sensitive periodic acid-Schiff positivity. They are treated by surgical resection. Pulmonary angiomyolipoma is also an extremely rare lesion and morphologically resembles its counterparts in other anatomic locations, though a lack of reactivity for HMB45 and melan-A was noted in a pulmonary lesion.

SICKLE CELL DISEASE

Sickle cell disease is associated with a spectrum of pulmonary complications. In the "acute chest syndrome," patients experience cough, fever, breathlessness, chest pain, and sputum production. This syndrome can be triggered by acute pneumonia and sepsis, often secondary to *Streptococcus pneumoniae, Haemophilus influenzae,* or *Mycoplasma pneumoniae* or, in younger children, infection with respiratory syncytial virus and other common respiratory viruses. Infarction due to in situ thrombosis and bone marrow embolism occurs in these patients, and thromboses and emboli can lead to pulmonary hypertension over time. Treatment consists of pain relief, oxygen, adequate fluid intake, and antibiotics.

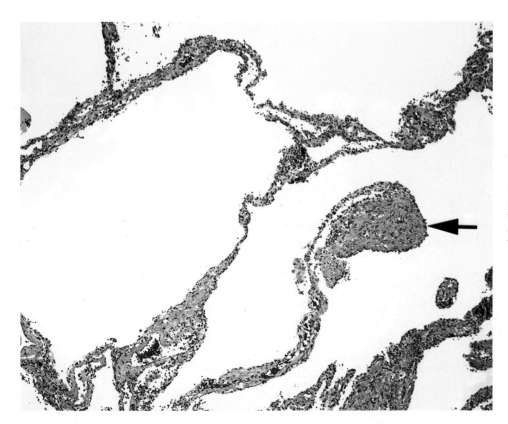

FIGURE 36-8

Lymphangioleiomyomatosis
The characteristic atypical smooth muscle cells (arrow) are found in the wall of this cystically distended air space.

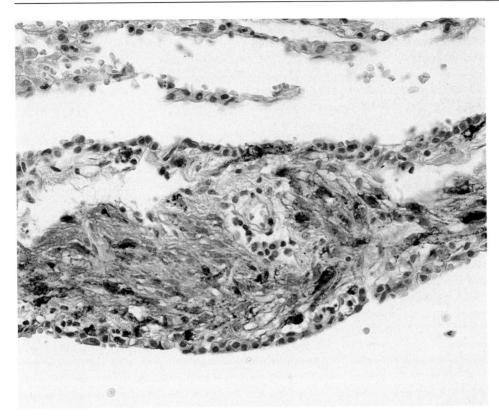

FIGURE 36-9

Lymphangioleiomyomatosis
The atypical smooth muscle cells stain for HMB45.

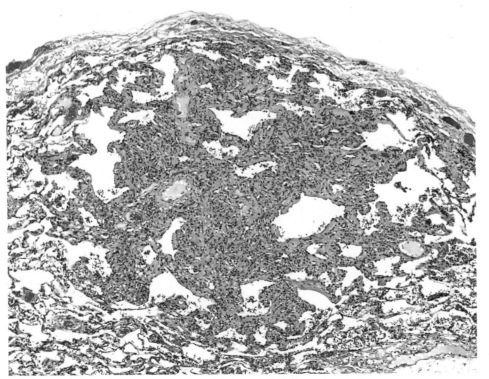

FIGURE 36-10

Micronodular pneumocyte hyperplasia
This well-demarcated nodule consists of a cytologically benign proliferation of type 2 pneumocytes lining thickened alveolar septa. (Generously contributed by Dr. Kevin Leslie, Mayo Clinic, Scottsdale, Arizona.)

FAMILIAL DYSAUTONOMIA

An autosomal recessive disease almost exclusively occurring in children of Ashkenazi Jewish descent, familial dysautonomia manifests itself with multiple problems related to autonomic dysfunction. Clinical symptoms include failure to make tears, excessive salivation, poor coordination of swallowing with recurrent aspiration, gastroesophageal reflux, recurrent lower respiratory tract infection, scoliosis, cardiovascular instability with varying blood pressure, and a blunted central hypoxic response that can potentially create a need for oxygen during aircraft flights and cause problems during underwater swimming with breath-holding.

STORAGE DISEASES

Although storage diseases are an infrequent cause of lung dysfunction, several of these rare disorders can cause clinically apparent lung disease. Interpretation of the histologic findings in patient samples is assisted in most cases, however, by the availability of a clinical history of one of these disorders.

NIEMANN-PICK DISEASE

Patients with pulmonary involvement by Niemann-Pick disease can manifest no respiratory symptoms or variable symptomatology including dyspnea, cough, and even respiratory failure. In three patients with type B disease reported by Nicholson et al, the lung was the only site of clinical disease. Histologically, foamy cells are found in aggregates in alveoli and alveolar septa (Figure 36-11) and ciliated epithelial cells can also demonstrate vacuolization in type B disease. The foamy cytoplasm is caused by intracellular accumulation of sphingomyelin. Ultrastructural examination reveals abnormal lamellar inclusions in lysosomes of affected cells. Whole lung lavage produced improvement in symptoms and lung function in two patients with type B disease, and two infants with type C disease died of respiratory failure, in this same series (Nicholson et al).

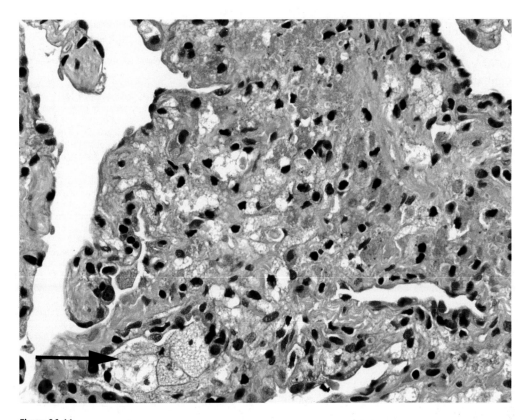

Figure 36-11
Niemann-Pick disease
The alveolar septum is expanded by a population of foamy macrophages. Similar cells are found in an alveolar space (arrow).
(Generously contributed by Dr. Carol Farver, Cleveland Clinic, Cleveland, Ohio.)

GAUCHER'S DISEASE

Gaucher's disease is a lysosomal storage disorder associated with an autosomal recessive deficiency of glucocerebrosidase activity. In this disorder, lipid-laden macrophages (Gaucher's cells) are found in a variety of tissues, particularly in the spleen, liver, bone marrow, lymph nodes, and central nervous system. Pulmonary involvement can develop in all subtypes, and involvement can be asymptomatic or associated with dyspnea or cough. Infiltrates can be seen on chest radiographs in a diffuse reticular, reticulonodular, or miliary pattern. Diffuse interstitial interlobular thickening and nodules are reportedly seen on high-resolution CT scan in approximately 17–30% of patients with Gaucher's disease. The microscopic patterns of pulmonary involvement by the Gaucher's cells have been described as intracapillary, patchy interstitial infiltrates with a lymphatic distribution, massive interstitial thickening, and intraalveolar infiltrates. Detection of the Gaucher's cells can be facilitated by periodic acid-Schiff staining and immunohistochemical staining for CD68.

FABRY'S DISEASE

Fabry's disease (angiokeratoma corporis diffusum universale) is an X-linked disorder of glycosphingolipid metabolism caused by a deficiency of α-galactosidase A activity, leading to increased glycosphingolipid accumulation in multiple anatomic sites. Airway obstruction thought to be due to accumulated glycolipids has been described, and symptoms can include dyspnea, wheezing, hemoptysis, and pneumothorax. Histologically, inclusions can be seen in respiratory epithelial cells, endothelial cells, and smooth muscle cells.

HERMANSKY-PUDLAK SYNDROME

Hermansky-Pudlak Syndrome, a rare autosomal recessive disease, encompasses the triad of albinism, a hemorrhagic predisposition due to a platelet storage pool defect, and systemic accumulation of ceroid. The responsible gene is believed to reside on chromosome 10, and encodes a transmembrane protein. Pulmonary involvement by this syndrome most often presents as a fibrotic lung disease. The distribution of fibrosis in this syndrome has been described as involving respiratory bronchioles and surrounding areas, in contrast to the more peripheral alveolar localization of the changes in usual intersitial pneumonia. Constrictive bronchiolitis, ceroid-containing macrophages and granulomatous inflammation have also been reported in association with this syndrome. Also characteristic is the accumulation of type 2 pneumocytes with foamy swelling and degeneration, which has been

termed "giant lamellar body degeneration," a feature corresponding to the giant lamellar bodies observed on ultrastructural examination.

CRYSTAL-STORING HISTIOCYTOSIS

Crystal-storing histiocytosis is a rare disorder that is usually (although not always) associated with multiple myeloma, lymphoma, plasma cell hyperplasia, or monoclonal gammopathy. Histiocytes containing eosinophilic immunoglobulin crystals form single or multiple lung masses. The histiocytes express CD68, but not S100. Similar lesions have been described in the head and neck, skin, bone, lymph nodes, and other sites.

SUGGESTED READINGS

Connective Tissue Diseases

1. Asherson RA, Cervera R, Piette JC, et al. Catastrophic antiphospholipid syndrome. Clinical and laboratory features of 50 patients. *Medicine (Baltimore)*. 1998;77:195-207.
2. Bouros D, Wells AU, Nicholson AG, et al. Histopathologic subsets of fibrosing alveolitis in patients with systemic sclerosis and their relationship to outcome. *Am J Respir Crit Care Med*. 2002;165:1581-6.
3. Bull TM, Fagan KA, Badesch DB. Pulmonary vascular manifestations of mixed connective tissue disease. *Rheum Dis Clin North Am*. 2005;31:451-64.
4. Castagnaro A, Chetta A, Marangio E, Zompatori M, Olivieri D. The lung in immune-mediated disorder: rheumatoid arthritis. *Curr Drug Targets Inflamm Allergy*. 2004;3:449-54.
5. Cha SI, Fessler MB, Cool CD, Schwarz MI, Brown KK. Lymphoid interstitial pneumonia: clinical features, associations and prognosis. *Eur Respir J*. 2006;28:364-9.
6. Colby TV. Pulmonary pathology in patients with systemic autoimmune diseases. *Clin Chest Med*. 1998;19:587-612.
7. Crestani B. The respiratory system in connective tissue disorders. Allergy. 2005;60:715-34.
8. Dawson JK, Fewins HE, Desmond J, Lynch MP, Graham DR. Fibrosing alveolitis in patients with rheumatoid arthritis as assessed by high resolution computed tomography, chest radiography, and pulmonary function tests. *Thorax*. 2001;56:622-7.
9. Fujita J, Tokuda M, Bandoh S, et al. Primary lung cancer associated with polymyositis/dermatomyositis, with a review of the literature. *Rheumatol Int*. 2001;20:81-4.
10. Hayakawa H, Sato A, Imokawa S, Toyoshima M, Chida K, Iwata M. Bronchiolar disease in rheumatoid arthritis. *Am J Respir Crit Care Med*. 1996;154:1531-6.
11. Hunninghake GW, Fauci AS. Pulmonary involvement in the collagen vascular diseases. *Am Rev Respir Dis*. 1979;119:471-503.
12. Johnston SL, Dudley CR, Unsworth DJ, Lock RJ. Life-threatening acute pulmonary haemorrhage in primary Sjögren's syndrome with cryoglobulinaemia. *Scand J Rheumatol*. 2005;34:404-7.
13. Lamblin C, Bergoin C, Saelens T, Wallaert B. Interstitial lung diseases in collagen vascular diseases. *Eur Respir J*. 2001;32:69s-80s.
14. Lee-Chiong TL Jr. Pulmonary manifestations of ankylosing spondylitis and relapsing polychondritis. *Clin Chest Med*. 1998;19:747-57.
15. Lynch JP III, Hunninghake GW. Pulmonary complications of collagen vascular disease. *Annu Rev Med*. 1992;43:17-35.
16. Murin S, Wiedemann HP, Matthay RA. Pulmonary manifestations of systemic lupus erythematosis. *Clin Chest Med*. 1998;19:641-65.
17. Parambil JG, Myers JL, Lindell RM, Matteson EL, Ryu JH. Interstitial lung disease in primary Sjögren syndrome. *Chest*. 2006;130:1489-95.
18. Park JH, Kim DS, Park IN, et al. Prognosis of fibrotic interstitial pneumonia: idiopathic versus collagen vascular disease-related. *Am J Respir Crit Care Med*. 2007;175:705-11.
19. Prakash UB. Respiratory complications in mixed connective tissue disease. *Clin Chest Med*. 1998;19:733-46.

20. Quismorio FP Jr. Pulmonary involvement in ankylosing spondylitis. *Curr Opin Pulm Med*. 2006;12:342-5.

21. Schwarz MI, Sutarik JM, Nick JA, Leff JA, Emlen JW, Tuder RM. Pulmonary capillaritis and diffuse alveolar hemorrhage. A primary manifestation of polymyositis. *Am J Respir Crit Care Med*. 1995;151:2037-40.

22. Schwarz MI, Zamora MR, Hodges TN, Chan ED, Bowler RP, Tuder RM. Isolated pulmonary capillaritis and diffuse alveolar hemorrhage in rheumatoid arthritis and mixed connective tissue disease. *Chest*. 1998;113:1609-15.

23. Swigris JJ, Berry GJ, Raffin TA, Kuschner WG. Lymphoid interstitial pneumonia: a narrative review. *Chest*. 2002;122:2150-64.

24. Tanaka N, Kim JS, Newell JD, et al. Rheumatoid arthritis-related lung diseases: CT findings. *Radiology*. 2004;232:81-91.

25. Tanoue LT. Pulmonary involvement in collagen vascular disease: a review of the pulmonary manifestations of the Marfan syndrome, ankylosing spondylitis, Sjögren's syndrome, and relapsing polychondritis. *J Thorac Imaging*. 1992;7:62-77.

26. Tansey D, Wells AU, Colby TV, et al. Variations in histological patterns of interstitial pneumonia between connective tissue disorders and their relationship to prognosis. *Histopathology*. 2004;44:585-96.

27. Travis WD, Colby TV, Koss MN, Rosado-de-Christenson ML, Muller NL, King TE. *Non-neoplastic Disorders of the Lower Respiratory Tract*. Washington, DC: American Registry of Pathology and the Armed Forces Institute of Pathology, 2002.

28. Warrington KJ, Moder KG, Brutinel WM. The shrinking lungs syndrome in systemic lupus erythematosus. *Mayo Clin Proc*. 2000;75:467-72.

29. White B. Interstitial lung disease in scleroderma. *Rheum Dis Clin North Am*. 2003;29:371-90.

30. White ES, Tazelaar HD, Lynch JP III. Bronchiolar complications of connective tissue diseases. *Semin Respir Crit Care Med*. 2003;24:543-66.

31. Yang Y, Fujita J, Tokuda M, Bandoh S, Ishida T. Lung cancer associated with several connective tissue diseases: with a review of literature. *Rheumatol Int*. 2001;21:106-11.

32. Yousem SA. The pulmonary pathologic manifestations of the CREST syndrome. *Hum Pathol*. 1990;21:467-74.

33. Yousem SA, Colby TV, Carrington CB. Follicular bronchitis/bronchiolitis. *Hum Pathol*. 1985;16:700-6.

34. Yousem SA, Colby TV, Carrington CB. Lung biopsy in rheumatoid arthritis. *Am Rev Respir Dis*. 1985;131:770-7.

35. Zamora MR, Warner ML, Tuder R, Schwarz MI. Diffuse alveolar hemorrhage and systemic lupus erythematosus. Clinical presentation, histology, survival, and outcome. *Medicine (Baltimore)*. 1997;76:192-202.

Marfan's Syndrome and Ehlers-Danlos Syndrome

36. Dinwiddie R, Sonnappa S. Systemic diseases and the lung. *Paediatr Respir Rev*. 2005;6:181-9.

Inflammatory Bowel Disease

37. Black H, Mendoza M, Murin S. Thoracic manifestations of inflammatory bowel disease. *Chest*. 2007;131:524-32.

38. Camus P, Piard F, Ashcroft T, Gal AA, Colby TV. The lung in inflammatory bowel disease. *Medicine (Baltimore)*. 1993;72:151-83.

39. Casey MB, Tazelaar HD, Myers JL, et al. Noninfectious lung pathology in patients with Crohn's disease. *Am J Surg Pathol*. 2003;27:213-9.

40. Foster RA, Zander DS, Mergo PJ, Valentine JF. Mesalamine-related lung disease: clinical, radiographic, and pathologic manifestations. *Inflamm Bowel Dis*. 2003;9:308-15.

41. Storch I, Sachar D, Katz S. Pulmonary manifestations of inflammatory bowel disease. *Inflamm Bowel Dis*. 2003;9:104-15.

42. Travis WD, Colby TV, Koss MN, Rosado-de-Christenson ML, Muller NL, King TE. *Non-neoplastic Disorders of the Lower Respiratory Tract*. Washington, DC: American Registry of Pathology and the Armed Forces Institute of Pathology, 2002.

Primary Biliary Cirrhosis

43. Amezcua-Guerra LM, Prieto P, Bojalil R, Pineda C, Amigo MC. Microscopic polyangiitis associated with primary biliary cirrhosis: a causal or casual association? *J Rheumatol*. 2006;33:2351-53.

44. Strobel ES, Bonnet RB, Werner P, Schaefer HE, Peter HH. Bronchiolitis obliterans organising pneumonia and primary biliary cirrhosis-like lung involvement in a patient with primary biliary cirrhosis. *Clin Rheumatol*. 1998;17:246-9.

45. Wallaert B, Bonniere P, Prin L, Cortot A, Tonnel AB, Voisin C. Primary biliary cirrhosis. Subclinical inflammatory alveolitis in patients with normal chest roentgenograms. *Chest*. 1986;90:842-8.

Tuberous Sclerosis Complex

46 Flieder DB, Travis WD. Clear cell "sugar" tumor of the lung: association with lymphangioleiomyomatosis and multifocal micronodular pneumocyte hyperplasia in a patient with tuberous sclerosis. *Am J Surg Pathol*. 1997;21:1242-7.

47. Glassberg MK. Lymphangioleiomyomatosis. *Clin Chest Med*. 2004;25:573-82.

48. Guinee D, Singh R, Azumi N, et al. Multifocal micronodular pneumocyte hyperplasia: a distinctive pulmonary manifestation of tuberous sclerosis. *Mod Pathol*. 1995;8:902-6.

49. Juvet SC, McCormack FX, Kwiatkowski DJ, Downey GP. Molecular pathogenesis of lymphangioleiomyomatosis: lessons learned from orphans. *Am J Respir Cell Mol Biol*. 2007;36:398-408.

50. Moss J, Avila NA, Barnes PM, et al. Prevalence and clinical characteristics of lymphangioleiomyomatosis (LAM) in patients with tuberous sclerosis complex. *Am J Respir Crit Care Med*. 2001;164:669-71.

51. Muir TE, Leslie KO, Popper H, et al. Micronodular pneumocyte hyperplasia. *Am J Surg Pathol*. 1998;22:465-72.

52. Ryu JH, Moss J, Beck GJ, et al. The NHLBI lymphangioleiomyomatosis registry: characteristics of 230 patients at enrollment. *Am J Respir Crit Care Med*. 2006;173:105-11.

53. Wu K, Tazelaar HD. Pulmonary angiomyolipoma and multifocal micronodular pneumocyte hyperplasia associated with tuberous sclerosis. *Hum Pathol*. 1999;30:1266-8.

Sickle Cell Disease

54. Prakash UB. Lungs in hemoglobinopathies, erythrocyte disorders, and hemorrhagic diatheses. *Semin Respir Crit Care Med*. 2005;26:527-40.

55. Dinwiddie R. The lung in multi-system disease. *Paediatr Respir Rev*. 2000;1:58-63.

Familial Dysautonomia

56. Dinwiddie R. The lung in multi-system disease. *Paediatr Respir Rev*. 2000;1:58-63.

Storage Diseases

57. Amir G, Ron N. Pulmonary pathology in Gaucher's disease. *Hum Pathol*. 1999;30:666-70.

58. Chung MJ, Lee KS, Franquet T, Müller NL, Han J, Kwon OJ. Metabolic lung disease: imaging and histopathologic findings. *Eur J Radiol*. 2005;54:233-45.

59. Kim W, Pyeritz RE, Bernhardt BA, Casey M, Litt HI. Pulmonary manifestations of Fabry disease and positive response to enzyme replacement therapy. *Am J Med Genet A*. 2007;143:377-81.

60. Nakatani Y, Nakamura N, Sano J, et al. Interstitial pneumonia in Hermansky-Pudlak syndrome: significance of florid foamy swelling/degeneration (giant lamellar body degeneration) of type-2 pneumocytes. *Virchows Arch*. 2000;437:304-13.

61. Nicholson AG, Florio R, Hansell DM, et al. Pulmonary involvement by Niemann-Pick disease. A report of six cases. *Histopathology*. 2006;48:596-603.

Crystal-Storing Histiocytosis

62. Fairweather PM, Williamson R, Tsikleas G. Pulmonary extranodal marginal zone lymphoma with massive crystal storing histiocytosis. *Am J Surg Pathol*. 2006;30:262-7.

63. Ionescu DN, Pierson DM, Qing G, Li M, Colby TV, Leslie KO. Pulmonary crystal-storing histiocytoma. *Arch Pathol Lab Med*. 2005;129:1159-63.

64. Jones D, Renshaw AA. Recurrent crystal-storing histiocytosis of the lung in a patient without a clonal lymphoproliferative disorder. *Arch Pathol Lab Med*. 1996;120:978-80.

65. Prasad ML, Charney DA, Sarlin J, Keller SM. Pulmonary immunocytoma with massive crystal storing histiocytosis: a case report with review of literature. *Am J Surg Pathol*. 1998;22:1148-53.

66. Sun Y, Tawfiqul B, Valderrama E, Kline G, Kahn LB. Pulmonary crystal-storing histiocytosis and extranodal marginal zone B-cell lymphoma associated with a fibroleiomyomatous hamartoma. *Ann Diagn Pathol*. 2003;7:47-53.

67. Wang CW, Colby TV. Histiocytic lesions and proliferations in the lung. *Semin Diagn Pathol*. 2007;24:162-82.

37

Respiratory Cytology
Jennifer Brainard

- **Techniques and Applications**
- **Normal Elements and Non-Cellular Components**
- **Non-Neoplastic Lung Diseases**
- **Benign Masses and Tumors**
- **Malignant Tumors**

TECHNIQUES AND APPLICATIONS

The major role of respiratory cytology is in diagnosis of malignant neoplasms involving the lung, both primary and metastatic. Cytologic techniques are also useful for staging primary lung carcinomas. Opportunistic infections, specific inflammatory processes, and some benign neoplasms may also be diagnosed cytologically. Before interpreting a cytologic sample from the respiratory tract, however, it is important to know how the specimen was collected. Sampling techniques greatly influence the cytologic appearance of the specimen (Figure 37-1). Respiratory cytology samples may be obtained using exfoliative methods or by fine needle aspiration (FNA).

Exfoliative respiratory cytology techniques include sputum cytology, bronchial cytology (washings and brushings), and bronchoalveolar lavage (BAL). Various factors influence the diagnostic yield of exfoliative techniques, including tumor location, size of the lesion, and histologic subtype. Overall, exfoliative methods have a reported sensitivity and specificity of 70% to 80%. False positive diagnoses are rare, and patients can be treated on the basis of the cytologic diagnosis alone.

Sputum samples are most commonly obtained from symptomatic patients. Although sputum cytology has been evaluated for screening for lung carcinomas, sputum screening programs have not realized a decrease in mortality from lung carcinoma. Cytologic examination of sputum has a number of advantages, however. Samples are easily obtained in a noninvasive manner,

and the samples reflect constituents from many regions of the lung. Sputum cytology is most useful in diagnosing centrally located malignancies (small cell carcinoma and squamous carcinoma). A spontaneously produced morning sputum sample has the highest diagnostic yield , and examination of 3 to 5 samples is desirable to increase the diagnostic yield. Techniques for inducing sputum samples in asymptomatic patients using a nebulizing solution have been reported. Induced sputum samples can also be used for assessing inflammation in patients with chronic respiratory conditions such as asthma, sarcoidosis, and chronic obstructive pulmonary disease and for diagnosing respiratory infections.

Sputum samples can be prepared by a variety of methods. The "pick and smear" method involves visual inspection of fresh specimens with selective smearing of strands or flecks of solid material. Sputum samples may also be prepared using the Saccomanno method in which sputum samples collected in 50% ethanol and 2% polyethylene glycol (carbowax) are placed in a blender, homogenized, and concentrated before smearing. Most commonly today, alcohol or another proprietary fixative is added to a fresh sputum sample, and the specimen is processed using cytospin or monolayer techniques. Numerous alveolar macrophages are required for a sputum sample to be considered adequate for evaluation, though there is no numeric standard. Ciliated bronchial epithelial cells are insufficient evidence of adequacy.

There are a number of disadvantages of sputum cytology. Sputum samples can be difficult to obtain or unsatisfactory if lower respiratory tract elements are not represented. Sputum evaluation does not help to localize a lung lesion. Sputum evaluation is less accurate for adenocarcinoma, metastases, and lymphoma. Most peripherally located tumors and most benign tumors cannot be diagnosed in sputum.

In many institutions, sputum cytology has been largely replaced by bronchial cytology. Indications for fiberoptic bronchoscopy include persistent cough, new solitary pulmonary nodule, persistent chest radiographic infiltrate, hemoptysis, bronchial obstruction, atelectasis, persistent localized wheezing, and confirmation of abnormal sputum cytology. Bronchial

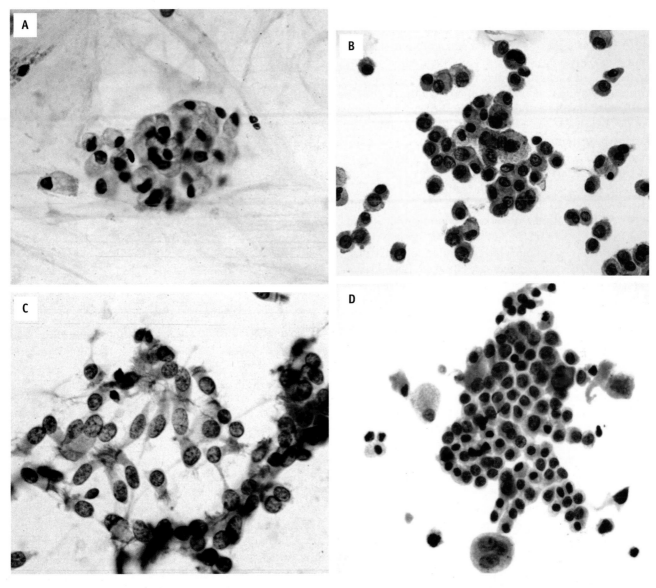

FIGURE 37-1

Respiratory cytology techniques
(A) Numerous alveolar macrophages are required for a sputum sample to be adequate for diagnosis **(B)** Bronchial washing and bronchoalveolar lavage samples consist predominantly of alveolar macrophages. Scattered ciliated bronchial epithelial cells may be seen. **(C)** Bronchial brushings consist predominantly of ciliated columnar respiratory epithelial cells. **(D)** Sheets of mesothelial cells are frequently seen in transthoracic fine needle aspiration samples.

cytologic specimens are collected during bronchoscopy and include bronchial washings and brushings. To obtain a bronchial washing sample, the bronchoscope is positioned in the area of the abnormality and repetitive installation and re-aspiration of 3 to 5 ml of a balanced saline solution is performed. The re-aspirated material can be sent fresh to the laboratory or placed in an appropriate cytologic fixative. Bronchial brushings are then obtained using a small circular stiff bristle brush with preparation of direct smears followed by rinsing of the brush in a preservative solution. Bronchial cytologic samples must be obtained before tissue biopsy procedures are performed to minimize peripheral blood contamination.

Advantages of bronchial cytology include the ability to localize and directly visualize a lung lesion and acquire a sample directly from this area. Bronchial techniques are better than sputum cytology for peripheral tumors and small tumors. Adequate bronchial specimens show large numbers of ciliated bronchial epithelial cells and alveolar macrophages. Bronchial specimens should be considered unsatisfactory for evaluation if there is heavy oral contamination or obscuring blood, inflammation, or drying. Disadvantages include the need to undergo the procedure, which can be unpleasant for the patient. Also, these techniques sample a limited area of the lung. Furthermore, benign tumors and extremely peripheral tumors are difficult to diagnose using these approaches.

BAL is a method used to evaluate the most distal air spaces. As such, it is a technique used to investigate diffuse disease processes. It is most commonly used in immunocompromised patients with pulmonary infiltrates due to suspected opportunistic infections. Cultures and special stains for microorganisms can be performed on the cytology sample. BAL is also useful in the setting of interstitial lung disease, pulmonary hemorrhage, lymphoproliferative disorders, and malignancy. To obtain a BAL sample, the bronchoscope is wedged into a subsegmental bronchus and a large volume (100-300 ml) of warm saline is instilled and re-aspirated in 20 to 100 ml aliquots. The first aliquot is discarded and the remaining aliquots are pooled. The resulting sample is sent fresh to the laboratory. Adequate BAL specimens have abundant alveolar macrophages. Excessive numbers (>75%) of ciliated respiratory epithelial cells or squamous cells indicate contamination and are not satisfactory. Specific rejection criteria exist but are not widely used.

FNA cytology of the respiratory tract can be performed through the bronchoscope or via a transthoracic approach. Percutaneous transthoracic FNA is most often used for peripheral lung lesions suspected to represent malignancies. This technique is superior to sputum and bronchial cytology for tumors that are not associated with airways. Percutaneous transthoracic FNA requires a sterile field and anesthesia. Radiographic guidance (CT, fluoroscopy) is needed to confirm needle position. The aspirate is performed, and direct smears with or without a needle rinse are prepared. Immediate assessment of specimen adequacy is optimal to minimize the number of needle passes. Repeat aspirations may be performed as needed. A major diagnostic pitfall using this technique is the misinterpretation of normal and reactive mesothelial cells as malignancy. Transbronchial (Wang needle) FNA is performed through the bronchoscope. This method is used as an adjunct to bronchoscopy to sample submucosal, necrotic, or highly vascular tumors. Transbronchial FNA is also quite useful for staging of lung tumors. Hilar, mediastinal, and subcarinal masses and lymph nodes may be sampled.

Overall, the sensitivity of lung FNA is 75% to 95%, and specificity is 95% to 100%. An exact classification of a malignant tumor is achieved in 70% to 85%. Diagnostic accuracy in separating small cell carcinoma from non-small cell carcinoma is reportedly 90% to 100%. FNA techniques are associated with more complications than sputum and bronchial cytology, particularly pneumothorax and hemoptysis. Only 5% to 10% of patients who develop a pneumothorax require treatment, however. Air embolism is a rare but fatal complication of FNA. The complication rate is related to the depth and size of the lesion, number of FNA passes, and operator experience. Also, needle size is important, with higher needle gauges associated with fewer complications.

FIBEROPTIC BRONCHOSCOPY—FACT SHEET

Indications for Fiberoptic Bronchoscopy

- ▸ Persistent cough
- ▸ New solitary pulmonary nodule
- ▸ Persistent chest radiographic infiltrate
- ▸ Hemoptysis
- ▸ Bronchial obstruction
- ▸ Atelectasis
- ▸ Persistent localized wheezing
- ▸ Confirmation of abnormal sputum cytology

NORMAL ELEMENTS AND NONCELLULAR COMPONENTS

The respiratory system is divided into the upper and lower respiratory tracts. Nonkeratinizing stratified squamous epithelium lines the upper portion of the respiratory tract, and respiratory epithelium lines the lower portion. Types of epithelial cells commonly encountered in respiratory tract samples include squamous cells, ciliated columnar bronchial epithelial cells, goblet cells, and alveolar pneumocytes (Figure 37-2). In the normal state, these cells are easily identified. It is important to become familiar with benign reactive changes in these normal cell types to avoid misinterpreting benign changes as malignancy (Figure 37-3). Reactive cells show enlarged nuclei with a mild to moderate degree of nuclear pleomorphism. Nucleoli are prominent. Overall, however, cohesion is maintained and cells are arranged in flat sheets. There is a range of cellular atypia, and there is not an identifiable discrete population of abnormal cells. The nuclear-to-cytoplasmic ratio is maintained. Importantly, any cells with cilia in respiratory cytology are benign cells. Reactive ciliated bronchial epithelial cells are commonly multinucleated.

It is also important to recognize benign cellular proliferations in respiratory cytology, including bronchial hyperplasia (Creola bodies), goblet cell hyperplasia, reserve cell hyperplasia, and squamous metaplasia (Figure 37-4). These changes occur in response to epithelial injury and if unrecognized, may be mistaken for malignancy. Epithelial injury by inflammation with airway remodeling occurs commonly in patients with asthma. Epithelial cell shedding may be pronounced in these patients, and it is estimated that asthmatic patients have a four-fold greater number of epithelial cells in BAL specimens than their normal counterparts. Ciliated columnar epithelial cells are preferentially denuded, and clusters of these sloughed epithelial cells are referred to as bronchial hyperplasia or Creola bodies. These cell clusters may have a rounded appearance, mimicking a cluster of adenocarcinoma cells. However, cells of bronchial hyperplasia have cilia, and

A

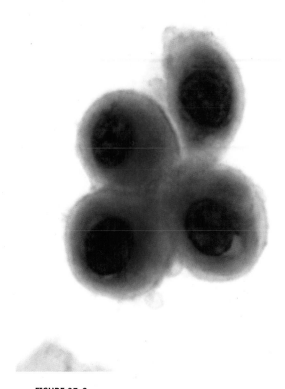

B

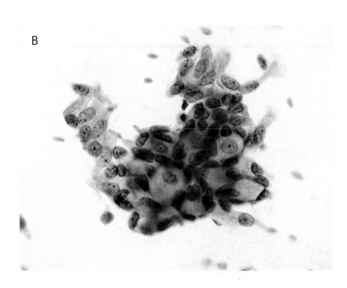

FIGURE 37-2

Normal cellular elements

(A) In addition to bronchial epithelial cells and alveolar macrophages, squamous metaplastic cells are frequently seen in respiratory samples, particularly in the setting of inflammation/airway injury. **(B)** Goblet cells are generally few in number in respiratory samples. They appear as large columnar cells with abundant cytoplasm distended by a large vacuole. The nuclei of goblet cells are small and pushed to the periphery of the cell.

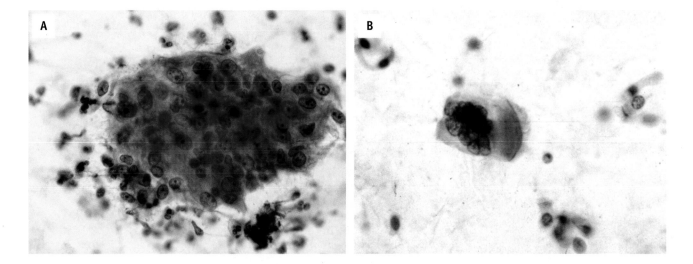

FIGURE 37-3

Reactive cellular changes

(A) Reactive epithelium occurs in flat cohesive sheets. There is a spectrum of nuclear changes present. The nuclear-to-cytoplasmic ratio is maintained. Nuclei are enlarged with pale chromatin and consistent nucleolation. **(B)** Reactive bronchial epithelial cells are typically multinucleated. Ciliated cells in respiratory cytology samples are benign.

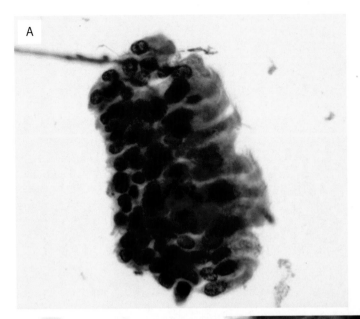

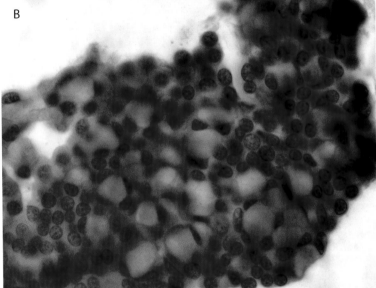

FIGURE 37-4

Benign cellular proliferations

(A) As a group, benign cellular proliferations in the lung are important to recognize to avoid an overdiagnosis of malignancy. Bronchial cell hyperplasia (Creola body) represents full-thickness sloughing of the respiratory mucosa. This is a common finding in chronic inflammatory conditions, particularly asthma. Cilia provide a clue to the correct interpretation. **(B)** Goblet cell hyperplasia also occurs in response to mucosal injury and consists of aggregates of numerous goblet cells, which are seen here as cells distended by a mucin vacuole that pushes the nucleus to the periphery of the cell. Careful attention to the nuclear features allows distinction from adenocarcinoma. **(C)** Reserve cells, the basal most cells of the epithelium, proliferate in response to mucosal injury and function to regenerate the epithelium. These cells can show nuclear molding and can mimic small cell carcinoma. They tend to show less pleomorphism than small cell carcinoma and are often found in groups, sometimes with respiratory epithelial cells or metaplastic squamous cells. Necrosis and apoptotic debris are absent.

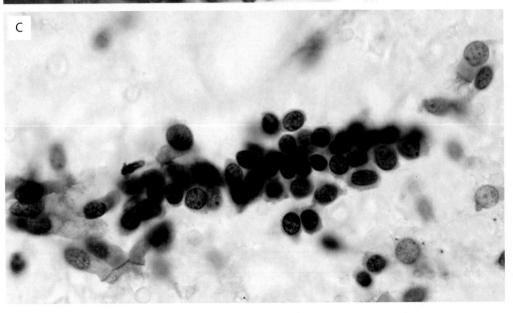

the nuclei in the cluster are normal and identical to the adjacent single bronchial epithelial cell nuclei. The presence of eosinophils and Charcot-Leyden crystals can also suggest a diagnosis of asthma. Numerous goblet cells may be seen in patients with chronic lung diseases, particularly chronic obstructive pulmonary disease and asthma. Goblet cell hyperplasia can also be mistaken for adenocarcinoma, particularly the bronchioloalveolar type, unless attention is paid to the bland nuclear features of the former. In response to an injury resulting in epithelial sloughing, reserve cell hyperplasia can be seen. It is the function of these reserve cells to regenerate the respiratory epithelium. Cells of reserve cell hyperplasia can mimic small cell carcinoma, and nuclear molding may be

seen. However, reserve cells have small condensed uniform nuclei, and the necrotic background and cellular discohesion of small cell carcinoma are absent. Squamous metaplasia, also a response to injury, can mimic squamous carcinoma, but usually demonstrates mild or minimal nuclear cytoatypia.

A variety of noncellular components are encountered with relative frequency in respiratory specimens. Some of these noncellular elements can serve as clues to an underlying disease process (amyloid, psammoma bodies, Charcot-Leyden crystals) (Figure 37-5). Others are important to recognize as contaminants to avoid overdiagnosis of malignancy (pollen, vegetable cells) (Figure 37-6).

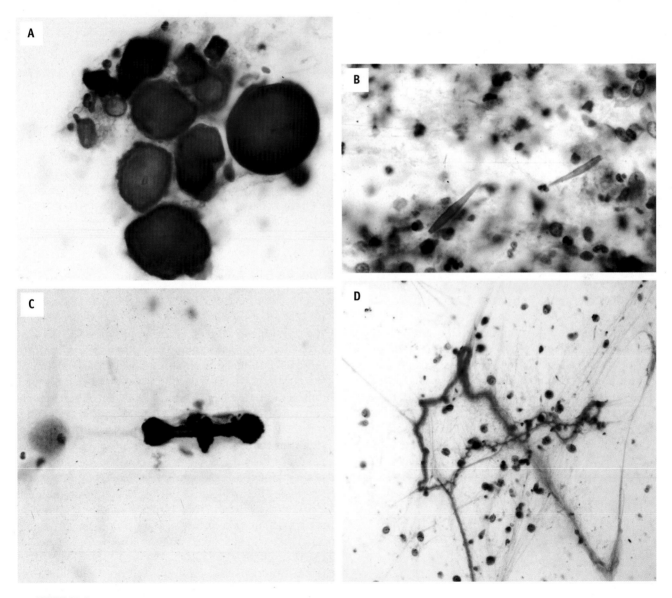

FIGURE 37-5

Noncellular elements

(A) Corpora amylacea appear as spherical acellular noncalcified concretions. **(B)** Charcot-Leyden crystals, seen in the setting of eosinophil degranulation, are sharp, angulated, needle-like crystals. **(C)** A ferruginous body is an asbestos fiber coated with iron salts. It appears as a brown rod-shaped structure with bulbous ends. **(D)** Curschmann spirals are coiled segments of inspissated mucus.

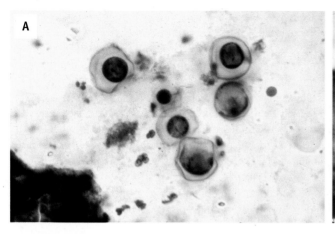
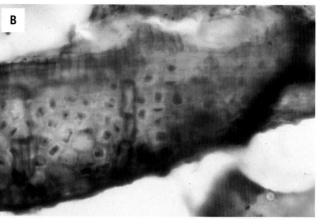

FIGURE 37-6
Vegetable cells
(A) Individual vegetable cells can be mistaken for cells of adenocarcinoma. The thickened cell border provides a clue. **(B)** An intact vegetable fragment is confirmatory.

NON-NEOPLASTIC LUNG DISEASES

INTERSTITIAL LUNG DISEASES

SARCOIDOSIS

The cytologic diagnosis of granulomatous inflammation in the lung and hilar or mediastinal lymph nodes is usually made by FNA. The diagnostic yield for combined transbronchial FNA of lung and lymph node reaches 80% to 90%, significantly higher than either of these procedures alone. The diagnosis of sarcoidosis requires both identification of non-necrotizing granulomatous inflammation and exclusion of an infectious etiology in a patient with an appropriate clinical history and radiologic findings. Granulomas of sarcoidosis are recognized as loose clusters of epithelioid histiocytes with elongate nuclei and fibrillar cytoplasm associated with variable numbers of small lymphocytes in a clean background (Figure 37-7). Multinucleated giant cells are characteristically present, and the identification of isolated multinucleated giant cells should prompt a search for granulomas elsewhere in the sample. A separate sample submitted for microbiologic culture is essential to exclude infectious etiologies for the granulomatous inflammation. Special stains to rule out acid fast bacilli and fungi may be performed on cell block material. A well-known diagnostic pit-fall is overdiagnosis of granulomatous inflammation as adenocarcinoma.

PULMONARY ALVEOLAR PROTEINOSIS

BAL is often the first diagnostic modality used in patients with pulmonary alveolar proteinosis. Grossly, BAL fluid from patients with pulmonary alveolar proteinosis is cloudy with granular debris. In stained preparations, this extracellular material usually predominates in the background of a paucicellular sample (Figure 37-8). Macrophages and scattered inflammatory cells are seen. The granular material represents surfactant and stains basophilic on Diff-Quik and Papanicolaou (Pap) stains, eosinophilic on hematoxylineosin stain, and is strongly periodic acid-Schiff (PAS)-positive. The cytologic differential diagnosis includes *Pneumocystis jiroveci* infection, amyloidosis, and organizing pneumonia. A fungal stain should be performed on all cases of suspected pulmonary alveolar proteinosis to exclude *Pneumocystis*. Other organism stains (Fite, Gram) may also be appropriate to evaluate for co-existing infections with *Nocardia* and other bacteria. Amyloid is a "waxy," smooth, and nongranular substance. It is usually only focally deposited and is rarely seen in BAL samples. Organizing pneumonia may show granular debris in the background, but

NONCELLULAR ELEMENTS IN RESPIRATORY CYTOLOGY SAMPLES
▸ Curschmann spirals
▸ Charcot-Leyden crystals
▸ Amyloid
▸ Ferruginous bodies
▸ Psammoma bodies
▸ Corpora amylacea
▸ Contaminants (pollen, food, etc.)

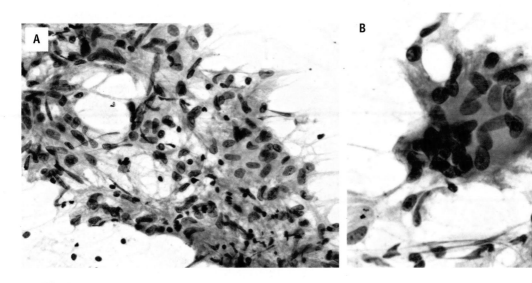

FIGURE 37-7

Sarcoidosis

(A) A granuloma appears as a loose aggregate of epithelioid histiocytes with fibrillar cytoplasm and interspersed small lymphocytes. Necrosis is absent, but microbiologic cultures are necessary to exclude infection. **(B)** Multinucleated giant cells are frequently seen in association with granulomas.

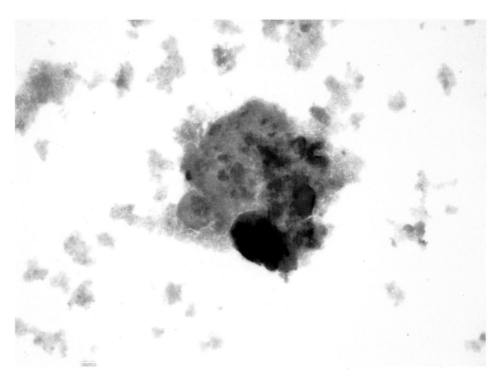

FIGURE 37-8

Pulmonary alveolar proteinosis
Granular material from bronchoalveolar lavage fluid in a patient with pulmonary alveolar proteinosis.

SARCOIDOSIS—CYTOLOGIC FEATURES

➧ Loose clusters of epithelioid histiocytes (granulomas)
➧ Multinucleated giant cells
➧ Lymphocytes
➧ Clean smear background
➧ Negative cultures and special stains

PULMONARY ALVEOLAR PROTEINOSIS—CYTOLOGIC FEATURES

➧ Paucicellular sample of mononuclear inflammatory cells
➧ Amorphous basophilic granular debris predominates
➧ Negative fungal stain

inflammatory cells (including neutrophils) usually predominate. The diagnosis of pulmonary alveolar proteinosis requires correlation with clinical and radiographic findings.

INFECTIONS

VIRAL INFECTIONS

Cytologic changes associated with viral infections include specific diagnostic inclusions, regenerative epithelial atypia, and ciliocytophthoria (Figure 37-9). Ciliocytophthoria refers to detachment of the ciliated portion of the columnar bronchial epithelial cell with resultant free-floating tufts of cilia in the background of the smear. Although not entirely specific, ciliocytophthoria is commonly associated with adenovirus infection. If specific viral inclusions are identified, a rapid diagnosis is possible (also discussed in chapter 13). Most viral infections are detected in BAL samples from immunocompromised hosts. Occasional cases are identified in FNA specimens.

Cytomegalovirus-infected cells appear enlarged, with maintenance of the nuclear-to-cytoplasmic ratio. There

is margination of nuclear chromatin with a large, central basophilic intranuclear inclusion surrounded by a pale halo. Granular, variably basophilic to eosinophilic cytoplasmic inclusions may also be seen. Cells infected with herpes simplex virus are enlarged and multinucleated. There is nuclear molding, margination of chromatin, and an intranuclear eosinophilic inclusion. Measles virus infection produces giant multinucleated cells with eosinophilic intranuclear and cytoplasmic inclusions. Similar giant cells may be seen in respiratory syncytial virus and parainfluenza infections.

FUNGAL INFECTIONS

Many fungal organisms are readily detectable in respiratory cytology samples. Some of these organisms are seen using conventional stains. Often, a specific morphologic

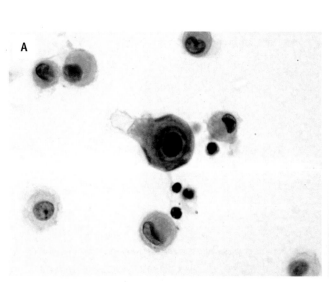

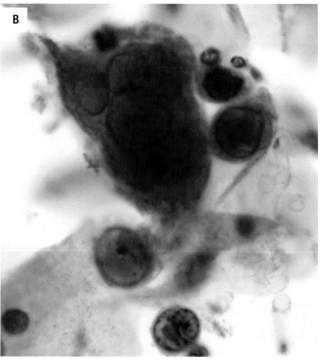

FIGURE 37-9

Viral infections

(A) Cytomegalovirus infection causes cellular enlargement with a large central basophilic intranuclear inclusion surrounded by a pale halo. Chromatin is marginated to the periphery of the nucleus. **(B)** Herpes simplex-infected cells show multinucleation with nuclear molding, margination of chromatin, and intranuclear inclusions.

diagnosis is possible. Diagnosis is generally more rapid than fungal culture.

CANDIDIASIS

Candida is normal flora of the oral cavity and the upper respiratory tract. *Candida* infection accounts for approximately 50% of opportunistic fungal infections. In severely immunocompromised patients, *Candida* infection presents with fever, cough, dyspnea, and lung infiltrates. Cytologic diagnosis requires an FNA specimen to exclude the possibility of a contaminant fungus (usually *C. albicans*). Morphologically, *Candida* species appear as budding yeasts with or without formation of pseudohyphae.

ASPERGILLOSIS

Aspergillus species cause a spectrum of pulmonary infections, including allergic bronchopulmonary, colonizing (fungus ball), and invasive forms. Manifestations of *Aspergillus* infection depend on immune status. *Aspergillus* organisms in cytology samples show septate hyphae with regular dichotomous branching at 45-degree angles (Figure 37-10). Birefringent calcium oxalate crystals may be seen. Fruiting heads can be seen with intracavitary growth. *Aspergillus fumigatus* is the most common organism identified. *Aspergillus niger* can be specifically identified if brown-black 3- to 5-μm conidia are present. Importantly, intracavitary *Aspergillus* (fungus ball) can be associated with marked cellular atypia of the lining cells

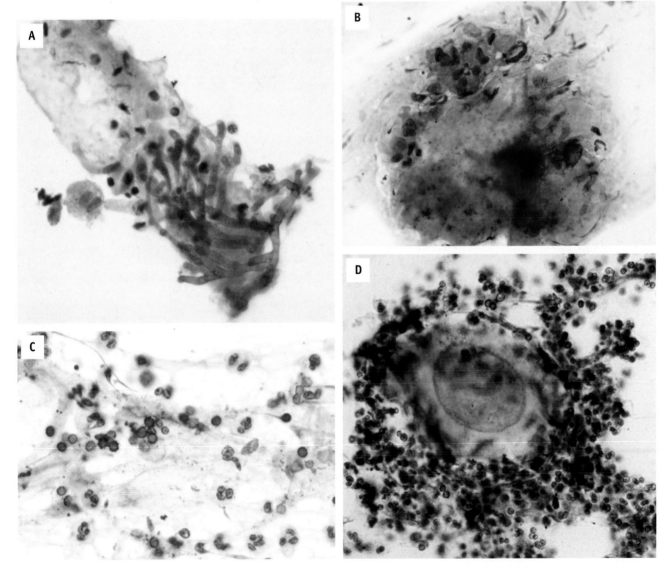

FIGURE 37-10

Aspergillus **infection**
(A) *Aspergillus* species show septate hyphae with regular, 45-degree dichotomous branching. These organisms are visible in routine cytologic stains. **(B)** *Aspergillus* commonly colonizes cavities in the lung. The squamous cells lining the cavity may show marked atypia. **(C)** Numerous brown black conidia are present in *Aspergillus niger* infection and allow specific identification. **(D)** Fruiting heads of *Aspergillus* may be seen in the setting of intracavitary growth.

of the cavity. Usually, this is squamous atypia, which may lead to an erroneous diagnosis of squamous cell carcinoma. Aspirates from squamous carcinomas should be highly cellular before a definitive diagnosis is made and should show at least a minor component of malignant cells that are not keratinizing. Caution should be exercised when making a diagnosis of squamous cell carcinoma when fungal elements are present in the background.

CRYPTOCOCCOSIS

Cryptococcus neoformans inhabits the soil and is found in bird droppings. It is a relatively common infection in immunocompromised hosts and can cause primary infection. In cytologic specimens, *Cryptococcus neoformans* appears as variably sized yeasts, measuring between 4 and 15 μm (Figure 37-11). Narrow-based budding is observed. These organisms have a mucin-rich capsule and a refractile center. They may be seen as pale yeasts on Pap stain but are difficult to detect. Silver stains highlight fungal organisms and mucin stains, such as mucicarmine, highlight the mucin-rich capsule.

PNEUMOCYSTIS JIROVECI

The taxonomy of *Pneumocystis* has been the subject of much debate, but this organism is currently classified as a fungus. It is a very common cause of pneumonia in immunocompromised hosts, causing bilateral pulmonary infiltrates, dry cough, fever and dyspnea. BAL has the highest diagnostic yield for this organism. On Pap-stained

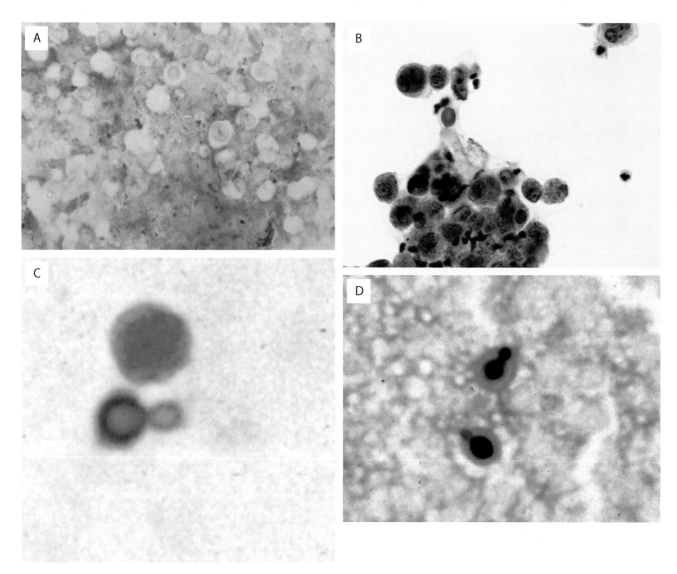

FIGURE 37-11

Cryptococcus neoformans
(A) *Cryptococcus neoformans* appears as variably-sized pale staining yeast forms in Diff-Quik-stained samples. The clear space around the yeast represents the capsule. (B) The yeast is also visible in Pap-stained preparations. (C) A mucicarmine stain highlights the mucin rich capsule surrounding the organisms. (D) A silver stain (GMS) highlights the organism and its narrow-based budding.

preparations, pale green-blue granular and vacuolated amorphous material is seen forming casts of alveolar spaces (Figure 37-12). Actual organisms are not seen using this stain and identification of alveolar casts should prompt special stains for fungus. On Gomori methenamine silver (GMS) stain, 6- to 8-μm cysts are seen. There is no budding. Trophozoites, with intracystic bodies, appear as blue dots on Giemsa stain.

DIMORPHIC FUNGI

The dimorphic fungal respiratory pathogens include *Blastomyces dermatitidis, Histoplasma capsulatum, Coccidioides immitis, Paracoccidioides brasiliensis* and *Sporothrix schenckii*. Respiratory infection is acquired by inhalation of dust or soil containing environmental conidia. These organisms grow as yeast forms in the body, and the yeast forms are observed in cytologic preparations (Figure 37-13) (see also chapter 12). Infection with these fungi is often associated with granulomatous inflammation, which is often suppurative.

Blastomyces dermatitidis is endemic in the regions surrounding the Great Lakes, adjacent the upper Mississippi River, and the Southeast. These yeast forms measure 6 to 15 μm in diameter and are round and thick walled. They exhibit broad-based budding.

Histoplasma capsulatum, which causes histoplasmosis, is the most common dimorphic fungal pathogen in the United States. This organism is found in moist soil, particularly when there is contamination with bird and bat droppings, and is endemic in the Ohio, Mississippi, and Missouri River valleys. The yeast form of *Histoplasma*

capsulatum measures 2 to 3 μm in diameter with a spherical or conical shape. Organisms are present within macrophages and may be surrounded by a clear halo. They are easily overlooked in routine preparations where they appear as pale blue-gray dots within macrophages. They are nicely highlighted with silver stains.

Coccidioides immitis lives in hot dry soil with an alkaline pH. It is endemic in the western and southwestern desert regions of the United States. *C. immitis* produces 10- to 60-μm diameter thick spherules. Endospores, measuring 2 to 4 μm mature within and populate the spherules. The capsule of the spherules eventually ruptures, causing release of endospores. Free endospores may be present in the background of the cytology sample, and may be confused with *Histoplasma capsulatum* or *Cryptococcus neoformans*. If this organism grows within a cavity, hyphae may be seen.

Paracoccidioides brasiliensis is the most common systemic fungal infection in Latin America. *P. brasiliensis* in cytologic samples shows 10- to 30-μm thick walled round yeast cells with multiple narrow-based daughter buds, giving this fungus its characteristic "mariner's wheel" appearance.

Sporothrix schenckii most commonly causes cutaneous and subcutaneous infection but is a rare cause of pulmonary disease in the immunocompromised. The yeast forms measure 2 to 4 μm, are oval to elliptical, and are present within macrophages, mimicking *Histoplasma capsulatum*. They may show a single bud. Larger cigar-shaped forms are also characteristically present and aid in identification.

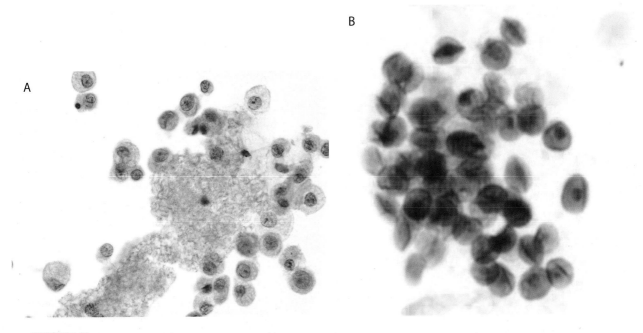

FIGURE 37-12

Pneumocystis jiroveci

(A) *Pneumocystis jiroveci* appears as frothy green-blue alveolar casts. **(B)** A silver stain (GMS) highlights the cysts of the organism with central depressions.

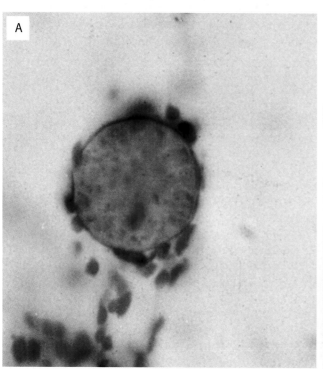

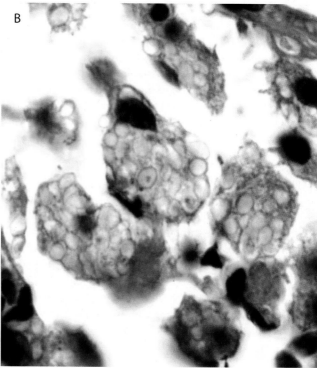

FIGURE 37-13

Dimorphic fungi

(A) Cysts of *Coccidioides immitis* containing numerous endospores are visible on routine cytologic stains. **(B)** Histiocytes containing *Histoplasma capsulatum* organisms. The organisms appear as blue dots in the cytoplasm of histiocytes.

PARASITIC INFECTIONS

STRONGYLOIDES STERCORALIS

Strongyloides stercoralis pulmonary involvement is seen in patients receiving high-dose steroids. The filariform larvae migrate through the intestinal wall of infected individuals into the bloodstream, ultimately penetrating alveolar spaces. A hemorrhagic pneumonia is the result of this migration. Larvae measure 400 to 500 μm in length and characteristically have a closed short gullet and a notched tail. This parasite may be grossly observed in bloody sputum.

BENIGN MASSES AND TUMORS

PULMONARY HAMARTOMA

Pulmonary hamartomas are the most common benign lung tumor. These tumors are typically well circumscribed round to oval radiographically stable masses located in the periphery of the lung. If diagnosis by FNA is achieved, hamartomas are usually left alone and thoracotomy avoided. Most of these tumors are noncalcified, but if calcification is present, it appears "popcorn-like" and is virtually diagnostic. Fatty densities may be seen within hamartomas on CT, and are also highly suggestive of the diagnosis.

Pulmonary hamartomas yield variably cellular aspirate samples consisting of benign mesenchymal and epithelial components (Figure 37-14). The mesenchymal component usually consists of myxoid, chondroid, or mature cartilage elements. Fat and smooth muscle may also be seen. Cytologically bland stellate and spindled mesenchymal cells are frequently embedded in chondromyxoid or fibromyxoid matrix. These mesenchymal cells are positive for S-100 protein, which may be useful in diagnosis. The epithelial cell component usually consists of benign cuboidal to low columnar glandular cells arranged in clusters and flat honeycomb sheets. The cytologic differential diagnosis includes chest wall elements, particularly in a paucicellular sample. Occasionally, the epithelial component is misinterpreted as malignancy if the background matrix material is overlooked.

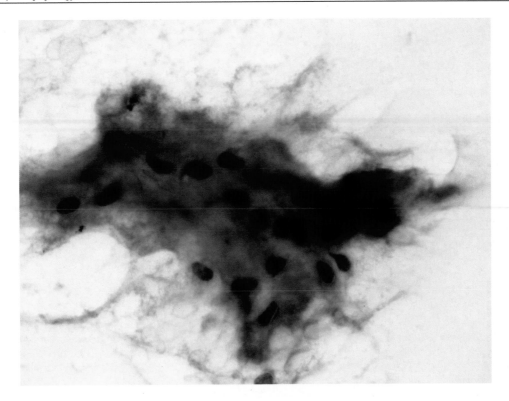

FIGURE 37-14

Pulmonary hamartoma

Cytologically bland spindled and stellate cells embedded in chondromyxoid matrix are frequently seen in fine needle aspiration specimens from pulmonary hamartoma. Mature cartilage, smooth muscle, and fat may be seen. A benign cuboidal epithelial cell component is common.

PULMONARY HAMARTOMA—CYTOLOGIC FEATURES

- ‣ Variably cellular aspirate
- ‣ Myxoid, chondroid matrix, or cartilage
- ‣ Bland spindled cells embedded in matrix
- ‣ Benign cuboidal glandular epithelium

AMYLOID TUMOR

Amyloid deposition in the lung is rare and occurs as part of systemic amyloidosis or as a process localized to the lung. Amyloid tumor is a form of localized amyloidosis of the lung, usually forming a parenchymal nodule, that is occasionally diagnosed by FNA. In aspirate samples, amyloid is an acellular material scattered in the background of the smears. It appears dense, smooth, and blue-green in Pap-stained preparations and has a scalloped border (Figure 37-15). The aspirate smears from amyloid tumor are generally of low cellularity and consist mostly of mononuclear inflammatory cells and occasional multinucleated giant cells. Smears and cell block material may be stained with Congo red to confirm the diagnosis. A careful search for associated tumor cells is warranted to exclude an amyloid-producing tumor.

INFLAMMATORY MYOFIBROBLASTIC TUMOR

Inflammatory myofibroblastic tumors usually present as solitary, well-circumscribed round to oval masses in the periphery of the lung. Most patients are under age 30 years. Aspirates from inflammatory myofibroblastic tumors are variably cellular and consist of spindled fibroblasts scattered singly and in small aggregates. A polymorphous inflammatory infiltrate accompanies the fibroblasts, consisting of lymphocytes, eosinophils, plasma cells, and histiocytes. Myxoid or fibrous background stromal fragments may be seen. The diagnostic specificity of this lesion on FNA is low, but the diagnosis may be suggested in the appropriate clinical setting.

MALIGNANT TUMORS

SQUAMOUS CELL CARCINOMA

Central necrosis with cavitation is common in squamous cell carcinomas of the lung. Because of this, cytologic sampling of squamous carcinomas typically produces large

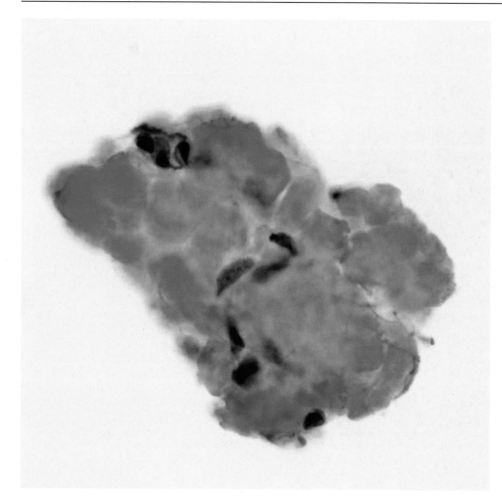

FIGURE 37-15
Amyloid tumor
Amyloid appears as waxy, smooth, acellular deposits with scalloped borders. A Congo red stain is confirmatory.

AMYLOID TUMOR—CYTOLOGIC FEATURES

‣ Paucicellular smears
‣ Dense waxy blue-green amyloid deposits
‣ Inflammatory cells and giant cells in background
‣ Congo red confirmatory

INFLAMMATORY MYOFIBROBLASTIC TUMOR—CYTOLOGIC FEATURES

‣ Spindled fibroblasts scattered singly and in small aggregates
‣ Open chromatin, inconspicuous nucleoli
‣ Polymorphous inflammatory infiltrate in background—eosinophils, plasma cells, and lymphocytes
‣ May see myxoid or fibrous stromal fragments

tissue fragments in an acutely inflamed and necrotic background. Squamous cell carcinomas show a spectrum of differentiation in cytologic preparations (Figure 37-16). There is evidence of cytoplasmic keratinization in better differentiated tumors. Keratinizing malignant cells have abnormal cytoplasmic morphology, including caudate, spindled, and tadpole forms. Anucleate keratinized cells are common. Chromatin is hyperchromatic and dense, and nucleoli are usually absent. Single malignant keratinizing cells are common, with dense orange cytoplasm in Pap-stained preparations. Nonkeratinizing malignant squamous cells have dense green-blue cytoplasm. Nuclear chromatin is dark and coarse, but nucleoli may be seen. In smaller tumor cell groups, sharp cytoplasmic borders may be observed. Malignant cells with a spindled morphology may be seen and occasionally predominate.

The differential diagnosis of squamous cell carcinoma in cytologic specimens includes atypical squamous metaplasia, small cell carcinoma, and metastases. The squamous metaplasia that occurs lining a fungal cavity may be quite atypical. To complicate matters, fungal organisms, particularly *Aspergillus*, may colonize

A

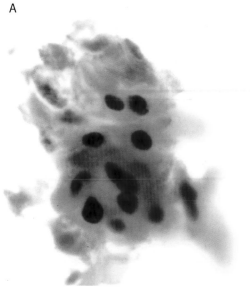

B

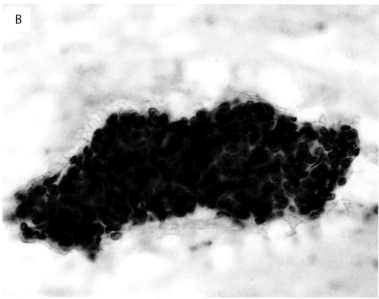

FIGURE 37-16

Squamous cell carcinoma

(A) Keratinizing squamous cell carcinoma is characterized by cells with dense orangeophilic cytoplasm and smudged, hyperchromatic nuclei without prominent nucleoli. An abnormal cytoplasmic morphology is common. (B) Squamous cell carcinomas often yield large cohesive tissue fragments in cytology specimens. Nuclear chromatin is dark and coarse. The cytoplasm is nonkeratinizing. (C) Squamous cell carcinomas may have a spindled morphology. Necrosis is commonly seen in the background.

C

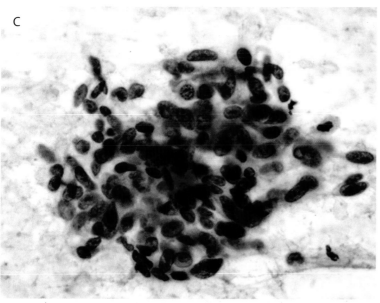

SQUAMOUS CELL CARCINOMA—CYTOLOGIC FEATURES

» Spectrum of differentiation; evidence of keratinization in better differentiated tumors
» Enlarged hyperchromatic nuclei
» Nucleoli less frequent than in other cancers
» Cells maintain dense cytoplasm, sharp borders
» Tissue fragments form monolayer sheets
» Necrotic inflamed background is common

---

the cavities formed by tumor. Care should be taken to exclude the possibility of atypical squamous metaplasia in the presence of fungus before a diagnosis of squamous carcinoma is made. A definitive diagnosis of malignancy is rarely warranted in this setting. Small cell carcinoma may be difficult to distinguish from poorly differentiated nonkeratinizing squamous carcinoma, and immunohistochemical staining to assist in resolving this differential diagnosis is discussed in chapter 38.

ADENOCARCINOMA

Adenocarcinomas typically yield tumor cells arranged in small three-dimensional clusters, acini, and singly. The tumor cell nuclei are enlarged and often eccentric, with prominent nuclear membrane irregularities. Columnar tumor cells or signet ring cells may be seen. Central macronucleoli are characteristic. The cytoplasm of tumor cells ranges from homogeneous to extreme vacuolation.

Bronchioloalveolar carcinoma (BAC) is a distinct subtype of pulmonary adenocarcinoma (Figure 37-17) that accounts for 1% to 5% of all lung carcinomas. The incidence of BAC is increasing. Histologically, there is preservation of lung architecture with tumor growth along alveolar septa (lepidic growth). Mucinous and nonmucinous variants are recognized. Most patients with BAC present with an asymptomatic solitary pe-

ripheral lung mass, but this tumor can also present as a region of consolidation resembling pneumonia. Invasive pulmonary adenocarcinomas may have areas with BAC-pattern growth.

Bronchioloalveolar carcinoma is characterized by cells in three-dimensional clusters with an extreme depth of focus, or in flat but crowded sheets (Figure 37-18). Papillary groups of tumor cells lacking fibrovascular cores may be seen. Nuclei are round to oval and relatively uniform, though nuclear folds, grooves, and other membrane irregularities may be found. Nuclear chromatin is fine and nucleoli are generally prominent. Intranuclear pseudoinclusions are frequently seen. Psammoma bodies are infrequently identified. BAC may yield deceptively bland tumor cells in cytologic preparations, leading to false negative diagnoses. The tumor cells of BAC may be misinterpreted as reactive pneumocytes, particularly in paucicellular specimens. BAC is most reliably diagnosed in highly cellular FNA samples. It is important to know the cytologic features of BAC in order that this deceptively bland malignancy is not overlooked. Also importantly, definitive distinction between pure BAC and invasive adenocarcinoma with a BAC component is not possible in cytologic samples.

SMALL CELL CARCINOMA

Cytologic samples of small cell carcinoma are more frequently diagnostic for small cell carcinoma than tissue biopsy (Figure 37-19). These tumors yield highly cellular specimens with cells arranged in small loose clusters and singly in a necrotic background with abundant karyorrhectic debris. Nuclear molding and numerous mitoses are characteristic. Individual tumor cells have scant cytoplasm, granular chromatin, and inconspicuous nucleoli. Tumor cells are approximately 1.5 times larger than a small lymphocyte. Differential diagnostic considerations include non-small cell carcinoma, non-Hodgkin lymphoma (NHL), and carcinoid tumor.

The distinction of small cell carcinoma from non-small cell carcinoma is clinically quite significant as therapy and prognosis differ greatly. Recognition of the

---

ADENOCARCINOMA—CYTOLOGIC FEATURES

» Relatively cohesive with cells arranged in three-dimensional clusters and acini
» Enlarged eccentric nuclei with nuclear membrane irregularities
» Central macronucleoli are characteristic
» Cytoplasm homogeneous to extreme vacuolation

BRONCHIOLOALVEOLAR ADENOCARCINOMA—CYTOLOGIC FEATURES

» Flat sheets, three-dimensional clusters or papillary groups
» Round to oval nuclei of uniform size
» Fine chromatin, small nucleoli
» Nuclear membrane folds and grooves
» Intranuclear pseudoinclusions
» Psammoma bodies are rare

A

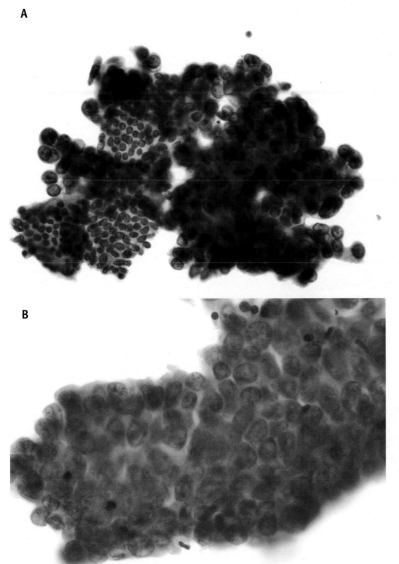

B

FIGURE 37-17

Pulmonary adenocarcinoma

(A) Adenocarcinoma appears as disorganized cohesive clusters of tumor cells. There is marked contrast with the normal epithelium in this field. Nuclear membrane irregularities and cytoplasmic vacuoles are seen. **(B)** The cells of adenocarcinoma often maintain nuclear polarity and have a columnar architecture. **(C)** High magnification demonstrates nuclear membrane irregularities, intranuclear inclusions and loose vacuolated cytoplasm.

C

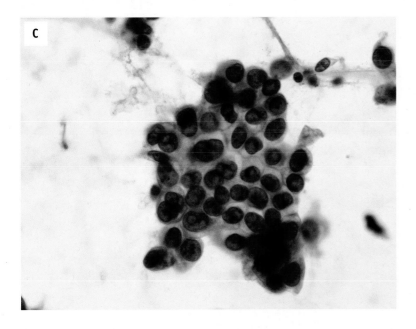

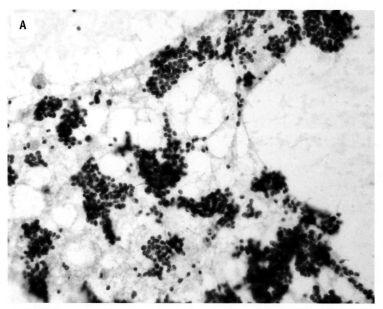

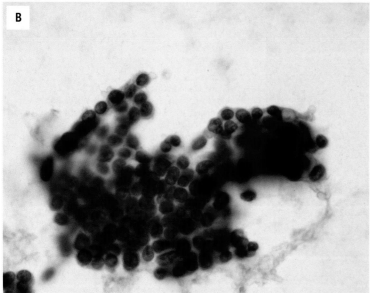

FIGURE 37-18

Bronchioloalveolar carcinoma
(A) At low magnification, this fine needle aspiration from a bronchioloalveolar carcinoma appears highly cellular with cells arranged in sheets and large clusters. The nuclei appear relatively uniform with minimal atypia. **(B)** At higher magnification, architectural disorder may be seen. There is mild nuclear pleomorphism, with several cells in this group showing nuclear membrane irregularities. A mucin vacuole is present in the cytoplasm of one tumor cell **(C)** Elsewhere in this sample, the tumor cells are arranged in sheets and display powdery chromatin, minimal nuclear atypia and inconspicuous nucleoli.

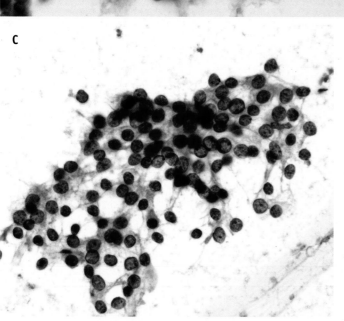

SMALL CELL CARCINOMA—CYTOLOGIC FEATURES

» Cells with scant cytoplasm in loose clusters and singly
» Nuclear molding and high mitotic rate
» Finely granular nuclear chromatin (salt and pepper)
» Inconspicuous nucleoli
» Background necrosis and karyorrhectic debris

small cell component of a mixed tumor is important in determining therapy. Most of the time, diagnosing small cell carcinoma is straightforward. In some cases, when tumor cells are better preserved, cells of small cell carcinoma may appear to have moderate amounts of cytoplasm. Pseudo-glandular formations may be seen in these areas. The characteristic nuclear features should lead to the correct diagnosis in these cases. Also, tumor

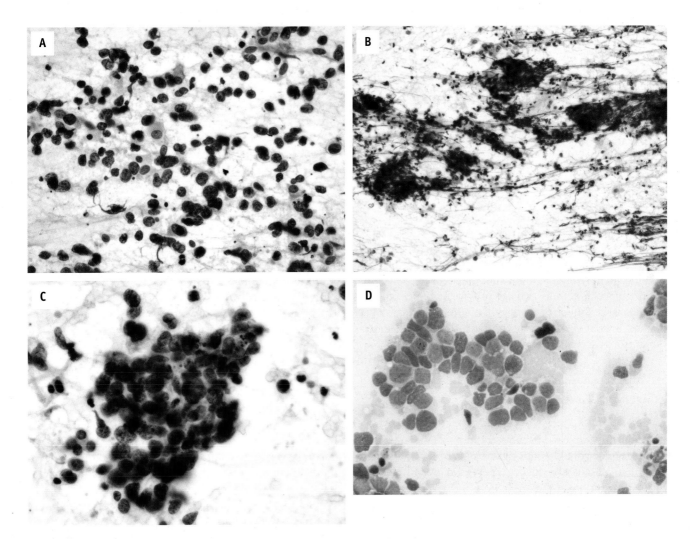

FIGURE 37-19

Small cell carcinoma

(A) Small cell carcinoma yields a highly cellular, discohesive tumor cell population. Occasional small aggregates of tumor cells are seen with nuclear molding within the groups. Apoptotic debris is present in the background. Individual tumor cells have minimal cytoplasm and stippled chromatin. Nucleoli are not seen. **(B)** At low magnification, nuclear material may show "streaming" against a background of necrosis. This finding is suggestive of small cell carcinoma and should prompt a search for diagnostic tumor cells. **(C)** Higher magnification of an aggregate of small cell carcinoma shows coarse stippled chromatin, inconspicuous nucleoli and nuclear molding. Apoptotic debris is present within the group. **(D)** On Diff-Quik stain, the cells of small cell carcinoma appear larger and some have appreciable cytoplasm. Nuclear molding is evident.

cells with increased cytoplasmic volume are usually a focal finding. Small cell carcinomas may have cytoplasmic globules, so-called paranuclear blue bodies, that may be misinterpreted as intracellular mucin. These are a characteristic feature of small cell carcinoma.

Differentiating small cell carcinoma from low-grade non-Hodgkin lymphoma can be quite difficult. There are important morphologic features that allow this distinction in the majority of cases. Ancillary studies including flow cytometry and immunohistochemistry may be helpful in difficult cases. Aspirates from both small cell carcinoma and NHL with a predominance of small cells yield highly cellular aspirates. The background of the smears is important. In small cell carcinoma, the background is characteristically necrotic with numerous apoptotic bodies/nuclear fragments. Lymphoglandular bodies are not seen. The smear background from an aspirate of a low-grade lymphoma usually shows prominent lymphoglandular bodies and an absence of necrosis. The pattern of cell arrangement is also important to evaluate at low magnification. Cells of small cell carcinoma tend to cluster. While a cellular aspirate of NHL may show occasional cell clusters, these are relatively infrequent. At intermediate and high magnification, nuclear molding is characteristically seen in small cell carcinoma and not seen in NHL. Also, small cell carcinoma cells may have a spindled morphology focally, also not a feature of NHL. Mitotic figures may be seen in small cell carcinoma and are usually not seen in NHL. If, from cytologic features, one cannot be certain of the cell lineage, simple immunophenotyping can be performed and will show a lack of expression of CD45 and other lymphoid markers such as CD2 and CD3 (T-cells) or CD19 and CD20 (B-cells) in small cell carcinomas. CD56, a common marker of NK-cell lineage in lymphoid malignancy, may be expressed in neuroendocrine tumors and can provide evidence of neuroendocrine differentiation when other hematologic makers are lacking. Differentiation of small cell carcinoma from carcinoid tumor is discussed below.

CARCINOID TUMOR

Cytologically, typical carcinoid tumors usually yield cellular samples consisting of tumor cells occurring singly and in small clusters (Figure 37-20). Stripped nuclei in the background are common. The individual cells are small and round to spindled. The nuclei have stippled, granular chromatin and inconspicuous nucleoli. The cells have scant to moderate amounts of cytoplasm. In many cases, the carcinoid tumor cells have a plasmacytoid appearance. Importantly, necrosis is absent. A streaming pattern of blood vessels with attached tumor cells may be present. Atypical carcinoid tumors show a greater degree of cellular pleomorphism, but overall cells are similar in appearance to those of a typical car-

cinoid tumor. However, the chromatin of atypical carcinoids is more uneven and coarsely granular than its typical counterparts. Nucleoli may be seen. Necrosis, mitotic figures and nuclear molding can also be seen in atypical carcinoid.

Carcinoid tumors may be misclassified as small cell carcinoma, particularly when a spindled morphology predominates. Importantly, carcinoid tumors usually lack necrosis and mitoses in cytology specimens, features almost invariably present in small cell carcinoma.

PULMONARY SARCOMA

Primary pulmonary sarcomas are rare. Most malignant spindle cell tumors in the lung are proven to be sarcomatoid carcinomas with immunohistochemical staining for cytokeratin. Furthermore, metastatic sarcomas involving lung are far more common than primary pulmonary sarcomas. Usually, recognizing a sarcoma as a malignant spindle cell lesion in a cytologic preparation is straightforward. Specifically classifying the neoplasm may be problematic. Virtually all types of sarcoma may be primary in the lung, and cytologic samples may have a variety of appearances depending on cell of origin. Most sarcomas yield cellular samples of discohesive malignant spindle cells with hyperchromatic irregular nuclei. A fascicular or sheet-like arrangement of cells is possible. Occasionally, osteoid, chondroid, or other matrix may be identified to aid in specific diagnosis. A cytology cell block should be attempted in cases of possible sarcoma to facilitate immunohistochemical staining. A careful review of a patient's clinical history is warranted to exclude the possibility of a sarcoma metastatic to lung. Importantly, malignant melanoma should also be considered whenever a malignant spindle cell neoplasm of the lung is encountered.

PULMONARY LYMPHOMA

Secondary involvement of the lung by lymphoma is quite common. In contrast, primary pulmonary lymphoma is relatively infrequent. The most common lymphoma to involve the lung is marginal zone lymphoma of MALT type, followed by diffuse large B-cell lymphoma. Primary pulmonary Hodgkin lymphoma is extremely rare, although secondary involvement of the lung in this disease is common.

MALT lymphomas, in general, are among the most difficult to diagnose definitively in cytologic samples. These lymphomas characteristically yield a polymorphous lymphoid sample dominated by small lymphoid

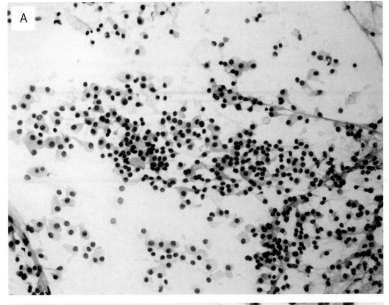

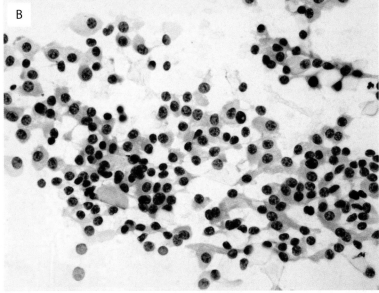

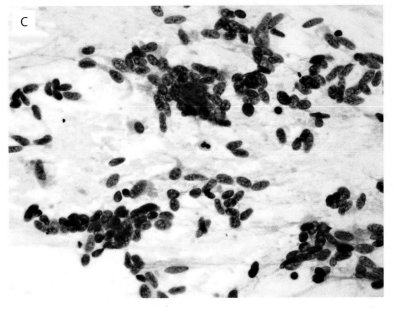

FIGURE 37-20

Carcinoid tumor

(A) An FNA from a typical carcinoid shows a highly cellular sample of plasmacytoid cells with moderate amounts of cytoplasm, arranged in loose clusters. A streaming pattern of blood vessels with attached tumor cells is seen. The background of the smear is clean. **(B)** At high magnification, the nuclei have stippled granular chromatin with inconspicuous nucleoli. No nuclear molding is seen. Occasional stripped nuclei are visible in this field. **(C)** Carcinoid tumors may have a spindled morphology. Numerous stripped nuclei are present. The cells are relatively bland and uniform. Necrosis is absent.

TYPICAL CARCINOID—CYTOLOGIC FEATURES

→ Cells occur singly and in clusters
→ Stripped nuclei common
→ Small plasmacytoid cells and/or spindled cells
→ Scant to moderate cytoplasm
→ Stippled granular chromatin
→ Inconspicuous nucleoli
→ Necrosis absent

ATYPICAL CARCINOID—CYTOLOGIC FEATURES

→ Greater cellular pleomorphism but overall cells similar to carcinoid
→ Nuclear molding and mitoses may be seen
→ More uneven coarsely granular chromatin
→ Small to prominent nucleoli
→ May see necrosis in background

cells (Figure 37-21). The small lymphocytes have variable amounts of cytoplasm. Plasmacytoid lymphocytes are common, and occasional transformed cells may be seen. Germinal center fragments may be seen. Based on this cellular polymorphism, MALT lymphomas are commonly misclassified as benign reactive lymphoid

proliferations. This can be avoided if material for flow cytometric immunophenotyping or for cell block preparation is prospectively collected.

Diffuse large B-cell lymphomas tend to be more diagnostically straightforward. These lymphomas yield highly cellular samples composed of sheets of large malignant lymphocytes (Figure 37-22). Lymphoglandular bodies are present in the background of the sample and offer a clue to the lymphoid origin of the malignant cells. Flow cytometry or immunohistochemistry is helpful to confirm the diagnosis and to exclude other large cell lung malignancies.

Cytologic diagnosis of Hodgkin lymphoma relies on the identification of Reed-Sternberg (RS) cells and RS variants in a benign inflammatory background. The first clue to the presence of RS cells or RS variants is the presence of scattered large cells that stand out because of their size on a low magnification scan of a reactive lymphoid or mixed inflammatory smear. Large stripped nuclei may also be seen. Granulomas may also be appreciated at low magnification. Classic RS cells have large, bilobed nuclei. Each nucleus has a large prominent inclusion-like nucleolus, which may approximate the size of a red blood cell. The mononuclear RS variants may be slightly smaller cells usually about 3 to 4 times the size of a small lymphocyte. Nuclei may be polylobated, and nucleoli are variable.

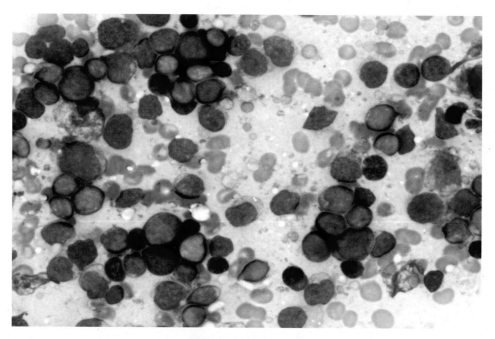

FIGURE 37-21

MALT lymphoma

Extranodal marginal zone lymphomas of MALT type yield a polymorphous population of lymphocytes. Plasma cells and transformed lymphocytes are commonly seen. Germinal center fragments are also frequently noted. This lymphoma is difficult to diagnose cytologically. Ancillary testing is required.

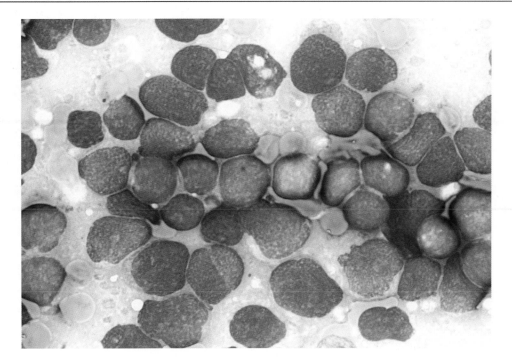

FIGURE 37-22

Diffuse large B-cell lymphoma

A monotonous population of large malignant lymphocytes characterizes diffuse large B-cell lymphoma. The cell population is discohesive. Nucleoli are prominent. Lymphoglandular bodies are scattered throughout the background of the smear, providing a clue to the lymphoid origin of the cells.

TUMORS METASTATIC TO THE LUNG

The lung is the most frequent site of metastasis for extrathoracic tumors. The most common adenocarcinomas metastatic to lung include renal cell carcinoma (Figure 37-23), breast carcinoma, prostate carcinoma, and colorectal adenocarcinoma (Figure 37-24). Melanoma, sarcoma, and germ cell tumors also commonly involve the lung. The most important factor in accurately diagnosing pulmonary metastasis is knowledge of the patient's clinical history. Review of prior material before diagnosing metastasis is essential.

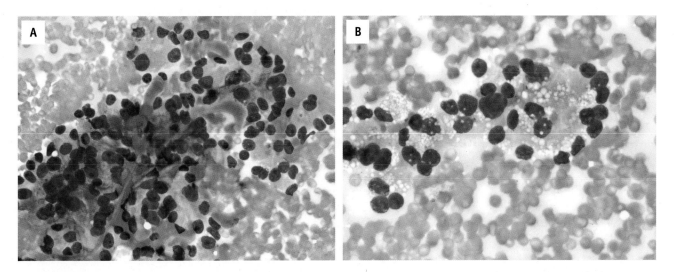

FIGURE 37-23

Metastatic renal cell carcinoma

(A) Metastatic renal cell carcinoma yields aggregates of round to polygonal tumor cells with a network of capillaries. On Diff-Quik stain, eosinophilic basement membrane material is prominent. **(B)** Cells with multiple variably sized cytoplasmic vacuoles are characteristic.

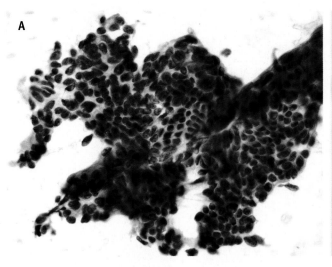

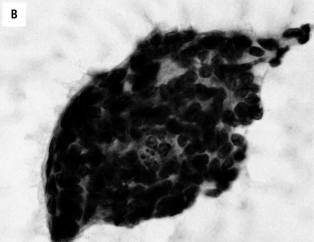

FIGURE 37-24

Metastatic colorectal adenocarcinoma
(A) Metastatic colorectal adenocarcinoma is composed of columnar tumor cells with nuclear stratification and pleomorphism. Nuclear polarity is maintained.
(B) Apoptotic debris (dirty necrosis) is visible within tumor cell groups.

SUGGESTED READINGS

Techniques, Applications, and Normal Cellular and Noncellular Elements

1. Bai TR, Knight DA. Structural changes in the airways in asthma: observations and consequences. *Clin Sci (Lond)*. 2005;108:463-77.
2. Cibas ES, Ducatman BS, eds. *Cytology: Diagnostic Principles and Clinical Correlates*. 2nd ed. Edinburgh, Scotland: Saunders; 2003.
3. Ehya H, Young NA. Cytologic approach to tumors of the tracheobronchial tree. *Chest Surg Clin N Am*. 2003;13:41-62.
4. Jeffrey PK. Remodeling in asthma and chronic obstructive lung disease. *Am J Respir Crit Care Med*. 2001;164:S28-38.
5. Rossi ED, Mule A, Maggiore C, et al. Cytologic diagnosis of pulmonary lesions. *Rays*. 2004;29:357-61.
6. Schreiber G, McCrory DC. Performance characteristics of different modalities for diagnosis of suspected lung cancer: summary of published evidence. *Chest*. 2003;123:115S-27S.
7. Yung RCW. Tissue diagnosis of suspected lung cancer: selecting between bronchoscopy, transthoracic needle aspiration and resectional biopsy. *Resp Care Clin*. 2003;9:51-76.

Interstitial Lung Diseases

8. Annema JT, Veseliç M, Rabe KF. Endoscopic ultrasound-guided fine needle aspiration for the diagnosis of sarcoidosis. *Eur Respir J*. 2005;25:405-9.
9. Gal AA, Koss MN. The pathology of sarcoidosis. *Curr Opin Pulm Med*. 2002;8:445-51.
10. Sosolik RC, Gammon RR, Julius CJ, Ayers LW. Pulmonary alveolar proteinosis: a report of two cases with diagnostic features in bronchoalveolar lavage specimens. *Acta Cytol*. 1998;42:377-83.

Infections

11. DiTomasso JP, Ampel NM, Sobonya RE, Bloom JW. Bronchoscopic diagnosis of pulmonary coccidiomycosis. Comparison of cytology, culture and transbronchial biopsy. *Diagn Microbiol Infect Dis*. 1994;18:83-7.
12. Hartmann B, Koss M, Hui A, Baumann W, Athos L, Boylen T. *Pneumocystis carinii* pneumonia in the acquired immunodeficiency syndrome (AIDS): diagnosis with bronchial brushings, biopsy and bronchoalveolar lavage. *Chest*. 1985;87:603-7.
13. Raag SS, Silverman JF, Zimmerman KG. Fine-needle aspiration biopsy of pulmonary coccidiomycosis: spectrum of cytologic findings in 73 patients. *Am J Clin Pathol*. 1993;99:582-7.

14. Silverman JF, Marrow HG. Fine needle aspiration cytology of granulomatous diseases of the lung including nontuberculous *Mycobacterium* infection. *Acta Cytol*. 1984;29:535-9.

Benign Pulmonary Masses

15. Dunbar F, Leiman G. The aspiration cytology of pulmonary hamartomas. *Diagn Cytopathol*. 1989;5:174-80.
16. Hummel P, Cangiarella JF, Cohen JM, Yang G, Waisman J, Chhieng DC. Transthoracic fine-needle aspiration biopsy of pulmonary spindle cell and mesenchymal lesions: a study of 61 cases. *Cancer*. 2001;93:187-98.
17. Machicao CN, Sorensen K, Abdul-Karim FW, Somrak TM. Transthoracic needle aspiration biopsy in inflammatory pseudotumors of the lung. *Diagn Cytopathol*. 1988;5:400-3.
18. Tomashefski JF, Cramer SF, Abramowsky C, Cohen AM, Horak G. Needle biopsy diagnosis of solitary amyloid nodule of the lung. *Acta Cytol*. 1980;24:224-7.
19. Wiatrowska BA, Yazdi HM, Matzinger FRK, MacDonald LL. Fine needle aspiration biopsy of pulmonary hamartomas. Radiologic, cytologic and immunocytochemical study of 15 cases. *Acta Cytol*. 1995;39:1167-74.

Malignant Lung Neoplasms

20. Cibas ES, Ducatman BS, eds. *Cytology: Diagnostic Principles and Clinical Correlates*. 2nd ed. Edinburgh, Scotland: Saunders; 2003.
21. Chilosi M, Zinzani PL, Poletti V. Lymphoproliferative lung disorders. *Semin Respir Crit Care Med*. 2005;26:490-501.
22. Hummel P, Cangiarella JF, Cohen JM, Yang G, Waisman J, Chhieng DC. Transthoracic fine-needle aspiration biopsy of pulmonary spindle cell and mesenchymal lesions: a study of 61 cases. *Cancer*. 2001;93:187-198.
23. MacDonald LL, Yazdi, HM. Fine-needle aspiration biopsy of bronchioloalveolar carcinoma. *Cancer*. 2001;93:29-34.
24. Michael CW, Richardson PH, Boudreaux CW. Pulmonary lymphoma of the mucosa-associated lymphoid tissue type: report of a case with cytological, histological, immunophenotypical correlation and review of the literature. *Ann Diagn Pathol*. 2005;9:148-52.
25. Nicholson SA, Ryan MR. A review of the cytologic findings in neuroendocrine carcinomas including carcinoid tumors with histologic correlation. *Cancer*. 2000;90:148-61.
26. Renshaw AA, Haja J, Lozano RL, Wilbur DC. Distinguishing carcinoid tumor from small cell carcinoma of the lung: correlating cytologic features and performance in the College of American Pathologists non-gynecologic cytology program. *Arch Pathol Lab Med*. 2005;129:614-8.

27. Renshaw AA, Voytek TM, Haja J, Wilbur DC. Distinguishing small cell car-
    cinoma from non-small cell carcinoma of the lung: correlating cytologic
    features and performance in the College of American Pathologists non-
    gynecologic cytology program. *Arch Pathol Lab Med.* 2005;129:619-23.
28. Saleh HA, Haapaniemi J, Khatib G, Sakr W. Bronchioloalveolar carci-
    noma: diagnostic pitfalls and immunocytochemical contribution. *Diagn
    Cytopathol.* 1998;18:301-6.
29. Sturgis CD, Nassar DL, D'Antonio JA, Raab SS. Cytologic features useful
    for distinguishing small cell from non-small cell carcinoma in bronchial
    brush and wash specimens. *Am J Clin Pathol.* 2000;114:197-202.
30. Szyfelbein WM, Ross JS. Carcinoids, atypical carcinoids and small-cell
    carcinomas of the lung: differential diagnosis of fine-needle aspiration
    biopsy specimens. *Diagn Cytopathol.* 1987;4:1-8.

38

Techniques and Applications to the Diagnosis of Lung Diseases: Immunohistochemistry

Dongfeng Tan • Dani S. Zander

INTRODUCTION

Immunohistochemistry (IHC) is a specialized technique for localizing expression of a variety of different substances, primarily proteins, by light microscopy. It is based on the creation of specific antigen-antibody reactions in tissues. Although IHC was developed in the early 1940s, the method has only found general application in surgical pathology since the late 1980s, when the technique became applicable to routinely formalin-fixed and paraffin-embedded sections. In the following years, technical advances in IHC have created sensitive detection systems, from the simplest one-step direct conjugate method to multiple-step detection techniques such as the avidin-biotin conjugate, peroxidase antiperoxidase, and biotin-streptavidin techniques, as well as the highly sensitive polymer-based labeling methods. Hybridoma technology has facilitated the manufacture of abundant, specific monoclonal antibodies. In addition, antigen retrieval methodologies have simplified pretreatment procedures, increased the in-

tensity of IHC staining, and provided a higher degree of reproducibility than traditional enzyme digestion methods.

Although the details of these techniques are beyond the scope of our discussion, one should be familiar with all steps in the "total IHC test" in order to detect, reduce, and correct deficiencies in IHC. Equally important, in order to achieve a successful result, one should be familiar with the antigen under investigation before performing IHC staining, particularly its subcellular localization, expected staining pattern, and sources of false-positive and false-negative staining. In recent years, the trend has been to move towards a panel approach to IHC evaluation. By using a roster of antibodies that includes antibodies expected to be positive and others to be negative for the specific differential diagnoses under consideration, the likelihood of error due to an aberrant result is reduced. This approach has enjoyed particular success in the evaluation of pleural neoplasms, as is discussed later in this chapter.

APPLICATIONS OF IMMUNOHISTOCHEMISTRY TO EVALUATION OF NON-NEOPLASTIC LUNG DISEASES

Applications of IHC to the diagnosis of non-neoplastic lung diseases have been focused primarily on detection of infectious agents. Traditionally, microbial identification in infectious diseases has been accomplished primarily by using serologic assays and culture techniques. However, serologic results can be difficult to interpret in a setting of immunosuppression or when only a single sample is available for evaluation. In addition, fresh tissue is not always available for culture, and culture of fastidious pathogens may take weeks or months to yield results. Alternatively, IHC can provide a rapid morphologic diagnosis, facilitating early treatment of serious infectious diseases. It also allows for microbiologic-morphologic correlation, establishing the pathogenic significance of microbiologic results by linking an isolated agent to one or more abnormalities in host tissues. The following

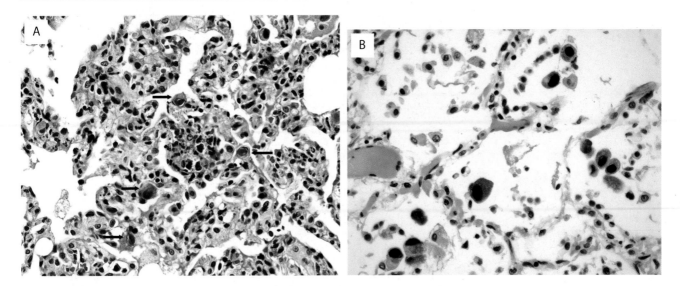

FIGURE 38-1
Cytomegalovirus
(A) Multiple CMV-infected cells (arrows) demonstrate characteristic cytologic features: intranuclear and cytoplasmic inclusions, cytomegaly, and nucleomegaly. A microabscess lies adjacent to the infected cells. **(B)** Immunohistochemistry using monoclonal anti-CMV antibody highlights CMV-infected cells.

paragraphs provide information about the use of IHC for diagnosis of viral agents, and additional information about the agents can be found in Chapter 13. Other applications of IHC to non-neoplastic lung diseases include the evaluation and classification of lymphoid processes, histiocytic and dendritic cell disorders, and selected interstitial lung diseases.

CYTOMEGALOVIRUS

Cytomegalovirus (CMV) is an important opportunistic pathogen in immunocompromised patients, particularly in those with malignancies, congenital immunodeficiency, transplants, or acquired immune deficiency syndrome (AIDS), and the lung is one of the primary sites infected. Histologic diagnosis of CMV in fixed tissues usually depends upon the identification of characteristic cytopathic effects, including intranuclear or cytoplasmic inclusions or both, cytomegaly, and nucleomegaly (Figure 38-1A). However, histologic examination does not always reveal the expected changes, especially in early or treated cases, and in some cases atypical cytopathic features can be confused with reactive or degenerative changes. IHC using monoclonal antibodies against CMV antigens allows for detection of CMV in infected cells (Figure 38-1B), and the sensitivity of IHC compares favorably with culture and in situ hybridization.

ADENOVIRUS

In immunocompromised patients, adenovirus is a less common pathogen than CMV but frequently behaves aggressively in this group and has occasionally been associated with fatal outcomes in transplant patients. In otherwise healthy individuals, upper respiratory tract infection is the usual presentation, and the incidence of serious pulmonary disease is very low. Characteristic adenovirus inclusions are amphophilic, intranuclear, homogeneous, and glassy. The inclusion can obscure the nuclear membranes, resulting in the designation "smudge cell." However, other viral inclusions, including those associated with CMV, herpes simplex virus (HSV), and varicella zoster virus (VZV), can be mistaken for adenovirus inclusions and vice versa. A monoclonal antibody reactive with 41 serotypes of adenovirus has been successfully used for IHC to confirm the presence of adenovirus in tissue (Figure 38-2).

HERPESVIRUSES

The diagnosis of HSV infection is relatively straightforward if there are abundant multinucleated giant cells and cells containing viral inclusions and showing "ground-

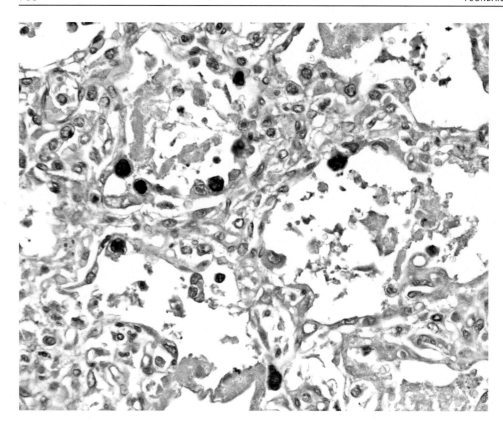

FIGURE 38-2
Adenovirus
Cells infected with adenovirus are stained by immunohistochemistry.

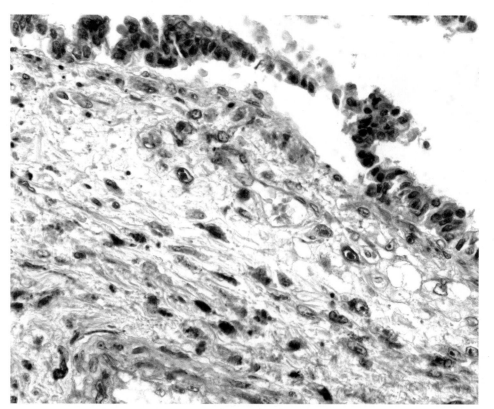

FIGURE 38-3
Herpes simplex virus
Numerous cells are immunopositive for HSV type 1. Several of these cells contain the characteristic intranuclear inclusions.

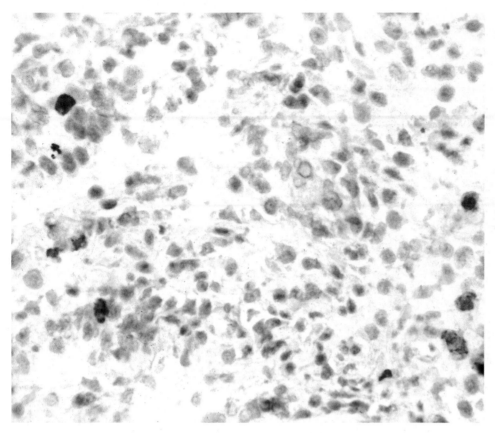

FIGURE 38-4
Varicella zoster virus
Use of a monoclonal antibody against the VZV envelope glycoprotein allows for distinction between VZV and HSV infections. (Courtesy of Gerhard Krueger, University of Texas, Houston, Texas.)

glass" chromatin. However, the detection of HSV infection can be difficult when the characteristic intranuclear inclusions or multinucleated giant cells, or both, are absent. Furthermore, the cytopathic changes associated with HSV infection are not specific and can also occur in association with VZV. IHC has not only proved to be a sensitive and specific technique to detect HSV infections but also is sufficiently sensitive and specific to enable distinction between HSV and VZV infections (Figures 38-3, 38-4). Recently, also, human herpesvirus type 8, also called Kaposi's sarcoma-associated herpesvirus, was identified by IHC in non-HIV-infected patients with interstitial pneumonitis.

OTHER VIRAL AGENTS

IHC has played a role in facilitating the identification of a number of emerging agents of viral hemorrhagic fevers, many of which present with hemorrhagic pneumonitis. For instance, IHC was central to the identification of viral antigens of previously unknown Hantavirus. Microbiologic-morphologic correlation demonstrated the distribution of viral antigen in endothelium of the microvasculature, particularly in the lung. IHC has been also used to confirm the diagnosis of respiratory viral diseases including influenza A virus (Figure 38-5), respiratory syncytial virus (Figure 38-6), and parainfluenza infections (Figure 38-7).

APPLICATIONS OF IMMUNOHISTOCHEMISTRY TO EVALUATION OF NEOPLASTIC LUNG DISEASES

Most common histologic types of lung carcinomas fall into two major groups: non-small cell lung cancers (NSCLCs) and small cell lung cancers (SCLCs). Treatment approaches to these categories of neoplasms differ substantially, so great importance attaches to accurate histopathologic diagnosis. Although diagnosis and classification of lung cancer is based primarily on histopathologic features, IHC is frequently used to support a morphologic diagnosis. IHC is particularly useful in several settings that are discussed below.

PULMONARY VERSUS EXTRAPULMONARY PRIMARY NEOPLASM

The lung is the most frequent site of involvement by metastatic neoplasms, and in fact, metastatic neoplasms to lung are more common than primary lung

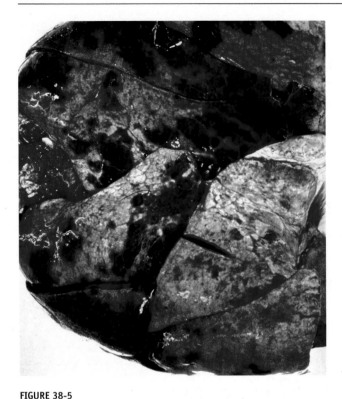

FIGURE 38-5
Viral hemorrhagic pneumonitis
Diffuse hemorrhage due to influenza A infection was noted in bilateral lobes. (Generously contributed by Dr. Gerhard Krueger, University of Texas Health Science Center at Houston, Houston, Texas.)

tumors. Based on clinicopathologic data, the lungs are involved by metastatic disease in one third to half of all malignant lesions. Although clinical history can be helpful in pointing towards a particular primary site, even in the absence of clinical data the pathologist must act with the consideration of metastatic disease in mind. Assessment of tumor morphology, evaluation for an in situ component, and comparison with earlier samples may be sufficient to answer the question of whether a tumor is primary or metastatic, but often more than one consideration exists for a potential primary site. IHC is extremely useful for differentiating primary pulmonary from metastatic carcinomas, particularly adenocarcinomas.

Among "specific" markers studied for pulmonary epithelium, thyroid transcription factor-1 (TTF-1) is the most widely used. TTF-1, a 38-kilodalton nuclear protein and a member of the *Nkx*2 homeodomain transcription factor family, was originally characterized as a promoter of thyroid-specific transcription of the thyroglobulin and thyroperoxidase genes. The distribution of TTF-1 in normal lung tissues includes alveolar cells, particularly type II pneumocytes, and nonciliated bronchiolar cells (Clara cells). TTF-1 is primarily expressed in neoplasms originating in the lung and thyroid. Up to 94% of pulmonary adenocarcinomas have been reported to express TTF-1 (Figure 38-8A). Studies have shown a lack of TTF-1 staining in adenocarcinomas of the colon and prostate, renal cell carcinomas, and breast carcinomas, and only rare gastric and endometrial adenocarcinomas have been

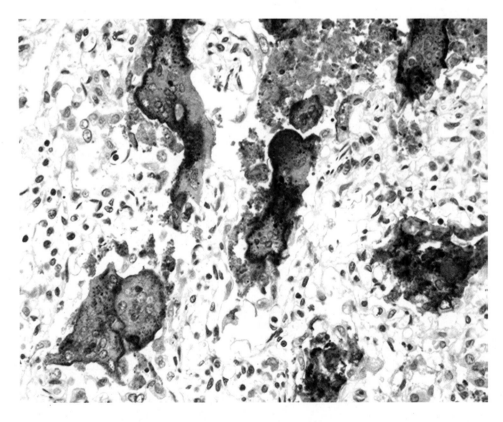

FIGURE 38-6
Respiratory syncytial virus
Multiple multinucleated cells stain strongly for respiratory syncytial virus.

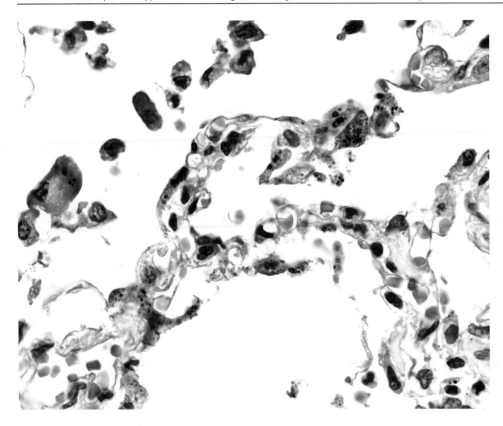

FIGURE 38-7

Parainfluenza type 3
Immunohistochemistry highlights infected cells in this culture-positive case of parainfluenza type 3.

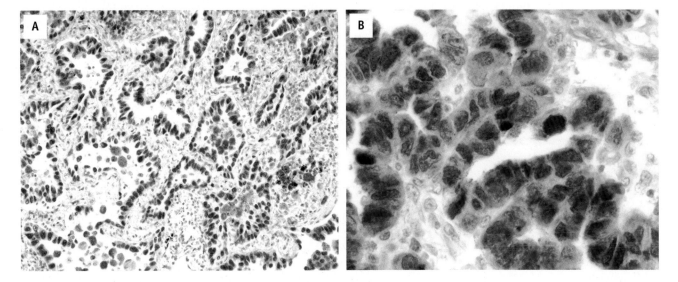

FIGURE 38-8

Thyroid transcription factor-1 (TTF-1) and surfactant precursor protein B
(A) Diffuse TTF-1 expression is evident in this pulmonary adenocarcinoma. **(B)** Dual staining of this adenocarcinoma reveals nuclear TTF-1 (brown) and cytoplasmic surfactant precursor protein B (red) expression.

reported as showing focal positivity. Furthermore, TTF-1 has been also proven useful in pulmonary FNA specimens. While the high specificity and relatively good sensitivity of TTF-1 make it a valuable antibody for differentiating primary pulmonary adenocarcinomas from metastatic adenocarcinomas, TTF-1 has limited value in

differentiating between pulmonary and extrapulmonary squamous cell carcinomas, since most pulmonary squamous cell carcinomas are immunonegative. It is also expressed by most SCLCs and many extrapulmonary small cell carcinomas, so it has little utility for determining the primary site of a small cell carcinoma.

Antibodies against surfactant proteins A and B (Figure 38-8B) have been evaluated in the differential diagnosis of pulmonary adenocarcinomas, but in general, they demonstrate sensitivities comparable to TTF-1 but lower specificities due to reactivity with carcinomas of the breast. Surfactant antibodies have a use, however, in the differential diagnosis of a TTF-1+ neoplasm in which lung and thyroid primaries are considered. Thyroglobulin is also helpful in this context.

IHC for CK7 and CK20 has been valuable for narrowing the list of potential primary sites of a variety of carcinomas (Table 38-1). CK7 is present in many simple and pseudostratified epithelia, including bronchogenic epithelium, and is generally strongly and diffusely positive in lung cancers. Colorectal carcinomas, hepatocellular carcinomas, renal cell carcinomas, and adrenal cortical carcinomas, on the other hand, are essentially always negative or minimally and weakly positive. Negative staining for CK7, combined with positive CK20 staining, is characteristic of colon cancer metastases in the lung (CK7-/CK20+). These stains can also help distinguish SCLC (CK7+or-/CK20-) from metastatic Merkel cell carcinoma (CK7-/CK20+).

Other carcinomas expressing the CK7+/CK20- immunoreactivity profile include breast carcinoma, endometrial adenocarcinoma, and nonmucinous ovarian carcinoma. For this reason, the authors usually perform TTF-1 staining with staining for CK7 and CK20, to differentiate between primary and metastatic carcinomas. Additional antibodies can also be added to this basic panel to tailor it for other potential primaries suggested by the histopathology and history (Table 38-1).

SMALL CELL LUNG CARCINOMA VERSUS NON-SMALL CELL LUNG CARCINOMA

Classification of a lung cancer as a SCLC or NSCLC is critical for determination of appropriate therapy. Although in most cases this is not an overly difficult task, occasional samples can be problematic due to intrinsic tumor characteristics (necrosis, morphologic features that seem to straddle both SCLC and NSCLC) or sampling effects (crush artifact, limited tumor representation). Differentiating between small cell squamous carcinomas of the lung and SCLCs can be particularly challenging.

Many antibodies have been tested for their potential utility for distinguishing between SCLCs and NSCLCs, and recent studies have revealed particularly good results with newer antibodies, including p63, high molecular weight keratin, and TTF-1 (Table 38-2). A recently discovered member of the p53 family of nuclear transcription factors, p63, is important for maintaining stem cell populations in squamous and other stratified epithelia and in normal lung, stains nuclei of bronchial reserve cells but not ciliated cells, alveolar epithelial

---

TABLE 38-1

Antibodies Commonly Used in the Evaluation of Adenocarcinomas and Their Usual Immunoreactivities

Site of Origin	CK7	CK20	Other Antibodies Frequently Immunopositive
Lung	+	Varies with histologic type	TTF-1
Colorectal	−	+	CDX-2, villin, CA 19-9
Pancreaticobiliary	+	+ or −	CA 125, CA 19-9
Breast	+	−	ER, PR, GCDFP
Prostate	−	−	PSA
Ovary	+	Varies with histologic type	CA 125
Endometrium	+	−	CA 125
Liver (hepatocellular)	−	−	HepPar-1
Kidney	−	−	CD10, RCC
Adrenal cortex	−	−	Inhibin

Abbreviations: + usually immunopositive; − usually immunonegative; ER = estrogen receptor; GCDFP = gross cystic disease fluid protein-15; PR = progesterone receptor; PSA = prostate specific antigen; RCC = renal cell carcinoma monoclonal antibody; TTF-1 = thyroid transcription factor-1

TABLE 38-2

Usual Immunoprofiles of Small Cell Lung Carcinoma (SCLC) and Poorly Differentiated Squamous Cell Carcinoma of Lung (PDSqCC)

Tumor Type	TTF-1	p63	HMWK	Synaptophysin	Chromogranin A
SCLC	+	−	−	+	+ or −
PDSqCC	−	+	+	−	−

Abbreviations: + usually immunopositive; − usually immunonegative; HMWK=high molecular weight keratin; TTF-1=thyroid transcription factor-1

cells, or non-epithelial cells. Studies have shown that most poorly differentiated squamous cell carcinomas will stain for p63 (Figure 38-9A), whereas SCLCs are p63-negative. Staining of adenocarcinomas and large cell carcinomas is more variable. Similarly, most poorly differentiated squamous cell carcinomas will stain for high molecular weight keratin (Figure 38-9B), whereas SCLCs will not stain. Furthermore, TTF-1 is rarely or only minimally expressed by poorly differentiated squamous cell carcinomas (Figure 38-9C). Conversely, SCLCs demonstrate the opposite pattern of immunoreactivities (p63-/high molecular weight keratin-/TTF-1+) (Figure 38-10A-C). This panel also facilitates diagnosis of combined small cell and non-small cell carcinomas by highlighting small populations of high molecular weight keratin-positive non-small carcinoma cells in a background of high molecular weight keratin-negative SCLC cells.

NEUROENDOCRINE NEOPLASM VERSUS NON-NEUROENDOCRINE NEOPLASM

Malignant pulmonary neuroendocrine tumors, as defined by the World Health Organization classification scheme, include the major categories of typical carcinoid, atypical carcinoid, large cell neuroendocrine carcinoma (LCNEC), and SCLC. Neuroendocrine differentiation can be demonstrated by electron microscopy or IHC in virtually all the lower grade tumors (typical and atypical carcinoid tumors) and lesser percentages of the higher grade neuroendocrine neoplasms (SCLC and LCNEC). Among the wide range of neuroendocrine IHC markers that are available, chromogranin, synaptophysin, and neural cell adhesion molecule (also referred to as CD56) appear to be the most reliable and widely used for detecting neuroendocrine differentiation (Figure 38-10D,E). CD57 (Leu-7) and neuron-

specific enolase have also been used to evaluate for neuroendocrine differentiation, but show less specificity than the other three markers.

Demonstration of neuroendocrine differentiation, while important for accurate classification, must be considered in the context of tumor morphology when determining the diagnosis for an individual neoplasm (see Chapter 27). In fact, immunohistochemical staining for neuroendocrine substances is not restricted to neuroendocrine neoplasms. Up to 20% of NSCLCs that lack light microscopic features of neuroendocrine morphology show evidence of neuroendocrine differentiation and should be classified according to their specific histologic type (i.e., squamous cell carcinoma) with a comment made regarding the presence of neuroendocrine differentiation. IHC can offer assistance, however, in differentiating between neuroendocrine neoplasms and other primary pulmonary neoplasms. For a differential diagnosis that includes a neuroendocrine tumor (LCNEC, SCLC, carcinoid) versus basaloid or poorly differentiated squamous cell carcinoma, the high molecular weight keratin antibody CK34βE12 is very helpful: it is reactive with most basaloid and poorly differentiated squamous cell carcinomas, but with substantially lower percentages of neuroendocrine neoplasms. Combined carcinomas, however, may show focal staining.

EPITHELIAL MESOTHELIOMA VERSUS ADENOCARCINOMA

The differential diagnosis of a malignant epithelial neoplasm in the pleura frequently includes adenocarcinoma (pulmonary or extrapulmonary) and malignant mesothelioma. IHC is the predominant ancillary technique used today to assist in resolution of this diagnostic question. It is usually not of value, however, for differentiating

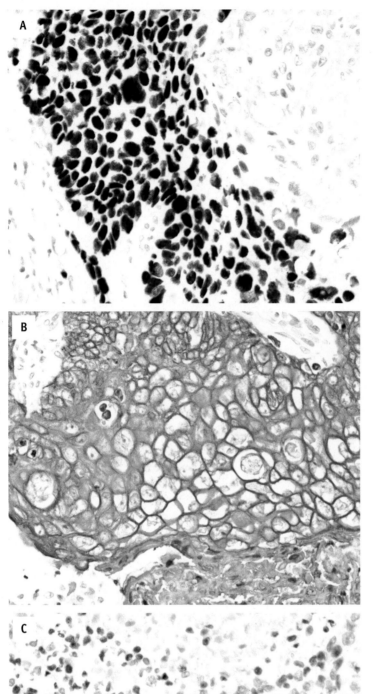

FIGURE 38-9

Squamous cell carcinoma

(A) p63 is expressed by the more poorly differentiated cells of this squamous cell carcinoma. (B) High molecular weight keratin staining is diffusely seen. (C) Lack of staining for TTF-1 is characteristic of poorly differentiated squamous cell carcinomas.

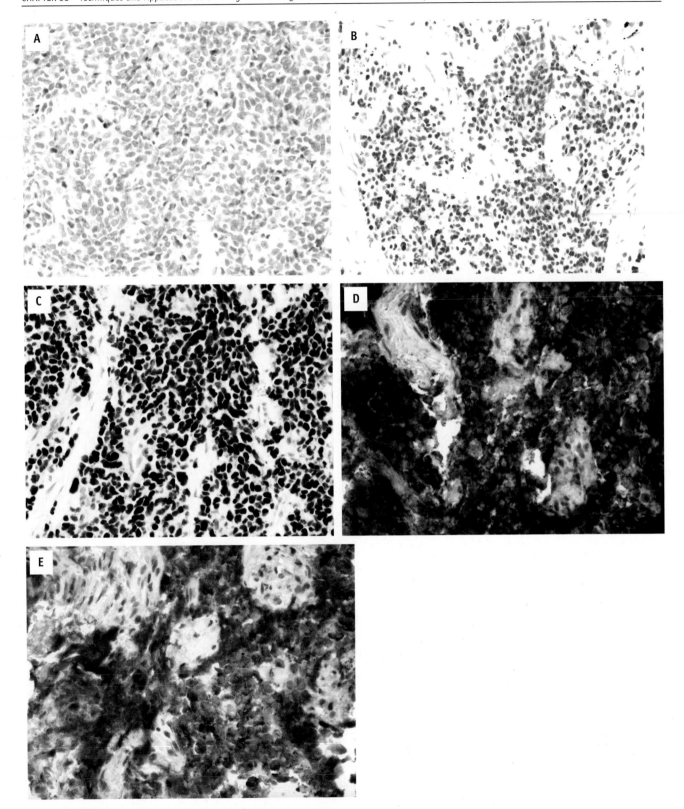

FIGURE 38-10

Small cell carcinoma
As expected, there is no staining for p63 **(A)** or high molecular weight keratin **(B)** in this tumor. TTF-1 **(C)** is strongly immunopositive, which is typical of small cell carcinomas. CD56 **(D)** and synaptophysin **(E)** staining are observed in this small cell carcinoma, despite crush artifact.

atypical reactive mesothelial proliferations from malignant mesothelioma.

A panel approach to IHC has been used with much success to distinguish adenocarcinoma from epithelial mesothelioma. The IHC panel is constructed to include several antibodies with high sensitivity and specificity for adenocarcinoma and several other antibodies with high sensitivity and specificity for mesothelioma (Table 38-3). This approach offers both positive and negative evidence for each entity and reduces the likelihood of an error in interpretation because of an aberrant staining result. Decision-making about the specific antibodies to include in the panel should also include consideration of which ones yield good staining results in a given laboratory.

Common choices for adenocarcinoma include carcinoembryonic antigen (CEA), CD15, B72.3, Ber-EP4, and MOC-31 (Figure 38-11). In general, these antibodies show low frequencies of reactivity with mesotheliomas. TTF-1 can also be included to provide evidence of a pulmonary origin for the adenocarcinoma, as opposed to an extrapulmonary origin (although thyroid neoplasms are frequently positive). Conversely, CK5/CK6 (Figure 38-12A) and calretinin (Figure 38-12B) are frequently selected for their high rates of reactivity with epithelial mesotheliomas and

TABLE 38-3

Immunohistochemical Differential Diagnosis Between Primary Lung Adenocarcinoma and Epithelial Mesothelioma

Tumor Type	CALR	CK5/6	TTF-1	CEA	CD15	Ber-EP4	B72.3
Adenocarcinoma of lung	−	−	+	+	+	+	+
Epithelial mesothelioma	+	+	−	−	−	−	−

Abbreviations: + often immunopositive; − usually immunonegative; CALR = calretinin; CEA = carcinoembryonic antigen; CK5/6 = cytokeratin 5/6; TTF-1 = thyroid transcription factor-1

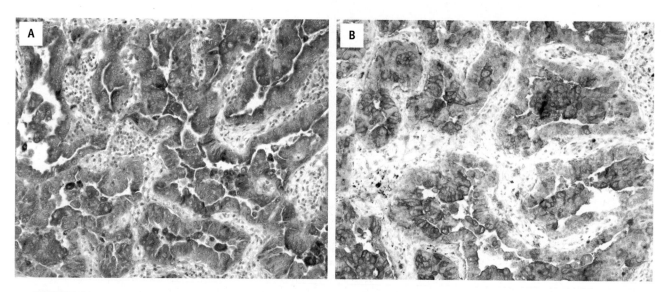

FIGURE 38-11

Adenocarcinoma involving the pleura
Diffuse staining for CEA **(A)** and CD15 **(B)** helps to confirm the diagnosis of adenocarcinoma rather than mesothelioma.

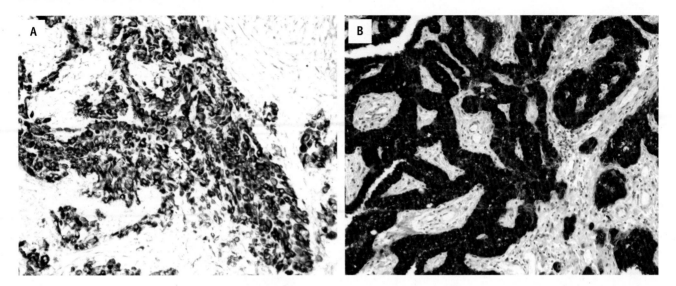

FIGURE 38-12

Malignant mesothelioma

These examples of epithelial mesotheliomas show characteristic staining for CK5/6 **(A)** (cytoplasmic staining) and calretinin **(B)** (nuclear and cytoplasmic staining).

their low levels of immunoreactivity with pulmonary adenocarcinomas. A recent study of IHC to distinguish epithelial mesotheliomas from lung adenocarcinomas yielded the following results: all (100%) of the mesotheliomas reacted with calretinin, cytokeratin 5/6, and mesothelin, 93% with WT1, 93% with EMA, 85% with HBME-1, 77% with thrombomodulin, 73% with CD44S, 73% with N-cadherin, 55% with vimentin, 40% with E-cadherin, 18% with Ber-EP4, 8% with MOC-31, 7% with BG-8, and none with CEA, B72.3, CD15, TTF-1, or CA 19-9. Of the adenocarcinomas, 100% were positive for MOC-31, Ber-EP4, and EMA, 96% for BG-8, 88% for CEA, 88% for E-cadherin, 84% for B72.3, 74% for TTF-1, 72% for CD15, 68% for HBME-1, 48% for CD44S, 48% for CA 19-9, 38% for mesothelin, 38% for vimentin, 30% for N-cadherin, 14% for thrombomodulin, 8% for calretinin, 2% for cytokeratin 5/6, and none for WT1.

MALIGNANT SPINDLE CELL NEOPLASMS OF THE LUNG

IHC can occasionally be of assistance in the diagnosis of malignant spindle cell neoplasms in the lung. Separation of spindle cell carcinomas from many primary or metastatic sarcomas and granulation tissue can be assisted by demonstration of keratin staining in the tumor cells (Figure 38-13). Addition of other antibodies can also be helpful, depending upon the differential diagnostic considerations (Table 38-4 and Figures 38-14, 38-15).

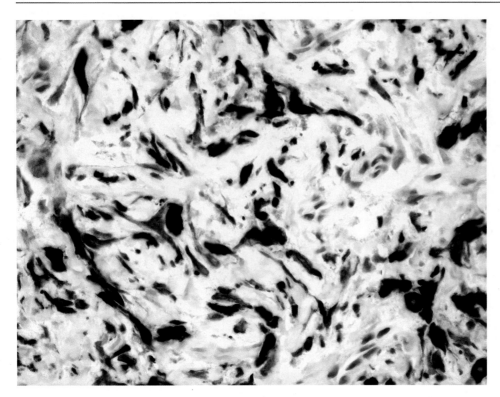

FIGURE 38-13
Spindle cell carcinoma
Pankeratin staining highlights the epithelial nature of a spindle cell carcinoma of the lung.

TABLE 38-4

Usual Immunoprofiles of Malignant Spindle Cell Neoplasms in the Lung

Tumor Type	Pankeratin	Other Antibodies Frequently Immunopositive
Spindle cell carcinoma	+	EMA, vimentin
Sarcomatoid malignant mesothelioma	+	CK7, calretinin, muscle markers, vimentin
Desmoid tumor	−	Muscle markers, vimentin
Malignant solitary fibrous tumor	−	CD34, CD99, bcl-2, vimentin
Sarcomatoid melanoma	−	S100, HMB45, Melan A, vimentin
Leiomyosarcoma	−	Muscle markers, vimentin
Kaposi's sarcoma	−	CD31, CD34, factor VIII related antigen, HHV8, vimentin
Angiosarcoma	−	CD31, CD34, factor VIII related antigen, vimentin
Malignant fibrous histiocytoma	−	A1ACT, A1AT, CD68, vimentin
Synovial sarcoma	+	EMA, CD99, bcl-2, vimentin

Abbreviations: + usually immunopositive; − usually immunonegative; A1ACT = alpha-1-antichymotrypsin; A1AT = alpha-1-antitrypsin; CK7 = cytokeratin 7; EMA = epithelial membrane antigen; HHV8 = human herpesvirus 8

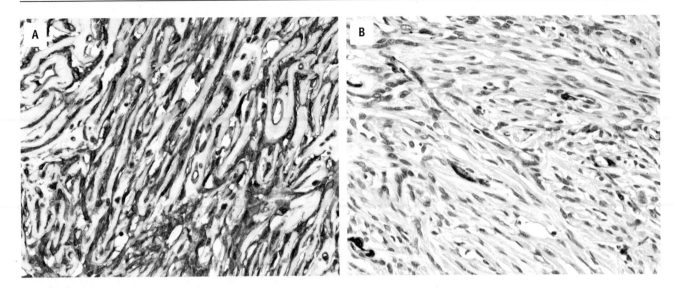

FIGURE 38-14

Solitary fibrous tumor

These neoplasms typically express CD34 **(A)** but usually not smooth muscle actin **(B)**.

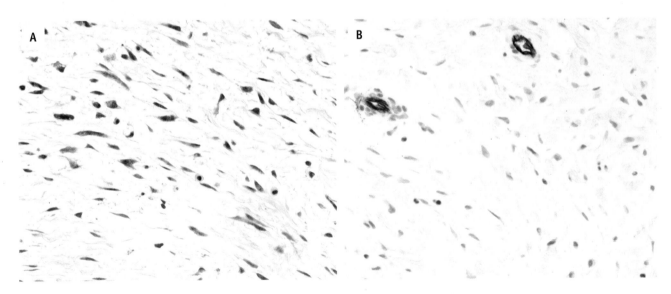

FIGURE 38-15

Desmoid tumor

Smooth muscle actin **(A)** is usually expressed by desmoid tumors, but CD34 staining is absent **(B)**.

SUGGESTED READINGS

Techniques of Immunohistochemistry (IHC)

1. Adams JC. Biotin amplification of biotine and horseradish peroxidase signals in histochemical stains. *J Histochem Cytochem.* 1992;40:1457-63.
2. Boon ME, Kok LP. Breakthrough in pathology due to antigen retrieval. *Mal J Med Lab Sci.* 1995;12:1.
3. Heras A, Roach CM, Key ME. Enhanced polymer detection system for immunohistochemistry. *Mod Pathol.* 1995;8:165A.
4. Taylor CR. An exaltation of experts: concerted efforts in the standardization of immunohistochemistry. *Hum Pathol.* 1994;25:2-7.
5. Werner M, Chott A, Fabiano A, et al. Effect of formalin tissue fixation and processing on immunohistochemistry. *Am J Surg Pathol.* 2000;24:1016-9.

Applications of IHC in Non-Neoplastic Diseases

6. Cartun RW. Use of immunohistochemistry in the surgical pathology laboratory for the diagnosis of infectious diseases. *Pathol Case Rev.* 1999;4:260-5.
7. Muller A, Franzen C, Klussmann P, et al. Human herpesvirus type 8 in HIV-infected patients with interstitial pneumonitis. *J Infection.* 2000;40:242-7.
8. Nolte KB, Feddersen RM, Foucar K, et al. Hantavirus pulmonary syndrome in the United States. A pathological description of a disease caused by a new agent. *Hum Pathol.* 1998;29:1393-1402.
9. Sheehan MM, Coker R, Coleman DV. Detection of cytomegalovirus (CMV) in HIV+ patients: comparison of cytomorphology, immunohistochemistry and in situ hybridization. *Cytopathology.* 1998;9:29-37.
10. Simsir A, Greenebaum E, Nuovo G, et al. Late fatal adenovirus pneumonitis in lung transplant recipient. *Transplantation.* 1998;65:592-4.

IHC in Distinguishing Primary Lung Cancer Versus Metastatic Carcinoma

11. Nakamura N, Miyagi E, Murata S, et al. Expression of thyroid transcription factor-1 in normal and neoplastic lung tissues. *Mod Pathol.* 2002;15:1058-67.
12. Oliveira AM, Tazelaar HD, Myers JL, et al. Thyroid transcription factor-1 distinguishes metastatic pulmonary from well-differentiated neuroendocrine tumors of other sites. *Am J Surg Pathol.* 2001;25:815-9.
13. Ordonez NG. Thyroid transcription factor-1 is a marker of lung and thyroid carcinomas. *Adv Anat Pathol.* 2000;7:123-7.
14. Raab SS, Sturgis CD, Wick MR. Metastatic tumors in the lung: a practical approach to diagnosis. In Leslie KO, Wick MR, eds. *Practical Pulmonary Pathology.* Philadelphia: Churchill Livingstone; 2005.
15. Yatabe Y, Mitsudomi T, Takahashi T. TTF-1 expression in pulmonary adenocarcinomas. *Am J Surg Pathol.* 2002;26:767-73.

IHC in Distinguishing Small Cell Carcinoma Versus Non-Small Cell Carcinoma

16. Irwin MS, Kaelin WG. P53 family update: p73 and p63 develop their own identities. *Cell Growth Differ.* 2001;12:337-49.
17. Pelosi G, Pasini F, Olsen SC, et al. P63 immunoreactivity in lung cancer: yet another player in the development of squamous cell carcinomas? *J Pathol.* 2002;198:100-9.
18. Wang BY, Gil J, Kaufman D, et al. P63 in pulmonary epithelium, pulmonary squamous neoplasms and other pulmonary tumors. *Hum Pathol.* 2002;33:921-6.
19. Wu M, Wang B, Gil J, et al. 63 and TTF-1 immunostaining. A useful marker panel for distinguishing small cell carcinoma of lung from poorly differentiated squamous cell carcinoma of lung. *Am J Clin Pathol.* 2003;119:696-702.
20. Zhang H, Liu J, Cagle PT, et al. Distinction of pulmonary small cell carcinoma from poorly differentiated squamous cell carcinoma: an immunohistochemical approach. *Mod Pathol.* 2005;18:111-8.

IHC in Distinguishing Neuroendocrine Neoplasms Versus Non-Neuroendocrine Tumors

21. Sturm N, Lantuéjoul S, Laverrière MH, Papotti M, Brichon PY, Brambilla C, Brambilla E. Thyroid transcription factor 1 and cytokeratins 1, 5, 10, 14 (34betaE12) expression in basaloid and large-cell neuroendocrine carcinomas of the lung. *Hum Pathol.* 2001;32:918-25.
22. Loy TS, Darkow GV, Quesenberry JT. Immunostaining in the diagnosis of pulmonary neuroendocrine carcinomas. An immunohistochemical study with ultrastructural correlations. *Am J Surg Pathol.* 1995;19:173-82.
23. Lyda MH, Weiss LM. Immunoreactivity for epithelial and neuroendocrine antibodies are useful in the differential diagnosis of lung carcinomas. *Hum Pathol.* 2000;31:980-7.
24. Sturm N, Rossi G, Lantuéjoul S, et al. 34BetaE12 expression along the whole spectrum of neuroendocrine proliferations of the lung, from neuroendocrine cell hyperplasia to small cell carcinoma. *Histopathology.* 2003;42:156-66.
25. Travis WD, Rush W, Flieder DB, et al. Survival analysis of 200 pulmonary neuroendocrine tumors with clarification of criteria for atypical carcinoid and its separation from typical carcinoid. *Am J Surg Pathol.* 1998;22:934-44.

IHC in Distinguishing Primary Lung Cancer Versus Mesothelioma

26. Clover J, Oates J, Edwards C. Anti-cytokeratin 5/6: A positive marker for epithelial mesothelioma. *Histopathology.* 1997;31:140-3.
27. Granville LA, Younes M, Churg A, et al. Comparison of monoclonal versus polyclonal calretinin antibodies for immunohistochemical diagnosis of malignant mesothelioma. *Appl Immunohistochem Mol Morphol.* 2005;13:75-9.
28. Moran CA, Wick MR, Suster S. The role of immunohistochemistry in the diagnosis of malignant mesothelioma. *Semin Diagn Pathol.* 2000;17:178-83.
29. Ordonez NG. Value of thyroid transcription factor-1, E-cadherin, BG8, WT1 and CD44S immunostaining in distinguishing epithelial pleural mesothelioma from pulmonary and nonpulmonary adenocarcinoma. *Am J Surg Pathol.* 2000;24:598-606.

IHC in Distinguishing Spindle Cell Malignant Neoplasms in the Lung

30. Andino L, Cagle PT, Murer B, et al. Pleuropulmonary desmoid tumors: immunohistochemical comparison with solitary fibrous tumors and assessment of ß-catenin and cyclin D1 expression. *Arch Pathol Lab Med.*, 2006;130:1503-9.
31. Granville L, Laga AC, Allen TC, et al. Review and update of uncommon primary pleural tumors: a practical approach to diagnosis. *Arch Pathol Lab Med.* 2005;129:1428-43.
32. Hammar SP. Lung and pleural neoplasms. In Dabbs DJ, ed. *Diagnostic Immunohistochemistry.* Philadelphia: Churchill Livingstone, 2002; 267-312.
33. Nappi O, Glasner SD, Swanson PE, Wick MR. Biphasic and monophasic sarcomatoid carcinomas of the lung: a reappraisal of "carcinosarcomas" and "spindle cell carcinomas." *Am J Clin Pathol.* 1994;102:331-40.
34. Wick M. Spindle cell neoplasms of the lung. *Semin Pathol.* 1999;17:142-7.

39

Techniques and Applications to the Diagnosis of Lung Diseases: Immunofluorescence

Cynthia M. Magro

- **Introduction**
- **Patterns of Direct Immunofluorescence and Their Correlations with Underlying Diseases**
  Localization of Immunoreactivity to Septal Capillary Endothelium
  Septal Wall Localization of Immunoreactivity
  Large Vessel Complement Localization
  Alveolar Basement Membrane Localization
  Deposition Along the Bronchial Basement Membrane Zone
  Deposition within Chondrocytes and Bronchial Epithelial Cells
- **Practical Tips Regarding the Interpretation of DIF of the Lung**

INTRODUCTION

Immunofluorescent (IF) testing is an important diagnostic adjunct in the assessment of immunologically mediated diseases, especially in the context of skin and renal disorders. The two main methods of IF testing are direct and indirect IF. The former involves the overlay of fluorescein-conjugated antibodies directed against immunoglobulin (IgG, IgM, and IgA) and complement fractions onto frozen sections of patient tissue. Indirect IF by definition employs a linking antibody; in its common usage, indirect IF refers to the use of patient serum in concert with fluorescein-conjugated human anti-IgG and a mucosal substrate, such as guinea pig, monkey esophagus, or rat bladder.

The utilization of either a direct or indirect IF assay is not considered routine practice in the assessment of most lung disorders. Interestingly, though, there are many disorders in the lung where an initial inciting trigger leading to pulmonary injury is clearly one related to an underlying immune-based etiology; hence, immunofluorescence would be of potential value. For example, oftentimes the septal microvasculature is the target, ei-

ther directly through antiendothelial cell antibodies or indirectly via circulating immune complexes. Evaluation of the IF profile in the context of a morphologic pattern indicating septal injury may allow for more specific diagnosis of a disease process.

The morphologic spectrum stemming from a septal capillary injury phenomenon is varied, but several patterns are recognized. These encompass pauci-inflammatory hemorrhage, including anti-glomerular basement membrane antibody disease (i.e., Goodpasture's syndrome) and idiopathic pulmonary hemosiderosis; a pauci-inflammatory endothelialitis characteristic of anti-Ro-associated lupus pneumonitis and dermatomyositis; and a neutrophil-rich septal capillaritis as seen within the spectrum of mixed cryoglobulinemia, microscopic polyangiitis, Wegener's granulomatosis, and Henoch-Schönlein purpura.

Transbronchial and wedge biopsies to undergo IF testing should be received fresh or placed in physiologic fixative such as Michel's medium. If fresh, one portion is fixed in formalin for routine light microscopic assessment while another piece is snap frozen in embedding medium for purposes of direct immunofluorescent testing, and stored at -70 degrees Celsius. The frozen or Michel's-fixed tissue sections are incubated with commercially prepared fluoresceinated antisera specific for human IgG, IgM, IgA, C3, C1q, C3d, C4d, and C5b-9. It is important to assess lung biopsy specimens under oil for optimal interpretation, since the deposition pattern is often very fine and may not be appreciated under ×400 magnification.

PATTERNS OF DIRECT IMMUNOFLUORESCENCE AND THEIR CORRELATION WITH UNDERLYING DISEASE

There are several patterns of IF staining that can be observed in specific disease processes, which are discussed below. Immunoglobulin and complement deposition can be either granular or homogeneous and can be observed in a variety of distributions (Table 39-1). Apparent fluorescence of elastic fibers or material within

TABLE 39-1

Major Immunoreactant Profiles

Site of Deposition	Pattern	Immunoreactant	Significance	Diseases
Alveolar basement membrane	Homogeneous	IgG, C1q, C3, C3d, and C4d; rarely IgA	Antibodies with specificity for the α3 chain of type IV collagen	Goodpasture's syndrome
Alveolar septae (endothelial cell or septal capillary wall)	Granular	IgG or IgA, C1q, C3d, C4d	Type II immune reaction directed at endothelium	Connective tissue diseases, idiopathic pulmonary fibrosis, lung allograft rejection
Alveolar septae	Granular	IgM, C3	Immune complex reaction or nonspecific trapping and reactivity	Mixed cryoglobulinemia, ANCA-associated vasculitic syndromes
Alveolar septae	Granular	IgA		Henoch-Schönlein purpura, rheumatoid arthritis

Abbreviation: ANCA = antineutrophil cytoplasmic antibody

alveolar spaces is unlikely to be of diagnostic significance. Also, in general, the more extensive the deposits, the more likely they are to be significant. Intensity is not as important as extensiveness.

LOCALIZATION OF IMMUNOREACTIVITY TO SEPTAL CAPILLARY ENDOTHELIUM

A finely speckled pattern showing cytoplasmic and/or nuclear endothelial cell localization (typically for IgG), classic components of complement activation (C1q and C4d), and other components of complement activation (C3d and C5b-9) (Figures 39-1, 39-2) can be seen in association with connective tissue diseases, including dermatomyositis, anti-Ro-associated systemic lupus erythematosus, scleroderma, and mixed connective tissue disease. There may be concomitant staining of other cells, including bronchial epithelium and macrophages, typically when there is a high-circulating antinuclear antibody (ANA). In addition, this pattern of fine endothelial cell staining can be found in idiopathic pulmonary fibrosis and lung allograft rejection. Another distinctive endothelial staining pattern is the oligodot or "nucleolar" pattern of decoration (Figure 39-3). It is an immunofluorescence pattern that is very characteristic of scleroderma and may be a clue to the existence of underlying scleroderma in patients whose lung biopsies show a compatible interstitial lung disease. This distinctive nucleolar pattern can also be seen in sclerodermatomyositis, reflecting antibodies to PM-Scl.

SEPTAL WALL LOCALIZATION OF IMMUNOREACTIVITY

This pattern can be encountered in the same spectrum of conditions in which there is localization of immunoreactivity within the endothelium and may include IgG, C1q, C4d, C3d, and C5b-9 (Figure 39-4). When the immunoreactants are represented by C3 and IgM, however, then the more likely basis is nonspecific microvascular injury whereby enhanced vascular permeability leads to nonspecific entrapment of immunoglobulin and C3 within the vessel wall. IgA-dominant deposition within the microvasculature is seen in two primary settings: Henoch-Schönlein purpura and rheumatoid arthritis.

LARGE VESSEL COMPLEMENT LOCALIZATION

Non-immunogenic lung injury syndromes including acute respiratory distress syndrome and radiation and chemotherapy pneumonitis can show C3 and C5b-9 deposition in larger vessels with lesser amounts of C5b-9 within the septal capillaries and venules.

ALVEOLAR BASEMENT MEMBRANE LOCALIZATION

Homogeneous linear staining along the alveolar basement membrane is typical for Goodpasture's syndrome (Figures 39-5, 39-6).

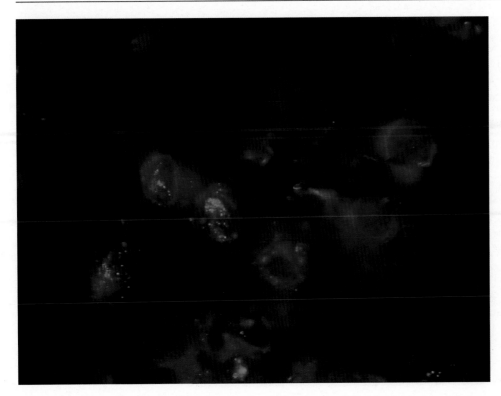

FIGURE 39-1

Septal capillary endothelial pattern
Granular DIF staining of the nucleus and cytoplasm of endothelial cells is visible. This immunofluorescence profile is characteristic of patients with pulmonary fibrosis in the setting of mixed connective tissue disease, anti-Ro-associated systemic lupus erythematosus, dermatomyositis, and idiopathic pulmonary fibrosis.

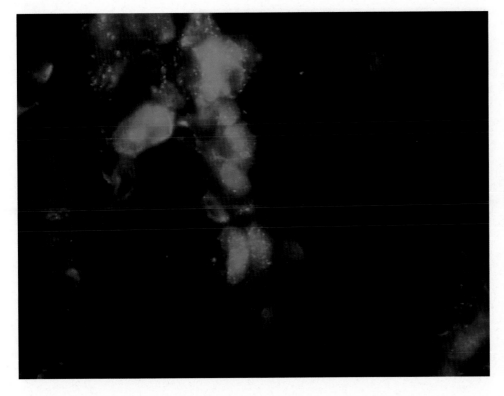

FIGURE 39-2

Septal capillary endothelial pattern
This pattern of immunofluorescence can also be seen in the setting of humoral lung allograft rejection.

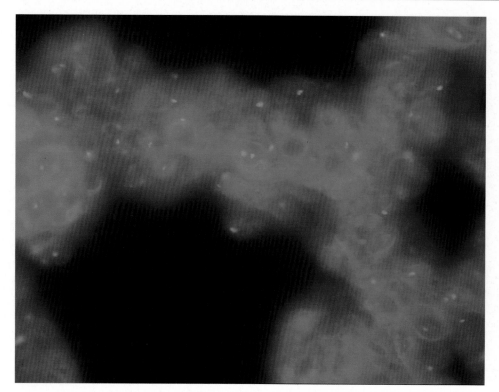

FIGURE 39-3

Nucleolar pattern

This image shows a nucleolar staining pattern involving the septal capillary endothelium. The nucleolar pattern correlates with antibodies to U3RNP, which is a serologic predictor of pulmonary fibrosis in patients with scleroderma.

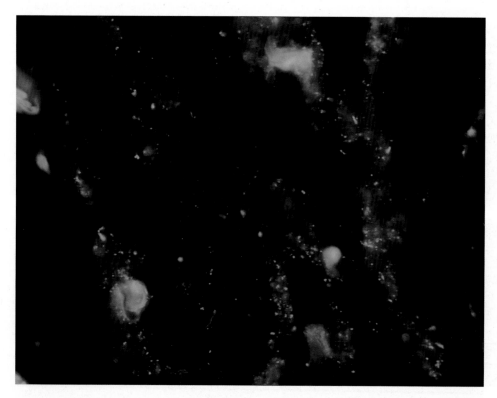

FIGURE 39-4

Septal granular pattern

There is granular deposition of IgG in the alveolar septae. There is no cellular localization per se. Despite the absence of obvious cellular localization, the pathogenetic implications are virtually identical, namely, one of a Gell and Comb's type II immune reaction directed at endothelium. Hence, this particular profile can be seen in the setting of collagen vascular diseases, humoral allograft rejection of the lung, and idiopathic pulmonary fibrosis.

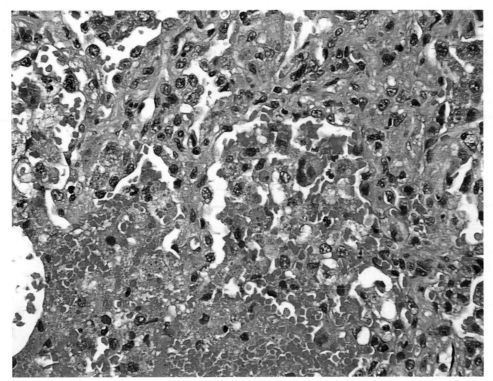

FIGURE 39-5

Goodpasture's syndrome

Alveolar hemorrhage with a relative dearth of inflammatory cells is characteristic but may also be encountered in idiopathic pulmonary hemosiderosis, humoral lung allograft rejection, and in association with collagen vascular diseases. Other pulmonary hemorrhage syndromes, such as Henoch-Schönlein purpura and the ANCA-positive vasculitic syndromes, are usually accompanied by significant interstitial neutrophilia.

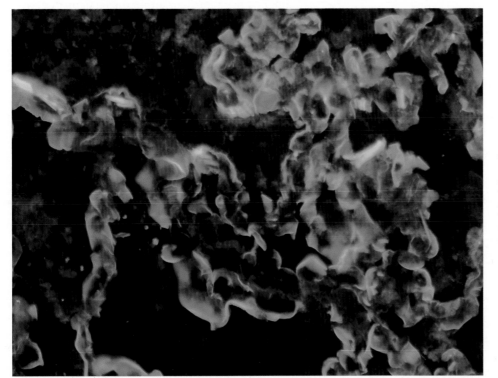

FIGURE 39-6

Goodpasture's syndrome

Linear DIF staining for IgG along the alveolar basement membrane zone is typical of Goodpasture's syndrome. The antibody is directed at a component of the basement membrane, namely, the noncollagenous component of the α3 domain of type IV collagen.

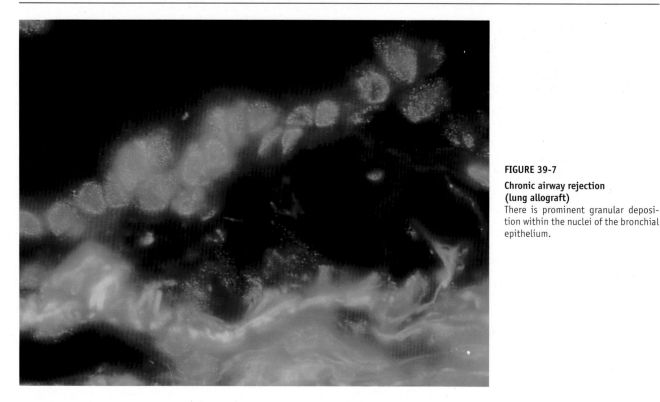

FIGURE 39-7

Chronic airway rejection (lung allograft)
There is prominent granular deposition within the nuclei of the bronchial epithelium.

DEPOSITION ALONG THE BRONCHIAL BASEMENT MEMBRANE ZONE

A granular deposition pattern within the basement membrane zone can be seen in association with collagen vascular diseases and chronic lung allograft rejection.

DEPOSITION WITHIN CHONDROCYTES AND BRONCHIAL EPITHELIAL CELLS

I have encountered staining of chondrocytes in patients with relapsing polychondritis and in the setting of chronic lung allograft rejection. Granular nuclear and/or cytoplasmic decoration of bronchial epithelium can be seen in collagen vascular diseases associated with antibodies to ribonucleoprotein (RNP) or Ro, and chronic lung allograft rejection (Figure 39-7).

PRACTICAL TIPS REGARDING THE INTERPRETATION OF DIAGNOSTIC IMMUNOFLUORESCENCE OF THE LUNG

Immunofluorescence techniques are less widely used as diagnostic adjuncts in pulmonary pathology than in dermatopathology and renal pathology. Interpretation of direct immunofluorescence on lung tissue specimens can be problematic for less experienced users. However, there are certain useful guidelines that can facilitate their interpretation.

1. The relevant deposition patterns are largely confined to the interstitium.
2. Deposition patterns observed in larger vessels or on the elastic fibers of the septae are unlikely to be of diagnostic significance.
3. The deposition patterns that are of pathogenetic importance represent either a coarse or fine granular pattern of deposition.
4. Any homogeneous deposition pattern within the septae, including in a mural vascular array, especially for IgA, can be nonspecific.
5. Deposition within the alveolar spaces does not constitute a significant pattern.
6. More extensive deposition is more likely to be significant than less extensive deposition. Focal deposition involving less than 20% of the lung parenchyma is likely to be not as significant as a similar deposition pattern involving more than 50% of the lung parenchyma.
7. Fluorescence intensity is not as important as the extensiveness of the deposition.

SUGGESTED READINGS

1. Beechler CR, Enquist RW, Hunt KK, et al. Immunofluorescence of transbronchial biopsies in Goodpasture's syndrome. *Am Rev Respir Dis.* 1980;121:869-72.
2. Bosch X, Lopez-Soto A, Mirapeix E, et al. Antineutrophil cytoplasmic autoantibody-associated alveolar capillaritis in patients presenting with pulmonary hemorrhage. *Arch Pathol Lab Med.* 1994;118:517-22.

3. Carette S, Macher AM, Nussbaum A, et al. Severe, acute pulmonary disease in patients with systemic lupus erythematosus: ten years of experience at the National Institutes of Health. *Semin Arthritis Rheum.* 1984;14:52-9.

4. Green RJ, Ruoss SJ, Kraft SA, Duncan SR, Berry GJ, Raffin TA. Pulmonary capillaritis and alveolar hemorrhage. Update on diagnosis and management. *Chest.* 1996;110:1305-16.

5. Hogan PG, Donald KJ, McEvoy JD. Immunofluorescence of lung biopsy tissue. *Am Rev Respir Dis.* 1978;118:537-45.

6. Kathuria S, Cheifec G. Fatal pulmonary Henoch-Schönlein syndrome. *Chest.* 1982;82:654-6.

7. Leatherman JW, Sibley RK, Davies SF. Diffuse intrapulmonary hemorrhage and glomerulonephritis unrelated to anti-glomerular basement membrane antibody. *Am J Med.* 1982;72:401-10.

8. Lombard CM, Colby TV, Elliot CG. Surgical pathology of the lung in anti-basement membrane antibody-associated Goodpasture's syndrome. *Hum Pathol.* 1989;20:445-51.

9. Magro CM, Morrison C, Pope-Harman A, Rothrauff SK, Ross P Jr. Direct and indirect immunofluorescence as a diagnostic adjunct in the interpretation of non-neoplastic lung disease. *Am J Clin Pathol.* 2003;119:279-89.

10. Magro CM, Ross P Jr, Kelsey M, Waldman WJ, Pope-Harman A. Association of humoral immunity and bronchiolitis obliterans syndrome. *Am J Transplant.* 2003;3:1155-66.

11. Markus HS, Clark JV. Pulmonary haemorrhage in Henoch-Schönlein purpura. *Thorax.* 1989;44:525-6.

12. Myers JL, Katzenstein AL. Wegener's granulomatosis presenting with massive pulmonary hemorrhage and capillaritis. *Am J Surg Pathol.* 1987;11:895-8.

13. Nakano H, Suzuki A, Tojima H, et al. A case of Goodpasture's syndrome with IgA antibasement membrane antibody. *Gakkai Zasshi.* 1990;28:634-8.

14. Schwarz M, Sutarik JM, Nick JA, et al. Pulmonary capillaritis and diffuse alveolar hemorrhage. A primary manifestation of polymyositis. *Am J Respir Crit Care Med.* 1995;151:2037-40.

40 Laboratory Diagnosis of Lung Diseases: Immunologic Tests

Semyon A. Risin

INTRODUCTION

There are strong rationales for immunologic testing in noninfectious pulmonary pathology. First, there is growing evidence of involvement of immunologic mechanisms in the pathogenesis of multiple primary lung conditions, including the allergic and obstructive lung diseases, pulmonary hemorrhage syndromes, and some of the interstitial lung diseases. A major thrust of some emerging treatment approaches is to modulate immune responses to ameliorate these diseases. There is also substantial overlap in the clinical presentations of primary pulmonary diseases and systemic autoimmune disorders, and immunologic testing is extremely important for establishing the correct diagnosis. Considering this, the intent of this chapter is to provide an overview of currently available immunologic tests and their applications to pulmonary pathology.

SYSTEMIC IMMUNITY IN PATIENTS WITH LUNG DISEASES

ASSESSMENT OF SYSTEMIC IMMUNITY

Assessment of systemic immunity includes testing of innate and adaptive cellular and humoral immune mechanisms. Innate immunity (phagocytosis, complement, pattern-recognition molecules, etc.) is antigen-nonspecific, provides a rapid response, and does not have memory. On the other hand, adaptive immunity (lymphocytes, T- and B-cell receptors, and secreted antibodies) is antigen-specific, requires time to develop a response, and has memory.

ASSESSMENT OF CELL-MEDIATED IMMUNITY

Assessment of cell-mediated immunity is a very complex task. It includes *in vivo* tests that are based on introduction of antigenic substances and observation of an inflammatory response; evaluation of the absolute and relative numbers of circulating T-lymphocytes and their subpopulations, B-lymphocytes, natural killer cells, neutrophils, eosinophils, and monocytes; and measurement of the cellular expression of activation markers and of numerous biologically active molecules (cytokines, chemokines) in circulation. It also includes the assessment of the functional activity of isolated immune cells and their responses to different stimulants *ex vivo*.

IN VIVO AND EX VIVO TESTS FOR ASSESSMENT OF CELL-MEDIATED IMMUNITY

The tests performed *in vivo* are limited to testing of cutaneous hypersensitivity reactions (type IV) to recall (tetanus, purified protein derivative, *Candida albicans*) and new (dinitrochlorobenzene) antigens. The antigens are introduced intradermally or applied on the skin as a patch. The results are read after 48 to 72 hours based on the measurement of a papular-type skin infiltration. Absence of a response indicates a lack of a type IV hypersensitivity response (anergy) to the antigen. Generalized anergy can be associated with immunodeficiency states, sarcoidosis, collagen vascular diseases, and other conditions. The purified protein derivative test for detection of infection by *Mycobacterium tuberculosis* is the most commonly used test in this group.

Assessment of the absolute and relative numbers of circulating immune cells of innate and adaptive immunity (natural killer cells, neutrophils, eosinophils, monocytes, T- and B-lymphocytes, CD4/CD8 cell ratio) is usually done by automatic cell count, cell microscopy, and flow cytometry. Flow cytometry is currently the most commonly used approach, and it is also the main approach for testing cellular expression of activation markers, integrins, other cell adhesion molecules, cytokines, and cytokine receptors. On the tissue level, cellular expression of many of these same molecules can be assessed by immunohistochemistry. Circulating biologically active molecules are measured by highly sensitive enzyme-linked immunosorbent assays (ELISAs) or immunofluorescent and chemiluminescent techniques. Testing of the functional activity of immune cells *ex vivo* involves numerous technical approaches (Table 40-1). Although most of these tests are too cumbersome and time consuming for clinical use and are generally limited to selected cases and research settings, some of the serologic tests are quite easy to perform and have broader clinical application.

SEROLOGIC PARAMETERS OF MONOCYTE/MACROPHAGE AND LYMPHOCYTE ACTIVATION

Measurement of the key molecules associated with activation of the T-lymphocyte/macrophage axis, which are released into systemic circulation (Table 40-2), is considered an appropriate and practical way to assess cell-mediated immunity. Several such molecules (neopterin, IL-13, sIL-2R, sICAM-1, interferon-γ) are currently favored, and commercial ELISAs have been developed for their testing.

TH1 AND TH2 IMMUNE RESPONSES IN LUNG DISEASES AND THEIR ASSESSMENT

CD4+ T-helper cells play a major immunoregulatory role in both cellular and humoral immune responses. They are divided into Th1 and Th2 cells based on the spectrum of cytokines they produce. Th1 and Th2 cells also show different patterns of expression of chemokine receptors that can be assessed by flow cytometry. Th1 cells express CXCR3 and CCR5, while Th2 cells express

---

TABLE 40-1

***Ex Vivo* Testing of the Functional Activity of Immune Cells**

Assessment of phagocytic activity (neutrophils, monocytes/ macrophages)

Cytotoxicity testing (NK, Tc)

Assessment of antigen- and/or mitogen-induced proliferation

Measurement of the synthesis and release of cytokines, soluble cytokine receptors and other soluble molecules (peripheral blood mononuclear cells)

   a. immediately *ex vivo*

   b. after stimulation (including stimulation by chemicals bypassing the ligand-receptor interaction [PMA, ionomycin])

Testing of expression of activation markers and adhesion molecules

Assessment of activation terminating mechanisms

Assessment of programmed cell death (apoptosis)

Evaluation of regulatory pathways

Gene expression studies

TABLE 40-2

Lymphocyte- and Monocyte-Derived Activation Molecules Assessed in Systemic Circulation

INTERFERON-γ

- Released by activated T-lymphocytes (antigen-primed Th0 and Th1 cells)
- Stimulates human monocytes/macrophages and induces production of other cytokines and soluble molecules
- Skews cell mediated immunity towards a Th1 response by suppressing Th2 differentiation

IL-13

- Produced mainly by Th2 cells
- Interferon-γ/IL-13 ratio is used as a measure of the Th1/Th2 balance

SOLUBLE IL-2R (sIL-2R) AND ICAM-1 (sICAM-1)

- Produced in large amounts by activated T-lymphocytes
- Soluble ICAM-1 is also produced by endothelial cells
- Serum ICAM-1 and ICAM-2 (but not ICAM -3) elevation is found in idiopathic pulmonary fibrosis and in secondary interstitial fibrosing conditions

NEOPTERIN

- Low-molecular-weight substance produced by monocytes/ macrophages stimulated by interferon-γ
- Serum level reflects monocyte/macrophage activation status
- Elevated in Wegener's granulomatosis, sarcoidosis, idiopathic pulmonary fibrosis, and chronic obstructive pulmonary disease
- Can be measured in serum and urine

CCR3, CCR4, and CCR8. These receptors interact with different ligands that are expressed by cells at sites of inflammation.

In the early 1990s, the idea was put forth that maintaining a balance between Th1 and Th2 stimulation in normal immune responses was important. It was postulated that in immunopathologic processes, there is a shift towards preferential stimulation of either a Th1 or Th2 type of response. Since then, a significant amount of evidence supporting this concept has accumulated. Moreover, it has become a leading principle influencing the development of immunomodulatory therapies. It must be noted, however, that the information regarding the division into Th1 and Th2 processes is sometimes quite controversial, and the concept of an imbalance does not completely account for disease manifestations, even in the best-studied lung diseases (e.g., asthma and sarcoidosis). The most convincing examples of successful practical applications of this concept, however, are the new treatments for rheumatoid arthritis (RA) and asthma.

Assessment of the type of T-helper response is based on measurement of specific sets of cytokine molecules. A Th1 response is associated with increased production of interferon-γ, IL-2, IL-3, TNF-α, and TNF-β, and a Th2 response with increased production of IL-4, IL-5, IL-10, IL-13, and TGF-β. Measurement of these cytokines and estimation of the ratios between them (e.g., interferon-γ/IL-13) is currently widely performed for clinical evaluation of the T-helper immune status. Interferon-γ inhibits the Th2 response, and the IL-10 produced by Th2 cells suppresses Th1 responses.

Asthma is the prototypic example of a lung disease in which cell-mediated immunity is skewed towards a Th2 response, whereas sarcoidosis is a disease characterized by Th1 responses. Increasing evidence indicates that eosinophil airway inflammation in asthma is due to a shift to Th2 cytokine production (IL-4, IL-5, and IL-13). These cytokines cause B-cell switching to IgE synthesis (IL-4), significant elevation in eosinophilopoiesis (IL-5), and recruitment of eosinophils to the site of inflammation (IL-4). They also upregulate the expression of vascular cell adhesion molecule -1 (VCAM-1) and P-selectin, facilitating selective eosinophil recruitment to the airways and mucus hypersecretion. Although there is clearly a significant role for these Th2 responses in promotion of airway inflammation in asthma, it appears that other mechanisms may also be involved in the pathogenesis of airway hyper-reactivity and airway obstruction. Infiltration of the airway smooth muscle by mast cells occurs in asthma, but not in eosinophilic bronchitis that is unaccompanied by airway hyper-reactivity and airway obstruction, and it has been suggested that this mast cell-induced myositis, rather than the Th2 activation, may be responsible for the airway hyper-reactivity and airway obstruction that characterize asthma. Also, the roles of the recently discovered T-regulatory cells in asthma are being actively explored.

Assessment of Humoral Immunity

Assessment of humoral immunity usually includes measurement of serum immunoglobulins and complement components. Polyclonal hypergammaglobulinemia is commonly present in sarcoidosis and collagen vascular diseases, and changes in complement levels can also be found in collagen vascular diseases. Skin tests assessing for type I hypersensitivity to a variety of potential allergens are commonly used to identify allergens in patients with asthma. Increases in IgE are found in asthma and Churg-Strauss syndrome. IgA deficiency predisposes to recurrent airway infections and bronchiectasis.

Autoimmunity and Lung Diseases

Autoimmune diseases are associated with impairment of the mechanisms responsible for self-tolerance. Assessment of autoimmunity generally includes a search for organ-specific and non-organ-specific autoantibodies, and sometimes for autoreactive T- and B-cell clones, depending upon the clinical situation. Autoantibodies of different specificities are present in numerous diseases with pulmonary manifestations. Detection of autoantibodies plays a pivotal role in differential diagnosis, particularly for the pulmonary hemorrhage syndromes. Diffuse pulmonary hemorrhage is associated with numerous immunologic disorders and nonimmunologic causes for which the therapeutic approaches differ. In a setting of pulmonary hemorrhage, detection of autoantibodies can be valuable for diagnosis and differentiation between the antineutrophil cytoplasmic antibody (ANCA)-associated systemic vasculitides (Wegener's granulomatosis, microscopic polyangiitis, Churg-Strauss syndrome), Goodpasture's syndrome, and pulmonary hemorrhage associated with a connective tissue disease, as well as other potential etiologies. Autoimmunity is also currently believed to be involved in the pathogenesis of alveolar injury and fibrogenesis in idiopathic and secondary forms of pulmonary fibrosis, and it may play a role in chronic obstructive pulmonary disease and cystic fibrosis.

Autoantibody Testing Methods: Overview of the Basic Principles

Indirect Immunofluorescence

This assay is based upon applying tested sera to fixed and permeabilized target cells or tissue sections on a glass slide. The antibodies, if present in the serum, bind to cell targets, and their binding is detected by applying secondary antibodies against human immunoglobulins, labeled with a fluorescent tag. The fluorescence is visualized with a fluorescent microscope. Antibody titers can be determined by serial dilution of the sera. The titers provide a semi-quantitative measurement of antibody levels and can be used for monitoring of disease activity in some cases.

IMMUNOBLOTTING

The extracted tissue antigens are separated on a gel by electrophoresis and then transferred and fixed on a cellulose membrane. The membrane is cut into strips and the strips are used for immunoblotting. The patient's sera is applied to the membrane strips, and time is allowed for the antibodies to bind to the antigens on the strips. After that, a secondary antibody conjugated to an enzyme (e.g., alkaline phosphatase, horseradish peroxidase) and an appropriate substrate for the enzymatic reaction are added. Binding of specific antibodies present in the patient's serum is manifested by stained dots or lines that highlight the position of the corresponding reactive antigenic components. Staining is due to the colored product of the enzymatic reaction.

IMMUNOPRECIPITATION

Radioactively labeled (S^{35}-methionine) proteins and/or labeled (P^{32}) nucleic acids from cell extracts (HeLa cells or others) are precipitated by the patient's sera and separated by gel electrophoresis. After separation and transfer to a nitrocellulose membrane, they are detected by radiography and further identified by comparison with known markers.

DOUBLE IMMUNODIFFUSION

Immunodiffusion implies migration towards each other of an antigen(s) and antibody(ies) in a semi-solid medium (usually agar or agarose gel). When equivalence in concentration of these components is achieved at a certain point, a visually detectable precipitate is formed. When testing mixtures of antigens and antibodies, the technique also allows one to determine nonidentity, complete identity, or partial identity of the components in the mixture. It also allows one to obtain quantitative results by titrating the tested sera.

ENZYME-LINKED IMMUNOSORBENT ASSAY

Enzyme-linked immunosorbent assays (ELISAs) utilize the same principle as immunoblotting. The difference is that the antigens or capture antibodies are attached to a solid phase that allows separation of the bound components from the liquid phase. The solid phase can be either the well bottom of a plastic plate or particulate material (beads). The patient's sera, the enzyme-conjugated sec-

ondary antibody, and the substrate for the enzymatic reaction are added in an appropriate sequence with intermediate washings to exclude nonspecific binding. The color product of the enzymatic reaction is measured by a spectrophotometer at the appropriate wave length. An optical density measurement above the cut-off value defines a positive reaction. Within a certain range, the obtained optical density values correlate with the levels of antibodies in the sera and can be used for quantitative measurements based on a calibration curve.

ANTINEUTROPHIL CYTOPLASMIC ANTIBODY TESTING IN DIAGNOSIS OF PULMONARY VASCULITIDES

The classic primary small vessel vasculitic syndromes include Wegener's granulomatosis, microscopic polyangiitis, and Churg-Strauss syndrome, diseases that often involve multiple organs but frequently involve the lung. Their morphologies are discussed in Chapter 8. Serologic testing can be very valuable for supporting or confirming one of these diagnoses, specifically by the assessment for ANCAs. ANCAs probably play a pathogenic role in these disorders as well as serving an important diagnostic function. They have been shown to cause inappropriate activation of neutrophils, resulting in endothelial cell and vascular damage. In patients with ANCA-associated systemic vasculitides, neutrophils have a higher rate of apoptosis and necrosis, which can be observed histologically in the necrotizing lesions of Wegener's granulomatosis. Continuing investigation into their roles in disease causation is under way, but their utility for assisting in diagnosis of ANCA-associated systemic vasculitides has been proven.

ANTINEUTROPHIL CYTOPLASMIC ANTIBODY TESTING: METHODOLOGY AND INTERPRETATION

ANCAs in ANCA-associated systemic vasculitides primarily target two substances: proteinase 3 (PR3) and myeloperoxidase (MPO). The classical approach to ANCA testing is based on indirect immunofluorescence (IIF). The tested sera are applied to fixed and permeabilized human leukocytes attached to a glass slide. The antibodies, if present in the serum, bind to a potential target, usually PR3 or MPO. Two patterns of IIF (Figure 40-1) are distinguished: cytoplasmic (cANCA) and perinuclear (pANCA). The cytoplasmic pattern is characterized by homogeneous or finely granular staining of the cytoplasm, corresponds primarily to anti-PR3 specificity, and is highly associated with Wegener's granulomatosis (Table 40-3). The perinuclear pattern demonstrates staining only at the periphery of the nuclei, corresponds primarily to anti-MPO specificity of the ANCAs, and is more closely associated with microscopic polyangiitis and Churg-Strauss syndrome (Table 40-3).

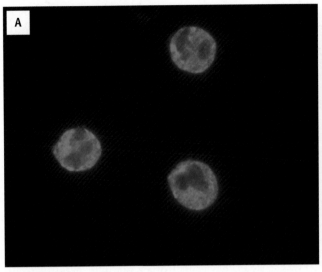

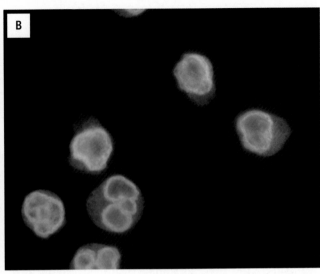

FIGURE 40-1

Indirect immunofluorescence test for ANCA
(A) Cytoplasmic staining (cANCA). **(B)** Perinuclear staining (pANCA).

TABLE 40-3

ANCA Sensitivities in ANCA-Associated Vasculitides

Disease	Sensitivity of Anti-Proteinase 3 (%) (most cANCA)	Sensitivity of Anti-Myeloperoxidase (%) (most pANCA)
WG	66%-85%	10%-21%
MPA	26%-45%	45%-58%
CSS	10%-33%	50%-60%

Abbreviations: CSS = Churg-Strauss syndrome; MPA = microscopic polyangiitis; WG = Wegener's granulomatosis

In ANCA-positive sera, the described IIF patterns should be seen only in neutrophils and monocytes—not in lymphocytes or eosinophils. The lymphocytes present on the slide serve as internal controls. If the lymphocytes, especially those that are distant from the positively stained neutrophils and monocytes, show perinuclear staining, it is usually suggestive of antinuclear antibodies and should trigger additional investigation. Cytoplasmic staining in lymphocytes indicates the presence of non-organ-specific anticytoplasmic antibodies, such as anti-Jo-1 or anti-ribosomal RNP, for example, that are associated with other autoimmune conditions. The fact that MPO is capable of diffusing into nearby cells and binding to their nuclear membranes explains perinuclear staining occasionally seen in adjacent lymphocytes in the absence of antinuclear antibodies.

Antibodies to other cationic components (elastase, cathepsin G, lactoferrin, and lysozyme) of neutrophils can also produce a pANCA pattern when antibodies to these components are present in the serum. However, microscopic polyangiitis and Churg-Strauss syndrome are associated only with MPO pANCA. On rare occasions, anti-MPO autoantibodies can produce a cANCA pattern. A cANCA pattern can also occur with antibodies to antigens that have partial homology with PR3 (neutrophil elastase, cathepsin G, heparin-binding protein, azurocidin, etc.). However, in most situations anti-PR3 and anti-MPO recognize conformational epitopes and do not show cross-reactivity with other substances.

For maximal diagnostic accuracy, it is recommended to combine standard IIF with target antigen-specific ELISA. In fact, when either a cANCA or pANCA pattern is detected by IIF, the presence of anti-PR3 or anti-MPO antibodies should be confirmed by antigen-specific ELISA. On the other hand, if the screening is performed by ELISA and the test is found to be positive, it is recommended to confirm specificity by IIF. It is claimed that the diagnostic specificity of ANCA detection by IIF reaches 99.6%.

In this context, it is appropriate to mention that ANCA-positivity by IIF and ELISA was reported recently in pulmonary tuberculosis patients. Considering the diagnostic difficulties in differentiating Wegener's granulomatosis from tuberculosis, this could represent a significant problem. In a small series, ANCA-positivity in patients with tuberculosis reached almost 40%. It was suggested, however, that considering the high prevalence of tuberculosis in the country where the study was conducted, the ANCA-positivity in these patients most likely represents an epiphenomenon rather than a true disease-associated finding. In another study, none of the ANCA-positive patients with tuberculosis demonstrated both cANCA IIF and anti-PR3 ELISA positivity; either one or the other test was found to be positive. This again underscores the importance of testing by both techniques for accurate diagnosis.

ANTINUCLEAR ANTIBODY TESTING IN PULMONARY DISORDERS

Connective tissue diseases (CTDs) are commonly associated with pathologic changes in the lungs. Although the CTDs are usually diagnosed antecedent to the development of lung disease, this is not always the case, and lung manifestations may represent the first clue to the presence of these disorders. Morphologic changes associated with CTDs are discussed in Chapter 36, and the following paragraphs will provide information about clinical laboratory testing that can contribute to the diagnosis of pulmonary involvement by a CTD. Detection of antinuclear antibodies (ANAs) of different specificities that are known to be associated with certain CTDs can be very helpful in such situations (Table 40-4).

TABLE 40-4

Indirect Immunofluorescence Patterns, Major Antigenic Targets, and Disease Associations

IIF Pattern	Major Antigenic Targets	Disease Associations
Homogeneous and peripheral	dsDNA, histones	SLE, Drug-induced lupus (histones)
Speckled	Nuclear matrix proteins, Smith, U1-snRNP, SS-A and SS-B antigens, RNA polymerases 2 and 3	SLE, SS, MCTD, SCL, RA, PM/DM
Nucleolar	PM-Scl multiprotein complex, fibrillarin	SCL, SLE, Raynaud's
Centromere	CENP - A, B, C	CREST, PBC, MCTD, Raynaud's

Abbreviations: CREST = calcinosis, Raynaud's, esophageal dysmotility, sclerodactyly, and telangiectasia syndrome; IIF = indirect immunofluorescence; MCTD = mixed connective tissue disease; PBC = primary biliary cirrhosis; PM/DM = polymyositis and dermatomyositis; RA = rheumatoid arthritis; SCL = scleroderma, systemic sclerosis; SLE = systemic lupus erythematosus; SS = Sjögren's syndrome

ANTINUCLEAR ANTIBODY TESTING: METHODOLOGY AND INTERPRETATION

The first step in the usual diagnostic algorithm for CTDs is detection of ANAs by IIF and identification of the staining pattern (Figure 40-2). The observed patterns provide guidance for further testing for identification of specific ANAs. In the current IIF test, human epithelioma (Hep-2) cells that are fixed and permeabilized by alcohol treatment are used as the targets. These cells have the advantages of large size and high mitotic index that allow easy viewing of the binding of antibodies to cellular structures both in interphase and mitotic cells. Several IIF patterns are distinguished, which correlate with ANAs of different specificities. These IIF patterns and ANA specificities have varying degrees of association with different disease entities. The homogeneous and peripheral patterns, for example, have the strongest association with systemic lupus erythematosus because they correlate with the presence of anti-dsDNA antibodies that show high specificity for lupus. The anti-dsDNA antibodies are usually confirmed by an IIF test utilizing a unicellular organism, *Crithidia luciliae*, as a target. There is also an ELISA test for anti-dsDNA antibodies.

Initial screening of sera for ANAs can also be done by generic ELISA utilizing a crude extract from calf thymus nuclear material as an antigen. The test is very sensitive and specific. ELISA-positive sera need to be additionally tested by IIF, however, for confirmation and pattern evaluation. Further identification of specific antibodies is performed either by double immunodiffusion or by specific ELISAs. More detailed analysis of ANAs can also be done by immunoblotting and immunoprecipitation methodologies.

RHEUMATOID FACTOR AND ANTIBODIES AGAINST CYCLIC CITRULLINATED PEPTIDE IN DIAGNOSIS OF RHEUMATOID ARTHRITIS

Pulmonary manifestations are common in patients with RA and span a broad spectrum of interstitial, airway, vascular, and pleural abnormalities (Chapter 36). Two serologic tests are currently considered the most informative for diagnosis of RA: detection of rheumatoid factor (RF) and detection of antibodies against cyclic citrullinated peptides (anti-CCP).

RHEUMATOID FACTOR

RF is defined as an autoantibody, most often of IgM isotype, against epitopes of the Fc fragment of IgG. The most common binding sites for RF are the $C\gamma2$ and/or $C\gamma3$ domains of IgG. RF participates in formation of immune complexes and therefore plays a pathogenic role. The presence of RF, however, is not totally limited to RA.

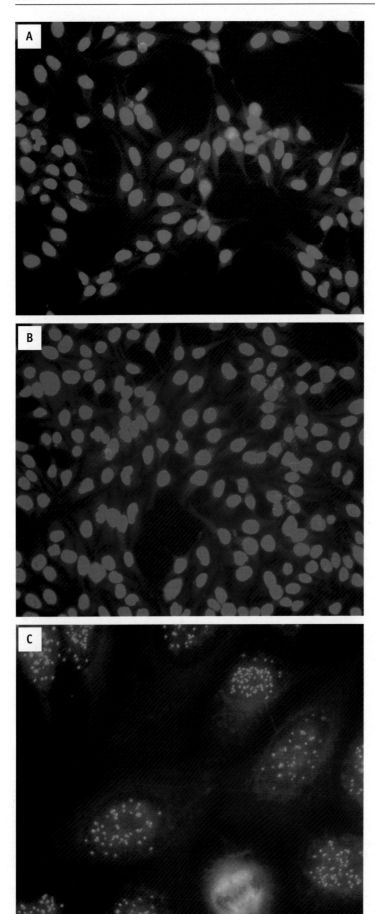

FIGURE 40-2

Indirect immunofluorescence test for ANA
(A) Homogeneous staining pattern. **(B)** Speckled staining pattern.
(C) Centromere staining pattern.

Detection of RF can be approached using several different methodologies. The agglutination technique has long been employed for this purpose and is based on observing agglutination of immunoglobulin-covered particles by testing the patient's sera. For targets, it uses either sheep red blood cells sensitized by rabbit antibodies against the sheep red blood cells (classical Waaler and Rose technique) or inert beads (bentonite, latex, etc.) covered by rabbit or human IgG (Singer and Plotz techniques). More commonly used now is the nephelometric technique that utilizes fluid-phase IgG aggregates or IgG-coated microparticles and measures their precipitation by the sera based on changes in light scattering. Finally, ELISA is also available for detecting RF. A significant advantage of ELISA testing is its ability to determine the isotype of the RF by applying isotype-specific secondary antibodies.

ANTI-CYCLIC CITRULLINATED PEPTIDE

This autoantibody is directed towards citrulline, a derivative of the amino acid arginine, which results from post-translational modification. Historically, it was first detected by IIF as an anti-perinuclear factor and/or anti-keratin antibody. Later, citrulline was proven to be the target antigen and an ELISA test was developed. It was discovered that the ELISA test shows much higher sensitivity (80%) and specificity (98%) for RA when selected cyclic citrullinated peptides are used as antigens. For comparison, the sensitivity and specificity of the IgM-RF ELISA are about 66% and 82%, respectively. Some studies have shown that anti-CCP appears early and can predict the development of RA. It can also predict erosive disease progression. Considering the early appearance of anti-CCP in RA, this marker could potentially be helpful in the differential diagnosis between RA with early lung manifestations and primary lung diseases. However, its presence in non-RA lung disease must also be studied.

ANTI-GLOMERULAR BASEMENT MEMBRANE ANTIBODY TESTING IN GOODPASTURE'S SYNDROME

In Goodpasture's syndrome, another important pulmonary hemorrhage syndrome, detection of antibodies with specificity for the glomerular basement membrane (anti-GBM) is crucial. Anti-GBM plays an important role in Goodpasture's syndrome pathogenesis by initiating injury to the glomerular and alveolar basement membranes, which ultimately leads to renal failure and pulmonary hemorrhage in most patients with this syndrome. Anti-GBM antibodies are directed towards defined epitopes of the alpha-3 chain of collagen 4, which is a major structural component of the glomerular basement membrane (GBM) and the alveolar basement membrane. These antibodies can be detected by IIF, using human kidney as a test system, or by immunoblotting, immunoprecipitation, or ELISA. In patients with Goodpasture's syndrome, the sensitivity of ELISA for anti-GBM is 87% and the specificity is 98%. Anti-GBM is not entirely specific for Goodpasture's syndrome, however, and can also be found in 12% of patients with systemic lupus erythematosus, 9% of patients with mixed connective tissue disease, and 4% of patients with other systemic vasculitides. Anti-GBM can also be demonstrated by immunofluorescence staining of the patient's renal or lung biopsies (Chapter 39).

ANTIPHOSPHOLIPID ANTIBODY TESTING IN LUNG DISEASE

Antiphospholipid antibody (APA) syndrome can occur as an isolated process or in the setting of a connective tissue disease, particularly systemic lupus erythematosus. In the lung, it is a cause of thromboembolism, acute respiratory distress syndrome, and pulmonary hemorrhage. APA targets acidic phospholipids—cardiolipin, phosphatidylserine, phosphatidylinositol, and phosphatidylglycerol. Beta-2-glycoprotein 1 (β2GP1), also known as apolipoprotein H, serves as a co-factor. The isotype of the antibody is an important predictive factor for thrombotic events; IgG APA (alone or with IgM or IgA) identifies patients prone to complications. Detection of APA can be approached using the nontreponemal tests for syphilis (VDRL, RPR), the test for lupus anticoagulant, or an ELISA. The ELISA allows determination of the isotype of APA, which is important for prognosis.

CRYOGLOBULINS IN LUNG DISEASE

Cryoglobulins are occasionally responsible for diffuse alveolar hemorrhage. Cryoglobulins are immunoglobulins that precipitate out of solution below body temperature. The thermal amplitudes of cryoglobulins differ and this can influence clinical presentation. There are three types of cryoglobulins. Type I (simple) cryoglobulins include clonal immunoglobulins and free light chains, which are associated with multiple myeloma, Waldenstrom's macroglobulinemia, and Bence Jones proteinuria. Type II and type III (mixed) cryoglobulins are immune complexes in which both the antigen and the antibody are immunoglobulins. The antigen is usually a polyclonal immunoglobulin and the antibody is either monoclonal (type II) or polyclonal (type III). In mixed cryoglobulins, the antigen is commonly IgG. There is a significant association of mixed cryoglobulinemia with RA, systemic sclerosis, vasculitis, glomerulonephritis, and other autoimmune conditions. Hepatitis C infection is also commonly present in patients with type II cryoglobulinemia; a high percentage of patients positive by second-generation ELISA for mixed cryoglobulins are also positive for hepatitis C antibody, and many of them show viremia. Type III mixed cryoglobulinemia shows associations with a variety of chronic infections and autoimmune processes.

ASSESSMENT OF LOCAL IMMUNITY AND/OR LOCAL MANIFESTATIONS OF SYSTEMIC IMMUNE RESPONSES

Analysis of local immune responses in the lung can provide valuable information about the pathogenesis, differential diagnosis, and progression of a number of lung diseases. Approaches include assessment of cellular composition, cytokine milieu, expression of activation markers, and soluble factor production in specimens obtained directly from the respiratory tract.

CELLULAR COMPOSITION

The cellular composition of induced sputum and bronchoalveolar lavage fluid is highly influenced by the nature of any pathologic processes present in the respiratory tract. Inflammatory cell influx and extravasation requires interactions between leukocytes and endothelial cells, which are mediated primarily by cell adhesion molecules and regulated by locally produced cytokines and systemic mechanisms. Cellular composition can be assessed by differential counting on stained smears, with or without immunohistochemistry to help identify specific cell populations, or by flow cytometry using a constellation of specific lineage markers. Neutrophil accumulation can also be assessed based on the neutrophil enzyme activity (myeloperoxidase, elastase) in liquid specimens.

Certain lung diseases are linked to changes in cellular composition. Sputum and/or bronchoalveolar lavage fluid neutrophilia is associated with bacterial infections, cystic fibrosis, and idiopathic pulmonary fibrosis. Increased eosinophils are observed in asthma, eosinophilic pneumonia, allergic bronchopulmonary aspergillosis, and Churg-Strauss syndrome. In patients with allergic airway disease, evaluation of percentages of eosinophils and neutrophils can aid in distinguishing between an asthma exacerbation and a superimposed infection. Lymphocytosis is found with hypersensitivity pneumonia, sarcoidosis, chronic infections, drug reactions, and a wide spectrum of other conditions. Immunophenotypic evaluation of the lymphocytes can help in differentiating between hypersensitivity pneumonitis and sarcoidosis, with increased CD8+ T-cells in the former and increased CD4+ T-cells in the latter disease. In chronic obstructive pulmonary disease, exacerbations can be associated with increased neutro-

phils, eosinophils and lymphocytes. There is also an increase in CD20+ and CD8+ cells with reduction in CD4+/CD8+ and Tc1/Tc2 (CD8+ interferonγ+/CD8+ IL4+) ratios. These changes in cellular composition during exacerbations of chronic obstructive pulmonary disease also correlate with increased proteolysis (elevated matrix metalloproteinase-9 activity and decreased tissue inhibitor of metalloproteinase-1 activity).

ACTIVATION MARKERS, CYTOKINES, AND ADHESION MOLECULES

Changes in expression of adhesion molecules, activation markers, and cytokines are recognized in many pathologic processes involving the lungs, and their measurement, both on the cellular level (by flow cytometry and immunohistochemistry) and in fluids (by ELISA), is becoming more widespread in research and clinical evaluation. The functional roles of IL-4 and IL-5 in asthma were discussed above, and other commonly studied molecules include the pro-inflammatory cytokines IL-1, IL-6, IL-8, and TNF-α. IL-1 plays a key role in promoting inflammatory responses and induces synthesis of IL-8. IL-8 in turn serves as an important neutrophil chemoattractant and activator. IL-6 shows a wide range of biological properties including the stimulation of B-cells and activation of immunoglobulin production. IL-6 and IL-8 are also produced by alveolar type II cells *in vitro*, and their production can be stimulated by pathogenic factors (e.g., asbestos). TNF-α is a multifunctional proinflammatory cytokine that causes induction of IL-1, IL-6, and macrophage inflammatory protein-1a (MIP-1a), and promotes recruitment of inflammatory cells and platelets. Local production of fibrogenic factors (platelet-derived growth factor (PDGF) and transforming growth factor-beta (TGF-β) promotes fibrogenesis in airways (asthma, obliterative bronchiolitis) and in the distal lung parenchyma. An association has been shown between (a) poor outcomes in the acute respiratory distress syndrome and (b) lung transplantation and persistently increased levels of pro-inflammatory cytokines (IL-1, IL-6, IL-8, TNF-α) in bronchoalveolar lavage fluid and plasma.

Another group of molecules that are detectable in cells and in the fluid phase, in induced sputum and bronchoalveolar lavage fluid, are the selectins and their ligands. The selectin family of cell adhesion molecules includes three structurally related carbohydrate-binding proteins. Two of them (E-selectin and P-selectin) are expressed on endothelial cells, and the third (L-selectin) is expressed on leukocytes. Leukocytes also express the P-selectin glycoprotein ligand-1 (PSGL-1) that also binds with lesser affinity to E-selectin. Interactions between these molecules play an essential role in primary leukocyte-endothelial cell adhesive contact. In chronic obstructive pulmonary disease, upregulation of PSGL-1 has been demonstrated on cell surfaces of neutrophils, eosinophils, monocytes, and lymphocytes, with increased expression of E- and P-selectins on endothelial cells of the submucosal blood vessels. There is also an increase in the plasma levels of soluble selectins (E- and P-). Elevated expression of Mac-1 (a molecule responsible for neutrophil migratory capacity) on circulating neutrophils has also been demonstrated. Mac-1 is a member of the β2-integrin family and is involved in adhesion and migration of neutrophils. Its expression is regulated by TNF-α.

SUGGESTED READINGS

General Immunology Textbooks and Laboratory Manuals

1. Coico R, Sunshine G, Benjamini E. *Immunology: A Short Course.* 5th ed. Hoboken, NJ: John Wiley and Sons, Inc.; 2003.
2. Male D. *Immunology. An Illustrated Outline.* 4th ed. Philadelphia, PA: Mosby; 2004.
3. Rose NR, Hamilton RG, Detrick B, eds. *Manual of Clinical Laboratory Immunology.* 6th ed. Washington, DC: ASM Press; 2002.

General Reviews on Immune Responses in Pulmonary Pathology

4. Curtis JL. Cell-mediated adaptive immune defense of the lungs. *Proc Am Thorac Soc.* 2005;2:412-6.
5. Martin TR, Frevert CW. Innate immunity in the lungs. *Proc Am Thorac Soc.* 2005;2:403-11.
6. Twigg HL III. Humoral immune defense (antibodies). *Proc Am Thorac Soc.* 2005;2:417-21.
7. Verhagen J, Taylor A, Blaser K, Akdis M, Akdis CA. T regulatory cells in allergen-specific immunotherapy. *Int Rev Immunol.* 2006;24:533-48.
8. Vliagoftis H, Befus AD. Mast cells at mucosal frontiers. *Curr Mol Med.* 2005;5:573-89.

Immune Responses in Pulmonary Diseases

Allergic Inflammation and Asthma

9. Barrios RJ, Kheradmand F, Batts L, Corry DB. Asthma. Pathology and pathophysiology. *Arch Pathol Lab* Med. 2006;130:447-51.
10. Bradding P, Walls AF, Holgate ST. The role of the mast cell in the pathophysiology of asthma. *J Allergy Clin Immunol.* 2006;117:1277-84.
11. Hawrylowicz CM. Regulatory T cells and IL-10 in allergic inflammation. *J Exp Med.* 2005;202:1459-63.
12. Kay AB. The role of T lymphocytes in asthma. *Chem Immunol Allergy* 2006;91:59-75.
13. Pease JE. Asthma, allergy and chemokines. *Curr Drug Targets.* 2006;7:3-12.
14. Van Oosterhout AJM, Bloksma N. Regulatory T-lymphocytes in asthma. *Eur Resp J.* 2005;26:918-32.

Interstitial Lung Diseases

15. Jindal SK, Agarwal R. Autoimmunity and interstitial lung disease. *Curr Opinion Pulm Med.* 2005;11:438-46.
16. Noble PW, Homer RJ. Idiopathic pulmonary fibrosis: new insights into pathogenesis. *Clin Chest Med.* 2004;25:749-58.
17. Papiris SA, Kollintza A, Kitsanta P, et al. Relationship of BAL and lung tissue CD4+ and CD8+ T lymphocytes, and their ratio in idiopathic pulmonary fibrosis. *Chest.* 2005;128:2971-7.
18. Reynolds HY, Gail DB, Kiley JP. Interstitial lung diseases—where we started from and are now going. *Sarcoidosis Vasc Diffuse Lung Dis.* 2005;22:5-12.

Chronic Obstructive Pulmonary Diseases

19. Cossman MM, Willemse BW, Jansen DF, et al. Increased number of B-cells in bronchial biopsies in COPD. *Eur Respir J.* 2006;27:60-4.
20. Takabatake N, Sata M, Abe S, et al. Impaired systemic cell-mediated immunity and increased susceptibility to acute respiratory tract infections in patients with COPD. *Resp Med.* 2005;99:485-92.

ANCA-Associated Vasculitides

21. Dean KD, West SG. Antiphospholipid antibodies as a cause of pulmonary capillaritis and diffuse alveolar hemorrhage: a case series and literature review. *Semin Arthritis Rheum.* 2005; 35:138-42.
22. Hagen EC, Daha MR, Hermans J, et al. Diagnostic value of standardized assays for anti-neutrophil cytoplasmic antibodies in idiopathic systemic vasculitis. EC/BCR Project for ANCA Assay Standardization. *Kidney Int.* 1998;53:743-53.
23. Kallenberg CG, Brouwer E, Weening JJ, Tervaert JW. Anti-neutrophil cytoplasmic antibodies: current diagnostic and pathophysiological potential. *Kidney Int.* 1994;46:1-15.
24. Khan AM, Elahi F, Hashmi SR, et al. Wegener's granulomatosis: a rare, chronic and multisystem disease. *Surgeon.* 2006;4:45-52.
25. Pesci A, Pavone L, Buzio C, Manganelli P. Respiratory system involvement in ANCA-associated systemic vasculitides. *Sarcoidosis Vasc Diffuse Lung Dis.* 2005;Suppl 1:S40-8.

Index

Page numbers in italic indicate figures. Page numbers followed by *b* indicate boxes. Page numbers followed by *t* indicate tables.

Q